National Institute of Allergy and Infectious Diseases, NIH

Volume 2

Impact on Global Health

Infectious Disease

Vassil St. Georgiev

For further volumes, go to
www.springer.com/series/7646

National Institute of Allergy and Infectious Diseases, NIH

Volume 2

Impact on Global Health

Vassil St. Georgiev, PhD

Office of Global Research, National Institute of Allergy and Infectious Diseases, NIH, Bethesda, MD, USA

Foreword by Anthony S. Fauci, MD

Director, National Institute of Allergy and Infectious Diseases, NIH, Bethesda, MD, USA

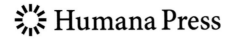 Humana Press

Vassil St. Georgiev, Ph.D.
National Institutes of Health
Department of Health and Human Services
6610 Rockledge Drive
Bethesda MD 20892
USA
vgeorgiev@niaid.nih.gov

ISBN 978-1-60327-296-4   e-ISBN 978-1-60327-297-1
DOI 10.1007/978-1-60327-297-1

Library of Congress Control Number: 2009920698

Printed on acid-free paper

springer.com

Dedication

*To the National Institute of Allergy and Infectious Diseases, NIH,
a world leader in supporting biomedical research in service to humanity
for more than 50 years.*

Foreword

The NIH speaks the universal language of humanitarianism . . . [it] has recognized no limitations imposed by international boundaries; has recognized no distinctions of race, or creed, or of color.
—U.S. President Franklin D. Roosevelt, National Institute of Health,
Bethesda, Maryland, 31 October 1940

In dedicating the NIH campus in 1940, President Roosevelt could look back to a proud scientific era that began around the time of his birth in 1882. In those days of Koch and Pasteur, the causes of important infectious diseases, such as cholera, tuberculosis, and diphtheria, were discovered, and many vaccines and therapeutics were rapidly developed. It was clear to Roosevelt and to scientists of his time that infectious diseases were an important global problem. Many of the most significant infectious disease discoveries of the late 19th and early 20th centuries had come from Africa, the Middle East, South America, and elsewhere in the developing world. For example, the discovery of the cause of yellow fever and the first successes in its control came from partnerships between American and foreign scientists working in Cuba, Panama, and other locales.

Roosevelt's inspiring words on that autumn day on the NIH campus indicate that he was looking not just to the past, but boldly ahead to the future as well. Viewing the future with optimism, rather than trepidation, he expected significant new challenges and imagined that NIH would do whatever necessary to meet them. Nearly seven decades later, the world's population has grown to more than 6 billion people, from 2.3 billion in Roosevelt's day, and the world is significantly more complicated. Hundreds of new diseases have emerged, and they have created an enormous burden on humankind. AIDS, emerging influenza strains, and drug-resistant malaria and tuberculosis have collectively killed hundreds of millions of people. Immunologic and immunodeficiency diseases have assumed a much greater role in creating human misery, while such neglected tropical diseases as schistosomiasis continue to exact an immense toll on morbidity, mortality and the economies of developing nations. At the same time, human movement has increased and become more efficient, transporting microorganisms from continent to continent within hours. Technological advances, such as vaccines and drugs, have been countered by the rapid emergence of microbial resistance. Biological warfare has been reborn from its military graveyard as a civilian threat. And the gap between rich and poor has widened, leading to health disparities so glaring that one might divide the world into the healthy and the unhealthy. The challenge for the National Institute of Allergy and Infectious Diseases (NIAID), now the second largest NIH institute, is to respond to the founding vision of President Roosevelt and to the hopes and expectations of those scientists and leaders who came before us.

We hope that this detailed summary of NIAID's global research efforts will be useful to both scientists and historians of science and also remind us of the spirit and optimism that led to the creation of NIH, including NIAID and its forebears. While examining the many specific details describing the approaches, initiatives, programs, and scientific activities related to our global research mission, we also remember the larger world within which we work. We wish to make several points that address not only what we do scientifically, but how and why we do it.

We are global citizens, and our world view remains humanitarian. President Roosevelt's dedication of NIH many years ago reflected not only an understanding of American science but also a national commitment to global citizenship. For seven decades, this global commitment has been manifested in NIH's global scientific efforts, including those of NIAID. For example, NIAID played a leading role in finding the causes of, and understanding the pathogenic mechanisms of AIDS and in developing, testing, and bringing into use an armamentarium of drugs that have improved and prolonged the lives of millions of patients. Because these remarkable achievements were most urgently needed in the developing world, NIAID drew upon the international AIDS research infrastructure it had created and fostered, partnering with other governments and philanthropic organizations to begin the slow process of saving lives and preventing new infections in every region of the world. These efforts were integral to The President's Emergency Plan for AIDS Relief (PEPFAR), a large-scale humanitarian commitment to developing nations to prevent and treat HIV/AIDS and to care for infected people. Although much remains to be done in the fight against AIDS, PEPFAR has been a triumph. The program is an affirmation of traditional American values and a strong confirmation that scientific accomplishment can also be a humanitarian instrument.

In a global village, it is no longer possible to geographically compartmentalize biomedical research. The spread of West Nile virus into the Western Hemisphere in 1999; the 2003 American outbreak of the imported African disease monkeypox; and widely publicized cases of multidrug-resistant tuberculosis remind us that the "our disease/their disease" paradigm is untenable. Most infectious disease threats Americans have faced in the past few decades, from exotic tropical diseases to antibiotic-resistant strains of bacteria to emerging strains of influenza viruses, have come wholly or partially from abroad. Obviously, to understand these diseases and the threats they pose, we must be able to study the causative organisms in their natural environments and to work collaboratively with foreign scientists who have the capacity to isolate microbial strains and conduct studies in their own endemic areas. In the past decade, NIH has embarked upon an unprecedented globalization of its research by focusing on specific diseases, such as AIDS, tuberculosis, and malaria, by more than quadrupling direct foreign research awards and foreign components of domestic awards, by doubling the foreign visitor program, and by joining forces with many developing nations to create a number of new and innovative research partnerships, such as NIAID's International Centers for Excellence in Research (ICER) and the Indo-U.S. HIV/STD Program, among many others.

The roles of microbial agents and of human hosts in disease occurrence are inextricably intertwined. The sequencing of the human genome and that of a large number of microbial pathogens and disease vectors is leading us to a much better understanding of how and why diseases occur and what can be done to control them. Humans themselves and their behaviors, actions, movements, commerce, and environmental perturbations are the selection pressures that drive pathogen emergence and evolution. Genomics and proteomics offer new opportunities not only for pathogen discovery, diagnostics, and drug/vaccine development, but also for understanding microbial emergence and host-switching at the genome level. Studying the host response to microbes is critical for a number of reasons: Understanding the genetics of the immune response to infections allows more rational design of drugs and vaccines and provides clues to therapy with existing drugs. Host responses may themselves be overexuberant and even pathogenic, and we need to better understand these immunopathogenic phenomena in order to prevent and treat them. Moreover, a better understanding of the genetic variations in host targets may allow us to predict and even prevent disease emergence.

Complex problems require complex approaches and creative partnerships; new challenges can be met by taking advantage of new opportunities. Many major human infectious diseases are complex and difficult to prevent and control with traditionally successful scientific approaches. For example, each of the three major infectious disease killers worldwide, HIV, *Plasmodium falciparum* malaria, and *Mycobacterium tuberculosis*, all have complex "life cycles," all cause chronic and persistent or recurrent disease, and none has been controlled by a successful vaccine. The great burden of mortality from these three diseases falls disproportionately on the poor, who live in resource-poor countries. What little money is available to address such overwhelming problems locally is spent in treatment and prevention, while many drug and vaccine manufacturers in wealthy nations remain unmotivated to invest multimillion-dollar efforts to produce vaccines and drugs that few can afford to buy. It therefore makes sense for biomedical research, public health, public policy, and philanthropy to engage each other in new and creative ways. Although NIH is the preeminent funder of global infectious disease and immunology research, important philanthropic organizations, such as the Bill & Melinda Gates Foundation, and many small and large nongovernmental organizations (NGOs) have recently appeared and expanded. These developments provide new opportunities to address medical, social, and humanitarian aspects of human health, and they bring science closer to the front lines of the war against infectious diseases. Increasingly, NIAID has been working collaboratively with foreign governments and scientists, NGOs, and philanthropic organizations to coordinate comprehensive approaches to important health problems in the developing world. As the world "shrinks" due to increased travel and more efficient communication, and as concentrations of wealth are brought about by the emerging and realigning economies of nations such as China and India, new opportunities for scientific progress will undoubtedly continue to appear. We must remain flexible and retain a capacity to form new alliances with a variety of partners in pursuit of ever-changing disease threats.

The biomedical science pathway begins with basic research findings and ends with their translation into life-saving tools and approaches. As Pasteur famously observed, "there does not exist a category of science to which one can give the name *applied science*. There are science and the applications of science, bound together as the fruit of the tree which bears it." In recent decades, biomedical science has been driven by technological advances, but basic science discovery itself is only the beginning of a process. An example of the successful progress of scientific endeavor in addressing an important problem, noted above, is the sequential clinical-epidemiologic recognition of AIDS, followed by the discovery of the etiologic agent, HIV, followed by the development of a screening diagnostic test, followed by scientific characterization of the virus, the development of antiviral drugs, the development of treatment strategies, and ultimately to the organization of large-scale programs based on accumulated scientific knowledge and effective drugs to prevent and treat HIV infections. The "products" of science include not only the diagnostic tests, vaccines, drugs, and prevention strategies we have developed, but also the knowledge and experience we have acquired to use them wisely. NIAID's efforts are part of a larger process that extends beyond the purely scientific to include the medical, societal, and humanitarian. Science is not a value system but a rational mechanism for discovering truths; it acquires meaning and value when we use it to serve humanity.

For the 54 years of our existence, NIAID has carried on the tradition of NIH and its antecedent organizations in maintaining a global and humanitarian perspective and in viewing and supporting biomedical science as an instrument of human progress. In recent decades, we have made enormous strides in eradicating and controlling diseases, but we have also suffered discouraging setbacks in the emergence of new diseases and the re-emergence of old ones. We are in an era in which enormous challenges, both old and new, are likely to confront us, but also an era in which we will find new opportunities to meet these challenges. As documented in the pages of this volume, our approach to the challenges of infectious diseases remains broad, flexible, and energetic. We deal with highly complex and technical issues at the level of the cell, the gene, and the molecule. But we seek also to understand the ways in which infectious organisms interact with, and evolve in response to, their human hosts; and we coordinate our research findings with colleagues in public health and with partners in society at large. In doing so, we remain focused on alleviating human suffering wherever it occurs and committed to our founding principles, articulated in the universal language of humanitarianism.

Bethesda, Maryland   Anthony S. Fauci, M.D.

Acknowledgments

Deep appreciation and gratitude is expressed to the following colleagues from NIAID for their help and encouragement during the preparation of this volume:

Anthony S. Fauci, MD, Director, National Institute of Allergy and Infectious Diseases (NIAID), NIH
Hugh Auchincloss, Jr., MD, Principal Deputy Director, NIAID, NIH
John J. McGowan, PhD, Deputy Director, NIAID, NIH
F. Gray Handley, MSPH, Associate Director for International Research Affairs, NIAID, NIH, and Steven Smith, JD, Director, Office of Global Research, NIAID, NIH, for their understanding and constant support during the preparation of this volume;

Division of Microbiology and Infectious Diseases (DMID), NIAID, NIH: Carole Heilman, PhD, Director, for her comments and support of Part I of this volume;

Division of AIDS (DAIDS), NIAID, NIH: Carl Dieffenbach, PhD, Director, and Jeff Nadler, PhD, Joan Romaine, MPH, Vanessa Elharrar, MD, Fulvia Veronese, PhD, Carla Pettinelli, MD, and Marjorie Dehlinger, DNSc, for their comments and support of Part II of this volume;

Division of Allergy, Immunology, and Transplantation (DAIT), NIAID, NIH: Daniel Rotrosen, MD, Director, and Charles Hackett, PhD, Deputy Director, for their comments and support of Part III of this volume;

Office of Communications and Government Relations (OCGR), NIAID, NIH: Dr. Veda Charrow for editing of Parts I and II of this volume;

Office of Cyber Infrastructure and Computational Biology, Customer Service Branch: James T. Mitchell for his timely help in solving computer issues.

In Memoriam

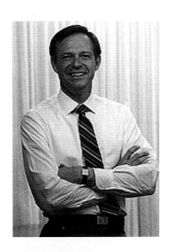

James C. Hill (1941–1997)

James C. Hill was NIAID's Deputy Director from 1987 until 1995. He played an important role in the early years of the AIDS epidemic as well as in the development of the *H. influenzae* type b (Hib) vaccines. His clear vision, dedication, and gentle humor helped steer the institute on its course.

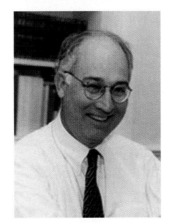

John R. La Montagne (1943–2004)

John R. La Montagne was former Director of the Division of Microbiology and Infectious Diseases and later NIAID's Deputy Director from 1998 until 2004. For his many years of dedicated service and contributions to public health, John La Montagne earned the respect of the biomedical community.

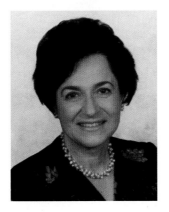

Elizabeth S. Georgiev (1937–2008)

Prior to her coming to the United States, Elizabeth S. Georgiev was an Assistant Professor in the Faculty of Pharmacy at the Medical University in Sofia, Bulgaria. In 1992, she joined the Pharmacy Department in the Clinical Center at NIH, where she worked on NIAID investigational drugs.

Contents

Part I
Microbiology and Infectious Diseases

Chapter 1

Introduction

The National Institutes of Health (NIH) is one of the world's foremost biomedical research centers. As an agency of the U.S. Department of Health and Human Services, NIH is the federal entity in charge of health research. NIH's mission to support biomedical research is achieved through its 27 institutes and centers.

The National Institute of Allergy and Infectious Diseases (NIAID) is one of the leading institutions at NIH. For more than 50 years, NIAID has supported research in immunology, allergy, and infectious diseases with the aim of understanding, treating, and ultimately preventing those diseases (http://www.usmedicine.com/article.cfm?articleID=122&issueID=20). To meet the challenges of the new millennium and take advantage of unprecedented scientific opportunities, the institute has developed a strategic research plan for the 21st century focused on four major areas:

- Immune-mediated diseases, including allergy and asthma
- HIV/AIDS
- Global health and emerging infectious diseases
- Vaccines

In its mission to reduce the burden of human disease, NIAID is committed to encouraging and supporting accelerated translation of biomedical discoveries into new treatments on a global scale, especially in the areas of HIV/AIDS, tuberculosis, and malaria (www.niaid.nih.gov/publications/globalhealth/global.pdf).

Immune-Mediated Diseases. The burden of immune-mediated diseases is staggering. In the United States, these conditions result in direct and indirect costs that exceed US$100 billion. Autoimmune diseases, such as rheumatoid arthritis, type 1 diabetes, and multiple sclerosis, together affect approximately 5% of the U.S. population. At least 7% of American children are asthmatic, and more than 1 in 5 individuals in the United States are affected by allergies. In addition, immune-mediated graft rejection remains a significant obstacle to the potentially life-saving transplantation of organs. Recent advances in basic and clinical immunology, many accomplished with NIAID funding and support, hold great promise for developing new treatments for individuals with immune-mediated diseases.

Among the most exciting areas of inquiry—and a major goal for the treatment of immune-mediated disorders—is the induction of immune tolerance; that is, selectively blocking (for a specific antigen) harmful immune responses while leaving protective immune responses intact. By inducing immune tolerance, it may be possible to prevent graft rejection in transplant patients without the long-term use of immunosuppressive drugs that dampen protective immune responses as well as destructive ones, thereby placing patients at increased risk of infection and malignancies.

The ability to block the immune response selectively also holds great promise for the treatment of many other immune-mediated conditions, including autoimmune diseases and asthma and allergic diseases. NIAID has developed a multifaceted research effort in immune tolerance. In autumn 1999, NIAID established the Immune Tolerance Network (ITN) in collaboration with the Juvenile Diabetes Foundation International and the National Institute of Diabetes and Digestive and Kidney Diseases (NIDDK) (http://www.usmedicine.com/article.cfm?articleID=122&issueID=20).

HIV/AIDS. Acquired immunodeficiency syndrome (AIDS), caused by the human immunodeficiency virus (HIV), is one of the greatest threats to global health and one of the most destructive scourges in human history. Since the beginning of the HIV pandemic, an estimated 58 million people worldwide have been infected with HIV, of whom approximately 22 million have died. In the United States, approximately 800,000 to 900,000 people are living with HIV/AIDS; 430,000 deaths among people with AIDS had been reported to the Centers for Disease Control and Prevention by the end of 1999.

The global HIV-infected population continues to expand: in 2000 alone, there were 5.3 million new infections worldwide, half of which occurred among people younger than 25 years of age. In the United States, the rate of new HIV infections has reached an unacceptable plateau of 40,000 per year, with minority communities

V. St. Georgiev, *National Institute of Allergy and Infectious Diseases, NIH: Impact on Global Health*, vol. 2, DOI 10.1007/978-1-60327-297-1_1, © Humana Press, a part of Springer Science+Business Media, LLC 2009

disproportionately affected (http://www.usmedicine.com/article.cfm?articleID=122&issueID=20).

Although potent combinations of anti-HIV drugs (highly active antiretroviral therapy, or HAART) have reduced the number of AIDS deaths and new AIDS cases in many Western countries, the utility of these medications is limited by their substantial cost, toxicities, complicated and disruptive dosing regimens, and the development of drug resistance. Therefore, an important NIAID research priority is the development of new, less toxic therapies to control HIV replication and boost, rebuild, or replace immunity lost in HIV infection. Other methods of preventing HIV transmission, such as education, behavior modification, and the social marketing and provision of condoms, have also proved effective, both in the United States and in developing countries such as Uganda, Senegal, and Thailand. To build on these successes, NIAID recently launched the international *HIV Prevention Trials Network (HPTN)* to develop and test promising non-vaccine strategies to prevent the spread of HIV. The HPTN, a collaborative effort with the National Institute of Child Health and Human Development, the National Institute of Mental Health, and the National Institute on Drug Abuse, includes research sites in the United States and countries in Latin America, Europe, Africa, and Asia. The institute recently launched the *HIV Vaccine Trials Network (HVTN)*, an international network to develop and test preventive HIV vaccines. The HVTN will conduct all phases of clinical trials, from evaluating candidate vaccines for safety and ability to stimulate immune responses to testing the efficacy of vaccines. In addition to sites in the United States, HVTN sites are located in sub-Saharan Africa, Asia, Latin America, and the Caribbean. The network's international sites are critical in helping to identify vaccines appropriate for those regions hit hardest by AIDS.

Global Health and Emerging Infectious Diseases. The NIAID research program is predicated on the view that we live in an interconnected, global community; indeed, the institute's international research programs span the globe. As a nation, the interest of the United States in global health stems both from humanitarian concerns and what has been called "enlightened self-interest." An area's poor health status can have a profound negative impact on its social and economic development and frequently contributes to political instability.

The globalization of health problems—and their relevance to the United States—was brought emphatically to the attention of the public and policymakers by the AIDS epidemic. In the past few years, global health problems, particularly those related to emerging infectious diseases, are being recognized at the highest levels. For example, in 2000 the United Nations Security Council for the first time devoted an entire session to a health issue—AIDS in Africa—recognizing the enormous threat that the disease poses to the security not only of that continent but also to that of the world. Despite many important advances in prevention and therapy, infectious diseases remain a leading impediment to global health. The World Health Organization (WHO) estimates that 1,500 people die each hour from an infectious disease. Half of these deaths occur in children under 5 years of age, and most of the rest are working adults who frequently are breadwinners and parents.

Adding to the burden of endemic infectious diseases are newly recognized diseases (e.g., HIV, Nipah virus) and the re-emergence of well-known diseases (e.g., tuberculosis, malaria) that have become increasingly problematic because of drug resistance, social conditions, and other factors. In addition, the international community now faces the specter of a new kind of emerging disease: one deliberately spread by a bioterrorist. These and other emerging disease threats are an important focus of NIAID efforts to improve global health. The NIAID's research efforts in this regard are directed toward three broad goals:

- Strengthening basic and applied research on the multiple host, pathogen, and environmental factors that influence the emergence of disease
- Supporting the development of diagnostics, vaccines, and therapies necessary to detect and control infectious diseases
- Maintaining and expanding the national and international scientific expertise required to respond to health threats

Many of the challenges posed by emerging infectious diseases lend themselves to research in a relatively new field: genomics. The sequencing of the entire human genome and the anticipated assignment, over the next few years, of function to the estimated 60,000 to 100,000 human genes will have an enormous impact on all of medicine, including our understanding of the host response to microbial pathogens. Parallel with the *Human Genome Project*, the many projects under way to sequence microbial pathogens will be a critical component of 21st-century strategies for developing diagnostics, therapeutics, and vaccines for endemic as well as emerging pathogens. The first microbial sequencing project, *Haemophilus influenzae*, was completed in July 1995 with extraordinary speed. Using newly developed techniques, investigators used a "shotgun" approach to sequence thousands of fragments of the bacterium's genome. Special computer programs read these sequences and stitched them together by comparing overlapping sequences. The result was the complete DNA sequence containing all of the genetic information of this bacterium. Encouraged by this success, NIAID has funded projects to sequence the full genomes of many medically important microbes, including the bacteria that cause tuberculosis, gonorrhea, chlamydia, and cholera, as well as individual chromosomes of important organisms such as the malaria parasite, *Plasmodium falciparum*. Many of these microorganisms have been completely sequenced and are now being annotated and analyzed. Currently, the NIAID-funded researchers deposit the sequence data in specialized and public databases such as *GenBank*, operated by the National Center for Biotechnology Information, where they can be accessed by anyone through the Internet. Access to the sequence data, before they are published in peer-reviewed journals, enables the broader research community to jump-start and accelerate its experimental studies.

Vaccine Development. Vaccination has been recognized as the greatest public health achievement of the 20th century, and vaccine research has long been a vital part of the NIAID research portfolio. NIAID-supported research has been instrumental in the development of many new and improved vaccines, such as those against hepatitis A and B, *Haemophilus influenzae* type b, pertussis, typhoid, varicella, and pneumococcal disease (http://www.usmedicine. com/article.cfm?articleID=122&issueID=20). The rapidly evolving science base in pathogen genomics, immunology, and microbiology will facilitate further progress in developing new or improved vaccines. The use of currently available and future technologies in the 21st century promises to bring about a renaissance in an already vital field. In particular, the availability of the genomic sequences of major microbial pathogens will make it easier to identify a wide array of new antigens for vaccine targets.

Vaccines that target mucosal surfaces, such as those in the intestine or respiratory tract, are of great importance, because many pathogens gain entry to the host via mucosal sites. Vaccines administered orally, nasally, or transdermally are easy to administer and therefore have potentially great utility in developing countries and for mass immunization programs. The development of new adjuvants, which boost the immune response to vaccines, is another important area of research that has progressed rapidly in recent years.

In addition to the development of vaccines against classic infectious diseases, vaccines are being investigated to fight potential agents of bioterrorism, chronic diseases with infectious origins, and autoimmune diseases and other immune-mediated conditions.

Addressing Health Disparities. Much of the NIAID research effort is aimed at the health disparities that exist in the United States, as well as at the growing gap in health status between developed and developing countries. One example of this is the development of vaccines to prevent infectious diseases that disproportionately affect the poor, both in the United States and abroad. Other research addresses conditions that exact a significant toll in minority communities, such as research on HIV treatment and prevention, hepatitis C, and asthma, as well as tissue typing and other transplantation research and research into certain autoimmune diseases. In addition, NIAID has a long-standing commitment to increasing the number of minority investigators involved in

biomedical research and to education and outreach activities. As part of a broad NIH effort to eliminate health disparities, NIAID has developed a strategic plan for addressing health disparities in the new millennium. As discussed in this plan, NIAID will continue to strengthen its efforts to help eliminate health disparities due to infectious and immunologic diseases.

1.1 Primary NIAID Research Areas in Microbiology and Infectious Diseases (Non-HIV/AIDS)

NIAID is continuing its support of research in microbiology and infectious diseases primarily through the Division of Microbiology and Infectious Diseases (DMID). In general, DMID supports research to control and prevent diseases caused by virtually all human infectious agents except HIV/AIDS (http://www3.niaid.nih.gov/ about/organization/dmid/overview/).

Major research areas in microbiology and infectious diseases supported by NIAID include:

- *Bacteriology and Mycology.* Research areas in basic bacteriology and mycology include molecular structure and functions, genetics, biochemical composition, and physiologic and biochemical processes. Studies on infectious human pathogens would extend basic insights to identify candidate antigens for vaccines and drug targets and to examine mechanisms of infections, pathogenicity, and virulence. Areas of particular interest include tuberculosis, streptococci, pneumonia, hospital-caused nosocomial infections, fungal/opportunistic infections, antibiotic resistance, bacterial sexually transmitted diseases, and bacterial diarrheas (http:// www3.niaid.nih.gov/about/organization/dmid/overview/).
- *Biodefense.* As concern grows about the use of biological agents as weapons in acts of terrorism and war, the U.S. federal agencies are evaluating and accelerating measures to protect the public from health consequences of such an attack. The ability of the U.S. government to detect and prevent infections that emerge as a result of bioterrorist incidents depends to a large degree on the state of biomedical science in general and the support NIAID is providing to the NIH's biodefense efforts and those of other federal agencies by funding and conducting research ranging from basic biology of pathogenic microorganisms (including those that could be intentionally introduced) and their interactions with the human immune system to preclinical and clinical evaluation of new diagnostics, therapeutics, and vaccines. One of the integral components of NIAID's Biodefense

Program is its Biodefense Vaccine and other Biologicals Product Development Section (BVBPDS), which is responsible for overseeing the creation, implementation, and execution of research focusing on the development of vaccines and other biological products (http://www3.niaid.nih.gov/about/organization/dmid/overview/).

- *Drug Development.* NIAID maintains an extensive drug development program that supports research at three levels: drug discovery (which encompasses the pathogenesis of the disease and identifying, characterizing, and screening the target on the pathogen); preclinical evaluation by testing drug candidates in models of human infections; and clinical trials evaluating new therapies. For most human pathogens, there are resources for identifying and validating the pathogen target and for developing the assay. For selected viruses and other pathogens, such as tuberculosis, hepatitis B and C, and the NIAID biodefense priority pathogens, there are additional resources for acquiring compounds, screening them, performing *in vitro* and *in vivo* assays, evaluating efficacy in animals and conducting preliminary drug exposure studies, and performing safety testing and pharmacokinetic/pharmacodynamic analyses. In addition, NIAID is involved in multiple public-private partnerships—arrangements that innovatively combine skills and resources from institutions in the public and private sectors to advance drug development (http://www3.niaid.nih.gov/about/organization/dmid/overview/).

- *Emerging and Re-emerging Infectious Diseases.* Despite remarkable advances in medical research and treatment, infectious diseases remain among the leading causes of death worldwide, resulting, in part, from the emergence of new infectious diseases, the re-emergence of old infectious diseases, and the persistence of intractable diseases, sometimes as the result of drug resistance. In addition, the finding that chronic diseases may develop as consequences of acute illness, the challenge of opportunistic infections, and the discovery of viral infections associated with malignancies are presenting new challenges to the scientific community. As a result, NIAID is continuing its support to basic and clinical research—in particular microbial genomics—to better understand the pathogenesis, microbiology, and epidemiology of emerging and re-emerging infectious diseases with the goal of developing more effective diagnostics, vaccines, and therapeutics (http://www3.niaid.nih.gov/about/organization/dmid/overview/).

- *Global Health Research.* A 2002 WHO report on the impact of infectious diseases on public health identifies the following leading infectious diseases with the highest mortality rates: respiratory diseases (pneumonia, influenza), diarrheal diseases, AIDS, malaria, measles, and tuberculosis (http://www.who.int/infectious-disease-report/2002/). Recognizing that infectious diseases spread without regard to national boundaries, NIAID will continue to make international research in infectious diseases a high priority by supporting research aimed at all aspects of infectious pathogens that present, or potentially present, a significant public health threat—research ranging from basic biology and pathology to vaccine development and improved diagnostics. One fundamental part of the NIAID international program is its emphasis on strengthening research capacity for infectious diseases in endemic areas. To achieve this goal, NIAID participates in a number of international partnerships, including the establishment of research programs in tropical medicine, country-to-country bilateral agreements, and interagency agreements with the U.S. Agency of International Development (USAID), the Centers for Disease Control and Prevention (CDC), the National Aeronautics and Space Administration (NASA), and the Department of State, as well as multilateral programs with WHO, the United Nations Children's Fund (UNICEF), the Global Alliance for Vaccines and Immunization (GAVI), and the Multilateral Initiative on Malaria (MIM) (http://www3.niaid.nih.gov/about/organization/dmid/overview/).

- *Microbial Genomics.* One important area of interest for NIAID is funding of research projects to sequence the full genomes of medically important microorganisms. Genome sequencing can make it easier to define targets for vaccine and drug development, identify mutations that contribute to drug resistance, help trace microbial evolution, and provide information for forensic studies by differentiating among strains of organisms (http://www3.niaid.nih.gov/about/organization/dmid/overview/).

- *Parasitology.* NIAID continues its support of research on human parasites using biochemical, genetic, and immunologic approaches to identify protective and diagnostic antigens and to develop more effective drugs. In addition, studies on insect vectors will help control the transmission of pathogens, such as malaria, that are responsible for inflicting significant morbidity and mortality worldwide. Because parasitic and other tropical diseases are international health problems, the NIAID support extends to clinical trials in regions where these infections are endemic through the Tropical Medicine Research Centers and the International Collaboration in Infectious Diseases Research programs (http://www3.niaid.nih.gov/about/organization/dmid/overview/).

- *Respiratory Diseases.* NIAID's Respiratory Diseases Program is aimed at supporting research on effective diagnosis, prevention, and treatment of respiratory infections. This includes developing vaccines and treatments, understanding the long-term health impact that respiratory pathogens have in various populations, stimulating basic research on the pathogenesis, immunity, and structural biology of these pathogens, and developing better diagnostics (http://www3.niaid.nih.gov/about/organization/dmid/overview/). To this end, major areas of interest remain research on influenza and severe acute respiratory syndrome (SARS).

- *Vaccine Development for Sexually Transmitted Infections.* Sexually transmitted infections (STIs) represent a critical global health priority because of their devastating impact on women and infants and their interrelationships with HIV/AIDS. The NIAID research funding is aimed at vaccine development as well as clinical, epidemiologic, and behavioral investigations to identify strategies for primary and secondary prevention of STIs and conditions associated with them. Such conditions include pelvic inflammatory disease (PID), infertility, ectopic pregnancy, cervical cancer, fetal wastage, prematurity, congenital infections, and the spread of HIV. NIAID is also supporting research on topical microbicides in an effort to prevent further spreading of STIs by funding basic product development and clinical research (http://www3.niaid.nih.gov/about/organization/dmid/overview/).

- *Vaccine Development.* One goal of primary importance to NIAID is the development of new and improved vaccines and strategies for vaccine delivery for the entire spectrum of infectious agents: viruses, bacteria, parasites, and fungi. To this end, since 1981, NIAID has been supporting a program for the accelerated development of new vaccines using advances in molecular biology, immunology, genetics, and epidemiology. An important part of these efforts is to conduct studies on vaccine safety through clinical trials sponsored by NIAID (http://www3.niaid.nih.gov/about/organization/dmid/overview/).

- *Virology.* NIAID continues its long-standing support of basic and applied research in virology ranging from vaccine development and gene therapy to drug target identification, as well as the study of virus-host interactions, especially those involved in pathogenesis and immune evasion. Basic information derived from these studies is being used to control the impact of significant viral diseases, such as polio, rabies, diseases caused by herpesviruses, emerging viral infections, and viruses important for biodefense, as well as to develop crucial public health tools, such as antiviral therapeutics (http://www3.niaid.nih.gov/about/organization/dmid/overview/).

Chapter 2

NIAID International Research Programs: Global Impact

NIAID conducts and supports a global program of research aimed at improving diagnosis, treatment, and prevention of immunologic, allergic, and emerging infectious diseases. This research has led to new therapies, vaccines, diagnostic tests, and other technologies that have improved the health of millions of people in the United States and around the world (http://www3.niaid.nih.gov/topics/GlobalResearch/default.htm).

Note: Whenever relevant, further detailed information on NIAID international research programs is described in the separate book chapters that follow.

Several unique NIAID international programs designed to promote scientific advances and cooperation on important infectious diseases and pathogens include:

- *International Research In Infectious Diseases (IRID).* The International Research In Infectious Diseases (IRID) initiative is intended to encourage the submission of *R01 applications of investigators from institutions in eligible foreign countries* (who do not currently have NIAID-funded research grant awards) to conduct studies and establish and/or extend collaborative infectious diseases research among investigators and institutions at international sites where NIAID has significant investment in research and/or infrastructure, including such international research programs as: (i) The International Centers of Excellence in Research (ICERs); (ii) International Collaborations for Infectious Diseases Research (ICIDRs); (iii) The Tropical Medicine Research Centers (TMRCs); and (iv) The Tuberculosis Research Program. Clinical trials will not be supported through IRID.

- *International Collaborations for Infectious Diseases Research (ICIDR).* The International Collaborations for Infectious Diseases (ICIDR) program is designed to promote collaborative research between U.S. investigators and scientists in about 15 countries where *tropical infections are endemic.* In 1999, the ICIDR program was re-competed to include a companion program from the Fogarty International Center, entitled *"Actions for Building Capacity (ABC),"* which supports training of foreign

investigators in the context of the ICIDR program. There are 14 NIAID-supported sites and 4 additional sites with support from NICHD and NIDA. There are nine ABC awards in the ICIDR program.

- *Tropical Disease Research Units (TDRU).* The Tropical Disease Research Units (TDRU) program is a *domestic grants award program* intended to provide support for multiproject, interdisciplinary studies that seek to develop new strategies to control diseases by *protozoa and helminths.*

- *Tropical Medicine Research Centers (TMRC).* The Tropical Medicine Research Centers (TMRC) is a program that is intended to support 4 foreign institutions—currently located in Mali, China, Colombia, and Brazil—in conducting research of direct relevance to the health of the people in tropical environments and to promote collaborations and exchange of information between foreign and U.S. scientists (http://grants.nih.gov/grants/guide/rfa-files/RFA-AI-06-006.html). This program was initiated in 1991 to support International Centers located in disease endemic areas in conducting research in major tropical diseases. The 2006 initiative solicited applications in the areas of leishmaniasis, Chagas' disease, and human African trypanosomiasis to facilitate translational research using the recently published genomes of the trypanosomatids.

- *International Centers for Tropical Diseases Research (ICTDR).* Institutions supported by grants from TDRU, ICIDR, and the TMRC programs and other large international research sites, along with the NIAID's Division of Intramural Research (DIR), comprise the NIAID Network of International Centers for Tropical Diseases Research (ICTDR). The ICTDR program incorporates NIAID-supported intramural and extramural tropical disease research centers into an interactive network focused on tropical infectious disease problems.

- *Tuberculosis Research Unit (TBRU).* The Tuberculosis Research Unit (TBRU) is a contract to Case Western Reserve University intended to develop surrogate markers of disease and human protective immunity and to conduct clinical trials of potential new TB therapeutic, preventive, and diagnostic strategies. In addition, well-characterized clinical samples will be available for distribution to TBRU investigators and their collaborators through a newly established repository. The activities of the TBRU are coordinated with other major organizations involved in tuberculosis research, including CDC, U.S. Department of Agriculture (USDA), U.S. Food and Drug Administration (FDA), WHO, Global Alliance for TB Drug Development, and the International Union Against Tuberculosis and Lung Disease (IUATLD), and with interested industrial partners.

- *Vaccine Action Program (VAP).* The Indo-U.S. Vaccine Action Program (VAP) was initiated in 1987 as a bilateral program that focuses on the development of safe and effective vaccines for major communicable diseases of interest to India and the United States through joint research and development. Currently, the focus of VAC is on HIV/AIDS, malaria, and tuberculosis.

- *U.S.-Japan Cooperative Medical Science Program.* This is a 36-year-old bilateral, cooperative research program involving U.S. and Japanese scientists who convene on a regular basis to address *public health priorities in Asia*; for example, the U.S.-Japan Workshops in Medical Mycology (http://www.niaid.nih.gov/dmid/fungal#2e). The goals of these workshops have been to initiate interactions; build collaborations; identify research needs; turn needs into opportunities; stimulate molecular research in medical mycology; and summarize recommendations emerging from workshop proceedings *(1)*.

- *International Training and Research in Emerging Infectious Diseases (ITREID).* The International Training and Research in Emerging Infectious Diseases (ITREID) has been established as collaboration between NIAID and the Fogarty International Center (FIC) to support international training and research. The intent of this program is to enable NIH grant recipients to enhance laboratory, epidemiologic, clinical, and social sciences research and to train scientists and public health workers from developing countries and their U.S. counterparts in research, control, and prevention strategies.

- *International Malaria Research Training Program (IMRTP).* The IMRTP initiative is a joint collaborative program of the Fogarty International Center and NIAID aimed at training and/or expanding the capabilities of scientists and health professionals from developing countries in which malaria is endemic and to engage in research relevant to severe malarial anemia (http://grants.nih.gov/grants/guide/rfa-files/RFA-TW-01-006.html).

- *International Cooperative Biodiversity Groups Program (ICBG).* The International Cooperative Biodiversity Groups is a program with a threefold mission: conservation of biodiversity, economic growth for developing countries (e.g., Central and South America, Nigeria, Cameroon, Madagascar, Jordan, Central Asia, Papua New Guinea, Laos, and Vietnam), and discovery of pharmaceuticals from natural products. NIAID, together with the National Cancer Institute (NCI), National Institute of Mental Health (NIMH), National Heart, Lung, and Blood Institute (NHLBI), National Institute on Drug Abuse (NIDA), FIC, the National Science Foundation, and the USDA, are the co-sponsors of ICBG. The current awards are given to multidisciplinary research groups that also include in-country, research-capacity collections, and *partnerships with a pharmaceutical company.* The ICBG program has been widely recognized as a model for research partnerships that acknowledge intellectual property ownership of indigenous communities.

- *International Clinical Studies Support Centers (ICSSC).* The primary goal of the International Clinical Studies Support Centers (ICSSC) is to enhance the capacity of *international clinical sites* to perform clinical research in accordance with international standards, such as the International Conference on Harmonization's (ICH) Good Clinical Practices (GCP), and to facilitate the planning and conduct of clinical epidemiologic studies and clinical trials that range from small, early-phase trials to large, multicenter efficacy trials. These studies are conducted throughout the world, primarily in Africa, South and Central America, and Asia.

- *Ethical Aspects of Research in Developing Countries.* NIAID sponsors workshops on the Ethical Aspects of Research in Developing Countries with the participation of the NIH Department of Bioethics. To date, there have been workshops held in Malawi and Ghana.

- *U.S.-South Africa Science and Technology Agreement.* A Framework Agreement between the U.S. government and the government of the Republic of South Africa concerning cooperation in scientific, technologic, and environmental fields, including areas of public health, was signed on December 5, 1995. This agreement is still in effect.

2.1 Global Research: Africa

As operationally defined by WHO, the African Region (WHO/AFRO) comprises 46 countries. Other countries in the African continent belong to another operationally defined region of WHO (http://www3.niaid.nih.gov/topics/GlobalResearch/Africa/default.htm).

As Africa confronts the 21st century, it faces several challenges. Some of the major challenges are in the interrelated areas of economic development and health. According to WHO, an estimated 45% of the population of Africa lives below the poverty line, on less than US$1.00 per day. As WHO reports, life expectancy is only 47 years, and people suffer from a wide range of diseases, several of which are NIAID's highest priorities for research:

- The majority of cases of malaria each year occur in Africa, primarily in children under 5 years of age
- HIV/AIDS has had a more devastating effect on Africa than on any other region of the world
- Tuberculosis (TB) is a major cause of death among people living with HIV/AIDS, and Africa bears the brunt of the HIV-fueled TB epidemic

2.1.1 Countries with NIAID-Funded Research Activities

African countries with current NIAID-funded activities (Fig. 2.1) include:

Benin	Malawi
Botswana	Mali
Burkina Faso	Mauritius
Cameroon	Mozambique
Central African Republic	Nigeria
Côte d'Ivoire	Republic of the Congo
Democratic Republic of the Congo (DRC)	Rwanda
Gabon	Senegal
Gambia, The	South Africa
Ghana	Tanzania
Kenya	Uganda
Liberia	Zambia
Madagascar	Zimbabwe

Additional countries where NIAID is conducting and supporting research will continue to be added. However, this information is not meant to be a complete list of NIAID research and NIAID-sponsored activities. It is intended to serve as an overview.

Research Focus. NIAID has funded research activities in 26 African countries, mostly in southern and eastern Africa. However, NIAID has also developed a major research presence in Mali in West Africa (http://www3.niaid.nih.gov/topics/GlobalResearch/Africa/default.htm).

HIV/AIDS, TB, and malaria are three of the most serious infectious diseases in Africa, causing millions of deaths each year. These three diseases are a major cause of poverty through their debilitating impact on the workforce and significantly affect the economic development and stability of the region. NIAID supports HIV/AIDS research in all of these 26 countries, with most projects conducted in areas with the highest incidence of infection and disease, namely Botswana, Kenya, Malawi, Rwanda, South Africa, Zambia, and Zimbabwe.

The recent emergence of multidrug-resistant TB (MDR TB) and extensively drug-resistant TB (XDR TB), especially in the context of HIV/AIDS infection, is being addressed by NIAID-funded projects conducted in South Africa, Tanzania, and Uganda.

Malaria remains a major threat, and NIAID conducts clinical, epidemiologic, drug, and vaccine research in east African countries such as Kenya, Malawi, Tanzania, and Uganda, and in Mali, Cameroon, Ghana, and The Gambia in central and West Africa.

Neglected diseases such as filariasis and schistosomiasis are receiving renewed attention, with NIAID projects in Kenya, Malawi, and South Africa. Diarrheal and respiratory diseases and vector-borne diseases, such as African trypanosomiasis (sleeping sickness), are also of concern.

2.1.1.1 The Gambia

The largest NIAID investment in The Gambia is in malaria, particularly severe malaria in children, and methods of controlling mosquito larvae. NIAID also has a program on *Helicobacter pylori* and two programs on HIV/AIDS. A major program on a Phase III pneumococcal conjugate vaccine study in Basse, The Gambia, involved collaboration among NIAID, the British Medical Research Council (MRC), Wyeth Pharmaceuticals, WHO, the Program for Appropriate Technology in Health (PATH), and the United States Agency for International Development (USAID). This study was successfully completed in 2005 and has provided data to show that serious infections and deaths can be prevented by the incorporation of a pneumococcal conjugate vaccine into the local expanded program on immunization (EPI) (http://www3.niaid.nih.gov/research/topics/bacterial/clinical/GambiaPneumococcalVaccineTrial.htm).

The MRC facility has offered the U.S. researchers the opportunity to undertake human clinical vaccine trials that comply fully with FDA regulations. Among these trials were a Phase II pneumococcal vaccine trial and a malaria vaccine involving the U.S. Department of Defense. Vector-borne diseases, including dengue, Crimean-Congo hemorrhagic fever, and yellow fever, remain endemic. Water-borne diseases include bacterial and protozoal diarrhea, hepatitis A, and typhoid fever.

Selected Current and Recent NIAID-Funded Research (Non-HIV/AIDS). The following information is not necessarily a complete list of NIAID research and NIAID-sponsored activities. It is intended to serve as an overview.

- *Malaria*

  (i) Severe malaria in African children—Michigan State University
  (ii) Antilarval measures in malaria control—University of Durham, United Kingdom

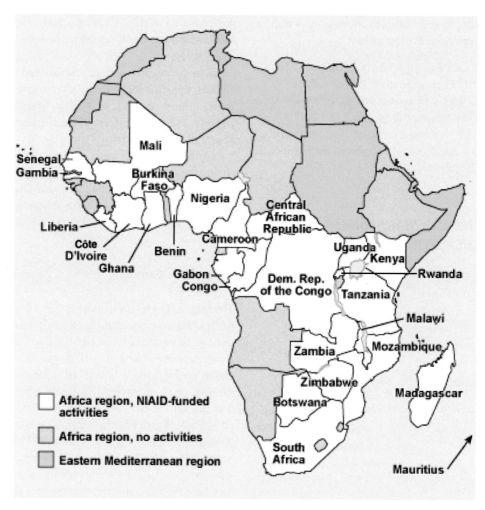

Fig. 2.1 Map of African countries with NIAID-funded activities—world regions as defined by WHO

- *Helicobacter pylori*

    (i) Genotypes of *Helicobacter pylori* in The Gambia—
         MRC, Banjul, The Gambia

2.1.1.2 Kenya

Kenya is a major site of NIAID funding, with 29 recently
funded activities. The heaviest investments are in HIV/AIDS,
malaria, schistosomiasis, and vector studies. There are
opportunities for further research in TB (especially in the
context of HIV/AIDS) and vector-borne diseases, especially
Rift Valley fever (RVF), a serious zoonosis (a disease that
primarily affects animals, but occasionally causes disease in
humans) (http://www3.niaid.nih.gov/topics/GlobalResearch/
Africa/Kenya.htm).

According to WHO data, child mortality remains high
in the country. Kenya has a high risk of food- and water-
borne diseases, particularly bacterial and protozoal diarrhea,
hepatitis A, schistosomiasis, and typhoid fever. Malaria is
endemic in many areas, especially around Lake Victoria, and
vector-borne diseases in general remain a threat, particularly
RVF. HIV/AIDS prevalence is 7.4% and, according to WHO,
the incidence of TB is high. The appearance of MDR TB and
emergence of XDR TB are potential threats. Kenya reported
two cases of polio in 2006, although it is not regarded as a
highly endemic country.

*Selected Current and Recent NIAID-Funded Research
(Non-HIV/AIDS).* The following information is not necessarily a complete list of NIAID research and NIAID-sponsored
activities. It is intended to serve as an overview.

- *Malaria*

    (i)   Associating genetic variation with resistance in
          severe malaria in East Africa—Harvard University
          Medical School
    (ii) Human immunity to merozoite surface protein-1 in
          western Kenya—Case Western Reserve University
    (iii) Fetal immunity to falciparum malaria—Case West-
          ern Reserve University

(iv) Redefining cerebral malaria—Michigan State University

(v) Malaria transmission and immunity in highland Kenya—University of Minnesota

- *Schistosomiasis*

  (i) Toward a molecularly defined vaccine for schistosomiasis—Southwest Foundation for Biomedical Research

  (ii) Evo-epidemiology of *Schistosoma mansoni* in western Kenya—University of New Mexico

  (iii) Determinants of resistance in human schistosomiasis—University of Georgia

- *Vectors*

  (i) Population genomics of mosquito *Anopheles gambiae* in Africa—University of California at Davis

  (ii) Nutritional ecology of adult *Anopheles gambiae*—Ohio State University

  (iii) Microbial control of immature *Anopheles* mosquitoes—University of Illinois at Champagne-Urbana

  (iv) Insecticide mosaics and sustainability of treated nets—Michigan State University

- *Other*

  (i) Immunologic studies of Burkitt's lymphoma—Case Western Reserve University

  (ii) Clinical epidemiology of *Mycoplasma genitalium*—University of Washington, Seattle

2.1.1.3 Mali

NIAID maintains on-site staff in Bamako, Mali, working in close association with the Faculty of Medicine, Pharmacy, and Odonto-Stomatology (FMPOS) at the University of Bamako. The intramural research program has been active in Mali since the late 1980s; in 2002, the FMPOS/University of Bamako was selected as an NIAID International Center of Excellence in Research. Milestones in the intramural collaborations with the FMPOS include the establishment of the Malaria Research and Training Center at the University of Bamako; the development of clinical field sites to test candidate malaria vaccines and to conduct studies on malaria and lymphatic filariasis; the development of a collaborative program to study HIV/AIDS and tuberculosis co-infection; the renovation of a BSL-3 laboratory for use in the co-infection studies; and the establishment of the Mali Service Center.

Mali's climate is highly stratified: hot and arid in the north and wetter and more humid in the south. This affects vector-borne diseases such as malaria. Food- and water-borne diseases, particularly associated with the Niger River, include

bacterial and protozoal diarrhea, hepatitis A, typhoid fever, and schistosomiasis.

Selected Current and Recent NIAID-Funded Research (Non-HIV/AIDS). The following information is not necessarily a complete list of NIAID research and NIAID-sponsored activities. It is intended to serve as an overview.

- *Malaria Clinical Research*

  (i) Malaria Vaccine Trials in Mali—University of Maryland, Baltimore

  (ii) Vaccines: Phase II trials in children (Bandiagara, Donéguebougou, Bancoumana), and Phase I trial in adults (Donéguebougou)—NIAID intramural program

  (iii) Preterm and infant mortality observational study—Gabriel Toure Hospital, Bamako

  (iv) Multidisciplinary studies of malaria protection by hemoglobinopathies and glucose-6-phosphate dehydrogenase (G6PD) deficiency—NIAID intramural program

- *Malaria*

  (i) Genetic basis for natural resistance to malaria in *Anopheles gambiae*—NIAID intramural program

  (ii) Identification of genetically susceptible *Anopheles gambiae* to *Plasmodium falciparum* by location—NIAID intramural program

  (iii) Genomics of mosquito resistance to *Plasmodium*—University of Minnesota at Twin Cities

  (iv) Niono Irrigation Project and Malaria: A Computer Model—University of California at Los Angeles

- *Filariasis Clinical Research*

  (i) Albendazole dosage/frequency-ivermectin/albendazole trial—NIAID intramural program

  (ii) Doxycycline to reduce microfilaremia in co-infections, safety and efficacy—NIAID intramural program

- *HIV/TB Clinical Research*

  (i) CD4$^+$ T-cell immune responses to *Mycobacterium tuberculosis*—NIAID intramural program

  (ii) Establishment of normal parameters for blood and sputum with samples obtained from volunteers in Bamako—NIAID intramural program

2.1.1.4 Mozambique

NIAID supports three projects in Mozambique, all linked to the country's high prevalence of HIV/AIDS. However, Mozambique's health priorities are more complex.

Mozambique suffers from high infant mortality, an expanding HIV/AIDS epidemic, malaria (*Plasmodium falciparum*) as the primary cause of mortality among children under 5 years of age, and recent severe outbreaks of cholera. Extensive malnutrition among children and an increasing burden of TB, according to WHO, are also of concern (http://www3.niaid.nih.gov/topics/GlobalResearch/Africa/Mozambique.htm).

2.1.1.5 Rwanda

All of NIAID's current funding in Rwanda involves HIV/AIDS—the adult prevalence rate in Rwanda is approximately 5%.

However, malaria is a major problem and probably contributes to the country's high infant mortality rate (WHO). There was a regional outbreak of meningococcus that caused as many as 636 cases in 2002, leading to a mass immunization program. As in many other countries in this region, water-borne diseases, such as bacterial diarrhea, hepatitis A, and typhoid fever, are prevalent. In addition, TB is a problem (WHO) that has remained steady over several years, with emerging MDR TB. Immunization rates are generally low.

2.1.1.6 South Africa

Currently, NIAID is funding more than 50 projects in South Africa, most of them involving HIV/AIDS research. However, the institute is also supporting research on TB, malaria, and other diseases or vectors. These projects focus primarily on treatment and pathogenesis. NIAID also supports some prevention and epidemiology studies in these areas and provides direct funding to seven institutions in South Africa involving 17 projects (http://www3.niaid.nih.gov/topics/GlobalResearch/Africa/SouthAfrica.htm).

The incidence of TB in South Africa is high, according to WHO. The recent emergence of MDR TB, and now XDR TB, is a major and urgent new challenge. Better surveillance for drug resistance is urgently needed to determine the level and extent of MDR and XDR TB, especially in relation to HIV status. HIV-associated infections such as *Cryptococcus neoformans* are increasingly found. Drug-resistant *Staphylococcus aureus* is a major health problem. There has been a rapid resurgence of chloroquine-resistant malaria strains, and schistosomiasis is endemic in rivers in eastern South Africa. Crimean-Congo hemorrhagic fever is also endemic. Despite a low life expectancy at birth (WHO), diseases such as diabetes mellitus and obesity are expected to increase significantly.

Selected Current and Recent NIAID-Funded Research (Non-HIV/AIDS). The following information is not nec-

essarily a complete list of NIAID research and NIAID-sponsored activities. It is intended to serve as an overview.

- *Tuberculosis*

  (i) A smart microscope for the detection of tuberculosis in ZN-stained sputum smears—University of Cape Town, South Africa

  (ii) Diagnostic yield of induced sputum for rapid diagnosis of pulmonary tuberculosis—University of Cape Town, South Africa

  (iii) Inherited resistance in Beijing with isolates of *M. tuberculosis*—University of Stellenbosch, South Africa

  (iv) Protective immunity induced by newborn Bacillus Calmette-Guérin (BCG) vaccination—University of Cape Town, South Africa

  (v) Regulation of dormancy in *M. tuberculosis*—University of Pennsylvania

  (vi) Ecology, genetics, and physiology of insect vectors—Iowa State University

  (vii) Host and pathogen determinants of *M. tuberculosis* latency—Public Health Research Institute, Newark

  (viii) Molecular approaches for understanding TB dynamics—Harvard University Medical School

  (ix) A second-generation patch test for tuberculosis—Sequella, Inc., Rockville, Maryland

  (x) Development of novel resistance management strategies—Liverpool School of Tropical Medicine, United Kingdom

  (xi) The role of the granuloma in *M. tuberculosis* infections—Cornell University, New York

- *HIV/TB Research*

  (i) BCG as an HIV vaccine vector—University of Cape Town, South Africa

  (ii) Novel TB prevention regimens for HIV-infected adults—Johns Hopkins University

- *Malaria Research*

  (i) Development of novel resistance management strategies—Liverpool School of Tropical Medicine, United Kingdom

2.1.1.7 Tanzania

NIAID funds research programs in Tanzania related to HIV/AIDS, TB, and malaria, among other diseases (http://www3.niaid.nih.gov/topics/GlobalResearch/Africa/Tanzania.htm). In comparison with its neighboring countries, the child mortality rate in Tanzania is lower, but the HIV/AIDS prevalence rate is higher. Major infectious diseases including food- or water-borne diseases, such as bacterial diarrhea, hepatitis A, and typhoid fever, and vector-borne diseases, such as malaria, remain serious. There has also been plague and a March 2007 outbreak of Rift Valley fever with clusters of human cases. Schistosomiasis is an important water contact disease. TB prevalence is high according to WHO, with a small percentage of TB cases identified as MDR TB. Noncommunicable diseases such as diabetes mellitus are rising significantly.

Selected Current and Recent NIAID-Funded Research (Non-HIV/AIDS). The following information is not necessarily a complete list of NIAID research and NIAID-sponsored activities. It is intended to serve as an overview.

- *Tuberculosis*

    (i) Nutrition, immunology, and epidemiology of TB—Harvard University School of Public Health
    (ii) TB clinical research: training the next generation—Centralized HIV-1 genes as vaccines—Duke University
    (iii) Training African giant rats as a cheap diagnostic tool for early TB detection—APOPO vzw, Antwerp, Belgium, and Tanzania

- *HIV/TB*

    (i) Disseminated tuberculosis in HIV infection—Dartmouth College
    (ii) Adjunct vitamin A therapy for tuberculosis and HIV/AIDS—Johns Hopkins University

- *Malaria*

    (i) Severe falciparum malaria: mechanisms of hypoargininemia—University of Utah
    (ii) Hyperphenylalaninemia in cerebral malaria—University of Utah
    (iii) Pathogenesis of falciparum malaria in infancy—Seattle Biomedical Research Institute
    (iv) Preventing pregnancy malaria: maternal-infant outcomes—Seattle Biomedical Research Institute
    (v) Nitric oxide and severe malaria—Duke University

- *Other*

    (i) Effect of zinc supplementation on pneumonia in children—Muhimbili University College of Health Sciences, Dar-es-Salaam, Tanzania

2.1.1.8 Uganda

Currently, NIAID is funding approximately 28 projects in Uganda related to HIV/AIDS, malaria, and TB (http://www3.niaid.nih.gov/topics/GlobalResearch/Africa/Uganda.htm). Among them are the program at Tufts University on cryptococcus; four core activities to support HIV/AIDS research; work on the interactions of HIV/AIDS and TB and of HIV/AIDS and malaria; and malaria drug studies.

Despite expending 7.6% of the gross domestic product (GDP) on health in 2004, Uganda has a high infant mortality rate and low life expectancy (WHO). HIV prevalence declined from 15% in 1991 to 5% by 2001, but this decline has stopped. The government has announced a countrywide plan to implement male circumcision as an HIV/AIDS preventive method. As in neighboring countries, tuberculosis incidence is high (WHO), and cases of MDR TB have been found. Outbreaks of meningococcal meningitis have occurred in 2006 and 2007, cholera in 2003, and Ebola in 2000. In addition, bacterial diarrhea, hepatitis A, typhoid fever, vector-borne diseases—malaria and African trypanosomiasis (sleeping sickness)—and water-contact schistosomiasis are high risks in some locations.

Selected Current and Recent NIAID-Funded Research (Non-HIV/AIDS). The following information is not necessarily a complete list of NIAID research and NIAID-sponsored activities. It is intended to serve as an overview.

- *HIV Interactions with Other Diseases*

    (i) Associating genetic variation with resistance in severe malaria in East Africa—Harvard University Medical School
    (ii) Human immunity to merozoite surface protein-1 in western Kenya—Case Western Reserve University
    (iii) Clinical studies of interactions between HIV and malaria—University of California at San Francisco

- *Tuberculosis*

    (i) Tuberculosis immunity in young children—Oregon Health & Science University
    (ii) Sample processing cartridges for rapid polymerase chain reaction (PCR) TB detection—Cepheid, Sunnyvale, California

- *Malaria*

    (i) Clinical and molecular studies of drug resistant malaria—University of California at San Francisco
    (ii) Utility of rapid diagnostic tests for malaria—University of California at San Francisco

- *Cryptosporidium*

    (i) Studies on *Cryptosporidium parvum* type 1—Tufts University

- *Chlamydia*

    (i) Immunopathogenesis of *Chlamydia trachomatis* infection—NIAID intramural research

2.2 Global Research: Asia

International Collaboration in Influenza Research. Within the NIH, the NIAID is tasked with performing and supporting research to prevent, detect, and treat infectious diseases such as influenza. During the past 5 years, NIAID influenza research funding grew from US$16.8 million to US$196.3 million in fiscal year 2006.

The NIAID influenza research effort covers the spectrum from basic research to clinical trials, leading to the discovery and implementation of influenza vaccines, therapeutics, and diagnostics. Like research on other diseases, influenza research progress hinges upon collaboration and shared resources (http://www.usminstitute.org/spotlight_23.html).

Seasonal influenza is a fairly predictable annual occurrence. WHO estimates that influenza epidemics result in 250,000 to 500,000 deaths globally per year. In contrast, the impact of pandemic influenza, an unpredictable but historically proven threat, can range from fairly mild (1968) to catastrophic (1918).

An influenza virus that causes illness in humans, to which the majority of the human population has little or no immunity, and that is easily transmissible among humans, constitutes a pandemic virus. Of the existing potential pandemic viruses, the highly pathogenic avian influenza (HPAI) H5N1 virus that has become endemic in poultry in Southeast Asia, Eastern Europe, and several countries in Africa presents a source of concern to scientists and health officials around the world.

Not surprisingly, seasonal influenza preparedness and prevention are inherently linked to pandemic influenza preparedness and prevention. Both seasonal influenza research and pandemic influenza research depend on collaboration, especially at the international level. NIAID participates in several international influenza research efforts regarding pandemic preparedness. Several international partners identified the need for a clinical research network focused on therapeutics. Thus, in 2005 the NIAID Division of Clinical Research, with multilateral partners, established the *Southeast Asia (SEA) Influenza Clinical Research Network* to advance the scientific knowledge and management of human influenza through integrated, collaborative clinical research. Partners include hospitals and institutions in Vietnam, Indonesia, Thailand, the United Kingdom, and the United States. The network is committed to building independent research capacity within the SEA countries involved. NIAID and the Wellcome Trust provide financial support. Initial clinical studies will evaluate appropriate dosage levels of the influenza antiviral drug oseltamivir in patients with severe seasonal or avian influenza. Pharmacokinetics studies of oseltamivir in Asian subjects began in autumn 2006 at the Network Pharmacokinetics Unit at Mahidol University in Thailand.

NIAID Research on SARS. NIAID maintains a long-standing commitment to conducting and supporting research on emerging infectious diseases, such as SARS, with the goal of improving global health. In carrying out its global health research mission, the institute is supporting SARS research, including intramural and extramural research and collaborations with international agencies and organizations, to rapidly initiate the development of diagnostics, therapeutics, and vaccines against SARS.

Through a grant supplement to the Chinese Center of Disease Control (China CDC) and their collaborators, NIAID has funded three different SARS projects. Approaches undertaken include:

- Developing immune correlates of protection through study of pediatric and adult serum, stool, and cellular clinical samples obtained longitudinally from SARS patients
- Developing a panel of human SARS-associated coronavirus (SARS-CoV) antisera that can be used to standardize diagnostic assays. This project will be a collaboration with FDA and CDC
- Attempting to identify animal reservoirs of SARS-CoV through surveillance of live animal markets.

NIAID has assembled a multidisciplinary working group to develop a broad-based program that addresses the research needed to combat SARS. Key NIAID intramural laboratories have begun to pursue a range of research strategies to develop a SARS vaccine as well as therapeutics, including immune-based therapies, and the institute extramural programs are poised to help as well. NIAID has also initiated and expanded collaborations with other federal agencies, academia, and private industry. In addition, NIAID has released "Sources Sought" announcements, a special mechanism to rapidly identify contractors who can develop treatment strategies, vaccines, and antibody preparations to address SARS (http://energycommerce.house.gov/reparchives/108/Hearings/05072003hearing917/Fauci1435print.htm).

NIAID has purchased several hundred SARS microarrays—essentially a reference strain of the SARS coronavirus embedded in a quartz chip—and distributed the arrays at no cost to qualified researchers worldwide (http://findarticles.com/p/articles/mi_pnih/is_200306/ai_1336428103).

Seroprevalence Studies. As part of the international avian influenza effort, NIAID has funded several seroprevalence studies in Southeast Asia. A study of close contacts of infected individuals is being conducted by the China CDC. A case-control study of infected individuals is also planned to examine risks associated with infection. Basic research on the cross-reactivity of immune responses to the influenza H5N1 strain is also being carried out at the Chinese Academy of Medical Science. Bird isolates will be evaluated at the Chinese Academy of Science.

In addition, a population-based seroprevalence study will be conducted in three provinces of Vietnam. This study will be coordinated by the National Institute of Hygiene and Epidemiology in collaboration with the AFRIMS laboratory in Thailand.

Enteric Diseases. NIAID has established an Interagency Agreement with the U.S. Department of Defense to support the AFRIMS (Armed Forces Research Institute of Medical Sciences) site in Thailand to develop a non-human primate model of shigellosis and to conduct clinical trials of vaccines against shigellosis and other enteric pathogens.

2.3 Partnerships

- *Product Development Public-Private Partnerships (PDPPPs).* In 2006, a new initiative was announced by NIAID that calls attention to the vital role played by PDPPPs in developing new products directed against the neglected tropical diseases. NIAID is seeking to provide support to PDPPPs that have diagnostic or therapeutic products requiring additional targeted funding in order to complete the preclinical phase of development and enable an Investigational New Drug (IND) or Investigational Device Exemption (IDE) to be submitted for transition to clinical development.
- *The Global Alliance for TB Drug Development (GATB).* GATB is a nonprofit organization involving many public and private partners, which is contributing to the development of new drugs to shorten or simplify the treatment of TB and facilitate TB control in high-burden countries. More than 30 organizations are stakeholders in this public-private partnership, including the Bill & Melinda Gates Foundation, CDC, NIAID/NIH, the Rockefeller Foundation, USAID, the World Bank, and WHO (http://www.tballiance.org/).
- *Bill & Melinda Gates Foundation.* The Bill & Melinda Gates Foundation has collaborated with NIAID by funding a symposium at the larger NIAID-organized U.S. – Japan Cooperative Medical Sciences Program, Panel Meeting and Scientific Conference on Cholera and Related Bacterial Enteric Infections (the symposium title: "Challenges in Translational Research: Symposium on Vaccine Development—Pathways to Licensure," Boston, Massachusetts, December 1, 2005).
- To enhance dialogue between NIAID-funded scientists working on malaria and the implementing organizations of the President's Malaria Initiative (PMI), NIAID convened a 3-day meeting in Kampala, Uganda, entitled "Malaria Research into Practice: Research to Advise Policy, Policy to Advise Research." Twenty-eight scientists from Africa and the United States participated in the meeting, which began on April 25, 2006, the African Malaria Day.
- *Multilateral Initiative on Malaria (MIM).* NIAID continues to support the MIM through grants to African researchers at African institutions under the MIM/TDR Program (http://www.who.int/tdr/diseases/malaria/mimprojectsall.htm).
- *Federal Malaria Vaccine Coordinating Committee (FMVCC).* NIAID continues to participate in FMVCC and provides support to the *MIM/TDR Task Force* to advance malaria research and strengthen research capacity at African institutions. NIAID also participates in the *Malaria Vaccine Advisory Committee* established at the *WHO Initiative for Vaccine Research (WHO/IVR)* and in the External Scientific Advisory Committee of the *Medicines for Malaria Venture*, a public-private partnership that fosters the accelerated development of new antimalarial compounds.
- *The International Cooperative Biodiversity Groups.* This NIAID-sponsored initiative addresses the interdependent issues of biodiversity conservation, economic capacity, and human health through discovery and development of therapeutic agents for diseases of importance in developing countries, as well as those of importance in developed countries. Five comprehensive awards and seven planning grants were announced (http://www.nih.gov/news/pr/dec2003/fic-16.htm). Areas of research include discovery of natural products for treatment of HIV, TB, malaria, and other tropical diseases, with screening of extracts from Uzbekistan, Kyrgyzstan, Papua New Guinea, Laos, Vietnam, Panama, Jordan, and Costa Rica. Two additional comprehensive awards co-funded by NIAID were awarded in 2006 (http://www.nih.gov/news/pr/jan2006/fic-03.htm) from the planning grants.
- *2006 NIAID Research Conference.* As part of its mission to reduce the burden of human disease, NIH—and NIAID in particular—has committed to encouraging the accelerated translation of biomedical discoveries into new treatments outside the United States. One direction for NIAID has been to broaden research opportunities and collaborations with scientists and research and educational institutions in Europe and in particular of countries from Central and Eastern Europe, the Baltics, Russia, Ukraine, and other newly independent states of the former Soviet Union. To this end, the Office of Global Research at NIAID took the initiative to organize the 2006 NIAID Research Conference in Opatija, Croatia (June 26–30, 2006) (http://www3.niaid.nih.gov/program/croatia).

The Scientific Program of the Conference covered a wide range of sessions by invited speakers on topics reflecting the broad scope of scientific activities of NIAID. The 2006 NIAID Research Conference also featured plenary lectures delivered by distinguished scientists, roundtable discussions on a wide variety of topics, and poster sessions open to all participants *(2)*.

Prior to the conference (June 24–25, 2006), a Satellite Symposium was held on "Grants Opportunities and Preparation" (grantsmanship, technology transfer, regulatory affairs, and FDA regulations with concurrent workshops) and on training opportunities at NIH by the Fogarty International Center. The training courses were conducted by staff members from the Division of Extramural Activities at NIAID and the NIH Offices of Technology Transfer and Regulatory Affairs *(2)*.

About 300 participants from 39 countries in Europe, Asia, and North America have attended the 2006 NIAID Research Conference. As a direct result of the conference, 13 new collaborations in biomedical research were established by U.S. and foreign scientists.

References

1. Dixon, D. M. (2001) U.S.-Japan workshops in medical mycology: past, present and future, *Jpn. J. Med. Mycol.*, **42**, 75–80.
2. Georgiev, V. St., Western, K. A., and McGowan, J. J. (eds.) (2006) *National Institute of Allergy and Infectious Diseases, NIH: Frontiers in Research*, vol. 1, Humana Press, Totowa, NJ .

Chapter 3

Bacterial Diseases

Bacterial diseases continue to present a major threat to human health. Because bacteria are ubiquitous and have such diverse metabolic capabilities, knowledge of their capabilities influences essentially all disciplines of biomedical science and is instrumental for understanding fundamental life processes of all organisms. Bacteria provide readily usable experimental systems to shed light on the complex metabolic and regulatory networks that control these processes. Many of the success stories arising from new technologies, such as genomics and proteomics, have resulted from new research in microbial physiology and genetics, justifying increased investment in the study of these organisms *(1)*.

Tuberculosis, for instance, ranks among the world's leading causes of death. *Streptococcus* (GBS), another bacterium, continues to be a frequent cause of life-threatening infection during the first 2 months of life. Food-borne and water-borne bacteria, such as *Salmonella* and *Campylobacter*, are responsible for a recent troubling increase in diarrheal disease. Meanwhile, during the past decade, scientists have discovered many new organisms and new strains of many familiar bacteria, such as *Escherichia coli*. Such emerging bacterial diseases present a clear challenge to biomedical researchers (http://www3.niaid.nih.gov/research/topics/bacterial/introduction).

The complexity of this challenge is becoming even clearer as researchers begin to appreciate the many unsuspected mechanisms that bacteria have for causing health problems in humans. For example, gene transfer among different strains of bacteria, and even between different species of bacteria, is now understood to be a common means whereby these organisms acquire resistance to antibiotics. Basic research has also discovered that some bacteria may play a major role in certain chronic diseases not formerly associated with bacterial infection. Thus, *Helicobacter pylori* has been found to cause ulcers and may contribute to stomach cancer, whereas Guillain-Barré syndrome has been associated with prior diarrheal disease caused by *Campylobacter jejuni* (http://www3.niaid.nih.gov/research/topics/bacterial/introduction).

NIAID researchers are involved in all aspects of investigation to help solve the difficult challenges of bacterial diseases. Research in basic bacteriology includes investigating molecular structure and function, genomics, biochemical composition, and physiologic and biochemical processes. Studies of these bacterial pathogens extend basic insights to identifying vaccine candidate antigens and drug targets and to examining mechanisms of infection, pathogenicity, and virulence.

Areas of particular interest include streptococci, pneumonia, nosocomial (hospital-associated) infections, antibiotic resistance, bacterial sexually transmitted diseases, and bacterial diarrhea. The NIAID program for antibacterial research is facilitated through its intramural laboratories, technology and research resources, and extramural research support, including support for many bacterial genome sequencing projects.

NIAID Intramural Laboratories

- The Laboratory of Human Bacterial Pathogenesis (LHBP) studies the molecular basis of human bacterial pathogenesis in its broadest sense
- The Laboratory of Host Defenses, Tuberculosis Research Section, is putting special emphasis on understanding and interpreting the genomic information encoded within *Mycobacterium tuberculosis*
- The Laboratory of Clinical Infectious Diseases conducts clinical and basic studies of important human infectious and immunologic diseases
- The Laboratory of Zoonotic Pathogens studies several bacteria that cause diseases in humans, including *Neisseria gonorrhoeae* (gonorrhea), *Borrelia burgdorferi* (Lyme disease), *Borrelia hermsii* (relapsing fever), and *Yersinia pestis* (plague)

3.1 Resources for Researchers

The following resources are available to researchers through the NIAID-funded units (http://www3.niaid.nih.gov/research/topics/bacterial/resources):

V. St. Georgiev, *National Institute of Allergy and Infectious Diseases, NIH: Impact on Global Health*, vol. 2, DOI 10.1007/978-1-60327-297-1_3, © Humana Press, a part of Springer Science+Business Media, LLC 2009

- Bacterial Respiratory Pathogen Reference Laboratory
- Biodefense and Emerging Infections Research Resources Repository (BEI Resources)
- Bioinformatics Resource Centers (BRC)
- Food and Waterborne Diseases Integrated Research Network
- In Vitro and Animal Models for Emerging Infectious Diseases and Biodefense
- Microbial Sequencing Centers
- National and Regional Biocontainment Laboratories (NBL, RBL)
- Network on Antimicrobial Resistance in *Staphylococcus aureus* (NARSA)
- Pathogen Functional Genomics Resource Center (PFGRC)
- Proteomics Research Centers (PRC)
- Regional Centers of Excellence for Biodefense and Emerging Infectious Diseases (RCE)
- Reservoirs of Antibiotic Resistance Network (ROAR)
- Shiga Toxin Producing *Escherichia coli* (STEC) Strain and Data Repository
- Tuberculosis Animal Research and Gene Evaluation Taskforce (TARGET)
- Tuberculosis Antimicrobial Acquisition and Coordinating Facility (TAACF)
- Tuberculosis Research Unit (Case Western Reserve University)
- TB Vaccine Testing and Research Materials (Colorado State University)

3.2 Recent Scientific Advances

- *Rapid Quantitative Profiling of Complex Microbial Populations.* Little is known about the complex microbial ecosystems found in environments throughout the world. Generating a census of the bacteria that inhabit these microbial communities is essential for understanding the biology of these organisms and their interactions with one another and their environments, whether the environment is a thermal vent or the human body. A recent study has described a rapid method for the profiling complex populations of bacteria by using a DNA oligonucleotide microarray that was capable of detecting and quantifying individual bacterial species in complex mixtures when the species was present at levels of <0.1% *(2)*. This system should greatly enhance studies on diverse microbial communities, such as those present in the intestine, on the skin, and in the mouth. Understanding the components of "normal" microbial populations is crucial to our development of effective vaccines and therapeutics.

- *Vitamin D–mediated Antimicrobial Immune Response.* The human immune response to microbial pathogens depends on the activation of several pattern recognition receptors known as the Toll-like receptors. Once activated, these receptors may induce the expression of a series of antimicrobial peptides that then destroy the invading pathogens. Susceptibility to tuberculosis infection (*Mycobacterium tuberculosis*) is associated with vitamin D deficiency. The mechanism by which vitamin D regulates antimicrobial actions is unknown. In a recent publication, NIAID-supported investigators showed that by binding to Toll-like receptors, tuberculosis peptides induced the expression of pro-vitamin D converting enzyme and vitamin D receptors by human phagocytic cells *(3)*. However, the activation of the Toll-like receptors did not directly result in the expression of the antimicrobial peptides. Yet, when stimulated with vitamin D, normal phagocytes displayed an increase in the expression and production of a key antimicrobial peptide called *cathelicidin*. In subsequent experiments, the investigators documented that the upregulation of the pro-vitamin D converting enzyme regulated the available vitamin D to the phagocytes. Therefore, both vitamin D and the bacterial peptides needed to be present in order to fully activate the phagocytes for antimicrobial activity. Clinically, African Americans have an increased sensitivity and a more severe and rapid course of tuberculosis. When compared with a cohort of Caucasians, the researchers found that the serum levels of African Americans contained less pro-vitamin D and their cells were less likely to be activated by the tuberculosis peptides. When this serum was supplemented with exogenous pro-vitamin D to levels comparable with those of the Caucasians, it restored the cellular activation *(3)*. These findings may have implications for patients with *atopic dermatitis*, where the decrease in expression of cathelicidin and the availability of vitamin D has been speculated to contribute to the disease pathogenesis.

- *Granulobacter bethesdensis—A Novel Bacterium Associated with Lymphadenitis in Chronic Granulomatous Disease.* Chronic granulomatous disease (CGD) is a rare inherited disease of the phagocyte NADPH oxidase system causing defective production of toxic oxygen metabolites, impaired killing of bacteria and fungi, and recurrent life-threatening infections. A novel Gram-negative rod, *G. bethesdensis,* has been identified in excised lymph nodes from a patient with CGD *(4)*. To confirm its pathogenicity, the researchers have demonstrated specific immune reaction by high-titer antibody showing that *G. bethesdensis* was able to cause similar disease when introduced into CGD—but not wild-type—mice and have recovered the same organism from pathologic lesions in these mice. This is the first reported case of invasive human disease caused by any Acetobacteraceae organism, and polyphasic taxonomic analysis has confirmed that *G. bethesdensis* represents a new genus and species.

References

1. Report by the American Society of Microbiology and the National Institutes of Health. *Basic Research on Bacteria: The Essential Frontier*, Washington, DC, February 2007 (http://www.asm.org/Policy/index.asp?bid=49274).
2. Palmer, C., Bik, E. M., Eisen, M. B., Eckburg, P. B., Sana, T. R., Wolber, P. K., Relman, D. A., and Brown, P. O. (2006) Rapid quantitative profiling of complex microbial populations, *Nucleic Acids Res.*, **34**(1), e5.
3. Liu, P. T., Stenger, S., Li, H., Wenzel, L., Tan, B. H., Krutzik, S. R., Ochoa, M. T., Schauber, J., Wu, K., Meinken, C., Kamen, D. L., Wagner, M., Bals, R., Steinmeyer, A., Zugel, U., Gallo, R. L., Eisenberg, D., Hewison, M., Hollis, B. W., Adams, J. S., Bloom, B. R., and Modlin, R. L. (2006) Toll-like receptor triggering of a vitamin D-mediated human antimicrobial response, *Science*, **311**, 1770–1773.
4. Greenberg, D. E., Ding, L., Zelazny, A. M., Stock, F., Wong, A., Anderson, V. L., Miller, G., Kleiner, D. E., Tenorio, A. R., Brinster, L., Dorward, D. W., Murray, P. R., and Holland, S. M. (2006) A novel bacterium associated with lymphadenitis in a patient with chronic granulomatous disease, *PLoS*, **2**(4), e28.

Chapter 4

Emerging and Re-emerging Infectious Diseases

Emerging diseases include outbreaks of previously unknown diseases or known diseases whose incidence in humans has significantly increased in the past two decades. Re-emerging diseases are known diseases that have reappeared after a significant decline in incidence (http://www3.niaid.nih.gov/research/topics/emerging).

Within the past two decades, innovative research and improved diagnostic and detection methods have revealed a number of previously unknown human pathogens. For example, within the past decade chronic gastric ulcers, which were formerly thought to be caused by stress or diet, were found to be the result of infection by the bacterium *Helicobacter pylori*.

New infectious diseases continue to evolve and "emerge." Changes in human demographics, behavior, land use, and so forth are contributing to the emergence of new diseases by changing transmission dynamics to bring people into closer and more frequent contact with pathogens. This may involve exposure to animal or arthropod carriers of disease.

As a result of innovative research and improved diagnostic and detection methods, a number of previously unknown pathogens—very often through host switching—have been identified as the causative agents of emerging and re-emerging diseases (www.niaid.nih.gov/dmid/eid/). For example, the increasing trade in exotic animals for pets and as food sources has contributed to the rise in opportunity for pathogens to jump from animal reservoirs to humans. For example, close contact with exotic rodents imported to the United States as pets was found to be the origin of the recent outbreak of monkeypox in the United States, and use of exotic civet cats for meat in China was found to be the route by which the SARS coronavirus made the transition from animal to human hosts (http://www3.niaid.nih.gov/research/topics/emerging).

In addition to the continual discovery of new human pathogens, old infectious disease enemies are "re-emerging." Natural genetic variations, recombinations, and adaptations allow new strains of known pathogens to appear to which the immune system has not been previously exposed and is therefore not primed to recognize (e.g., influenza). Furthermore, human behavior plays an important role in the re-emergence of diseases. Increased and sometimes imprudent use of antimicrobial drugs and pesticides has led to the development of resistant pathogens, allowing many diseases that were formerly treatable with drugs to make a comeback (e.g., tuberculosis, malaria, nosocomial infections, and food-borne infections). Recently, decreased compliance with vaccination policy has also led the to re-emergence of diseases, such as measles and pertussis, that were previously under control. The use of deadly pathogens, such as smallpox or anthrax, as agents of bioterrorism is an increasingly acknowledged threat to the civilian population. Moreover, many important infectious diseases have never been adequately controlled on either the national or international level. Infectious diseases that have posed ongoing health problems in developing countries are re-emerging in the United States (e.g., food- and water-borne infections, dengue, West Nile virus) (http://www3.niaid.nih.gov/research/topics/emerging).

4.1 Recent Outbreaks of Emerging and Re-emerging Infectious Diseases

Individual statistics for morbidity and mortality of emerging and re-emerging infections are difficult to determine because of their limited outbreaks. Current information on international outbreaks of infectious diseases can be obtained from WHO (http://www.who.int/csr/don/en/) and the CDC (http://www.cdc.gov/mmwr).

Recent outbreaks include:

- *Human Metapneumovirus (hMPV)*. HMPV was first identified in The Netherlands in 2001 in samples from children with respiratory tract disease *(1)*. It is a new member of the Paramyxoviridae family (subfamily Pneumovirus). Although newly discovered, hMPV is not thought to be a newly evolved virus because it was also found in Dutch blood samples dating back to the 1950s. Instead, it is believed that this pathogen has long been

V. St. Georgiev, *National Institute of Allergy and Infectious Diseases, NIH: Impact on Global Health*, vol. 2, DOI 10.1007/978-1-60327-297-1_4, © Humana Press, a part of Springer Science+Business Media, LLC 2009

a common but undetected cause of many human respiratory illnesses. Moreover, it has been suggested that hMPV may be the second most common source of childhood respiratory infections after the respiratory syncytial virus (RSV), and its association with respiratory disease in adults and children has been reported in Canada, Australia, the United States, Hong Kong, Japan, and Finland. In addition, data from Hong Kong have indicated that half of the SARS patients tested during the recent outbreak were also co-infected with hMPV.

- *Borrelia hermsii*. A multicase tick-borne relapsing fever outbreak caused by *B. hermsii* has been reported in western Montana. *B. hermsii* is a pathogen closely related to the bacterium that causes Lyme disease, and its vector is *Ornithodoros hermsii (2)*. Though the tick-borne relapsing fever is endemic in the higher elevations and coniferous forests of the western United States and southern British Columbia, Canada, this is the first outbreak reported beyond the geographic range known previously in the United States. Patients usually become ill after sleeping in cabins infested with spirochete-infected ticks that feed quickly during the night.

- *Vibrio cholerae*. During spring 2002, a resurgence of cholera caused by *Vibrio cholerae* O139 was reported in Dhaka and adjoining areas in Bangladesh with an estimated 30,000 cases of cholera. The re-emerged O139 strains were found to belong to a single ribotype corresponding with one of two ribotypes that caused the initial O139 outbreak in 1993. This evidence suggested that the O139 strains continue to evolve and that the adult population continues to be more susceptible to O139 cholera, indicating the lack of adequate immunity against this serogroup *(3)*.

- *Norwalk-like Calciviruses (NLVs)*. The NLVs are an emerging group of pathogens of global importance that are frequently involved in food- and water-borne disease outbreaks. The human calciviruses belong to the genus Novovirus (NV) *(4)*. Whereas transmission of these viruses is primarily from person to person, numerous examples have illustrated that NVs are efficiently transmitted in food, water, or contaminated environmental surfaces *(5)*. Studies in which NVs were molecularly characterized have shown that numerous variants co-circulate in the community, but occasionally shifts did occur in which a single variant dominated over a wide geographic area *(6)*. During the period 1995–1996, a worldwide epidemic was observed *(7)*. The mechanism of emergence of these variants is unclear, but one hypothesis is that they represent widespread common-source events *(5)*.

- *Chikungunya*. Between March 28, 2005, and February 12, 2006, 1,722 cases of chikungunya have been reported in areas in the Indian Ocean, most notably in the French island of La Reunion *(8)*. Estimation from a mathematical model has indicated that as many as 110,000 people may have been infected by the chikungunya virus since March 2005. During the first week of February, other countries in the southwest Indian Ocean reported cases: Mauritius (206), the Seychelles (1,255 cases), and spreading further to Mayotte (France), India, China, and Europe. The disease is believed to have been first diagnosed in Tanzania in 1952 and then in Portklang in Malaysia in 1999. Warm and humid climate and water reservoirs serve as breeding grounds for chikungunya. The illness is considered to be a rare form of viral fever caused by an Alphavirus belonging to the group IV Togaviridae family *(9)*. The disease has a human-mosquito-human transmission. The mosquito vector is *Aedes aegyptii*. Chikungunya is not fatal but is associated with high morbidity (insomnia, severe headache, crippling joint and muscle pains) said to last for weeks. In a very recent development (September 6, 2007), the Ministry of Health of Italy confirmed about 160 cases of chikungunya in the Ravenna region of Northern Italy—the first reported outbreak of this tropical virus in Europe (http://news.bbc.co.uk/2/hi/health/6981476.stm).

- *Toxoplasma gondii*. Recently, several water-borne outbreaks of toxoplasmosis have been described *(10–15)*. Data from Brazil and North America have indicated that unfiltered drinking water contaminated with the parasite's oocysts is the main source of infection. However, transmission of toxoplasmosis has also resulted from consumption of food or water contaminated with oocysts from cat feces or soil or by eating undercooked meat that contained oocysts *(16, 17)*. In Latin America, seroprevalence of immunoglobulin G (IgG) to *T. gondii* was found to be generally high, ranging from 51% to 72% *(17)*.

4.2 Research Plans and Priorities

In response to the threat of emerging and re-emerging infectious diseases, NIAID has developed a strategy for addressing these issues through targeted research and training, initially outlined in 1999 in "A Research Agenda for Emerging Infectious Diseases" (http://www.niaid.nih.gov/publications/execsum/bookcover.htm), later updated in 2000 as "NIAID: Planning For the 21st Century" (http://www.niaid.nih.gov/strategicplan/pdf/splan.pdf), and in 2001 as "NIAID Global Health Research Plan for HIV/AIDS, Malaria, and Tuberculosis" (http://www.niaid.nih.gov/publications/globalhealth/global.pdf). This document outlines the institute's plans for the next decade for diagnosing, treating, and preventing these three infections and also lays out a plan for enhancing research capacity in-country (http://www3.niaid.nih.gov/research/topics/emerging).

The NIAID research plans and priorities include:

- Strengthening basic and applied research on the pathogen, host, and environmental factors that influence disease emergence
- Using knowledge of pathogen, host, and environment interactions to enhance the ability to predict and prevent conditions that lead to human disease
- Supporting development of diagnostics, vaccines, and therapies necessary to detect and control infectious diseases
- Supporting sequencing and postgenomics research of emerging infectious disease agents and animal vectors to reveal the genetic basis for the microbe or vector's evolution, adaptation, and pathogenicity
- Developing new strategies to control diseases that are re-emerging due to drug or insecticide resistance
- Identifying better control strategies for intractable infectious diseases that continue to challenge global health
- Maintaining and developing the national and international scientific expertise required to respond to future health threats by supporting research and training programs

4.3 Resources for Researchers

4.3.1 New Research Facilities and Resources

NIAID is planning and has established several facilities and research programs to enhance research on emerging infectious diseases, including both naturally occurring outbreaks and those that may emerge as a result of deliberate release (acts of bioterrorism):

- *Regional Centers of Excellence for Biodefense and Emerging Infectious Diseases Research (RCE).* RCE will provide the scientific information and translational research capacity to make the next generation of therapeutics, vaccines, and diagnostics effective against emerging infectious agents, including the NIAID Category A–C Agents.
- *New NIAID Intramural Biosafety Level 3 (BSL-3) Laboratories.* These laboratories will enable the institute to conduct BSL-3 animal studies and laboratory research on emerging infectious agents, such as multidrug-resistant *Mycobacterium tuberculosis* (MDR TB), *Borrelia*, *Yersinia*, influenza virus, West Nile virus, and dengue virus
- *Two National Biocontainment Laboratories (NBL) and 13 Regional Biocontainment Laboratories (RBL).* The NBLs and RBLs would provide Biosafety Level 3 and 4 facilities for biodefense and emerging infectious disease research.

- *NIAID's Biodefense and Emerging Infections Research Resources Program.* This program has been designed to support the acquisition, authentication, storage, and distribution to the scientific community of state-of-the-art research and reference reagents related to biodefense and emerging infectious diseases.
- *The In Vitro and Animal Models for Emerging Infectious Diseases and Biodefense Program.* This program provides a range of resources for preclinical testing of new therapies and vaccines including non-human primate models to be used in emerging infectious diseases and biodefense research.
- *The Food- and Water-borne Diseases Integrated Network.* This network expands the NIAID capacity to conduct clinical research studies of food- and water-borne enteric pathogens.

4.3.2 Other Resources

- *Malaria Research and Reference Reagent Resource (MR4) Center*
- *NIAID Animal Study Proposals*
- *Shiga Toxin Producing* Escherichia coli *(STEC) Strain and Data Repository*

4.4 List of NIAID Emerging and Re-emerging Diseases

Group I: Pathogens Newly Recognized in the Past Two Decades
Acanthamebiasis
Australian bat Lyssavirus
Babesia, atypical
Bartonella henselae
Ehrlichiosis
Encephalitozoon cuniculi
Encephalitozoon hellem
Enterocytozoon bieneusi
Helicobacter pylori
Hendra or equine morbilli virus
Hepatitis C
Hepatitis E
Human herpesvirus 8
Human herpesvirus 6
Lyme borreliosis
Parvovirus B19

Group II: Re-emerging Pathogens
Enterovirus 71
Clostridium difficile

Coccidioides immitis
Mumps virus
Prion diseases
Streptococcus, group A
Staphylococcus aureus
Coccidioides immitis

Group III: Agents with Bioterrorism Potential

NIAID: Category A
Bacillus anthracis (anthrax)
Clostridium botulinum toxin (botulism)
Yersinia pestis (plague)
Variola major (smallpox) and other related pox viruses
Francisella tularensis (tularemia)
Viral hemorrhagic fevers:
    Arenaviruses
        LCM, Junin virus, Machupo virus, Guanarito virus
        Lassa fever
    Bunyaviruses: Hantaviruses; Rift Valley fever
        Flaviviruses: Dengue
        Filoviruses: Ebola and Marburg viruses

NIAID: Category B
Burkholderia pseudomallei
Coxiella burnetii (Q fever)
Brucella species (brucellosis)
Burkholderia mallei (glanders)
Chlamydia psittaci (Psittacosis)
Ricin toxin (from *Ricinus communis*)
Epsilon toxin of *Clostridium perfringens*
Staphylococcus enterotoxin B
Typhus fever (*Rickettsia prowazekii*)
Food- and water-borne pathogens:
    Bacteria
        Diarrheagenic *E. coli*
        Pathogenic *Vibrio* species
        Shigella species
        Salmonella
        Listeria monocytogenes
        Campylobacter jejuni
        Yersinia enterocolitica
    Viruses (Calciviruses, hepatitis A)
    Protozoa
        Cryptosporidium parvum   *Giardia lamblia*
        Microsporidia   *Entamoeba histolytica*
        Toxoplasma   *Cyclospora cayetanensis*
Additional viral encephalitides:
    West Nile virus
    La Crosse virus
    California encephalitis
    Venezuelan equine encephalomyelitis (VEE)
    Eastern equine encephalomyelitis (EEE)
    Western equine encephalomyelitis (WEE)

Japanese encephalitis virus
Kyasanur Forest virus

NIAID: Category C
Emerging infectious disease threats such as Nipah virus and additional hantaviruses

NIAID Priority Areas

- Tick-borne hemorrhagic fever viruses
    Crimean-Congo hemorrhagic fever virus
- Tick-borne encephalitis viruses
- Yellow fever
- Multidrug-resistant tuberculosis
- Influenza
- Other *Rickettsia* species
- Rabies
- Prions
- Chikungunya virus
- Severe acute respiratory syndrome–associated coronavirus (SARS-CoV)
- Antimicrobial resistance, excluding research on sexually transmitted organisms
- Antimicrobial research, as related to engineered threats
- Innate immunity, defined as the study of nonadaptive immune mechanisms that recognize, and respond to, microorganisms, microbial products, and antigens

References

1. van den Hoogen, B. G., de Jong, J. C., Groen, J., Kuiken, T., de Groot, R., Fouchier, R. A. M., and Osterhaus, A. D. M. E. (2001) A newly discovered human pneumovirus isolated from young children with respiratory tract disease, *Nat. Med.*, **7**, 719–724.
2. Schwan, T. G., Policastro, P. F., Miller, Z., Thompson, R. L., Damrow, T., and Keirans, J. E. (2003) Tick-borne relapsing fever caused by *Borrelia hermsii*, Montana, *Emerg. Infect. Dis.*, **9**(9), 1151–1154.
3. Faruque, S. M., Chowdhury, N., Kamruzzaman, M., Ahmad, Q. S., Faruque, A. S. G., Salam, M. A., Ramamurthy, T., Nair, G. B., Weintraub, A., and Sack, D. A. (2003) Reemergence of epidemic *Vibrio cholerae* O139, Bangladesh, *Emerg. Infect. Dis.*, **9**(9), 1116–1122.
4. Koopmans, M., von Bonsdorff, C., Vinjé, J., de Medici, D., and Monroe, S. (2002) Foodborne viruses, *FEMS Microbiol. Rev.*, **26**, 187–205.
5. Koopmans, M., Vennema, H., Heersma, H., van Strien, E., van Duynhoven, Y., Brown, D., Reacher, M., and Lopman, B., for the European Consortium on Foodborne Viruses (2003) Early identification of common-source foodborne virus outbreaks in Europe, *Emerg. Infect. Dis.*, **9**(9), 1136–1142.
6. Koopmans, M., Vinjé, J., de Wit, M., Leenen, I., van der Poel, W., and van Duynhoven, Y. (2000) Molecular epidemiology of human enteric caliciviruses in The Netherlands, *J. Infect. Dis.*, **181**(Suppl. 2), S262–S263.
7. Noel, J. S., Fankhauser, R., Ando, T., Monroe, S., and Glass, R. (1999) Identification of a distinct common strain of "Norwalk-Like Viruses" having a global distribution, *J. Infect. Dis.*, **179**, 1334–1344.

8. WHO Report: Epidemic and Pandemic Alert and Response (EPR). (2006) Chikungunya in La Reunion Island (France), 17 February 2006.

9. Yadav, P., Shouche, Y. S., Munot, H. P., Mishra, A. C., and Mourya, D. T. (2003) Genotyping of chikungunya virus isolates from India during 1963–2000 by reverse transcription-polymerase chain reaction, *Acta Virol.*, **47**(2), 125–127.

10. Heukelbach, J., Meyer-Cirkel, V., Sabola Moura, R. C., Gomide, M., Nogueira Queiroz, J. A., Saweljew, P., and Liesenfeld, O. (2006) Waterborne toxoplasmosis, Northeastern Brazil, *Emerg. Infect. Dis.*, **13**(2), 287–289.

11. de Moura, L., Bahia-Oliveira, L. M., Wada, M. Y., Jones, J. L., Tuboi, S. H., Carmo, E. H., Massa Ramalho, W., Camargo, N. J., Trevisan, R., Graça, R. M. T., da Silva, A. J., Moura, I., Dubey, J. P., and Garrett, D. O. (2006) Waterborne toxoplasmosis, Brazil, from field to gene, *Emerg. Infect. Dis.*, **12**(2), 326–329.

12. Bahia-Oliveira, L. M. G., Jones, J. L., Azavedo-Silva, J., Alves, C. C., Oréfice, F., and Addiss, D. G. (2003) Highly endemic, waterborne toxoplasmosis in North Rio de Janeiro State, Brazil, *Emerg. Infect. Dis.*, **9**(1), 55–62.

13. Aramini, J. J., Stephen, C., Dubey, J. P., Engelstoft, C., Schwantje, H., and Ribble, C. S. (1999) Potential contamination of drinking water with *Toxoplasma gondii* oocysts, *Epidemiol. Infect.*, **122**, 305–315.

14. Bowie, W. R., King, A. S., Weker, D. H., Isaak-Renton, J. L., Bell, A., Eng, S. B., Marion, S. A., and the British Columbia Toxoplasma Investigation Team (1997) Outbreak of toxoplasmosis associated with municipal drinking water, *Lancet*, **350**, 173–177.

15. Eng, S. B., Werker, D. H., King, A. S., Marion, S. A., Bell, A., Issac-Renton, J. L., Irwin, G. S., and Bowie, W. R. (1999) Computer-generated dot maps as an epidemiologic tool: investigating an outbreak of toxoplasmosis, *Emerg. Infect. Dis.*, **5**(6), 815–819.

16. Montoya, J. G. and Liesenfeld, O. (2004) Toxoplasmosis, *Lancet*, **363**, 1965–1976.

17. Tenter, A. M., Heckeroth, A. R., and Weiss, L. M. (2000) *Toxoplasma gondii*: from animals to humans, *Int. J. Parasitol.*, **30**, 1217–1258.

Chapter 5

Fungal Diseases

During the past three decades or so, the incidence of fungal infections has increased dramatically. Deep-seated mycoses are creating serious problems for clinicians working with certain populations of patients, such as those with cancer, those who are immunocompromised, and those who are physiologically compromised *(1,2)*.

The ever-expanding application of immunosuppressive therapy and the role that host factors (the T-lymphocyte system) play in the defense against systemic fungal infections are currently the subject of intensive studies, and new approaches for antifungal therapies are being investigated.

The need for effective antifungal drugs has been felt more and more acutely with the emergence of the AIDS pandemic and the AIDS-related complex (ARC), which have nearly always been associated with opportunistic fungal infections. Another factor facilitating the spread of opportunistic mycoses has been the significant improvement achieved in the management of bacterial diseases. Clinicians have been particularly concerned that the increasing use of antifungal drugs would lead to drug-resistant fungi, especially in settings such as hospitals, where nosocomial (hospital-acquired) infections have been a growing problem. Recent studies have documented resistance of the *Candida* species to fluconazole and other azole and triazole drugs that are used widely to treat patients with systemic fungal infections. In addition, primary or inherent resistance would limit the activity of currently available antifungal drugs for fungi such as *Aspergillus* and other emerging molds (http://www3.niaid.nih.gov/research/topics/fungal/introduction).

The true incidence of human fungal infections is difficult to assess because fungal diseases can be difficult to diagnose. Historically, estimates of incidence have been made in association with periodic epidemics, positive skin tests, and a limited number of surveillance studies.

Furthermore, fungi present an especially complex challenge to researchers, in part because pathogenicity is often associated with certain morphologic forms or a certain part of the life cycle of a fungal species. For example, pathogens such as *Histoplasma capsulatum*, *Coccidioides immitis*, or *Sporothrix schenckii* convert from one morphologic form to another in the host tissue before they propagate to cause disease. *Cryptococcus neoformans* causes infection only in the asexual form of its life cycle (yeast cells). The molecular biological progress made in *Cryptococcus neoformans* over the past 5 years attests to the importance of collaborative research between medical and molecular researchers. Researchers are identifying a series of antigenic peptides from fungal pathogens that can generate immune responses, which may assist in developing an antifungal vaccine.

At present, the majority of antifungal agents available to clinicians, in addition to having some unacceptable side effects, are by mechanism of action fungistatic. Such a mode of action, for the most part, requires prolonged periods of treatment, and relapses are frequent after treatment has ceased. Because both the human and fungal cells are eukaryotic, prolonged antifungal chemotherapy would be damaging to the host cells, too. Overcoming an obstacle such as this presents a fundamental challenge to scientists in their quest for safer, more selective and effective antifungal agents *(3–8)*.

Primary fungal pathogens include *Coccidioides immitis*, *Blastomyces dermatitidis*, *Paracoccidioides brasiliensis*, *Histoplasma capsulatum*, and *Sporothrix schenckii*. All except *P. brasiliensis* are endemic in the United States.

The opportunistic fungal pathogens (e.g., *Aspergillus* spp., *Candida* spp., *Cryptococcus neoformans*, *Pneumocystis jirovecii*) are common causes of infection in immunocompromised hosts. The emergence of fungal diseases is noteworthy in hospital settings, especially with regard to some cancers, bone marrow and organ transplants, and surgical trauma patients. Recent serologic surveys of patients (Arizona) with community-acquired pneumonia (CAP) found that 29% of the patients were positive for coccidioidomycosis *(9)*.

Note: For an extensive discussion of fungal diseases, see Chapter 36 in Part II.

V. St. Georgiev, *National Institute of Allergy and Infectious Diseases, NIH: Impact on Global Health*, vol. 2, DOI 10.1007/978-1-60327-297-1_5, © Humana Press, a part of Springer Science+Business Media, LLC 2009

5.1 Plans, Priorities, and Goals

Major research goals and objectives include (http://www3.niaid.nih.gov/research/topics/fungal/introduction):

- *Molecular Biology.* Transferring the technology developed in model systems to the medically important fungi to address topics of clinical relevance, including vaccine candidates and new drugs and diagnostic targets.
- *Immunobiology.* Identifying immunologically protective antigens, antibodies, and pathways to plan new vaccine approaches and to improve therapies.
- *Pathogenesis.* Identifying mechanisms of pathogenesis to interrupt and/or prevent the infection.
- *Therapy.* Facilitating improvements in available treatments through studies, including clinical trials of new treatments and comparative treatments of systemic fungal diseases.
- *Genome Sequencing and Genomics.* Providing complete genomic sequencing and facilitating genomics/proteomics approaches to address key fungal pathogens in humans.

5.2 Resources for Researchers

NAID has made available to researchers the following resources (http://www3.niaid.nih.gov/research/topics/fungal/resources.htm):

- Invasive Aspergillosis Animal Model (IAAM) Contract
- Bacteriology and Mycology Study Group
- Mycology Research Units
- Peptide Synthesis and Analysis Unit
- Pathogen Functional Genomics Resource Center

5.3 Recent Scientific Advances

- *Novel Cryptococcus neoformans Virulence Factor with Therapeutic Potential.* The pathogen is transmitted through inhalation and causes the most common fungal meningoencephalitis in immunocompromised patients. A recent study *(10)* has shown that the glycosphingolipid glucosyl ceramide (GlcCer), which is present in *C. neoformans*, is essential for fungal growth in the host extracellular environments, such as in alveolar spaces and the bloodstream, and is required for the fungus to leave the lungs and reach the brain. In addition, GlcCer is required for the fungus to replicate in the tiny air sacs within the lungs. Because GlcCer is also present in other clinically important fungi (e.g., *Aspergillus fumigatus*),

it may become an attractive target for antifungal drug development.

- *Global Control of Dimorphism and Virulence in Fungi.* There are six dimorphic fungi that cause mycoses worldwide that can switch from nonpathogenic molds in soil to pathogenic yeast after spores are inhaled and exposed to elevated temperature. The mechanisms that regulate this switch remain obscure. However, recent data have indicated that a hybrid histidine kinase would sense host signals and trigger the transition from mold to yeast *(11)*. The kinase also regulates the cell-wall integrity, sporulation, and expression of virulence genes *in vivo*.
- *Apoptosis of Leukocytes During Infection with Histoplasma capsulatum Enhances Host Resistance.* A pathogen-induced apoptosis of lymphocytes is associated with increased susceptibility to infection. It has been determined that apoptosis was a critical element of immunity to *H. capsulatum* in that the level of apoptotic lymphocytes, predominantly T cells, progressively increased in the lungs of mice during the course of *H. capsulatum* infection *(12)*. Furthermore, in animal studies, infections became more severe when mice were treated with drugs that reduced apoptosis. Thus, contrary to experience in other pathogens, apoptosis was a critical element of protective immunity to *H. capsulatum*. The production of certain chemical signals was markedly elevated when apoptosis had been blocked, and the release of these cytokines exacerbated the severity of infection.
- *Extra Chromosomal Material Increases Antifungal Resistance in Candida albicans.* Resistance to antifungal drugs is a serious problem in the treatment of *Candida albicans*. Data have shown that aneuploidy in general, and a specific segmental aneuploidy consisting of an isochromosome composed of the two left arms of chromosome 5, were associated with azole resistance *(13)*. It was found that the isochromosome will form around a single centromere flanked by an inverted repeat and was found as an independent chromosome or fused at the telomere to a full-length homologue of chromosome 5. Increases and decreases in drug resistance were strongly associated with gain and loss of this isochromosome, which bears genes expressing the enzyme in the ergosterol pathway targeted by azole drugs, efflux pumps, and a transcription factor that positively regulates a subset of efflux pump genes *(13)*.
- *Two Fused Antigens Protect Against Lethal Dose of Coccidioides posadasii.* Although no licensed vaccine exists yet for a fungus, evidence suggests that protective immunity can be induced in animal models. Thus, a number of fungal proteins have been found that impart at least partial immunity in mouse models. In an effort to boost the efficacy of these potential vaccines, two recombinant antigens that individually protect mice from lethal

infection were studied in combination, either as a mixture of two separately expressed proteins or as a single chimeric expression product containing both antigens *(14)*. The results have shown that mice vaccinated with either combination survived a lethal dose of *C. posadasii*–induced infection longer than did mice given single antigens. The immunized mice also exhibited *Coccidioides*-specific antibodies (IgG immunoglobulins) and yielded splenocytes that produced interferon-γ in response to either antigen. The chimeric antigen had the practical advantage of offering enhanced protection from multiple components without increasing production costs.

- *Genome Sequencing of Fungal Pathogens.* NIAID has funded studies to determine the genome sequence of *Aspergillus fumigatus* as part of an international consortium. The studies were successfully completed in 2005. The genome sequences of two other related *Aspergillus* species were also part of the same project. In addition, support was provided for the sequencing of *Coccidioides immitis* (the strain being sequenced has been renamed *C. posadasii*) and *Histoplasma capsulatum*. A functional/comparative genomic study of *H. capsulatum* and *Blastomyces dermatitidis* that includes low-level sequencing of *B. dermatitidis* was funded in 2003.

References

1. Georgiev, V. St. (1997) *Infectious Diseases in Immunocompromised Hosts*, CRC Press, Boca Raton, FL, pp. 739–1189.
2. Georgiev, V. St. (2001) *Opportunistic Infections: Treatment and Prophylaxis*, Humana Press, Totowa, NJ.
3. Georgiev, V. St. (1992) Treatment and developmental therapeutics in aspergillosis. 1. Amphotericin B and derivatives, *Respiration*, **59**, 291–302.
4. Georgiev, V. St. (1992) Treatment and developmental therapeutics in aspergillosis. 2. Azoles and other antifungal drugs, *Respiration*, **59**, 303–313.
5. Georgiev, V. St. (1993) Opportunistic/nosocomial infections. Treatment and developmental therapeutics. I. Cryptococcosis, *Med. Res. Rev.*, **13**, 493–506.
6. Georgiev, V. St. (1993) Opportunistic/nosocomial infections. Treatment and developmental therapeutics. II. Cryptococcosis, *Med. Res. Rev.*, **13**, 507–527.
7. Georgiev, V. St. (1993) Opportunistic infections: treatment and developmental therapeutics of cryptosporidiosis and isosporiasis, *Drug Dev. Res.* **28**, 445–459.
8. Georgiev, V. St. (1995) Treatment and developmental therapeutics of blastomycosis, *Int. J. Antimicrob. Agents*, **6**, 1–12.
9. Valdivia, L., Nix, D., Wright, M., Lindberg, E., Fagan, T., Lieberman, D., Stoffer, T. P., Ampel, N. M., and Galgiani, J. N. (2006) Coccidioidomycosis as a common cause of community-acquired pneumonia, *Emerg. Infect. Dis.*, **12**(6), 958–962.
10. Ritterhous, P. C., Kechchian, T. B., Allegood, J. C., Merrill, A. H., Jr., Hennig, M., Luberto, C., and Del Poeta, M. (2006) Glucosylceramide synthase is an essential regulator of pathogenicity of *Cryptococcus neoformans*, *J. Clin. Invest.*, **116**(6), 1651–1659.
11. Nemecek, J. C., Wuthrich, M., and Klein, B. C. (2006) Global control of dimorphism and virulence in fungi, *Science*, **312**(5773), 583–588.
12. Allen, H. L. and Deepe, G. S., Jr. (2005) Apoptosis modulates protective immunity to the pathogenic fungus *Histoplasma capsulatum*, *J. Clin. Invest.*, **115**(10), 2875–2885.
13. Selmecki, A., Forche, A., and Berman, J. (2006) Aneuploidy and isochromosome formation in drug-resistant *Candida albicans*, *Science*, **313**(5785), 367–370.
14. Shubitz, L. F., Yu, J.-J., Hung, C.-Y., Kirkland, T. N., Peng, T., Perrill, R., Simons, J., Xue, J., Herr, R. A., Cole, G. T., and Galgiani, J. N. (2006) Improved protection of mice against lethal respiratory infection with *Coccidioides posadasii* using two recombinant antigens expressed as a single protein, *Vaccine*, **24**(31–32), 5904–5911.

Chapter 6

Tropical Medicine and Parasitic Diseases

Tropical diseases, especially those of infectious etiology, are particularly prevalent in areas defined geographically as tropical and subtropical (loosely defined as the area between 30° north and 30° south of the equator). Tropical infections include bacterial infections, such as tuberculosis and typhoid, and viral infections, such as measles, dengue, and a host of parasitic diseases (http://www.niaid.nih.gov/dmid/pdf/factsheet.pdf).

Diseases caused by protozoan and helminth parasites are among the leading causes of death and disease in tropical and subtropical regions of the world. Efforts to control the invertebrate vector (carrier, such as the mosquito) of these diseases are often difficult because of resistance to pesticides, concerns regarding environmental damage, and lack of adequate infrastructure to apply existing vector control methods.

No vaccines are currently licensed to prevent or control the spread of parasitic diseases. Thus, control of these diseases depends heavily on the availability of drugs. Unfortunately, most existing therapeutics are either incompletely effective or toxic to the human host.

In a number of cases, even safe and effective drugs are failing as a result of the selection and spread of drug-resistant variants of the parasites. This is best dramatized by the global spread of drug-resistant *Plasmodium falciparum*, the organism responsible for the most lethal form of malaria (see Chapter 20). New therapeutic agents are therefore urgently needed (http://www3.niaid.nih.gov/research/topics/parasitic/introduction.htm).

deaths are directly attributable to infectious and parasitic diseases (WHO Report, "Scaling up the Response to Infectious Diseases; http://www.who.int/infectious-disease-report/2002/framesintro.html). Taken together, HIV/AIDS, tuberculosis, and malaria accounted for 5.6 million deaths, or approximately 30% of the mortality resulting from infectious and parasitic diseases. Lower respiratory infections and diarrheal diseases accounted for a further 3.9 million and 1.8 million deaths, respectively (http://www.who.int/whr/2004/en).

In addition, the scale of individual pain and suffering inflicted by these diseases is immense. At any one time, hundreds of millions of people, mainly in developing countries, are disabled by infectious and parasitic diseases. Thus, in 2002 alone, infectious and parasitic diseases were responsible for 356,824,000 Disability Adjusted Life Years (DALYs; healthy life years lost due to disability and premature mortality). These included acute respiratory infections (90 million); diarrheal diseases (61 million); HIV/AIDS (86 million); malaria (48 million); measles (27 million); tuberculosis (35 million); and tropical parasitic diseases (12 million) (http://www.who.int/whr/2004/en).

Individuals living in poverty are more susceptible to infection, in part because of concomitant malnutrition. Addressing malnutrition and the control and treatment of malaria were identified by the Copenhagen Consensus as two of the top priority areas for advancing global welfare (http://www.copenhagenconsensus.com).

6.1 Incidence and Prevalence of Morbidity and Mortality

Infectious diseases continue to account for a large proportion of the world's death and disability. According to the most recent World Health Report, infectious and parasitic diseases in 2002 were responsible for 18,324,000 deaths, or 19.1% of global mortality (http://www.who.int/whr/2004/en). In the developing world, however, more than 40% of

6.1.1 Tropical Parasitic Diseases: Statistical Data

Disease-specific estimates for tropical parasitic diseases (see various WHO reports cited above; CDC Health Topics, http://www.cdc.gov/health/default.htm; and Section 6.2:

- *Malaria.* 300 million to 500 million cases of malaria occur each year, and more than 1 million people die of malaria each year; 90% in Africa with 0.5 million to 3.0 million deaths, primarily children under 5 years of age in sub-Saharan Africa.

- *Schistosomiasis*. 600 million people at risk in 74 countries; 200 million infected; mortality relatively low but tens of millions with debilitating chronic morbidity.

- *Lymphatic/Bancroftian Filariasis, Elephantiasis*. 905 million people at risk in 73 countries throughout the tropics and subtropics; 120 million infected (45 million in India; 32 million in Africa, and populations in other countries Asia, the Western Pacific, and Central and South America); 1 million severely disabled; prevalence is increasing in many countries due to urbanization.

- *Onchocerciasis (River Blindness)*. 90 million at risk in 34 countries mainly in Africa with additional foci in Latin America and the Middle East; 18 million infected; more than 300,000 blinded, reducing life expectancy by 65% (Final Report on the Conference on the Eradicability of Onchocerciasis; http://www.cartercenter.org/documents/1047.pdf).

- *African Trypanosomiasis (Sleeping Sickness)*. 60 million at risk in 36 countries mostly in sub-Saharan Africa; estimated 300,000 to 500,000 infected; disease is invariably fatal if untreated, and the available treatment produces severe side effects in 10% of patients. Major epidemics are a constant threat to the economic development of Central and East Africa (http://www.cdc.gov/ncidod/eid/vol4no3/gubler.htm).

- *American Trypanosomiasis (Chagas' Disease)*. 100 million at risk in 21 countries in Central and South America; 16 million to 18 million infected; 1 million new cases of chronic disease and more than 45,000 deaths annually; transfusion-acquired infection is common, and recent cases of disease after organ transplantation in the United States have led to consideration of screening the U.S. blood supply for American trypanosomiasis (http://www.cdc.gov/mmwr/preview/mmwrhtml/mm5110a3.htm).

- *Leishmaniasis*. 350 million people at risk in 88 countries; 12 million infected. One million to 1.5 million cases/year of cutaneous disease; 500,000 cases and more than 50,000 deaths/year from visceral disease. More than 90% of the world's cases of visceral leishmaniasis are in India, Bangladesh, Nepal, Sudan, and Brazil. The incidence of HIV/*Leishmania* co-infections is increasing, especially in southern Europe.

- *Intestinal Helminths (Roundworms)*. The most common infections in humans, especially in tropical and subtropical countries, and the leading cause of disease burden in children aged 5 to 14 years (World Bank World Development Report, 1993). One billion persons are infected with *Ascaris*, 900 million with *Trichuris*, and 500 million with hookworms *(1)* (Albonico, M. and Savioli, L., WHO Doc-

ument CTD/MIP/WP.93.7, 1993). Even moderate infection is associated with poor physical and mental development. More intense infection results in severe anemia (hookworms), intestinal obstruction (ascariasis), and chronic colitis (trichuriasis). Recent estimates of clinical disease: 12 million to 59 million with *Ascaris*; 7 million to 26 million with *Trichuris*; and 35 million to 148 million with hookworm (Bundy et al., *Health Priorities and Burden of Disease*, Harvard University Press, 1997).

- *Mycobacterial Diseases (Tuberculosis, Leprosy, and Buruli Ulcer)*. These diseases are of global concern (see Chapter 14).

- *Diarrheal Diseases*. The vicious cycle of infection and malnutrition is responsible for millions of cases per year of acute and persistent diarrhea in children living in developing countries with contaminated food and water and poor hygiene. The causative agents of diarrhea with an infectious origin may be parasitic, bacterial, or viral (http://www.cdc.gov/ncidod/dpd/parasites/diarrhea/factsht_chronic_diarrhea.htm). Despite the development of oral rehydration therapies, persistent diarrhea still accounts for substantial losses in children under age 5. Amebiasis has a global distribution of more than 50 million cases worldwide, with estimated 40,000 to 110,000 deaths annually. Giardiasis is found in every region of the world and is one of the most common causes of water-borne disease. *Cryptosporidium parvum* is increasingly recognized as a pathogen, in both immunocompetent and immunocompromised individuals. In some studies from developing countries, it is the organism identified with the greatest frequency in diarrheal stools (WHO Division of Communicable Diseases Report on Intestinal Parasitic Infections, 1991). The first reports of *Cyclospora* infections appeared in the medical literature in 1979. Since that time, and with improved diagnostics, there are increasing numbers of reports of diarrheal disease associated with this and other protozoan parasites such as *Isospora*. Also, parasites of the phylum *Microsporidia* (http://www.dpd.cdc.gov/dpdx/HTML/Microsporidiosis.htm) are being increasingly recognized as opportunistic infections worldwide, particularly in the tropical and subtropical countries where AIDS therapies are not widely available.

- *Food-borne Parasitic Diseases*. Toxoplasmosis, which is caused by a coccidian parasite, accounts for billions of dollars in medical costs as a result of productivity and disability losses. Infection with the pig tapeworm, *Taenia solium,* is responsible for central nervous system disorders in humans and is a common occurrence in the tropics, where it is a leading cause of seizures. Prevalence rates of 8% and 10.8% have been reported in epidemiologic surveys in Peru and Mexico, respectively *(2)*.

6.2 Neglected Tropical Diseases

The neglected tropical diseases are a group of 13 major disabling conditions that are among the most common chronic infections in the world's poorest people *(3)*. Through the newly established *Global Network for Neglected Tropical Diseases*, with updated guidelines for drug administration issued by WHO, partnerships are coordinating their activities in order to launch a more integrated assault on these conditions.

The parasitic and bacterial infections known as the neglected tropical diseases include three soil-transmitted helminth infections (ascariasis, hookworm infection, and trichuriasis), lymphatic filariasis, onchocerciasis, dracunculiasis, schistosomiasis, Chagas' disease, human African trypanosomiasis, leishmaniasis, Buruli ulcer, leprosy, and trachoma *(4–6)*. An expanded list could include dengue fever, the treponematoses, leptospirosis, strongyloidiasis, foodborne trematodiasis, neurocysticercosis, and scabies *(6)*, as well as other tropical infections. The parasitic and bacterial diseases identified as being neglected are among some of the most common infections in the estimated 2.7 billion people who live on less than US$2 per day *(3)*. These diseases occur primarily in rural areas and in some poor urban settings of low-income countries in sub-Saharan Africa, Asia, and Latin America. The neglected tropical diseases lead to long-term disability and poverty *(4–8)*. The poverty results from disfigurement or other sequelae of long-term illness, impaired childhood growth and development, adverse outcomes of pregnancy, and reduced productive capacity. These features contrast with those of emerging acute infections, such the avian influenza, Ebola virus infection, and the West Nile virus infection *(7)*.

The Millennium Declaration, adopted by world leaders at the United Nations in September 2000, has established an ambitious set of eight millennium development goals to eliminate extreme poverty, hunger, and disease by 2015. The sixth goal, "to combat HIV/AIDS, malaria, and other diseases," specifically addresses the health and economic impact of infectious diseases. This goal has led to considerable and welcomed large-scale financial support through ambitious initiatives sponsored by the Group of Eight (G8) governments to fight HIV/AIDS and malaria. These initiatives include the U.S. President's Emergency Plan for AIDS Relief, the U.S. President's Malaria Initiative, and the Global Fund to Fight AIDS, Tuberculosis, and Malaria *(3)*.

A foundation was led in the latter part of the 20th century for the establishment of international partnerships to control or eliminate these infections *(3)*. A critical step occurred in the late 1980s, when the first partnership was created to control a neglected tropical disease by delivering donated ivermectin to treat onchocerciasis *(5)*. To date, more than 300 million treatments have been provided, initially through the *Onchocerciasis Control Program* and subsequently through the *African Programme for Onchocerciasis Control* and the *Onchocerciasis Elimination Program for the Americas (9)*.

To catalyze the integration of measures to control neglected tropical diseases, a group of partnerships that have been committed to combating the seven most prevalent of these diseases are cooperating with each other in the Global Network for Neglected Tropical Diseases. This network operates according to WHO treatment guidelines and algorithms and with vector management and other environmental control measures *(10)*.

Despite its enormous benefits, preventive chemotherapy with the rapid-impact package will not affect the three neglected tropical diseases with the highest rates of death—Chagas' disease, human African trypanosomiasis, and visceral leishmaniasis. Strategies to control these diseases are based on surveillance, early diagnosis and treatment, and vector control *(3,11–13)*. These criteria for effective control present challenges because of the lack of appropriate diagnostic tools and safe drugs. To date, the greatest successes in the control of Chagas' disease and human African trypanosomiasis have occurred as a result of vector control. Vector control has dramatically reduced the transmission of Chagas' disease in five South American countries *(12)*. The transmission of human African trypanosomiasis has been reduced through the use of simple, impregnated tsetse-fly traps that supplement surveillance and diagnostic measures *(11)*.

Although strategies to control and eliminate human African trypanosomiasis, leishmaniasis, and Chagas' disease are available *(14, 15)*, ultimately, success will almost certainly depend on access to new and cost-effective products for improved control *(3)*. However, in the absence of commercial markets for drugs for neglected tropical diseases, the pipeline of new drugs for these diseases has virtually dried up during the past three decades *(16)*. In response to this crisis, partnerships have been established to address product development for neglected tropical diseases *(17)*. These partnerships for product development have been either exploiting newly completed genome projects for protozoan parasites *(18)* in order to identify potential drug targets for high-throughput screening or taking more traditional approaches to drug development and clinical testing *(19)*. As a result of these activities, several new antiprotozoan drugs are under development for Chagas' disease, leishmaniasis, and human African trypanosomiasis, including miltefosine, paromomycin, sitamaquine, imiquimod, a pentamidine analogue known as DB289, and a vinyl sulfone known as K777, as well as combinations such as nifurtimox-eflornithine and paromomycin combined with antimonial agents *(13,17,19,20)*. However, highly efficacious drugs for the treatment of Buruli ulcer have not yet been developed *(3)*.

Nevertheless, even with regard to the proposed rapid-impact package, challenges remain *(3)*. These challenges include integrated and rapid mapping of the seven targeted diseases; careful assessment of safety, compatibility, and compliance; integrated monitoring and evaluation that are compatible with the capacity of the health system, on the one hand, and with scientific need on the other; cost-effectiveness and cost-benefit studies; and analyses to determine the effect of integrated control on health systems *(3,6,21)*.

6.3 NIAID Involvement in Tropical Medicine and Parasitic Diseases

Over the years, NIAID has continued its support of research to develop more effective prevention approaches, diagnostics, and treatments for tropical infectious diseases, primarily through the traditional investigator-initiated research grant mechanism. Such research is targeted at; (i) developing a better understanding of the pathogenesis of infections; (ii) developing more effective prevention approaches, diagnostics, and treatments; (iii) focusing on microbial pathogens and their interactions with their hosts; and (iv) focusing on vectors that transmit many of these pathogens. In this context, aspects of the NIAID-supported research will depend upon easy access to populations of patients, vectors, and pathogens *available only* in endemic areas of resource-poor countries. Hence, an important complementary objective of the NIAID programs is to strengthen the regional research capacity for institutions and scientists working in those countries.

Major areas of research include (http://www3.niaid.nih.gov/research/topics/parasitic/research activities.htm):

- *Diagnosis*. New technologies are being applied to understand disease pathology and develop cost-effective, sensitive, and specific tests for the infectious agent that are useful and applicable in field situations in the tropics. Such tests would make it possible to determine disease epidemiology and to identify the risk of disease. Improved diagnostics are also being developed for detecting drug-resistant pathogens to improve treatment regimens and to form national and regional control policies.
- *Drug Discovery and Development*. Basic biochemical/molecular studies are being carried out to identify enzymes, metabolic pathways, and pathogen components that are targets for chemotherapeutic intervention. Funding of genome initiatives and databases for many of the organisms above has also expanded the chemotherapeutic and vaccine targets. Studies are also being conducted to determine the mode of action of existing drugs and the mechanisms of drug resistance. Further development

requires studies in animal models and in field and clinical settings to assess efficacy and safety.
- *Immunologic Interventions*. Basic and applied studies are being undertaken to identify the role of the host's immune response in protection and disease. Such studies will provide the foundation for developing vaccines that protect the individual from infection and disease, as well as for the design of intervention strategies that block immunopathologic processes. Moreover, these studies would have wider applicability because parasite systems have served as important models for the role of immune cells and factors in other diseases.
- *Vector Biology and Control*. Basic and applied research on arthropod vectors and their interactions with pathogens and humans are being undertaken to develop tools for interrupting pathogen transmission to humans. Specific emphasis is placed on vector ecology, the pathogen-vector interaction, population genetics, and on genetic and genomic studies. Sequencing efforts are ongoing for some of the most important vectors of pathogens to humans. The research seeks to develop novel, environmentally sound, insect control strategies.

6.3.1 Recent Programmatic Accomplishments and Developments

- Recognizing the enormous public health burden of malaria, NIAID has put considerable efforts into its malaria-related activities, as follows (see Chapter 20):

  ○ *Malaria Research and Reference Reagent Resource Center (MR4)*
  ○ *Multilateral Initiative on Malaria (MIM)*
  ○ *NIAID Plan for Research to Accelerate Development of Malaria Vaccines*
  ○ Establishment of field sites in endemic malaria areas for clinical studies and trials
  ○ Co-sponsorship of a consensus meeting on the design of Phase III clinical trials of new antimalarial drug combinations

- In 2004, NIAID issued a renewal of the *Tropical Diseases Research Units (TDRU)* program (http://grants2.nih.gov/grants/guide/rfa-files/RFA-AI-03-018.html). Initiated in 1980, this program continues to support multiproject, multidisciplinary research programs for the preclinical development of (i) new chemotherapeutic agents that inhibit parasite targets to treat or prevent infection and disease; or (ii) innovative approaches to limit transmission of the parasite at the level of the pathogen's invertebrate vector. Each research program will focus on one parasitic disease or one target in closely related pathogens or vectors and on either drug- or vector-control interventions. The objective is to support translational research leading to the discovery and preclinical development of new drugs or vector control methods to reduce or eliminate morbidity and mortality resulting from parasitic infections.

- In 2006, NIAID announced the renewal of the *Tropical Medicine Research Centers* (http://grants.nih.gov/grants/guide/rfa-files/RFA-AI-06-006.html). This program was initiated in 1991 for the purpose of supporting international centers located in disease endemic areas to conduct research in major tropical diseases. The 2006 Request for Applications (RFA) solicited applications in the areas of leishmaniasis, Chagas' disease, and human African trypanosomiasis to facilitate translational research using the recently published genomes of the trypanosomatids. Applications were received from a diverse set of endemic areas in North and South America, Africa, and Asia.
- For more than 30 years, NIAID has supported two helminth resources that serve the research community. The *Schistosome Resource Center* (http://www.schisto-resource.org) is maintained by the Biomedical Research Institute, and the *Filaria Research Center* (http://www.filariasiscenter.org) is maintained by the University of Georgia. Investigators worldwide may obtain from the two centers schistosome or filaria life stages for research or teaching purposes. Selected materials, including molecular and genomic reagents, are made available to biochemists, immunologists, vector biologists, and other scientists who cannot reasonably maintain the helminths' life cycles, due to lack of space, time, funding, or requisite expertise. Investigators may obtain parasites, vectors, and mammalian hosts free of charge, excluding shipping costs. In addition to fostering schistosomiasis and filaria research, these two NIAID resources have served as valuable backup facilities for investigators who have experienced problems with their own established parasite life cycles. In 2006, both resource centers were in their second year of a 7-year contract.
- In 2006, NIAID continued and extended its support and management of genome projects relevant to parasites and vectors of diseases to humans (http://www.niaid.nih.gov/research/topics/pathogen):

  ○ The genome sequencing of *Plasmodium falciparum*, the most lethal malaria parasite, and of its mosquito vector *Anopheles gambiae* were published in the October 3 and 4, 2002, issues of the journals *Nature* and *Science*, respectively. The *Plasmodium vivax* genome is also nearing completion (see also Chapter 20 for further details). NIAID also continues to support *PlasmodB* for bioinformatic analysis of

the *Plasmodium* genome and also contracts resources to support bioinformatic and proteomic analysis of parasite genomes and vectors of biodefense and emerging disease concern, including *Cryptosporidium* and *Toxoplasma* (http://www.niaid.nih.gov/dmid/genomes/prc/centers.htm).

  ○ Resources such as microarray slides representing the genomes of *P. falciparum* and *An. gambiae* are available to malaria researchers studying gene expression of parasites/vectors (see also Chapter 20 for further details). Microarrays are also available for *Trypanosoma cruzi and Trypanosoma brucei* from the *Pathogen Functional Genomics Resource Center* (http://www.niaid.nih.gov/dmid/genomes/pfgrc/guidelines.htm) (see also Chapter 25 for further details).
  ○ The three genomes of *Leishmania major*, *Trypanosoma brucei*, and *Trypanosoma cruzi (22)* were published in 2005.
  ○ The genome of *Entamoeba histolytica* was published in 2005 *(23)*, and the genome sequences of other amitochondrial protists (*Giardia lamblia* and *Trichomonas vaginalis*) were nearing completion as of 2007.
  ○ The genome of the mosquito *Aedes aegyptii*, the main vector of dengue and yellow fever, has been completed. A computational annotation assembly is now available in GenBank (AAGE00000000) and at VectorBase. Functional assignments and gene accessions are also available. Ongoing sequencing efforts include the genome of the mosquito *Culex pipiens*, an important vector of West Nile virus, and of the tick *Ixodes scapularis* (the main vector of Lyme disease).

- NIAID also is continuing to co-fund several relevant trans-NIH initiatives. The *International Cooperative Biodiversity Groups* initiative addresses the interdependent issues of biodiversity conservation, economic capacity, and human health through the discovery and development of therapeutic agents for diseases of importance in developing countries, as well as those important to developed countries (http://www.nih.gov/news/pr/dec2003/fic-16.htm). Areas of research include discovery of natural products for treating HIV, tuberculosis, malaria, and other tropical diseases by screening extracts from Uzbekistan, Kyrgyzstan, Papua New Guinea, Vietnam, Panama, Jordan, and Costa Rica. Two additional comprehensive awards co-funded by NIAID were awarded in 2006 from the planning grants (http://www.nih.gov/news/pr/jan2006/fic-03.htm).
- NIAID continues its support for the *U.S.-Japan Cooperative Medical Science Program*. Communication across panels and establishment of triangular collaborative projects among scientists from the United States, Japan,

and endemic areas have been encouraged through the annual joint conferences of this program. Participants are actively working on obtaining funding for such triangular collaborations.

6.3.2 Resources for Researchers

The following NIAID-supported resources are available for researchers (http://www3.niaid.nih.gov/research/topics/parasitic/resources):

- Schistosoma Resource Center
- Malaria Research and Reference Reagent Resource Center (MR4)
- Parasitic Infection Research Center
- The Plasmodium falciparum Genome Database (PFDB)—J. Craig Venter Institute
- Malaria Genome Sequence Tag Projects—University of Florida

6.3.3 Partners

A critical aspect of NIAID's future ability to control parasitic diseases will depend on the skills and expertise of biomedical scientists, clinicians, and other health care workers, as well as on public health specialists working in endemic regions. Therefore, strengthening the research capability of scientists in their own countries is an important focus of NIAID efforts. *The International Centers for Tropical Disease Research (ICTDR) Network* consists of NIAID-supported centers focused on research in tropical diseases and includes international research sites in more than 20 countries.

NIAID researchers work closely with national and international organizations involved in research and control of parasitic diseases. NIAID was a founding member of the Multilateral Initiative on Malaria (MIM), which emphasizes strengthening research capacity against malaria in Africa. Other NIAID collaborations include federal agencies, such as USAID and the CDC, WHO, the Bill & Melinda Gates Foundation, the World Bank, the Rockefeller Foundation, the European Commission, and the *Program for Appropriate Technology in Health (PATH)*.

6.4 Recent Scientific Advances

- *Annual Mass Administration of Two Drugs Dramatically Reduced Lymphatic Filariasis in Endemic Areas.*

Lymphatic filariasis (a disabling disease caused by the mosquito-borne nematode parasite *Wuchereria bancrofti*) is a major public health problem in many tropical and subtropical regions. Filariasis has been endemic in Egypt for centuries. In 2000, the Egyptian Ministry of Health and Population initiated one of the first national programs to eliminate filariasis based on WHO's new mass treatment strategy, which aims to eliminate filariasis in all endemic countries by the year 2020. The Egyptian program called for mass drug administration (MDA) of two medicines (*diethylcarbamazine* and *albendazole*) to all people living in infected areas once a year for 5 years. The program is supported by a broad-based publicity campaign, and excellent MDA coverage rates were achieved. This study assessed the impact of five rounds of MDA on filariasis infection and transmission rates in sentinel Egyptian villages. It also explored the value of different tests for monitoring the effect of MDA and for assessing progress in national filariasis elimination programs. These tests—a test that detects parasite waste products in human blood, an antibody test that shows whether young children have been exposed to the parasite, and a sensitive test for detection of parasite DNA in mosquitoes—were developed in previous NIAID-supported projects *(24)*.

The study showed that MDA had a dramatic impact on filariasis infection and transmission rates in the villages studied; very little evidence of infection was detected after the fifth round of MDA. These results suggest that MDA has probably eliminated lymphatic filariasis in most endemic areas in Egypt. It provides important early data to demonstrate the feasibility of global elimination of lymphatic filariasis based on a MDA strategy *(24)*.

- *Identification of a Novel Pathway of Immune-mediated Protection Against Intestinal Worm Infections.* Infections with helminthic parasites are a leading cause of global morbidity. No vaccines are currently available for any helminthic infections of humans, and the mechanisms of immunologically mediated protection against helminthic parasites remain elusive. Like allergens, helminth parasites induce T-helper type 2 (Th2) cytokine responses, resulting in arginase-1 expression by alternatively activated macrophages (AAMacs). Examination of intestinal tissues of mice after primary and secondary infections by a natural gastrointestinal parasite led to the discovery that AAMacs functioned as important effector cells of the protective memory response directed against the parasites *(25)*. Furthermore, whereas previous studies demonstrated that arginase blockade *in vivo* promotes intracellular parasite killing by enhancing classic macrophage activation, the recent studies demonstrated that arginase itself also mediated protective responses by the host against extracellular intestinal parasites by a novel mechanism for immunologically mediated protection against intestinal helminths *(25)*.

- *Transcriptome, Proteome, and Genome Analysis of the Asian Schistosome Provides New Targets for Drugs, Vaccines, and Diagnostics.* The Asian blood fluke, *Schistosoma japonicum*, is a water-borne pathogen, and the disease it causes, schistosomiasis japonica, is a major public health problem in southern and southwestern China. An international group of scientists has collaborated to analyze the proteome, transcriptome, and genome of *S. japonicum*. Approximately 100,000 transcript sequences have been determined, along with more than 3,000 protein sequences. In addition, a sixfold coverage of the draft genome sequence of *S. japonicum* has been completed and is publicly accessible (http://lifecenter.sgst.cn/sj.do) *(26,27)*. The completion of the genome sequence of *S. japonicum* will represent a landmark achievement in schistosomiasis research, enabling scientists to better understand the biology of the microbe and the host response and to develop improved diagnostics, vaccines, and therapeutics.

- *Identification of Novel Fatty Acid Metabolic Pathways May Provide New Targets for Drugs Against African Sleeping Sickness.* Eukaryotic and prokaryotic organisms typically synthesize fatty acids using either type I or type II synthase enzyme. In addition, eukaryotes extend preexisting long-chain fatty acids using microsomal elongase (ELO) enzyme. It has been determined that *Trypanosoma brucei*, an eukaryotic human parasite that causes sleeping sickness, uses an unconventional method to synthesize nearly all its fatty acids *(28)*. In particular, it uses three elongases instead of type I or type II synthases. Trypanosomes encounter diverse environments with different fatty acid requirements during their life cycle. The tsetse vector form, for example, requires one type of fatty acid, whereas the bloodstream form needs another. The results of the study showed that trypanosome fatty acid synthesis is modular and is regulated up or down based on the exogenous environment. The unusual pathway of fatty acid synthesis in *T. brucei* displays modified enzyme functions to provide for the extensive growth requirements of distinct fatty acids during the parasite's life cycle. These enzymes may provide targets for novel interventions.

- *Diapause Triggers a Molecular Switch That Promotes Sugar Versus Blood Feeding in the Mosquito Culex pipiens.* Diapause (or overwintering dormancy) allows certain mosquito species to survive during the cold winter months. In the mosquito *Culex pipiens*, a vector for West Nile virus and other diseases, diapause triggers a change in female feeding behavior from blood feeding to sugar feeding. In this study, it was demonstrated that

genes involved in the digestion of a blood meal are down-regulated and that genes associated with the accumulation of lipid reserves were upregulated in females that were about to undergo diapause. The cessation of host-seeking behavior (and therefore, of blood feeding) and the increase in nectar and other sugar feeding are a consequence of the diapause process *(29)*. By understanding the molecular triggers that result in this change in feeding behavior, scientists may be able to target this process to avoid the transmission of parasites by mosquitoes through blood feeding.

References

1. Bethony, J., Brooker, S., Albonico, M., Geiger, S., Loukas, A., Diemert, D., and Hotez, P. (2006) Soil-transmitted helminth infections: ascariasis, trichuriasis, and hookworm, *Lancet*, **367**(9521), 1521–1532.
2. Tsang, V. C. W. and Wilson M. (1995) *Taenia solium* cysticercosis: an under-recognized but serious public health problem, *Parasitol. Today*, **11**, 124–126.
3. Hotez, P. J., Molyneux, D. H., Fenwick, A., Kumaresam, J., Erhlich Sachs, S., Sachs, J. D., and Savioli, L. (2007) Control of neglected tropical disease, *N. Engl. J. Med.*, **357**(10), 1018–1027.
4. Molyneux, D. H., Hotez, P. J., and Fenwick, A. (2005) Rapid-impact interventions: how a policy of integrated control for Africa's neglected tropical diseases could benefit the poor, *PLoS Med.*, **2**, e336–e336.
5. Hotez, P. J., Ottesen, E., Fenwick, A., and Molyneux, D. (2006) The neglected tropical diseases: the ancient afflictions of stigma and poverty and the prospects for their control and elimination, *Adv. Exp. Biol. Med.*, **582**, 22–33.
6. Hotez, P. J., Molyneux, D. H., Fenwick, A., Ottesen, E., Ehrlich Sachs, S., and Sachs, J. D. (2006) Incorporating a rapid-impact package for neglected tropical diseases with programs for HIV/AIDS, tuberculosis, malaria, *PLoS Med.*, **2**, e102–e102.
7. Hotez, P. J. (2006) The "biblical diseases" and U.S. vaccine diplomacy, *Brown World Aff. J.*, **12**, 247–258.
8. Lammie, P. J., Fenwick, A., and Utzinger, J. (2006) A blueprint for success: integration of neglected tropical disease control programmes, *Trends Parasitol.*, **22**, 313–321.
9. Boatin, B. A. and Richards, F. O., Jr. (2006) Control of onchocerciasis, *Adv. Parasitol.*, **61**, 349–394.
10. World Health Organization. (2006) *Preventive Chemotherapy in Human Helminthiasis*, World Health Organization, Geneva.
11. Févre, E. M., Picozzi, K., Jannin, J., Welburn, S. C., and Maudlin, I. (2006) Human African trypanosomiasis: epidemiology and control, *Adv. Parasitol.*, **61**, 167–221.
12. Yamagata, Y. and Nakagawa, J. (2006) Control of Chagas disease, *Adv. Parasitol.*, **61**, 129–165.
13. Alvar, J., Croft, S., and Olliaro, P. (2006) Chemotherapy in the treatment and control of leishmaniasis, *Adv. Parasitol.*, **61**, 223–274.
14. World Health Organization (2006) Human African trypanosomiasis (sleeping sickness): epidemiological update, *Wkly Epidemiol. Rec.*, **81**, 71–80.
15. Pan American Health Organization (2006) *XVth Meeting of the Southern Cone Intergovernmental Commision to Eliminate Triatoma Infestans and Interrupt the Transmission of Transfusional Trypanosomiasis (INCOSUR-Chagas)*, Brasília,

Brazil, 6–9 June, 2006. Accessed August 10, 2007, at http://www.paho.org/English/AD/DPC/CD/dch-incosur-xv.htm.

16. Chirac, P. and Torreele, E. (2006) Global framework on essential health R&D, *Lancet*, **367**, 1560–1561.

17. Croft, S. L., Barrett, M. P., and Urbina, J. A. (2005) Chemotherapy of trypanosomiases and leishmaniasis, *Trends Parasitol.*, **21**, 508–512.

18. El Sayed, N. M., Myler, P. J., Blandin, G., et al. (2005) Comparative genomics of trypanosomatid parasitic protozoa, *Science*, **309**, 404–409.

19. Renslo, A. R. and McKerrow, J. H. (2006) Drug discovery and development for neglected parasitic diseases, *Nat. Chem. Biol.*, **2**, 701–710.

20. Croft, S. L., Seifert, K., and Yardley, V. (2006) Current scenario of drug development for leishmaniasis, *Indian J. Med. Res.*, **123**, 399–410.

21. Laxminarayan, R., Mills, A. J., Breman, J. G., et al. (2006) Advancement of global health: key messages from the Disease Control Priorities Project, *Lancet*, **367**, 1193–1208.

22. El-Sayed, N. M., Myler, P. J., Bartholomeu, D. C., et al. (2005) The genome sequence of *Trypanozome cruzi*, the etiologic agent of Chagas' disease, *Science*, **309**(5733), 409–415.

23. Loftus, B., Anderson, I., Davies, R., et al. (2005) The genome of the protist parasite *Entamoeba histolytica*, *Nature*, **433**, 865–868.

24. Ramzy, R. M. R., El Setouhy, M., Helmy, H., Ahmed, E. S., Abd Elaziz, K. M., Farid, H. A., Shannon, W. D., and Weil, G. J. (2006) Effect of yearly mass drug administration with diethylcarbamazine and albendazole on bancroftian filariasis in Egypt: a comprehensive assessment, *Lancet*, **367**, 992–998.

25. Anthony, R. M., Urban, J. F., Jr., Alem, F., Hamed, H. A., Rozo, C. T., Boucher, J. L., Van Rooijen, N., and Gause, W. C. (2006) Memory T(H)2 cells induce alternatively activated macrophages to mediate protection against nematode parasites, *Nat. Med.*, **12**(8), 955–960.

26. Liu, F., Lu, J., Hu, W., Wang, S.-Y., Cui, S.-J., Chi, M., Yan, Q., Wang, X.-R., Song, H.-D., Xu, X.-N., Wang, J.-J., Zhang, X.-L., Zhang, X., Wang, Z.-Q., Xue, C.-L., Brindley, P. J., McManus, D. P., Feng, Z., Chen, Z., and Han, Z.-G. (2006) New perspectives on host-parasite interplay by comparative transcriptomic and proteomic analyses of *Schistosoma japonicum*, *PLoS Pathogens*, **2**(4), e29.

27. Wang, L., Yang, Z., Li, Y., Yu, F., Brindley, P. J., McManus, D. P., Wei, D., Han, H., Feng, F., Li, X., and Hu, W. (2006) Reconstruction and *in silico* analysis of the MAPK signaling pathways in the human blood fluke, *Schistosoma japonicum*, *FEBS Lett.*, **580**, 3677–3686.

28. Lee, S. H., Stephens, J. L., Paul, K. S., and Englund, P. T. (2006) Fatty acid synthesis by elongases in trypanosomes, *Cell*, **126**(4), 691–699.

29. Robich, R. M. and Denlinger, D. L. (2005) Diapause in the mosquito *Culex pipiens* evokes a metabolic switch from blood feeding to sugar gluttony, *Proc. Natl. Acad. Sci. U.S.A.*, **102**, 15912–15917.

Chapter 7

Virology

NIAD supports a broad spectrum of both basic and applied research in virology to expand the understanding of the biology, pathogenesis, and the immunology of viral diseases, leading to their prevention, control, and treatment, including research on (i) the viral replication cycle; (ii) the structure and function of the viral components; (iii) host virus interactions, including pathogenesis, immune evasion, and immune enhancement; (iv) viral genetics and evolution; (v) viral interference and defective interfering particles; (vi) virus vector relationships; (vii) epidemiology and natural history; and (viii) preclinical and clinical research to develop vaccines, adjuvants, therapeutics, immunomodulators, and diagnostics (http://www3.niaid.nih.gov/research/topics/viral/introduction).

In addition, research on the emergence of new epidemic viruses through *host switching* has become a major priority for NIAID-supported research (http://www3.niaid.nih.gov/research/topics/viral/newepi_wkshp.pdf).

7.1 Resources for Researchers

The most important task of the *NIAID Antiviral Testing Program* is the evaluation of the efficacy and toxicity of new antiviral agents using a broad array of *in vitro* assays and *in vivo* animal models (http://www3.niaid.nih.gov/research/topics/viral/resources.htm). The main objective of this program is to identify antiviral agents with the potential to treat viral infections of public health importance, including those for newly emerging infections and those that are not a high priority for the pharmaceutical industry. NIAID ensures that the intellectual property rights of the compound supplier are protected. The viruses and models covered under this program include:

In Vitro Screens

- *Herpesviruses*: herpes simplex virus-1 (HSV-1); herpes simplex virus-2 (HSV-2); varicella-zoster virus (VZV); Epstein-Barr virus (EBV); cytomegalovirus (CMV); human herpes virus-6 (HHV-6); and human herpes virus-8 (HH-8)
- *Respiratory Viruses*: Influenza A and B; respiratory syncytial virus (RSV); parainfluenza virus (PIV); measles; rhinoviruses; adenoviruses; and severe acute respiratory syndrome (SARS) virus
- *Papillomaviruses and BK virus*
- *Biodefense*: orthopoxviruses (vaccinia, cowpox); Venezuelan equine encephalomyelitis virus (VEE); Punta Toro virus; Pichinde virus; Yellow fever virus; West Nile virus; and dengue virus

Animal Models

- HCV/-SCID/bg/uPA chimeric model
- *Herpesviruses*: HSV-1, HSV-2, murine cytomegalovirus (MCMV), guinea pig cytomegalovirus (GPCMV), human cytomegalovirus (HCMV$_{SCID-hu}$)
- *Respiratory Viruses*: Influenza A and B, RSV, PIV-3, Maedi-Visna virus (MV)
- *Hepatitis Viruses*: woodchuck hepatitis virus (WHV) and hepatitis B (HBV$_{transgenic}$)
- *Papillomaviruses*: Shope, HPV$_{SCID-hu}$
- Hamster scrapie in hamster-prion transgenic mice
- *Biodefense*: orthopoxviruses (vaccinia, cowpox, ectromelia), Punta Toro virus, Pichinde virus, Banzi virus, Semliki Forest virus, and West Nile virus

7.1.1 The Collaborative Antiviral Study Group (CASG)

CASG is a multi-institutional collaborative network funded by NIAID to conduct clinical trials and evaluate experimental therapies for viral infections. It comprises investigators at nearly 50 clinical research institutions and a Central Unit that serves as the core administrative, research, laboratory, biostatistical, and data management component of CASG. The CASG infrastructure would allow researchers to respond expeditiously to promising new therapies and

V. St. Georgiev, *National Institute of Allergy and Infectious Diseases, NIH: Impact on Global Health*, vol. 2, DOI 10.1007/978-1-60327-297-1_7, © Humana Press, a part of Springer Science+Business Media, LLC 2009

to unanticipated emerging clinical priorities (http://www3. niaid.nih.gov/research/topics/viral/resources.htm).

7.2 Recent Scientific Advances

- *Insulin-Degrading Enzyme Is a Cellular Receptor Mediating Varicella-Zoster Virus Infection and Cell-to-Cell Spread.* The varicella-zoster virus (VZV), which causes chickenpox and shingles, is likely spread to susceptible hosts as a cell-free virus. However, its cell-to-cell transmission in the body and *in vitro* is facilitated by the interaction of the VZV glycoprotein E (gE) with the insulin-degrading enzyme (IDE). IDE serves as a receptor through an extracellular domain. Cell-to-cell spread of the virus has been impaired by blocking IDE *(1)*. This finding suggests that IDE may become a valid target for new shingles and chickenpox treatments.

- *Structure of the Parainfluenza Virus 5 F Protein in Its Metastable, Prefusion Conformation.* Enveloped viruses have evolved complex glycoprotein machinery that drives the fusion of viral and cellular membranes, permitting the viral genome to enter the cell. For the paramyxoviruses, the fusion (F) protein catalyzes this membrane merger and entry step, and it has been postulated that the F protein undergoes complex refolding during this process. The crystal structure of the parainfluenza virus 5 F protein in its prefusion conformation and stabilized by the addition of a carboxy-terminal trimerization domain has been elucidated *(2)*. The positions and structural transitions of key parts of the fusion machinery, including the hydrophobic fusion peptide and two helical heptad repeat regions, clarified the mechanism of the F protein–mediated membrane fusion.

- *Development of a Humanized Monoclonal Antibody with Therapeutic Potential Against West Nile Virus.* Neutralization of West Nile virus (WNV) *in vivo* correlates with the development of an antibody response against the viral envelope (VE) protein. Using random mutagenesis and yeast surface display, the individual contact residues of 14 newly generated monoclonal antibodies against domain III of the WNV E protein have been defined *(3)*. One of them, a humanized version of E16 (HV-E16) retained antigen specificity, avidity, and neutralizing activity. In postexposure therapeutic trials in mice, a single dose of HV-E16 protected mice against WNV-induced mortality and may, therefore, be considered a viable treatment option against WNV infection in humans.

- *NIAID West Nile Virus (WNV) Vaccine Clinical Trial.* A small clinical trial to test the safety of an experimental vaccine against WNV was initiated in 2005 at the NIH Clinical Center. The experimental vaccine is composed of a small, circular piece of DNA plasmid that contains genes that code for two key surface proteins of WNV (niaidnews@niaid.nih.gov).

References

1. Li, Q., Ali, M. A., and Cohen, J. I. (2006) Insulin degrading enzyme is a cellular receptor mediating varicella-zoster virus infection and cell-to-cell spread, *Cell*, **127**(2), 305–316.
2. Yin, H.-S., Wen, X., Paterson, R. G., Lamb, R. A., and Jardetzky, T. S. (2006) Structure of the parainfluenza virus 5 F protein in its metastable, prefusion confirmation, *Nature*, **439**, 38–44.
3. Oliphant, T., Engle, M., Nybakken, G. E., Doane, C., Johnson, S., Huang, L., Gorlatov, S., Mehlhop, E., Marri, A., Chung, K. M., Ebel, G. D., Kramer, L. D., Fremont, D., H., and Diamond, M. S. (2005) Development of a humanized monoclonal antibody with therapeutic potential against West Nile virus, *Nat. Med.*, **11**, 522–530.

Chapter 8

Sexually Transmitted Infections

Sexually transmitted infections (STIs) are critical global and national health priorities because of their devastating impact on women and infants and their interrelationships with HIV/AIDS. The number of STIs, commonly known as sexually transmitted diseases (STDs), is continuing to increase dramatically worldwide. STIs and HIV are linked both by biological interactions and because both infections occur in the same populations. Infection with certain STIs can increase the risk of acquiring and transmitting HIV as well as altering the progression of the disease. In addition, STIs can cause long-term health problems, particularly in women and infants. Some of the sequelae of STIs include pelvic inflammatory disease (PID), infertility, tubal or ectopic pregnancy, cervical cancer, and perinatal or congenital infections in infants born to infected mothers (http://www3.niaid.nih.gov/research/topics/STI/introduction).

National figures for chlamydia, gonorrhea, and syphilis, each of them a notifiable infectious disease, are available from the CDC (http://www.cdc.gov/std/stats/toc2004.htm). However, reporting by the states to the CDC is voluntary and therefore not always complete. In addition, because STIs are often asymptomatic, the CDC and other clinic-based data underestimate the true burden of disease. Estimates for nonnotifiable STIs are drawn from targeted and, in some cases, population-based studies, as indicated.

8.1 Chlamydia

Chlamydia is one of the most widespread bacterial STIs in the United States, and *Chlamydia trachomatis* is the etiologic agent of the disease. The CDC estimates that in the United States, 2.8 million people are infected by chlamydia. Chlamydial infection, which is curable, can be transmitted by vaginal, oral, or anal sexual contact with an infected partner. It can cause serious problems in men and women, such as penile discharge and infertility, respectively, as well as infections in newborn babies of infected mothers. Furthermore, in women, chlamydial infections may result in

PID, which is a major cause of infertility, ectopic pregnancy, and chronic pelvic pain. The rate of reported chlamydial infection is greater among women than among men, and adolescent women are at the highest risk of infection. Asymptomatic infection is common among both men and women (http://www.niaid.nih.gov/factsheets/stdclam.htm).

The complete DNA sequences of *Chlamydia trichomatis* and *Chlamydia pneumoniae* have been recently determined and published (1). Although both species live inside the host cell, which distinguishes them from most other bacteria, they differ from each other by the diseases they cause. *C. trichomatis* causes trachoma, a preventable form of blindness in infants and infections of the genital tracts of adults, whereas *C. pneumoniae* causes pneumonia, bronchitis, and, more rarely, sore throats and sinus infections.

8.2 Gonorrhea

Gonorrhea is the second most commonly reported notifiable disease in the United States. The disease is caused by the bacterium *Neisseria gonorrhoeae*, which can infect the genital tract, mouth, and rectum of both men and women. In women, the first place of infection is the opening of the uterus (cervix). The infection is transmitted by vaginal, oral, and anal sex with an infected partner (http://www.niaid.nih.gov/factsheets/stdgon.htm).

In 2004, 330,132 cases of gonorrhea were reported in the United States. The rate of 113.5 cases per 100,000 was the lowest rate of reported gonorrhea ever. Gonorrhea rates are greatest among women aged 15 to 19 years and 20 to 24 years (610.9 per 100,000 and 569.1 per 100,000, respectively) and among men aged 20 to 24 years (430.6 per 100,000). When examining race and ethnicity, age, and gender, the highest rate in the United States was found among African Americans, 15 to 24 years of age, and among women, respectively. As with chlamydia, gonorrhea can infiltrate the uterus and fallopian tubes, resulting in pelvic inflammatory disease. The latter affects more than 1 million women in the United States and can cause ectopic pregnancy and infertility in as many as 10% of infected women (http://www.niaid.nih.gov/factsheets/stdgon.htm).

8.3 Syphilis

Syphilis is a genital ulcerative disease caused by *Treponema pallidum*. Untreated early syphilis in pregnant women results in perinatal death in up to 40% of cases and if acquired during the 4 years preceding pregnancy may lead to infection of the fetus in more than 70% of cases. Although the syphilis rates in the United States declined dramatically by 90% from 1990 to 2000, the number of cases rose from 5,979 in 2000 to 7,980 in 2004. In a single year from 2003 to 2004, the number of cases increased by 8%. The disease is contracted most often through sexual contact, and the bacterium is passed from infected skin or mucous membrane (genital area, lips, mouth, or anus) of an infected partner. Syphilis can also be passed by an infected mother to an infant during pregnancy, causing congenital syphilis (http://www3.niaid.nih.gov/healthscience/healthtopics/syphilis/default.htm).

8.4 Chancroid

Chancroid is an acute genital ulcerative disease caused by *Haemophilus ducreyi*. It is endemic in many parts of the developing world and is an important risk factor for heterosexual spread of HIV. The Joint United Nations Programme on HIV/AIDS (UNAIDS) and WHO have estimated that the annual global incidence of chancroid is approximately 6 million cases *(2)*. Chancroid usually occurs in discrete outbreaks in the United States, although the disease is endemic in some areas and often is not recognized.

In addition to the morbidity associated with chancroid, the disease is also a public health problem because *H. ducreyi* and HIV facilitate each other's transmission; per individual sexual act, chancroid is estimated to enhance HIV transmission 10- to 100-fold *(2)*.

H. ducreyi is a strictly human pathogen and naturally infects genital and nongenital skin, mucosal surfaces, and regional lymph nodes. It is thought to enter the skin through breaks in the epithelium that occur during intercourse, with a high transmission rate *(2)*.

8.5 Trichomoniasis

Trichomoniasis is a common STI that affects both women and men, although symptoms are more common in women. It is the most common curable STI in young, sexually active women (http://www3.niaid.nih.gov/healthscience/healthtopics/vaginitis/trichmoniasis). According to the CDC, an estimated 7.4 million new cases occur in men and women every year in the United States (http://www.cdc.gov/std/Trichomonas/STDFact-Trichomoniasis.htm).

Trichomoniasis is caused by a parasite called *Trichomonas vaginalis*. The genome sequence of *T. vaginalis* has been determines and published recently *(3)*.

Trichomoniasis is primarily an infection of the urogenital tract. The vagina is the most common place for infection in women, and the urethra (urine canal) is the most common place for infection in men. Transmission occurs through sexual intercourse with an infected partner. Although some infected women have minor or no symptoms, many do have symptoms, which usually appear within 5 to 28 days after they come in contact with the parasite. The symptoms in women include heavy, yellow-green or gray vaginal discharge, discomfort during sex, vaginal odor, and painful urination. Women also may have irritation and itching of the genital area and, on rare occasions, lower abdominal pain. Most infected men do not have symptoms. If they do, the symptoms include a thin, whitish discharge from the penis and painful or difficult urination and ejaculation (http://www3.niaid.nih.gov/healthscience/healthtopics/vaginitis/trichmoniaisis).

8.6 Oral and Genital Herpes

There are two types of herpes simplex viruses (HSVs), and both can cause genital herpes. HSV type 1 (HSV-1) most commonly infects the lips, causing sores known as fever blisters or cold sores, but it also can infect the genital area and produce sores. HSV type 2 (HSV-2) is the usual cause of genital herpes, but it also can infect the mouth (http://www.niaid.nih.gov/factsheets/stdherp.htm). Serious consequences of genital HSV infection include lifelong recurrent episodes of painful genital lesions, increased likelihood of HIV transmission and acquisition, and, for women, possible transmission to fetus or neonate, which can result in neonatal brain damage or death. Genital HSV-2 infection is more common in women (approximately 1 of 4 women) than in men (almost 1 of 5) (http://www.cdc.gov/std/Herpes/STDFact-Herpes.htm).

8.7 Human Papillomavirus

Human papillomavirus (HPV) is the name of a group of viruses that includes more than 100 different strains or types. More than 30 of these viruses are sexually transmitted, and they can infect the genital area of men and women. Most people who become infected with HPV will not have any symptoms and will clear the infection on their own. Some of these viruses are called "high-risk" types and can lead to cancer of the cervix, vulva, vagina, anus, or penis in addition to Pap test abnormalities. Others are called "low-risk" types, and they may cause mild Pap test abnormalities or genital warts. Genital warts are single or multiple growths or bumps that appear in the genital area and sometimes are cauliflower shaped (http://www.cdc.gov/std/HPV/STDFact-HPV.htm). Approximately 20 million people worldwide are currently infected with HPV. At least 50% of sexually active men and women acquire genital HPV infection at some point in their lives. By age 50, at least 80% of sexually active women will have acquired a genital HPV infection.

HPV is of clinical and public health importance because persistent infection with certain oncogenic types can lead to cervical cancer. Cervical cancer is one of the most common cancers in women worldwide. On June 8, 2006, an HPV vaccine was licensed by the FDA for use in females aged 9 to 26 years. Another HPV vaccine is in the final stages of clinical testing, but not yet licensed. These vaccines offer a promising new approach to the prevention of HPV and associated conditions.

8.7.1   Cervical Cancer

Cancer of the cervix (also known as cervical cancer) begins in the lining of the cervix. The causative agent is HPV. It does not form suddenly; normal cervical cells gradually develop precancerous changes (cervical intraepithelial neoplasia, squamous intraepithelial lesion, and dysplasia) that turn into cancer. There are two main types of cervical cancer: squamous cell carcinoma (80% to 90% of cervical cancers) and adenocarcinoma. Only some women with precancerous changes of the cervix will develop cancer. For most women, precancerous cells will remain unchanged and go away without treatment. Most HPV infections do not progress to cervical cancer. And whereas some types of HPV can cause cervical cancer, other types are associated with vulvar cancer, anal cancer, and cancer of the penis (a rare cancer). In women with abnormal cervical cells, a Pap smear will detect HPV (http://www3.niaid.nih.gov/healthscience/healthtopics/human_papilomavirus/complications.htm).

8.7.2   Pregnancy and Childbirth

Genital warts may cause a number of problems during pregnancy. Because genital warts can multiply and become brittle, one option is for their removal, if necessary.

Genital warts also may be removed to ensure a safe and healthy delivery of the newborn. Sometimes these warts get larger during pregnancy, making it difficult to urinate if they are in the urinary tract. If the warts are in the vagina, they can make the vagina less elastic and cause obstruction during delivery.

Rarely, infants born to women with genital warts develop warts in their throats (*respiratory papillomatosis*). Although uncommon, it is a potentially life-threatening condition for the child, requiring frequent laser surgery to prevent blocking of the breathing passages. Research on the use of interferon therapy with laser surgery indicates that this drug may show promise in slowing the course of the disease (http://www3.niaid.nih.gov/healthscience/healthtopics/human_papilomavirus/complications.htm).

8.7.3   Human Papillomavirus Vaccines

The FDA recently approved Gardasil, a vaccine produced by Merck & Co., Inc. It is called a quadrivalent vaccine because it protects against four HPV types: 6, 11, 16, and 18. Gardasil is given through a series of three *injections* into muscle *tissue* over a 6-month period.

Another promising vaccine, Cervarix, is produced and is being tested by GlaxoSmithKline but is not yet approved by the FDA. This vaccine is called a bivalent vaccine because it targets two HPV types: 16 and 18. Early findings have shown that this vaccine also protects against persistent infection with these two types of HPV. It is also given in three doses over a 6-month period.

Neither of these HPV vaccines has been proved to provide complete protection against persistent infection with other HPV types, some of which cause cervical cancer. Therefore, about 30% of cervical cancers and 10% of genital warts will not be prevented by these vaccines. In addition, the vaccines do not prevent other sexually transmitted diseases, nor do they treat HPV infection or cervical cancer. Because the vaccines will not protect against all infections that cause cervical cancer, it is important for vaccinated women to continue to undergo cervical cancer screening as is recommended for women who have not been vaccinated (http://www.cancer.gov/cancertopics/factsheets/risk/HPV-vaccine.htm).

8.8   Bacterial Vaginosis

Bacterial vaginosis is the name of a condition in women where the normal balance of bacteria in the vagina is disrupted and replaced by an overgrowth of certain bacteria. It is sometimes accompanied by discharge, odor, pain, itching, or burning. Bacterial vaginosis is the most common vaginal infection in women of childbearing age (http://www. cdc.gov/std/BV/STDFact-Bacterial-Vaginosis.htm). In most cases, bacterial vaginosis causes no complications. However, bacterial vaginosis has been associated with an increased risk of HIV acquisition and transmission. Furthermore, bacterial vaginosis can increase a woman's susceptibility to other STIs, such as chlamydia and gonorrhea. It is also associated with adverse outcomes of pregnancy (http://www.cdc. gov/std/BV/STDFact-Bacterial-Vaginosis.htm).

8.9 Impact of STIs on Women and Infants

8.9.1 Pelvic Inflammatory Disease

Each year millions of women worldwide will experience an episode of acute PID and hundred of thousands will become infertile as a result of it. In addition, large proportions of ectopic pregnancies that occur every year are due to the consequences of PID (http://www.cdc.gov/std/PID/STDFact-PID.htm).

If not adequately treated, 20% to 40% of women infected with chlamydia and 10% to 40% of women infected with gonorrhea may develop PID. Among women with PID, scarring will cause infertility in 20%, ectopic pregnancy in 9%, and chronic pelvic pain in 18%. Approximately 70% of chlamydial infections and 50% of gonococcal infections in women are asymptomatic. These infections are detected primarily through screening programs. The vague symptoms associated with chlamydial and gonococcal PID cause 85% of women to delay seeking medical care, thereby increasing their risk of infertility and ectopic pregnancy. Data from a randomized controlled trial of chlamydia screening in a managed care setting suggest that such screening programs can reduce the incidence of PID by as much as 60% (http://www.cdc.gov/std/PID/STDFact-PID.htm).

Having bacterial vaginosis has been associated with an increase in the development of PID after surgical procedures such as a hysterectomy or abortion (http://www.cdc.gov/ std/BV/STDFact-Bacterial-Vaginosis.htm).

8.9.2 Adverse Outcomes of Pregnancy

A pregnant woman with an STI may experience early onset of labor, premature rupture of membranes surrounding the fetus in the uterus, and uterine infection after delivery (http://www.cdc.gov/std/STDFact-STDs&Pregnancy.htm).

The harmful effects of STIs on babies may include stillbirth, low birth weight, conjunctivitis (eye infection), pneumonia, neonatal sepsis (infection in the bloodstream), neurologic damage (such as brain damage or motor dis-

order), congenital abnormalities (including blindness, deafness, or other organ damage), acute hepatitis, meningitis, chronic liver disease, and cirrhosis. Some of these problems can be prevented if the mother receives routine prenatal care, which includes screening tests for STIs starting early in pregnancy and repeated close to delivery, if necessary. Other problems can be treated if the infection is found at birth (http://www.cdc.gov/std/STDFact-STDs&Pregnancy.htm).

Genital HSV can cause potentially fatal infections in newborns. Initial infection during pregnancy causes a greater risk of transmission to the infant. If a woman has active genital herpes at delivery, a cesarean delivery is usually performed (http://www.cdc.gov/std/Herpes/STDFact-Herpes.htm).

The syphilis bacterium can infect the fetus of a woman during her pregnancy. Depending on how long a pregnant woman has been infected, she may have a high risk of having a stillbirth or of giving birth to an infant who dies shortly after birth. An infected infant may be born without signs or symptoms of disease. However, if not treated immediately, the infant may develop serious problems within a few weeks. Untreated newborns may become developmentally delayed, have seizures, or die (http://www.cdc.gov/ std/syphilis/STDFact-Syphilis.htm).

In pregnant women, there is some evidence that untreated chlamydial infections can lead to premature delivery. Babies who are born to infected mothers can get chlamydial infections in their eyes and respiratory tracts. Chlamydia is a leading cause of early infant pneumonia and conjunctivitis (pinkeye) in newborns (http://www. cdc.gov/std/chlamydia/STDFact-Chlamydia.htm).

Pregnant women with trichomoniasis may have babies who are born early or with low birth weight (less than 5 lb) (http://www.cdc.gov/std/Trichomonas/STDFact-Trichomoniasis.htm).

Pregnant women with bacterial vaginosis more often have babies who are born prematurely or with low birth weight (less than 5 lb) (http://www.cdc.gov/std/bv/STDFact-Bacterial-Vaginosis.htm).

8.10 Impact of STIs on HIV/AIDS

The presence of an STI increases the likelihood of acquiring and transmitting HIV. Recent studies indicate that the more prevalent nonulcerative STIs (chlamydial infection, gonorrhea, bacterial vaginosis, and trichomoniasis) as well as the ulcerative diseases (genital herpes, syphilis, and chancroid) increase the risk of HIV transmission at least two- to fivefold.

There is substantial biological evidence demonstrating that the presence of other STIs increases the likelihood of both acquiring and transmitting HIV (http://www. cdc.gov/std/hiv/STDFact-STD&HIV.htm). Women infected with chlamydia are three to five times more likely to become infected with HIV if exposed (http://www.cdc.gov/std/chlamydia/STDFact-Chlamydia.htm). Furthermore, persons with gonorrhea can more easily contract HIV, and HIV-infected people with gonorrhea are more likely to transmit HIV to someone else (http://www.cdc.gov/std/Gonorrhea/STDFact-gonorrhea.htm). Chancroid is a co-factor for HIV transmission (http://www.cdc.gov/STD/treatment/2-2002TG.htm#Chancroid).

There is an estimated two- to fivefold increased risk of acquiring HIV infection when syphilis is present (http://www.cdc.gov/std/syphilis/STDFact-Syphilis.htm). Another STI, herpes, may also play a role in the spread of HIV. Herpes can make persons more susceptible to HIV infection, and it can make HIV-infected individuals more infectious (http://www.cdc.gov/std/Herpes/STDFact-Herpes.htm). The genital inflammation caused by trichomoniasis can increase a woman's susceptibility to HIV infection if she is exposed to the virus. Having trichomoniasis may increase the chance that an HIV-infected woman passes HIV to her sex partner(s) (http://www.cdc.gov/std/Trichomonas/STDFact-Trichomoniasis.htm). Finally, bacterial vaginosis can increase the susceptibility and transmissibility of HIV and other STIs (http://www.cdc.gov/std/BV/STDFact-Bacterial-Vaginosis.htm).

STI treatment reduces an individual's ability to transmit HIV. Studies have shown that treating STDs in HIV-infected individuals decreases both the amount of HIV they shed and how often they shed the virus *(4)*.

8.11 NIAID Involvement in STI Research

8.11.1 Plans, Priorities, and Goals

NIAID supports research designed to prevent and control STIs. Major research goals and objectives include (http://www3.niaid.nih.gov/research/topics/STI/introduction): (i) developing and licensing safe and effective vaccines, topical microbicides, therapeutics, and strategies for preventing and treating STIs and sequelae; (ii) understanding the long-term health impact of a sexually transmitted pathogen on various populations; and (iii) developing better and more rapid diagnostics.

8.11.2 Research Activities

NIAID supports a broad STI research portfolio, which addresses these diseases through individual investigator-initiated research grants, contracts, and a variety of research programs (http://www3.niaid.nih.gov/research/topics/STI/research.htm), including:

- *The STD Cooperative Research Centers (CRCs).* The CRCs have been established to: (i) bridge basic biomedical, clinical, behavioral, and epidemiologic research; (ii) promote productive collaborations among academic researchers; and (iii) facilitate the development of intervention-oriented research. This program has been broadened to include topical microbicides.

- *The STD Clinical Trials Unit (STD CTU).* The STD CTU conducts clinical trials to test the safety and efficacy of biomedical and behavioral interventions aimed at preventing and controlling STIs.

- *The Topical Microbicides Program.* This program conducts basic research, product development, and clinical evaluation activities aimed at developing female-controlled barrier methods for the prevention of HIV/AIDS and other STIs.

- The sequencing of the genomes of sexually transmitted pathogens, including *Chlamydia trachomatis*, *Neisseria gonorrhoeae*, and *Haemophilus ducreyi*.

- Support for databases of genomic and postgenomic information and analysis tools on sexually transmitted pathogens. This information has provided new insights into the pathogenesis of numerous STIs and is paving the way for new opportunities to develop diagnostics, drugs, vaccines, and microbicides.

- A pivotal Phase III double-blind clinical efficacy trial of an investigational vaccine for the prevention of genital herpes, which opened in November 2002, will enroll 7,550 women at approximately 25 sites across the United States. This study, which is called the *Herpevac Trial for Women*, is being conducted as a public-private partnership with GlaxoSmithKline.

- *The STD Prevention Primate Unit (STD PPU).* STD PPU was established to carry out preclinical evaluation of topical microbicides and vaccines at the University of Washington, which over the past year has evaluated several candidate microbicides for safety (effects on surface tissues and microenvironment of the cervix and vagina) in pig-tailed macaques. Results from a DMID-supported testing contract have been coordinated with testing conducted by the Division of Acquired Immunodeficiency Syndrome (DAIDS) to facilitate product development and safety and efficacy testing in clinical trials.

8.11.3 Resources for Researchers

The Computer Retrieval of Information on Scientific Projects (CRISP). CRISP is a searchable database of federally funded biomedical research projects conducted at universities, hospitals, and other research institutions.

8.12 Recent Scientific Advances

- *Condom Use Reduces the Risk of Genital Human Papillomavirus Infection in Young Women.* HPV is a common sexually transmitted infection that can lead to cervical cancer. Most new cases of HPV infection occur in 15- to 24-year-old women, but risk continues even in older sexually active women. Data have demonstrated that the incidence of genital HPV infection was 37.8 per 100 patient-years at risk among women whose partners used condoms for all instances of intercourse compared with 89.3 per 100 patient-years at risk in women whose partners used condoms less than 5% of the time *(5)*.

- *Chlamydia trachomatis Protein Offers a Species-Common Pan-Neutralizing Antigen. C. trachomatis* serovariants are the leading cause of bacterial STIs and infectious preventable blindness (blinding trachoma). To date, there is no vaccine against this pathogen. Recent research has shown that all *C. trachomatis* reference serotypes responsible for disease and blinding trachoma synthesize a highly conserved surface-exposed antigen termed polymorphic membrane protein D (PmpD) *(6)*. Moreover, antibodies specific to PmpD were neutralizing *in vitro*, and antibodies against serovariable-neutralizing targets, such as the major outer membrane protein, block PmpD neutralization. Collectively, this and other evidence suggested that PmpD is a previously uncharacterized *C. trachomatis* species-common pan-neutralizing target, and that a vaccine protocol using recombinant PmpD to elicit neutralizing antibodies in the absence of immunodominant type-specific antibodies might be highly efficacious and surpass the level of protection achieved through natural immunity *(6)*.

- *Immunization with the Haemophilus ducreyi Hemoglobin Receptor HgbA Protects Against Infection in the Swine Model of Chancroid.* To fulfill its obligate requirement for heme, *H. ducreyi*, the etiologic agent of chancroid, uses two TonB-dependent receptors: the hemoglobin receptor (HgbA) and a receptor for free heme (TdhA). Expression of HgbA is necessary for the pathogen to survive and initiate disease in a human model of chancroid. By using a swine model of *H. ducreyi*, researchers have demonstrated that an experimental HgbA vaccine efficiently prevented chancroid *(7)*. Antibodies from sera of HgbA-immunized animals bound to and initiated antibody-dependent bactericidal activity against homologous *H. ducreyi* strain 35000HP and heterologous strain CIP542 ATCC. However, an isogenic *hgbA* mutant of 35000HP was not killed, indicating specificity. Anti-HgbA immunoglobulin G blocked hemoglobin binding to the HgbA receptor, suggesting a novel mechanism of protection

through the limitation of heme/iron acquisition by *H. ducreyi (7)*.

8.13 Clinical Trials

Several clinical trials have been initiated:

1. *The Sexually Transmitted Infections Clinical Trial Group (STICTG)* is initiating a Phase I trial to evaluate the safety of a twice-daily, vaginally applied microbicide gel (SPL 7013) to prevent genital herpes. This microbicide is being tested in conjunction with NIAID's Division of AIDS (DAIDS) where it will be assessed for the prevention of HIV transmission (http://www.fhi.org/stictg.about.htm).

2. A pivotal Phase III double-blind clinical trial is designed to evaluate the efficacy of an investigational vaccine for the prevention of genital herpes, enrolling women at approximately 42 sites in United States and Canada. The study, called the Herpevac Trial for Women (http://niaid.nih.gov/dmid/stds/herpevac), is being conducted as a public-private partnership with the GlaxoSmithKline Company.

3. The STICTG is conducting a randomized Phase III clinical trial to evaluate the equivalency of oral azithromycin versus injectable benzathine penicillin for treating primary syphilis.

References

1. Read, T. D., Brunham, R. C., Shen, C., et al. (2000) Genome sequences of *Chlamydia trichomatis* MoPn and *Chlamidia pneumoniae* Ar39, *Nucleic Acids Res.*, **28**(6), 1397–1406.
2. Spinoal, S. M., Bauer, M. E., and Munson, R. S., Jr. (2002) Immunopathogenesis of *Haemophilus ducreyi* infection (chancroid), *Infect. Immun.*, **70**(4), 1667–1676.
3. Carlton, J. M., Hirt, R. P., Silva, J. C., et al. (2007) Draft genome sequence of the sexually transmitted pathogen *Trichomonas vaginalis*, *Science*, **315**(5809), 207–212.
4. Fleming, D. T. and Wasserheit, J. N. (1999) From epidemiological synergy to public health policy and practice: the contribution of other sexually transmitted diseases to sexual transmission of HIV infection, *Sex. Transm. Infect.*, **72**(1), 3–17.
5. Winer, R. L., Hughes, J. P., Feng, Q., O'Reilly, B. S., Kiviat, N. B., Holmes, K. K., and Koutsky, L. A. (2006) Condom use and the risk of genital human papilomavirus infection in young women, *N. Engl. J. Med.*, **354**(25), 2645–2654.
6. Crane, D. D., Carlson, J. H., Fischer, E. R., Bavoil, P., Hsia, R.-C., Tan, C., Kuo, C.-C., and Caldwell, H. D. (2006) Chlamydia trachomatis polymorphic membrane protein D is a species-common pan-neutralizing antigen, *Proc. Natl. Acad. Sci. U.S.A.*, **103**(6), 1894–1899.
7. Afonina, G., Leduc, I., Nepluev, I., Jeter, C., Routh, P., Almond, G., Orndorff, P. E., Hobbs, M., and Elkins, C. (2006) Immunization with the *Haemophilus ducreyi* hemoglobin receptor HgbA protects against infection in the swine model of chancroid, *Infect. Immun.*, **74**(4), 2224–2232.

Chapter 9

Enteric Diseases

The gastrointestinal (GI) tract is the largest lymphoid organ in the human body and, therefore, any defects in the cellular and/or humoral immune responses may be indicators of a strong disposition to a multitude of enteric viral, bacterial, protozoan, and fungal pathogens (1). The identification of enteric pathogens in the GI tract has been especially important in patients with AIDS, where the HIV-induced immunodeficiency greatly increases the possibility of opportunistic infections (2).

The great majority of enteric infections occur after pathogens from contaminated food or water have been ingested, as well as through fecal-oral transmission. In addition to acute illness, which is usually characterized by diarrhea of varying morbidity, some of the enteric pathogens may be associated with chronic infection and more serious complications, including life-threatening systemic infections and severe dehydrating diarrhea. Long-term complications include malnutrition, malabsorption of vital drugs, and immunologic complications. In the United States, diarrhea is the second most common infectious illness, accounting for 16% of diagnoses. WHO has estimated that diarrheal diseases account for 15% to 34% of all deaths in certain countries and has placed the death toll worldwide at 4 million to 6 million people, with most cases occurring in children of preschool age, the elderly, and the immunocompromised. In addition to naturally acquired infection, the potential for food- and water-borne pathogens to be used as weapons for mass poisoning has been recognized by their inclusion in the List of NIAID Category B Priority Pathogens (http://www3.niaid.nih.gov/research/topics/enteric/introduction.htm).

A major part of the research activities of NIAID in the area of enteric diseases is carried out through the *Food and Waterborne Diseases Integrated Research Network (FWD IRN)* (http://www3.niaid.nih.gov/reesrach/topics/enteric/research.htm). The network facilitates the integration of research programs to develop products to rapidly identify, prevent, treat, and diagnose food- and water-borne diseases that threaten public health. The FWD IRN comprises seven contracts providing expertise in the areas of clinical research, immunology, microbiology, and zoonoses to address priority research and product development needs for food- and water-borne pathogens. To this end, the FWD IRN includes (i) the capabilities to develop and evaluate vaccines, therapeutics, and rapid detection methods; (ii) integration of human mucosal immunity with clinical research; and (iii) definition of the ecology and microbiology of food- and water-borne zoonoses, as well as drug-resistant pathogens. The Research Units and the Coordinating and Biostatistics Center (CoBC) of FWD IRN (http://web.emmes.com/study/fwd) are

(i) Clinical Research Unit—University of Maryland
(ii) Immunology Research Unit—University of Maryland
(iii) Microbiology Research Unit—Michigan State University
(iv) Microbiology and Botulism Research Unit—Tufts University
(v) Zoonoses Research Unit—Cornell University
(vi) Zoonoses Research Unit—Washington State University
(vii) Coordination and Biostatistics Center—The EMMES Corp., Rockville, Maryland

9.1 Epidemiology of Enteric Diseases

In its "State of the Art of New Vaccines: Research and Development" report published in January 2006 (http://www.who.int/vaccines-documents), WHO estimated the global mortality from diarrheal diseases to be 4 million to 6 million annually. Worldwide:

- *Rotavirus* is estimated to account for almost 40% of all cases of severe diarrhea and has accounted for 600,000 deaths each year, mostly in children under age 2 (http://www.who.int/vaccine_research/diseases/rotavirus/en/).
- *Caliciviruses* appeared to be the most common cause of gastroenteritis outbreaks and accounted for 18% to 20%

V. St. Georgiev, *National Institute of Allergy and Infectious Diseases, NIH: Impact on Global Health*, vol. 2, DOI 10.1007/978-1-60327-297-1_9, © Humana Press, a part of Springer Science+Business Media, LLC 2009

of diarrheal episodes worldwide (http://www.who.int/immunization/topics/caliciviruses/en/print.html).

- *Enterotoxigenic Escherichia coli (ETEC)* is the most common cause of diarrhea in the developing world, with 280 million to 500 million diarrheal episodes in children annually, and an estimated 300,000 to 500,000 deaths each year, mostly in young children *(3)*.

- *Campylobacter jejuni* is the most common bacterial cause of diarrhea in many developed countries and represents the second leading cause of traveler's diarrhea after ETEC, with an estimated 400 million cases per year worldwide (http://www.who.int/topics/campylobacter/en/).

- *Shigella* causes an estimated 165 million cases of severe dysentery annually, resulting in more than 1 million deaths, primarily in young children (http://www.who.int/vaccine_research/diseases/shigella/en/).

- *Cholera* is an important disease in regions where poor sanitation and population overcrowding are common. Global estimates are close to 1 million cases with 100,000 to 300,000 deaths annually, mostly in Asia and Africa (http://www.who.int/topics/cholera/en/).

- *Typhoid fever*, caused by *Salmonella typhi*, also remains a serious health problem in developing countries. WHO estimates 16 million to 33 million cases and 500,000 to 600,000 deaths each year, with the incidence highest in children 5 to 19 years of age (http://www.who.int/topics/salmonella/en/; http:// www.cdc.gov/ncidod/dbmd/diseaseinfo/ typhoid-fever_g.htm).

In the United States, according to estimates by the CDC, 76 million people contract *food-borne* infections annually, leading to 325,000 hospitalizations and 5,000 deaths. In 2004, CDC reported 251 national food-borne disease outbreaks, with Novovirus and *Salmonella* as the most common pathogens.

During the period 1996–2004, the incidence of *Campylobacter*, Shiga toxin–producing *Escherichia coli* (STEC) 0157, *Listeria*, *Salmonella*, and *Yersinia* declined substantially, with the number of reported cases of *Campylobacter*, enterohemorrhagic *E. coli*, and *Listeria* approaching the national objective levels. However, the incidence of *Vibrio* infections increased in 2004, while the rate of *Shigella* infections remained relatively stable. The percentage of persons hospitalized and the case-fatality rates were highest for *Listeria* infections (97% and 16%, respectively) (http://www.cdc.gov/foodnet/).

In its 2005 Final Report of Notifiable Diseases *(4)*, CDC listed the reported number of cases (given in parentheses) in the United States for the following food- and water-borne diseases: salmonellosis (45,322), shigellosis (16,168), *E. coli* O157:H7 (2,621), listeriosis (896), *E. coli* Shiga

toxin (+) non-O157:H7 (501), *E. coli* Shiga toxin (+) not serogrouped (407), typhoid fever (324), hemolytic uremic syndrome (HUS) (221), botulism (135), and cholera (8). However, these national statistics can be influenced by large individual disease outbreaks, such as the 2006 *Salmonella* outbreak associated with tomatoes in Maryland (http://www.cdc.gov/salmonella/) and several regional incidences of acute gastroenteritis in 2005 after Hurricane Katrina (http://www.cdc.gov/mmwr/preview/mmwrhtml/mm5440a3.htm).

9.2 Shigella spp.

Shigella is a genus of Gram-negative facultatively anaerobic bacteria of the family Enterobacteriaceae *(1)*. On the basis of biochemical and antigenic studies, *Shigella* is differentiated into four distinct species: *S. dysenteriae* (subgroup A), *S. flexneri* (subgroup B), *S. boydii* (subgroup C), and *S. sonnei* (subgroup D). *S. dysenteriae* is highly pathogenic, causing severe dysentery that can be fatal in children. In fact, bacillary dysentery is considered to be one of the major factors in childhood mortality, especially in developing countries, in some cases causing more deaths than does watery diarrhea *(1)*. *Shigella* bacteremia may lead to complications such as hematologic disorders (hemoglobinopathy), disseminated intravascular coagulation, paroxysmal atrial tachycardia, leukopenia, and hypogammaglobulinemia.

In terms of therapy, in addition to oral rehydration, antimicrobial agents still remain an important part in the treatment of shigellosis. However, for several decades the steady and continuing increase in drug resistance toward commonly prescribed antimicrobial agents has remained a problem for the effective management of shigellosis *(1)*. In spite of continuing research, a vaccine against shigellosis is still not available.

9.3 Salmonella spp.

Salmonella is a genus of Gram-negative facultatively anaerobic bacteria of the family Enterobacteriaceae *(1)*. *Salmonella* is divided into species or serotypes on the basis of O (somatic), Vi (capsular), and H (flagellar) antigens. There are several species of *Salmonella* that are pathogenic to humans, causing enteric fever (typhoid and paratyphoid), septicemias, and gastroenteritis. The most frequent clinical manifestation has been food poisoning.

Some of the most common species of *Salmonella* species include:

(i) *S. arizonae*, the causative agent of gastroenteritis, enteric fever, bacteremia, and local infection in humans. It is considered to be an opportunistic pathogen in immunocompromised patients, causing systemic infections in subjects with underlying diseases.

(ii) *S. choleraesuis*, a group C species associated with paratyphoid fever, gastroenteritis, and septicemia in humans. It is a highly invasive serotype that is most often recovered from blood but not stools. It is considered to be one of the most virulent *Salmonella* spp. responsible for the highest incidence of fatal infections in humans.

(iii) *S. enteritidis*, which in humans may produce paratyphoid fever, septicemia, and gastroenteritis. *S. enteritidis* serotype *dublin* is a group D *Salmonella* species that could present high risk for immunocompromised hosts causing severe illness with fever, diarrhea, and bacteremia.

(iv) *S. typhi*, a group D serotype that has been associated with typhoid fever in humans and is transmitted by water or food contaminated by human excreta. *S. typhi* is further subdivided into V strains containing the Vi (virulence) antigen, V-W strains that have partially lost their Vi antigen, and W strains, which do not contain the Vi antigen.

(v) *S. heidelberg*. By some accounts, it is the third most common serotype implicated in salmonellosis.

Immunity to salmonella infections is usually short lived, and susceptibility to identical serotypes has been documented. Enhanced severity of salmonella disease has been observed in patients with different hemolytic anemias (e.g., sickle cell anemia), collagen vascular disease, immunosuppression, malaria, and HIV infection. Bacteremia and dissemination occur only rarely in adolescent children and adults but has been diagnosed in 5% to 40% of infants with gastroenteritis *(1)*.

Rarely a cause of meningitis in adults, *Salmonella*-associated meningitis is predominately a disease in infants. Even though the overall incidence of *Salmonella* meningitis is low, the mortality rate has been exceedingly high, mostly because of difficulties in sterilizing the cerebrospinal fluid, disease-related complications (cerebral abscesses, subdural empyema, and ventriculitis), hydrocephalus, and frequent relapses *(1)*. Treatment of *Salmonella* meningitis has not been well defined, but ampicillin and chloramphenicol seem to be the most effective drugs.

In general, treatment of *Salmonella* infections usually involves antibiotics, such as oral ciprofloxacin. Treatment of *S. arizonae* has been guided by the susceptibility of the organism, but most commonly the use of ampicillin or trimethoprim-sulfamethoxazole (TMP-SMX).

To further complicate treatment, drug resistance by *S. dublin* has been well documented, especially against antibiotics (chloramphenicol). The high frequency of resistance to *S. dublin* and the potential for serious head and neck

infection in immunocompromised patients make early diagnosis and treatment of this pathogen very important *(1)*.

Several vaccines against *S. typhi* have already been developed *(1)*.

9.4 Yersinia enterocolitica

Like other Enterobacteriaceae species, *Yersinia enterocolitica* is a facultatively anaerobic, Gram-negative coccoid bacterium *(1)*. It is a rapidly emerging human enteric pathogen associated with a wide spectrum of clinical and immunologic manifestations. *Y. enterocolitica* has been isolated worldwide from both clinical and nonclinical specimens but seems to be more commonly distributed in cooler climatic regions. Different *Yersinia* serotypes vary in their virulence. Serotypes O:3, O:8, and O:9 are considered the most virulent, causing outbreaks of disease worldwide. For reasons still not well understood, it seems that serotypes O:3 and O:9 have predominated in Europe, whereas serotype O:8 has been the causative agent of most infections in the United States *(1)*. Transmission of *Y. enterocolitica* to humans occurs primarily by ingestion of contaminated food (especially pork meat), water, and milk.

Y. enterocolitica is known to invade peritoneal macrophages and the epithelial cells in the intestinal mucosa. Consequently, the bacteria will proliferate within the macrophages and then eventually will infiltrate the regional lymph nodes by transport to these cells.

9.4.1 Iron as Bacterial Growth Factor

For the majority of bacteria, iron is an essential growth factor that is obtained by most microorganisms through the release of high-affinity, low-molecular-weight iron chelators, known as siderophores. After binding ferric iron (Fe^{3+}), the siderophores reenter the bacteria *(5)*. However, *Y. enterocolitica* is one bacterium that cannot synthesize siderophores *(6)*. Instead, it is endowed with siderophore receptors and can use as growth factors siderophores delivered by other bacteria (such as deferoxamine B), exogenous siderophores, or hemin *(6)*. This enables *Y. enterocolitica* to grow in the intestine where siderophores of bacterial origin are abundant. However, in tissue and organic fluid, the bacterium must compete with other iron-binding protein (transferrin, lactoferrin), and multiplication is only possible when there is an iron overload and supply is adequate, or when there are exogenous siderophores present. Because both iron overloading and increased levels of deferoxamine were found to substantially increase the virulence of *Yersinia*, these two conditions are considered to be independent predisposing factors for systemic infection with *Y. enterocolitica*. Studies on the iron-repressible outer membrane proteins (Irp) and siderophore production of *Y. enterocolitica* (serotype 8) have shown that its virulence was closely associated with the siderophore production, expression of an iron-repressible outer membrane polypeptide (65,000 Da), and the pesticin sensitivity of *Y. enterocolitica (7)*.

9.5 Campylobacter spp.

Campylobacter is a genus of motile Gram-negative microaerophilic to anaerobic bacteria *(1)*. In humans and animals, the bacterium is found in the oral cavity, the GI tract, and the reproductive organs. Some of the *Campylobacter* species are pathogenic in humans causing enteritis and systemic diseases. Such factors as advanced age, a dysfunctional GI tract, or underlying immune deficiency would enhance the risk of infections. Among the *Campylobacter* species, *C. coli* is the cause of diarrhea in humans; *C. cinaedi* and *C. fennelliae* are known to effect proctitis and diarrhea in immunocompromised homosexual men. *C. fetus* (also known as *Vibrio fetus*) is associated with febrile illness as well as thrombophlebitis, endocarditis, infected aortic aneurysm, septic arthritis, and osteomyelitis. *C. fetus* subsp. *jejuni* (*C. jejuni*, *Vibrio coli*, *V. jejuni*) is a common pathogen associated with acute bacterial gastroenteritis in humans. Currently, *C. coli* and *C. jejuni* are recognized to be among the most important causes of diarrhea in both immunocompetent and immunocompromised hosts *(1)*.

C. pyloti (*Helicobacter pylori*) is a species associated with gastritis and pyloric ulcers in humans.

9.5.1 Campylobacter jejuni/coli–Associated Enteritis

Campylobacter jejuni/coli–associated enteritis has been commonly diagnosed among children in developing countries, where *C. jejuni* may be excreted by up to 40% of children under 5 years of age *(8)*. Their transmission in humans has most often been caused by drinking contaminated water or ingesting unpasteurized milk and by contact with domestic animals suffering from diarrhea *(1)*.

Although in the majority of cases fluid replacement without antibiotics may be sufficient treatment, in more serious cases specific therapy may be indicated. Macrolide antibiotics and fluoroquinolone antibacterials (ciprofloxacin, norfloxacin, ofloxacin) have been shown to be effective either prophylactically or as therapy, where they may shorten the duration of diarrhea by 1 to 2 days. The combination of trimethoprim-sulfamethoxazole, which has been used extensively in other enteric infections (shigellosis, severe traveler's diarrhea), has not been found effective against *C. jejuni* because of drug resistance *(9)*. It is not unusual that *C. jejuni* enteritis (as many as 3% of patients) may be followed by Reiter's syndrome or reactive arthritis *(10)*.

9.5.2 Campylobacter jejuni Bacteremia and the Guillain-Barré Syndrome

There have been an increasing number of reports of patients developing Guillain-Barré syndrome after *C. jejuni* gastrointestinal infection *(1)*. In the observed cases, usually symptoms of *C. jejuni*–associated diarrhea had preceded the onset of the Guillain-Barré syndrome by 5 to 10 days, and the severity of the syndrome varied greatly. The exact pathologic mechanism of *C. jejuni*–associated Guillain-Barré syndrome is still unclear. According to some studies, the pathophysiology of the *C. jejuni*–associated Guillain-Barré syndrome may involve an human leukocyte antigen (HLA)-related predisposition to develop immune responses against antigens shared by *C. jejuni* and elements of the nervous system *(11)*. These data, together with the clinical response observed in some patients treated intravenously with immunoglobulin and plasmapheresis, supported a key role for the humoral response in the *C. jejuni*–associated Guillain-Barré syndrome.

9.5.3 Drug Resistance by Campylobacter spp.

C. jejuni/coli resistance to macrolide antibiotics (erythromycin, tetracycline) is plasmid-mediated. It has also been found that erythromycin resistance can occur independently of tetracycline resistance *(1)*.

Although generally susceptible to fluoroquinolones (ciprofloxacin, ofloxacin, norfloxacin), both *C. jejuni* and *C. coli* have developed resistance (sometimes spontaneous) to these agents. There have also been data indicating the development of spontaneous resistance to fluoroquinolones. The development of spontaneous resistance against fluoroquinolones may be explained either as a result of a spontaneous mutation in the bacterial chromosome or as a secondary cross-resistance to therapy with unrelated antibiotics *(12)*.

Detailed understanding of the mechanisms of *Campylobacter* resistance to fluoroquinolones is important for developing preventive strategies. Currently, two major mechanisms have been defined: (i) alterations in the bacterial DNA gyrase, the molecular target of the quinolone action; and (ii) reduction of drug accumulation in the cells.

9.5.3.1 Alterations in Bacterial DNA Gyrase

The bacterial DNA gyrase is a type II topoisomerase, an enzyme common for eubacteria, Archaebacteria, viruses, and eukaryotes. In general, the role of topoisomerase enzymes is essential for DNA replication and recombination. In this regard, the DNA gyrase has been unique in its ability to insert superhelical turns (negative supercoils) into covalently closed double-stranded bacterial DNA molecules *(13)*. The process of supercoiling involves the concerted action of two gyrase subunits A, which mediate transient double-strand breakage and rejoining, and two subunits B, which provide energy by ATP hydrolysis for regenerating the enzyme conformation to initiate the next cycle of DNA cleavage, strand passage, and rejoining of the broken strands *(14)*. What the fluoroquinolones do is to suppress the rejoining of the broken strands by forming stable ternary complexes with the bacterial gyrase and DNA; the subunits A will attach covalently to the cleaved DNA ends through tyrosine ester bonds.

This unique feature of bacterial type II topoisomerases, such as DNA gyrase, to insert negative supercoils into DNA may well account for the *selective* action of the fluoroquinolones on bacteria, as isolated mammalian topoisomerase enzymes studied to date have been highly resistant to inhibition by quinol-4-ones.

Two genes, *gyr*A and *gyr*B, are coding for subunits A and B, respectively. To date, several mutations, namely *nal*A, *nfx*A, *nor*A, and *cfx*A, resulting in resistance to nalidixic acid (a nonfluorinated 1,8-naphthyridine derivative) and fluoroquinolones, have been mapped at the *gyr*A locus *(1)*. All mutations were found to be confined within a highly conserved region, the "quinolone resistance-determining region" (QRDR). However, despite increasing the resistance toward quinolones, these mutations did not change the bacterial susceptibilities to several structurally unrelated drugs.

The isolation of DNA gyrase that was less sensitive to inhibition by ciprofloxacin from a ciprofloxacin-resistant *C. jejuni* isolate did signify that ciprofloxacin resistance in this organism has also been associated with alteration in the DNA gyrase *(15)*. Further data on quinolone-resistant *C. jejuni* mutants also strongly implied that alteration of the subunit A of DNA gyrase has been responsible for the observed resistance *(16)*.

In contrast with mutations in *gyr*A, the *gyr*B gene mutations have been shown to be of lesser importance for the formation of drug resistance *(14)*.

9.5.3.2 Reduction of Quinolone Accumulation

To reach the intracellular DNA gyrase as their target, the quinolones must penetrate the bacterial cell wall. Clinical resistance because of reduced drug accumulation has been associated with at least one of two different mechanisms: (i) an energy-independent, passive mechanism that is based either on structural alterations or on a reduced expression of outer membrane protein (OMP) porins (water-filled protein pores) that facilitate the passage of hydrophilic quinolone compounds (e.g., ciprofloxacin, ofloxacin) through the outer bacterial membrane (e.g., Gram-negative organisms); and/or (ii) an energy-requiring, active efflux mechanism of quinolones *(14)*.

Impaired Permeability of Outer Cell Membrane

Most studies to determine the mechanism of reduced quinolone accumulation have been done on *E. coli*. *E. coli* has two major porins, OMP F and OMP C, forming pores of 1.2 and 1.0 nm, respectively *(17)*. Although loss of either porin by inactivation of the respective structural genes (*omp*F and *omp*C) would diminish the accumulation of hydrophilic quinolones, in *E. coli* the major portal of entry is OMP F. Moreover, because the OMP F porin lacks specificity, other unrelated drugs (tetracycline, chloramphenicol, β-lactams), besides quinolones, may also use it to enter the bacterial cell; consequently, the loss of OMP F resulted in parallel resistance to all of these compounds. In addition to mutations in the structural *omp*F gene, mutations at several unrelated loci have also been proved to reduce the amount of the OMP F porin, thereby decreasing drug accumulation *(1)*.

Regarding *C. jejuni*, the mechanism of its resistance to fluoroquinolones appeared not to be related to the acquisition of plasmids or to alteration in OMPs, including the 45-kDa OMP that is considered the major porin of this organism *(15)*.

Increased Out-of-Cell Efflux

Studies using energized inverted membrane vesicles of *E. coli* provided the first evidence for reduced accumulation of quinolones due to increased efflux out of the cells *(18)*. Evidence was shown that accumulation of hydrophilic (but not hydrophobic) quinolones did occur. The observed process was saturable, thereby indicating carrier-mediated transport.

9.6 Clostridium botulinum

Clostridium botulinum, the causative pathogen of botulism, is a Gram-positive, spore-producing, obligate anaerobic bacterium. It is found in the soil, where it produces spores able to survive in a dormant state until exposed to conditions that can support their growth. There are seven types of neurotoxic botulism toxins, designated by the letters A through G, which are produced as a single-chain protein (protoxin) with a molecular weight of 150 kDa. The toxins are released from the bacteria as part of a noncovalent multimeric complex that may protect the toxins at low pH in the GI tract, but which will dissociate spontaneously at physiologic pH. Only types A, B, E, and F are pathogenic to humans. Two other *Clostridium* species, *C. baratii* and *C. butyricum,* are also known to produce toxins (types F and E, respectively) that can cause illness in humans.

Botulism is a rare but serious disease caused by the nerve toxins produced by *C. botulinum*. There are three main kinds of botulism: (i) *food-borne botulism* is caused by eating foods that contain the botulism toxin; (ii) *wound botulism* is caused by toxin produced from a wound infected with *C. botulinum*; and (iii) *infant botulism* is caused by consuming the spores of the botulinum bacteria, which then grow in the intestines and release toxin. *All forms of botulism can be fatal and are considered medical emergencies.* Food-borne botulism can be especially dangerous because many people can be poisoned by eating a contaminated food. Used as a biological weapon, an aerolized or food-borne botulinum toxin will cause acute symmetric, descending flaccid paralysis with prominent bulbar palsies such as diplopia, dysarthria, dysphonia, and dysphagia, which would typically present 12 to 72 hours after exposure (http://www.bt.cdc.gov) *(19)*.

In the United States, 110 cases of botulism, on average, are reported each year. Of these, approximately 25% are food-borne, 72% are infant botulism, and the rest are wound botulism. Whereas the number of cases of food-borne and infant botulism in recent years has changed little, cases of wound botulism have increased because of the use of black-tar heroin, especially in California (http://www.cdc.gov/ncidod/dbmd/diseaseinfo/botulism_g.htm).

9.6.1 Symptoms of Botulism and Treatment

The classic symptoms of botulism include double vision, blurred vision, drooping eyelids, slurred speech, difficulty swallowing, dry mouth, and muscle weakness. Infants with botulism appeared lethargic, feed poorly, are constipated, and have a weak cry and poor muscle tone. All symptoms are the result of muscle paralysis caused by the bacterial toxin. If untreated, these symptoms may progress to cause paralysis of the arms, legs, trunk, and respiratory muscles. In food-borne botulism, symptoms can occur as early as 6 hours or as late as 10 days after exposure.

Regarding the diagnosis of botulism, it is important to note that symptoms of other diseases such as Guillain-Barré syndrome, stroke, and myasthenia gravis can appear similar to those of botulism, and special tests (brain scan, spinal fluid examination, nerve conduction tests, and Tensilon test for myasthenia gravis) may be needed to exclude these other conditions. The most direct way to confirm the diagnosis of botulism is to demonstrate the botulinum toxin in the patient's serum or stools (http://www.cdc.gov/ncidod/dbmd/diseaseinfo/botulism_g.htm).

Botulism can result in death due to respiratory failure. However, in the past 50 years the mortality rate has decreased from about 50% to 8%. The respiratory failure and paralysis that occur with severe botulism may require a patient to be on a breathing machine (ventilator) for weeks, plus intensive medical and nursing care. If diagnosed early, food-borne and wound botulism can be treated with an antitoxin that will block the action of the botulinum toxin circulating in the blood.

9.7 Listeria monocytogenes

Listeria monocytogenes, the etiologic agent of listeriosis, is a Gram-positive bacterium with pathogenic activity to humans. It exhibits marked tropism for the central nervous system (CNS) and the placenta. As many as 5% of the general population harbor *Listeria* in their intestinal tracts *(20)*.

Listeriosis is a rare but serious infectious disease in immunocompromised patients *(1)*. Primarily, listeriosis affects individuals with deficient cell-mediated immunity, often the very young, the elderly, patients on immunosuppressive therapy, cancer patients, and pregnant women. In the latter case, listeriosis may occur even in the absence of overt immune deficiency. AIDS patients, because of their severe immunodeficiency, may be highly susceptible to invasive *Listeria* infections, especially those with CD4$^+$ cell counts bellow 50/μL. A preceding gastrointestinal infection or disruption causing inflamed bowel mucosa may facilitate invasion of the bloodstream by the pathogen.

In adults, listeria infection, either sporadic or as the result of an outbreak, has been primarily food-borne. It is typically associated with meningitis, endocarditis, and disseminated granulomatous lesions.

Listeriosis usually responds to antimicrobial therapy, with no reports of recurrent infection. In general, treatment with antibiotics (penicillin, ampicillin, amoxicillin), alone or in combination with aminoglycoside (gentamicin), is usually recommended *(1)*. On several occasions, TMP-SMX was reported to be effective when administered at concentrations attainable in serum and cerebrospinal fluid *(1)*.

9.8 Escherichia coli Diarrheal Diseases

Escherichia coli are Gram-negative bacilli of the family Enterobacteriaceae and a common member of the normal flora of the human large intestine. As long as these bacteria do not acquire genetic elements encoding for virulence factors, they remain benign commensals. Strains that acquire bacteriophage or plasmid DNA encoding enterotoxins or invasion factors become virulent and can cause noninflammatory diarrhea (watery diarrhea) or inflammatory diarrhea (dysentery with stools usually containing blood, mucus, and leukocytes). These diseases are most familiar as the "traveler's diarrhea," although they may cause major health problems in endemic countries, especially among infants.

Several groups of *E. coli* are associated with diarrheal diseases:

(i) *Enterotoxigenic E. coli (ETEC)*. These *noninvasive* strains produce enterotoxins that can be either cytotoxic (damaging the mucosal cells) or cytotonic (inducing only the secretion of water and electrolytes).

(ii) *Enteropathogenic E. coli (EPEC)* strains are *noninvasive* and are usually associated with outbreaks of diarrhea in newborn nurseries but do not produce recognizable toxins or invasion factors.

(iii) *Enteroinvasive (Shigella-Type) E. coli (EIEC)* strains produce *invasion factors* and cause destruction and inflammation resembling the effects of *Shigella*. Like *Shigella* species, they are typically lactose nonfermenting and invade the colonic mucosa, where they spread laterally and induce a local inflammatory response.

(iv) *Shiga Toxin–Producing E. coli (STEC)* (formerly known as *enterohemorrhagic E. coli* or *verotoxin-producing E. coli*) strains such as O157:H7 are capable of causing *invasive* human illness by releasing large quantities of one or more potent toxins that cause severe damage to the lining of the intestines.

(v) *Enteroaggregative E. coli (EAEC)* strains are defined by their characteristic "stacked brick" adherence pattern in cell culture–based assays. These organisms elaborate one or more enterotoxins and elicit hemorrhagic damage to the intestinal mucosa.

9.8.1 Enterotoxigenic Escherichia coli

The ETEC-produced toxins stimulate the lining of the intestines, causing them to secrete excessive fluid, thus producing diarrhea.

First recognized as a cause of human diarrheal disease in the 1960s, ETEC emerged as a major bacterial source of diarrhea among travelers and children in the developing world.

Among children age 5 or under in the developing world, the annual burden of diarrhea is estimated to be 1.5 billion episodes, accounting for 3 million deaths. In children in these settings, ETEC is the most frequent enteropathogen, accounting for approximately 210 million diarrhea cases and approximately 380,000 deaths annually (http://www.who.int/vaccine_research/diseases/e_e_coli.en).

ETEC is also increasingly being recognized as an important cause of food-borne illness in developed nations, including the United States (http://www.cdc.gov/ncidod/dbmd/diseaseinfo/etec_g.htm). Infection occurs when a person eats food, or drinks water or ice, contaminated with ETEC bacteria. Human or animal wastes (e.g., feces) are the ultimate source of ETEC contamination.

ETEC produces two toxins, a heat-stable toxin known as ST, and a heat-labile toxin (LT). Although different strains of ETEC can secrete either one or both of these toxins, the illness caused by both toxins are similar.

9.8.1.1 Symptoms/Treatment of ETEC Disease

Infection with ETEC can produce profuse watery diarrhea and abdominal cramping. Fever, nausea with or without vomiting, chills, loss of appetite, headache, muscle pain, and bloating can also occur but are less common. Illness develops 1 to 3 days after exposure and usually lasts 3 to 4 days. Symptoms rarely last more than 3 weeks. Most patients recover with supportive measures alone and do not require hospitalization or antibiotics. Clear liquids are recommended to prevent dehydration and loss of electrolytes. Antimotility medications should be avoided by persons with high fever or bloody diarrhea and should be discontinued if the diarrhea symptoms persist more than 48 hours. Antibiotics can shorten the duration of diarrheal illness and discomfort, especially when given early, but they are usually not required. It should be noted that ETEC is frequently resistant to common antibiotics, including TMP-SMX and ampicillin. Because of the worldwide increase of resistance, the decision to use antibiotics should be carefully weighed against the severity of the illness and the risk of adverse reactions (http://www.cdc.gov/ncidod/dbmd/diseaseinfo/etec_g.htm).

9.8.2 Enteropathogenic Escherichia coli

EPEC is a leading cause of infantile diarrhea in developing countries. In industrialized countries, the frequency of EPEC infections, though decreasing, still continues to be an important cause of diarrhea *(21)*. Dual infections involving both ETEC and EPEC have been frequently observed worldwide.

9.8.2.1 Pathogenesis: Typical and Atypical EPEC

The central mechanism of the EPEC pathogenesis is a bacterium-produced lesion called "attaching and effacing" (A/E), which is characterized by destruction of microvilli, intimate adherence of bacteria to the intestinal epithelium, pedestal formation, and aggregation of polarized actin and other elements of the cytoskeleton at sites of bacterial attachment *(22)*. The ability to produce A/E lesions has also been detected in strains of Shiga toxin–producing *E. coli* (enterohemorrhagic *E. coli*; EHEC) and in strains of other bacterial species *(21)*.

The genetic determinants for the production of A/E lesions are located on the locus of enterocyte effacement (LEE), a pathogenicity island that contains the genes encoding intimin, a type III secretion system, a number of secreted (Esp) proteins, and the *translocated intimin receptor* named Tir. Two LEE insertion sites have been described on the *E. coli* chromosome, and a third unidentified insertion site has been reported *(22,23)*.

During the 2nd International Symposium on EPEC (Sao Paulo, 1995), after recognizing that EPEC are diarrheagenic *Escherichia coli* that produce a characteristic histopathology known as A/E on intestinal cells and that do not produce Shiga, Shiga-like, or verocytotoxins, most participants accepted the following definition of typical and atypical EPEC:

(i) *Typical EPEC* of human origin possesses a virulence plasmid known as the EAF (EPEC adherence factor) plasmid that encodes localized adherence on cultured epithelial cells mediated by the Bundle Forming Pilus. The majority of the typical EPEC strains fall into certain well-recognized O:H serotypes.
(ii) *Atypical EPEC* does not possess the EAF plasmid.

In general, typical EPEC strains are more homogeneous in their virulence characteristics than the atypical ones by producing (with few exceptions) only virulence factors encoded by the LEE region and the EAF plasmid. Typical and atypical EPEC strains also differ in their adherence patterns and intimin types *(22)*.

Typical EPEC serotypes are strongly associated with diarrhea in children under age 1 where, in several well-controlled studies *(23)*, these serotypes have been found to be the main cause of endemic diarrhea.

A remarkable epidemiologic difference between typical and atypical EPEC serotypes is their geographic distribution. Typical EPEC serotypes have traditionally been associated with outbreaks of infantile diarrhea (serotypes O55:H5 and O111:H2). In the past, these epidemic serotypes were frequently identified in industrialized countries as the cause of outbreaks and sporadic cases of diarrhea, but at present they are very rare; currently, serotypes without the EAF plasmid predominate *(22)*. The reason for these changes is still not clear, but the decline in the frequency of the EAF-positive serotypes that has occurred in Europe and the United States (and is beginning to take place in other countries such as Brazil) may be the result of improvements in therapy, sanitary conditions, and control of hospital infections *(22)*.

9.8.3 *Shiga Toxin–Producing Escherichia coli*

The STEC strains are associated with diarrhea, hemorrhagic colitis, hemolytic-uremic syndrome (HUS), and postdiarrheal thrombotic thrombocytopenic purpura (TTP). The Shiga-producing *E. coli* O157:H7 is the prototype and the most virulent member of this *E. coli* pathotype. The STEC toxins (verotoxin, Shiga-like toxin) are closely related or identical to the toxin produced by *Shigella dysenteriae*.

The STEC strains are highly virulent—oral exposure to a very small number of these invasive bacteria causes severe illness. The site of the infection is the colon, where adherence is rapidly followed by invasion of the intestinal epithelial cells. Illness caused by STEC often begins with an acute inflammatory response and destruction of tissue producing initially a nonbloody diarrhea that progresses to diarrhea with visible or occult blood and sheets of mucus containing polymorphonuclear cells. Severe abdominal pain (cramping) is typical; fever occurs in less than one third of the episodes. The action of Shiga toxin on the intestinal cells results in hemorrhagic colitis, and the absorption of the toxin in the circulation leads to systemic complications, including HUS and neurologic sequelae (http://www.cfsan.fda.gov/~mow/chap15.html). The illness is usually self-limited and lasts for an average of 8 days. Some persons may exhibit watery diarrhea only.

STEC, including *E. coli* O157:H7, are increasingly common in the United States, especially in children, causing hemorrhagic colitis. Outbreaks of hemorrhagic colitis have been linked to contaminated apple cider, raw vegetables, salami, yogurt, and ingestion of water in recreational areas. Person-to-person transmission is common during outbreaks. The frequency of HUS as a complication of *E. coli* O157:H7 in children has been estimated to be 5% to 10% but can be higher during outbreaks. Diarrhea and sometimes HUS caused by STEC strains other than O157:H7 are common outside the United States.

9.8.3.1 Hemolytic-Uremic Syndrome

The hemolytic-uremic syndrome (HUS) is a disorder associated with hemolytic anemia, thrombocytopenia, and acute renal failure *(24)*. There have been observations that hemolytic anemia, which was often preceded by diarrhea, was associated with thrombocytic renal microangiopathy and mild disseminated intravascular coagulopathy. These findings suggested the possibility of an endotoxin derived from the GI tract, which produced a Schwartzman-like reaction in the renal microvasculature *(1)*.

In many children with diarrhea caused by *E. coli* O157:H7, HUS is mild and self-limited—microangiopathic hematologic changes, thrombocytopenia and/or nephropathy will develop during the 2 weeks after the onset of diarrhea.

Prior treatment with several drugs (mitomycin and penicillins) has been suggested to be a potential risk factor for HUS by either direct (triggering HUS) or indirect means (to allow time for the HUS to develop from the release of bacterial endotoxins from dying bacteria, or the absorption of endotoxins or other bacterial products from luminal bacteria through the ulcerated mucosa) *(1)*.

9.8.3.2 Thrombotic Thrombocytopenic Purpura

Thrombotic thrombocytopenic purpura (TTP; thrombotic microangiopathy) is a syndrome characterized by microangiopathic hemolytic anemia, thrombocytopenia, neurologic disorders, fever, and renal dysfunction *(1)*. In adults, TTP may have a more gradual onset than does HUS and is part of a disease spectrum often designated as TTP-HUS.

The pathophysiology of TTP seemed to correlate with the presence of circulating immune complexes that promote formation of microthrombi. For the latter to occur, endothelial cell damage leading to platelet adhesion and aggregation and a decrease in prostaglandin I_2 production play an important role. The etiology of such a potentially fatal hematologic abnormality may well involve the patient's immune deficiency *(25, 26)* and/or pathogen-related endotoxins *(26)*. Thus, endothelial damage or direct platelet aggregation by endotoxins during infection, and immune-related endothelial damage, have been postulated to play a role in the pathogenesis of secondary thrombotic microangiopathy *(1)*.

9.8.4 Enteroinvasive Escherichia coli

The EIEC strains are biochemically, genetically, and pathogenically closely related to *Shigella* species. It appears that the EIEC category is not a taxonomic entity but a group of isolates restricted to certain serotypes that cause a dysentery-like illness *(27,28)*. The most frequent serotypes within EIEC are O28ac, O29, O112ac, O124, O136, O143, O144, O152, O159, O164, and O167 *(21)*. Several of the serotypes represented in the EIEC group are either identical (e.g., O-antigens of *E. coli* O124 and *Shigella dysenteriae*

type 3; O-antigens of *E. coli* O143 and *Shigella boydii* type 8) or cross-reactive with some *Shigella* serotypes *(29)*. The cross-reactivity between *E. coli* O164 and *Shigella dysenteriae* type 3 has been described to be of the *a,b–a,c* type, indicating that both common and unique epitopes are present in both strains *(29)*.

The EIEC infection is similar clinically to infection caused by *Shigella* species. Although dysentery can occur, diarrhea usually is watery, without blood or mucus. Patients are often febrile, and stools may contain leukocytes.

Outbreaks associated with EIEC and EAEC (see below) have occurred, usually secondary to contaminated food, among people of all ages. The period of communicability is for the duration of excretion of the specific pathogen.

9.8.5 Enteroaggregative Escherichia coli

Since first described in 1987, EAEC strains have been recognized increasingly as pathogens of diarrhea in developing countries and, more recently, in the industrialized world *(30)*.

EAEC is currently defined as *E. coli* strains that do not secrete heat-labile or heat-stable enterotoxins and that adhere to HEp-2 cells in an aggregative (AA) pattern. This definition may encompass both pathogenic and nonpathogenic clones that share a factor(s) conferring a common phenotype.

A three-stage model has been proposed for the EAEC pathogenesis: (i) Stage I involves initial adherence to the intestinal mucosa and the mucus layer. (ii) Stage II comprises enhanced mucus production, apparently leading to a deposit of a thick mucus-containing biofilm encrusted with EAEC. The blanket may promote persistent colonization and nutrient malabsorption. (iii) Stage III, as suggested from histopathologic and molecular evidence, includes the elaboration of toxins of inflammation, which result in damage to the mucosa and intestinal secretion. Malnourished hosts may be unable to repair the mucosal damage and may thus become prone to the persistent diarrhea syndrome *(30)*.

EAEC causes watery diarrhea, predominately in infants and young children in resource-limited countries, but all ages can be affected. The clinical course of the illness is usually associated with a prolonged diarrhea (over 14 days). Asymptomatic infection may be accompanied by subclinical inflammatory enteritis, which may cause growth disturbances. *The long duration of EAEC diarrhea is its most striking feature, longer than that associated with any other enteric pathogen.*

A large percentage of patients excreting EAEC have detectable fecal lactoferrin and supranormal levels of IL-8 in the stool. Although this observation suggests that EAEC infection may be accompanied by mucosal inflammation, most patients lack overt clinical evidence of inflammation *(30)*.

9.8.6 *Shigella spp. and Escherichia coli: The Relationships*

Shigella spp. cause an estimated 150 million cases and 600,000 deaths annually and can cause disease after ingestion of as few as 10 bacterial cells *(31)*. The *Shigella*-like strains that cause an invasive, dysenteric, diarrheal illness were first described in 1971, more than a decade before the appearance in 1982 of the enterohemorrhagic *E. coli* strains (such as the *E. coli* O157:H7) that launched the interest in the *E. coli–Shigella* connection *(27)*.

Shigellosis is a locally invasive colitis in which bacteria invade and proliferate within colonocytes and mucosal macrophages, trigger apoptosis of macrophages, and spread through the mucosa from cell to cell (see also Section 9.2). Despite their local invasiveness, shigellae rarely cause bacteremia. However, shigellosis occasionally precipitates the HUS, which is characterized by vaso-occlusive renal failure, consumptive thrombocytopenia, microangiopathic anemia, and neurologic dysfunction. These manifestations result in part from the actions of the Shiga toxin, the distinctive cytotoxin produced by *S. dysenteriae* type 1, on neurons and the renal and cerebral endothelial cells *(27)*.

Ever since the initial discovery of *Shigella dysenteriae,* shigellae have generally been regarded on both microbiological and clinical grounds as distinct from *Escherichia coli*. Whereas most *E. coli* are motile, lactose-, lysine decarboxylase-, and indole-positive, and mostly avirulent, shigellae are nonmotile, are typically lactose-, lysine decarboxylase-, and indole-negative, and are obligate pathogens.

However, the emergence of *E. coli* O157:H7 and other Shiga toxin–producing *E. coli* strains that, like shigellae, caused food- and water-borne outbreaks of hemorrhagic colitis, a dysentery-like illness (sometimes complicated by HUS), has prompted *a reconsideration of the relationship between these two genera.* Thus, *Shigella*-like strains of *E. coli*, such as the EIEC, like shigellae, are able to invade and proliferate within intestinal epithelial cells, eventually causing cell death. Thus, EIEC share with shigellae an ~140-MDa plasmid (pINV) *(31)* that encodes several outer-membrane proteins involved in the invasion of host cells. In addition, like shigellae, EIEC are usually nonmotile and lactose-negative. Furthermore, EIEC are usually lysine decarboxylase-negative, a characteristic that, in both EIEC and shigellae, is due to large deletions ("black holes") in the genome that correspond with chromosomal regions present in *E. coli* K-12. These

deleted genes encode enzymes involved in metabolic reactions that produce compounds such as cadaverine that interfere with the uptake of shigellae and EIEC by the host cells. Hence, these deletions may enhance the ability to invade host cells. EIEC and shigellae also exhibit considerable antigenic cross-reactivity. On the other hand, EIEC do not produce Shiga toxins and are not known to cause HUS *(27)*.

The STEC (*E. coli* O157:H7) and shigellae exhibit a number of clinical and pathogenic differences. The prototypical STEC-associated syndrome is hemorrhagic colitis, a passage of a large volume of grossly bloody stools without obvious pus or mucus, accompanied by abdominal pain, but not tenesmus or fever. These manifestations differ from classic dysentery and probably reflect the pancolitis of STEC in contrast with (i) the more focal proctocolitis of shigellosis and EIEC infection; (ii) the toxigenic but noninvasive nature of the STEC disease; and (iii) the mucosal invasion of shigellosis. Furthermore, STEC share with *S. dysenteriae* type 1 the production of bacteriophage-encoded Shiga toxin(s) and expression of a type III secretion apparatus. However, in contrast with shigellae, STEC (O157:H7) produce a unique enterohemolysin and exhibit A/E adherence to enterocytes, similar to that exhibited by the EPEC. In addition, whereas in shigellae the type III secretion apparatus is encoded on the 140-MDa, a virulence plasmid, in both STEC (O157:H7) and EPEC it is encoded on a chromosomal pathogenicity–associated island termed *"locus of enterocyte effacement."* Moreover, the virulence plasmid of STEC is distinct from that of *Shigella* spp., EIEC, and EPEC *(27)*.

These and other findings *indicate that STEC, EIEC, and EPEC all share with one another, and with shigellae, one or more important clinical or pathogenic features.* These perplexing similarities and differences would be best understood in the context of the population structure of *E. coli* and *Shigella* spp. *(27)*.

The first direct genetic insights into the evolutionary relationships between *Shigella* spp. and *E. coli* were provided by DNA-DNA reassociation studies, which showed that shigellae exhibit more than 75% nucleotide similarity to *E. coli* (within the range observed among different *E. coli* strains, *strongly justifying that shigellae could be part of the genus Escherichia proper (32).*

Indeed, comparative DNA sequence analysis and multilocus enzyme electrophoresis (MLEE) subsequently showed unequivocally that from a population genetics standpoint, shigellae were better regarded as pathotypes or clones of *E. coli* *(33–36)*. These data showed that the four *Shigella* species constituted two related clusters within the larger *Escherichia coli* population, one comprising representatives of three of the four putative *Shigella* species, the other comprising representatives of all four species *(27,33,36)*.

9.9 Novoviruses

Novoviruses (genus Novovirus, family Calciviridae) are a group of related, single-stranded RNA, nonenveloped viruses that cause acute gastroenteritis in humans. Novovirus was recently approved as the official name for the group of viruses previously known as the Norwalk-like calciviruses (NLVs). Gastroenteritis caused by the novoviruses, including Norwalk, Snow Mountain, and Hawaii viruses, is an inflammation of the stomach and the intestines, which is sometimes misnamed as "stomach flu." In fact, it is not related to the flu (influenza), which is a respiratory illness caused by the influenza virus.

Novoviruses are usually found in contaminated food or drink, but they can also live on surfaces or be spread through contact with an infected person. Each year in the United States, 23 million Novovirus infections result in an estimated 50,000 hospitalizations and 310 deaths (http://www.cdc.gov/ncidod/dvrd/revb/gastro/novovitus.htm).

Discovered in 1972, the novoviruses were the first to be definitively associated with acute gastroenteritis (37). During the next two decades, researchers were unable to develop a simple methodology to detect these viruses and define them as the etiologic agents of nonbacterial gastroenteritis. The single, positive strand of the Norwalk virus DNA contains three open reading frames, one of which is known to encode the single capsid protein.

Today, the novoviruses are recognized as the most common cause of infectious gastroenteritis among persons of all ages (38) and are a major contributor to illness in nursing homes, hospitals, and lately on cruise ships.

Symptoms of acute gastroenteritis include nausea, abdominal cramps, vomiting, diarrhea, headache, fatigue, fever, and muscle ache. Novoviruses do not invade the colon; therefore fecal leukocytes are typically absent and hematochezia is rare. Symptoms can develop within hours or a few days after infection, and the illness typically lasts 24 to 48 hours.

The best treatment for Novovirus infection is to get plenty of bed rest and rehydration with fluids. Antibiotics should not be taken since they are ineffective against novoviruses.

9.10 Rotaviruses

The rotaviruses are nonenveloped, double-shelled viruses. Their genome is composed of 11 segments of double-stranded RNA, which code for six structural and five nonstructural proteins. Rotaviruses have a characteristic wheel-like appearance when viewed under electron microscope (the name "rota" in Latin means "wheel").

Rotaviruses are the most common cause of severe diarrhea among children, resulting in the hospitalization of approximately 55,000 children each year in the United States and the death of more than 600,000 children annually worldwide (http://www.cdc.gov/ncidod/dvrd/revb/gastro/toravirus.htm). Adults can also be infected, although the disease tends to be mild.

The primary mode of transmission is fecal-oral, although there is evidence of low titers of virus in respiratory tract secretions and other fluids. Because the virus is stable in the environment, transmission can also occur through ingestion of contaminated water or food and contact with contaminated surfaces. In the United States and other countries with a temperate climate, the disease has a winter seasonal pattern, with annual epidemics occurring from November to April.

The incubation period for Rotavirus disease is approximately 2 days. The illness is characterized by vomiting and watery diarrhea for 3 to 8 days, and fever and abdominal pain occur frequently. Immunity after infection is incomplete, but repeat infections tend to be less severe than the original illness.

For persons with healthy immune systems, Rotavirus gastroenteritis is a self-limiting illness, lasting only a few days. Treatment is nonspecific and consists of oral rehydration therapy to prevent dehydration. About 1 of 40 children will require hospitalization for intravenous fluids (http://www.cdc.gov/ncidod/dvrd/revb/gastro/toravirus.htm).

9.11 Recent Scientific Advances

- *Bacterial-Host Communication Through Host Hormones.* The quorum-sensing system is the cell-to-cell signaling mechanism by which bacteria respond to hormone-like molecules called *autoinducers* (AIs). The AI-3 quorum-sensing system is also involved in interkingdom signaling with the eukaryotic hormones epinephrine/norepinephrine. However, this signaling system has never been shown to be involved in virulence *in vivo*, and the bacterial receptor for these signals had not been identified. Recently, it has been shown that *E. coli* O157:H7 can respond to the human hormones epinephrine/norepinephrine, leading to the activation of the pathogen's virulence genes (39). In addition, QseC sensor kinase was found to be the bacterial receptor for the host epinephrine/norepinephrine and the AI-3 produced by the gastrointestinal microbial flora. Furthermore, it has also been demonstrated that an α-adrenergic antagonist can specifically block the QseC response to these signals. Given the role that the quorum-sensor system plays in bacterial virulence, further characterization of this unique signaling mechanism may become important for developing novel classes of antimicrobial drugs.

- *Impact of Listeria monocytogenes in Pregnancy.* Infection with *Listeria monocytogenes* is a significant health problem during pregnancy. In a recent study, the *L. monocytogenes* trafficking between maternal organs and the placenta in a pregnant guinea pig model of listeriosis was investigated *(40)*. It was shown that only a single bacterium is sufficient to cause infection of the placenta and that the placenta represents a protected site for bacterial growth. The inability of the maternal host to eradicate bacteria in the placental compartment permitted *Listeria* to be disseminated to the maternal organs. Once colonized, the placenta becomes a nidus of infection resulting in massive reseeding of maternal organs, where *L. monocytogenes* cannot be cleared until trafficking is interrupted by expulsion of the infected placenta tissues *(40)*.

- *Mutual Enhancement of Virulence by Enterotoxigenic and Enteropathogenic Escherichia coli.* The incidence and importance of co-infections with multiple pathogens have been recognized recently. This study was focused on the interactions of two globally prevalent enteric pathogens, enterotoxigenic *E. coli* (ETEC) and enteropathogenic *E. coli* (EPEC), both common causes of diarrhea—ETEC typically causes traveler's diarrhea, and EPEC causes disease mostly in children. Dual infections with both pathogens have been noted fairly frequently in studies worldwide. Furthermore, the cholera toxin and forskolin markedly potentiated the EPEC-induced ATP release from the host cell, and this potentiated release was found to be mediated by the cystic fibrosis transmembrane conductance regulator. To this end, both crude and purified ETEC toxins also potentiated the EPEC-induced ATP release *(41)*. This finding demonstrated that ETEC toxins and EPEC-induced damage to the host cell both enhance the virulence of the other type of *E. coli*, thus revealing a molecular basis for a microbial interaction that could increase the severity of the disease in persons infected with ETEC and EPEC.

- *Rapid Quantitative Profiling of Complex Microbial Populations.* A comprehensive identification and quantitation of the constituents of the microbial communities is an essential foundation for understanding their biology. To address this requirement, a new, simple, reliable, and optimized DNA oligonucleotide microarray assay has been developed *(42)*. It comprised ten 462 small subunit (SSU) ribosomal DNA (rDNA) probes (7,167 unique sequences) selected to provide quantitative information on the taxonomic composition of diverse microbial populations. Using this microarray enabled individual bacterial species to be detected and qualified when present at fractional abundances of less than 0.1% in complex synthetic mixtures. The estimates of dissemination of the abundance of bacterial species obtained by using this microarray were similar to those obtained by phylogenetic analysis of SSU

rDNA sequences from the same samples—the currently accepted method for profiling microbial communities. Furthermore, probes designed to represent higher order taxonomic groups of bacterial species reliably detected microorganisms for which there were no species-specific probes.

- *SV2 is the Protein Receptor for Botulinum Neurotoxin A (BoNT/A).* The botulinum toxins (BoNT) rank among the most toxic substances known and are responsible for food poisoning with high morbidity and mortality. It is still not very well understood how the widely used botulinum neurotoxin A (BoNT/A) will recognize and enter the neurons. However, in a recent study it was discovered that BoNT/A enters neurons by binding to the synaptic vesicle protein SV2 (isoforms A, B, and C) *(43)*. The findings that fragments of SV2 that harbor the toxin interaction domain inhibited BoNT/A from binding to neurons and that mice lacking an SV2 isoform (SV2B) displayed reduced sensitivity to BoNT/A, indicated that SV2 acted as the protein receptor for BoNT/A.

9.12 NIAID Involvement in Enteric Diseases Research

Bacterial and viral infections of the GI tract account for a greatly underappreciated burden of morbidity and mortality domestically and overseas. The enteric pathogens cause disease symptoms ranging from mild gastroenteritis to life-threatening systemic infections and severe dehydrating diarrhea. In addition to the acute risks of disease, long-term complications of enteric diseases include malnutrition, malabsorption of vital drugs, and immunologic complications. In the United States, diarrhea is the second most common infectious illness, accounting for 1 of every 6 (16%) diagnoses. Data compiled by WHO indicate that diarrheal diseases account for 15% to 34% of all deaths in certain countries. Conservative estimates place that death toll at 4 million to 6 million per year, with most of these occurring in children of preschool age, the elderly, and the immunocompromised, all of whom are particularly vulnerable. In developing countries particularly, acute diarrheal disease is also associated with significant delays in physical and intellectual development. Travelers, relief workers, and the U.S. military are at greatly heightened risk of incapacitating illness. In addition to naturally acquired infection, the potential for food- and water-borne pathogens to be used as weapons for mass poisoning has been recognized by their inclusion in the list of NIAID Category B priority pathogens.

To combat this tremendous disease burden, NIAID supports active research aimed at better understanding the pathogenic mechanisms employed by these organisms, more comprehensive and accurate surveillance, and better ways to prevent, diagnose, and treat these diseases.

9.12.1 Major Goals and Objectives

NIAID research plans and priorities against enteric infections include:

- Develop improved safe and efficacious vaccines and treatments for bacterial and viral enteric infections
- Expand vaccine testing into international arenas where disease burden and consequent benefit to the public health may be greater
- Understand fully the natural history, pathogenesis, and host responses to infection by enteric pathogens
- Develop high-performance methods and reagents capable of diagnosing currently unattributed enteric infections
- Look for an infectious etiology of enteric diseases with no known cause
- Characterize and understand the role of the normal intestinal flora in disease and disease prevention
- Promote interagency collaborations, both national and international

9.12.2 Resources for Researchers

- Food and Waterborne Diseases Integrated Research Network (FWD IRN)
- Shiga Toxin–Producing *Escherichia coli* (STEC) Strain and Data Repository
- Biodefense and Emerging Infections Research Resources Repository (BEI Resources)
- Rotavirus serotyping monoclonal reagents, which have been made available to qualified researchers for non-human use

9.12.3 Clinical Trials

The following clinical studies in enteric diseases are ongoing or were completed in 2006:

- *Ongoing evaluation of a New Challenge Pool of Norwalk Virus Inocula (Lot 42399).* A second study entitled: "Evaluation of a New Challenge Pool of Norwalk Virus Inocula" (Lot 42399) in human subjects. The study is testing the third dilution of Lot 42399 in order to determine the ID_{50} values. (http://www.clinicaltrials. gov/ct/show/NCT00138476?order=1)

- Reactogenicity and immunogenicity of live attenuated Indian neonatal Rotavirus vaccine candidate strains 116E and I321 in healthy, nonmalnourished infants 8 to 12 weeks of age. The trial was carried out and completed in the All-India Institute of Medical Sciences, New Delhi (http:// www.clinicaltrials.gov/ct/show/NCT00280111?order=1).
- Safety and immunogenicity Phase I trial of a live, attenuated *Salmonella typhi* vaccine (Ty800) developed by Avant Immunotherapeutics, Inc. (www.hhs.gov/ nvpo/research/Schmitt%(N54).
- Phase I randomized, double-blind, heterologous prime-boost study of the safety and immunogenicity of Vi Polysaccharide typhoid vaccine after priming by live attenuated oral Vi + *Salmonella typhi* strain CVD 909 (http://clinicaltrials.gov/ct/show/NCT00326443; jsessionid=A0AE2973592FE35F674B9ECE959FFF0D? order=5).

9.13 Enteric Vaccines for Pediatric Use

Diarrheal diseases continue to pose a major health problem, especially among young children in developing nations. In addition to immediate morbidity and mortality, the future growth and cognitive development of millions of children are compromised by repeated intestinal diseases. Malnutrition stemming from early diarrheal diseases is a major factor that is correlated with profound developmental delays, cognitive deficits, diminished immunologic function, and a sharp increase in susceptibility to other diseases, often observed at around 6 months of age. To this end, enteric vaccines for pediatric use represent a valuable approach to equitable protection of millions of children worldwide *(44)* (http://www3. niaid.nih.gov/research/topics/enteric/meetings.htm).

The current inventories of approved vaccines for diarrheal pathogens include *(44)*:

(i) Rotavirus vaccine Rotashield (withdrawn).
(ii) Typhoid vaccines Ty21 and Vi capsular polysaccharide.
(iii) Cholera: CVD 103HgR and inactivated whole *V. cholerae* O1 in combination cholera toxin B subunit.

Although licensed vaccines against *V. cholerae* and *S. typhi* do exist, they are often underutilized *(44)*.

Vaccine development and deployment strategies are often complicated by the difference among regions in relation to populations and the major etiologic agents of endemic and epidemic disease. Thus, mortality from diarrheal disease is concentrated in relatively few countries and is attributed to relatively few major pathogen species *(44)*.

Major initiatives of NIAID-supported research on enteric vaccines for pediatric use include vaccines against bacterial and viral agents affecting childhood health in developing nations: ETEC, *Shigella* species, *Salmonella enterica* serovar Typhi, *Vibrio cholerae*, *Campylobacter jejuni*, and Rotavirus *(44)*.

In addition to basic research, a number of specific research and technical gaps remain that have been deemed critical for vaccine development *(44)*:

- Small animal models of colonization, disease, and immunogenicity (ETEC, shigellae, *Campylobacter*, *Salmonella typhi*, and *Vibrio cholerae*)
- Genomic sequence analysis of multiple serovar isolates for each genus, and production of the corresponding microarray reagents
- Identification of antigens that provide protection genus-wide (shigellae) and species-wide (ETEC and cholera)
- Identification of the human-specific colonization factor(s) of *S. typhi*
- Mechanism of autoimmune sequelae, such as reactive arthritis caused by shigellae, *Campylobacter*, nontyphoidal *Salmonella*, as well as the Guillain-Barré syndrome caused by *Campylobacter*
- Epidemiologic data on the burden of disease in developing countries for all pathogens down to the level of antigen expression by specific etiologic agents
- Role of human genetic polymorphisms in susceptibility to disease and response to vaccines
- Mechanisms of induction and enhancement of mucosal immunity, particularly in malnourished populations
- Optimization of adjuvant efficacy; systematic and direct comparisons of adjuvants and delivery problems
- Rapid diagnostics to assess prevalence, asymptomatic carriage, vaccine efficacy, and appropriate treatment
- Role of malnutrition, endogenous intestinal flora, chronic infection, intestinal inflammation, and nutritional supplements on the efficacy of vaccines in endemic areas, to include better understanding of the intestinal and immunologic status of children in endemic areas
- Access to field sites and clinical samples
- Correlates of pathology and immunogenicity between North Americans and individuals in endemic areas

Multiple agents should be addressed because numerous enteric pathogens coexist in endemic areas and co-infections are common. Combined or conjugated vaccines can be developed that protect against more than one antigenic type. This will be particularly important for pathogens like ETEC and shigellae because there are 41 *Shigella* serotypes and numerous combinations of surface antigens in ETEC. Protective vaccines need to address at least the most prevalent combinations of antigens *(44)*.

Many of the experiences of the 1990s have translated to new approaches for vaccination generally. Among the enteric infections, the most innovative and integrated program to accelerate the development and introduction of enteric vaccines in recent years has been the *Diseases of the Most Impoverished (DOMI)* program of the International Vaccine Institute, funded by the Bill & Melinda Gates Foundation. The DOMI program began in 2000 and in the past 6 years has made significant progress in identifying the barriers to implementing vaccination. By adopting a new approach to vaccine implementation, the initial focus of the DOMI program has been to seek the introduction of already licensed vaccines against cholera (orally administered killed whole cell vaccine) and typhoid fever (parenteral Vi purified polysaccharide vaccine). Both locally produced and internationally sourced vaccines were to be promoted. To date, the DOMI program showed the efficacy of the typhoid Vi polysaccharide vaccine in endemic areas to have 70% protective efficacy under outbreak conditions and that the protection lasted over 3 years. A DOMI clinical trial in China showed re-injection to be safe *(44)*.

9.14 Mucosal Immunity

Depending on the pathogen and the site of the infection, mucosal immunity plays an important role in preventing, clearing, or containing infection. The induction of the immune response is carried out through M cells, and secretory IgA (sIgA) is an important barrier to infection.

Different routes of administration may be protective for different pathogens. One advantage of using the nasal route is that 10-fold less antigen is required to induce an immune response. One caveat to this approach is that mucosal studies in mice have not always translated to humans. For example, intranasal immunization of mice resulted in distant mucosal immunity, but this result has not been reproduced in humans. In addition, whereas oral delivery to mice resulted in good vaginal antibody response, this finding was not replicated in humans *(44)*.

Natural mucosal barriers to vaccine delivery included (i) degradation and inactivation; (ii) mucosal clearance and capture in mucin gels; (iii) epithelial barriers and inefficiency of uptake; (iv) preexisting immunity from natural exposure; and (v) mucosal inflammation *(44)*.

9.14.1 Mucosal Adjuvants

Although replicating antigens usually do not require an adjuvant to induce an immune response, mucosal immunity adjuvants are used to link innate and acquired immunity.

Mucosal delivery offers several advantages, including (i) multivalent delivery and (ii) an easily administered/

needle-free and potentially less expensive route capable of inducing both mucosal and systemic immune responses. However, disadvantages also exist, such as the mucosally administered antigens, in general, are not immunogenic and may result in a default type 2 response. Concern regarding oral tolerance induction and safety, especially for nasal delivery, may also become an issue *(44)*.

In addition, mucosal delivery will require safe and effective adjuvants. The two main types of mucosal adjuvants are the ADP-ribosylating toxins (LT, Choleratoxin (CT)) and the toll-like receptors (TLR) agonists (CpG, trade name (Corixa Corp.) (MPL), and flagellin). Because both LT and CT are very potent enterotoxins, research in this field is somewhat inhibited. LT mutants have been studied as adjuvants. LT mutants promote both humoral and cellular immunity and are effective via various routes: mucosal (oral, intranasal, rectal), parenteral, and topical (transdermal). However, there is an agreement that some ADP-ribosylating activity is required for effective adjuvanticity of LT/CT formulations *(44)*. Furthermore, whether the adjuvanticity of mutant LT can be separated from enterotoxigenicity should be explored in a clinical trial to compare the adjuvanticity of mutant versus active LT or CT *(44)*.

The TLR agonists activate NF-κB, which leads to an inflammatory response.

The mucosal response induced by biological response modulators (BRMs) is too unbalanced to make BRMs good adjuvants candidates.

The mechanisms of adjuvanticity are still not well understood and are likely pathogen-dependent. Likewise, the targeting of antigens to dendritic cells remains to be elucidated. Mechanism(s) of adjuvanticity may include *(44)* (i) enhanced luminal permeability; (ii) upregulation of co-stimulatory molecules (B7-1, B7-2) on antigen-presenting cells (APCs); (iii) depletion of CD8$^+$ intraepithelial lymphocytes; (iv) induction of antigen-specific T-cell responses; (v) increased antigen uptake and presentation by intestinal epithelial cells; (vi) enhanced/suppressed cytokine secretion; (vii) induction of apoptosis; and (viii) induction of epithelial cells to produce/release cytokines.

9.15 Live Bacteria Vectors

Live attenuated bacterial vaccines offer several advantages. They are safe, effective, and require no cold chain, if lyophilized. In addition, no use-of-needle costs or associated biohazards are associated with live attenuated bacterial vaccines *(44)*.

Among the live attenuated bacterial vaccines, research on the *recombinant attenuated Salmonella vaccines (RASV)* has been well documented *(44)*. Thus, desired attributes

of RASV include (i) complete attenuation but invasive to lymphoid tissue; (ii) enhanced immunogenicity to protective antigen; (iii) diminished immune response to *Salmonella* antigens; (iv) maximized either Th1 or Th2 response to foreign antigen; and (v) provision of biological containment (i.e., programmed death).

Another advantage of live attenuated bacterial vectors for enteric vaccines is their potential use to deliver other pathogenic antigens. Thus, *Salmonella* could be used to deliver *Campylobacter* antigens. In addition, the *Salmonella* vector might also prove useful for expression of parasitic or *Clostridium difficile* antigens. However, protective protein antigens have not yet been identified for many enteric pathogens *(44)*.

9.16 Delivery Platforms

The advantages and disadvantages of different vaccine delivery platforms may be summarized as follows *(44)*.

Parenteral administration ensures delivery of a known dose. However, the compliance rates for a complete immunization schedule are usually poor. Mucosal, specifically oral, delivery poses problems regarding the accuracy of the delivery dose and secondary transmission/biocontainment issues. In addition, other factors must also be considered: consistency, taste, stability in the stomach, and the potential for development of tolerance.

Other delivery platforms include microencapsulation. Issues related to this include the state of the technology, the very large amounts of immunogen required, as well as stability and reproducibility issues. Transdermal prime, followed by an oral boost, has been showing promising results. In another delivery approach, genetically modified plants may offer an alternative, as use of these plants has moved from edible vaccine to antigen production *(44)*.

Bacterial spores have also been explored as delivery vehicles for antigens. Preliminary studies have shown induction of systemic antibody response to antigen delivered by *Bacillus subtilis* spores. Advantages offered by a spore-delivery system include the potential to combine multiple antigens, very inexpensive production, and commensal organisms to be used as carriers *(44)*.

References

1. Georgiev, V. St. (1998) Gastrointestinal infections in the immunocompromised hosts. In: *Infectious Diseases in Immunocompromised Hosts*, CRC Press, Boca Raton, FL, pp. 473–480.
2. Smith, P. D. and Janoff, E. N. (1988) Infectious diarrhea in human immunodeficiency virus infection, *Gastrointerol. Clin. North Am.*, **17**, 587.

3. World Health Organization. (2006) *Wkly Epidemiol. Rec. (WER)*, **81**, 97–104 [March 17, 2006].

4. Centers for Disease Control and Prevention (2005) Final 2005 reports of notifiable diseases, *Morb. Mortal. Wkly Rep.*, **55**(32), 880–881.

5. Finkelstein, R. A., Sciortino, C. V., and McIntosh, M. A. (1983) Role of iron in microbe–host interactions, *Rev. Infect. Dis.*, **5**(Suppl. 4), S759–S577.

6. Perry, R. D. and Brubaker, R. R. (1979). Accumulation of iron in *Yersinia, J. Bacteriol.*, **137**, 1290–1298.

7. Heesemann, J., Hantke, K., Vocke, T., Saken, E., Rakin, A., Stojilkovic, I., and Berner, R. (1993) Virulence of *Yersinia enterocolitica* is closely associated with siderophore production, expression of an iron-repressible outer membrane polypeptide of 65,000 Da and pesticin sensitivity, *Mol. Microbiol.*, **8**(2), 397–408.

8. Richardson, N. J., Koornhof, H. J., and Bokkenheuser, V. D. (1981) Long-term infections with *Campylobacter fetus* subsp. *jejuni, J. Clin. Microbiol.*, **13**(5), 846–849.

9. DuPont, H. L., Ericsson, C. D., Robinson, A., and Johnson, P. C. (1987) Current problems in antimicrobial therapy for bacterial enteric infection, *Am. J. Med.*, **82**(Suppl. 4A), 324–328.

10. Keat, A. (1983) Reiter's syndrome and reactive arthritis in perspective, *N. Engl. J. Med.*, **309**(26), 1606–1615.

11. Hagensee, M. E., Benyunes, M., Miller, J. A., and Spach, D. H. (1994) *Campylobacter jejuni* bacteremia and Guillain-Barré syndrome in a patients with GVHD after alogeneic BMT, *Bone Marrow Transplant.*, **13**(3), 349–351.

12. Cohen, S. P., McMurry, L. M., Hooper, D. C., Wolfson, J. S., and Levy, J. S. (1989) Cross-resistance to fluoroquinolones in multiple-antibiotic resistant (Mar) *Escherichia coli* selected by tetracycline or chloramphenicol decreased drug accumulation associated with membrane changes in addition to OmpF reduction, *Antimicrob. Agents Chemother.*, **33**(8), 1318–1325.

13. Cozzarelli, N. R. (1980) DNA gyrase and supercoiling of DNA, *Science*, **207**(4434), 953–960.

14. Wiedemann, B. and Heisig, P. (1994) Mechanisms of quinolone resistance, *Infection*, **22**(Suppl. 2), S73–S79.

15. Segreti, J., Gootz, T. D., Goodman, L. J., Parkhurst, G. W., Quinn, J. P., Martin, B. A., and Trenholme, G. M. (1992) High-level quinolline resistance in clinical isolates of *Campylobacter jejuni, J. Infect Dis.*, **165**(4), 667–670.

16. Gootz, T. D. and Martin, B. A. (1991) Characteristics of high-level quinolone resistance in *Campylobacter jejuni, Antimicrob. Agents Chemother.*, **35**(5), 840–845.

17. Nikaido, H. and Rosenberg, E. Y. (1983) Porin channels in *Escherichia coli*: studies with liposomes reconstituted from purified proteins, *J. Bacteriol.*, **153**(1), 241–252.

18. Cohen, S. P., Hooper, D. C., Wolfson, J. S., Souza, K. S., McMurry, L. M., and Levy, S. B. (1988) Endogenous active efflux of norfloxacin in susceptible *Escherichia coli, Antimicrob. Agents Chemother.*, **32**(8), 1187–1193.

19. Arnon, S. S., Schechter, R., Inglesby, T. V., Henderson, D. A., Bartlett, J. G., Ascher, M. S., Eitzen, E., Fine, A. D., Hauer, J., Layton, M., Lillibridge, S., Osterholm, M. T., O'Toole, T., Parker, G., Perl, T. M., Russell, P. K., Swerdlow, D. L., and Tonat, K. for the Working Group on Civillian Defense (2001) Botulinum toxin as a biological weapon: medical and public health management, *N. Engl. J. Med.*, **285**(8), 1059–1070.

20. Schuchat, A., Deaver, K. A., Wenger, J. D., Plikaytis, B. D., Mascola, L., Pinner, R. W., Reingold, A. L., and Broome, C. V. (1992) Role of food in sporadic listeriosis. I. Case-control study of dietary risk factors. The Listeria Study Group, *J. Am. Med. Assoc.*, **267**, 2041–2045.

21. Nataro, J. P. and Kaper, J. B. (1998) Diarrheagenic *Escherichia coli, Clin. Microbiol. Rev.*, **11**, 142–201.

22. Trabulsi, L. R., Keller, R., and Tardelli Gomes, T. A. (2002) Typical and atypical enteropathogenic *Escherichia coli, Emerg. Infect. Dis.*, **8**(5), 508–513.

23. Sperandio, V., Kaper, J. B., Bortolini, M. R., Neves, B. C., Keller, R., and Trabulsi, L. R. (1998) Characterization of the locus of enterocyte effacement (LEE) in different enteropathogenic *Escherichia coli* (EPEC) and Shiga toxin-producing *Escherichia coli* (STEC) serotypes, *FEMS Microbiol. Lett.*, **164**, 133–139.

24. Gasser, C., Gautier, E., Steck, A., Siebenmann, R. E., and Oechslin, R. (1955) Hämolytisch-urämische syndrome: bilaterale nierenrindennekrosen bei akuten erworben hämolytischen anämien, *Schweiz. Med. Wochenschr.*, **85**(38–39), 905–909.

25. Leaf, A. N., Laubenstein, L. J., Raphael, B., Hochster, H., Baez, L., and Karpatkin, S. (1988) Thrombotic thrombocytopenic purpura associated with human immunodeficiency virus type 1 (HIV-1) infection, *Ann. Intern. Med.*, **109**(3), 194–197.

26. Beris, P., Dunand, V., Isoz, C., and Reynard, C. (1990) Association of thrombotic thrombocytopenic purpura and human immunodeficiency virus infection, *Nouv. Rev. Fr. Hematol.*, **32**(4), 277–280.

27. Johnson, J. R. (2000) *Shigella* and *Escherichia coli* at the crossroads: Machiavellian masqueraders or taxonomic treachery? *J. Med. Microbiol.*, **49**, 583–585.

28. Linnenborg, M., Weintraub, A., and Widmalm, G. (1999) Structural studies of the O-antigen polysaccharide from the enteroinvasive *Escherichia coli* O164 cross-reacting with *Shigella dysenteriae* Type 3, *Eur. J. Biochem.*, **266**, 460–466.

29. Cheasty, T. and Rowe, B. (1983) Antigenic relationships between the enteroinvasive *Escherichia coli* O-antigens O28c, O112ac, O124, O136, O143, O144, O152, and O164 and *Shigella* O-antigens, *J. Clin. Microbiol.*, **17**, 681–684.

30. Nataro, J. P., Steiner, T., and Guerrant, R. L. (1998) Enteroaggregative *Escherichia coli, Emerg. Infect. Dis.*, **4**(2), 251–261.

31. Sansonetti, P. I., d'Hauteville, H., Formal, S. B., and Toucas, M. (1982) Plasmid-mediated invasiveness of "*Shigella*-like" *Escherichia coli, Ann. Microbiol. (Paris)*, **133**(3), 611–617.

32. Brenner, D. J., Fanning, G. R., Skerman, F. J., and Falkow, S. (1975) Polynucleotide sequence divergence among strains of *Escherichia coli* and closely related organisms, *J. Bacteriol.*, **109**, 953–965.

33. Whittam, T. S., Ochman, H., and Selander, R. K. (1983) Multilocus genetic structure in natural populations of *Escherichia coli, Proc. Natl. Acad. Sci. U.S.A.*, **80**, 1651–1755.

34. Hartl, D. L. and Dykhuizen, D. E. (1984) The population genetics of *Escherichia coli, Annu. Rev. Genet.*, **18**, 31–68.

35. Pupo, G. M., Kariolis, D. K. R., Lan, R., and Reeves, P. R. (1997) Evolutionary relationships among pathogenic and nonpathogenic *Escherichia coli* strains inferred from multilocus enzyme electrophoresis and *mdh* sequence studies, *Infect. Immun.*, **65**, 2685–2692.

36. Ochman, H., Whittam, T. S., Caugant, D. A., and Selander, R. K. (1983) Enzyme polymorphism and genetic population structure in *Escherichia coli* and *Shigella, J. Gen. Microbiol.*, **129**, 2715–2726.

37. Widdowson, M.-A., Monroe, S. S., and Glass, R. I. (2005) Are novoviruses emerging? *Emerg. Infect. Dis.*, **11**(5), 735–737.

38. Mead, P. S., Slutsker, L., Dietz, V., McCaig, L. F., Breese, J. S., Shapiro, C., Griffin, P. M., and Tauxe, R. V. (1999) Food-related illness and death in the United States, *Emerg. Infect. Dis.*, **11**(5), 607–625.

39. Clarke, M. B., Hughes, D. T., Zhu, C., Boedeker, E. C., and Sperandio, V. (2006) The QseC sensor kinase: a bacterial adrenergic receptor, *Proc. Natl. Acad. Sci. U.S.A.*, **103**(27), 10420–10425.

40. Bakardjiev, A. I., Theriot, J. A., and Portnoy, D. A. (2006) *Listeria monocytogenes* traffics from maternal organs to the placenta and back, *PLoS Pathogens*, **2**(6), e80.

41. Crane, J. K., Choudhari, S. S., Naeher, T. M., and Duffey, M. E. (2006) Mutual enhancement of virulence by enterotoxigenic and enteropathogenic *Escherichia coli*, *Infect. Immun.*, **74**(3), 1505–1515.

42. Palmer, C., Bik, E. M., Eisen, M. B., Eckburg, P. B., Sana, T. R., Wolber, P. K., Relman, D. A., and Brown, P. O. (2006) Rapid quantitative profiling of complex microbial populations, *Nucleic Acids Res.*, **34**(1), e5.

43. Dong, M., Yeh, F., Tepp, W. T., Dean, C., Johnson, E. A., Janz, R., and Chapman, E. R. (2006) SV2 is the protein receptor for botulinum neurotoxin A, *Science*, **312**(5773), 595–596.

44. Enteric Vaccines for Pediatric Use. (2004) NIAID Workshop Report, Airlie Center, Warrenton, VA, April 24–26, 2004.

Chapter 10

Respiratory Diseases

Upper respiratory tract infections are the most common type of infectious diseases and a leading cause of outpatient illness (1,2).

Serious pneumococcal infections are a major global health problem. The World Health Organization estimates that more than 1.6 million people—including more than 800,000 children under the age of 5—die every year from pneumococcal infections. Nearly all of these deaths occur in the world's poorest countries. Pneumococcal meningitis is the most severe form of pneumococcal disease and one of the most fatal childhood illnesses. In developing countries, it kills or disables 40% to 70% of children who get it (http://www3.niaid.nih.gov/research/topics/bacterial/AboutPneumococcalDisease.htm).

The primary causes of death from pneumococcus are pneumonia, in which fluid fills the lungs, hindering oxygen from reaching the bloodstream; meningitis, an infection of the fluid surrounding the spinal cord and brain; and sepsis, an overwhelming infection of the bloodstream by toxin-producing bacteria.

It is estimated that each adult in the United States will experience two to four respiratory infections annually (1). Persons older than 65 have the highest rate of pneumonia admissions.

Although serotypes of the rhinoviruses account for 20% to 30% of episodes of the common cold, the specific causes of most upper respiratory infections are still undefined.

Pneumonia remains an important cause of morbidity and mortality for nonhospitalized adults despite the widespread use of antimicrobial therapy. There are no accurate numbers of episodes of pneumonia occurring annually in ambulatory patients. However, pneumonia ranks as the sixth leading cause of death in the United States. In younger adults, the atypical pneumonia syndrome is the most common clinical presentation (1).

Mycoplasma pneumoniae is the most frequently identified causative agent. Other less common agents include *Legionella pneumophila*, influenza viruses, adenoviruses, and *Chlamydia*.

The pathogens responsible for community-acquired pneumonias are changing. Thus, about four decades ago, *Streptococcus pneumoniae* accounted for the majority of community-acquired infections. Today, a broad array of community-acquired pathogens have been implicated as etiologic agents for respiratory infections, including *Legionella* species, Gram-negative bacilli, *Haemophilus influenzae*, *Staphylococcus aureus*, and nonbacterial pathogens (1).

10.1 Adenoviruses

The adenoviruses represent a group of pathogens found in all regions of the world (3). In addition to human adenovirus types, there are simian types, and there are other types, such as bovine, avian, canine, and murine (rodent). Many of them have induced malignancy in certain species.

A family of more than 42 serotypes of human adenoviruses has been associated with a wide variety of infections, including respiratory infections, conjunctivitis, hemorrhagic cystitis, and gastroenteritis.

Primary adenovirus infections with serotypes 1, 2, and 5 (parts of subgenus C) are common in infancy. The infection is usually restricted to the upper respiratory tract, and the adenovirus may persist after infancy in tonsillar, adenoidal, and other lymphoid tissues. Although not very common, infections of the central nervous system such as meningoencephalitis have been reported as complicating infections of the respiratory tract.

Nosocomial hospital outbreaks of adenovirus infections have been reported in both pediatric and adult units. In addition, acute respiratory disease associated with adenovirus in the military is also well documented (2).

10.1.1 Adenovirus Modulation of the Immune Response

Several interesting *in vitro* studies have revealed the ability of some adenovirus early proteins to modulate the host's immune responses by interfering with the expression of major histocompatibility complex (MHC) class I

V. St. Georgiev, *National Institute of Allergy and Infectious Diseases, NIH: Impact on Global Health*, vol. 2,
DOI 10.1007/978-1-60327-297-1_10, © Humana Press, a part of Springer Science+Business Media, LLC 2009

antigens *(4)*. Taken into account, these protein-protein inter-actions indicate that inhibition of the normal processing and transport of the MHC antigens would result in their reduced expression on the cell surface *in vivo*. Because class I MHC antigens are necessary for cytotoxic T-lymphocyte recognition of virus-infected cells, a reduction in the level of cell surface MHC antigens may not only modulate acute adenovirus pathogenicity *(5)* but also play a role in the establishment of viral persistence and latency *(4)*.

10.1.2 Adenovirus Infections in Immunocompromised Hosts

Although immunocompromised patients are no more at risk for adenovirus infections than are immunocompetent persons, in immunocompromised patients these infections are manifested by higher morbidity and mortality *(3)*. Patients (renal transplant recipients, hematologic malignancies, and AIDS) have shown increased incidence of infections involving serotypes 11, 34, 35 (subgenus B1), and 43 (subgenus D). Other studies have revealed serotype 5 (subgenus C) as the frequent cause of serious infections in patients undergoing chemotherapy, in severe combined immunodeficiency (SCID), and in children receiving liver transplants *(3)*. In addition, adenoviruses of subgenus C have been implicated in cases of disseminated infections in immunocompromised host disease.

Although cell-mediated immune deficiency appears to be a major predisposing factor for severe adenovirus disease, overwhelming infection cannot be limited to a particular immune defect, and the diagnosis should be considered in a broad range of immunocompromised hosts. Adenovirus infections can also be a consequence of reactivation of persistent infection acquired during childhood.

Clinical manifestations include pharyngitis, pneumonia, hematuria, diarrhea, liver dysfunction, disseminated intravascular coagulation, hepatitis, and multiorgan involvement *(3)*. Fulminant hepatitis has been diagnosed in association with AIDS and inherited immunodeficiency syndromes and after liver or bone marrow transplantation. Frequent co-infections with HSV, CMV, or both have been recognized.

10.2 Mycoplasma pneumoniae

Mycoplasma pneumoniae is among the smallest free-living microorganisms, being intermediate in size between bacteria and virus *(6)*. Its small genome and small size is the cause of diagnostic difficulties. The organism is not visible on Gram stains and does not grow on standard bacteriologic media.

Based on cultural isolation directly from the affected site, in combination with one or more additional diagnostic tests, there can no longer be doubt that *M. pneumoniae* causes pneumonia that can be fatal in all age groups and that in some persons this same organism has the ability to produce invasive infection resulting in protean clinical manifestations. A common cause of pharyngitis and bronchopneumonia, *M. pneumoniae* may also cause fulminant pneumonia, cardiac disease, arthritis, dermatologic conditions, and CNS disease *(7)*.

10.3 Bordetella pertussis

Bordetella pertussis, the causative agent of pertussis (whooping cough), is a very small Gram-negative aerobic coccobacillus that appears singly or in pairs. The bacterium colonizes the cilia of the mammalian respiratory epithelium. In general, it is thought that the bacterium does not invade the tissues. However, recent evidence has shown the presence of *B. pertussis* in alveolar macrophages.

Whooping cough is a relatively mild disease in adults, although it can in some cases become incapacitating *(8)*. On the other hand, it has a significant mortality rate in infants *(8)*. Until immunization was introduced in the 1930s, whooping cough was one of the most frequent and severe diseases in infants. However, since the early 1980s, the reported cases of whooping cough have increased steadily *(9–11)*.

10.4 Respiratory Syncytial Virus

The respiratory syncytial virus (RSV) remains the most common cause of viral lower airway disease in infants and children *(12)*. It is a medium-sized membrane-coated RNA virus that can exert a significant immunosuppressive effect, thereby preventing the development of effective immunity by the host *(13)*.

Although symptomatic RSV-induced disease is most often associated with the very young, the virus may be found in the respiratory secretion of infected persons at any age.

Compared with immunocompetent hosts, immunocompromised patients, either children or adults, are at greater risk of developing much more severe lower respiratory tract infection due to RSV *(12–15)*. Underlying conditions include solid organ (kidney, pancreas) and bone marrow transplantations and hematologic malignancies (T-cell lymphoma) *(15)*.

In HIV-related immunodeficiency in children, the RSV infection frequently resulted in pneumonia, whereas bronchiolitis with wheezing occurred rarely *(16)*.

The use of aerolized ribavirin in the treatment of RSV-induced infections, particularly in severe disease, has been well documented *(12,16)*.

10.5 Human Metapneumovirus

The human metapneumovirus (hMPV) is a recently discovered virus from the Metapneumovirus genus *(17)*. Genetically, hMPV is similar to avian pneumovirus. Serologic studies have provided evidence that hMPV is not a newly evolved virus. Instead, it has been the common but undetected cause of many human respiratory diseases for at least 50 years.

The clinical symptoms of the children from whom the virus was isolated were similar to those caused by human RSV infection, ranging from upper respiratory tract disease to severe bronchiolitis and pneumonia *(17)*. However, although initial studies have involved children, hMPV infection has been detected in adults of all ages and may account for a significant portion of persons hospitalized with respiratory infections *(18)*.

10.6 Human Parainfluenza Viruses

The human parainfluenza viruses (HPIVs) are negative-sense, single-stranded RNA viruses that possess fusion and hemagglutinin-neuraminidase glycoprotein "spikes" on their surface. There are four serotypes of HPIV (1 through 4) and two subtypes (4a and 4b) *(19, 20)*.

The HPIVs are second to RSV as common causes of lower respiratory tract infections in young children *(21)*. Like RSV, HPIVs can cause repeated infections throughout life, usually manifested by an upper respiratory tract illness (e.g., cold and/or sore throat). However, HPIVs can also cause serious lower respiratory tract disease with repeat infection (e.g., pneumonia, bronchitis, bronchiolitis), particularly in elderly and/or immunocompromised patients.

Each of the four HPIVs has different clinical and epidemiologic features. The most distinctive clinical manifestation of HPIV-1 and HPIV-2 is croup (i.e., laryngotracheobronchitis). HPIV-1 is most common in children, whereas HPIV-2 is less frequently detected. In addition, both HPIV-1 and HPIV-2 can cause other upper and lower respiratory tract illnesses. Of the other two HPIVs, HPIV-3 is more often associated with bronchiolitis and pneumonia, whereas HPIV-4 in general is less frequently detected, possibly because it is less likely to cause severe illness.

Currently, there is no vaccine to protect against HPIV infections. However, research efforts are being directed at developing vaccines against HPIV-1 and HPIV-3 infections.

10.7 Respiratory Diphtheria

Diphtheria is an acute bacterial disease caused by toxigenic strains of *Corynebacterium diphtheriae* and occasionally *C. ulcerans (22)*. The disease affects the mucous membranes of the respiratory tract (respiratory diphtheria), skin (cutaneous diphtheria), and occasionally other sites (eyes, nose, vagina).

In the prevaccine era, children were at higher risk for respiratory diphtheria. Recently, diphtheria has primarily affected older children and adults in the sporadic cases reported in the United States (0 to 5 cases annually) and in the largest outbreaks in Russia and the newly independent states of the former Soviet Union *(23)*. The latter have reported outbreaks such as the one that began in 1990 involving more than 150,000 cases.

Myocarditis, polyneuritis, and airway obstruction are common complications of respiratory diphtheria. Unlike cutaneous diphtheria, death occurs in 5% to 10% of the respiratory cases *(23)*.

10.8 Chlamydia pneumoniae

Chlamydia pneumoniae is an important cause of an acute respiratory infection but can also be associated with chronic disease *(24)*. Because *Chlamydia pneumoniae* is distinct from other *Chlamydia* species, a new name has been proposed for this bacterium, *Chlamydophila pneumoniae*.

According to CDC estimates, although the overall incidence is unknown, each year an estimated 2 million to 5 million cases of pneumonia and 500,000 pneumonia-related hospitalizations occur in the United States. Although all ages are at risk, the infection is most common in school-age children. Re-infection throughout life appears to be common (http://www.cdc.gov/ncidod/dbmd/diseaseinfo/chlamydiapneumoniae_t.htm).

The clinical manifestations of *Chlamydia* pneumonia or bronchitis will start with little or no fever and the gradual onset of cough. Less common presentations include pharyngitis, laryngitis, and sinusitis. The spectrum of illness can range from asymptomatic infection to severe disease. In addition, according to some investigators, *C. pneumoniae* infection may be associated with atherosclerotic vascular disease, as well as with Alzheimer's disease, asthma, and reactive arthritis.

10.9 Pseudomonas aeruginosa and Cystic Fibrosis

Pseudomonas aeruginosa is a hydrophilic bacterium that is commonly found in moist environments, such as sink drains and vegetables.

P. aeruginosa is the predominant respiratory pathogen in patients with cystic fibrosis (CF), but means by which the organism is acquired is controversial *(24)*. Most patients with CF are ultimately infected with *P. aeruginosa*, and once acquired the infection is not readily eradicated *(25)*. The unique tropism of *P. aeruginosa* for the CF respiratory tract has not been adequately explained: competing and complementary hypotheses have been postulated, but none of these theories has been widely accepted as the single unifying explanation for the peculiar propensity of *P. aeruginosa* to infect the CF airway *(25)*.

It has been suggested that the peculiar "CF phenotype" of *P. aeruginosa* evolves in the CF respiratory tract during chronic infection after patients become culture-positive for a more typical phenotype—nonmucoid, lipopolysaccharide, smooth, and motile. Therefore, it seems logical to postulate that patients with CF can acquire bacteria with the typical phenotype from the environment and that transition to the "CF phenotype" will occur under the conditions found in the CF endothelial space *(26)*.

It is estimated that more than 90% of cystic fibrosis patients colonized with *P. aeruginosa* will succumb to the disease. The median age of survival is in the mid-thirties, and 40% of cystic fibrosis patients are age 18 and over *(27)*.

10.10   Bacterial Meningitis

Meningitis is a serious infection of the fluid in the spinal cord and the fluid that surrounds the brain caused by either a virus or a bacterium. Knowing whether meningitis is caused by a virus or a bacterium is important because of differences in the seriousness of the illness and the treatment needed.

Viral meningitis is usually a mild illness. It clears up within 1 to 2 weeks without specific treatment. Viral meningitis is also known as *aseptic meningitis.*

Bacterial meningitis, also known as *meningococcal meningitis*, is a much more serious, even severe, disease that can result in brain damage and even death. It is most commonly caused by one of three types of bacteria: *Haemophilus influenzae* type b (Hib), *Neisseria meningitides,* and *Streptococcus pneumoniae*. Worldwide, there are estimates of 1.2 million cases annually with a death toll of about 135,000. Especially dangerous is meningococcal meningitis in sub-Saharan Africa, where the disease causes severe epidemics, as well as in Europe, the Americas, and New Zealand *(28)*.

The bacteria are spread by direct close contact with the discharges from the nose or throat of an infected individual (http://www.cdc.gov/ncidod/dbmd/diseaseinfo/meningococcal_g.htm).

Before the 1990s, Hib was the leading cause of bacterial meningitis, but new vaccines being given to children as part of their routine immunizations have reduced the occurrence of serious Hib disease. Today, together with *Streptococcus pneumoniae, Neisseria meningitidis* are the leading source of bacterial meningitis worldwide that results in serious morbidity and mortality, mainly in children and young adults *(23)*. New data have shown an increased risk for freshman college students living on campus.

Meningitis caused by *Neisseria meningitides* is also called *meningococcal meningitis,* whereas meningitis caused by *Streptococcus pneumoniae* is known as *pneumococcal meningitis.*

The bacteria often live harmlessly in a person's mouth and throat. In rare instances, however, bacteria can break through the body's immune defenses and travel to the fluid surrounding the brain and the spinal cord. There they began to multiply quickly. Soon thereafter, the thin membrane that covers the brain and spinal cord (meninges) becomes swollen and inflamed, leading to the classic symptoms of meningitis.

In persons over age 2, common symptoms include high fever, headache, and stiff neck. In advanced illness, bruises will develop under the skin and spread quickly. In newborns and infants, the typical symptoms of fever, headache, and neck stiffness may be difficult to detect. Other signs in infants may be inactivity, irritability, vomiting, and poor feeding. As the disease progresses, *patients of any age* can have seizures. Advanced bacterial meningitis can lead to brain damage, coma, and death.

10.10.1   Treatment of Bacterial Meningitis

Pneumococcal infections are becoming more difficult to treat as bacteria become resistant to some of the most commonly used antibiotics. Antibiotic resistance has economic as well as clinical consequences. Overuse of antibiotics leads to increased resistance and threatens the effectiveness of existing therapy, which in turn increases the cost of treatment by requiring the use of more expensive antibiotics.

Data from a recently published study suggest that the problem of pneumococcal disease will increase in the wake of increasing HIV infection. Data from a South African study show that children with HIV/AIDS are 20 to 40 times more likely to get pneumococcal disease than are children without HIV/AIDS (http://www3.niaid.nih.gov/research/topics/bacterial/AboutPneumococcalDisease.htm).

If detected early, bacterial meningitis may be treated effectively with vaccines. New, lifesaving pneumococcal vaccines are safe and highly effective in preventing pneumococcal disease.

Since 2000, when infants in the United States began receiving routine vaccination against pneumococcal disease, the country has nearly eliminated childhood pneumococcal disease caused by vaccine serotypes. In addition, vaccination of infants has reduced the spread of pneumococcal bacteria, so that adults have less contact with pneumococci and are thus indirectly protected from pneumococcal disease.

There are vaccines against Hib, some strains of *N. meningitides*, and many types of *S. pneumoniae*. The vaccines against Hib are very safe and effective. The vaccine against *N. meningitides* (meningococcal vaccine) is not routinely used in adults and is relatively ineffective in children under age of 2. It is used mainly to control outbreaks of some types of meningococcal meningitis. The vaccine against *S. pneumoniae* (pneumococcal meningitis) is not effective in persons under 2 years of age but is recommended for all persons over age 65 and younger persons with certain medical problems.

Routine vaccination with meningococcal vaccine is recommended for college students, as well as other high-risk populations (29).

10.11 Recent Scientific Advances

Novel Cytotoxin of Mycoplasma pneumoniae May Explain the Cause of Clinical Signs and Symptoms. Unlike many bacterial pathogens, *Mycoplasma pneumoniae* is not known to produce classic toxins, and precisely how *M. pneumoniae* injures the respiratory epithelium has remained unknown. However, recently the identification of a virulence factor (MPN372) has been reported *(30)* that is possibly responsible for the airway cellular damage and other sequelae associated with *M. pneumoniae* infections in humans. MPN372 encodes a 68-kDa protein that possesses ADP-ribotransferase (ART) activity. Furthermore, a dramatic seroconversion to MPN372 was observed in patients diagnosed with *M. pneumoniae*–associated pneumonia, indicating that this toxin is synthesized *in vivo* and possesses highly immunogenic epitopes *(30)*.

10.12 NIAID Involvement in Respiratory Diseases Research

The NIAID supports research on more effective prevention and treatment approaches to control pneumonia and its causes (http://www3.niaid.nih.gov/healthscience/ healthtopics/pneumonia/research.htm), including:

- Developing and testing vaccines and treatments for the disease-causing microbes that cause pneumonia
- Stimulating research on the structure and function of these microorganisms
- Developing better and more rapid diagnostic tools

- Understanding the long-term health impact respiratory pathogens have in various populations
- Examining the effect of vaccines in high-risk populations
- Determining how pneumococcus causes disease and becomes resistant to antibiotics

NIAID research has made important contributions to developing the pneumococcal conjugate vaccine for children. This vaccine helps to prevent pneumococcal diseases in newborns and toddlers and is the latest advance in developing vaccines against common bacterial infections.

10.12.1 The Gambia Pneumococcal Vaccine Trial

NIAID also supports studies to develop and evaluate improved pneumococcal vaccines for children worldwide. In one such study, NIAID researchers worked with the government of The Gambia and scientists from several international research institutions to test a pneumococcal conjugate vaccine. Health care experts have consistently identified pneumococcus as the most common cause of bacterial pneumonia in The Gambia. In a pattern typical of many developing areas, infant and child mortality rates in The Gambia are high, acute respiratory infections are a leading cause of death, and pneumococcus is the most common cause of these infections. Results of a 4-year, randomized, controlled clinical trial showed that the vaccine reduced childhood mortality by 16% in children who received the pneumococcal conjugate vaccine. The vaccine contained 9 of the pneumococcal serotypes (subtypes) that are most common in The Gambia. The vaccine was 77% effective in preventing infections caused by the vaccine serotypes (www.niaid.nih.gov/dmid/gambia).

The Gambia Pneumococcal Vaccine Trial was the first major randomized, controlled vaccine clinical trial in nearly 20 years to show a statistically significant reduction in overall child mortality. Findings indicate that vaccinating infants against *Streptococcus pneumoniae* could substantially reduce death and illness among children in developing countries, including in rural areas with limited access to public health systems. If used widely, a pneumococcal conjugate vaccine could prevent hundreds of thousands of child deaths each year.

The Gambia Pneumococcal Vaccine Trial Partners. The study was supported by a broad coalition of international partners including the National Institute of Allergy and Infectious Diseases/National Institutes of Health; the British Medical Research Council/United Kingdom; the London School of Hygiene and Tropical Medicine; WHO; the U.S. Agency for International Development; the U.S. Centers for Disease

Control and Prevention; Wyeth-Lederle Vaccines; and the Program for Appropriate Technology in Health (PATH) Children's Vaccine Program.

10.13 Clinical Trials

- Since 2003, NIAID continues to support preclinical and clinical studies to control selected human respiratory pathogens through two 7-year contracts (Bacterial Respiratory Pathogens Research Unit; BRPRU) to the University of Iowa and the Baylor College of Medicine. Studies at the University of Iowa involve pneumococci, meningococci, group A streptococci, pseudomonas, *Chlamydia pneumoniae*, and nontypeable *Haemophilus influenzae* (http://www.uihealthcare.com/news/news/2003/09/15respiratory.html). Studies at the Baylor College of Medicine involve viral pathogenesis and evaluation of new viral vaccines and therapeutics against influenza, RSV, and SARS (http://www.bcm.edu/molvir/eidbt/eidbt-mvm-flu.htm).

- A randomized, double-blind, placebo-controlled trial to evaluate the effects of zinc supplementation in children age 6 to 36 months hospitalized with acute pneumonia is under way at the Mohimbili Hospital in Dar-es-Salaam, Tanzania. The presence of pneumonia will be radiographically confirmed (http://www. clinicaltrials.gov/ct/show/NCT00133432;jsessionid=02E7D36B 5FAD07DE08E3546B86B4D78A?order=9).

- A randomized, controlled, Phase III efficacy trial (co-sponsored by NIAID, WHO, USAID, Children's Vaccine Program at PATH, and the MRC in London) was successfully completed in The Gambia in 2005 (http://www.niaid.nih.gov/dmid/gambia/default.htm).

- Rhinosinusitis is a common health problem with significant patient morbidity and lost productivity, in which antibiotics are frequently prescribed, often unnecessarily. A randomized clinical trial is under way to evaluate the effectiveness of a 10-day course of amoxicillin versus placebo in patients with a clinical diagnosis of acute bacterial rhinosinusitis. The study will evaluate symptoms, disease recurrence, satisfaction with health care, and direct costs (http://clinicaltrials.gov/ct/show/NCT00377403;jsessionid=34221EDAA8A E01841C7B59D0D21EC014?order=10).

References

1. Garibaldi, R. A. (1985) Epidemiology of community-acquired respiratory tract infections in adults. Incidence, etiology, and impact, *Am. J. Med.*, **78**(6B), 32–37.

2. Gray, G. C., Callahan, J. D., Hawksworth, A. W., Fisher, C. A., and Gaydos, J. C.(1999) Respiratory diseases among U.S. military personnel: countering emerging threats, *Emerg. Infect. Dis.*, **5**(3), 379–387.

3. Georgiev, V. St. (1998) Adenoviruses. In: *Infectious Diseases in Immunocompromised Hosts*, CRC Press, Boca Raton, FL, pp. 171–179.

4. Flomenberg, P. R., Chen, M., and Horwitz, M. S. (1987) Characterization of a major histocompatibility complex class I antigen-binding glycoprotein from adenovirus type 35, a type associated with immunocompromised hosts, *J. Virol.*, **61**(12), 3665–3671.

5. Doherty, P. C. and Zinkernagel, R. M. (1975) H-2 compatibility requirement for T-cell-mediated lysis of target cell infected with lymphocytic choriomeningitis virus, *J. Exp. Med.*, **141**, 1427–1436.

6. Cassell, G. H., Clyde, W. A., and Davis, J. K. (1985) Mycoplasmal respiratory infections. In: *The Mycoplasmas*, vol 4 (Razin, S. and Barile, M. F., eds), Academic Press, Orlando, FL, pp. 65–106.

7. Cassell, G. (1995) Severe mycoplasma disease—rare or underdiagnosed? *West. J. Med.*, **162**(2), 172–175.

8. Jenkinson, D. (1995) Natural cause of 500 consecutive cases of whooping cough: a general practice population study, *Lancet*, **310**, 299–302.

9. Cherry, J. D., Brunell, P. A., Golden, G. S., and Karzon, D. T. (1988) Report of the task force on pertussis and pertussis immunization-1988, *Pediatrics*, **81**(6), 933–984.

10. Pertussis Report (2005), *Morb. Mortal. Wkly Rep.*, **53**(52), 1213–1220.

11. Tanaka, M. (2003) Trends in pertussis among infants in the United States, 1980–1999, *J. Am. Med. Assoc.*, **290**, 2968–2975.

12. Georgiev, V. St. (1998) Respiratory syncytial virus. In: *Infectious Diseases in Immunocompromised Hosts*, CRC Press, Boca Raton, FL, pp. 191–198.

13. Stark, J. M. (1993) Lung infections in children, *Curr. Opin. Pediatr.*, **5**, 273–280.

14. Ogra, P. L. and Patel, J. (1988) Respiratory syncytial virus infection and the immunocompromised host, *Pediatr. Infect. Dis. J.*, **7**, 246–249.

15. Englund, J. A., Sullivan, C. J., Jordan, M. C., Dehner, L. P., Vercillotti, G. M., and Balfour, H. H., Jr. (1988) Respiratory syncytial virus infection in immunocompromised adults, *Ann. Intern. Med.*, **109**, 203–208.

16. Chandwani, S., Borkowsky, W., Krasinski, K., Lawrence, R., and Welliver, R. (1990) Respiratory syncytial virus infection in human immunodeficiency virus-infected children, *J. Pediatr.*, **117**, 251–254.

17. van den Hoogen, B. G., de Jong, J. C., Groen, J., Kuiken, T., de Groot, R., Fouchier, R. A. M., and Osterhaus, A. D. M. E. (2001) A newly discovered human pneumovirus isolated from young children with respiratory tract disease, *Nat. Med.*, **7**, 719–724.

18. Falsey, A., Erdman, D., Anderson, L. J., and Walsh, E. E. (2003) Human metapneumovirus infections in young and elderly adults, *J. Infect. Dis.*, **187**, 785–790.

19. Collins, P. L., Chanock, R. M., and McIntosh, K. (1995) Parainfluenza viruses. In: *Fields Virology*, 3rd ed. (Fields, B. N., Knipe, D. M., and Howley, P. M. eds.), Lippincott-Raven, Philadelphia, pp. 1205–1241.

20. Glezen, W. P. and Denny, F. W. (1997) Parainfluenza viruses. In: *Viral Infections in Humans: Epidemiology and Control*, 4th ed. (Evans, A. and Kaslow, R. eds.), Plenum, New York, pp. 551–567.

21. Counihan, M. E., Shaym D. K., Holman, R. C., Lowther, S. A., and Anderson, L. J. (2001) Human parainfluenza virus-associated hospitalizations among children less than five years of age in the United States, *Pediatr. Infect. Dis. J.*, **20**(7), 646–653.

22. Respiratory Diphtheria Caused by *Corynebacterium ulcerans*—Terre Haute, Indiana, 1996 (1997) *Morb. Mortal. Wkly Rep.* **46**(15), 330–332.

23. Morbidity and Mortality Report for Pertussis Disease (2002) *Morb. Mortal. Wkly Rep.*, **51**(04), 73–76.

24. Govan, J. R. W. (2000) Infection control in cystic fibrosis: methicilin-resistant *Staphylococcus aureus,Pseudomonas aeruginosa* and the *Burkholderia cepacia* Complex, *J. R. Soc. Med.*, **93**, 40–45.

25. Speert, D. P., Campbell, M. E., Henry, D. A., Milner, R., Taha, F., Gravelle, A., Davidson, A. G. F., Wong, L. T. K., and Mahenthiralingam, E. (2002) Epidemiology of *Pseudomonas aeruginosa* in cystic fibrosis in British Columbia, Canada, *Am. J. Respir. Clin. Care Med.*, **166**, 988–993.

26. Speert, D. P., Farmer, S. W., Campbell, M. E., Musser, J. M., Selander, R. K., and Kuo, S.(1990) Conversion of *Pseudomonas aeruginosa* to the phenotype characteristic of strains from patients with cystic fibrosis, *J. Clin. Microbiol.*, **28**, 188–194.

27. Saiman, L. and Siegel, J. (2004) Infection control in cystic fibrosis, *Clin. Microbial. Rev.*, **17**(1), 57–71.

28. Rosenstein, N. E., Perkins, B. A., Stephens, D. S., Popovic, T., and Hughes, J. M. (2001) *Meningococcal* diseases, *N. Engl. J. Med.*, **344**(18), 1378–1388.

29. Centers for Disease Control and Prevention (2005) Prevention and control of *meningococcal* disease: recommendations of the Advisory Committee on Immunization Practices (ACIP), *Morb. Mortal. Wkly Rep.*, **54**(RR-7), 1–21.

30. Kannan, T. R. and Baseman, J. B. (2006) ADP-ribosylating and vacuoling cytotoxin of *Mycoplasma pnaumoniae* represents unique virulence determinant among bacterial pathogens, *Proc. Natl. Acad. Sci. U.S.A.,* **103**(17), 6724–6729.

Chapter 11

Streptococcus pneumoniae (Pneumococcal) Disease

Streptococcus is a genus of nonmotile (with few exceptions), nonspore-forming, aerobic to facultatively anaerobic bacteria (family Lactobacillaceae) that occur in pairs (diplococci) or short or long chains and that contain Gram-positive, spherical or ovoid cells. The type species is *Streptococcus pyogenes*. The *Streptococcus* bacteria are divided into two major groups, A and B. Group A *streptococci* (GAS) causes a broad spectrum of diseases that range from uncomplicated pharyngitis ("strep throat") to life-threatening illnesses, including pneumonia, bacteremia, necrotizing fasciitis (soft tissue disease), and streptococcal toxic shock syndrome (multiorgan failures). In addition, acute rheumatic fever and rheumatic heart disease can be potential complications after untreated strep throat infections. Group B *streptococci* (GBS) causes serious illness in newborns, pregnant women, postpartum women, and adults with chronic medical conditions (http://www3.niaid.nih.gov/research/topics/bacterial/AboutPneumococcalDisease.htm).

Streptococcus pneumoniae (also known as pneumococcus) is a group A, lancet-shaped bacterium (cocci) usually seen in pairs (diplococci), but it also may be observed as a single organism and in short chains. It is often found in the noses and throats of healthy persons and is spread person-to-person through close contact. Pneumococcus is a common cause of mild illness, such as sinus and ear infections (otitis media), but can also cause life-threatening infections, such as pneumonia, meningitis, and infections of the bloodstream. Many strains are resistant to antibiotics.

Severe, sometimes life-threatening GAS disease may occur when bacteria get into parts of the body where bacteria usually are not found, such as blood, muscle, or the lungs. These infections are termed *invasive GAS disease*. Two of the most severe, but least common, forms of invasive GAS disease are necrotizing fasciitis and streptococcal toxic shock syndrome (STSS). Necrotizing fasciitis (occasionally described by the media as "the flesh-eating bacteria") destroys muscles, fat, and skin tissue. STSS causes blood pressure to drop rapidly and organs (e.g., kidney, liver, lungs) to fail. It should be noted that STSS *is not* the same as the "toxic shock syndrome" frequently associated with tampon usage. About 20% of patients with necrotizing fasciitis and more than half with STSS die. About 10% to 15% of patients with other forms of invasive GAS disease die. Severe invasive GAS disease is believed to have re-emerged during the past 10 to 20 years. It is estimated that 9,600 to 9,700 cases of invasive GAS disease occur in the United States each year, resulting in 1,100 to 1,300 deaths (http://www.cdc.gov/ncidod/dbmd/abcs/survreports/gbs05.pdf) *(1)*.

Pneumonia is a disease of the lung that is caused by a variety of bacteria, including *Streptococcus, Staphylococcus, Pseudomonas, Haemophilus, Chlamydia,* and *Mycoplasma,* several viruses, and a certain fungi and protozoans. The disease may be divided into two forms: *bronchial pneumonia* and *lobar pneumonia*. Bronchial pneumonia is most prevalent in infants, young children, and aged adults. It is caused by various bacteria, including *Streptococcus pneumoniae,* and involves the alveoli contiguous to the larger bronchioles of the bronchial tree. Lobar pneumonia is more prone to occur in younger adults. More than 80% of all cases of lobar pneumonia are caused by *Streptococcus pneumoniae.* Lobar pneumonia involves all of a single lobe of the lungs (although more than one lobe may be affected), wherein the entire area of involvement tends to become a consolidated mass (http://www3.niaid.nih.gov/research/topics/bacterial/AboutPneumococcalDisease.htm).

According to estimates by WHO, *S. pneumoniae* kills worldwide close to 1 million children under 5 years of age annually, especially in developing countries where pneumococcus is one of the most important bacterial pathogens in early infancy. In developed countries, virtually every child becomes a nasopharyngeal carrier of *S. pneumoniae* during the first year of life. Many go on to develop one or more episodes of otitis media, and a smaller number develop more serious invasive pneumococcal infections.

Data from the CDC have shown a 70% decrease in the incidence of GBS infections among newborn infants when antibiotics have been administered to pregnant women at the time of labor (http://www.cdc.gov/ncidod/dbmd/abcs/survreports/gbs05.pdf) *(2,3)*.

Acute rheumatic fever (ARF) is the major cause of heart disease in children worldwide. Whereas the incidence of ARF has declined in industrialized countries since the 1950s, in developing countries ARF remains an endemic disease with estimated annual median incidences ranging from 20 to 374 per 100,000 school-aged children. Global estimates for rheumatic heart disease include 16 million existing cases, 282,000 new cases each year, and 233,000 deaths each year *(4)*.

In supporting research for streptococcal diseases, the major thrust of the NIAID Streptococcal Program is toward developing and testing new streptococcal vaccines that are safe, immunogenic, and provide prolonged protective immunity. An important emphasis will be placed on the immunologic response of infants, the elderly, and other high-risk populations. Examples of current vaccine development and testing relate to prevention of pharyngitis, sinusitis, bronchitis, chronic obstructive pulmonary disease, pneumonia, meningitis, bacteremia, neonatal sepsis, arthritis, epiglottitis, and rheumatic fever. Although the most mature area is the development and clinical evaluation of protein-polysaccharide conjugate vaccines, NIAID will actively support research to develop alternative vaccines that might provide immunity at an earlier age or that are more broadly protective than the conjugate vaccines. Toward this goal, NIAID is also supporting research on the pathogenesis, immunity, genomics, and structural biology of streptococcal bacteria (http://www3.niaid.nih.gov/research/topics/bacterial/AboutPneumococcalDisease.htm).

11.1 Streptococcal Vaccines

Currently, two vaccines are available to prevent pneumococcal disease: the pneumococcal conjugate vaccine (PCV) (Prevnar; Wyeth Vaccines) and the pneumococcal polysaccharide vaccine (PPV) (Pneumovax; Merck & Co.). Both vaccines provide protection by inducing antibodies to specific types of the pneumococcal capsule (90 different serotypes of pneumococcal capsule have been identified). The conjugate vaccine protects against the 7 serotypes most common in young children in the United States; the 23-valent polysaccharide vaccine includes 23 serotypes. Both vaccines are effective in preventing invasive disease (the severe form of pneumococcal disease in which the pathogen is found in the blood, spinal fluid, or other typically sterile bodily fluids). The conjugate vaccine, licensed for use in young children, also prevents some pneumonia and ear infections (http://www2.ncid.cdc.gov/travel/yb/utils/ybGet.asp?section=dis&obj=strep.htm).

11.1.1 Pneumococcal Conjugate Vaccine

The pneumococcal conjugate vaccine is part of the routine *infant* immunization schedule (all children younger than 2 years old). It is also administered to children 2 to 4 years of age who have (i) sickle cell hemoglobinopathies; (ii) functional or anatomic asplenia; (iii) received or will receive a cochlear implant; (iv) HIV infection; (v) chronic disease, including chronic cardiac and pulmonary disease excluding asthma, diabetes mellitus, or cerebrospinal fluid leak; and (vi) immunocompromising conditions, including hematologic or other disseminated malignancies, chronic renal failure or nephritic syndrome, ongoing immunosuppressive therapy, and solid organ transplant (http://www2.ncid.cdc.gov/travel/yb/utils/ybGet.asp?section=dis&obj=strep.htm).

Pneumococcal conjugate vaccine should also be considered for healthy children 2 to 4 years of age, especially those 24 to 35 months old, those attending group child care, and those in the United States who are of African American, Alaskan Native, or Native American descent.

11.1.2 Pneumococcal Polysaccharide Vaccine

The pneumococcal polysaccharide vaccine is part of the routine *adult* immunization schedule, but many adults who should have received the vaccine have not. In 2003, only 62% of adults 62 years of age or older had received the vaccine.

The pneumococcal polysaccharide vaccine is recommended for all adults age 65 or older and for persons 2 to 64 years of age with certain chronic illnesses or immunocompromised conditions, including (i) chronic cardiovascular disease (e.g., congestive heart failure or cardiomyopathies); (ii) chronic pulmonary disease (e.g., chronic obstructive pulmonary disease or emphysema, but not asthma); (iii) diabetes mellitus; (iv) alcoholism; (v) chronic liver disease (cirrhosis); (vi) cerebrospinal fluid leaks; (vii) functional or anatomic asplenia; (viii) cochlear implant (or those planning to receive a cochlear implant); (ix) HIV infection; (x) multiple myeloma; or (xi) immunocompromising conditions, including hematologic or other generalized malignancies, chronic renal failure or nephritic syndrome, ongoing immunosuppressive therapy, and bone marrow or solid organ transplantation.

The polysaccharide vaccine should also be given to those 2 to 64 years of age who are living in settings in which the risk for invasive pneumococcal disease is increased, such as certain Native American communities (e.g., Alaskan Natives and certain American Indian populations) and residents of nursing homes and other long-term care facilities.

A single dose of pneumococcal polysaccharide vaccine should be given at age 65 or at the time a high-risk condition is recognized. Children 2 to 4 years of age with indications for pneumococcal polysaccharide vaccine should receive the vaccine at least 2 months after receiving doses of the conjugate vaccine. Persons with an indication of polysaccharide vaccine but with unknown vaccination history should receive one dose. A second dose of vaccine should be used for the following populations: (i) persons age 65 or older who received the vaccine at least 5 years before and were less than 65 years of age at the time of initial vaccination and (ii) persons with sickle cell disease, asplenia, renal disease, hematologic or generalized malignancy, or other immunocompromising condition.

For children under age 10, the second dose may be given 3 or more years after the first dose; for older persons, revaccination may be done after 5 years. Because of limited data on the safety of multiple doses and on the duration of protection provided by the polysaccharide vaccine, recommendations are for a single revaccination 3 to 5 years after the initial dose. These recommendations *have been misinterpreted as suggesting revaccination every 5 years* (http://www2.ncid.cdc.gov/travel/yb/utils/ybGet.asp?section=dis&obj=strep.htm).

11.1.3 Safety and Side Effects

Mild local reactions such as redness, swelling, or tenderness occur in 10% to 23% of infants after receiving the conjugate vaccine. Larger areas of redness or swelling or limitations in arm movement may occur in 1% to 9%. After conjugate vaccine, low-grade fever can occur in up to 24% of children, and fever higher than 102.2°F may occur in up to 2.5%.

For pneumococcal polysaccharide vaccine, mild, local side effects occur in approximately half of vaccine recipients and are more common after revaccination. Local reactions usually resolve by 48 h after vaccination. More severe local reactions are rare. Systemic symptoms, including myalgias and fever, are rare after polysaccharide vaccine (http://www2.ncid.cdc.gov/travel/yb/utils/ybGet.asp?section=dis&obj=strep.htm).

11.2 Recent Scientific Advances

- *Identification of Novel Conserved Protein Structures as Potential Vaccine Candidates for Preventing Group B Streptococcal Infections.* GBS are the major cause of bacterial infections in newborns, causing sepsis and meningitis. Recently, GBS have been implicated as the cause of invasive disease in the elderly. To be effective, capsular polysaccharide-conjugate vaccines need to include multiple components (capsular polysaccharides) to protect against numerous types of GBS. An alternative approach for the development of an efficacious vaccine against GBS will require identifying conserved proteins that will provide cross-protection against all GBS. Genomic analysis of eight different GBS strains identified genes in each of the strains that encode pilus-like structures. These are long surface structures made of proteins that extend out from the cell wall and capsular polysaccharide of GBS *(5)*. Protein components from these pilus-like structures were shown to be antigenic and induce protective immunity in mouse models. The similarities of these proteins with pili in other bacteria indicate that they may provide a way for the bacteria to attach to human tissue and may therefore be important in colonization *(5)*.

- *Evolution and Global Dissemination of Macrolide-Resistant Group A Streptococci.* Macrolide resistance by *S. pneumoniae* has emerged as a serious threat for the therapy of GAS. However, the strain typing information that is currently available has been insufficient for estimating the total number of macrolide-resistant clones, their geographic distribution, and their evolutionary relationships. In a recent study, sequence-based strain typing was used to characterize 212 macrolide-resistant GAS (MRGAS) isolates from 34 countries *(6)*. Evaluation of clonal complexes, *emm* type, and resistance gene content [*erm*(A), *erm*(B), *mef*(A), and undefined] indicated that macrolide resistance was acquired via ≥49 independent genetic events. In contrast with other collections of mostly susceptible GAS, genetic diversification of MRGAS clones has occurred primarily by mutation rather than by recombination. This and other findings have suggested that horizontal transfer of macrolide resistance genes to numerous genetic backgrounds, as well as global dissemination of resisting clones and their descendants, were both major components of the present-day macrolide resistance problem found in these species *(6)*.

- *Validation of a New Semiautomated Serotyping Assay for Streptococcus pneumoniae.* A recently developed rapid pneumococcal serotyping method (multibed assay) has been used to identify 36 pneumococcal serotypes. The multibed assay, which represents a multiplex immunoassay for capsular polysaccharides in lysates of pneumococcal cultures, was validated by examining 495 clinical isolates of pneumococci obtained in Brazil, Denmark, and Mexico *(7)*. The bacterial strains represented all 23 serotypes included in the licensed polysaccharide vaccine. The results of the study have shown that the new semiautomated technology will have to use a large number of clinical isolates from different geographic locations in order to validate any new *S. pneumoniae* serotyping assay.

11.3 Antimicrobial Drug Resistance

Antimicrobial drug resistance is a common global problem. During the 1970s–1980s, drug resistance was considered a hospital-based problem mainly related to nosocomially acquired resistant organisms *(8)*. Throughout the 1990s, there was recognition that many community-acquired microorganisms were resistant to first-line antibiotics, thereby prompting the use, in some clinical situations, of broader spectrum agents. Toward the late 1990s and currently, the realization is that community-acquired pathogens may be multiresistant.

11.3.1 Overview of Antimicrobial Drug Resistance

In general terms, the antimicrobial resistance may be broadly categorized as intrinsic, acquired, and *de novo*. For *intrinsic resistance*, the microorganism either lacks the specific target to which the antimicrobial agent must bind to exert a biological effect or the target is present but not readily accessible by the drug. For *acquired resistance*, a microorganism becomes less susceptible to the drug than it initially was. Acquisition of resistance may occur by transmissible genetic elements, such as plasmids or transposons. Finally, *de novo* resistance arises from the bacterial population and results from mutation in the host chromosome that affects genes encoding for proteins targeted by various antimicrobial agents.

The major mechanisms of antimicrobial resistance include:

(i) Decreased uptake/altered membrane permeability.
(ii) Efflux.
(iii) Enzymatic modification of the antimicrobial compound.
(iv) Altered target/binding sites.

A single pathogen may have only one mechanism of resistance or may simultaneously possess multiple mechanisms, thereby conferring multidrug resistance (8).

11.3.2 Drug Resistance of Streptococcus pneumoniae

A major advance in the treatment of streptococcal infections was made with the introduction of penicillin nearly 60 years ago. In the following years, pneumococci were considered so uniformly sensitive to penicillin (with a minimum inhibitory concentration <0.2 mg/L) that sensitivity tests were usually not performed and it remained the drug of choice for ther-

apy *(8)*. Erythromycin and tetracycline were alternatives for therapy in patients with β-lactam–related allergies.

It was in Australia in 1967 that the first clinically significant isolate of penicillin-resistant pneumococcus was reported *(9)*. Subsequently, penicillin-resistant *S. pneumoniae* isolates were reported in South Africa *(10)*. Concurrently, a number of reports described pneumococcal resistance to tetracycline *(11)*, erythromycin *(12)*, and clindamycin *(13)*. Resistance to quinolones *(14)* and third-generation cephalosporins was reported in the 1980s *(15)* and throughout the 1990s. In 1999, strains showing tolerance to vancomycin have been described *(16)*.

The rapid emergence of penicillin-resistant *S. pneumoniae* (particularly in the 1990s) and the concomitant cross-resistance to many other antimicrobial agents *has demanded that routine susceptibility testing be performed on each isolate deemed clinically significant.*

11.3.2.1 Emergence of Resistance

The β-lactamase resistance enzyme has not been associated with pneumococcal resistance, and no other enzymatic mechanism has been described *(8)*. However, pneumococci are naturally transformable, a property that appears essential to the evolution of antimicrobial resistance. Thus, resistance will occur after mutations in native DNA as a result of the incorporation of externally acquired naked DNA, which may come either from other strains of pneumococci, α-hemolytic streptococci, or other organisms colonizing the oral-pharyngeal surfaces. Subsequently, alterations in the native DNA will result in changes to the *penicillin-binding proteins (PBPs)*, such as modifications of the high molecular weight proteins 1A, 2B, and 2X *(8)*.

PBPs are important structural proteins located in the peptidoglycan layer of the bacterial cell wall. They play an essential role in cell wall formation as they mediate the cross-linking of peptidoglycan, which, in turn, provides structural integrity and rigidity to the cell wall. PBPs are the targets for the β-lactam antimicrobial agents. These antimicrobial agents act by binding to the PBPs, thereby preventing cross-linking of the peptidoglycan layer. Instability of the bacterial cell wall because of interference with peptidoglycan formation will lead to autolysis and death of the microorganism *(8)*.

The resistance of the pneumococci to macrolides, clindamycin, and lincosamides is the result of either constitutive or inducible methylation of the 23SrRNA *(17)*. *S. pneumoniae* demonstrating multiple resistant phenotypes, including erythromycin, streptomycin, kanamycin, tetracycline, and chloramphenicol, are likely because of the transposable element Tn1545 *(18)*.

Vancomycin is a soluble, complex glycopolypeptide. It was released in the mid-1950s and was effective against penicillin-resistant *S. pneumoniae*. Its activity has made this antibiotic necessary when penicillin resistance is suspected and alternative agents are not available. The mechanism of action of vancomycin involves the inhibition of synthesis of the second stage of cell wall peptidoglycan polymers by binding with the *D*-alanyl-*D*-alanine precursor. A second mechanism of action involves damage to protoplasts by altering the cytoplasmic membrane permeability. In addition, vancomycin may also impair the RNA synthesis *(8)*.

11.3.2.2 Drug-Resistant *S. pneumoniae* Meningitis

Pneumococci reach the central nervous system (CNS) either by a hematogenous route from a distant focus of infection—usually the lower airways with or without pneumonia—or, even more frequently, by direct entrance of bacteria to the cerebrospinal fluid (CSF) from an infectious focus near the CNS, such as acute otitis media, acute sinusitis, or a cranial fistula *(19)*.

Except for epidemics or hyperendemic situations of meningococcal disease, *S. pneumoniae* has long been and continues to be the most frequent cause of community-acquired bacterial meningitis in adults older than age 30, causing most morbidity and mortality *(19)*. In industrialized countries, the mortality rate of pneumococcal meningitis in adults ranges from 25% to 30%, and these figures remained constant throughout the antibiotic era in spite of improved critical care medicine. In view of the current loss of susceptibility of many *S. pneumoniae* strains to β-lactam antibiotics, that situation could become even worse. The prognosis of pneumococcal meningitis, especially in adults, is depending more on early diagnosis and early preventive treatment of neurologic complications than on antibiotic failure *(19)*.

Initially, the solution to the problem of resistance to β-lactam antibiotics seemed to be the use of vancomycin, to which all pneumococci remained (and still remain) susceptible, with minimal inhibitory concentrations (MICs) between 0.25 and 1.0 µg/mL. However, several clinical failures have been documented when vancomycin was used in conjunction with dexamethasone *(19)*. Those failures were mainly due to insufficient antibiotic penetration into the CSF because of individual variability in its passing through the blood-brain barrier and to the effect of dexamethasone, which is shown to reduce CSF vancomycin penetration *(20)*. Therefore, the recommendation is that vancomycin is not to be used alone for the treatment of pneumococcal meningitis, but rather, combined antibiotic regimens are recommended for both empirical treatment and treatment of those cases caused by β-lactam–resistant pneumococcal strains *(21)*.

11.4 NIAID Involvement in International Research on Pneumococcal Disease

- A NIAID-sponsored randomized, double-blind, placebo-controlled trial is under way in Dar-es-Salaam, Tanzania, to evaluate the effects of zinc supplementation in children age 6 to 36 months hospitalized with acute pneumonia. The enrolled children will receive zinc (or a placebo) daily during the hospitalization phase, and the study will essentially conclude at the day they are discharged from the hospital. Pneumonia will be radiographically confirmed.

- In conjunction with WHO, USAID, the Bill & Melinda Gates Foundation's Children's Vaccine Program at PATH, and the MRC in London, NIAID is continuing its support of randomized, controlled, Phase III efficacy trials in The Gambia to evaluate a nine-valent pneumococcal conjugate vaccine (Wyeth-Lederle Vaccines) administered with an adjuvant, DPT/Hib. The trial should be able to detect a 20% to 25% reduction in radiographic pneumonia.

References

1. O'Brien, K. L., Beall, B., Barrett, N. L., Ciesak, P. R., Reingold, A., Farley, M. M., Danila, R., Zell, E. R., Facklam, R., Schwartz, A., and Schuchat, A. (2002) Epidemiolgy of invasive group A *Streptococcus* disease in the United States, 1995–1999, *Clin. Infect. Dis.*, **35**(3), 268–276.
2. Centers for Disease Control (2002) Prevention of perinatal GBS disease, *Morb. Mortal. Wkly Rep.*, **51**(RR-11), 5.
3. Schrag, S. J., Zywicki, S., Farley, M. M., Reingold, A. L., Harrison, L. H., Lefkowitz, L. B., Hadler, J. L., Danila, R., Cieslak, P. R., and Schuchat, A. (2000) Group B streptococcal disease in the era of intrapartum antibiotic prophylaxis, *N. Engl. J. Med.*, **342**(1), 15–20.
4. Carapetis, J. R., Steer, A. C., Mulholland, E. K., and Weber, M. (2005) The global burden of group A streptococcal diseases, *Lancet Infect. Dis.*, **5**(11), 685–694.
5. Rosini, R., Rinaudo, C. D., Soriani, M., Lauer, P., Mora, M., Maione, D., Taddei, M., Santi, I., Ghezzo, C., Brettoni, C., Buccato, S., Margarit, I., Grandi, G., and Telford, J. L. (2006) Identification of novel genomic island coding for antigenic pilus-like structures in *Streptococcus agalactiae*, *Mol. Microbiol.*, **61**, 126–141.
6. Robinson, D. A., Sutcliffe, J. A., Tewodros, W., Manoharan, A., and Bessen, D. E. (2006) Evolution and global dissemination of macrolide-resistant group A streptococci, *Antimicrob. Agents Chemother.*, **50**, 2903–2911.
7. Lin, J., Kaltoft, M. S., Brandao, A. P., Echaniz-Aviles, G., Brandileone, M. C., Hollingshead, S. K., Benjamin, W. H., and Nahm, M. H. (2006) Validation of a multiplex pneumococcal serotyping assay with clinical samples, *J. Clin. Microbiol.*, **44**, 383–388.
8. Blondeau, J. M. (2004) Emerging resistance to vancomycin, rifampin, and fluoroquinolones in *Streptococcus pneumoniae*. In: *Management of Multiple Drug-Resistant Infections* (Gillespie, S. H., ed.), Humana Press, Totowa, NJ, pp. 49–78.

9. Hansman, D. and Bullen, M. (1967) A resistant pneumococcus, *Lancet*, **2**, 264–265.

10. Appelbaum, P. C., Bhamjee, A., Scragg, J. N., Hallett, A. F., Bowen, A. J., and Cooper, R. C. (1977) *Streptococcus pneumoniae* resistant to penicillin and chloramphenicol, *Lancet*, **2**, 995–997.

11. Evans, W. and Hansman, D. (1963) Tetracycline-resistant pneumococcus, *Lancet*, **1**, 451.

12. Francis, R. S., May, J., and Spicer, C. C. (1964) Influence of daily penicillin, tetracycline, erythromycin and sulphamethoxypyridazine on exacerbations of bronchitis: a report to the research committee of the British Tuberculosis Association, *Br. Med. J.*, **1**, 728–732.

13. Kislak, J. W. (1967) Type 6 pneumococcus resistant to erythromycin and lincomycin, *N. Engl. J. Med.*, **276**, 852.

14. Klugman, K. P. (1990) Pneumococcal resistance to antibiotics, *Clin. Microbiol. Rev.*, **3**(2), 171–196.

15. Asensi, F., Perez-Tamarit, D., Otero, M. C., Gallego, M., Llanes, S., Abadia, C., and Canto, E. (1989) Imipenem-cilastin therapy in a child with meningitis caused by a multiply resistant pneumococcus, *Pediatr. Infect. Dis. J.*, **399**, 590–593.

16. Novak, R., Henriquies, B., Charpentier, E., Normark, S., and Tuomanen, E. (1999) Emergence of vancomycin tolerance in *Streptococcus pneumoniae*, *Nature*, **399**, 590–593.

17. Leclercq, R. and Courvalin, P. (1991) Bacterial resistance to macrolide, lincosamide and streptogramin antibiotics by target modification, *Antimicrob. Agents Chemother.*, **35**, 1267–1272.

18. Courvalin, P. and Carlier, C. (1986) Transposable multiple antibiotic resistance in *Streptococcus pneumoniae*, *Mol. Gen. Genet.*, **205**, 291–297.

19. Fernández Viladrich, P. (2004) Management of meningitis caused by resistant *Streptococcus pneumoniae*. In: *Management of Multiple Drug-Resistant Infections* (Gillespie, S. H., ed.), Humana Press, Totowa, NJ, pp. 31–48.

20. Paris, M., Hickey, S. M., Uscher, M. I., Shelton, S., Olsen, K. D., and McCracken, G. H., Jr. (1994) Effect of dexamethazone on therapy of experimental penicillin- and cephalosporin-resistant pneumococcal meningitis, *Antimicrob. Agents Chemother.*, **38**, 1320–1324.

21. Kaplan, S. L. (2002) Management of pneumococcal meningitis, *Pediatr. Infect. Dis. J.*, **21**, 589–591.

Chapter 12

Severe Acute Respiratory Syndrome

Early in 2003, an outbreak of the until then unknown severe acute respiratory syndrome (SARS) was reported in southeastern People's Republic of China. The outbreak was thought to have first emerged in the Guangdong province in November 2002. Subsequently, the infections spread to Hong Kong (February 2003) and other countries of Southeast Asia, including Vietnam, Taiwan, and Singapore, as well as to Canada and the United States (http://www.fda.gov/oc/opacom/hottopics/sars/).

Epidemiologic studies have shown that the disease disproportionately affected health care workers (21% of all cases) and close contacts of SARS patients, such as family members. No new cases of SARS have been reported since April, 2004 (http://www.who.int/scr/don/2004_04_30/en). There has been some evidence from research to suggest the presence of a variation in an immune system gene that may make people with the variation much more vulnerable to the SARS-associated coronavirus (SARS-CoV). This genetic variation is more common among people of Southeast Asian descent but is rare in other populations. This may help explain why most SARS cases have occurred in China and Southeast Asia.

According to statistics by WHO, a total of 8,098 people worldwide contracted SARS during the 2003 outbreak. Of these, 774 died (overall fatality rate: 9.6%). In the United States, only 8 people had laboratory evidence of SARS—all of them had traveled to other parts of the world where SARS was present. Higher mortality has been observed in older patients and in patients with comorbid conditions, such as diabetes, lymphopenia, and liver dysfunction (http://www.cdc.gov/ncidod/sars).

The novel SARS-CoV was identified as the cause of SARS. Previously identified human coronaviruses (named for their spiky, crown-like appearance) are known to cause only mild respiratory infections (e.g., common cold). It now seems likely that SARS-CoV had evolved from one or more animal viruses into a completely new strain.

The SARS-CoV spreads primarily through close human contact (e.g., droplets, airborne particles in face-to-face contacts). Touching a SARS-CoV–infected surface and subsequently touching the eyes, nose, or mouth may also lead to infection. SARS typically begins with flu-like symptoms, including high fever (100.4°F/38°C, or higher) that may be accompanied by headache and muscle aches, cough, and shortness of breath. In some cases, the fever may not appear for up to 10 days. Up to 20% of people infected may develop diarrhea. Most patients with SARS subsequently will develop pneumonia. Between 10% and 20% of SARS patients will become progressively worse and develop breathing problems so severe that they may require the help of a mechanical respirator. SARS is fatal in some cases, often due to respiratory failure. Other possible complications include heart and liver failure.

12.1 NIAID Agenda for SARS Research

In spite of a concerted global effort, there is still no effective treatment for SARS. A combination of antiviral drugs normally used to treat AIDS—lopinavir-ritonavir along with ribavirin—have been shown in clinical studies to prevent serious complications and deaths from SARS. However, further studies are needed. In August 2004, the SARS-CoV was added to NIAID's List of Category C Priority Pathogens for Biodefense (http:// www2.niaid.nih.gov/biodefense/bandc_priority.htm). Funding opportunities are listed under NIAID's biodefense programs (http://www2.niaid.nih.gov/biodefense/research/funding.htm).

On May 30, 2003, NIAID convened an international meeting on SARS to develop a robust research agenda focused on the discovery of effective therapies to control the disease.

A number of research goals and objectives have been recommended:

- Expand research efforts on the basic biology of the virus, including studies on replication, biodiversity, factors that influence transmission to humans, and the development of animal models

V. St. Georgiev, *National Institute of Allergy and Infectious Diseases, NIH: Impact on Global Health*, vol. 2, DOI 10.1007/978-1-60327-297-1_12, © Humana Press, a part of Springer Science+Business Media, LLC 2009

- Determine the basis of SARS-associated immunopathology and identify the components of innate and protective immunity, and the impact of polymorphisms on the disease outcome
- Support the rapid development of multiple vaccine strategies
- Expand capacity for *in vitro* evaluation of antiviral drugs with activity against SARS, and identify viral and host targets for therapeutic intervention
- Develop diagnostics that are rapid, sensitive, and easy to use and that can be widely distributed
- Define SARS disease progression, persistence, correlates of immunity and susceptibility, or resistance to reinfection
- Expand surveillance to identify the animal reservoir(s) and factors that influence the spread of the virus, and assess whether immunocompromised individuals, children, and pregnant women are at an increased risk
- Provide the research community with resources, including opportunities to upgrade biocontainment facilities, and provide standardized reference reagents, including microarrays and tetramers

12.1.1 Research Programmatic Developments

In response to the need for a rapid increase in research on the SARS coronavirus, NIAID has initiated a vigorous program to support the development of diagnostics, vaccines, and therapeutics for SARS (http://www.google.com/search?hl=en&q=niaid+infergen+sars). Several major programs of NIAID-supported SARS research include:

- A clinical protocol to evaluate interferon-alfacon-1 (Infergen, Amgen, Inc.), an engineered recombinant interferon molecule that has a potent anti-SARS-CoV activity in an *in vitro* assay for cytopathic activity. Infergen has previously been known for its anti-hepatitis C activity.
- NIAID's Vaccine Research Center (VRC) has contracted with Vical, Inc., to manufacture a single-dosed, circular DNA plasmid-based vaccine encoding the S protein of the SARS-CoV. *In vitro* studies have demonstrated that this vaccine induces T-cell and neutralizing antibody responses, as well as protective immunity. A Phase I open-label clinical study to evaluate safety, tolerability, and immune responses was completed in May 2006. In the study, healthy subjects were administered 4.0 mg DNA vaccine doses at three 1-month intervals. The vaccine was well tolerated.
- Several animal models have been developed for SARS, including mouse, hamster, and non-human primates. None of the animals tested exhibited clinical disease after

intranasal administration of the virus but rather exhibited antibodies against SARS-CoV and cleared the virus.
- NIAID Biodefense Proteomics Research Program Contract "Identifying Targets for Therapeutic Interventions Using Proteomic Technology" has been implemented, and seven centers have been funded (http://www.niaid.nih.gov/dmid/genomes/prc/default.htm).
- A NIAID grant supplement to China's CDC and its collaborators has initiated the development of three different SARS projects: (i) development of immune correlates of protection through the study of pediatric and adult serum, stool, and cellular clinical samples obtained longitudinally from SARS patients; (ii) development of a panel of human SARS-CoV antisera that can be used to standardize diagnostic assays (in collaboration with CDC and FDA); and (iii) identification of animal reservoirs of SARS-CoV.

12.2 Recent Scientific Advances

- *Identification of SARS-CoV ORF Structures.* To date, the three-dimensional structures of seven open reading frames (ORF) structures have been elucidated, namely (i) ORF 1a/nsp3b (phosphatase); (ii) ORF 1a/nsp5 (3CL-pro); (iii) ORF 1a/nsp7 (with four-helix bundle); (iv) ORF 1a/nsp9 (RNA binding domain); (v) ORF1a/sars7a (unknown function); (vi) ORF 1a/nsp10 (contains zinc finger); and (vii) ORF 1a/nsp3d (PLpro-protease with deubiquitinating activity). Their determinations have been accomplished after cloning, expression, and x-ray crystallography (http://www.proteomicsresource.org/Meeting/May2007/presentations/2007_May_PRC2007_FSPS_SSS.pdf).
- *Inhibition, Escape, and Attenuated Growth of SARS-CoV Demonstrated with Antisense Oligomers.* Peptide-conjugated antisense morpholino oligomers (P-PMOs) were designed to bind by base pairing to specific sequences in the SARS-CoV (Tor2 strain) genome *(1)*. The P-PMOs were tested for their capacity to inhibit the production of infectious virus, as well as to probe the function of conserved viral RNA motifs and secondary structures. The P-PMOs tested were found effective when administered at any time prior to peak viral synthesis and exerted sustained antiviral effects. After several viral passages in the presence of regulatory sequence-targeted P-PMO, partially drug-resistant SARS-CoV mutants arose that grew more slowly than did wild-type SARS-CoV. These results suggested that the P-PMO compounds tested exhibited a powerful therapeutic potential against SARS-CoV.
- *Supramolecular Architecture of Severe Acute Respiratory Syndrome Coronavirus Revealed by Electron*

Cryomicroscopy. In a recent report *(2)*, the two-dimensional images of the S, M, and N proteins of SARS-CoV and two other coronaviruses at a resolution of approximately 4 nm have been described. Trimeric glycoprotein S proteins were in register with four underlying ribonuclear densities. The ribonuclear particles displayed coiled shapes when released from the viral membrane. This is the first detailed view of coronavirus ultrastructure and will help in understanding the coronavirus assembly pathway.

- *The SARS-CoV Cysteine Protease, the Papain-like Protease (PLpro), Is Identified and Structurally Characterized.* The replication of SARS-CoV and other coronaviruses is dependent on processing of replicase polyproteins by two cysteine proteases, one of which is the papain-like protease (PLpro). By using bioinformatics analyses of multiple SARS-CoVs, researchers have been able to identify a putative catalytic triad and a zinc-binding site *(3, 4)*. Furthermore, molecular modeling of PLpro suggested deubiquitinating activity. The 1.85 Å crystal structure of the PLpro catalytic core was then elucidated, demonstrating an intact zinc-binding motif, a catalytically competent active site that includes a ubiquitin-like amino terminal domain, as well as overall resemblance to known deubiquitinating enzymes. Sites within the catalytic cleft were well defined and accounted for strict substrate-recognition motifs. The detailed understanding of the SARS-CoV Plpro enzymatically active domain is critical to the development of antiviral drugs and to better understanding of the role of PLpro in the biogenesis of the SARS-CoV replicase complex.

- *Human Antibodies That Block Human and Animal SARS Viruses Identified.* An international team of investigators has identified the first human antibodies that can neutralize different strains of virus responsible for outbreaks of SARS *(5)*. The researchers used a mouse model and *in vitro* assays to test the neutralizing activity of the antibodies. The study is important because the viral strain that caused the outbreak in people in 2002 probably no longer exists in nature, and what is needed is a proof that the antibodies are effective not only against the strain of SARS virus isolated from people but also against a variety of animal strains, because animals will be a likely source for re-emergence of the SARS virus. The investigators' research into the spike glycoprotein—the part of the virus that binds and allows entry into human cells—provided the knowledge needed to identify several human antibodies against the SARS virus. In particular, the researchers identified two human antibodies that bind to a region on the SARS virus' spike glycoprotein, which is called the receptor-binding domain (RBD). One of the antibodies, called S230.15, was found in the blood of a patient who had been infected with SARS and later recovered. The second antibody, m396, was taken from a library of human antibodies the researchers developed from the blood of 10 healthy volunteers. Because humans already have immune cells that express antibodies that are very close to those that can effectively neutralize the SARS virus, m396 could be fished out of healthy volunteers. The investigators next solved the structure of m396 and its complex with the SARS RBD and showed that the antibody binds to the region on the RBD that allows the virus to attach to host cells. If the antibodies were successful in binding to the SARS RBD, they would prevent the virus from attaching to the SARS coronavirus receptor, ACE2, on the outside of human cells, effectively neutralizing it. When tested in cells in the laboratory, both antibodies potently neutralized samples of the virus from both outbreaks. The antibodies also neutralized samples of the virus taken from wild civets (a cat-like mammal in which strains of the virus were found during the outbreaks), although with somewhat lower potency. The discovery of two effective antibodies has the advantage that a newly emergent variation of the SARS coronavirus might be insensitive to neutralization with one, but still susceptible to the other. The results of the study have demonstrated novel, potential antibody-based therapeutics against SARS that could be used alone or in combination *(5)*.

References

1. Neuman, B. W., Stein, D. A., Kroeker, A. D., Churchill, M. J., Kim, A. M., Kuhn, P., Dawson, P., Moulton, H. M., Bestwick, R. K., Iversen, P. L., and Buchmeier, M. J. (2005) Inhibition, escape, and attenuated growth of severe acute respiratory syndrome coronavirus treated with antisense morpholino oligomers, *J. Virol.*, **79**(15), 9665–9676.
2. Neuman, B. W., Adair, B. D., Yoshioka, C., Quispe, J. D., Orca, G., Kuhn, P., Milligan, R. A., Yeager, M., and Buchmeier, M. J. (2006) Supramolecular architecture of severe acute respiratory syndrome coronavirus revealed by electron cryomicroscopy, *J. Virol.*, **80**(16), 7918–7928.
3. Barretto, N., Jukneliene, D., Ratia, K., Chen, Z., Mesecar, A. D., and Baker, S. C. (2005) The papain-like protease of severe acute respiratory syndrome coronavirus has deubiquinating activity, *J. Virol.*, **79**(24), 15189–15198.
4. Ratia, K., Saikatendu, K. S., Santarsiero, B. D., Barretto, N., Baker, C., Stevens, R. C., and Mesecar, A. D. (2006) Severe acute respiratory syndrome coronavirus papain-like protease: structure of a viral deubiquitinating enzyme, *Proc. Natl. Acad. Sci. U.S.A.*, **103**(15), 5717–5722.
5. Zhu, Z., Chakraborti, S., He, Y., Roberts, A., Sheahan, T., Xiao, X., Hensley, L. E., Prabakaran, P., Rockx, B., Sidorov, I. A., Corti, D., Vogel, L., Feng, Y., Kim, J., Wang, L., Baric, R., Lanzavecchia, A., Curtis, K. M., Nabel, G. J., Subbarao, K., Jiang, S., and Dimitrov, D. (2007) Potent cross-reactive neutralization of SARS coronavirus isolates by human monoclonal antibodies, *Proc. Natl. Acad. Sci. U.S.A.*, **104**(29), 12123–12128.

Chapter 13

Influenza

Influenza is a highly contagious, acute respiratory illness afflicting humans. Although influenza epidemics occur frequently, their severity varies (1). Not until 1933, when the first human influenza virus was isolated, was it possible to define with certainty which pandemics were caused by influenza viruses. In general, influenza A viruses are more pathogenic than are influenza B viruses. Influenza A virus is a zoonotic infection, and more than 100 types of influenza A viruses infect most species of birds, pigs, horses, dogs, and seals. It is believed that the 1918–1919 pandemic originated from a virulent strain of H1N1 from pigs and birds.

The natural reservoir of influenza viruses was identified as wild aquatic birds, from whose populations viruses with new surface proteins could emerge through reassortment. However, it is still not possible to predict how and when new influenza strains will emerge or how virulent a new strain will prove (2).

Currently, influenza A viruses of subtypes H1N1 and H3N2 and influenza B viruses of two antigenically distinct hemagglutinin lineages are present in human populations. The occurrence of sporadic avian influenza subtypes (e.g., H9, H7, and particularly H5) in human populations have led to widespread concerns about the possibility of an influenza pandemic.

Since 1889, at least five major pandemics have been recorded, when new hemagglutinin and/or neuraminidase subtypes have been introduced into human populations. The pandemic of 1918–1919 was by far the worst of its kind. It was followed by pandemics of decreasing severity in 1957 (Asian flu; subtype H2N2), 1968 (Hong Kong flu; subtype H3N2), and 1977 (Russian flu; subtype H1N1).

13.1 Pathophysiology

Based on the antigenic differences between their nucleoprotein (NP) and matrix (M) protein antigens, the influenza viruses are divided into types A, B, and C (1). The influenza A viruses are further divided into subtypes.

The influenza viruses are single-stranded RNA viruses and share structural and biological similarities. The viral RNA core consists of 8 gene segments surrounded by a coat of 10 (influenza A) or 11 (influenza B) proteins. Immunologically, the most important surface proteins are hemagglutinin and neuraminidase, as the influenza viruses are typed on the basis of these proteins. For example, influenza A subtype H3N2 expresses hemagglutinin 3 and neuraminidase 2. The most prevalent human influenza A strains are H1N1 and H3N2.

Although the morphologic characteristics of the influenza viruses are a genetic trait, the spherical morphology appears to be dominant on passage in chicken embryos or tissue culture systems. The most distinct feature of the influenza virions is the presence of a layer of spikes projecting radially outward over the surface. The surface spikes are of two distinct types, corresponding with the hemagglutinin and neuraminidase components of the virus.

13.1.1 Hemagglutinin

The hemagglutinin (HA) is the surface glycoprotein, which accounts for approximately 25% of viral protein and is distributed evenly on the virion surface. It is responsible for the virus's binding to the host receptor, internalization of the virus, and subsequent membrane-fusion events within the endosomal pathway in the infected cell. Furthermore, HA is also the most abundant antigen on the viral surface and harbors the primary neutralizing epitopes for antibodies (1).

Structurally, HA is a glycoprotein consisting of two polypeptide chains, HA1 and HA2. HA1 and HA2 are linked by a single disulfide bond, and each HA "spike" contains three of these HA1 and HA2 chains. Furthermore, HA contains up to seven oligosaccharide chains (six in HA1 and one in HA2) linked to asparagine. The majority of these carbohydrate chains are on the lateral surface of the trimer. No obligatory function has been assigned to these side chains (1).

V. St. Georgiev, *National Institute of Allergy and Infectious Diseases, NIH: Impact on Global Health*, vol. 2,
DOI 10.1007/978-1-60327-297-1_13, © Humana Press, a part of Springer Science+Business Media, LLC 2009

13.1.2 Neuraminidase

The neuraminidase (NA) exists as a mushroom-shaped spike containing a hydrophobic region by which it is embedded in the viral membrane in the opposite way to the HA. NA is the second subtype-specific glycoprotein on the influenza virion and is composed of a single polypeptide chain *(1)*. It is not evenly distributed on the virion surface but rather found in patches. The principal biologic role of NA protein of the influenza A virus is the cleavage of the terminal sialic acid residues that are receptors of the virus's HA protein. Removal of these residues from the surface of infected cells and from newly formed viruses will prevent the budding viruses from clumping to each other or to the cell surfaces. In addition, the ability to cleave sialic acid is also thought to help the virus to penetrate mucus *(3)*.

Because NA functions largely in the release of newly formed viral particles, antibodies against it do not prevent initial infection. However, they sharply limit its spread and therefore, in humans, selection favors NA variants with mutations that hinder antibody recognition *(antigenic shift) (3)*.

13.1.3 Nucleoprotein

The nucleoprotein (NP) is one of the type-specific antigens of influenza viruses that distinguish among types A, B, and C viruses *(1)*. The nucleoproteins are basic proteins that constitute the backbone of the helical internal complex and have a putative role in transcription and replication. During infection, the NP accumulates in the nucleus, and karyophilic sequences have been identified that are partially conserved among the influenza A, B, and C viruses.

13.1.4 Matrix Proteins (M)

The RNA segment 7 of influenza A viruses codes for two proteins M1 and M2 *(1)*. The basic organization of RNA segment 7 is present in all influenza A and B viruses sequenced.

The M1 protein is a virion structural protein that is intimately associated with the lipid bilayer. It is believed to be a multifunction protein having a role in the downregulation of the activity of the virion-associated transcriptase. It is located in the nucleus, cytoplasm, and plasma membrane of infected cells. Passively transferred monoclonal antibodies to the M1 protein did not confer resistance to infection.

The M2 protein of influenza A virus is an integral membrane protein that is expressed on the surface of infected cells with an extracellular domain *(1)*. The M2 protein is present in high copy number in infected cells and thus appears to be actively excluded from the virions.

13.2 Influenza A (H1N1) Pandemic of 1918–1919

In just 8 months, the 1918–1919 pandemic known as the "Spanish influenza" killed between 20 million and 40 million people worldwide *(2)*. The virus causing this influenza pandemic was not isolated at the time. However, its enhanced severity, multiple waves in just 1 year, and its predilection for the young and healthy all suggested that this influenza pandemic was unique. As the most deadly influenza virus ever experienced, the 1918 strain offers a unique opportunity to understand the connection between genotype and virulence *(2)*.

From preserved autopsy samples of two U.S. soldiers and from the frozen lungs of an Inuit woman, fragments of the deadly virus have been isolated, copied, and analyzed. The strains from these three cases have been named: (i) A/South Carolina/1/18; (ii) A/New York/1/18; and (iii) A/Brevig Mission/1/18. For the first time, it has become possible to test hypotheses about where the 1918 influenza virus came from and what made it so deadly *(2,3)*.

Advances in molecular biology techniques have allowed scientists to get a closer look at the virus that caused the 1918 pandemic *(3–7)*. *It was defined as influenza virus A H1N1 strain.*

13.2.1 Structural Elucidation of the 1918 Influenza A Hemagglutinin

The crystal structure of the 1918 influenza HA has been elucidated from a second human subtype (H1) derived from reassembling the extinct 1918 influenza virus *(8, 9)*. In addition, two closely related HAs in complex with receptor analogues have also been determined *(9)*. These two related HAs may explain how the 1918 HA, while retaining receptor binding site amino acids characteristic of an avian precursor HA, was able to bind human receptors and how, as a consequence, the virus was able to spread in human populations *(9)*.

The primary event in influenza infection is the binding of the virus to the host receptor. The crystal structure of HA has shown that its receptor-binding site is situated in a shallow pocket in the membrane-distal HA1 domain in each subunit of the HA trimer *(8, 9)*.

The nature of the receptor's sialic acid linkage to the vicinal galactose is the primary determinant in lung epithelial cells that differentiates avian viruses from mammalian. Sialic acids are usually found in either α2,3- or α2,6-linkages to galactose, which is the predominant penultimate sugar of the *N*-linked carbohydrate side chains. The binding preference of a given HA for one or other of these linkage types correlates with the species specificity for infection (*species barrier*). Thus, avian viruses preferentially bind to receptors with an α2,3-linkage to galactose, whereas human-adapted viruses are specific for the α2,6-linkage *(9)*. For example, the HAs of all 15 antigenic subtypes found in avian influenza viruses bind preferentially to sialic acid in α2,3-linkage, and it is this form of the sialosaccharide that predominates in the avian enteric tract where these viruses replicate. Human viruses of the H1, H2, and H3 subtypes that are known to have caused pandemics in 1918, 1957, and 1968, respectively, recognize α2,6-linked sialic acid, the major form found on cells of the human respiratory tract *(9)*.

Because an avian origin has been proposed for the HAs of swine and human viruses, changes in the binding specificity of HAs will be required for cross-species transfer.

13.2.2   Characterization of the 1918 Influenza Neuraminidase Gene

The complete coding sequence of the 1918 influenza virus A neuraminidase gene has been determined and compared with other N1 subtype NA genes, including nine N1 newly sequenced strains *(3)*. In general, the 1918 NA shares many sequences and structural characteristics with avian strains, including the conserved active site, wild-type stalk length, glycosylation sites, and antigenic sites. Phylogenetically, the 1918 NA gene appears to be intermediate between mammals and birds, suggesting that it was introduced into mammals just before the 1918 pandemic *(3)*.

The active catalytic site of the NA protein consists of a pocket in the top surface of each subunit of the tetrameric protein. The pocket contains 15 charged amino acids that are conserved in all influenza A viruses *(3)*.

13.2.3   Characterization of the 1918 Influenza Virus Polymerase Genes

The influenza A viral heterotrimeric polymerase complex (PA, PB1, PB2) is known to be involved in many aspects of viral replication and to interact with host factors, thereby having a role in host specificity. Recently, an additional small open reading frame has been identified that codes for a peptide (PB1-F2) that is thought to play a role in the virus-induced cell death. It is not yet clear how the polymerase complex must change to adapt to a new host. However, a single amino acid change in PB2, E627K, was shown to be important for adaptation in mammals.

The polymerase protein sequences from the 1918 human influenza virus differ from avian consensus sequences at only a small number of amino acids; that is consistent with the hypothesis that they derived from an avian source shortly before the 1918 pandemic. However, when compared with avian sequences, the nucleotide sequences of the 1918 polymerase genes have more synonymous differences than expected, suggesting evolutionary distance from known avian strains *(10)*.

In 2005, the sequence and phylogenetic analyses of the complete genome of the 1918 influenza virus were determined *(10)*. The data suggested that the 1918 virus was not a reassortant virus like those of the 1957 and 1968 pandemics. More likely, the 1918 virus was an entirely avian-like virus that had adapted to humans.

One interesting feature found in the polymerase complex of the 1918 virus and subsequent human isolates as well was the presence of a Lys residue at position 627. This residue has been implicated in host adaptation and has been previously shown to be critical for high pathogenicity in mice infected with the 1997 H5N1 virus *(11)*.

13.2.4   Virulence of the 1918 Influenza A Virus

One of the characteristics of the 1918 influenza pandemic was its unusual virulence, reflected in the dramatic increase in the severity of the illness and the prevalence of pneumonic complications *(2,3)*. The virulence of the influenza viruses is a complicated function of the genetic characteristics of the virus itself, the immune status of the infected person, and the dose and route of transmission. The severity of the 1918 pandemic suggested that both the HA and NA were *antigenically novel* as supported by sequence and phylogenetic analyses of both 1918 HA and NA proteins *(5)*, as well as that the virus had not circulated widely in the human population before spring 1918 *(3)*.

The relationship between virulence and the genetic structure of the influenza virus is complex. There have been several examples where simple changes in a single gene resulted in dramatic changes in virulence. Thus, one of these changes is the insertion of basic amino acids in the HA cleavage site, which will allow the virus to grow in many tissues outside its normal host cells. Although this change has been found in the H5 and H7 subtypes in birds, it *was not found* in the 1918 HA *(5)*. In another change observed in the NA gene, the loss of a glycosylation site at amino acid 146 in WSN/33 contributed to making the virus exceptionally virulent as well as neurotropic in mice. This change was also *not observed* in the 1918 virus strain *(3)*.

13.3 Asian Influenza A Pandemics of 1957 and 1968

Although milder than the 1918 Spanish H1N1 influenza pandemic, both the 1957 Asian influenza H2N2 pandemic and the 1968 Hong Kong influenza H3N2 pandemic caused significant morbidity and mortality worldwide (1,2).

The 1957 influenza pandemic was caused by a reassortant virus that was derived from the HA (H2), NA (N2), and PB1 (polymerase basic protein 1) genes from an avian influenza virus infecting ducks and the remaining gene segment from the previously circulating human H1N1 virus (12–14).

The H3N2 virus that caused the 1968 pandemic consisted of avian HA (H3) and PB1 genes in a background of other internal protein genes of the human H2N2 virus that was circulating at the time (12–14). The presence of an avian HA H3 glycoprotein made the reassortant virus antigenically novel to humans, and it spread in the susceptible human population causing a pandemic (12, 13).

Studies on the origin and evolutionary pathways of the PB1 genes of influenza A viruses responsible for the 1957 and 1968 human pandemics and the variable or conserved region of the PB1 protein have shown that the evolutionary tree constructed from nucleotide sequences suggested that (i) the PB1 gene of the 1957 human pandemic strain, A/Singapore/1/57 (H2N2), was probably introduced from avian species and was maintained in humans until 1968; (ii) in the 1968 pandemic strain, A/NT/60/68 (H3N2), the PB1 gene was not derived from the previously circulating virus in humans but probably from another avian virus; and (iii) a current human H3N2 virus inherited the PB1 gene from an A/NT/60/68-like virus (12). Nucleotide sequence analysis also showed that the avian PB1 gene was introduced into pigs. Hence, transmission of the PB1 gene from avian to mammalian species is a relatively frequent event. Comparative analysis of deduced amino acid sequences disclosed highly conserved regions in PB1 proteins, which may be key structures required for PB1 activities (12).

The RNA of the human influenza virus Singapore (H2N2) strain has been labeled *in vivo* by phosphorus-32 and separated by polyacrylamide gel electrophoresis into eight segments, which were correlated to the corresponding gene functions and/or proteins (2). The base sequence homology between the individual genes (segments) of the H2N2 virus and those of different influenza A strains has been determined by molecular hybridization. Segments 1, 5, 7, and 8 of the Singapore strain exhibit a base sequence homology of almost 100% compared with those of the FM1 strain (H1N1), whereas the homology between the other segments was significantly lower (24% to 76%). For the Singapore and Hong Kong (H3N2) strains, all segments except that coding for the HA (24%) exhibit a homology close to 100%. The ^{32}P-labeled segment 4 (HA gene) of the avian influenza A strain duck Ukraine (Hav7Neg2) showed a homology of 92% to Hong Kong, whereas the homology of at least two other segments was significantly lower. These results were interpreted as an indication that the H2N2 subtype is derived from the H1N1 subtype by a recombination event retaining four H1N1 segments, whereas the other four segments were gained from another yet unknown strain. The H3N2 subtype is presumably derived from a H2N2 subtype, retaining seven segments of the H2N2 subtype, whereas the gene coding for the HA is obtained from the duck Ukraine or another highly related strain (13).

13.4 Avian Influenza A (H5N1)

An unprecedented epizootic avian influenza A (H5N1) virus that is highly pathogenic has crossed the species barrier in Asia to cause human fatalities and thus poses an increased threat of pandemic (15). In 1997, an avian subtype, H5N1, was first described in Hong Kong. The infection was confirmed in only 18 people, but 6 of them died. Subsequent, although sporadic, cases of avian (bird flu) influenza continued to be recorded, mainly in southern China, but also in other regions of Southeast Asia. The H5N1 influenza, in nearly all cases, has been transmitted to humans from birds. Other routes of transmission include possibly environment-to-humans, and limited, nonsustained, human-to-human transmission. Transmission to felids has been observed by feeding raw infected chicken to tigers and leopards in zoos in Thailand and to domestic cats under experimental conditions. Transmission between felids has been found under such conditions.

Because of the poultry outbreaks and bird-to-human transmission, hundreds of new cases of avian influenza have been reported, stretching from Southeast Asia (mainly China, Vietnam, Thailand, and Indonesia) through Mongolia, Kazakhstan, and Russia to Turkey, raising the concern that a slight mutation may convert subtype H5N1 into a strain that would be easily transmitted from human to human. To date, human-to-human transmission of influenza A virus (H5N1) has been suggested in several household clusters (11) and in one case of apparent child-to-mother transmission (16). There has been a WHO report suggesting that local virus H5N1 strains (northern Vietnam) *may be adapting to humans* (17) (http://www.who.int/csr/resources/publications/influenza/WHO_CDS_CSR_GIP_2005_7/en/). However, epidemiologic and virologic studies will be needed to confirm these findings.

13.4.1 Pathogenesis

Studies of isolates of avian influenza A (H5N1) from patients in 1997 have shown that the virulence factors included (i) the highly cleavable hemagglutinin that can be activated by multiple cellular proteases; (ii) a specific substitution in the polymerase basic protein 2 (Glu627Lys) that enhances replication; and (iii) a substitution in nonstructural protein 1 (Asp92Glu) that confers increased resistance to inhibition by interferons and tumor necrosis factor α (TNF-α) *in vitro* and prolonged replication in swine, as well as greater elaboration of cytokines, particularly TNF-α, in human macrophages exposed to the virus *(15)*.

Since 1997, studies of influenza A (H5N1) have indicated that these viruses continue to evolve, including (i) changes in antigenicity and internal gene constellations; (ii) an expended host range of avian species and the ability to infect felids; (iii) enhanced pathogenicity in experimentally infected mice and felids, in which they caused systemic infections; and (iv) increased environmental stability *(15)*.

Phylogenetic analyses have demonstrated that the Z genotype has become dominant *(18)* and that the virus has evolved into two distinct clades, one encompassing isolates from Cambodia, Laos, Malaysia, and Vietnam, and the other isolates from China, Indonesia, Japan, and South Korea *(17)*. Recently, a separate cluster of isolates has appeared in northern Vietnam and in Thailand, which included variable changes near the receptor-binding site and one fewer arginine residue in the polybasic cleavage site of the hemagglutinin *(12)*. However, the importance of these genetic and biologic changes with respect to human epidemiology or virulence is uncertain.

13.4.2 Host Immune Responses to Avian Virus A (H5N1)

The relatively low frequency of influenza A (H5N1) illness in humans despite widespread exposure to infected poultry has suggested that the *species barrier* to acquisition of this avian virus is substantial. Clusters of cases in family members may be caused by common exposures, although the genetic factors that may affect a host's susceptibility to disease will require more studies *(15)*.

The innate immune responses to influenza A (H5N1) may contribute to disease pathogenesis. In the 1997 outbreaks, elevated blood levels of interleukin-6, TNF-α, interferon-γ, and soluble interleukin-2 receptor were observed in individual patients *(19)*, and in patients in 2003, elevated levels of the chemokines interferon-inducible protein 10, mono-

cyte chemoattractant protein 1, and monokine induced by interferon-γ were found 3 to 8 days after the onset of illness *(20)*. Recently, plasma levels of inflammatory mediators (interleukin-6, interleukin-8, interleukin-1β, and monocyte chemoattractant protein 1) were found to be higher among patients who died than among those who survived, and the average levels of plasma interferon-α were about three times as high among patients with avian influenza A who died as among healthy controls *(15)*. Among survivors, specific humoral immune responses to influenza A (H5N1) are detectable by microneutralization assay 10 to14 days after the onset of illness.

13.4.3 Clinical Features

The clinical spectrum of influenza A (H5N1) in humans has been based on descriptions of hospitalized patients *(15)*. The frequencies of milder illness, subclinical infections, and atypical presentations (e.g., encephalopathy, gastroenteritis) have not been determined, but case reports indicated that each have occurred. Most of the hospitalized patients were previously healthy young children or adults.

Incubation. The incubation period of the avian influenza A (H5N1) may be longer compared with those of other known human influenzas—in most cases it is within 2 to 4 days after exposure but occasionally up to 8 days *(15)*. The case-to-case intervals in household clusters have generally been 2 to 5 days with a upper limit between 8 and 17 days (possibly resulting from unrecognized exposure to infected animals or environmental sources).

Initial Symptoms. Most patients have initial symptoms of high fever (38°C or higher) and an influenza-like illness with lower respiratory tract symptoms *(21)* (http://www.who.int/csr/disease/avian_influenza/guidelines/Guidelines_Clinical%20Management_H5N1_rev.pdf). Upper respiratory tract symptoms are manifested only occasionally. Also, unlike patients with infections caused by avian influenza A (H7N7) viruses, patients with avian influenza A (H5N1) rarely have developed conjunctivitis *(22)*. Diarrhea, vomiting, abdominal pain, pleuritic pain, and bleeding from the nose and gums have also been reported early in the course of illness. Watery diarrhea may precede the respiratory manifestations by up to 1 week *(15)*.

Clinical Course and Management. Lower respiratory tract manifestations develop early in the course of the disease—respiratory distress, tachypnea, and inspiratory crackles are common. Sputum production is variable and occasionally bloody. Nearly all patients have clinically apparent pneumonia. Progression to respiratory failure has been associated with diffuse, bilateral, ground-glass infiltrates and manifestations of acute respiratory distress syndrome (ARDS).

Multiorgan failure with signs of renal dysfunction, and sometimes cardiac compromise including cardiac dilatation and supraventricular tachyarrhythmias, have been common *(15)*.

Most hospitalized patients with avian influenza A (H5N1) have required ventilatory support within 48 hours after admission, as well as intensive care for multiorgan failure and sometimes hypotension. Empirical treatment with broad-spectrum antibiotics, antiviral agents—alone or with corticosteroids—has been tried in most patients, although their effects have not been rigorously assessed *(15)*. Early initiation of antiviral drugs appears to be beneficial *(11)*.

Mortality. Death has occurred an average of 9 or 10 days after the onset of illness (range, 6 to 30 days), and most patients have died of progressive respiratory failure *(15)*. The mortality rate among hospitalized patients has been high although the overall rate has probably been much lower *(17)*. In contrast with 1997, when most deaths occurred among patients older than 13 years of age, recent infections have caused high rates of death among infants and young children (89% among children younger than 15 years of age in Thailand).

13.5 Avian Influenza A (H9N2)

Since the late 1990s, several cases of human infections with the avian influenza A (H9N2) virus have been reported *(23)*. However, despite concerns after the initial cases of human infections with the H9N2 strain occurred, no virulent outbreak of human H9N2 infection did occur. As with influenza A (H5N1) virus outbreaks, there has been considerable apprehension that a virulent H9N2 strain might still mutate to allow human-to-human infection and that such a strain might also possess the triad of infectivity, lethality, and transmissibility.

13.5.1 *Molecular Characterization of Avian Influenza A (H9N2) Virus*

The avian H5N1 influenza virus that was transmitted from poultry to humans in 1997 and caused high mortality in both species is unusual in having a large proportion of amino acid substitutions in all gene products except in the surface antigen, thus suggesting that the H5N1 virus may be a *reassortant (24)*. Phylogenetic and antigenic analyses of the H9N2 and H5N1 viruses and a quail H9N2 virus, all isolated from Hong Kong, provided evidence that the H5N1 and H9N2 influenza viruses were indeed reassortants, and that the quail H9N2 virus may have been the internal gene donor *(25,26)*. The reassortment between N5N1 and N9N2 had occurred

prior to the human infection by H5N1 in 1997. Further results have indicated the presence of multiple lineages of H9N2 viruses in Asia and at least three distinguishable subgroups in Hong Kong poultry *(25)*, as well as that H9N2 influenza viruses possessing H5N1-like internal genomes continue to circulate in poultry in southeastern China *(27)*.

In another study *(28)*, the H9N2 influenza viruses were found to have receptor specificity similar to that of human H3N2 viruses. In addition, the neuraminidase of poultry H9N2 viruses has mutations in its hemadsorbing site, a characteristic resembling that of human H2N2 and N3N2 viruses, but differing from that of other avian viruses. These *peculiar features* of the surface glycoproteins of H9N2 viruses from Hong Kong suggest an *enhanced propensity for introduction into humans* and emphasize the importance of poultry in the zoonotic transmission of influenza viruses.

13.6 NIAID and Influenza Research

The influenza infection (flu) is a contagious respiratory illness that can cause mild to severe illness, which at times can lead to death. The best way to prevent influenza is by getting a flu vaccination each year. According to statistics by the CDC, every year in the United States, on average: (i) 5% to 20% of the population will contract flu; (ii) more than 200,000 people are hospitalized from flu complications; and (iii) about 36,000 people die from flu *(29)* (http://www. cdc.gov/flu/keyfacts.htm). Recent studies have revealed that children 6 to 23 months of age have a substantially higher risk for influenza-associated morbidity *(30,31)*. Despite the high annual rates of influenza in children, preventive vaccines are given infrequently *(27)*. For the influenza season 2003–2004, 92 pediatric deaths were reported to the CDC (http://www.cdc.gov/mmwr/preview/mmwrhtml/mm5253a4.htm).

Upon recommendations of the Blue Ribbon Panel on Influenza Research *(32)*, major goals and objectives of the NIAID's Influenza Program involve research in the following areas (http://www3.niaid.nih.gov/about/directors/congress/2004/02122004.htm):

- *Basic Biology.* NIAID supports many basic research projects aimed at understanding how the influenza virus replicates, interacts with the host, stimulates an immune response, and evolves into new strains. Results from these studies lay the foundation for the design of new antiviral drugs, diagnostics, and vaccines.
- *Antiviral Drugs.* NIAID currently supports the identification, development, and evaluation of new antiviral drugs against influenza, including the screening of new drug candidates to see if they have activity against the virus

both in laboratory cells and in animals. NIAID is also focused on developing novel broad-spectrum therapeutics intended to work against many influenza virus strains; some of these target viral entry into human cells, whereas others specifically attack and degrade the viral genome. Development and evaluation of a combination antiviral regimen against potential pandemic influenza strains is also now under way.

- *Diagnostics.* NIAID supports the development of rapid, ultrasensitive devices to detect influenza virus infection. Although early in development, these devices will allow detection of newly emerging viral mutants and discrimination between different antigenic subtypes.

- *Surveillance and Epidemiology.* The threat from influenza, like virtually all emerging and re-emerging infectious disease threats, is global in scope. For this reason, in recent years NIAID has expanded its activities in other countries. Through a contract for pandemic influenza preparedness, NIAID supports a long-standing program in Hong Kong to detect the emergence of influenza viruses with pandemic potential in animals. Under this program, scientists had detected the re-emergence of highly pathogenic H5N1 avian strains in this area in 2002 and 2003 and were instrumental in the early detection and characterization of the SARS coronavirus in 2003. This approach has underscored the concept that research on one type of infectious disease often supports or can be applied to research on other types of infectious diseases, whether newly emerging, re-emerging, or deliberately introduced.

- *Vaccine Development and Evaluation.* Because influenza is so easily transmitted, effective vaccines are essential to controlling annual influenza epidemics. The current egg-based system used to produce licensed influenza vaccines—despite being reliable for more than 40 years—can still be improved. Limitations of the current system include (i) a lengthy manufacturing process; (ii) the need to select which virus strains will be in the vaccine at least 6 months in advance of the influenza season; (iii) the need to produce nearly 90 million doses of a new influenza vaccine each year; and (iv) the need for hundreds of millions of fertilized chicken eggs to manufacture the vaccine. The early decision about which strains to include in the influenza vaccine will not always be correct, and the long lead time required to produce the vaccine makes midstream corrective action impossible. Additional limitations may also include allergenicity of eggs in some individuals, and the inability to use eggs for propagating viruses lethal to chickens. NIAID is currently supporting several research projects aimed at developing vaccines that can be manufactured more rapidly, are more broadly cross-protective, and are more effective. The use of reverse genetics—a genetic tool developed by

NIAID-supported scientists—holds the promise of more rapid generation of high-yielding vaccine candidates that match the anticipated epidemic strain. Reverse genetics can also be used to turn highly pathogenic influenza viruses into vaccine candidates more suitable for manufacturing of vaccine by removing or modifying certain virulence genes; laboratories around the world are using the technique to prepare vaccine candidates against the H5N1 viruses emerging in Asia. NIAID also is funding the development of new influenza vaccine technologies. Recently, NIAID supported a Phase II clinical trial of a new influenza vaccine produced in a cell culture system as an alternative to manufacturing the vaccine in eggs. Another approach has focused on improving the effectiveness of current inactivated virus vaccines by giving increasing doses of influenza vaccine to elderly individuals, the population that frequently accounts for up to 90% of influenza deaths each year in the United States. NIAID is also funding the development of new technologies for the production of influenza vaccines; these involve DNA-based approaches and broadly protective vaccines based on influenza virus proteins that are shared by multiple strains of the influenza virus.

13.6.1 Research Programmatic Developments

- *The Broad Agency Announcement (BAA).* BAA was issued in 2006 to continue and to expand influenza surveillance activities, such as the *Pandemic Preparedness in Asia* contract held by the St. Jude Children's Research Hospital in Memphis (N01-AI-95357), to carry out surveillance and characterization of avian influenza viruses with pandemic potential in Hong Kong, Thailand, Vietnam, and Indonesia.

- *Vaccine Development and Optimization.* Major accomplishments of the program include:

  (i) NIAID's continuing support for the development of novel vaccination strategies for the elderly. Thus, a study conducted to assess the immunogenicity and reactogenicity of a current U.S. vaccine formulation at increased doses in the elderly population (65 years and older; n=202) has shown that at the increased dose (60 μg), higher levels were observed for the mean serum hemagglutination inhibition and neutralizing antibody levels (44% to 71% and 54% to 79%, respectively) compared with the standard dose (15 μg) of the vaccine *(33)*. Increasing the antigen content of inactivated vaccines may provide a straightforward approach to improving protection in the elderly.

(ii) In 2006, a multicenter clinical trial to evaluate the safety and immunogenicity of trivalent inactivated influenza vaccine (produced by CSL, Ltd.) was completed (DMID-06-0016) (http://vaccines.stanford.edu/completed_studies.html).

(iii) In 2006, NIAID initiated or completed a number of multicenter Phase I/II clinical trials to study the safety and immunogenicity of H5N1 A/Vietnam/1203/2004 inactivated influenza vaccines from pharmaceutical companies (Sanofi-Pasteur, Novartis/Chiron, and Baxter). The studies, carried out in children, adults, and the elderly, were aimed at investigating dose ranges, routes of administration, and the use of adjuvants (e.g., aluminum hydroxide, MF59) (http://www.clinicaltrials.gov). Results from the Sanofi-Pasteur vaccine trial showed that the vaccine was well tolerated, and 54% of the subjects (n = 99) receiving the higher dose (90 μg) achieved a neutralizing antibody response to the vaccine at serum dilutions of 1:40 or greater, whereas only 22% of the subjects (n = 100) who received the 15-μg dose developed a similar response to the vaccine *(34)*.

(iv) Results from a Phase I randomized, double-blind clinical trial to assess the safety and immunogenicity of a 2-dose schedule (administered on days 0 and 28) of 4 dose levels (3.73, 7.5, 15, and 30 μg hemagglutinin) of inactivated influenza A/chicken/Hong Kong/G9/97 (H9N2) vaccine with and without adjuvant have shown that the combination of MF59 adjuvant with a subunit vaccine was associated with improved immune responses to the H9N2 virus *(35)*. The adjuvanted vaccine was immunogenic even after a single dose, raising the possibility that 1-dose vaccination strategy may be attainable with the use of adjuvanted vaccine.

(v) NIAID's Vaccine Research Center (VRC) has undertaken an initiative to develop a protective vaccine that is effective against multiple influenza strains (see Section 13.8). The proposed approach is to incorporate both conserved and variable genes into DNA and adenoviral (AdV) vectors that can be readily produced by existing methodologies. In particular, the VRC has been involved in developing three new vaccines, each comprising a single plasmid DNA encoding hemagglutinin protein from H1N1, H3N2, and H5N1 subtypes isolated from recent human outbreaks of influenza. Adenoviral construct expressing the same inserts are also being constructed. In addition, protein subunit vaccines based on production from insect and mammalian cells are being developed and tested.

- *Surveillance and Influenza Genetics.* In 2004, NIAID initiated the *Genome Sequencing Project*, which is providing influenza sequence data, thereby enabling scientists to further study how influenza viruses evolve, spread, and cause disease. To this end, in 2006, the *Global Initiative on Sharing Avian Influenza Data (GISAID)*, an international consortium to promote data sharing, was created. By March 2006, 1,553 human and avian isolates were completely sequenced and released to the public (GenBank).

- *Immunity to Influenza.* NIAID is currently involved in supporting a robust program that will further broaden the knowledge regarding immunity to influenza, as follows:

  (i) *NIH Tetramer Facility at Emory University.* Since 1999, the tetramer facility has prepared nearly 2,400 unique tetramers, of which 459 have been directly related to monitoring T-cell functions against infectious diseases; of those, 45 tetramers were produced specifically for influenza-related studies.

  (ii) *Immune Epitope Database and Analysis Resource (IEDB) at La Jolla Institute of Allergy and Immunology.* In 2005, IEDB became publicly available (http://www.immuneepitope.org). The IEDB contains extensively curated information from the published literature on antibody and T-cell epitopes, as well as tools to predict antibody and T-cell epitopes or visualization/mapping of epitopes onto known protein structures. There are currently 17,868 unique epitopes within the database, including all published influenza antibody and T-cell epitopes.

  (iii) *Modeling Pulmonary Immunity.* This program, conducted at the University of Pittsburgh, involves analysis of innate and adaptive immunity in the lungs and draining lymph nodes of mice (various ages) either infected with or vaccinated against influenza viruses. The computational models to be developed may be used to simulate human innate responses to adjuvants or immune modulators, as a method for screening novel compounds against influenza.

  (iv) *Biodefense Immune Modeling.* Scientists from the University of Rochester will conduct a comprehensive examination of B- and T-cell–mediated immunity to influenza vaccination in healthy adults and influenza A infection or vaccination in mouse model systems. The major goal of these studies is to produce computational models capable of predicting human immune responses to natural variants or genetically engineered influenza viruses and can be used to test novel vaccine strategies or immune modulators *in silico*, prior to further testing in animal models and humans.

(v) *Pathways in the Interferon Signaling Cascade.* This NIAID-supported program is aimed at creating computational models to decipher the type 1 interferon signaling networks in primary human dendritic cells that are modulated by viral proteins.

13.6.2 Centers of Excellence for Influenza Research and Surveillance

NIAID has had a long history of supporting research activities to provide more effective approaches to controlling influenza virus infections. These activities include both basic and applied research on the influenza virus basic biology and replication, pathogenesis, immunology, epidemiology, and clinical research to develop new and improved diagnostics, antiviral drugs, and vaccines. Because of the ever-present threat of an influenza pandemic, NIAID has initiated a program to establish NIAID *Centers of Excellence for Influenza Research and Surveillance (CEIRS)* to support the research agenda of the *HHS Pandemic Influenza Plan*. The overall goal of this program is to provide the government with the information and public health tools and strategies needed to control and lessen the impact of epidemic influenza and the increasing threat of pandemic influenza.

The activities undertaken by the NIAID Centers of Excellence for Influenza Research and Surveillance will lay the groundwork for developing new and improved control measures for emerging and re-emerging influenza viruses, including determining the prevalence of avian influenza viruses in animals in close contact with humans, understanding how influenza viruses evolve, adapt, and transmit, and identifying immunologic factors that determine disease outcome. In the event of an urgent public health emergency involving the emergence and rapid spread of an influenza pandemic in humans, the network of centers will also develop and implement a *NIAID Pandemic Public Health Research Response Plan*.

Each of the NIAID Centers of Excellence for Influenza Research and Surveillance has a focus on one or both of the following research areas:

- *Research Area 1: Animal Influenza Surveillance.* This is designed to conduct prospective international and/or domestic surveillance of animal influenza for the rapid detection and characterization of influenza viruses with pandemic potential.
- *Research Area 2: Pathogenesis and Host Response Research.* This is designed to enhance understanding of the molecular, ecologic, and environmental factors that influence pathogenesis, transmission, and evolution of influenza viruses, as well as to characterize the protective immune response.

On March 30, 2007, NIAID awarded six Centers of Excellence for Influenza Research and Surveillance to the following institutions:

- Emory University: Research Area 2: Pathogenesis and Host Response Research
- Mount Sinai School of Medicine: Research Area 2: Pathogenesis and Host Response Research
- St. Jude Children's Research Hospital: Research Areas 1 and 2: Animal Influenza Surveillance; and Pathogenesis and Host Response Research
- University of California, Los Angeles: Research Area 1: Animal Influenza Surveillance
- University of Minnesota: Research Area 1: Animal Influenza Surveillance
- University of Rochester: Research Area 2: Pathogenesis and Host Response Research

13.6.3 NIAID Involvement in International Influenza Research

(i) NIAID has awarded two contracts for the production of inactivated H5N1 vaccine to Aventis Pasteur (Swiftwater, Pennsylvania) and Chiron (Liverpool, United Kingdom).

(ii) NIAID is also supporting the production of inactivated H9N2 vaccine manufactured with and without adjuvant by Chiron (Sienna, Italy).

(iii) *Clinical Trials of Pandemic Influenza Vaccine.* In 2003, NIAID conducted a Phase I/II clinical trial to evaluate increasing doses of inactivated influenza vaccine made by using the H9N2 virus isolated in 1999 from two infected children in Hong Kong. Immunogenicity assays have been generated and data analysis is ongoing. The preliminary data showed that the vaccine was well tolerated.

In 2004, NIAID expanded its "Pandemic Preparedness in Asia" contract to St. Jude Children's Research Hospital (N01-AI-95357). Activities conducted under this expansion include (i) establishing animal influenza surveillance sites in Asia; (ii) generating high-yielding vaccine candidates against influenza strains with pandemic potential accompanying reagents; (iii) supporting an international animal surveillance training course in Hong Kong; and (iv) studying newly emerging influenza strains infecting swine in the United States. In 2004, NIAID launched the *Influenza Genome Sequencing Project*, which will rapidly provide influenza sequence data to the scientific community to enable further studies of how the influenza viruses evolve, spread, and cause disease, and which may ultimately lead to improved methods of treatment and prevention.

13.7 Influenza Vaccine Research

During the past several years, there have been increasing reports of direct transmission of avian influenza viruses to humans (36–38). Furthermore, the continuing outbreaks of H5N1 influenza virus infections in avian species and humans in several countries (36,39,40) has emphasized the considerable threat posed by highly pathogenic avian influenza (HPAI) and low pathogenic avian influenza LPAI viruses to human health (14). This, coupled with the difficulty to predict which subtype of avian influenza virus will cause the next human pandemic means that an ideal vaccine would elicit an immune response that protects the host from infection with a broad range of influenza viruses from the same or different subtypes (14).

The HA and NA glycoproteins of influenza viruses undergo genetic and antigenic variation to escape the immune response (14,41,42). Whereas the presence of neutralizing antibodies specific for the HA glycoprotein at systemic or mucosal sites of infection would provide immediate protection against infection with influenza viruses, the clearance of human influenza viruses depends mainly on cell-mediated immunity (43). Although antibodies specific for the NA glycoprotein do not neutralize infectivity, they restrict virus replication by preventing the release of new virus particles, a process that requires viral NA proteins. Therefore, antibodies specific for NA can decrease the severity of the disease (44, 45). Epitopes recognized by cytotoxic T lymphocytes (CTLs) are present on NP, PB2, and PA proteins of human influenza viruses. Therefore, if a virus with a new HA and/or NA glycoprotein emerges in the human population, cell-mediated immunity directed against the highly conserved internal proteins could have a role in protection at the time of a pandemic (14). The principle underlying the currently licensed vaccines against human influenza viruses is the induction of protective antibodies specific for the HA glycoprotein of the predicted epidemic strain. The concentration of HA glycoprotein in licensed, inactivated virus vaccines for seasonal influenza is standardized, but the concentration of NA glycoprotein is not standardized (14).

Although most influenza vaccines are designed to induce HA-specific antibody responses to protect the host from infection, the biology of avian influenza viruses presents several unique challenges compared with human influenza viruses. These challenges include the presence of different subtypes of HA and NA glycoproteins and the genetic and antigenic diversity within each subtype (14).

Whereas the antigenic diversity has consequences for pandemic vaccines that must be considered in the design of a protective vaccine, not all of the 16 HA and 9 NA subtypes of avian influenza viruses have similar pandemic potential. Although HPAI H5N1 viruses are the main focus of global attention, LPAI H9N2 viruses are also widespread in poultry in Asia (46) and HPAI H7 viruses have caused large outbreaks in poultry in Europe (47), North America (48), and South America (49). Although HPAI viruses cause morbidity and mortality in poultry, HPAI viruses might not be intrinsically more likely to cause a human pandemic than would LPAI viruses. To this end, there are no known examples of a pandemic caused by an H5 or H7 HPAI virus, although virologic data are limited to those from the three influenza pandemics that occurred in the past century (38).

Because of this uncertainty, it would be highly desirable to develop vaccines against each of the subtypes of avian influenza virus, although the order of development can be prioritized on the basis of epidemiologic data (14).

A comparison of the predicted protein structures of HA glycoprotein subtypes 1 to 15 has led to the classification of these subtypes into four different clades: clade 1 (H1, H2, H5, H6, H11 and H13), clade 2 (H8, H9 and H12), clade 3 (H3, H4 and H14), and clade 4 (H7, H10 and H15) (51).

Phylogenetic analysis of the genes encoding certain subtypes of HA glycoprotein reveals a separation into lineages that correspond with the geographic separation of the birds that they infect. These genetic lineages are referred to as the Eurasian and North American lineages, and they generally correspond with the flight paths of migratory birds (51–53). Viruses from these two lineages might also be antigenically distinguishable, but the consequences of these genetic and antigenic differences for vaccine development are not known (14).

Circulating human influenza viruses undergo rapid mutation owing to the low fidelity of the viral RNA-dependent RNA polymerase (54). Antigenic drift occurs when the genes encoding the HA and/or NA glycoproteins undergo stepwise mutations, resulting in variant viruses with amino acid changes at one or more antibody-binding sites of HA and/or NA (55) that allow the viruses to evade neutralization by antibodies generated as a result of previous natural infection or vaccination. The internal protein genes of avian influenza viruses are not under positive immune selection in waterfowl and shorebirds. However, the use of veterinary vaccines to protect poultry from infection with avian influenza viruses might drive evolution of the HA glycoprotein if such vaccines do not induce sterilizing immunity (14).

The viral determinants of pathogenicity of avian influenza viruses in humans are multigenic. Further studies are required to understand how the pathogenicity of avian influenza viruses affects the infectivity and transmissibility of these viruses in humans and to establish whether these factors have implications for vaccine design (14).

13.7.1 Types of Influenza Vaccines

Inactivated virus vaccines and live attenuated virus vaccines that are being developed for pandemic influenza are based on technologies that are licensed for the existing seasonal human influenza vaccines (14). Vaccines based on various other platforms, such as live virus vectors expressing influenza virus proteins and DNA vaccines, are also being developed and have shown promise in preclinical studies (see Table 2 in Ref. 14).

The currently licensed vaccines against human influenza viruses are produced in embryonated chicken eggs, and the manufacturing process can take 6 to 9 months (14). Consequently, for vaccines that are based on the currently licensed technologies, the availability of embryonated eggs is a crucial factor, and if the pandemic virus causes widespread morbidity and mortality in poultry, the supply of embryonated eggs might be compromised. Therefore, alternative substrates, including mammalian cell lines, such as Madin-Darby canine kidney (MDCK) cells and Vero cells, have been developed for the production of influenza viruses for use in vaccines. To this end, considerable progress was made in the development of vaccines based on inactivated influenza viruses and live cold-adapted influenza viruses grown in these cell lines in microcarrier fermentors (56–58).

Influenza A viruses replicate in several experimental animals, including chickens, mice, cotton rats, ferrets, hamsters, guinea pigs, and non-human primates. The use of mouse models for the study of influenza is limited because intranasally administered influenza A viruses do not cause symptoms of respiratory tract disease in mice, although some influenza A viruses are lethal in some other animal models (14). Ferrets are generally thought to be the best available model for influenza research. Unlike mice, ferrets develop fever, rhinorrhea, and sneezing after infection with intranasally administered human influenza viruses and the virus replicates in the respiratory tract of these animals. Seronegative ferrets develop a strain-specific immune response to human influenza viruses. Currently, preclinical studies of pandemic influenza vaccines are carried out in mice and ferrets (14).

13.7.1.1 Inactivated Virus Vaccines

In preclinical studies, parenterally administered, inactivated whole-virus H9 and H5 subtype vaccines were shown to be effective in mice against challenge with homologous and heterologous viruses (14,59–63). Recombinant H5 influenza viruses—which contain a modified HA glycoprotein, a wild-type NA glycoprotein from the 1997 or 2003 H5N1 viruses or from an LPAI H5N3 virus, and internal protein genes from the PR8 H1N1 influenza virus (A/Puerto Rico/8/34) that confer high yield in eggs—have been generated by reverse genetics (64–68). The removal of the multibasic amino acid motif in HA that makes the HA0 precursor of HPAI viruses highly cleavable attenuated the virus for infection of chickens, mice, and ferrets without altering the antigenicity of the HA glycoprotein (38). Two doses of these inactivated virus vaccines provided complete protection from lethal challenge with homologous and heterologous H5N1 viruses in mice and ferrets (64–68).

Data from Phase I clinical trials of inactivated virus vaccines against H9N2, H5N3, H5N1, and H2N2 viruses have been reported and other vaccines are still under evaluation (see Table 2 in Ref. 14). Studies that were carried out to date indicated that inactivated split-virion vaccines against avian influenza viruses—in which the virions were disrupted or split by detergent treatment and the surface glycoproteins were then partially purified—were not optimally immunogenic (69) and required multiple doses (70) or the inclusion of an adjuvant (71–74) to induce a protective immune response (14).

Whole-virus vaccines are more immunogenic than are split-virion vaccines, but they are likely to be more reactogenic (75). Adjuvants are required to increase the immunogenicity of inactivated virus vaccines and to decrease the concentration of viral proteins that is required to induce protective immunity, and several adjuvants for this purpose are under investigation, including aluminum salts, the squalene-oil-water emulsion (MF59), and other proprietary compounds (14).

An inactivated whole-virus H9N2 vaccine was found to be immunogenic in individuals who had circulating antibodies induced by prior exposure to H2N2 viruses that cross-reacted with H9N2 viruses, but the vaccine was not immunogenic in individuals who were born after 1968, when H2N2 viruses stopped circulating in humans (76). This observation is consistent with findings from studies of an H1N1 vaccine in 1976–1977, when prior exposure to H1N1 viruses that had circulated in the population earlier ("priming") was found to be a determinant of the response to vaccination (75, 77). These studies also emphasized the need for two doses of vaccine in "unprimed" individuals. In other studies of vaccines against H9N2 viruses, aluminum hydroxide and MF59 adjuvants improved immunogenicity (71, 73).

Inactivated virus vaccines prepared from recombinant PR8 viruses that consisted of a modified HA glycoprotein and wild-type NA glycoproteins from H5N1 viruses isolated in 2004 were evaluated as *subvirion vaccines* or whole-virus vaccines, with or without adjuvants (68,72,78,79). The subvirion vaccines were safe and well-tolerated in healthy adults, and the antibody response that was induced could be enhanced by increasing the dose of antigen used or by the addition of an adjuvant (72, 79). A whole-virus vaccine was also well-tolerated by humans, and when administered with an adjuvant, this vaccine was immunogenic at a lower dose than that of the subvirion vaccines (74). However, the available data indicate that inactivated H5 influenza virus vaccines are poorly immunogenic and require a large concentration of HA glycoprotein or co-administration with an adjuvant to achieve the desired antibody response (14).

13.7.1.2 Live Attenuated Virus Vaccines

Live attenuated, cold-adapted influenza virus vaccines against human influenza viruses elicit both systemic immunity and mucosal immunity at the primary portal of infection (14).

These vaccine strains are generated by the reassortment of a wild-type influenza virus carrying the HA and NA genes of interest with a cold-adapted donor AA (H2N2) influenza virus (A/Ann Arbor/6/60), which was generated by serial passage of the wild-type AA virus at successively lower temperatures (80). The temperature-sensitive, attenuated, cold-adapted donor AA virus has five mutations in three gene segments that contribute to the temperature-sensitive or attenuation phenotype (81), and the virus has a high degree of phenotypic and genotypic stability (82). Candidate live attenuated virus vaccines against H9N2 and H5N1 avian influenza viruses generated on this cold-adapted donor backbone using reassortment and plasmid-based reverse genetics, respectively (see Fig. 3 in Ref. 14), were safe and effective in mice and ferrets (83–85). Phase I clinical evaluation of these vaccines is currently in progress (14).

Generally, live attenuated virus vaccines must retain some infectivity to be immunogenic. Hence, virus shedding during clinical testing of these vaccines must be closely monitored (14). There are potential challenges in the development of live attenuated virus vaccines for pandemic influenza, namely, (i) to generate reassortant viruses that are sufficiently infectious when the HA glycoprotein is derived from an avian influenza virus, in particular if the HA used has a preference for α2,3-linked oligosaccharides; (ii) to reproducibly achieve the desired level of viral attenuation with different combinations of HA and NA genes; and (iii) to minimize the risk of reassortment with circulating human influenza viruses. The evaluation of live attenuated virus vaccines of different subtypes in preclinical studies in appropriate animal models and in clinical studies will address the first two challenges. The standard approach of preclinical evaluation that is applied to vaccines against human influenza viruses might not be uniformly applicable to avian influenza viruses, because the infectivity, immunogenicity, and protective efficacy of avian influenza viruses of different subtypes have not been studied extensively (86). The risk of reassortment of the live attenuated vaccine virus with human influenza viruses

during clinical trials can be minimized by conducting vaccine studies in isolation units when human influenza viruses are not circulating in the community. In the event of an influenza pandemic, the potential benefits of a live attenuated virus vaccine will have to be balanced against the risks associated with it, and this type of vaccine will only be introduced judiciously when a pandemic is imminent (14).

13.7.1.3 Recombinant Subunit, DNA, and Vectored Vaccines

The use of recombinant or expressed proteins of the influenza virus in a vaccine is an attractive option for vaccine development because these approaches do not require handling of HPAI or infectious viruses for vaccine production (6).

Preclinical studies of recombinant HA, NA, and M2 proteins as vaccine antigens (see Table 2 in Ref. 14) showed that the proteins were poorly immunogenic and required multiple doses (87) or the inclusion of adjuvants (88, 89) for improved immunogenicity and efficacy. DNA vaccines encoding the HA and NA glycoproteins of avian influenza viruses or conserved internal virus proteins, such as matrix proteins and nucleoproteins, induced protective immunity in mice and chickens (90–93). The protective efficacy of a nucleoprotein-encoding DNA vaccine was increased by a booster vaccination in the form of a recombinant replication-defective adenovirus (rAdV) expressing the nucleoprotein (94). In two recent studies, intramuscular or intranasal immunization of mice with a human rAdV vaccine expressing the influenza virus HA glycoprotein induced both humoral and cell-mediated immune responses and conferred protection against challenge with the wild-type virus in mice and chickens (95, 96). A recombinant baculovirus-expressed H5 glycoprotein subunit vaccine was well tolerated but was poorly immunogenic in humans, indicating the need for an adjuvant (97). The production of recombinant proteins and DNA vaccines is safe and economical, but clinical studies of their safety and immunogenicity in humans are awaited (14).

13.7.1.4 Universal Influenza Virus Vaccines

An ideal influenza vaccine would be effective against a range of virus subtypes and could be useful during pandemic and interpandemic periods. One approach to creating a universal vaccine would be to target an antigenically stable protein or an antigenically stable part of a variable protein that is essential for virus replication (14). The high degree of conservation of the M2 protein makes it a prime candidate for a universal influenza vaccine. The M2 protein induced cross-reactive immunity that decreased the severity of disease in animal models after challenge with wild-type virus (98, 99).

However, the emergence of immune-escape mutants of the M2 protein in mice in the presence of specific antibodies raised concerns regarding the usefulness of the M2 protein as a target for a universal vaccine *(100)*. Clinical studies would be required to evaluate the immunogenicity of the M2 protein in humans *(14)*.

It has been suggested that the use of the NA glycoprotein, which is less variable than the HA glycoprotein, to induce cross-protective immunity should be explored *(101)*. NA-specific immunity in mice provides significant cross-protection against antigenically distinct viruses of the same subtype *(102, 103)*. Although NA-specific antibodies do not prevent infection with influenza viruses, they decrease the severity and duration of illness in humans by limiting the release and spread of the virus *(44, 45)*.

Furthermore, if common immunogenic epitopes are identified within the four clades of HA glycoprotein subtypes, HA-based immunogens could induce widely cross-reactive immunity *(104)*. Alternatively, genetically engineered viruses that have several conserved immunogenic epitopes on the viral envelope could be developed and evaluated for use as a universal influenza vaccine *(101)*. Recombinant viruses expressing chimeric HA glycoproteins have also been described recently *(105)*. Although universal influenza vaccines are still in preclinical development, the potential benefits of such vaccines are so great that strategies to develop them must be encouraged *(14)*.

13.7.2   Immunogenicity of Pandemic Influenza Vaccines

The evaluation of vaccines against potential pandemic strains of avian influenza viruses presents a unique challenge because vaccines developed against these viruses can only be evaluated for safety and immunogenicity, and not for protection, in clinical trials because challenge studies to assess the efficacy of the vaccines cannot be undertaken in humans *(14)*. In addition, when the immunogenicity of candidate pandemic vaccines is assessed, the data can be difficult to interpret because specific information on the nature and magnitude of the antibody response that correlates with protection is lacking. If a vaccine is immunogenic, it might be possible to assess its efficacy by testing the vaccine in a large group of people who are at high risk from infection with avian influenza virus, such as poultry farmers in areas with severe epizootics *(14)*.

Serum and mucosal antibodies can independently mediate immunity to influenza viruses. Live viruses and inactivated virus vaccines differ in the induction of protective antibodies, but there are no standardized methods for evaluating the mucosal antibody response. The conventional assay for assessing the immunogenicity of a human influenza vaccine is the *hemagglutination-inhibition assay*. Although the standard hemagglutination-inhibition assay, which uses chicken or turkey erythrocytes, is relatively insensitive for the detection of antibodies specific for H5N1 viruses, there is a modified assay using horse erythrocytes that was found to be more sensitive because horse erythrocytes exclusively express the α2,3-linked oligosaccharide side chains that are preferred for binding by avian influenza viruses. However, the horse erythrocyte hemagglutination-inhibition assay has not been well standardized, and the antibody titers determined by this assay that correlate with protection are not known. Therefore, the choice of assays by which the immune response is assessed poses a practical challenge for the evaluation of pandemic influenza vaccines*(14)*.

An alternative to the hemagglutination-inhibition assay that might be more biologically relevant is a neutralization assay, in which the ability of antibodies to neutralize the infectivity of the avian influenza virus is assessed *(14)*. Using paired sera from individuals infected with H5N1 influenza virus in 1997 in Hong Kong collected at the acute and convalescent stages of infection, a neutralizing antibody titer of 1:80 was shown to be indicative of infection with an H5N1 virus *(106)*. However, it is not known whether this antibody titer correlates with protection from re-infection. Other barriers to the use of the neutralization assay are the requirement for appropriate biosafety containment measures, as the assay requires handling of the infectious virus, and the fact that the test has not yet been standardized *(107)*.

13.8   Recent Scientific Advances

- *Sialidase Fusion Protein as a Novel Inhibitor of Influenza Virus Infection.* A recombinant fusion protein (DAS181) composed of a sialidase catalytic domain derived from *Actinomyces viscosus* was fused with a cell surface–anchoring sequence. When applied topically via inhalation, DAS181 effectively removed the influenza viral receptors, sialic acids, from the airway epithelium *(108)*. By effectively cleaving the sialic acid receptors used by both the human and avian influenza viruses, DAS181 prevented the virus from binding to and entering the host cells. This is an innovative antiviral strategy because DA181 acts on the receptors used by the influenza virus rather than targeting the virus itself.

- *Large-Scale Sequence Analysis of Avian Influenza Isolates.* Avian influenza is a significant human health threat globally because of its potential to infect humans and result in a global influenza pandemic; however, very little sequence information for avian influenza virus (AIV) has been publicly available. A more comprehensive collection of publicly available sequence data for AIV is necessary for research in influenza to understand how flu evolves, spreads, and causes disease to shed light on the emergence of influenza epidemics and pandemics and to uncover new targets for drugs, vaccines, and diagnostics. A team of NIAID-supported scientists has released genomic data from the first large-scale sequencing of AIV isolates, doubling the amount of AIV sequence data in the public domain *(109)*. These sequence data include 2,196 AIV genes and 169 complete genomes from a diverse sample of birds. The preliminary analysis of these sequences, along with other AIV data from the public domain, revealed new information about AIV, including the identification of a genome sequence that may be a determinant of virulence. This study provides valuable sequencing data to the scientific community and demonstrates how informative large-scale sequence analysis can be in identifying potential markers of disease.

- *Architecture of Ribonucleoprotein Complexes in Influenza A Virus Particles.* Data from transmission electron microscopy of serially sectioned virions of influenza A viruses have shown that the ribonucleoprotein complexes (RNPs) of the virus are organized in a distinct pattern: seven segments of different lengths surrounding a central segment *(110)*. Furthermore, the individual RNPs are suspended from the interior of the viral envelope at the distal end of the budding virion and are oriented perpendicular to the budding tip. These findings have argued against a random incorporation of RNPs into virions, supporting instead a model in which each segment contains specific incorporation signals that would enable the RNPs to be recruited and packaged as a complete set. The selective mechanism of RNP incorporation into virions and the unique organization of the eight RNP segments may be crucial to maintaining the integrity of the viral genome during repeated cycles of replication *(110)*.

- *Structure and Receptor Specificity of the Hemagglutinin from an H5N1 Influenza Virus.* The hemagglutinin structure at 2.9 Å resolution from a highly pathogenic Vietnamese H5N1 influenza virus (Viet04) has been elucidated *(111)*. Its structure was found to be more related to that of the 1918 *(8)* and other human H1 hemagglutinins than to a 1997 duck H5 hemagglutinin. Glycan microarray analysis of the Viet04 virus revealed an avian $\alpha 2,3$ sialic acid receptor binding preference. Introduction of mutations that can convert H1 serotype hemagglutinins to human $\alpha 2,6$ receptor specificity only enhanced or reduced affinity for the avian-type receptors. However, mutations that can convert avian H2 and H3 hemagglutinins to human receptor specificity, when inserted onto the Viet04 hemagglutinin framework, permitted binding to a natural $\alpha 2,6$ glycan, thereby suggesting a path for this H5N1 virus to *gain a foothold in the human population (111)*.

- *NS1-Truncated Modified Live-Virus Vaccine.* Swine influenza viruses (SIVs) naturally infect pigs and can be transmitted to humans. Furthermore, in the pig, genetic reassortment to create novel influenza subtypes by mixing avian and human influenza viruses *is possible.* Therefore, a vaccine against SIV and inducing cross-protective immunity between different subtypes and strains circulating in pigs will be highly advantageous. To this end, an H3N2 SIV (A/swine/Texas/4199-2/98) (labeled TX98) containing a deleted NS1 gene expressing a truncated NS1 protein of 126 amino acids (NS1/126) was attenuated in swine. Subsequently, 4-week-old pigs were vaccinated with the TX98 NS1/126 modified live-virus (MLV) vaccine. The highly attenuated MVL completely protected against challenge with the homologous SIV *(112)*. Vaccinated pigs challenged with the heterosubtypic N1N1 virus demonstrated macroscopic lung lesions similar to those of the unvaccinated H1N1 control pigs. Remarkably, vaccinated pigs challenged with the H1N1 SIV had significantly less microscopic lung lesions and less virus shedding from the respiratory tract than did unvaccinated, H1N1-challenged pigs. Furthermore, all vaccinated pigs developed significant levels of hemagglutination inhibition and enzyme-linked immunosorbent assay titers in serum and mucosal immunoglobulin A antibodies against H3N2 SIV antigens *(112)*.

- *Immunization by H5 Avian Influenza Hemagglutinin Mutants with Altered Receptor Binding Specificity.* Scientists from NIAID's VRC have developed a strategy to generate vaccines and therapeutic antibodies that could target predicted H5N1 mutants before these viruses evolve naturally. This advance was made possible by creating mutations in the region of the H5N1 hemagglutinin protein that directs the virus to bird or human cells and eliciting antibodies to it *(113)*.

- *Protective Immunity to Lethal Challenge of the 1918 Pandemic Influenza Virus by Vaccination.* Using the genetic sequence information for the 1918 flu virus, VRC scientists have created plasmids— small strands of DNA designed to express specific characteristics—carrying genes for the virus's hemagglutinin protein, the surface protein found in all flu viruses that allows the virus to stick to a host cell and cause infection *(114)*. The researchers created two types of plasmids: one to reflect the HA found in the original 1918 flu virus; the other an altered HA protein designed to attenuate the virus. Mice were then injected with a DNA vaccine containing both types of plasmids to determine whether they would generate immune responses to the 1918 virus. The researchers found significant responses both in terms of the production of T cells and the production of neutralizing antibodies.

References

1. Murphy, B. R. and Webster, R. G. (1990) Orthomyxoviruses. In: *Fields Virology*, 2nd ed. (Fields, B. N., Knipe, D. M., Chanock, R. N., Hirsch, M. S., Melnick, J. L., Monath, T. P., and Roizman, B., eds.), Raven Press, New York, pp. 1091–1152.

2. Reid, A. H., Taubenberger, J. K., and Fanning, T. G. (2001) The 1918 Spanish influenza: integrating history and biology, *Microb. Infect.*, **3**(1), 81–87.

3. Reid, A. H., Fanning, T. G., Janczewski, T. A., and Taubenberger, J. K. (2000) Characterization of the 1918 "Spanish" influenza virus neuraminidase gene, *Proc. Natl. Acad. Sci. U.S.A.*, **97**(12), 6785–6790.

4. Taubenberger, J. K., Reid, A. H., Krafft, A. E., Bijwaard, K. E., and Fanning, T. G. (1999) Initial genetic characterization of the 1918 "Spanish" influenza virus, *Science*, **275**, 1793–1796.

5. Reid, A. H., Fanning, T. G., Hultin, J. V., and Taubenberger, J. K. (1999) Origin and evolution of the 1918 "Spanish" influenza virus hemagglutinin gene, *Proc. Natl. Acad. Sci. U.S.A.*, **96**, 1651–1656.

6. Basler, C. F., Reid, A. H., Dybing, J. K., Janczewski, T. A., Fanning, T. G., Zheng, H., Salvatore, M., Perdue, M. L., Swayne, D. E., Garcia-Sastre, A., Palese, P., and Taubenberger, J. K. (2001) Sequence of the 1918 pandemic influenza virus nonstructural gene (NS) segment and characterization of recombinant viruses bearing the 1918 NS gene, *Proc. Natl. Acad. Sci. U.S.A.*, **98**(5), 2746–2751.

7. Reid, A. H., Fanning, T. G., Janczewski, T. A., McCall, S., and Taubenberger, J. K. (2002) Characterization of the 1918 "Spanish" influenza virus matrix gene segment, *J. Virol.*, **76**(21), 10717–10723.

8. Stevens, J., Corper, A. L., Basler, C. F., Taubenberger, J. K., Palese, P., and Wilson, I. A. (2004) Structure of the uncleaved human H1 hemagglutinin from the extinct 1918 influenza virus, *Science*, **303**(5665), 1866–1870.

9. Gamblin, S. J., Haire, L. F., Russell, R. J., Stevens, D. J., Xiao, B., Ha, Y., Vasisht, N., Steinhauer, D. A., Daniels, R. S., Elliot, A., Wiley, D. C., and Skehel, J. J. (2004) The structure and receptor binding properties of the 1918 influenza hemagglutinin, *Science*, **303**(5665), 1838–1842.

10. Taubenberger, J. K., Reid, A. H., Lourens, R. M., Wang, R., Jin, G., and Fanning, T. G. (2005) Characterization of the 1918 influenza virus polymerase genes, *Nature*, **437**, 889–893.

11. Hien, T. T., Liem, N. T., Dung, N. T., San, L. T., Mai, P. P., van Vinh Chau, N., Suu, P. T., Dong, V. C., Mai, L. T. Q., Thi, N. T., Khoa, D. B., Phat, L. P., Truong, N. T., Long, H. T., Tung, C. V., Giang, L. T., Tho, N. D., Nga, L. H., Tien, N. T. K., San, L. H., Tuan, L. V., Dolecek, C., Thanh, T. T., de Jong, M., Schultsz, C., Cheng, P., Lim, W., Horby, P., and Farrar, J., for The World Health Organization International Avian Influenza Investigative Team (2004) Avian influenza A (H5N1) in 10 patients in Vietnam, *N. Engl. J. Med.*, **350**(12), 1179–1188.

12. Kawaoka, Y., Krauss, S., and Webster, R. G. (1989) Avian-to-human transmission of the PB1 gene of influenza A viruses in the 1957 and 1968 pandemics, *J. Virol.*, **63**, 4603–4608.

13. Scholtissek, C., Rohde, W., Von Hoyningen, V., and Rott, R. (1978) On the origin of the human influenza virus subtypes H2N2 and H3N2, *Virology*, **87**, 13–20.

14. Subbarao, K. and Joseph, T. (2007) Scientific barriers to developing vaccines against avian influenza viruses, *Nat. Rev. Immunol.*, **7**, 267–278.

15. The Writing Committee of the World Health Organization (WHO) Consultation on Human Influenza A/H5 (2005) Avian influenza A (H5N1) infection in humans, *N. Engl. J. Med.*, **353**(13), 1374–1385.

16. Ungchusak, K., Auewarakul, P., Dowell, S. F., Kitphati, R., Auwanit, W., Puthavathana, P., Uiprasertkul, M., Boonnak, K., Pittayawonganon, C., Cox, N. J., Zaki, S. R., Thawatsupha, P., Chittaganpitch, M., Khontong, R., Simmerman, J. M., and Chunsutthiwat, S. (2005) Probable person-to-person transmission of avian influenza A (H5N1), *N. Engl. J. Med.*, **352**(4), 333–340.

17. World Health Organization (2005) WHO Inter-Country-Consultation: Influenza A/H5N1 in Humans in Asia: Manila, Philippines, 6–7 May 2005.

18. Li, K. S., Guan, Y., Wang, J., Smith, G. J. D., Xu, K. M., Duan, L., Rahardjo, A. P., Puthavathana, P., Buranathai, C., Nguyen, T. D., Estoepangestie, A. T. S., Chaisingh, A., Auewarakul, P., Long, H. T., Hahn, N. T. H., Webby, R. J., Poon, L. L. M., Chen, H., Shortridge, K. F., Yuen, K. Y., Webster, R. G., and Peiris, J. S. M. (2004) Genesis of a highly pathogenic and potentially pandemic H5N1 influenza virus in Eastern Asia, *Nature*, **430**, 209–213.

19. To, K. F., Chan, P. K., Chan, K. F., Lee, W. F., Lam, W. Y., Wong, K. F., Tang, N. L. S., Tsang, D. N. C., Sung, R. Y. T., Buckley, T. A., Tam, J. S., and Cheng, A. F. (2001) Pathology of fatal human infection associated with avian influenza A H5N1 virus, *J. Med. Virol.*, **63**, 242–246.

20. Peiris, J. S., Yu, W. C., Leung, C. W., Cheung, C. Y., Ng, W. F., Nicholls, J. M., Ng, T. K., Chan, K. H., Lai, S. T., Lim, W. L., Yuen, K. Y., and Guan, Y. (2004) Re-emergence of fatal human influenza A subtype H5N1 disease, *Lancet*, **363**(9409), 617–619.

21. World Health Organization (2004) WHO Interim Guidelines on Clinical Management of Humans Infected by Influenza A(H5N1), February 20, 2004.

22. Fouchier, R. A. M., Schneeberger, P. M., Rozendaal, F. W., Broekman, J. M., Kemink, S. A. G., Munster, V., Kuiken, T., Rimmelzwaan, G. F., Schutten, M., van Doornum, G. J. J., Koch, G., Bosman, A., Koopmans, M., and Osterhaus, A. D. M. E. (2004) Avian influenza A virus (H7N7) associated with human conjunctivitis and a fatal case of acute respiratory distress syndrome, *Proc. Natl. Acad. Sci. U.S.A.*, **101**(5), 1356–1361.

23. Butt, K. M., Smith, G. J. D., Chen, H., Zhang, L. J., Leung, Y. H. C., Xu, K. M., Lim, W., Webster, R. G., Yuen, K. Y., Peiris, J. S. M., and Guan, Y. (2005) Human infection with and avian H9N2 influenza A virus in Hong Kong in 2003, *J. Clin. Microbiol.*, **43**(11), 5760–5767.

24. Zhou, N. N., Shortridge, K. F., Claas, E. C. J., Krauss, S. L., and Webster, R. G. (1999) Rapid evolution of H5N1 influenza viruses in chickens in Hong Kong, *J. Virol.*, **73**, 3366–3374.

25. Guan, L., Shortridge, K. F., Krauss, S., and Webster, R. G. (1999) Molecular characterization of H9N2 influenza viruses: were they the donors of the "internal" genes of H5N2 viruses in Hong Kong? *Proc. Natl. Acad. Sci. U.S.A.*, **96**, 9363–9367.

26. Xu, K. M., Li, K. S., Smith, G. J. D., Li, J. W., Tai, H., Zhang, J. X., Webster, R. G., Peiris, J. S. M., Chen, H., and Guan, Y. (2007) Evolution and molecular epidemiology of H9N2 influenza A viruses from quail in southern China, 2000 to 2005, *J. Virol.*, **81**(6), 2635–2645.

27. Guan, Y., Shortridge, K. F., Krauss, S., Chin, P. S., Dyrting, K. C., Ellis, T. M., Webster, R. G., and Peiris, M. (2000) H9N2 Influenza viruses possessing H5N1-like internal genomes continue to circulate in poultry in southeastern China, *J. Virol.*, **74**(20), 9372–9380.

28. Matrosovich, M. N., Krauss, S., and Webster, R. G. (2001) H9N2 influenza A viruses from poultry in Asia have human virus-like receptor specificity, *Virology*, **281**(2), 156–162.

29. Thompson, W., Shay, D. K., Weintraub, E., Brammer, L., Bridges, C. B., Cox, N. J., and Fukuda, K. (2004) Influenza-associated hospitalizations in the United States, *J. Am. Med. Assoc.*, **292**(11), 1333–1340.

30. Neuzil, K. M., Mellen, B. G., Wright, P. F., Mitchel, E. F., and Griffin, M. R. (2000) The effect of influenza on hospitalizations, outpatient visits and courses of antibiotics in children, *N. Engl. J. Med.*, **342**(4), 225–231.

31. Izurieta, H. S., Thompson, W. W., Kramarz, P., Shay, D. K., Davis, R. L., DeStefano, F., Black, S., Shinefield, H., and Fukuda, K. (2000) Influenza and the rates of hospitalization for respiratory disease among infants and young children, *N. Engl. J. Med.*, **342**(4), 232–239.

32. National Institute of Allergy and Infectious Diseases (2007) Report of the Blue Ribbon Panel on Influenza Research, September 11–12, 2006 (http://www3.niaid.nih.gov/health-science/healthtopics/Flu/default.htm).

33. Keitel, W. A., Atmar, R. L., Cate, T. R., Petersen, N. J., Greenberg, S. B., Ruben, F., and Couch, R. B. (2006) Safety of high doses of influenza vaccine and effect on antibody responses in elderly persons, *Arch. Intern. Med.*, **166**(10), 1121–1127.

34. Treanor, J. J., Campbell, J. D., Zangwill, K. M., Rowe, T., and Wolff, M. (2006) Safety and immunogenicity of an inactivated subvirion influenza A (H5N1) vaccine, *N. Engl. J. Med.*, **354**(13), 1343–1351.

35. Atmar, R. L., Keitel, W. A., Patel, S. M., Katz, J. M., She, D., El Sahly, H., Pompey, J., Cate, T. R., and Couch, R. B. (2006) Safety and immunogenicity of nonadjuvanted and MF59-adjuvanted influenza A/H9N2 vaccine preparation, *Clin. Infect. Dis.*, **43**, 1135–1142.

36. Gillim-Ross, L. and Subbarao, K. (2006) Emerging respiratory viruses: challenges and vaccine strategies, *Clin. Microbiol. Rev.*, **19**, 614–636.

37. Lewis, D. B. (2006) Avian flu to human influenza, *Annu. Rev. Med.*, **57**, 139–154.

38. Stephenson, I., Nicholson, K. G., Wood, J. M., Zambon, M. C., and Katz, J. M. (2004) Confronting the avian influenza threat: vaccine development for a potential pandemic, *Lancet Infect. Dis.*, **4**, 499–509.

39. Beigel, J. H., Farrar, J., Han, A. M., Hayden, F. G., Hyer, R., de Jong, M. D., et al. (2005) Avian influenza A (H5N1) infection in humans, *N. Engl. J. Med.*, **353**, 1374–1385.

40. de Jong, M. D. and Hien, T. T. (2006) Avian influenza A (H5N1), *J. Clin. Virol.*, **35**, 2–13.

41. Couch, R. B. and Kasel, J. A. (1983) Immunity to influenza in man, *Annu. Rev. Microbiol.*, **37**, 529–549.

42. Potter, C. W. and Oxford, J. S. (1979) Determinants of immunity to influenza infection in man, *Br. Med. Bull.*, **35**, 69–75.

43. Gerhard, W. (2001) The role of the antibody response in influenza virus infection, *Curr. Top. Microbiol. Immunol.*, **260**, 171–190.

44. Kilbourne, E. D., Laver, W. G., Schulman, J. L., and Webster, R. G. (1968) Antiviral activity of antiserum specific for an influenza virus neuraminidase, *J. Virol.*, **2**, 281–288.

45. Murphy, B. R., Kasel, J. A., and Chanock, R. M. (1972) Association of serum anti-neuraminidase antibody with resistance to influenza in man, *N. Engl. J. Med.*, **286**, 1329–1332.

46. Choi, Y. K., Ozaki, H., Webby, R. J., Webster, R. G., Peiris, J. S., Poon, L., Butt, C., Leung, Y. H. C., and Guan, Y. (2004) Continuing evolution of H9N2 influenza viruses in Southeastern China, *J. Virol.*, **78**, 8609–8614.

47. Fouchier, R. A., Schneeberger, P. M., Rozendaal, F. W., Broekman, J. M., et al. (2004) Avian influenza A virus (H7N7) associated with human conjunctivitis and a fatal case of acute respiratory distress syndrome, *Proc. Natl. Acad. Sci. U.S.A.*, **101**, 1356–1361.

48. Hirst, M., Astell, C. R., Griffith, M., Coughlin, S. M., Moksa, M., Zeng, T., et al. (2004) Novel avian influenza H7N3 strain outbreak, British Columbia, *Emerg. Infect. Dis.*, **10**, 2192–2195.

49. Suarez, D. L., Senne, D. A., Banks, J., Brown, I. H., Essen, S., et al. (2004) Recombination resulting in virulence shift in avian influenza outbreak, Chile, *Emerg. Infect. Dis.*, **10**, 693–699.

50. Russell, R. J., Gamblin, S. J., Haire, L. F., Stevens, D. J., et al. (2004) H1 and H7 influenza haemagglutinin structures extend a structural classification of haemagglutinin subtypes, *Virology*, **325**, 287–296.

51. Webster, R. G., Bean, W. J., Gorman, O. T., Chambers, T. M., and Kawaoka, Y. (1992) Evolution and ecology of influenza A viruses, *Microbiol. Rev.*, **56**, 152–179.

52. Banks, J., Speidel, E. C., McCauley, J. W., and Alexander, D. J. (2000) Phylogenetic analysis of H7 haemagglutinin subtype influenza A viruses, *Arch. Virol.*, **145**, 1047–1058.

53. Makarova, N. V., Kaverin, N. V., Krauss, S., Senne, D., and Webster, R. G. (1999) Transmission of Eurasian avian H2 influenza virus to shorebirds in North America, *J. Gen. Virol.*, **80**, 3167–3171.

54. Cox, N. J. and Bender, C. A. (1995) The molecular epidemiology of influenza virus, *Semin. Virol.*, **6**, 359–370.

55. Wilson, I. A. and Cox, N. J. (1990) Structural basis of immune recognition of influenza virus hemagglutinin, *Annu. Rev. Immunol.*, **8**, 737–771.

56. Ghendon, Y. Z., Markushin, S. G., Akopova, I. I., Koptiaeva, I. B., Nechaeva, E. A., Mazurkova, L. A., Radaeva, I. F., and Kolokoltseva, T. D. (2005) Development of cell culture (MDCK) live cold-adapted (CA) attenuated influenza vaccine, *Vaccine*, **23**, 4678–4684.

57. Oxford, J. S., Manuguerra, C., Kistner, O., Linde, A., Kunze, M., Lange, W., et al. (2005) A new European perspective of influenza pandemic planning with a particular focus on the role of mammalian cell culture vaccines, *Vaccine*, **23**, 5440–5449.

58. Palker, T., Kiseleva, I., Johnston, K., Su, Q., Toner, T., et al. (2004) Protective efficacy of intranasal cold-adapted influenza A/New Caledonia/20/99 (H1N1) vaccines comprised of egg- or cell culture-derived reassortants, *Virus Res.*, **105**, 183–194.

59. Lu, X., Tumpey, T. M., Morken, T., Zaki, S. R., Cox, N. J., Katz, J. M., et al. (1999) A mouse model for the evaluation of pathogenesis and immunity to influenza A (H5N1) viruses isolated from humans, *J. Virol.*, **73**, 5903–5911.

60. Wood, J. M., Major, D., Daly, J., Newman, R. W., Dunleavy, U., et al. (1999) Vaccines against H5N1 influenza, *Vaccine*, **18**, 579–580.

61. Chen, H., Subbarao, K., Swayne, D., Chen, Q., Lu, X., Katz, J., Cox, N., and Matsuoka, Y. (2003) Generation and evaluation of a high-growth reassortant H9N2 influenza A virus as a pandemic vaccine candidate, *Vaccine*, **21**, 1974–1979.

62. Lu, X., Renshaw, M., Tumpey, T. M., Kelly, G. D., Hu-Primmer, J., and Katz, J. M. (2001) Immunity to influenza A H9N2 viruses induced by infection and vaccination, *J. Virol.*, **75**, 4896–4901.

63. Takada, A., Kuboki, N., Okazaki, K., Ninomiya, A., Tanaka, H., Ozaki, H., Itamura, S., et al. (1999) Avirulent avian influenza virus as a vaccine strain against a potential human pandemic, *J. Virol.*, **73**, 8303–8307.

64. Subbarao, K., Chen, H., Swayne, D., Mingay, L., Fodor, E., Brownlee, G., et al. (2003) Evaluation of a genetically modified reassortant H5N1 influenza A virus vaccine candidate generated by plasmid-based reverse genetics, *Virology*, **305**, 192–200.

65. Govorkova, E. A., Webby, R. J., Humberd, J., Seiler, J. P., and Webster, R. G. (2006) Immunization with reverse-genetics-produced H5N1 influenza vaccine protects ferrets against homologous and heterologous challenge, *J. Infect. Dis.*, **194**, 159–167.

66. Lipatov, A. S., Hoffmann, E., Salomon, R., Yen, H. L., and Webster, R. G. (2006) Cross-protectiveness and immunogenicity of influenza A/Duck/Singapore/3/97 (H5) vaccines against infection with A/Vietnam/1203/04 (H5N1) virus in ferrets, *J. Infect. Dis.*, **194**, 1040–1043.

67. Nicolson, C., Major, D., Wood, J. M., and Robertson, J. S. (2005) Generation of influenza vaccine viruses on Vero cells by reverse

genetics: an H5N1 candidate vaccine strain produced under a quality system, *Vaccine*, **23**, 2943–2952.

68. Webby, R. J., Perez, D., Coleman, J., Guan, Y., Knight, J., Govorkova, E., et al. (2004) Responsiveness to a pandemic alert: use of reverse genetics for rapid development of influenza vaccines, *Lancet*, **363**, 1099–1103.

69. Nicholson, K. G., Colegate, A., Podda, A., et al. (2001) Safety and antigenicity of non-adjuvanted and MF59-adjuvanted influenza A/Duck/Singapore/97 (H5N3) vaccine: a randomised trial of two potential vaccines against H5N1 influenza, *Lancet*, **57**, 1937–1943.

70. Stephenson, I., Nicholson, K. G., Colegate, A., Podda, A., Wood, J., Ypma, E., and Zambon, M. (2003) Boosting immunity to influenza H5N1 with MF59-adjuvanted H5N3 A/Duck/Singapore/97 vaccine in a primed human population, *Vaccine*, **21**, 1687–1693.

71. Atmar, R. L., Keitel, W. A., Patel, S. M., Katz, J. M., She, D., El Sahly, H., Pompey, J., et al. (2006) Safety and immunogenicity of nonadjuvated and MF59-adjuvanted influenza A/H9N2 vaccine preparations, *Clin. Infect. Dis.*, **43**, 1135–1142.

72. Bresson, J. L., Perronne, C., Launay, O., Gerdil, C., Saville, M., Wood, J., et al. (2006) Safety and immunogenicity of an inactivated split-virion influenza A/Vietnam/1194/2004 (H5N1) vaccine: phase I randomised trial, *Lancet*, **367**, 1657–1664.

73. Hehme, N., Engelmann, H., Kunzel, W., Neumeier, E., and Sanger, R. (2002) Pandemic preparedness: lessons learnt from H2N2 and H9N2 candidate vaccines, *Med. Microbiol. Immunol. (Berlin)*, **191**, 203–208.

74. Lin, J., Zhang, J., Dong, X., Fang, H., Chen, J., et al. (2006) Safety and immunogenicity of an inactivated adjuvanted whole-virion influenza A (H5N1) vaccine: a phase I randomised controlled trial, *Lancet*, **368**, 991–997.

75. Wright, P. F., Thompson, J., Vaughn, W. K., Folland, D. S., Sell, S. H., and Karzon, D. T., (1977) Trials of influenza A/New Jersey/76 virus vaccine in normal children: an overview of age-related antigenicity and reactogenicity, *J. Infect. Dis.*, **136**, S731-S741.

76. Stephenson, I., Nicholson, K. G., Gluck, R., Mischler, R., Newman, R. W., et al. (2003) Safety and antigenicity of whole virus and subunit influenza A/Hong Kong/1073/99 (H9N2) vaccine in healthy adults: phase I randomised trial, *Lancet*, **362**, 1959–1966.

77. Parkman, P. D., Hopps, H. E., Rastogi, S. C., and Meyer, H. M., Jr. (1977) Summary of clinical trials of influenza virus vaccines in adults, *J. Infect. Dis.*, **136**, S722–S730.

78. Ozaki, H., Govorkova, E. A., Li, C., Xiong, X., et al. (2004) Generation of high-yielding influenza A viruses in African green monkey kidney (Vero) cells by reverse genetics, *J. Virol.*, **78**, 1851–1857.

79. Treanor, J. J., Campbell, J. D., Zangwill, K. M., Rowe, T., and Wolff, M. (2006) Safety and immunogenicity of an inactivated subvirion influenza A (H5N1) vaccine, *N. Engl. J. Med.*, **354**, 1343–1351.

80. Maassab, H. F. and Bryant, M. L. (1999) The development of live attenuated cold-adapted influenza virus vaccine for humans, *Rev. Med. Virol.*, **9**, 237–244.

81. Jin, H., Lu, B., Zhou, H., Ma, C., Zhao, J., et al. (2003) Multiple amino acid residues confer temperature sensitivity to human influenza virus vaccine strains (FluMist) derived from cold-adapted A/Ann Arbor/6/60, *Virology*, **306**, 18–24.

82. Cha, T. A., Kao, K., Zhao, J., Fast, P. E., Mendelman, P. M., and Arvin, A. (2000) Genotypic stability of cold-adapted influenza virus vaccine in an efficacy clinical trial, *J. Clin. Microbiol.*, **38**, 839–845.

83. Li, S., Liu, C., Klimov, A., Subbarao, K., Perdue, M. L., et al. (1999) Recombinant influenza A virus vaccines for the pathogenic human A/Hong Kong/97 (H5N1) viruses, *J. Infect. Dis.*, **179**, 1132–1138.

84. Chen, H., Matsuoka, Y., Swayne, D., Chen, Q., Cox, N. J., et al. (2003) Generation and characterization of a cold-adapted influenza A H9N2 reassortant as a live pandemic influenza virus vaccine candidate, *Vaccine*, **21**, 4430–4436.

85. Suguitan, A. L., Jr., McAuliffe, J., Mills, K. L., Jin, H., Duke, G., Lu, B., et al. (2006) Live, attenuated influenza A H5N1 candidate vaccines provide broad cross-protection in mice and ferrets, *PLoS Med.*, **3**, e360.

86. Luke, C. J. and Subbarao, K. (2006) Vaccines for pandemic influenza, *Emerg. Infect. Dis.*, **12**, 66–72.

87. Nwe, N., He, Q., Damrongwatanapokin, S., Du, Q., Manopo, I., et al. (2006) Expression of hemagglutinin protein from the avian influenza virus H5N1 in a baculovirus/insect cell system significantly enhanced by suspension culture, *BMC Microbiol.*, **6**, 16.

88. de Wit, E., Munster, V., Spronken, M., Bestebroer, T. M., Baas, C., et al. (2005) Protection of mice against lethal infection with highly pathogenic H7N7 influenza A virus by using a recombinant low-pathogenicity vaccine strain, *J. Virol.*, **79**, 12401–12407.

89. Rimmelzwaan, G. F., Claas, E. C., van Amerongen, G., de Jong, J. C., and Osterhaus, A. D. (1999) ISCOM vaccine induced protection against a lethal challenge with a human H5N1 influenza virus, *Vaccine*, **17**, 1355–1358.

90. Bright, R. A., Ross, T. M., Subbarao, K., Robinson, H. L., and Katz, J. M. (2003) Impact of glycosylation on the immunogenicity of a DNA-based influenza H5 HA glycoprotein vaccine, *Virology*, **308**, 270–278.

91. Epstein, S. L., Tumpey, T. M., Misplon, J. A., Lo, C.-Y., Cooper, L. A., et al. (2002) DNA vaccine expressing conserved influenza virus proteins protective against H5N1 challenge infection in mice, *Emerg. Infect. Dis.*, **8**, 796–801.

92. Kodihalli, S., Kobasa, D. L., and Webster, R. G. (2000) Strategies for inducing protection against avian influenza A virus subtypes with DNA vaccines, *Vaccine*, **18**, 2592–2599.

93. Qiu, M., Fang, F., Chen, Y., Wang, H., Chen, Q., Chang, H., et al. (2006) Protection against avian influenza H9N2 virus challenge by immunization with hemagglutinin- or neuraminidase-expressing DNA in BALB/c mice, *Biochem. Biophys. Res. Commun.*, **343**, 1124–1131.

94. Epstein, S. L., Kong, W., Misplon, J. A., Lo, C.-Y., Tumpey, T. M., et al. (2005) Protection against multiple influenza A subtypes by vaccination with highly conserved nucleoprotein, *Vaccine*, **23**, 5404–5410.

95. Gao, W., Soloff, A. C., Lu, X., Montecalvo, A., Nguyen, D. C., et al. (2006) Protection of mice and poultry from lethal H5N1 avian influenza virus through adenovirus-based immunization, *J. Virol.*, **80**, 1959–1964.

96. Hoelscher, M. A., Garg, S., Bangari, D. S., Belser, J. A., Lu, X., et al. (2006) Development of adenoviral-vector-based pandemic influenza vaccine against antigenically distinct human H5N1 strains in mice, *Lancet*, **367**, 475–481.

97. Treanor, J. J., Wilkinson, B. E., Masseoud, F., Hu-Primmer, J., Battaglia, R., O'Brien, D., et al. (2001) Safety and immunogenicity of a recombinant hemagglutinin vaccine for H5 influenza in humans, *Vaccine*, **19**, 1732–1737.

98. Ernst, W. A., Kim, H. J., Tumpey, T. M., Jansen, A. D. A., Tai, W., et al. (2006) Protection against H1, H5, H6 and H9 influenza A infection with liposomal matrix 2 epitope vaccines, *Vaccine*, **24**, 5158–5168.

99. Gerhard, W., Mozdzanowska, K., and Zharikova, D. (2006) Prospects for universal influenza virus vaccine, *Emerg. Infect. Dis.*, **12**, 569–574.

100. Zharikova, D., Mozdzanowska, K., Feng, J., Zhang, M., and Gerhard, W. (2005) Influenza type A virus escape mutants emerge *in vivo* in the presence of antibodies to the ectodomain of matrix protein 2, *J. Virol.*, **79**, 6644–6654.

101. Palese, P. (2006) Making better influenza virus vaccines? *Emerg. Infect. Dis.*, **12**, 61–65.

102. Chen, J., Fang, F., Li, X., Chang, H., and Chen, Z. (2005) Protection against influenza virus infection in BALB/c mice immunized with a single dose of neuraminidase-expressing DNAs by electroporation, *Vaccine*, **23**, 4322–4328.

103. Kilbourne, E. D., Pokorny, B. A., Johansson, B., Brett, I., et al. (2004) Protection of mice with recombinant influenza virus neuraminidase, *J. Infect. Dis.*, **189**, 459–461.

104. Subbarao, K., Murphy, B. R., and Fauci, A. S. (2006) Development of effective vaccines against pandemic influenza, *Immunity*, **24**, 5–9.

105. Li, Z. N., Mueller, S. N., Ye, L., Bu, Z., Yang, C., et al. (2005) Chimeric influenza virus hemagglutinin proteins containing large domains of the *Bacillus anthracis* protective antigen: protein characterization, incorporation into infectious influenza viruses, and antigenicity, *J. Virol.*, **79**, 10003–10012.

106. Rowe, T., Abernathy, R. A., Hu-Primmer, J., Thompson, W. W., Lu, X., et al. (1999) Detection of antibody to avian influenza A (H5N1) virus in human serum by using a combination of serologic assays, *J. Clin. Microbiol.*, **37**, 937–943.

107. Stephenson, I. (2006) H5N1 vaccines: how prepared are we for a pandemic? *Lancet*, **368**, 965–966.

108. Malakhov, M. P., Aschenbrenner, L. M., Smee, D. F., Wandersee, M. K., Sidwell, R. W., Gubareva, L. V., Mishin, V. P., Hayden, F. G., Kim, D. H., Ing, A., Campbell, E. R., Yu, M., and Fang, F. (2006) Sialidase fusion protein as a novel broad-spectrum inhibitor of influenza virus infection, *Antimicrob. Agents Chemother.*, **50**, 1470–1479.

109. Obenauer, J. C., Denson, J., Mehta, P. K., Su, X., Mukatira, S., Finkelstein, D. B., Xu, X., Wang, J., Ma, J., Fan, Y., Rakestraw, K. M., Webster, R. G., Hoffman, E., Krauss, S., Zheng, J., Zhang, Z., and Naeve, C. W. (2006) Large-scale sequence analysis of avian influenza isolates, *Science*, **311**(5767), 1576–1580.

110. Noda, T., Sagara, H., Yen, A., Takada, A., Kida, H., Cheng, R. H., and Kawaoka, Y. (2006) Architecture of ribonucleoprotein complexes in influenza A virus particles, *Nature*, **439**(7075), 490–492.

111. Stevens, J., Blixt, O., Tumpey, T. M., Taubenberger, J. K., Paulson, J. C., and Wilson, I. A. (2006) Structure and receptor specificity of the hemagglutinin from an H5N1 influenza virus, *Science*, **312**(5772), 404–410.

112. Richt, J. A., Lekcharoensuk, P., Lager, K. M., Vincent, A. L., Loiacono, C. M., Janke, B. H., Wu, W.-H., Yoon, K.-J., Webby, R. J., Solórzano, A., and García-Sastre, A. (2006) Vaccination of pigs against swine influenza viruses by using an NS1-truncated modified live-virus gene, *J. Virol.*, **80**(22), 11009–1118.

113. Yang, Z.-Y., Wei, C.-J., Kong, W.-P., Wu, L., Xu, L., Smith, D. F., and Nabel, G. J. (2007) Immunization by avian H5 influenza hemagglutinin mutants with altered receptor binding specificity, *Science*, **317**(5839), 825–828.

114. Kong, W. P., Hood, C., Yang, Z.-Y., Wu, C.-J., Xu, L., Garcia-Sestre, A., Tumpay, T. M., and Nabel, G. J. (2006) Protective immunity to lethal challenge of the 1918 pandemic influenza virus by vaccination, *Proc. Natl. Acad. Sci. U.S.A.*, **103**(43), 15987–15991.

Chapter 14

Tuberculosis

Pulmonary tuberculosis (consumption; phthisis; TB) is considered to be one of the most devastating human diseases, causing death and prolonged disability among people worldwide over many centuries *(1, 2)*. *Mycobacterium tuberculosis* (Mtb), the causative agent of tuberculosis, was discovered by Robert Koch in 1882, and since then tuberculosis has become one of the most intensely studied infectious diseases. After a decline in prevalence during the latter part of the 20th century, the incidence of tuberculosis has risen substantially in recent years.

For 2004, WHO reported an estimated 1.7 million deaths from TB, which included TB deaths in HIV-infected patients (http://www.who.int/mediacentre/ factsheets/fs104/en/). Both the largest number of deaths and the greatest number per capita occur in Africa, where HIV has led to rapid growth of the TB epidemic.

According to estimates by WHO, one third of the world's population (1.86 billion) is infected with *M. tuberculosis*, and 16.2 million people are currently suffering from tuberculosis (http://www.who.int/mediacentre/ factsheets/fs104/en/).

In Europe in 2004, an East-West gradient was shown to exist among new cases of tuberculosis, with 12.6 per 100,000 reported in the European Union and Western Europe, 50.7 per 100,000 in Central Europe, and 104 per 100,000 in Eastern Europe *(3)* (http://www.eurotb.org/rapports/ 2004/report_2004.htm).

A century ago, tuberculosis was the leading cause of death in the United States. However, after the introduction of effective antibiotic therapeutics and improvement in living conditions, the number of persons with TB disease and TB deaths declined steadily from the turn of the 20th century (death rate: 195 per 100,000) until 1985 (death rate: 0.7 per 100,000). However, from 1985 to 1992, case rates of tuberculosis in the United States unexpectedly increased, largely due to the HIV epidemic, cutbacks in public health infrastructure and treatment programs, increased poverty, homelessness, and drug abuse. Since 1992, a large influx of federal funds and renewed emphasis on antituberculosis therapy, prevention, and control have led again to declining tuberculosis cases and death rates in the United States (http://

www.cdc.gov/nchstp/tb/pubs/IOM/iomreport.htm). Foreign-born persons composed 54.3% of the new tuberculosis cases in the United States in 2005. The tuberculosis rate (21.8 per 100,000) among foreign-born individuals is nearly nine times the rate (2.5 per 100,000) among persons born in the United States (http://cdc.gov/mmwr/preview/ mmwrhtm/mm5511a3.htm).

The pattern of tuberculosis has also changed, and in recent years the incidence of extrapulmonary TB has become more common. Cases of extrapulmonary tuberculosis most commonly involve cerebral tuberculosis. Among the various contributing factors responsible for this disturbing trend, special attention has been given to the continuously increasing population of immunocompromised patients, especially those with HIV/AIDS. A small but statistically significant increase of tuberculosis in intravenous drug users has also been observed *(4)*.

Outbreaks of multidrug-resistant tuberculosis (MDR TB), initially reported to occur in hospitals and prisons, are characterized by high mortality rates, disease transmission within institutions, and high transmission rates to healthy health care workers *(5)*. MDR TB is a re-emerging infectious disease that has recently been included on the NIAID's Category C biodefense list.

Recently, a new and very disturbing trend has been taking place: the emergence of *Extensively Drug-Resistant Tuberculosis (XDR TB)*. XDR TB is defined as a multidrug (isoniazid, rifampin)-resistant tuberculosis (MDR TB) that is also resistant to fluoroquinolones and at least one of the three second-line injectable drugs (capreomycin, kanamycin, and amikacin).

14.1 Mycobacterium tuberculosis Co-infection in AIDS Patients

Worldwide, *M. tuberculosis* is the most common co-infection in persons with HIV/AIDS and is the leading cause of death in this population *(6)*. These two pathogens have a deadly synergy *(7)*:

(i) HIV infection promotes progression from latent or recurrent TB infection to disease *(8)*. There is a 5% to 10% annual risk of reactivation of latent infection in individuals co-infected with HIV and tuberculosis compared with a 10% lifetime risk in the HIV-negative population *(9)*.

(ii) HIV-infected patients are at increased risk of new infection with *M. tuberculosis (10)*.

(iii) The presence of tuberculosis can accelerate the course of HIV infection in individuals co-infected with *M. tuberculosis (11)*.

It has been well documented that HIV-infected patients are at particular risk of developing *M. tuberculosis* infection, and the course of the disease in such patients is accelerated as co-infected patients rapidly progressed from *M. tuberculosis* infection to active TB disease. Furthermore, co-infection with *M. tuberculosis* accelerates the progression of AIDS by increasing the replication rate of the HIV virus in *M. tuberculosis* co-infected patients *(12)*.

Although tuberculosis may be treatable and often preventable, it is believed that tuberculosis may be one of the most common opportunistic infections and *the leading cause of death among HIV-infected patients*, accounting for approximately 11% of all adult HIV/AIDS deaths worldwide *(3)*.

More than a quarter of the 42 million people infected with HIV worldwide are also infected with tuberculosis, and most live in countries with limited resources for health care (Africa and Asia). Thus, in some countries of sub-Saharan Africa, 50% to 80% of patients with tuberculosis are also HIV-positive, and high rates of tuberculosis (15% to 30%) are also observed in cohorts receiving highly active antiretroviral therapy (HAART) *(13)*. Tuberculosis caused 30% of AIDS-associated deaths in Africa in 1999 alone *(14)*.

Protective immunity to *M. tuberculosis* is dependent on an intact cellular immune system, with Th1-type CD4$^+$ T-lymphocytes being essential for the protective immunity against mycobacteria. Activation of macrophages by the release of interferon-γ (IFN-γ) from activated CD4$^+$ and CD8$^+$ T-lymphocytes is the primary mechanism by which *M. tuberculosis* replication is inhibited and by which *M. tuberculosis* is ultimately killed.

HIV infection, by impairing cell-mediated immunity, is the most potent known risk factor for reactivation of latent *M. tuberculosis*. HIV infects and kills CD4$^+$ T-lymphocytes, and as their concentration declines both the HIV infection and TB disease will progress *(6)*. Results from a recent study that modeled the effects of antiretroviral therapy on the incidence of tuberculosis in developing countries have estimated that the incidence of tuberculosis will increase by a factor of 2.1 for each reduction of 200/μL in the CD4$^+$ count *(15)*.

Although tuberculosis affects predominately the alveoli of the lung, extrapulmonary involvement is not unusual in HIV-positive patients, especially those with low CD4$^+$ counts where the extrapulmonary manifestations may occur in as many as half of the cases. In this situation, the lymphatic system has frequently been involved *(16)*. The incidence of tuberculous meningitis has also been higher among HIV-infected patients, but the clinical outcome has been similar to that in non–HIV-infected patients *(1)*.

The atypical presentation of extrapulmonary TB disease in HIV-infected patients also interferes with its timely and effective diagnosis. Because tuberculosis is difficult to diagnose in HIV-positive patients, it is readily (and inadvertently) transmitted to those not infected with HIV, especially in settings where both diseases are common *(17)*.

A comparative study to determine the clinical characteristics of cerebral tuberculoma in patients with and without HIV infection has shown that whereas disease-associated seizures were observed in HIV-negative individuals, in HIV-positive patients this finding was absent *(18)*. Instead, all patients studied had headache and fever and their cerebrospinal fluid (CSF) specimens showed the presence of lymphocytic meningitis. HIV-infected patients, where the cerebral tuberculoma was the result of dissemination, presented with spontaneous hypodense cerebral lesions; in contrast, the HIV-negative patients showed hyperdense cerebral lesions.

One very serious problem confronting clinicians treating HIV-positive patients with tuberculosis has been the high incidence of multidrug-resistant strains of *M. tuberculosis* compounding the mortality rate, which can reach 80%. In addition, such cases usually progress very rapidly. Inadequate treatment has been thought to be one major reason for the development of MDR TB, which is especially likely to occur when single drugs have been added to a failing regimen *(19)*. To avoid potential pitfalls, when initiating treatment in patients with confirmed MDR TB both the treatment history and the *in vitro* susceptibilities of the patient's *M. tuberculosis* strains should be thoroughly evaluated—the selected regimen should include between four and seven antimycobacterial agents, including such drugs as pyrazinamide, ethambutol, streptomycin, ofloxacin, ciprofloxacin, ethionamide, cycloserine, capreomycin, and *p*-aminosalicylic acid.

14.2 Mycobacterium tuberculosis

In contrast with most pathogenic bacteria, which are either facultative aerobes or anaerobes, the human tuberculous bacillus, *M. tuberculosis*, is an obligate aerobe. In humans, *M. tuberculosis* is observed as slightly bent or curved slender rods, approximately 2 to 4 μm long and 0.2 to 0.5 μm wide. In culture media, the cells may vary from coccoid to filamentous. An interesting feature of the virulent *M. tuberculosis* strains is their ability to grow as intertwining "serpentine cords" in which the bacilli aggregate with their long axes parallel *(1, 2)*.

One of the most characteristic features of mycobacteria has been their unusually high lipid content (20% to 40% of dry weight). The mycobacteria, which replicate slowly and may remain dormant for prolonged periods of time, *can be eradicated by drugs only when the organisms are replicating.*

The well-known "Bacille Calmette-Guérin" (BCG) is an attenuated mutant of *Mycobacterium bovis* that has been carried through several hundred serial cultures on unfavorable, bile-containing media. As a result, it multiplies in the host to a limited extent, causing at most only minor and transient lesions. BCG has been used to immunize humans against tuberculosis and has remained avirulent for more than 40 years *(1)*.

In humans, *M. tuberculosis* can be found in open cavities, closed caseous lesions, and within macrophages. Unlike *Mycobacterium leprae*, *M. tuberculosis* is not found inside cells other than macrophages and polymorphonuclear cells. *In vitro*, however, *M. tuberculosis* readily penetrates all cell lines tested.

Within macrophages, *M. tuberculosis* produces large amounts of lipoarabinomannan, a highly immunogenic, cell wall–associated glycolipid *(19a)*. Lipoarabinomannan is a potent inhibitor of interferon (IFN)-γ–mediated activation of murine macrophages by scavenging cytotoxic oxygen-free radicals. In addition, lipoarabinomannan inhibits the protein kinase C activity and blocks the transcriptional activation of IFN-γ–inducible genes in human macrophage-like cells. The adverse activity of lipoarabinomannan may contribute to the observed persistence of mycobacteria within mononuclear phagocytes.

14.2.1 Mycobacteriophages

The study of *M. tuberculosis* is complicated by the fact that the bacterium is very pathogenic and has an extremely slow growth rate, with a doubling time of approximately 24 hours *(20, 21)*. On the positive side, *M. tuberculosis* can grow on defined medium and pure clonal cultures can be propagated; this will facilitate studying its microbiological, metabolic, and chemical characteristics.

The development of genetic approaches to study mycobacteria started to make rapid advances in the late 1980s *(22)*. Such approaches made it possible to define the role of the mycobacteriophages (i.e., viruses that infect mycobacterial hosts) as means to deliver DNA into *M. tuberculosis*, develop genetic selectable markers, and construct recombinant strains *(23–26)*.

Although simple to isolate from the environment, very few mycobacteriophages have been studied in any molecular detail until recently, when most of the sequenced mycobacteriophages were isolated using *M. smegmatis* as a host *(27)*. Using *M. smegmatis* to propagate is relatively simple and fast, and a subset of these mycobacteriophages is expected to also infect slow-growing strains of *M. tuberculosis*. It is noteworthy that the currently available mycobacteriophage genomes are all strikingly diverse at the nucleotide sequence level (no two are the same) but not homogenously diverse. Furthermore, although the phage genome architecture is quite varied, all were densely packed with protein-coding genes that appeared to be organized into long operons with many genes closely linked and transcribed in the same direction *(27)*.

Most bacteriophages appear to be double-stranded DNA (dsDNA)-tailed viruses, and all mycobacteriophages belong to this general group. However, the dsDNA-tailed phages can be generally classified into three types: Siphoviridae (with long flexible tails), Myoviridae (with contractile tails), and Podoviridae (with short stubby tails). Of the known 30 sequenced mycobacteriophages, all but two (Bxz1 and Catera) belong to the Siphoviridae type, and interestingly, there are none to date that belong to the Podoviridae type *(27, 28)*.

Genetic Mosaicism of Mycobacteriophages. Whereas the mycobacteriophages appeared genetically diverse when compared at the nucleotide sequence level, a comparative analysis of the putative encoded proteins at the amino acid sequence level *(27)* revealed the presence of many genes that have clearly arisen from a common ancestor but diverged sufficiently long ago that their shared history would only be recognizable at the amino acid sequence level and not at the nucleotide level *(20, 27)*. Thus, when comparing these genomes by looking at their shared genes as deduced by similarity of amino acid sequence, pervasive mosaicism stands out as a characteristic feature of the genomic architecture *(29)*. This mosaicism is amply manifested by the presence of modules (containing one or a few genes) that are related to genes in another genome; however, adjacent genes (to their immediate left and right) are not related to each other but are in turn related to genes in different "phams" that have gene members in other phages *(27)*. Fundamentally, each mycobacteriophage genome represents a unique assemblage of individual modules *(27)*.

There are two plausible models to explain how genetic mosaicism in bacteriophages is generated. One early model *(30)* suggested the presence of short conserved boundary sequences at module junctions, which help to target the homologous recombination system to those positions. Although some evidence supporting the validity of this model has been presented (the analysis of *E. coli* phage HK620) *(31)*, the examples given in support appeared to be relatively few compared with the vast number of module junctions that had been identified. A more recent second model, which seems to be generally more applicable, suggested that recombination events largely occur by illegitimate recombination and are not directed by sequence similarity beyond perhaps a few common nucleotides *(32, 33)*. In this model, most of the events would give rise to genomic garbage, and rare subsequent events would likely to be required to produce a viable virus. Nevertheless, this is expected to be a creative process that would generate new module junctions, which can then be subsequently moved around by homologous recombination between common genes *(20, 29)*.

Mycobacteriophage Phamilies (Phams). Whereas just over half of the approximately 3,300 genes are not related to other mycobacteriophage genes, the other half can be grouped in "phamilies" or "phams" of related genes *(27)*. The size and distribution of these phamilies represent an alternative representation of the genetic diversity of mycobacteriophages. Because, to date, only 20 of these phamilies were found present in 10 or more of the 30 mycobacteriophage genomes, it would be interesting to study whether there are any phamilies that are present in all 30 genomes and thus might represent a mycobacteriophage signature that would be useful for predicting mycobacteriophage hosts using metagenomic data *(20)*. However, though there are three phamilies that appear to be present in all 30 genomes, the composite genes in all three phamilies—which correspond with tail fiber and lysis genes—are themselves mosaically constructed, and there is no segment of amino acid sequence that is characteristic of the mycobacteriophages *(27)*.

Acquisition of Host Genes by Mycobacteriophages. A somewhat surprising aspect of the illegitimate recombination model for genetic mosaicism is that it suggests that participation in the recombinant events is not restricted to the phage genome. That is, extensive similarity is not required and thus the host chromosome can also be involved *(20)*. In fact, because the bacterial genome is about 100-fold larger than a typical phage genome, it is be likely that it would become an active participant in the process. In this context, for example, it is not surprising that among the 30 sequenced mycobacteriophage genomes there were numerous genes that have been previously identified as bacterial genes (although they are now "phage" genes) *(27)*. Such acquisition of host genes is especially noteworthy, because it seems to emphasize that phages had likely played a large role in the evolution of bacteria, by acquiring DNA and transferring it between bacterial hosts. To this end, whereas a specific role of phages in the evolution of mycobacterial virulence has yet to be elucidated, such a role does not seem implausible, nor does the possibility that phages could have played a role in the dissemination of other phenotypes such as drug resistance *(20)*.

Mycobacteriophage-Based Genetic Tools. The isolation and characterization of mycobacteriophages have been extremely important for the development of genetic tools to manipulate *M. tuberculosis* and provide useful insights that may not have occurred without these phage-based approaches:

- *Shuttle plasmids (SPs)* are among the most important mycobacteriophage-based genetic tools. They represent chimeric molecules that replicate in *E. coli* as a large cosmid molecule and in mycobacteria as phages *(23)*. SPs can be manipulated using their propagation in *E. coli* and then used for the efficient delivery of (i) DNA to their bacterial hosts; (ii) reporter genes, such as luciferase for use in diagnosis and drug susceptibility *(34, 35)*; (iii) transposons for random mutagenesis *(36)*; and (iv) for the creation of gene replacement mutants by specialized transduction *(37)*.

- *Integration-Proficient Plasmid Vectors.* The integration-proficient plasmid vectors can be constructed by inserting the phage attachment site (*attP*) and the integrase gene into a plasmid vector that can otherwise neither integrate nor replicate in mycobacteria *(38)*. When electroporated into mycobacteria, the integrase gene is expressed, and a site-specific recombination between the *attP* site and a unique chromosomal *attB* site is catalyzed by the phage-derived integrase, and transformants can be selected *(20)*. The stability of integration-proficient vectors is dependent on the specific integrase used, the mode in which it is delivered, and whether or not the phage-encoded *excise* [a member of the larger group of *Recombination Directionality Factors*, or RDFs *(39)*] is also present *(40)*.

- *tRNA Suppressors.* Whereas tRNA suppressors have proved to be very significant tools in *E. coli* genetics, isolating informational suppressors in mycobacteria has been largely unsuccessful, because these have only minimal sets of tRNA genes with little redundancy *(20)*. To overcome this, tRNA genes derived from phage L5 have been mutated and expressed in such a way that they can act as tRNA suppressors in *M. smegmatis*. One specific application of these tRNA suppressors has been in the identification of the RDF (*xis*) gene involved in regulating Bxb1 integration and excision *(32)*.

14.3 Diagnostic and Differentiation Procedures for Mycobacterium tuberculosis

Diagnostic and differentiation procedures for *M. tuberculosis* are usually based on the presence of antigens exclusive to the organism *(41)*. Among the several proteins present in *M. tuberculosis* but absent in the *M. bovis* BCG sonic extracts, the denoted MTP40 antigen has been extensively studied and found to be exclusive to *M. tuberculosis.*

In addition, several PCR-based assays have been developed for detecting mycobacteria. Using PCR, DNA amplification of three *M. tuberculosis*–specific DNA sequences, IS6110, the 65-kDa antigen, and the MPB64, have been developed and used for rapid diagnosis of tuberculous meningitis *(1).*

14.4   Host Defense Against Mycobacteria

The spread of the AIDS pandemic, coupled with the re-emergence of tuberculosis, has presented the scientific and medical communities with an enormous public health challenge that has rekindled interest in the mechanisms by which the immune system may control mycobacterial infections.

There is a sequence of events that follows the intracellular penetration of *M. tuberculosis* into phagocytic cells *(1).* This sequence includes the activation of accessory cells to trigger the host immune response, the activation of various effector cells and cytotoxic lymphocytes, and the enhanced production of cytokines. Two fractions of mycobacterial proteins (molecular weight of 20,000 and 46,000, respectively) that have consistently stimulated the production of interleukin-1 and the tumor necrosis factor-α (TNF-α) by monocytes have been identified *(42).* The increased levels of these two cytokines may cause the fever and cachexia that have been readily associated with tuberculosis.

Although the relationship between host and mycobacteria is still not very well understood, experimental evidence has shown that in the presence of antimycobacterial drugs and normal host defense mechanisms, the tubercle bacilli are converted into metabolically inactive, non–acid fast (NAF) granular forms. These forms represent cell wall–deficient variants that remain dormant but may also revert back to the parent, acid-fast bacilli in the case of immunocompromised patients, thus causing the disease to persist in spite of chemotherapy *(43).*

Experimental evidence has suggested that humoral (B cell) responses in tuberculosis will precede the protective cell-mediated immunity. In the majority of patients, the humoral response is characterized by an initial rise in specific IgM immunoglobulins, followed by an increase in the IgG production during the subclinical infection stage. Eventually, the B-cell responses are suppressed as protective cell-mediated immunity is established during the protracted subclinical phase of the infection *(44).*

In addition to the well-known immunologic role of T cells bearing the conventional $\alpha\beta$ T-cell receptor, research data have indicated that $\gamma\delta$ T-cells may also play a distinct role in generating the primary immune response to mycobacteria *(45).*

The growth of *M. tuberculosis* in human macrophages has been investigated at both ambient oxygen concentrations (5% CO_2 and 95% air, corresponding with 20% O_2 or 140 mmHg PO_2) and concentrations corresponding with tissue levels (5% CO_2 and 5% CO_2 in nitrogen balance, corresponding with 36 mmHg PO_2) *(46).* When cultivated at lower PO_2 concentrations, macrophages had an increased glycolytic (but decreased oxidative) metabolism. Upon stimulation, such macrophages had a better preserved ability to respond with an increased production of superoxide anion. After infection with *M. tuberculosis,* macrophages cultivated at lower PO_2 permitted significantly less growth of the bacterium than did macrophages cultured at higher PO_2 levels. Crude lymphokines, recombinant IFN-γ, or recombinant TNF-α have not consistently affected the growth of mycobacteria in macrophages cultured at either high or low oxygen pressure. The observed reduced growth of mycobacteria cultivated in macrophages at physiologic PO_2 levels may explain the preferential localization of tuberculosis lesions in body areas, such as the lung apex, where the tissue levels of PO_2 are high *(46).*

In the context of host immune responses against mycobacteria, the lymphocyte response has been an essential part of the immune defense against these organisms. Thus, in human pulmonary tuberculosis, CD4[+] lymphocytes were found in substantially increased numbers in the pleural fluid but relatively depleted in the blood. In the bronchoalveolar lavage fluid, their numbers varied widely in localized pulmonary and miliary tuberculosis but were highest in lavage fluid from patients with miliary tuberculosis. In the latter case, the increase was the result of an increase in CD8[+] lymphocytes, which were also increased in the blood *(47).*

14.5   Evolution of Therapies and Treatment of Mycobacterium tuberculosis

Specific chemotherapy against tuberculosis was started in the early 1940s *(2).* Soon after its discovery as an antituberculosis agent, isoniazid (isonicotinyl hydrazine; INH) became an essential agent of any antituberculosis therapy. Next, the introduction of the rifampicin antibiotics, streptomycin, pyrazinamide, and the fluoroquinolones made it possible that such therapy not only could be relatively short in duration but also could be given intermittently, thus allowing for closer supervision and monitoring. Isoniazid, rifampin, rifabutin, pyrazinamide, and ethambutol are the major antimycobacterial agents used to treat tuberculosis *(48, 49).*

The mechanisms of action of various antimycobacterial agents are different, as are their primary sites of action *(49)*. Thus, isoniazid and rifampin exert their bactericidal activity against all mycobacteria. By comparison, streptomycin is most effective against bacilli found in open cavities, whereas the bactericidal activity of pyrazinamide is most pronounced against bacilli within the macrophages.

In therapeutic doses, isoniazid, rifampin, and pyrazinamide usually achieve adequate tissue and body fluid concentrations to kill *M. tuberculosis* in all body sites. Ethambutol, ethionamide, and *p*-aminosalicylic acid are all bacteriostatic *(49)*.

Drug resistance is common among mycobacteria, and the number of drug-resistant mutants is usually proportional to the size of the mycobacterial population. The main rationale for antituberculosis treatment is to give a regimen combining drug(s) having bactericidal activity with bacteriostatic agents that suppress the emergence of drug-resistant mutants. Microbiologic cure usually requires between 18 and 24 months of therapy. It is generally accepted that using at least two bactericidal drugs against susceptible isolates is likely to provide cure in 6 to 9 months *(50)*.

One of the recommended chemotherapeutic regimens for newly diagnosed patients (both children and adults) involves a 6-month daily course of isoniazid and rifampicin, supplemented with pyrazinamide for the first 2 months *(51, 52)*.

The optional treatment of tuberculosis in HIV-positive patients is still being defined because patients' response to treatment of pulmonary tuberculosis may vary considerably. Although several studies have indicated that adverse outcomes are more likely to occur in patients with delayed sputum sterilization, there is limited methodology to identify such patients prospectively. In this regard, multivariate models have been developed to predict the response to therapy in a prospectively recruited cohort of HIV-negative subjects with drug-sensitive tuberculosis *(53)*.

Since 1986, powerful short-course regimens have also been commonly used *(54)*. One preferred combination has been isoniazid, rifampin, and pyrimidazine administered on a daily basis for 2 months, followed by isoniazid and rifampin for an additional 4 months. Also, a 9-month regimen of isoniazid and rifampin has been found equally effective. However, supplementation (in case of drug resistance) or extension (when immunosuppression has been present) of short-course regimens has been strongly recommended *(49)*.

In March 2007, WHO added four antituberculosis drugs to its list of *prequalified products*: cycloserine, ethambutol-isoniazid, ethambutol, and pyrazinamide. Cycloserine is particularly important because, as a second-line therapy, it can treat tuberculosis that is resistant to standard treatment.

14.5.1 Drug Interactions in HIV-Infected Patients

In cases of rifampin (rifampicin; Rifadin; Rimactane), although true intolerance to this antibiotic has been rare even among HIV-infected patients, discontinuation owing to thrombocytopenia, creatinine over 2.0 mg/mL, bilirubin over 2.0 mg/mL, or severe reactions (generalized rash, persistent drug fever, or severe interference with methadone metabolism) has been reported *(54)*.

In general, rifampin should not be administered with protease inhibitors or non-nucleoside reverse transcriptase inhibitors *(55, 56)*. Although rifabutin is an acceptable alternative, certain precautions must be taken. In particular, rifabutin should not be used with the hard-gel protease inhibitor saquinavir and the non-nucleoside reverse transcriptase inhibitor delavirdine, and caution should be applied when co-administered with the soft-gel saquinavir. In addition, rifabutin should be given to HIV-infected patients at one half the usual daily dose (from 300 to 150 mg daily) when co-administered with indinavir, nelfinavir, or amprenavir, and one fourth the usual daily dose (i.e., 150 mg every other day, or 3 times weekly) with ritonavir. In the latter case, adding ritonavir will facilitate the combined therapy of rifampin and saquinavir *(57)*. Based on pharmacokinetic data, rifabutin may be applied at an increased dose (450 mg daily) when co-administered with efavirenz *(56)*.

14.5.2 Highly Active Antiretroviral Therapy and Mycobacterial Infections in HIV-Positive Patients

Since its introduction, HAART has significantly reduced the incidence of opportunistic infections in HIV-positive patients in general, and mycobacterial infections in particular *(58)*. This, coupled with continuing prophylaxis against specific opportunistic infections, would definitely increase the survival benefits in this population *(2)*.

In a European report *(59)* using data from a EuroSIDA study (1994–1999) involving a multicenter observational cohort of more than 7,000 patients, there has been a marked decrease in the incidence of *M. tuberculosis* infections; the decrease has been attributed to favorable changes in the $CD4^+$ cell counts after the introduction of HAART.

Although the use of HAART exerted a remarkable impact on the course of HIV disease, because of potential drug interactions it has also raised several issues with respect to HIV-related tuberculosis and its treatment. In particular, such drug interactions will necessitate the need of either a non–rifamycin-based regimen or a rifabutin-based regimen in patients receiving HAART and treated for tuberculosis *(60)*.

14.5.3 Prophylaxis of Tuberculosis in HIV-Infected Patients

In a recent report *(61)*, the *Advisory Council for the Elimination of Tuberculosis* recommended a model for tuberculosis control programs to be implemented in the United States that includes three priority strategies for prevention and control: (i) identifying and treating persons with active tuberculosis; (ii) finding and screening persons who had contact with patients with tuberculosis to determine whether they have been infected with *M. tuberculosis* or have active disease and providing appropriate treatment if necessary; and (iii) screening populations at high risk for tuberculosis and providing therapy to prevent progression of active disease.

In general, although prophylaxis with isoniazid for 6 to 12 months has been very important, it is often a neglected preventive measure for patients latently infected but still without active disease *(62)*. Daily therapy with 300 mg of isoniazid for at least 9 months has been recommended for patients at high risk for tuberculosis *(63, 64)*.

In HIV-infected pregnant women, when the patients have not been exposed to drug-resistant tuberculosis, daily or twice-weekly prophylaxis with isoniazid is the recommended regimen of choice. However, because of concerns regarding teratogenicity, prophylaxis should be initiated after the first trimester. In addition, to reduce the danger of neurotoxicity, preventive therapy with isoniazid should be accompanied with pyridoxine *(55)*.

14.5.4 Adjunctive Immunotherapy of Tuberculosis

Modulation of the host response has the promise to become a powerful tool in the treatment of tuberculosis *(65)*. In a randomized, placebo-controlled trial, a cohort of HIV-negative Ugandan patients with newly diagnosed pulmonary tuberculosis was subjected to adjunctive immunotherapy with a heat-killed *Mycobacterium vaccae*. Patients were randomized to a single dose of *M. vaccae* or placebo 1 week after beginning of chemotherapy and were followed up for 1 year. The results have demonstrated an early increase in sputum-culture conversion after 1 month of chemotherapy and greater radiographic improvement (91% vs. 77% for placebo recipients at 6 months) among patients receiving *M. vaccae*, which was safe and well tolerated *(66)*.

Adjuvant cytokines such as interleukin 2 (IL-2), IL-12, interferon-γ, and granulocyte-macrophage colony-stimulating factor (GM-CSF) may also prove useful in shortening the duration of treatment and overcoming drug resistance *(65)*.

14.5.5 Vaccine Development Against Tuberculosis

As tuberculosis is continuing to emerge as a global health threat, there has been an urgent need to develop more effective tuberculosis vaccines because chemotherapy and BCG vaccine have failed to control the ever-growing tuberculosis epidemic *(7, 67)*. As more vaccines enter early clinical trials, there is a pressing need to identify correlates of protection to aid decisions about which vaccines should go forward into clinical testing *(67)*.

14.5.5.1 Bacille Calmette-Guérin Vaccine

The BCG is a live attenuated strain of *Mycobacterium bovis* obtained by passaging the microorganism in culture more than 230 times *(7, 67)*. It was first used in humans in 1921 by Calmette and Guérin, and in 1924, the Institut Pasteur began to mass produce and distribute the vaccine. Seed stock of BCG was distributed to other manufacturers and the process of attenuation continued, resulting in more than 16 *(68)* distinct strains of BCG worldwide.

Although BCG vaccine is one of the most widely used vaccines, there are still conflicting reports about its efficacy. Whereas there is evidence that the protection against disseminated forms of tuberculosis in childhood and tuberculous meningitis is approximately 80% *(69)*, an average efficacy of 50% (0 to 80%) was reported in a meta-analysis of literature covering 1,264 articles, from which 70 clinical trials were selected spanning a 46-year period *(70)*. Blocking or masking of the immune response by prior exposure to environmental mycobacteria remains the most plausible explanation for the variability in BCG efficacy *(71, 72)*.

14.5.5.2 Protective Immunity Against Mycobacterium tuberculosis

A T-helper (Th1) cell–mediated immune response with the release of IFN-γ is required for protection from disease *(73–77)*. However, even though IFN-γ is important for protective immunity, IFN-γ alone is not sufficient for protection. Because no other correlate has been identified, the release of IFN-γ from CD4$^+$ and CD8$^+$ T-cells would remain as the primary assay used to determine the immunogenicity of any new tuberculosis vaccine *(7, 67)*.

The importance of class II–restricted CD4$^+$ T-cells in immunity against tuberculosis has been demonstrated by adoptive transfer experiments and more recently confirmed by using CD4$^+$ knockout mice *(78, 79)*. There is also increasing evidence from both animal and human studies that class I–restricted CD8$^+$ T-lymphocytes have contributed to antimycobacterial immunity *(80–84)*. Furthermore, γ/δ cells and non–classically restricted T-lymphocytes, such as CD1-restricted T cells, may also play a protective role *(85, 86)*, but it is not yet fully understood how to induce these cell types by vaccination *(7)*.

The inhibition of apoptosis of infected host cells is a well-known but poorly understood function of pathogenic mycobacteria. It has been shown that inactivation of the *secA2* gene in *M. tuberculosis*, which encodes a component of a virulence-associated protein secretion system, enhanced the apoptosis of infected macrophages by diminishing secretion of mycobacterial superoxide dismutase *(87)*. Deletion of *secA2* markedly increased priming of antigen-specific CD8$^+$ T-cells *in vivo*, and vaccination of mice and guinea pigs with a *secA2* mutant significantly increased resistance to challenge by *M. tuberculosis* compared with standard *M. bovis* BCG vaccination. The results of the study have defined a mechanism for a *key immune evasion strategy* of *M. tuberculosis* that may provide a novel approach for improving mycobacterial vaccines.

14.5.5.3 Scientific Strategies

Depending on the disease stage, there are three main strategies that can be used for a vaccine intervention to reduce the incidence of tuberculosis *(67)*:

(i) *Preexposure Vaccines.* The vaccine is given before the person comes into contact with the pathogen. Because tuberculosis is endemic in many parts of the world and is easily transmissible by aerosol, a preexposure vaccine would be best administered at birth. BCG is currently administered at birth in many countries.

(ii) *Postexposure Vaccines.* The vaccine is administered after infection to prevent the development of the disease. Given that one third of the world's population is latently infected with *M. tuberculosis*, such a vaccine would have a more immediate impact on the incidence of disease.

(iii) *Therapeutic Vaccines.* The vaccine could be administered after the disease has developed, usually as an adjunct to chemotherapy. The aim of vaccination is to reduce relapse rates and possibly to reduce the length of treatment with chemotherapy.

Prime-Boost Immunization Strategy

The use of vaccines to induce a protective humoral immune response against subsequent exposure to a pathogen is a widely used principle in preventing infectious diseases. Furthermore, repeated vaccination with the same vaccine results in higher levels of antibodies than that after a single vaccination. However, whereas such *homologous* boosting is sufficient for organisms for which protective immune response depends on humoral immunity, the induction of a strong cellular immune response by vaccination is not as straightforward. Such intracellular pathogens as *M. tuberculosis*, HIV, and *Plasmodium falciparum* all require, at least in part, a strong cellular immune response for protective immunity *(88)*. The use of different antigen delivery systems (plasmid DNA vaccines; recombinant proteins together with a Th1-inducing adjuvant; recombinant viral and bacterial vectors) to induce high levels of cellular immunity, although promising, has shown certain limitations.

Furthermore, unlike the induction of antibodies, repeated homologous boosting with the same vaccine does not result in an increase in the magnitude of cellular immune response induced, as preexisting anti-vector immunity will inhibit processing of antigens.

Such shortcomings have led to the development of a new strategy, known as "heterologous prime-boost" to improve the immunogenicity of T-cell–inducing vaccines. This strategy involves administering two different vaccines, each one expressing the same antigen, and then giving the vaccines several weeks apart *(88)*. The heterologous prime-boost strategy has been demonstrated to induce substantially higher levels of T cells than does homologous boosting with the same vector in a wide variety of animal models against a wide variety of pathogens. Proof-of-principle of the immunogenicity and effectiveness of the heterologous prime-boost immunization has been further demonstrated in humans, in the case of *P. falciparum* *(89)*. Using the same approach in tuberculosis, priming with a DNA vaccine expressing both ESAT-6 and MPT63, and boosting with a recombinant modified vaccinia Ankara virus (MVA) expressing the same antigens, induced higher levels of antigen-specific CD4$^+$ T-cells than that seen with homologous boosting and protection against challenge equivalent to BCG *(90)*. Improved levels of CD4$^+$ and CD8$^+$ T-cells were seen when DNA and MVA constructs expressing antigen 85A were used in a prime-boost regime that was as protective as BCG *(91)*.

It should be emphasized, however, that in order to incorporate BCG into a heterologous prime-boost strategy, the antigen chosen for selection in the boosting subunit vaccine *must* be present in all strains of BCG and be highly conserved among all mycobacterial species *(88)*.

The exact mechanisms by which the heterologous prime-boost immunization strategy induced significantly higher antigen-specific T-cell responses than did the homologous boosting with the same vector have not been fully understood (88). It is likely that several different mechanisms contribute to the success of this strategy, and the mechanism may also depend in part on the nature of the boosting vector used. One mechanism that contributes to the success of prime-boost strategies is the *T-cell immunodominance*. That is, on first exposure to an antigen, in priming immunization, T-cell responses will be induced to the most immunodominant epitopes within the same antigen. The boosting vaccination, which shares only the relevant antigen with the priming vaccination, will preferentially expand the immunodominant memory T-cells induced by the priming vaccination, and hence focus the immune response on those responses (88). A second mechanism for prime-boost relates to the qualities of the vector. Thus, recombinant poxviruses and recombinant adenoviruses are particularly suitable for boosting previously primed T-cell responses by inducing nonspecific costimulated responses that facilitate the amplification of preexisting memory immune responses (88).

A third explanation for the enhanced immunogenicity of the prime-boost strategy is that it avoids the induction of antivector immunity (both T- and B-cell mediated) that occurs with homologous boosting with the same vaccine (88).

14.5.5.4   Vaccines in Preclinical or Clinical Evaluation

Currently, there are number of new vaccines in preclinical testing in animal models. Because of the complexity of working with *M. tuberculosis*, the majority of them are preexposure vaccines. Animal models for both postexposure and therapeutic vaccines are being developed but at present are less well established (67).

Vaccines can be live-attenuated organisms, heat-inactivated or chemically inactivated whole organisms, or consist of a subunit of DNA, protein, or lipid from the pathogen (67). Typically, live-attenuated vaccines are more immunogenic than are the inactivated vaccines, whereas the subunit vaccines are the least immunogenic. However, the immunogenicity of subunit vaccines can be increased by using multiple vaccinations or by including an adjuvant in the vaccine formulation.

When tested in mouse and guinea pig models, BCG (a live-attenuated vaccine) was highly immunogenic and conferred excellent protection against challenge. This finding has led to vaccination strategies that include BCG, either by boosting a BCG vaccination or by developing an improved strain of BCG. It has also been possible to improve the protective effects of BCG by giving a BCG vaccination followed by a subunit vaccine. Such a heterologous prime-boost strategy has relied on the subunit vaccine encoding an antigen present in both BCG and *M. tuberculosis*—the cellular

immune response to the mycobacterial antigen was primed by BCG and then boosted by the subunit vaccine (67).

At present, a number of tuberculosis vaccines are undergoing preclinical and clinical trials listed in the Investigational Drug Database (© 1997–2006 Thompson Scientific Ltd.) (http://www.iddb.com) (67):

- *Preclinical Evaluation*

  ○ *The Statens Serum Institute/Aeras/Intercell (HyVac4) Vaccine*. HyVac4 is a protein (TB10.40) in an antigen 85B fusion molecule) plus adjuvant, BCG prime-boost subunit vaccine (91a).

  ○ *Polymun TB Vaccine*. The Polymun TB vaccine is a protein-based (ESAT)-6-NS1 (influenza) vaccine that is administered as a nasal spray.

  ○ *Crucell/Aeras TB vaccine*. The Crucell/Aeras vaccine represents an adenovirus expressing Ag85B (antigen 85B), BCG prime-boost vaccine.

  ○ *BioSante (Bio-vant-TB) Vaccine*. The Bio-vant-TB vaccine is being tested as a BCG replacement vaccine comprising bacterial cells.

  ○ *Universitat Autonoma de Barcelona (RUTI) Vaccine*. The RUTI vaccine is also intended as a BCG replacement vaccine comprising *M. tuberculosis* fragments encapsulated in liposomes (92).

- *Clinical Evaluation*

  ○ *Aeras/UCLA (rBCG30) Vaccine*. rBCG30 represents a preexposure vaccine. Phase I clinical trials with a recombinant BCG Tice strain overexpressing antigen 85B began in 2004 (92a). It was designed as a replacement for BCG vaccine (93, 94).

  ○ *GlaxoSmithKline (Mtb72F/AS02A) Vaccine*. Mtb72F/AS02A is a BCG prime-boost vaccine consisting of the *M. tuberculosis* polyprotein Mtb72F delivered as recombinant protein (Mtb35:Mtb32) plus adjuvant (95, 96). It is a fusion of the Mtb39 (PPE protein) and Mtb32 (serine protease antigens from *M. tuberculosis*), and as these proteins are present in BCG, Mtb72F can be used in a heterologous prime-boost regimen with BCG (95). The vaccine entered Phase I trials in 2004, and vaccination of purified protein derivative-positive adults began in 2005 (http://www.clinicaltrials.gov/ct/show/nct00146744).

  ○ *The Statens Serum Institute/Aeras/Intercell/Chiron (Hybrid 1) Vaccine*. Hybrid 1 is BCG prime-boost vaccine. It is a recombinant fusion protein of the ESAT-6 and Ag85B antigens from *M. tuberculosis*. The vaccine entered clinical trials in 2005 and is being used in combination with the adjuvant IC-31, developed by Intercell, and nasal route of administration using adjuvant (LTK-63) (97). Antigen 85B is also present in BCG and would enable Hybrid 1 to be used in a prime-boost regimen with BCG. ESAT-6 is a highly immunogenic antigen from *M. tuberculosis* that is not present in BCG. Because ESAT-6 has been shown to be useful for the diagnosis of latent TB infection *(98)*, vaccination with the ESAT-6 antigen may compromise the value of ESAT-6 as a diagnostic marker for TB infection *(67)*.

○ *SR-Pharma (SLR-172) Vaccine.* SLR-172 is a therapeutic vaccine consisting of *M. vaccae* bacterial cells *(99)*. SLR-172 entered Phase II trial in 2002.

○ *The University of Oxford (MVA85A) Vaccine.* MVA85A was the first subunit TB vaccine to enter clinical trials and the only one for which published trial data are available *(93)*. The MVA85A vaccine comprises a recombinant viral vector (MVA; recombinant modified vaccinia Ankara virus) *(100, 101)* expressing antigen 85A (Ag85A) working in tandem with BCG, prime-boost vaccine *(102, 103)*. In the first Phase I study of MVA85A, it was found to induce high levels of antigen-specific IFN-γ–secreting T cells when used alone in BCG-naïve healthy volunteers. In volunteers who had been vaccinated 0.5 to 38 years previously with BCG, MVA85A induced substantially higher levels of antigen-specific IFN-γ–secreting T-cells, and at 24 weeks after vaccination these levels were 5 to 30 times greater than in those administered a single BCG vaccination.

The MVA85A vaccine has already passed safety tests in healthy volunteers in The Gambia. In clinical trials, MVA85A has been highly immunogenic. The magnitude of the CD4$^+$ T-cell response induced by BCG-MVA85A was greater than any response seen before using a viral vector boost *(93)*. Phase II clinical trials with MVA85A started in the Western Cape in South Africa, and in July 2007, a clinical Phase II trial involving adolescents and HIV-positive adult patients began in South Africa.

Other TB Vaccine Studies

• A Phase I trial was conducted to assess the safety and immunogenicity of inactivated *M. vaccae* as a candidate vaccine to prevent tuberculosis in AIDS patients *(104, 105)*. The trial, which was conducted in Zambia, involved a cohort of HIV-positive patients with lymphocytic counts at or below 200 cells/mm^3 and a cohort of healthy subjects (BCG-immunized and naïve). The patients received either a three-dose (HIV-negative) or a five-dose (HIV-positive) schedule of intradermal *M. vaccae* at 0, 2, 4, 11, and 13 months. The five-dose series of vaccinations was safe and induced lymphocytic proliferation responses to the vaccine antigen *(104)*.

• Using microarray DNA-chip technology, a study was initiated to determine the best candidate for a therapeutic *M. tuberculosis* vaccine *(106)*. In another study, the cell-mediated and protective immune responses to DNA vaccines encoding the *M. tuberculosis* proteins ESAT-6, MPT-64, Antigen85A, and KatG were administered intranasally or intramuscularly and evaluated *(107)*. At Day 28 after a low-dose aerosol challenge with *M. tuberculosis* Erdman, several of the DNA vaccine constructs demonstrated protective immune responses as measured by reduced lung and spleen colony-forming units.

• A mutant of *M. tuberculosis* deficient in antigen 85A expression acted as vaccine against experimental tuberculosis in mice *(108)*.

14.5.6 *Drug Resistance of Mycobacterium tuberculosis*

With the emergence of drug-resistant strains of *M. tuberculosis (109)*, the effective chemotherapy of the disease will require rapid assessment of drug resistance *(2)*. Until recently, the available methodology would not allow drug susceptibility to be determined for 2 to 18 weeks because of the 20- to 24-hour doubling time of *M. tuberculosis*. However, some newer techniques, such as the firefly luciferase-based assay, may remedy this situation by significantly shortening the ascertainment times. Phenotypic methods to identify drug-resistant *M. tuberculosis* are based on the measurement of the microbial growth on a nutritional supplement with antimicrobial agents. However, using this methodology (e.g., the Bactec radiometric method, mycobacterial growth indicator tube, and the method in solid medium) is time-consuming and would require 5 to 21 days to complete. In contrast, the genotype-based methodology, which uses the knowledge of genes involved in the resistance to identify the different mutations conferring the antimicrobial resistance, reduces the time to detect resistance from weeks to days *(110)*.

To avoid potential pitfalls when initiating treatment of patients with confirmed MDR TB, both the treatment history and the *in vitro* susceptibilities of the patient's tuberculosis strains should be thoroughly evaluated. The selected regimen should include between four and seven antimycobacterial agents, including such drugs as pyrazinamide, ethambutol, streptomycin, ofloxacin, ciprofloxacin, ethionamide, cycloserine, capreomycin, and *p*-aminosalicylic acid *(110a)*. Based on tuberculosis-susceptibility patterns, predictors of multidrug resistance, and implications for initial therapeutic regimens, a theoretically effective antituberculosis regimen was assumed to contain at least two drugs to which an *M. tuberculosis* isolate was susceptible *(111)*.

Historically, the majority of multidrug-resistant antituberculosis regimens contained isoniazid and rifampin as part of the same regimen *(2)*. As a consequence of this combined therapy, acquired rifampin resistance without preexisting isoniazid resistance is highly unusual in patients with tuberculosis *(112)*, and strains resistant only to rifampin have rarely been recovered. However, there has been increased evidence of HIV-positive patients infected with mono-rifampin-resistant *M. tuberculosis (113)*.

14.5.6.1 Multidrug-Resistant Tuberculosis

In recent years, the worldwide treatment of tuberculosis has been further hampered by the emergence of multidrug-resistant mutants of mycobacterium.

According to estimates by WHO, annually at least 300,000 new cases of multidrug-resistant tuberculosis (MDR TB) occur worldwide; 79% of them are resistant to at least three of the four main drugs used to cure tuberculosis *(114)*. (http://www.who.int/mediacentre/news/releases/2004/pr17/en/print.html).

In the United States, cases of MDR TB represent a relatively small percentage of total TB cases, with the most common form being caused by *M. tuberculosis* strains resistant to isoniazid (7.8% of cases in 2004) (http://www.cdc.gov/nchstp/tb/surv/surv2004/default.htm). Even though the latest national surveillance data show that tuberculosis rates in the United States reached an all time low in 2005 *(114, 115)*, TB drug resistance is increasing. Thus, tuberculosis that is resistant to at least two first-line therapies (isoniazid and rifampin) increased 13.3% from 2003 to 2004—the largest single-year increase in MDR TB since 1993.

The long duration and associated adverse side effects of the standard antituberculosis treatment often will result in patients not completing the full course of therapy, which allows for the emergence of single-drug and multidrug resistant *M. tuberculosis* strains. Drug-resistant tuberculosis may require up to 2 years of treatment depending on the pattern of resistance. This therapy will usually include the use of second-line drugs (SLDs) (e.g., cycloserine), which are less effective, sometimes more toxic, and often cost more than isoniazid- and rifampin-based regimens. In addition, drug-resistant patients may remain infectious for long periods, thereby increasing the possibility of transmission of drug-resistant *M. tuberculosis* strains (http://www.cdc.gov/nchstp/tb/pubs/tbfactsheets/250112.htm).

14.5.6.2 Extensively Drug-Resistant Tuberculosis

Since 2000, there have been worldwide reports of the emergence of extensively drug-resistance tuberculosis (XDR TB).

Because it is virtually untreatable, XDR TB represents a very serious threat to the control of tuberculosis and to public health worldwide (http://www.who.int/tb/en). From 2000 to 2004, 2% of tuberculosis patients whose isolates were tested in a survey of a worldwide laboratory network were classified as XDR TB *(114)*. Over the 5-year period in this survey, XDR TB increased from 5% of MDR TB cases in 2000 to 6.5% in 2004 (excluding South Korea). According to the survey, in the industrialized nations, including the United States, XDR TB increased from 3% of MDR TB cases in 2000 to 11% in 2004 *(114, 116)* (http://www.cdc.gov/od/oc/media/pressrel/fs060323.htm).

In a published report in March 2006, the CDC, in collaboration with the WHO and participating supranational reference laboratories, had agreed to define XDR TB as cases of tuberculosis in persons whose *M. tuberculosis* isolates were resistant to isoniazid and rifampin and at least three of six main classes of second-line drugs (aminoglycosides, polypeptides, fluoroquinolones, thioamides, cycloserine, and *p*-aminosalicylic acid) *(117, 118)*. Since that original publication, additional reports have documented the presence of XDR TB in Iran *(119)* and South Africa *(120)*, with high mortality among persons infected with HIV who are benefiting from antiretroviral therapy. The worldwide emergence and transmission of these *M. tuberculosis* strains highlighted the urgency of strengthening the national TB and HIV/AIDS control programs, particularly in settings with high HIV prevalence (http://www.mrc.ac.za/pressreleases/8pres2006.htm). Subsequently, a revised case definition of XDR TB has been adopted, based on observations that (i) whereas drug-susceptibility testing to fluoroquinolones and some second-line injectable drugs (i.e., the aminoglycosides, amikacin and kanamycin, and the polypeptide capreomycin) yields reproducible and reliable results, the drug-susceptibility testing to other second-line drugs is less reliable; and (ii) the resistance to fluoroquinolones and second-line injectable drugs has been associated with poor treatment results.

Hence, *the new agreed-upon definition of XDR TB (118) has been defined as the occurrence of tuberculosis in persons whose M. tuberculosis isolates are resistant to:*

(i)   Isoniazid and rifampin.
(ii) Any fluoroquinolone.
(iii) At least one of three injectable second-line drugs (i.e., amikacin, kanamycin, or capreomycin).

14.6 Recent Scientific Advances

- *Isoniazid Target in M. tuberculosis Is Identified*. Although INH is one of the most effective drugs against tuberculosis, *M. tuberculosis* resistance to this drug is increasing despite the use of multidrug regimens. Recently, a team of researchers using specialized linkage transduction have succeeded in introducing a small but defined change (mutation) in the protein InhA alone, which is thought to be the primary target of INH. This small change was found to be the same one that is seen in InhA when the bacteria become resistant to INH— *M. tuberculosis* with the changed protein InhA could no longer be killed with normal amounts of INH. When isolated, the altered InhA protein from *M. tuberculosis* lost its ability to effectively bind to INH *(121)*. With this information at hand, it will be possible to characterize the exact effect of INH on the bacterial metabolism, better understand how *M. tuberculosis* creates resistance toward INH, and design new drugs that will be effective against this mutated drug target.

- *Potent Twice-Weekly Rifapentine-Containing Regimens in Murine Tuberculosis.* Recent studies have demonstrated that intermittent administration of rifamycin-based regimens resulted in higher rates of tuberculosis relapse and treatment failure than did daily therapy. However, twice-weekly treatment of TB with rifampin, INH, and pyrazinamide may be improved by increasing the exposure of *M. tuberculosis* to rifamycin by substituting rifapentine for rifampin. To test this hypothesis, the activities of standard daily and twice-weekly rifampin plus INH-based regimens were compared with those of twice-weekly rifapentine plus INH- or moxifloxacin-containing regimens in the murine model of tuberculosis *(122)*. The obtained results have demonstrated that after 2 months of treatment, twice-weekly therapy with rifapentine (15 or 20 mg/kg), moxifloxacin, and pyrazinamide was significantly more active than the standard daily or twice-weekly therapy with rifampin, INH, and pyrazinamide. Stable cure was achieved after 4 months of twice-weekly rifapentine plus INH- or moxifloxacin-containing therapy, but only after 6 months of standard daily therapy, thereby *permitting the shortening of the currently accepted treatment duration by 2 months.* In addition, twice-weekly rifapentine (15 mg/kg) displayed more favorable pharmacodynamics than did daily rifampin (10 mg/kg).

- *Vitamin D–mediated Antimicrobial Immune Response.* The human immune response to microbial pathogens depends on the activation of several pattern recognition receptors known as the Toll-like receptors. Once activated, these receptors may induce the expression of a series of antimicrobial peptides that then destroy the invading pathogens. Susceptibility to infection by *M. tuberculosis* is associated with vitamin D deficiency; however, the mechanism by which vitamin D regulates its antimicrobial action is still unknown. In a recent study, evidence was obtained that by binding to Toll-like receptors, the *M. tuberculosis* peptides induced human phago-

cytic cells *(123)* to express pro-vitamin D converting enzyme and vitamin D receptors. However, the activation of the Toll-like receptors did not directly result in the expression of the antimicrobial peptides. Yet, when stimulated with vitamin D, normal phagocytes displayed an increase in the expression and production of a key antimicrobial peptide, *cathelicidin*. Subsequent experiments have documented that the upregulation of the pro-vitamin D converting enzyme regulated the available vitamin D to the phagocytes. Hence, both vitamin D and the bacterial peptides are needed to be present to fully activate the phagocytes for antimicrobial activity *(123)*.

- *Combining Prevention of Mother-to-Child Transmission of HIV with Active Case Finding for Tuberculosis.* Tuberculosis has become the preeminent manifestation of HIV infection and a leading cause of maternal mortality and morbidity in settings with high HIV prevalence. Furthermore, active tuberculosis in pregnant women has potentially serious consequences for fetuses and newborns. *Prevention of Mother-to-Child Transmission of HIV (PMTCT)* programs test large numbers of pregnant women for HIV annually and offer an opportunity for implementing a targeted TB screening program. In one such study conducted in Soweto, South Africa, a cohort of HIV-infected pregnant women was screened for symptoms of active TB by lay counselors at the post-test counseling sessions. If symptomatic, they were referred to nurses who investigated them further. The findings confirmed that the rates of tuberculosis in HIV-infected pregnant women were high, and screening for TB during routine antenatal care should be implemented in high HIV-prevalence settings *(124)*.

- *Interleukin 12p40 Is Required for Dendritic Cell Migration and T-Cell Priming After M. tuberculosis Infection.* Dendritic cell (DC) production of the cytokine interleukin-12 (IL-12) plays an important role during *M. tuberculosis* infection. In particular, the importance of IL-12p70 in the CD4$^+$ T-cell response to *M. tuberculosis* has been well documented both experimentally and by the increased susceptibility of humans deficient in the IL-12 pathway to tuberculosis and other mycobacterial infections. IL-12p70 is a heterodimer composed of two subunits, p40 and p35. It has been demonstrated in murine models of tuberculosis that IL-12p35 deficiency was less detrimental to the host response than was IL-12p40 deficiency, suggesting that IL-12p40 does have a role separate from IL-12p35. After *M. tuberculosis* infection, the dendritic cells that line the lung will migrate to the draining lymph nodes (DLN) and present the bacterial antigens to naïve T cells to initiate an adaptive immune response. T cells from IL-12p40–deficient mice were not activated after infection with *M. tuberculosis*. However, the IL-12p40 was needed for the dendritic cells' migration into the draining lymph nodes and the subsequent activation of the T cells. The failure to migrate to the DLN after *M. tuberculosis* exposure was related to the inability to respond to chemokines, signals needed for cell traffic from one area to another. This defect could be rescued by providing a homodimer of IL-12p40 to the IL-12p40–deficient mice. This novel role for IL-12p40 in the activation of naïve T cells in response to *M. tuberculosis* may also provide insights into how to activate T cells during lung infections *(125)*.

- *Improved Recovery of M. tuberculosis from Children Using the Microscopic Observation Drug Susceptibility Method.* The diagnosis of pulmonary tuberculosis presents challenges in children because symptoms are nonspecific, sputa are not accessible, and *M. tuberculosis* cultures and smears often are negative. The Microscopic Observation Drug Susceptibility (MODS) technique is a simple, inexpensive method for isolating *M. tuberculosis* with superior speed and sensitivity over the Lowenstein-Jensen culture in studies of adults with pulmonary tuberculosis. The MODS method was studied to determine whether it can improve the sensitivity and the speed of *M. tuberculosis* recovery among Peruvian children with symptoms suggestive of pulmonary tuberculosis *(126)*. The results have shown that isolating *M. tuberculosis* from children with suspected pulmonary tuberculosis using MODS resulted in greater yields and faster recovery than did the Lowenstein-Jensen method and significantly improved the local capabilities to detect pediatric tuberculosis in resource-poor countries *(126)*.

- *Transcription Factor T-bet Is a Key Factor in Host Susceptibility to M. tuberculosis.* It is critical to understand the immune system control points that affect the resistance to *M. tuberculosis* infection, because the molecules that are part of these control points may be defective in people who are not resistant to infection. In this regard, T-bet has been identified as a key transcription factor for the development of Th1 cells and the induction of IFN-production. When ectopically expressed, T-bet induces Th1 cell differentiation of Th precursor cells and of polarized Th2 cells. Recently, T-bet was found to control the function of macrophages, immune cells that play a key role in the response to *M. tuberculosis* infection. It has been shown that mice that do not produce the transcription factor T-bet were more likely to die from *M. tuberculosis* infection, to have more severe inflammation of the lungs after *M. tuberculosis* infection, and to have dysfunctional macrophages in response to *M. tuberculosis* infection compared with mice that produce normal levels of T-bet *(127)*. These findings indicate that T-bet is a key controller of the immune response to *M. tuberculosis* and could be an important new drug target for improving the immune response.

14.7 NIAID Research Agenda in Tuberculosis

The NIAID is leading in tuberculosis research at the NIH. NIAID supports studies to better understand how *M. tuberculosis* infects and causes disease in humans and how the human immune system responds to it. This research will help to develop new tools to diagnose tuberculosis and to find better vaccines and new medicines against tuberculosis. Listed below are some important directions of NIAID-supported tuberculosis research (http://www3.niaid.nih.gov/topics/tuberculosis/Research/researchOverview.htm):

- *Diagnostics*

  o Potential new tests may speed the diagnosis of TB from 4 weeks to 2 days
  o Differences found in the DNA of *M. tuberculosis* and the bacterium used in the BCG vaccine may lead to a test to tell the difference between people who really have TB and those who are merely reacting to previous BCG vaccination
  o Characterization of antibodies and other components of the immune response may potentially identify people who are infected with *M. tuberculosis* and are at the highest risk of developing active disease

- *Treatment*

  o Development of promising new drug candidates, some of which are currently are being tested in human clinical trials
  o Evaluation of shorter treatment regimens to make it easier for patients to complete drug therapy
  o Inclusion of antibiotics that are already available for treatment of other infections and have been shown to act on *M. tuberculosis,* which may make therapy more potent and easier to tolerate

- *Vaccines*: Three new vaccine candidates are now in clinical trials and several more are being analyzed in animal studies.

14.7.1 The 2007 NIAID Research Agenda for MDR and XDR Tuberculosis

In 2007, the NIAID released its *NIAID Research Agenda for Multidrug-Resistant and Extensively Drug-Resistant Tuberculosis.* Although the focus of this document has been on MDR/XDR TB, many of the research priorities identified here also relate to drug-sensitive tuberculosis. The research priorities identified in the agenda build on a foundation of ongoing NIAID-supported tuberculosis research, which currently comprises more than 300 research projects worldwide.

Diagnosing, treating, and controlling the spread of TB has become increasingly complicated because of the HIV/AIDS co-epidemic and the emergence of MDR and XDR TB, which threaten to set tuberculosis control efforts back to the preantibiotic era. Although NIAID is well prepared to foster the development of new TB diagnostics, drugs, and vaccines, given the realities of MDR/XDR TB, the 2007 research agenda has outlined those areas that need additional attention to enable public health officials to more effectively combat all forms of tuberculosis. The agenda is a Web-based "living document" that can be updated as scientific and public health needs and opportunities evolve.

NIAID collaborated with other government and non-government experts to prepare the MDR/XDR TB research agenda. In addition to its review by TB specialists in academia, advocacy groups, international organizations, and other government agencies, the draft agenda was presented to the National Advisory Allergy and Infectious Diseases Council, NIAID's main scientific advisory body.

The research agenda specifically describes six critical areas where additional investigation is needed to close gaps in the current understanding of MDR/XDR TB and to improve the clinical management of patients with tuberculosis:

- Finding new TB diagnostic tools
- Improving therapy for all forms of tuberculosis, including MDR/XDR TB
- Understanding basic biology and immunology of tuberculosis
- Studying MDR/XDR TB epidemiology
- Enhancing the clinical management of MDR/XDR TB in people with or without HIV/AIDS
- Improving tuberculosis prevention strategies, including vaccines

14.7.2 Research Areas of NIAID Support

Currently, the NIAID agenda in supporting research in tuberculosis encompasses a broad range of research initiatives carried out by the Division of Microbiology and Infectious Diseases (DMID), the Division of AIDS (DAIDS), and the Division of Allergy, Immunology, and Transplantation (DAIT). The primary NIAID research goals and objectives have been in the areas of basic research, prevention, and treatment (http://www3.niaid.nih.gov/topics/tuberculosis/Research/researchGoals.htm):

- *Basic Research.* NIAID is committed to encouraging and supporting meritorious investigator-initiated research directed toward improving knowledge about tuberculosis and how it afflicts humans. Research is aimed at com-

bining fundamental science and translational studies for developing and evaluating new health care interventions to combat and prevent multidrug-resistant and drug-sensitive TB strains, as emphasized in the strategic plan for NIAID Category C biodefense/emerging infections (http://www2.niaid.nih.gov/NR/rdonlyres/45F7F0F7-1E15-4B1C-A22D-5F35F370C259/0/categorybandc.pdf). NIAID will provide high-quality standardized research materials to qualified investigators to facilitate fundamental and translational research in tuberculosis, will provide expertise in TB immunology, genomics, and postgenomics, and will target identification and tools development to help select and characterize new TB health care interventions.

- *Vaccine Development and Evaluation.* NIAID will continue to support the development and evaluation of TB vaccines, including supporting fundamental and clinical research leading to the development and testing of (an) effective new vaccine(s) to prevent and control tuberculosis. The institute will provide facilities and resources for screening TB vaccine candidates in appropriate animal models and, as part of its public-private partnerships, will support developing and optimizing advance-stage vaccine candidates for preclinical and Investigative New Drug (IND) studies. NIAID will encourage research to enhance the effectiveness of the immune response to intracellular pathogenic organisms such as mycobacteria or related organisms.

- *Adjuvant/Antigen Identification.* NIAID is actively promoting vaccine-relevant research to identify dominant mycobacterial antigens and novel adjuvants that induce protective cellular immune responses. NIAID will support research to identify genes expressed in immune responses to mycobacterial infection, especially soluble proteins that might be used in vaccination or in treatment of the disease.

- *Diagnosis.* NIAID support includes the development of improved diagnostic tools for early diagnosis and monitoring of infection and disease progression for drug-resistant and drug-sensitive mycobacteria. NIAID also supports research on the development of immunologic reagents for early diagnosis and monitoring of TB disease.

- *Epidemiology.* Epidemiologic support will include research on the development of new molecular tools to assess the factors influencing the occurrence, distribution, and transmission of drug-sensitive and drug-resistant *M. tuberculosis* strains.

- *Animal Models.* Support will include research aimed at improved animal models for infection and disease for use in studying the virulence and pathogenicity of drug-sensitive and drug-resistant *M. tuberculosis* and for evaluating candidate antituberculosis therapies and vaccines.

- *Drug Discovery, Development, and Treatment of Tuberculosis.* NIAID continues to provide contract resources for evaluating new candidate antibiotics active against *M. tuberculosis* in laboratory assays and animal models of infection and disease. NIAID also continues to support research on the mechanisms of drug resistance and activity, early target identification and verification, and clinical testing of prophylactic and therapeutic antituberculosis regimens.
- *Clinical Research on Therapeutic Interventions in HIV/TB.* This area of NIAID support includes clinical research to evaluate and improve the effectiveness of regimens for the treatment and prophylaxis of *M. tuberculosis*, especially MDR TB, in the setting of HIV co-infections.
- *Technology Transfer.* Support for technology transfer is aimed at accelerating the development and commercialization of candidate TB treatments identified through NIAID TB drug screening contracts or otherwise developed at NIH, universities, and nonprofit laboratories.
- *Training.* NIAID is committed to promoting training to increase the number, and improve the skills, of basic and clinical researchers on TB.

14.7.2.1   Major NIAID Programs in Tuberculosis Research

- *Tuberculosis Research Unit (TBRU).* The major focus of the TBRU contract (N01-AI-95383 to Case Western Reserve University) is to make progress in developing surrogate markers of disease and human protective immunity and in conducting clinical trials of potential new TB therapeutics, preventive, and diagnostic strategies (http://www.tbresearchunit.org). Furthermore, well-characterized clinical samples will be available for distribution to TBRU investigators and their contract collaborators. *The activities of the TBRU are coordinated with other major organizations involved in tuberculosis research, including the CDC, USAID, FDA, WHO, Global Alliance for TB Drug Development, and the International Union Against Tuberculosis and Lung Disease (IUATLD), and with interested industrial partners.*
- *Clinical Studies: Enrollment and Data Analysis: Completed*

   o Phase II: "Study of Safety and Preliminary Evidence for Microbiologic and Immunologic Activity of rhIL-2 (Proleukin®) in HIV-non-infected Adults with Pulmonary Tuberculosis." *Site*: Uganda.

- *NIAID-Supported Clinical Trials: Currently Enrolling* (http://www3.niaid.nih.gov/topics/tuberculosis/Research/clinicalTrials.htm)

   o Immune Response to *Mycobacterium tuberculosis* Infection
   o Multi-Drug Resistant Tuberculosis in Korea
   o Metronidazole for Pulmonary Tuberculosis (South Korea)
   o Tuberculosis Immunity in Children
   o Anti-HIV Drugs for Ugandan Patients with HIV and Tuberculosis
   o Daily Isoniazid to Prevent Tuberculosis in Infants Born to Mothers with HIV
   o Effect of Multivitamin Supplements on Clinical and Immunological Response in Childhood Tuberculosis
   o Immune Responses to *Mycobacterium tuberculosis*
   o Early Bacterial Activity (EBA)
   o Treatment of Latent TB Infection for Jailed Persons
   o Paucibacillary TB Natural History and Resistance Diagnostic

- *Clinical Studies: Ongoing*

   o Phase I: "Randomized, Open Label, Multiple Dose Phase I Study of the Early Bactericidal Activity of Linezolid, Gatifloxacin, Levofloxacin, and Moxifloxacin in HIV-non-infected Adults with Initial Episodes of Sputum Smear-Positive Pulmonary Tuberculosis." *Site*: Brazil.
   o Phase III: "A Prospective Study of Shortening the Duration of Standard Short Course Chemotherapy from 6 Months to 4 Months in HIV-non-infected Patients with Fully Drug-susceptible, Non-cavitary Pulmonary Tuberculosis with Negative Sputum Cultures after 2 Months of Anti-TB Treatment." *Sites*: Uganda, Brazil, and the Philippines.
   o *Kawempe Community Health Study (KCHS)*: The study will determine the critical host factors associated with tuberculosis infection, re-infection, and reactivation from latency and the progression of clinical disease. KCHS will also identify and track *M. tuberculosis* strains, as well as track transmission dynamics to provide background information for Phase II/III vaccine or therapeutic clinical trials. *Site*: Uganda.
   o Children's Health: "Immune Response to BCG Vaccination in HIV-Infected Infants." *Site*: South Africa.
   o Pilot Immunology Studies: "A Longitudinal Study of the Immune Response to Different Stages of Tuberculosis." *Site*: Uganda.
   o Pilot Study: "Assess Immunologic and Microbiologic Predictors of Response to Short Course Anti-TB Treatment in HIV-non-infected Adults with Initial Episodes of Smear Positive Pulmonary Tuberculosis." TBRU investigators have shown that examining whole blood bactericidal activity against *M. tuberculosis* during treatment of pulmonary tuberculosis may be useful for

assessing the sterilizing activity of new anti-TB drugs. *Site*: Brazil.

- *Therapeutic Clinical Studies in HIV-Infected Populations.* NIAID is participating as scientific coordinators and medical officers for ongoing *international* research project grants and cooperative agreements for co-infection research as follows: *Clinical Studies: Active Enrollments*

  o University of Natal, South Africa: "Collaborative AIDS Programme of Research in South Africa-CAPRISA."

  o Johns Hopkins University: "Novel TB Prevention Regimens for HIV-Infected Adults in South Africa."

  o Tulane University: "Practical Diagnostics for AIDS-Related Pediatric Tuberculosis in Peru." It is not a therapeutic trial, but a clinical study to evaluate diagnostic tests for detection of *M. tuberculosis* in HIV-positive and HIV–negative children.

  o Johns Hopkins University: "Adjunct Vitamin Therapy for Tuberculosis and HIV/AIDS in Malawi." This is a placebo-controlled Phase III study to determine whether daily micronutrient supplementation can reduce mortality, anemia, wasting, and relapse (antituberculosis therapy versus antituberculosis therapy plus multivitamins).

  o Cambodian Health Committee: "A Cambodian Clinical Research Network for HIV/TB." This is an exploratory, developmental study (CIPRA) to determine whether early initiation of antiretroviral therapy will affect tuberculosis cure, survival, relapse, and control of HIV in urban and rural settings.

  o Dartmouth-Hitchcock Medical Center: "Disseminated Tuberculosis in HIV Infection: Epidemiology and Prevention in Tanzania." The study is aimed at testing a tuberculosis vaccine versus placebo vaccine in a Phase II trial. It will measure time of development of disseminated or pulmonary tuberculosis after vaccination.

  o Case Western Reserve University: "A Randomized, Phase II Study of Punctuated Antiretroviral Therapy for HIV-Infected Patients with Active Pulmonary Tuberculosis and CD4$^+$ Count Greater Than 350 cells/mm^3." This is a study to determine whether antiretroviral therapy during treatment of active tuberculosis will delay HIV disease progression in HIV-positive patients with active tuberculosis and CD4$^+$ counts greater than 350 cells/mm^3.

  o Duke University: "International Studies of AIDS-Associated Co-Infections (ISAAC)." The aims of this project are to establish an ISAAC unit in Tanzania to develop critical research infrastructure; to catalyze interactions across the ISAAC unit scientific programs; and to foster an independent and sustainable research

enterprise within the Kilimanjaro Christian Medical Center HIV/AIDS Program.

  o University of California: "A Strategy Study of Immediate Versus Deferred Initiation of Antiretroviral Therapy for HIV-Infected Persons Treated for Tuberculosis with CD4$^+$ Counts of Less Than 200 cells/mm^3." This study will compare whether the strategy of starting antiretroviral therapy 2 weeks versus 8 to 12 weeks after initiation of antituberculosis therapy will reduce mortality and AIDS-defining events in patients being treated for tuberculosis.

  o Stanford University: "Optimizing NNRTI Doses in Patients with HIV and Tuberculosis." This study will compare two different doses of one of two non-nucleoside reverse transcriptase inhibitors (NNRTI) used as an initial triple-drug active antiretroviral regimens in patients co-infected with HIV and tuberculosis.

- *Training*

  o NIAID continues to collaborate with the Fogarty International Center to award and administer a training program, "The International Centers for Excellence in Research (ICER): Clinical Research and Management Training Program." Awards made outside the United States include: Chennai, India; Uganda; and Mali.

  o NIAID continues to support *International Clinical Science Workshops for Asian Scientists*. Sites: Thailand and India.

  o NIAID is continuing its funding of the *International Clinical Studies Support Center*, currently run by the Family Health International, to provide training and assistance related to clinical studies to foreign scientists.

- *Networks, Consortia, and Partnerships*

  o NIAID participates in public-private partnerships to stimulate the development of new drug/treatments against tuberculosis with the (i) American Lung Association; (ii) American Thoracic Society; (iii) CDC Division of Tuberculosis Elimination; (iv) Global Alliance for TB Drug Development (GATB); (v) Bill & Melinda Gates Foundation; (vi) Rockefeller Foundation; (vii) J. Craig Venter Institute; (viii) International Union Against Tuberculosis and Lung Disease; (ix) National Center for Biotechnology Information (National Library of Medicine, NIH); (x) U.S. Agency for International Development (USAID); (xi) Wellcome Trust Sanger Institute; (xii) Stop TB Partnership; (xiii) World Bank; (xiv) World Health Organization (http://www3.niaid.nih.gov/ topics/tuberculosis/Research/partners.htm) (for a comprehensive list, see: http://www.tballiance.org).

- *Vaccine Treatment and Evaluation Unit (VTEU), St. Louis*: "Phase I Studies of the Safety and Immunogenicity of Primary and Secondary BCG Vaccination Delivered Intradermally, Orally, and by Combined Routes of Administration in Healthy and Previously Immunologically Naïve Volunteers."
- *Research Resources Support*

  ○ *Tuberculosis Research Materials and Vaccine Testing Contract (N01 AI 75320)* to Colorado State University. Through this contract, NIAID is providing TB research reagents to qualified investigators throughout the world, enabling them to work with consistent, high-quality reagents prepared from the virulent and difficult to handle pathogen, *M. tuberculosis*. Screening potential tuberculosis vaccine candidates in appropriate animal models is also offered as a resource through this contract. In addition, DNA-based TB microarrays and, in collaboration with DMID's Pathogen Functional Genomics Resource Center, *M. tuberculosis* clones are available for qualified applicants. Information, reagent request forms, and microarray applications are available at: http://www.cvmbs.colostate.edu/microbiology/tb/top.htm. This contract was re-competed in 2005. At the end of FY2006, more than 150 new TB vaccine candidates had been tested under this contract, one of which recently entered human clinical trials, with several others progressing through various stages of preclinical development.

  ○ *Tuberculosis Animal Research and Gene Evaluation Task Force* (to Johns Hopkins University through RFP-NIH-NIAID-DMID-03-09, Part A). The goal of the contract is to determine, in animal models, the biological function of *M. tuberculosis* gene products that may have utility as drug, vaccine, or diagnostic targets. Transposon mutants developed under the contract are provided, upon request, to the research community. Services can be accessed at: http://www.hopkinsmedicine.org/TARGET.

  ○ *NIAID Tetramer Facility (TF)*. NIAID oversees the contract supporting this reagent resource that has provided more than 1,500 class I peptide/major histocompatibility complex (MHC) tetramer reagents to the scientific community and that now offers human and mouse CD1d monomers and tetramers, a limited set of premade class II MHC tetramers, and custom class II HLA tetramer synthesis. This contract will collaborate with the TB Research Reagents and Vaccine Testing contract to produce TB-specific tetramers using reagents produced by the TB contract. The NIAID Tetramer Facility can be accessed at: http://www.niaid.nih.gov/reposit/tetramer/index.html.

  ○ *Immune Epitope Database and Analysis Program.* This program supports a comprehensive database of antigenic determinants recognized by antibodies and T cells, which will include epitopes of *M. tuberculosis*. This publicly available database and associated analytical and predictive tools will facilitate vaccine development in many areas, including tuberculosis. One contract was awarded to La Jolla Institute of Allergy and Immunology. The database can be accessed at: http://immuneepitope.org/home.do.

  ○ *Modeling Immunity for Biodefense.* This program supports interactive, multidisciplinary teams focused on the development of innovative and functional mathematical models of immunity to infectious diseases. The teams will conduct basic and applied research to develop tools that can accurately model host immunity to specific infections. In 2005, one award was made to the University of Pittsburgh for modeling host immunity to tuberculosis infection in mouse and non-human primate models *in vivo* and human macrophages *in vitro*.

  ○ *Anti-infective Drug Development Contracts.* Research and development contracts supported by NIAID are actively testing new candidate compounds for efficacy against mycobacterial complications of AIDS in culture and in animals, a critical component in new drug development and approval. The contract resources allow NIAID to (i) support investigator-initiated drug discovery; (ii) stimulate private sector sponsorship of new drugs; (iii) perform comparison or confirmatory studies from different sponsors; and (iv) provide information for selecting anti-opportunistic infections and anti-hepatitis C virus drug candidates for designing clinical studies. Specifics on contract-generated publications and meeting presentations can be accessed at: http://www.taacf.org/.

  ○ *Tuberculosis Technology Transfer Support.* Tuberculosis Technology Transfer Support has been contracted to the Research Triangle Institute (RFP NIH-NIAID-DAIDS-99-16). The Research Triangle Institute (RTI) will assist the GATB as the project manager for the development of drug candidate PA-824. In their capacity as the PA-824 project manager, RTI will coordinate discussions among GATB and more than 12 other research organizations worldwide, including Chiron Corp, involved in this project. In addition, RTI will provide technical advice to facilitate nonclinical studies on the efficacy of PA-824, including Material Transfer Agreements, and will assist in the overall planning and management of key nonclinical studies as well as the Phase I human clinical trial.

  ○ *Technical Advice and Contract Resources to Sequella, Inc.* NIAID is providing technical advice and contract resources to Sequella, Inc., for the preclinical development of a new chemical entity, SQ-109, which is an adamantyl ethane-diamine derivative. With support from two separate NIAID Challenge Grant Programs and the NCI-NIAID Inter-Institute Program for the Development of AIDS-Related Therapeutics, Sequella, Inc., is developing SQ-109 as a promising new therapeutic candidate for treating drug-resistant and drug-susceptible tuberculosis. In 2006, SQ-109 received FDA clearance to enter Phase I clinical trials.

○ *Technical Advice and Contract Resources to GATB.* NIAID is assisting the GATB in developing a new anti-tuberculosis drug, PA-824. A nitroimidazole antibiotic compound, PA-824, whose preclinical development was supported through NIAID resources, successfully completed Phase I safety clinical trials in humans. The following clinical studies were initiated to assess the safety, tolerability, and pharmacokinetics of PA-824: (i) a multiple-dose (7 days), ascending dose study in healthy males and females; (ii) a multiple-dose (8 days) renal effects study in healthy males and females; and (iii) a single-dose study to assess pharmacokinetics, metabolism, and excretion of [^{14}C]PA-824 in healthy males. Nonclinical studies included a single-dose pharmacokinetics and Absorption, Distribution, Metabolism, Excretion (ADME) study of [^{14}C]PA-824 in rats. Results obtained to date have indicated an adequate bioavailability of PA-824 in a tablet formulation.

The GATB is a nonprofit organization involving many public and private partners that is contributing to the development of new drugs to shorten or simplify the treatment of tuberculosis and facilitate TB control in high-burden countries. More than 30 organizations are stakeholders in this public-private partnership, including the Bill & Melinda Gates Foundation, CDC, NIAID/NIH, the Rockefeller Foundation, USAID, the World Bank, and the WHO (for a comprehensive list, see: www.tballiance.org).

○ *Millennium Vaccine Initiative—Novel Vaccines for Tuberculosis and Malaria.* The goal of this contract is to increase collaboration between industry and the public sector to promote the development of new vaccines to prevent tuberculosis and malaria in developing countries using existing technology platforms. Awarded initially in 2003 to Corixa Corporation for an initial feasibility and early development phase, in 2006 this contract was transitioned to the Infectious Disease Research Institute (IDRI) in Seattle under a contract innovation agreement for the advanced development phase of this contract.

○ *NIH Roadmap.* NIAID program staff are serving as the NIAID liaison to two NIH Roadmap initiatives:

(i) The Molecular Libraries Screening Centers Network (MLSCN) NIH Roadmap Initiative (http://grants1.nih.gov/grants/guide/rfa-files/RFA-RM-04-017. html).

(ii) NIH-RAID Translational Cores Resources Pilot Project (http://grants.nih.gov/grants/guide/notice-files/NOT-RM-05-004.html).

○ NIAID program staff serve as external consultants or liaisons to national and international TB-related groups. These collaborative activities communicate NIAID's strategic directions for the Tuberculosis Program to ensure maximum utilization of NIAID resources. National groups include the Advisory Council for the Elimination of Tuberculosis (ACET), CDC's TB Clinical Trials Consortium and TB Epidemiologic Studies Consortium, and the Infectious Disease Society of America. International groups include the STOP TB Vaccine Partnership's Diagnostic, Vaccine, and Drug Development and the HIV/TB Working Groups, the WHO's Special Programme for Research and Training in Tropical Diseases (TDR), the International Union against Tuberculosis and Lung Disease (IUATLD), the Global Alliance for TB Drug Development, the Bill & Melinda Gates Foundation, and several European research consortia.

○ *IUALTD Pediatric Tuberculosis Working Group.* NIAID is serving as program liaison to coordinate research activities in pediatric tuberculosis, including studies on vaccine response, and diagnostic and therapeutic needs.

○ *Federal TB Task Force.* NIAID is participating in the Federal TB Task Force activities including the International, Diagnostic and Basic Research Working Groups.

References

1. Georgiev, V. St. (1997) *Mycobacterium tuberculosis.* In: *Infectious Diseases in Immunocompromised Hosts*, CRC Press, Boca Raton, FL, pp. 269–299.
2. Georgiev, V. St. (2003) *Mycobacterium tuberculosis.* In: *Opportunistic Infections and Prophylaxis*, Humana Press, Totowa, NJ, pp. 81–91.
3. Dye, C., Scheele, S., Dolin, P., Pathania, V., and Raviglione, M. C. (1999) Consensus statement. Global burden of tuberculosis: estimated incidence, prevalence, and mortality by country. WHO Global Surveillance and Monitoring Project, *J. Am. Med. Assoc.*, **282**(7), 677–686.
4. Huebner, R. E. and Castro, K. G. (1995) The changing face of tuberculosis, *Annu. Rev. Med.*, **46**, 47–55.
5. Pearson, M. L., Jereb, J. A., Frieden, T. R., Crawford, J. T., Davis, B. J., Dooley, S. W., and Jarvis, W. R. (1992) Nosocomial transmission of multiple drug resistant *Mycobacterium tuberculosis*: a risk to patients and health care workers, *Ann. Intern. Med.*, **117**(3), 191–196.

6. McShane, H. (2005) Co-infection with HIV and TB: double trouble, *Int. J. STD AIDS*, **16**, 95–101.

7. McShane, H. (2004) Developing an improved vaccine against tuberculosis, *Expert Rev. Vaccines*, **3**(3), 299–306.

8. Markowitz, N., Hansen, N. I., Hopewell, P. C., et al. (1997) Incidence of tuberculosis in the United States among HIV-infected persons. The pulmonary complications of HIV infection study group, *Ann. Intern. Med.*, **126**(2), 123–132.

9. Corbett, E. L. and De Cock, K. M. (1996) Tuberculosis in the HIV-positive patient, *Br. J. Hosp. Med.*, **56**(5), 200–204.

10. Daley, C. L., Small, P. M., Schecter, G. F., et al. (1992) An outbreak of tuberculosis with accelerated progression among persons infected with the human immunodeficiency virus. An analysis using restriction-fragment-length polymorphisms, *N. Engl. J. Med.*, **326**(4), 231–235.

11. Whalen, C., Horsburgh, C. R., Horn, D., Lahart, C., Simberkoff, M., and Ellner, J. (1995) Accelerated course of human immunodeficiency virus infection after tuberculosis, *Am. J. Respir. Crit. Care Med.*, **151**(1), 129–135.

12. Goletti, D., Weissman, D., Jackson, R. W., Graham, N. M., Vlahov, D., Klein, R. S., Munsiff, S. S., Ortona, L., Cauda, R., and Fauci, A. S. (1996) Effect of *Mycobacterium tuberculosis* on HIV replication. Role of immune activation, *J. Immunol.*, **157**(3), 1271–1278.

13. Corbett, E. L., Watt, C. J., Walker, N., Maher, D., Williams, B. G., Raviglione, M. C., and Dye, C. (2003) The growing burden of tuberculosis. Global trend and interaction with the HIV epidemic, *Arch. Intern. Med.*, **163**(9), 1009–1021.

14. Zumla, A., Malon, P., Henderson, J., and Grange, J. M. (2000) Impact of HIV infection on tuberculosis, *Postgrad. Med.*, **76**(895), 259–268.

15. Williams, B. G. and Dye, C. (2003) Antiretroviral drugs for tuberculosis control in the era of HIV/AIDS, *Science*, **301**, 1535–1537.

16. Greten, T., Hautmann, H., Trauner, A., and Huber, R. M. (1994) Esophagomediastinal fistulae as a rare complication of tuberculosis in an HIV-infected patient, *Dtsch. Med. Wochenschr.*, **119**(47), 1613–1617.

17. Hopewell, P. (1992) Impact of human immunodeficincy virus infection on the epidemiology, clinical features, management, and control of tuberculosis, *Clin. Infect. Dis.*, **18**(3), 540–547.

18. Martinez-Vazquez, C., Bordon, J., Rodriguez-Gonzalez, A., de la Fuente-Aguado, J., Sopeña, B., Gallego-Rivera, A., and Martinez-Cueto, P. (1995) Cerebral tuberculoma – a comparative study in patients with and without HIV infection, *Infection*, **23**(3), 149–153.

19. Mahmoudi, A. and Iseman, D. (1993) Pitfalls in the care of patients with tuberculosis: common errors and their association with the acquisition of drug resistance, *J. Am. Med. Assoc.*, **270**(1), 65–68.

19a. Chan, J., Fan, X. D., Hunter, S. W., Brennan, P. J., and Bloom, B. R. (1991) Lipoarabinomannan, a possible virulence factor involved in persistence of *Mycobacterium tuberculosis* within macrophages, *Infect. Immun.*, **59**(5), 1755–1761.

20. Hatfull, G. F. (2008) What can mycobacteriophages tell us about *Mycobacterium tuberculosis*. In: *National Institute of Allergy and Infectious Diseases, NIH: Frontiers in Research*, vol 1 (Georgiev, V. St., Western, K. A., and McGowan, J. J., eds.), Humana Press, Totowa, NJ, pp. 67–76.

21. Bloom, B. R. (1992)*Tuberculosis: Pathogenicity, Protection, and Control*, ASM Press, Washington, DC.

22. Jacobs, W. R., Jr. (2000) *Mycobacterium tuberculosis*: a once genetically intractable organism. In: *Molecular Genetics of the Mycobacteria* (Hatfull, G. F. and Jacobs, W. R., Jr., eds.), ASM Press, Washington, DC, pp. 1–16.

23. Jacobs, W. R., Jr., Tuckman, M., and Bloom, B. R. (1987) Introduction of foreign DNA into mycobacteria using a shuttle plasmid, *Nature*, **327**, 532–535.

24. Jacobs, W. R., Jr., Snapper, S. B., Tuckman, M., and Bloom, B. R. (1989) Mycobacteriophage vector systems, *Rev. Infect. Dis.*, **11**(Suppl. 2), S404–S410.

25. Snapper, S. B., Lugosi, L., Jekkel, A., Melton, R. E., Kieser, T., Bloom, B. R., and Jacobs, W. R., Jr. (1988) Lysogeny and transformation in mycobacteria: stable expression of foreign genes, *Proc. Natl. Acad. Sci. U.S.A.*, **85**, 6987–6991.

26. Hatfull, G. F. (2004) Mycobacteriophages and tuberculosis. In: *Tuberculosis* (Eisenach, K., Cole, S. T., Jacobs, W. R., Jr., and McMurray, D., eds.), ASM Press, Washington, DC, pp. 203–218.

27. Hatfull, G. F., Pedulla, M. L., Jacobs-Sera, D., Cichon, P. M., Foley, A., Ford, M. E., Gonda, R. M., Houtz, J. M., Hryckowian, A. J., Kelchner, V. A., Namburi, S., Pajcini, K. V., Popovich, M. G., Schleicher, D. T., Simanek, B. Z., Smith, A. L., Zdanowicz, G. M., Kumar, V., Peebles, C. L., Jacobs, W. R., Jr., Lawrence, J. G., and Hendrix, R. W. (2006) Exploring the mycobacteriophage metaproteome: phage genomics as an educational platform, *PLoS Gent.*, **2**, e92.

28. Hatfull, G. F. (2006) Mycobacteriophages. In: *The Bacteriophages* (Calendar, R., ed.), Oxford University Press, New York, pp. 602–620.

29. Pedulla, M. L., Ford, M. E., Houtz, J. M., Karthikeyan, T., Wadsworth, C., Lewis, J. A., Jacobs-Sera, D., Falbo, J., Gross, J., Pannunzio, N. R., Brucker, W., Kumar, V., Kandasamy, J., Keenan, L., Bardarov, S., Kriakov, J., Lawrence, J. G., Jacobs, W. R., Jr., Hendrix, R. W., and Hatfull, G. F. (2003) Origins of highly mosaic mycobacteriophage genomes, *Cell*, **113**, 171–182.

30. Susskind, M. M. and Botstein, D. (1978) Molecular genetics of bacteriophage P22, *Microbiol. Rev.*, **42**, 385–413.

31. Clark, A. J., Inwood, W., Cloutier, T., and Dhillon, T. S. (2001) Nucleotide sequence of coliphage HK620 and the evolution of lambdoid phages, *J. Mol. Biol.*, **311**, 657–679.

32. Ghosh, P., Kim, A. I., and Hatfull, G. F. (2003) The orientation of mycobacteriophage Bxb1 integration is solely dependent on the central dinucleotide of attP and attB, *Mol. Cell*, **12**, 1101–1111.

33. Hendrix, R. W. (2003) Bacteriophage genomics, *Curr. Opin. Microbiol.*, **6**, 506–511.

34. Jacobs, W. R., Jr., Barletta, R. G., Udani, R., Chan, J., Kalkut, G., Sosne, G., Kieser, T., Sarkis, G. J., Hatfull, G. F., and Bloom, B. R. (1993) Rapid assessment of drug susceptibilities of *Mycobacterium tuberculosis* by means of luciferase reporter phages, *Science*, **260**, 819–822.

35. Sarkis, G. J., Jacobs, W. R., Jr., and Hatfull, G. F. (1995) L5 luciferase reporter mycobacteriophages: a sensitive tool for the detection and assay of live mycobacteria, *Mol. Microbiol.*, **15**, 1055–1067.

36. Bardarov, S., Kriakov, J., Carriere, C., Yu, S., Vaamonde, C., McAdam, R. A., Bloom, B. R., Hatfull, G. F., and Jacobs, W. R., Jr. (1997) Conditionally replicating mycobacteriophages: a system of transposon delivery to *Mycobacterium tuberculosis*, *Proc. Natl. Acad. Sci. U.S.A.*, **94**, 10961–10966.

37. Bardarov, S., Bardarov, S., Jr., Pavelka, M. S., Jr., Sambandamurthy, V., Larsen, M., Tufariello, J., Chan, J., Hatfull, G., and Jacobs, W. R., Jr. (2002) Specialized transduction: an efficient method for generating marked and unmarked targeted gene disruptions in *Mycobacterium tuberculosis*, *M. bovis* BCG, and *M. smegmatis*, *Microbiology*, **184**, 3007–3017.

38. Lee, M. H., Pascopella, L., Jacobs, W. R., Jr., and Hatfull, G. F. (1991) Site-specific integration of mycobacteriophage L5: integration-proficient vectors for *Mycobacterium smegmatis*, *Mycobacterium tuberculosis*, and Bacille Calmette-Guérin, *Proc. Natl. Acad. Sci. U.S.A.*, **88**, 3111–3115.

39. Lewis, J. A. and Hatfull, G. F. (2001) Control of directionality in integrase-mediated recombination: examination of recombination directionality factors (RDFs) including Xis and Cox proteins, *Nucleic Acids Res.*, **29**, 2205–2216.

40. Lewis, J. A. and Hatfull, G. F. (2003) Control of directionality in L5 integrase-mediated site-specific recombination, *J. Mol. Biol.*, **326**, 805–821.

41. Leao, S. C. (1993) Tuberculosis: new strategies for the development of diagnostic tests and vaccines, *Braz. J. Med. Biol. Res.*, **26**(8), 827–833.

42. Wallis, R. S., Amir-Tahmasseb, M., and Ellner, J. J. (1990) Induction of interleukin-1 and tumor necrosis factor by mycobacterial proteins: the monocyte Western blot, *Proc. Natl. Acad. Sci. U.S.A.*, **87**, 3348–3352.

43. Chandrasekhar, S. and Ratnam, S. (1992) Studies on cell-wall deficient non-acid fast variants of *Mycobacterium tuberculosis*, *Tuber. Lung Dis.*, **73**(5), 273–279.

44. David, H. L., Papa, F., Cruaud, P., Berlie, H. C., Moroja, M. F., Salem, J. I., and Costa, M. F. (1992) Relationships between titers of antibodies immunoreacting against glycolipid antigens from *Mycobacterium leprae* and *M. tuberculosis*, the Mitsuda and Mantoux reactions, and bacteriological loads: implications in the pathogenesis, epidemiology and serodiagnosis of leprosy and tuberculosis, *Int. J. Lepr. Other Mycobact. Dis.*, **60**(2), 208–224.

45. Janis, E. M., Kaufmann, S. H., Schwartz, R. H., and Pardoll, D. M. (1989) Activation of gamma delta T cells in the primary immune response to *Mycobacterium tuberculosis*, *Science*, **244**(4905), 713–716.

46. Meylan, P. R., Richman, D. D., and Kornbluth, R. S. (1992) Reduced intracellular growth in human macrophages cultivated at physiologic oxygen pressure, *Am. Rev. Respir. Dis.*, **145**(4 Pt. 1), 947–953.

47. Ainslie, G. M., Solomon, J. A., and Bateman, E. D. (1992) Lymphocyte and lymphocyte subset numbers in blood and in bronchoalveolar lavage and pleural fluid in various forms of human pulmonary tuberculosis at presentation and during recovery, *Thorax*, **47**, 513–518.

48. Van Scoy, R. E. and Wilkowske, C. J. (1999) Antimycobacterial therapy, *Mayo Clin. Proc.*, **74**, 1038–1048.

49. Georgiev, V. St. (1994) Treatment and developmental therapeutics of *Mycobacterium tuberculosis* infections, *Int. J. Antimicrob. Agents*, **4**, 157–173.

50. Committee on Infectious Diseases (1992) Chemotherapy for tuberculosis in infants and children, *Pediatrics*, **89**, 161–165.

51. Blom-Bülow, B. (1990) Dosing regimens in the treatment of tuberculosis, *Scand. J. Infect. Dis., Suppl.*, **74**, 258–261.

52. Doganay, M., Calangu, S., Turgut, H., Bakir, M., and Aygen, B. (1995) Treatment of tuberculous meningitis in Turkey, *Scand. J. Infect. Dis.*, **27**, 135–138.

53. Wallis, R. S., Perkins, M. D., Phillips, M., Joloba, M., Namale, A., Johnson, J. L., Whalen, C. C., Teixeira, L., Demchuk, B., Dietze, R., Mugerwa, R. D., Eisenach, K., and Ellner, J. J. (2000) Predicting the outcome of therapy for pulmonary tuberculosis, *Am. J. Respir. Crit. Care Med.*, **161**(4 Pt. 1), 1076–1080.

54. Cook, S. V., Fujiwara, P. L., and Frieden, T. R. (2000) Rates and risk factors for discontinuation of rifampicin, *Int. J. Tuberc. Lung Dis.*, **4**, 118–122.

55. U.S. Public Health Service and Infectious Diseases Society of America (2000) 1999 USPHS/IDSA guidelines for the prevention of opportunistic infections in persons infected with human immunideficiency virus, *Infect. Dis. Obstet. Gynecol.*, **8**(1), 3–74.

56. Centers for Disease Control (1998) Prevention and treatment of tuberculosis among patients infected with human immunodeficiency virus: principles of therapy and revised recommendations, *Morb. Mortal. Wkly Rep.*, **47**(RR-20), 1–58.

57. Veldkamp, A. I., Hoetelmans, R. M., Beijnen, J. H., Mulder, J. W., and Meenhorst, P. L. (1999) Ritonavir enables combined therapy with rifampin and sequinavir, *Clin. Infect. Dis.*, **29**, 1586.

58. Centers for Disease Control (1998) Report of the NIH panel to define principles of therapy of HIV infection and guidelines for use of antiretroviral agents in HIV-infected adults and adolescents, *Morb. Mortal. Wkly Rep.*, **47**(RR-5), 39–82.

59. Kirk, O., Gatell, J. M., Mocroft, A. (2000) Infections with *Mycobacterium tuberculosis* and *Mycobacterium avium* among HIV-infected patients after the introduction of highly active antiretroviral therapy, EuroSIDA Study Group JD, *Am. J. Respir. Crit. Care Med.*, **162**(3 Part 1), 865–872.

60. Perlman, D. C., El-Helou, P., and Salomon, N. (1999) Tuberculosis in patients with human immunodeficiency virus infection, *Semin. Respir. Infect.*, **14**, 344–352.

61. Essential Components of a Tuberculosis Prevention and Control Program (1995) Recommendation of the Advisory Council for the Elimination of Tuberculosis, *Morb. Mortal. Wkly Rep.*, **44**(RR-11), 1–34.

62. Pust, R. E. (1992) Tuberculosis in the 1990s: resurgence, regimens, and resources, *South. Med. J.*, **85**(5), 584–593.

63. Stearn, B. F. and Polis, M. A. (1994) Prophylaxis of opportunistic infections in persons with HIV infection, *Cleve. Clin. J. Med.*, **61**(3), 187–194.

64. Graham, N. M., Galai, N., Nelson, K. E., Astemborski, J., Bonds, M., Rizzo, R. T., Sheeley, L., and Vlahov, D. (1996) Effect of isoniazid chemoprophylaxis on HIV infection, *Arch. Intern. Med.*, **156**(8), 889–894.

65. Holland, S. M. (2000) Cytokine therapy of mycobacterial infections, *Adv. Intern. Med.*, **45**, 431–452.

66. Johnson, J. L., Kamya, R. M., Okwera, A., Loughlin, A., Nyole, S., Hom, D. L., Wallis, R. S., Hirsch, C. S., Wolski, K., Foulds, J., Mugerwa, R. D., and Ellner, J. J. (2000) Randomized controlled trial of *Mycobacterium vaccae* immunotherapy in nonhuman immunodeficiency virus-infected Ugandan adults with newly diagnosed pulmonary tuberculosis. The Ugandan-Case Western Reserve University Research Collaboration, *J. Infect. Dis.*, **181**, 1304–1312.

67. Fletcher, H. and McShane, H. (2006) Tuberculosis vaccines: current status and future prospects, *Expert Opin. Emerging Drugs*, **11**(2), 207–215.

68. Behr, M. A., Wilson, M. A., Gill, W. P., et al. (1999) Comparative genomic of BCG vaccines by whole-genome DNA microarray, *Science*, **284**, 1520–1523.

69. Rodrigues, L. C., Diwan, V. K., and Wheeler, J. G. (1993) Protective effect of BCG against tuberculous meningitis and milliary tuberculosis: a meta-analysis, *Int. J. Epidemiol.*, **22**(6), 1154–1158.

70. Colditz, G. A., Brewer, T. F., Berkey, C. S., et al. (1994) Efficacy of BCG vaccine in the prevention of tuberculosis. Meta-analysis of published literature, *J. Am. Med. Assoc.*, **271**, 698–702.

71. Wilson, M. E., Fineberg, H. V., and Colditz, G. A. (1995) Geographic latitude and the efficacy of Bacillus Calmette-Guérin vaccine, *Clin. Infect. Dis.*, **20**, 982–991.

72. Brandt, L., Feino Cunha, J., Weinreich Olsen, A., et al. (2002) Failure of the *Mycobacterium bovis* BCG vaccine: some species of environmental mycobacteria block multiplication of BCG and induction of protective immunity to tuberculosis, *Infect. Immun.*, **70**, 672–678.

73. Geluk, A., van Meijgaarden, K. E., Franken, K. L., et al. (2000) Identification of major epitopes of *Mycobacterium tuberculosis* AG85B that are recognized by *HLA-A*0201*-restricted CD4^{+} T cells in HLA-transgenic mice and humans, *J. Immunol.*, **165**, 6463–6471.

74. Mutis, T., Cornelisse, Y. E., and Ottenhoff, T. H. (1993) Mycobacteria induce CD4^{+} T cells that are cytotoxic and display T_H1-like

cytokine secretion profile: heterogeneity in cytotoxic activity and cytokine secretion levels, *Eur. J. Immunol.*, **23**, 2189–2195.

75. Altare, F., Durandy, A., Lammas, D., et al. (1998) Impairment of mycobacterial immunity in human interleukin-12 receptor deficiency, *Science*, **280**, 1432–1435.

76. Jouangue, E., Altare, E., Lamhamedi, S., et al. (1996) Interferon-gamma-receptor deficiency in an infant with fatal Bacille Calmette-Guérin infection, *N. Engl. J. Med.*, **335**, 1956–1961.

77. Kaufmann, S. H. (2001) How can immunology contribute to the control of tuberculosis? *Nat. Rev. Immunol.*, **1**, 20–30.

78. Caruso, A. M., Serbina, N., Klein, E., et al. (1999) Mice deficient in CD4 T-cells have only transiently diminished levels of IFN-γ, yet succumb to tuberculosis, *J. Immunol.*, **162**(9), 5407–5416.

79. Orme, I. M. and Collins, F. M. ((1984) Adoptive protection of *Mycobacterium tuberculosis*-infected lung. Dissociation between cells that passively transfer protective immunity and those that transfer delayed-type hypersensitivity to tuberculin, *Cell. Immunol.*, **84**(1), 113–120.

80. Flynn, J. L., Goldstein, M. M., Triebold, K. J., Koller, B., and Bloom, B. R. (1992) Major histocompatibility complex class I-restricted T-cells are required for resistance to *Mycobacterium tuberculosis* infection, *Proc. Natl. Acad. Sci. U.S.A.*, **89**(24), 12013–12017.

81. Lalvani, A., Brookes, R., Wilkinson, R. J., et al. (1998) Human cytolytic and interferon-γ-secreting CD8$^+$ T-lymphocytes specific for *Mycobacterium tuberculosis*, *Proc. Natl. Acad. Sci. U.S.A.*, **95**(1), 270–275.

82. Lazarevic, V. and Flynn, J. (2002) CD8$^+$ T-cells in tuberculosis, *Am. J. Respir. Crit. Care Med.*, **166**(8), 1116–1121.

83. Turner, J., D'Souza, C. D., Pearl, J. E., et al. (2001) CD-8- and CD95/95L-dependent mechanisms of resistance in mice with chronic pulmonary tuberculosis, *Am. J. Respir. Cell Mol. Biol.*, **24**(2), 203–209.

84. van Pinxteren, L. A., Cassidy, J. P., Smedegaard, B. H., Agger, E. M., and Andersen, P. (2000) Control of latent *Mycobacterium tuberculosis* infection is dependent on CD8 T-cells, *Eur. J. Immunol.*, **30**(12), 3689–3698.

85. Kaufmann, S. H. (1996) γ/δ and other unconventional T-lymphocytes: what do they see and what do they do? *Proc. Natl. Acad. Sci. U.S.A.*, **93**(6), 2272–2279.

86. Moody, D. B., Ulrich, T., Muhlbecker, W., et al. (2000) CD1c-mediated T-cell recognition of isoprenoid glycolipids in *Mycobacterium tuberculosis* infection, *Nature*, **404**(6780), 884–888.

87. Hinchey, J., Lee, S., Jeon, B. Y., Basaraba, R. J., Venkataswamy, M. M., Chen, B., Chan, J., Braunstein, M., Orme, I. M., Derrick, S. C., Sheldon L., Morris, S. L., Jacobs, W. R., Jr., and Porcelli, S. A. (2007) Enhanced priming of adaptive immunity by a proapoptotic mutant of *Mycobacterium tuberculosis*, *J. Clin. Invest.*, **117**, 2279–2288.

88. McShane, H. and Hill, A. (2005) Prime-boost immunisation strategies for tuberculosis, *Microbes Infect.*, **7**, 962–967.

89. McConkey, S. J., Reece, W. H. H., Moorthy, V. S., Webster, D., et al. (2003) Enhanced T-cell immunogenicity of plasmid DNA vaccines boosted by recombinant modified vaccinia virus Ankara in humans, *Nat. Med.*, **9**(6), 729–735.

90. McShane, H., Brookes, R., Gilbert, S. C., and Hill, A. V. S. (2001) Enhanced immunogenicity of CD4(+) T-cell responses and protective efficacy of a DNA-modified vaccinia virus Ankara prime-boost vaccination regimen for murine tuberculosis, *Infect. Immun.*, **69**(2), 681–686.

91. McShane, H., Behboudi, S., Goonetilleke, N., Brookes, R., and Hill, A. V. S. (2002) Protective immunity against *M. tuberculosis* induced by dendritic cells pulsed with both CD4(+) and CD8(+)-T-cell epitopes from antigen 85A, *Infect. Immun.*, **70**(3), 1623–1626.

91a. Dietrich, J., Aagard, C., Leah, R., et al. (2005) Exchanging ESAT6 with RB10.4 in Ag85B fusion molecule-based tuberculosis subunit vaccine: efficient protection and ESAT6-based sensitive monitoring of vaccine efficacy, *J. Immunol.*, **174**, 6332–6339.

92. Cardona, P. J., Amat, I., Gordillo, S., et al. (2005) Immunotherapy with fragmented *Mycobacterium tuberculosis* cells increases the effectiveness of chemotherapy against a chronical infection in a murine model of tuberculosis, *Vaccine*, **23**, 1393–1398.

92a. Horwitz, M. A. (2005) Recombinant BCG expressing *Mycobacterium tuberculosis* major extracellular proteins, *Microbes Infect.*, **7**, 947–954.

93. Horwitz, M. A. and Harth, G. (2003) A new vaccine against tuberculosis affords greater survival after challenge than the current vaccine in the guinea pig model of pulmonary tuberculosis, *Infect. Immun.*, **71**, 1672–1679.

94. Horwitz, M. A., Harth, G., Dillon, B. J., and Maslesa-Galic, S. (2000) Recombinant Bacillus Calmette-Guérin (BCG) vaccines expressing the *Mycobacterium tuberculosis* 30-kDa major secretory protein induce greater protective immunity against tuberculosis than conventional BCG vaccines in a highly susceptible animal model, *Proc. Natl. Acad. Sci. U.S.A.*, **97**, 13853–13858.

95. Skeiky, Y. A., Alderson, M. R., Ovendale, P. J., et al. (2004) Differential immune responses and protective efficacy induced by components of a tuberculosis polyprotein vaccine. Mtb72F, delivered as naked DNA or recombinant protein, *J. Immunol.*, **172**, 7618–7628.

96. Brandt, L., Skeiky, Y. A., Alderson, M. R., et al. (2004) The protective effect of the *Mycobacterium bovis* BCG vaccine is increased by coadministration with the *Mycobacterium tuberculosis* 72-kilodalton fusion polyprotein Mtb72F in *M. tuberculosis*-infected guinea pigs, *Infect. Immun.*, **72**, 6622–6632.

97. Langermans, J. A., Doherty, T. M., Vervenne, R. A., et al. (2005) Protection of macaques against *Mycobacterium tuberculosis* infection by a subunit vaccine based on a fusion protein of antigen 85B and ESAT-6, *Vaccine*, **23**, 2740–2750.

98. Mazurek, G. H., Jereb, J., Lobue, P., et al. (2005) Guidelines for using the QuantiFERON-TB Gold test for detecting *Mycobacterium tuberculosis* infection, United States, *Morb. Mortal. Wkly Rep.*, **54**, 49–55.

99. Mwinga, A., Nunn, A., Clark, S. O., et al. (2002) *Mycobacterium vaccae* (SRL-172) immunotherapy as an adjunct to standard anti-tuberculosis treatment in HIV-infected adults with pulmonary tuberculosis: a randomized placebo-controlled trial, *Lancet*, **360**, 1050–1055.

100. Mayr, A., Stickl, H., Muller, H. K., Danner, K., and Singer, H. (1978) The smallpox vaccination strain MVA: marker, genetic structure, experience gained with the parenteral vaccination and behavior in organisms with a debilitated defense mechanisms [trans. from German], *Zentralbl. Bakteriol. [B]*, **167**, 375–390.

101. Meyer, H., Sutter, G., and Mayr, A. (1991) Mapping of deletions in the genome of the highly attenuated vaccinia virus MVA and their influence on virulence, *J. Gen. Virol.*, **72**(Pt. 5), 1031–1038.

102. McShane, H., Pathan, A. A., Sander, C. R., Keating, S. M., Gilbert, S. C., Huygen, K., Fletcher, H. A., and Hill, A. V. (2004) Recombinant modified vaccinia virus Ankara expressing antigen 85A boosts BCG-primed and naturally acquired antimycobacterial immunity in humans, *Nat. Med.*, **10**(11), 1240–1244 [erratum: *Nat. Med.*, **10**(12), 1397].

103. McShane, H., Pathan, A. A., Sander, C. R., et al. (2005) Boosting BCG with MVA85A: the first candidate subunit vaccine for tuberculosis in clinical trials, *Tuberculosis (Edinb)*, **85**, 47–52.

104. Waddell, R. D., Chintu, C., Lein, A. D., Zumla, A., Karagas, M. R., Baboo, K. S., Habbema, J. D. F., Tosteson, A. N. A., Morin, P., Tvaroha, S., Arbeit, R. D., Mwinga, A., and von Reyn, F. C. (2000) Safety and immunogenicity of a five-dose series of inactivated *Mycobacterium vaccae* vaccination for the prevention of HIV-associated tuberculosis, *Clin. Infect. Dis.*, **30**(Suppl. 3), S309–S315.

105. Lein, A. D., Waddell, R. D., Chintu, C., Baboo, K. S., Zumla, A., Morin, P. M., Karagas, M. R., and von Reyn, C. F. (1998) Phase I trial of *Mycobacterium vaccae* immunization in HIV infected and healthy adults in Lusaka, Zambia, *5th Conf. Retroviruses Opportunistic Infect.*, Feb. 1–5, 217, abstract 736.

106. Tallat, A. M., Lyons, R., and Johnson, S. A. (1999) Towards therapeutic *Mycobacterium tuberculosis* vaccine using DNA microarray technology, *Abstr. Gen. Meet. Am. Soc. Microbiol.*, May 30–June 3, 652, abstract U-98.

107. Howard, A., Li, Z., Kelley, C., Collins, F., and Morris, S. (1999) Protecion and cytokine production associated with DNA vaccines against tuberculosis, *Abstr. Gen. Meet. Am. Soc. Microbiol.*, May 30–June 3, 651, abstract U-93.

108. Jagannath, C., Copenhanver, R., Armitige, L., Wanger, A., Norris, S., Actor, J. K., and Hunter, R. L. (1999) A mutant of *Mycobacterium tuberculosis* H37Rv deficient in antigen 85A expression, acts as vaccine against experimental tuberculosis in mice, *Abstr. Gen. Meet. Am. Soc. Microbiol.*, May 30–June 3, 652, abstract U-96.

109. Riska, P. F., Jacobs, W. R., Jr., and Alland, D. (2000) Molecular determinants of drug resistance in tuberculosis, *Int. J. Lung Dis.*, **4**(2 Suppl. 1), S4–S10.

110. Loiez-Durocher, C., Vachee, A., and Lamaitre, N. (2000) Drug resistance in *Mycobacterium tuberculosis*: diagnostic methods, *Ann. Biol. Clin. (Paris)*, **58**, 291–297.

110a. Iseman, M. D. (1993) Treatment of multidrug-resistant tuberculosis, *N. Engl. J. Med.*, **329**(11), 784–791.

111. Weltman, A. C. and Rose, D. N. (1994) Tuberculosis susceptibility patterns, predictors of multidrug resistance, and implication for initial therapeutic regimens at a New York City Hospital, *Arch. Intern. Med.*, **154**(19), 2161–2167.

112. Nolan, C. M., Williams, D. L., Cave, M. D., Eisenach, K. D., el-Hajj, H., Hooton, T. M., Thompson, R. L., and Goldberg, S. V. (1995) Evolution of rifampin resistance in human immunodeficiency virus-associate tuberculosis, *Am. J. Respir. Crit. Care Med.*, **152**(3), 1067–1071.

113. Lutfey, M., Della-Latta, P., Kapur, V., Palumbo, L. A., Gurner, D., Stotzky, G., Brudney, K., Dobkin, J., Moss, A., Musser, J. M., and Kreiswirth, B. N. (1996) Independent origin of mono-rifampin-resistant *Mycobacterium tuberculosis* in patients with AIDS, *Am. J. Respir. Crit. Care Med.*, **153**(2), 837–840.

114. Centers for Disease Control and Prevention (2006) Trends in tuberculosis – United States (2005), *Morb. Mortal. Wkly Rep.*, **55**(RR-11), 305–308.

115. Centers for Disease Control (2007) Trends in Tuberculosis – United States (2006), *Morb. Mortal. Wkly Rep.*, **56**(RR-11), 245–250.

116. Centers for Disease Control (2007) Extensively drug-resistant tuberculosis – United States (1993–2006), *Morb. Mortal. Wkly Rep.*, **56**(RR-11), 250–253.

117. Centers for Disease Control (2006) Emergence of *Mycobacterium tuberculosis* with Extensive resistance to second-line drugs – worldwide (2000–2004), *Morb. Mortal. Wkly Rep.*, **55**(RR-11), 301–305.

118. Notice to readers: revised definition of extensively drug-resistant tuberculosis (2006) *J. Am. Med. Assoc.*, **296**(23), 2792.

119. Masjedi, M. R., Farnia, P., Sorooch, S., Pooramiri, M. V., Mansoori, S. D., Zarifi, A. Z., Velayati, A. A., and Hoffner, S. (2006) Extensively drug-resistant tuberculosis: 2 years of surveillance in Iran, *Clin. Infect. Dis.*, **43**, 841–847.

120. Gandhi, N. R., Moll, A., Sturm, A. W., Pawinski, R., Govender, T., Lalloo, U., Zeller, K., Andrews, J., and Friedland, G. (2006) Extensively drug-resistant tuberculosis as a cause of death in patients co-infected with tuberculosis and HIV in a rural area of South Africa, *Lancet*, **368**(9547), 1575–1580.

121. Vilchese, C., Wang, F., Arai, M., Hazbon, M. H., Colangeli, R., Kremer, L., Weisbrod, T. R., Alland, D., Sacchetini, J. C., and Jacobs, W. R., Jr. (2006) Transfer of a point mutation in *Mycobacterium tuberculosis inhA* resolves the target of isoniazid, *Nat. Med.*, **12**, 1027–1029.

122. Rosenthal, I. M., Williams, K., Tyagi, S., Peloquin, C. A., Vernon, A. A., Bishai, W. R., Grosset, J. H., and Nuermberger, E. L. (2006) Potent twice-weekly rifapentine-containing regimens in murine tuberculosis, *Am. J. Respir. Crit. Care Med.*, **174**, 94–101.

123. Liu, P. T., Stenger, S., Li, H., Wenzel L., Tan, B. H., Krutzik, S. R., Ochoa, M. T., Schauber, J., Wu, K., Meinken, C., Kamen, D. L., Wagner, M., Bals, R., Steinmeyer, A., Zugel, U., Gallo, R. L., Eisenberg, D., Hewison, M., Hollis, B. W., Adams, J. S., Bloom, B. R., and Modlin, R. L. (2006) Toll-like receptor triggering of a vitamin D-mediated human antimicrobial response, *Science*, **311**, 1770–1773.

124. Kali, P., Gray, G. E., Violari, A., Chaisson, R. E., McIntyre, J. A., and Martinson, N. A. (2006) Combing PMTCT with active case finding for tuberculosis, *J. Acquir. Immune Defic. Syndr.*, **42**(3), 379–381.

125. Khader, S. A., Partida-Sanchez, S., Bell, G., Jelley-Gibbs, D. M., Swain, S., Pearl, J. E., Ghilardi, N., deSauvage, F. J., Lund, F. E., and Cooper, A. M. (2006) Interleukin 12p40 is required for dendritic cell migration and T cell priming after *Mycobacterium tuberculosis* infection, *J. Exp. Med.*, **203**, 1805–1815.

126. Oberhelman, R. A., Soto-Castellares, G., Caviedes, L., Castillo, M. E., Kissinger, P., Moore, D. A. J., Evans, C., and Gilman, R. H. (2006) Improved recovery of *Mycobacterium tuberculosis* from children using the microscopic observation drug susceptibility method, *Pediatrics,* **188**, e100–e106.

127. Sullivan, B., Jobe, O., Lazarevic, V., Vasquez, K., Bronson, R., Glimcher, L. H., and Kramnik, I. (2006) Increased susceptibility of mice lacking T-bet to infection with *Mycobacterium tuberculosis* correlates with increased IL-10 and decreased IFN-γ production, *J. Immunol.*, **175**, 4593–4602.

Chapter 15

Viral Hepatitis

Although the development of acute hepatitis after percutaneous exposure to human serum or blood has been known for more than a century, it was not until the 1960s that the actual etiologic agent of hepatitis was identified, when the hepatitis virus B surface antigen (HBsAg) was discovered and recognized as the viral antigen associated with acute hepatitis B (1).

Viral hepatitis, a general term that has been reserved for liver infections caused by one of at least five distinct hepatic agents, continues to be one of the major health problems worldwide. The causative agents of hepatitis are nonopportunistic hepatotropic viruses, known as hepadnaviruses, including hepatitis A virus, hepatitis B virus, hepatitis D virus, hepatitis C virus, and the non-A non-B hepatitis virus (1). Although not directly opportunistic, some hepadnaviruses, such as hepatitis B virus, have been implicated as potential cofactors in the development and progression of HIV infection.

15.1 Hepatitis A

In most cases, the hepatitis A virus (HAV) (family Picornaviridae) causes a subclinical disease. HAV, which has no known carrier state and plays no role in the production of chronic active hepatitis or cirrhosis, disappears after acute infection. Transmission of the disease has been primarily through oral-fecal contact (1).

Hepatitis A vaccine is now universally recommended for all children at age 1 year (12 to 23 months). Two doses of the vaccine should be administered at least 6 months apart. Since the adoption of childhood vaccination in high-risk areas, the overall incidence of hepatitis A infections has declined steadily.

15.2 Hepatitis B

Hepatitis B virus (HBV) is the prototype virus of the Hepadnaviridae family that exhibits striking tropism for hepatocytes but may also be detected in peripheral blood mononuclear cells and tissues (1). The majority of the worldwide hepatitis burden, with subsequent chronic hepatitis, cirrhosis, and liver cancer, has been due to HBV.

Studies in recent years have renewed interest in HBV as a possible cofactor in the progression of HIV disease to AIDS (1). It has been estimated that more than 84% of HIV-infected patients have presented with HBV markers. Thus, as a lymphotropic virus, infections caused by HBV have been common among HIV-infected patients, as evidenced by HBV DNA being recovered from lymphoid cells of patients co-infected with HBV and HIV. Furthermore, the HBV protein X was shown to activate the long terminal repeat (LTR) of HIV and thus to enhance its replication *in vitro* (2, 3). However, other studies, such as the Multicenter AIDS Cohort Study (4) and the Vancouver Lymphadenopathy-AIDS Study (5), have not found previous or current HBV infection to be associated with progression to AIDS, and that in HIV-positive patients, co-infection with HBV made no difference in the clinical outcome of the HIV disease (6).

A measurable and steady decline in hepatitis B rates in the United States has coincided with the implementation of a national strategy to eliminate HBV infection including routine childhood immunization (7–10).

15.3 Hepatitis C

In 1989, a new virus that has been responsible for most of the posttransfusion hepatitis and a large proportion of sporadic or community-acquired non-A non-B hepatitis was cloned by using a recombinant immunoscreening approach and identified as hepatitis C virus (HCV) (family Flaviviridae) (11). As with chronic hepatitis B infection, evidence has been emerging that liver damage may be mediated by the immune reaction to infected hepatocytes rather than by HCV itself. Nevertheless, there have also been reports suggesting a direct HCV cytopathic effect on liver cells (1). In contrast with HBV, HCV has rarely been the cause of fulminant hepatitis.

One of the main routes of transmission of HCV and hepatitis C infection has been through infected blood and blood products. Other risk factors include injection drug use, tattooing, needle-stick accidents, blood exchanges during ritual ceremonies, organ transplantation involving HCV-infected donors, and the use of folk medicines. Although uncommon, vertical transmission of HCV has been well documented *(1)*.

The frequency of heterosexual co-transmission of HCV and HIV has been studied *(12)*. The results have shown that HCV transmission to sexual partners was five times higher when HIV was also transmitted, suggesting that HIV may be a cofactor for the sexual transmission of HCV. Furthermore, liver failure occurred more frequently in HCV-seropositive hemophiliacs co-infected with HIV than in those who were HCV-seropositive but without HIV infection. This finding has strongly indicated that the HIV-induced immune deficiency may promote increased HCV replication *(13)*.

Monitoring acute hepatitis C has been challenging because no serologic marker for acute infection exists, and many health departments do not have the resources to determine whether a positive laboratory report for HCV represents acute infection (http://www3.niaid.nih.gov/research/topics/hepatitis/hepcfacts.htm).

Worldwide, some 180 million people are chronically infected with HCV, with more than 4 million in the United States. The Institute of Medicine has classified hepatitis C as an emerging infectious disease.

15.3.1 The HCV Disease

HCV can be contracted through the transmission of infected blood or body fluids (e.g., by transfusions, needle-sharing, sexual intercourse, or from an infected mother to her infant) (http://www3.niaid.nih.gov/research/topics/hepatitis/hepcfacts.htm). However, since the availability and mandatory adoption of reliable blood screening regimens in 1992, the risk of transmission of HCV via blood transfusion has fallen to less than one per million units of transfused blood, according to the Centers for Disease Control and Prevention (CDC). The majority of new HCV infections now occur among intravenous drug users.

Most acutely and chronically infected people are relatively free of physical symptoms and, in fact, are not even aware of their being infected. HCV causes damage to the liver, the extent of which can only be determined by microscopic examination of a liver biopsy. Symptoms of liver damage may not be apparent for several years and, unfortunately, by the time serious liver disease is diagnosed, the liver damage can be considerable and even irreversible—often resulting in end-stage liver disease, cirrhosis, and primary liver cancer. The rate of progression of chronic HCV-related liver disease is variable, and slow for most individuals (i.e., approximately 20% of individuals progress to cirrhosis after 20 years of chronic infection). Alcohol and other hepatitis viruses are associated with faster progression of the disease; therefore, infected individuals are advised to avoid alcohol consumption and to be vaccinated against hepatitis A and B. At present, commercially vaccines are unavailable for HCV and hepatitic E virus (HEV).

15.3.2 Treatment

The current standard of treatment for hepatitis C is a combination of pegylated interferon and ribavirin, which is intended to achieve a sustained elimination of HCV from the blood. However, the response to this treatment is variable, depending on the variant (genotype) of the infecting virus. Moreover, this therapy is associated with significant side effects. Although treatment responses are unpredictable, they are best in patients infected with HCV genotypes 2 or 3 ($\sim$75%), but considerably less in those infected with HCV genotype 1 ($\sim$ 45%), the predominant strain in the United States (http://www3.niaid.nih.gov/research/topics/hepatitis/hepcfacts.htm).

15.3.3 Challenges and Research Priorities

Hepatitis C virus infection is an increasing public health concern. Without more effective antiviral and immunologic therapies, the CDC has estimated that deaths due to HCV will double or triple in the next 15 to 20 years simply because of the length of time most people in the United States have been infected.

Better treatment strategies will stem from better understanding of the mechanisms of virus replication and pathogenesis. One of the remaining great research challenges is to identify the immune responses that are responsible for the clearance of an acute infection, which occurs spontaneously in a small subset of infected individuals. The successful development of vaccines will depend on overcoming this challenge.

Importance of Increasing Awareness. The fact that most people who are infected with HCV lack symptoms even though they may have been infected several years earlier makes it important for individuals at high risk—in particular, those who have had transfusions of blood or blood products before the routine implementation of blood testing, and others who have a greater risk of exposure, such as health care professionals, hemodialysis patients, and those with intimate contact with infected persons—to be tested for HCV, so that treatment may be initiated as early as possible.

15.4 Hepatitis D (Delta)

The hepatitis delta virus (HDV) is a unique RNA virus that requires for its replication a helper function provided by HBV, during which the HBsAg will actually envelop the infectious HDV RNA. Consequently, HDV may only replicate in patients who have already been infected with HBV *(1)*.

The clinical course of HDV infection, which may present as either acute or chronic disease, has been variable but is usually more severe than that of other forms of hepatitis. The acute HDV infection may be manifested as fulminant hepatitis, a rare sequela of the acute hepatitis caused by other hepatitis viruses. The chronic form of HDV infection is a serious and rapidly progressive liver disease *(1)*.

15.5 Recent Scientific Advances

- *High-Throughput Screen Can Identify Novel Hepatitis B Virus Treatments at a New Target Site.* A new high-throughput screen has been developed that would allow selection of compounds that prevent newly replicated HBV viral components from forming and assembling intact virus particles *(14)*. This assembly step, which is also common to other viruses, is crucial and represents a new target for drug development.
- *High-Density Lipoproteins Stimulate Cell Entry of Hepatitis C Virus and Inhibit Neutralizing Antibodies.* In normal circumstances, in reaction to a viral infection, the human body will produce neutralizing antibodies to inhibit the viral replication and help clear the infection. However, this is not the case in most HCV infections, which result in chronic virus persistence, despite the presence of neutralizing antibodies. This is because HCV exploits serum-dependent mechanisms that inhibit neutralizing antibodies. Recent data *(15)* have provided evidence that a high-density lipoprotein (HDL)—a normal serum component and ligand of the scavenger receptor BI (SR-BI)—will accelerate the entry of virions into the host cell. SR-BI is also a putative HCV coreceptor and their interaction will minimize the time for antibodies to interact, thereby attenuating neutralization. Consequently, compounds that inhibit the lipid transfer functions of SR-BI can restore neutralization by antibodies, thus opening the possibilities of new therapeutic intervention.
- *Oxidized Low-Density Lipoproteins Inhibit Cell Entry by Hepatitis C Virus.* Several studies have demonstrated that serum lipoproteins play an integral part in HCV entry and infection. In contrast with the stimulatory activity of the HDL, oxidized low-density lipoproteins (oxLDL)—also ligands of SR-BI—potently inhibit the entry of HCV

into the liver cells *(16)*. Native LDL does not have this effect. Furthermore, oxidized LDL will alter the biophysical properties of the virus, indicating a ternary interaction with both virus and target cells that inhibits the entry of the virus. This new finding suggests yet another anti-HCV drug target involving the SR-BI receptor and its lipid binding functions.

- *Peginterferon α-2a Plus Ribavirin Versus Interferon α-2a Plus Ribavirin for Chronic Hepatitis C in HIV Co-infected Persons.* Chronic hepatitis C infection is a major cause of complications in patients who were also infected with HIV. Results from a multicenter, randomized trial comparing peginterferon α-2a plus ribavirin with interferon plus ribavirin for the treatment of chronic hepatitis C in patients co-infected with HIV have demonstrated that using peginterferon α-2a instead of interferon in combination with ribavirin has been superior and may provide clinical benefit even in the absence of virologic clearance *(17)*.

15.6 NIAID Involvement in Viral Hepatitis Research

NIAID's involvement in viral hepatitis research focuses on (i) basic and/or clinical research on viral replication and pathogenesis, virus-host interactions involved in pathogenesis and immune responses; (ii) development of cell culture and small animal model systems for virus replication; (iii) development of vaccines and therapeutics, especially new targets and novel therapeutic approaches for HBV and vigorous programs to develop and test vaccines against hepatitis C virus; and (iv) support of preclinical and clinical development resources (see Section 15.6.3 below). Notably, in addition to individual investigator-initiated grant awards, cooperative agreements and interagency agreements have been established (http://www3.niaid.nih.gov/research/topics/hepatitis/research.htm). These include:

- Eight new cooperative *Research Centers* for the study of HCV, each engaged in various aspects of the host's immunologic response to infection as it pertains to successful control of virus (RFA AI 04-028)
- Three partnership awards to industry partners for the development of vaccines for HCV
- An interagency agreement with the National Institute of Diabetes and Digestive and Kidney Diseases (NIDDK) through which NIAID provides support for the virology and immunology ancillary study conducted via NIDDK's Hepatitis C Antiviral Long Term Treatment against Cirrhosis (HALT-C) clinical trial

(i)   http://www.niddk.nih.gov/fund/program/f-llist.htm
      (summary of HALT-C trial)
(ii) http://www.niddk.nih.gov/fund/ancillary-studies/
      studies.htm (ancillary studies)

15.6.1   Plans, Priorities, and Goals

The NIAID Hepatitis Research Program supports research
on all hepatitis viruses. However, commensurate with the
magnitude of the medical burdens imposed by these viruses,
the greatest emphasis is placed on the study of hepatitis C and hepatitis B viruses (http://www3.niaid.nih.gov/
research/topics/hepatitis/introduction.htm). These studies are
focused on

- Understanding the pathogenesis and immunology of hepatitis viruses
- Developing novel therapeutics and vaccines against diseases caused by the hepatitis viruses

15.6.2   Resources for Researchers

NIAID has made available the following resources for
researchers (http://www3.niaid.nih.gov/research/topics/ hep-
atitis/research.htm):

(i)   NIH AIDS Research and Reference Reagents Program
(ii) HCV Sequence Database
(iii) Lamivudine (Epivir) (information from NIAID and
      Clinical Center Research Program)

15.6.2.1   Preclinical Product Development

- NIAID supports contract resources that provide preclinical *in vitro* screening of candidate drugs for hepatitis B
  and hepatitis C. These systems have been further standardized by government contractors and are available to
  academic and pharmaceutical company sponsors free of
  charge. The HBV model *(18)* with human hepatoma cells
  transfected with HBV is under contract to Georgetown
  University. One HCV model is an enhanced 1b replicon
  with stable luciferase reporter expression, supported by
  a contract to the Southern Research Institute (SRI), and
  a second HCV culture model is a 1a replicon with similar readout. A third HCV *in vitro* screen uses a SEAP
  reporter replicon. For several years, NIAID has provided
  two preclinical animal models for evaluating therapeutic candidates for hepatitis B. The Utah State University
  contract has refined the HBV transgenic mouse model

developed initially at Scripps Research Institute for use by
academic and pharmaceutical sponsors. Also available is
the woodchuck animal model contract at Cornell University. Woodchucks, infected with a well-characterized pool
of woodchuck hepatitis virus, are the closest infection
model to humans for preclinical testing of therapies for
hepatitis B.

- Recently, NIAID added a contract focused on preclinical evaluation of therapies and vaccines for HCV. It provides access to the SCID-Alb-uPA chimera mouse model
  engrafted with human livers housed at KMT Hepatech, in
  Edmonton, Alberta, Canada.

15.6.3   Clinical Trials

- A Phase I study to evaluate the safety of HCV E1E2 vaccine with two different adjuvants, MF59.1 and/or CPG
  7909.
- A Phase I study in patients chronically infected with
  HCV and who have failed conventional treatment to
  determine whether autologous monocyte-derived dendritic cells (DCs) pulsed with HCV-specific lipopeptides
  in vitro generate any adverse events after autologous
  transfusion and to determine (i) whether DC therapy can
  generate a cell-mediated immune response in subjects; (ii)
  whether DC therapy can increase the titer of HCV-specific
  antibodies; and (iii) whether DC therapy can reduce the
  viral load or eliminate the virus.
- A pilot study aimed at characterizing interferon β–
  induced gene expression in liver cells and peripheral
  blood lymphocytes, using high-density oligonucleotide
  microarray expression analysis in patients with chronic
  HCV disease.

References

1. Georgiev, V. St. (1998) Hepatitis. In: *Infectious Diseases in
   Immunocompromised Hosts*, CRC Press, Boca Raton, FL, pp.
   205–220.
2. Seto, E., Yen, T. S., Peterlin, B. M., and Ou, J. H. (1988) Transactivation of the human immunodeficiency virus long terminal repeat
   by the hepatitis B virus X protein, *Proc. Natl. Acad. Sci. U.S.A.*, **85**,
   8286–8290.
3. Twu, J.-S., Chu, K., and Robinson, W. S. (1989) Hepatitis B virus
   gene activates KB-like enhancer sequences in the long terminal
   repeat of the human immunodeficiency virus, *Proc. Natl. Acad. Sci.
   U.S.A.*, **86**, 5168–5172.
4. Solomon, R. E., VanRaden, M., Kaslow, R. A., Lyter, D., Vissher,
   B., Farzadegan, H., and Phair, J. (1990) Association of hepatitis B
   surface antigen and core antibody with acquisition and manifestation of human immunodeficiency virus type 1 (HIV-1) infection,
   Am. J. Publ. Health, **80**, 1475–1478.

5. Schechter, M. T., Craib, K. J. P., Le, T. N., Willoughby, B., Douglas, B., Sestak, P., Montaner, J. S., Weaver, M. S., Elmslie, K. D., and O'Shaughnessy, M. V. (1989) Progression to AIDS and predictors of AIDS in seroprevalent and seroincident cohorts of homosexual men, *AIDS*, **3**, 347–353.

6. Stevenson, M., Natin, D., Fernando, R., and Shahmanesh, M. (1993) Hepatitis B markers do not predict decline in CD4 counts, *Proc. IVth Conf. AIDS,* Berlin, Abstr. PO-B02-0947.

7. Centers for Disease Control and Prevention (2006) Recommended childhood and adolescent immunization schedule, *Morb. Mortal. Wkly Rep.*, **54**(52), Q1–Q4.

8. Lavanchy, D. (2004) WHO: Communicable Disease Surveillance and Response, Geneva, Switzerland, *J. Vir. Hep.*, **11**, 97–107.

9. Centers for Disease Control and Prevention (2004) Incidence of acute hepatitis B-United States, 1990–2002, *Morb. Mortal. Wkly Rep.*, **52**(51–52), 1252–1254.

10. Centers for Disease Control and Prevention (1991) Hepatitis B virus: a comprehensive strategy for eliminating transmission in the United States through universal childhood vaccination: recommendations of the immunization practices advisory committee, *Morb. Mortal. Wkly Rep.*, **40**(RR-13), 1–19.

11. Cuthbert, J. A. (1994) Hepatitis C: progress and problems, *Clin. Microbiol. Rev.*, **7**, 505–532.

12. Eyster, M. E., Alter, H. J., Aledorf, L. M., Quan, S., Hatzakis, A., and Goedert, J. J. (1991) Heterosexual co-transmission of hepatitis C virus (HCV) and human immunodeficiency virus (HIV), *Ann. Intern. Med.*, **115**, 764–768.

13. Eystert, M. E., Fried, M. W., Di Bisceglie, A. M., and Goedert, J. J. (1994) Increasing hepatitis C virus RNA levels in hemophiliacs: relationship to human immunodeficiency virus infection and liver disease. Multicenter Hemophilia Cohort Study, *Blood*, **84**, 1020–1023.

14. Stray, J. S., Johnson, J. M., Kopek, B. G., and Zlotnick, A. (2006) An in vitro fluorescence screen to identify antivirals that disrupt hepatitis B virus capsid assembly, *Nat. Biotechnol.*, **24**(3), 358–362.

15. Dreux, M., Pietschmann, T., Granier, C., Voisset, C., Ricard-Blum, S., Mangeot, P. E., Keck, Z., Fong, S., Vu-Dae, N., Dubuisson, J., Bartenschlager, R., Lavillette, D., and Cossett, F. I. (2006) High density lipoprotein inhibits hepatitis C virus neutralizing antibodies by stimulating cell entry via activation of the scavenger receptor BI, *J. Biol. Chem.*, **281**(27), 18285–18295.

16. von Hahn, T., Lindenblach, B. D., Boullier, A., Quehenberger, O., Paulson, M., Rice, C. M., and McKeating, J. A. (2006) Oxidized low-density lipoprotein inhibits hepatitis C entry in human hepatoma cells, *Hepatology*, **43**(5), 932–942.

17. Chung, R. T., Andersen, J., Volberding, P., Robbins, G. K., Liu, T., Sherman, K. E., Peters, M. G., Koziel, M. J., Bhan, A. K., Alston, B., Colquhoun, D., Nevin, T., Harb, G., van der Horst, C., for the AIDS Clinical Trials Group A5071 Study Team (2004) Peginterferon alfa-2a plus ribavirin versus interferon alfa-2a plus ribavirin for chronic hepatitis C in HIV-coinfected persons, *N. Engl. J. Med.*, **351**(5), 451–459.

18. Korba, B. E. and Milman, G. (1999) A cell culture assay for compound which inhibit hepatitis B virus replication, *Antiviral Res.*, **15**(3), 217–228.

Chapter 16

West Nile Virus

The West Nile virus (WNV) belongs to the genus Flavivirus (family Flaviviridae) and was previously classified as a group B arbovirus. These disease-causing pathogens are spread to humans by insects, usually mosquitoes. Other flaviviruses include the Yellow fever virus, Japanese encephalitis virus, dengue virus, and the Saint Louis encephalitis virus (see sections on flaviviruses in Chapters 19 and 23). The West Nile virus was isolated first in Uganda in 1937 and then in other parts of the Eastern Hemisphere (Africa, Asia, the Middle East, and Europe). Since 1999, when it emerged in the Western Hemisphere (for the first time in the New York City area), it has been classified as an emerging infectious disease in the United States (http://cdc.gov/ncidod/dvbid/westnile/surv&control05Maps.htm). The WNV infection is considered to be zoonotic by nature because the first step in the transmission of WNV usually takes place when a mosquito bites an infected bird, and the virus primarily cycles between mosquitoes and birds, which are highly susceptible to infection; more than 40 species of mosquitoes are capable of transmitting the virus. However, infected mosquitoes can also transmit WNV to humans and other incidental hosts [other mammals, birds, and even reptiles (e.g., alligators)]. Although the vast majority of human WNV infections (about 80%) do not cause serious disease (mild symptoms of fever, headache, body aches, and occasionally skin rash and swollen lymph glands), when the virus enters the brain it may cause life-threatening encephalitis or meningitis. Such complications usually are associated with elderly people and/or immunocompromised persons. Recovery from severe illness can be very slow, and cognitive and functional disabilities can linger for months or years after the acute phase; some of the neurologic effects—such as paralysis—may be permanent.

In 1999, the first incidence of WNV in the United States occurred in the New York City metropolitan area; the outbreak affected 62 people, resulting in 7 deaths. Since 2002, WNV has become the most prevalent mosquito-borne infectious disease in the United States. In 2003, 9,862 human cases and 264 deaths were reported from 45 states and the District of Columbia. In the subsequent years, the incidence and mortality rates from WNV infections dropped, with the majority of cases occurring in California. Fewer cases were reported in 2006, which likely reflected the heightened awareness and precautions taken to prevent mosquito bites (www.cdc.gov/ncidod/dvbid/westnile/index.htm).

16.1 NIAID Involvement in West Nile Virus Research

When the West Nile virus appeared on the East Coast of the United States in 1999, NIAID immediately initiated a program to develop specific countermeasures (http://www3.niaid.nih.gov/healthscience/healthtopics/westNile/default.htm). Fortunately, there already had been in place an active basic research program on flaviviruses that served as a solid foundation for the West Nile virus research effort and that allowed research to move forward rapidly. Research funding has increased approximately 10-fold since the virus first appeared in North America. With this infusion of resources, scientific progress over the past 5 years has been swift (http://www.niaid.nih.gov/factsheets/westnile.htm).

16.1.1 Basic Research

Complex interactions among the virus, birds and other animals, mosquitoes, and the environment have influenced the pattern of WNV emergence and distribution across the United States, and specific factors contributing to the emergence of WNV are poorly understood. Understanding of these factors is essential in planning strategies to prevent, treat, and control this disease. The goal of NIAID basic research on WNV is to develop a knowledge base to enable medical countermeasures to be developed against WNV. To this end, NIAID is supporting basic research at universities and other institutions to better understand the infection in animals and humans, the virus itself, and

V. St. Georgiev, *National Institute of Allergy and Infectious Diseases, NIH: Impact on Global Health*, vol. 2, DOI 10.1007/978-1-60327-297-1_16, © Humana Press, a part of Springer Science+Business Media, LLC 2009

the environmental factors that influence the emergence of disease (http://www.niaid.nih.gov/factsheets/westnile.htm). Topics of research interest include:

- Determining how the virus replicates and spreads throughout the body to develop vaccines and drugs to prevent and treat disease
- Determining which viral proteins contribute to the virus' ability to cause disease
- Investigating how the immune system responds to the most serious form of the disease, West Nile encephalitis
- Examining the ecology and year-to-year maintenance of mosquito-borne encephalitis viruses and how genetic variation affects the spread and virulence of the virus
- Studying whether migrating bird populations carry the virus to points in Central and South America

The emergence of WNV in Central and South America, which harbor abundant mosquito populations, could set up conditions for a potentially severe epidemic.

Researchers also are working to better understand other insects and ticks that transmit other flaviviruses. Such an understanding will allow improved monitoring and surveillance and enable the development and preliminary testing of strategies to control carriers of the virus.

16.1.2 Research to Prevent West Nile Virus Disease

NIAID provides major funding to support the development of several WNV vaccine approaches, including chimeric vaccines (which combine genes from more than one virus into a single vaccine), naked DNA vaccines, and vaccines containing cocktails of individual West Nile proteins (http://www.niaid.nih.gov/factsheets/westnile.htm). Projects include the following:

- In November 2003, Acambis PLC started the first human clinical trial of a WNV vaccine. The Acambis vaccine is based on work performed under a fast-track project funded by NIAID in 2000. Scientists based the vaccine on one already licensed for preventing yellow fever, which is caused by another Flavivirus. Called a chimeric virus vaccine, the Acambis vaccine contains genes from two different viruses—yellow fever and West Nile. Researchers have replaced some of the yellow fever virus genes with genes for a surface protein of WNV. Acambis is also developing similar chimeric vaccines for dengue fever and Japanese encephalitis. The Acambis West Nile vaccine performed well in hamsters, mice, monkeys, and horses, and has now entered human clinical trials.

- NIAID intramural scientists pioneered the concept of creating chimeric vaccines for flaviviruses in 1992. A chimeric West Nile vaccine was developed and tested in monkeys, with promising results. This experimental vaccine, which uses an attenuated dengue virus as a backbone to carry WNV protective antigens, is in an ongoing Phase I human trial (for more details see the NIAID press release at www.niaid.nih.gov/newsroom/releases/wnv).

- Researchers at the NIAID Vaccine Research Center (VRC) have also developed an investigational vaccine for preventing WNV infection, in collaboration with Vical, Inc. The vaccine is based on an existing codon-modified gene-based DNA plasmid vaccine platform designed to express WNV proteins. In April 2005, after preclinical safety studies and viral challenge studies, VRC initiated a Phase I clinical trial to evaluate safety, tolerability, and immune responses of this recombinant DNA vaccine in human volunteers. Also in collaboration with Vical, Inc., VRC is currently developing a second-generation DNA vaccine using an improved expression vector expressing the same WNV proteins.

- In 2002, NIAID-supported researchers developed a hamster model of WNV infection that closely mimics the human disease. This animal model has proved useful in evaluating ways to prevent serious complications associated with this emerging infectious disease. Using the hamster model, researchers were able to determine that prior infection with other related viruses may provide complete or partial immunity to West Nile virus.

16.1.3 Research on West Nile Virus Treatments

No specific therapies for WNV infection currently exist; supportive care is generally the only treatment for those infected. NIAID has been supporting research to develop and test antiviral drugs, antibody products, and other therapies to prevent or treat severe complications of WNV infection that may develop, such as encephalitis and meningitis (http://www.niaid.nih.gov/factsheets/westnile.htm). For example, currently NIAID is funding a nationwide clinical trial to test whether antibodies from persons who have recovered from WNV infection can be used to treat those with severe West Nile neurologic disease. Investigators are comparing this treatment to placebo treatments to assess safety and to determine whether these antibodies help overcome the severe disease symptoms (www.casg.uab.edu).

Because some drugs are effective against related viruses in laboratory tests, scientists are optimistic that they will be able to develop drugs to treat WNV disease. Over the past several years, NIAID has expanded its *in vitro* and *in vivo* antiviral screening program to screen chemical compounds for possible effectiveness against WNV (www.niaid.nih.gov/dmid/viral). Promising antiviral drugs identified *in vitro* have been subsequently tested in hamster or mouse models of the disease. These animal models allow scientists to evaluate a drug's safety and efficacy before possible human trials. Since October 2003, more than 2,500 drugs have been screened *in vitro* and about 1% to 2% have shown promise for additional testing in animals.

In addition, NIAID clinicians are studying how WNV disease progresses in people who have or are at risk of developing its most serious complications. This research study, conducted through the Collaborative Antiviral Study Group and at the National Institutes of Health Clinical Center, measures the neurologic function of people hospitalized with WNV and will continue to monitor them as they recover. Data collected in this study will give researchers a better understanding of West Nile encephalitis and will assist in designing better treatments for this form of WNV disease.

16.1.4   Research to Improve the Diagnosis of West Nile Virus

NIAID is also sponsoring research to develop methods that will more quickly and accurately detect WNV in humans, animals, and mosquitoes. NIAID has awarded Small Business Innovation Research grants to small biotechnology companies to support development of new diagnostic tests for WNV. At least one such test under development has shown promise for more accurate diagnosis of WNV in humans and animals.

16.1.5   Resources for Researchers

The following resources funded by NIAID are currently available to scientists:

- *The World Reference Center for Emerging Viruses and Arboviruses* at the University of Texas Medical Branch at Galveston. This international program characterizes numerous viruses spread by mosquitoes, ticks, and other insects and animals to people and domestic animals. It also investigates the epidemiology of the diseases these viruses cause. The center stores various strains of the WNV as well as samples of sera containing WNV antibodies. Researchers in the United States and other countries may request samples for use in experiments.
- Sets of overlapping peptides for 11 WNV proteins were made available in 2005 through the NIAID Biodefense and Emerging Infections Research Resources Program

(www.beiresources.org). The peptides will be useful for vaccine research as well as immunologic research to assess the body's response after exposure to WNV. NIAID has expanded its funding of WNV research in academic and private sector laboratories. This includes establishing two Emerging Viral Diseases Research Centers in New York and Texas with collaborating laboratories in Colorado, Massachusetts, and several other states. These centers focus on West Nile and other emerging viruses.

16.2   Recent Scientific Advances

- During the past 2 years, NIAID-supported research resulted in the development of several high-throughput anti-WNV assays by engineering WNV replicons and the full-length viral genome into cells in culture *(1)*; and in the design and synthesis of several classes of small molecules with anti-WNV activity *(2, 3)*.
- *RNA Interference as a Potential Antiviral Therapy Against West Nile Virus.* RNA interference (RNAi) is a recently discovered cellular mechanism in which small pieces of double-stranded RNA (small interfering RNAs (siRNAs)) have suppressed the expression of genes with sequence homology *(4)*. Recent research data *(5)* have demonstrated that the RNA interference could be harnessed to protect laboratory animals against lethal infections from WNV and Japanese encephalitis virus (JEV) by having a single siRNA targeting a conserved sequence present in both WNV and JEV.
- *A Nonreplicating Recombinant West Nile Virus Subunit Vaccine.* The development of WNV vaccine is in progress. In a recent study, the production, purification, and immunogenicity in mice of a nonreplicating recombinant subunit WNV vaccine have been described and the protective efficacy of the vaccine in a hamster model of WNV encephalitis demonstrated *(6)*. Compared with replicating vaccines (live-attenuated or chimeric), the nonreplicating vaccines have the advantage of being safer in elderly and/or immunocompromised populations where live virus vaccines may be contraindicated because of the risks of adverse side effects.
- *Immunosuppressed Hamster Model of West Nile Virus Infection.* A recently developed immunosuppressed hamster model has shown much more severe WNV disease and a higher fatality rate compared with that in immunocompetent animals *(7)*. Whereas the WNV infection in untreated immunocompetent hamsters was confined to the brain and spinal cord, WNV infection in immunosuppressed animals was much more extensive and diffuse, involving the adrenal, kidney, heart, and lung, as well as

the brain and spinal cord. As with humans, the immuno-suppressed hamsters failed to develop antibodies against WNV.

16.3 Clinical Trials

- In September 2003, the FDA cleared a Phase I/II randomized, placebo-controlled clinical trial in the United States and Canada to evaluate the safety, tolerability, and potential efficacy of intravenous immunoglobulin G(Omr-IgG-am, Omrix Biopharma-ceuticals Ltd.) against WNV. This product has been shown to contain high levels of anti-WNV antibodies that had been isolated from patients who recovered from WNV disease. This study was performed under the NIAID Collaborative Antiviral Study Group (CASG) (http://clinicaltrials.gov/show/NCT00068055) and (http:// www.casg.uab.edu/adult/index.htm).
- NIAID has also been supporting a Phase I/II clinical trial initiated in September 2003 to assess the natural history of WNV encephalitis and to evaluate potential prognostic indicators of disease progression. This trial is also being performed under the CASG (www3.niaid.nih.gov/about/overview/profile/fy2005/pdf/research_drug.pdf).
- *NIAID Biodefense and Emerging Infections Research Resources Program.* As of September 2003, sets of WNV peptides have been made available to the research community through the NIAID Biodefense and Emerging Infections Research Resources Program (BEI Resources: http://www. beiresources.org) and managed by American Type Culture Collection (ATCC). These sets of peptides are useful in vaccine and immunology research, epitope mapping, and assessing the cytotoxic T lymphocyte (CTL) reactivity in individuals exposed to WNV.

References

1. Puig-Basagoiti, F., Deas, T. S., Ren, P., Tilgner, M., Ferguson, D. M., and Shi, P.-Y. (2005) High-throughput assays using a luciferase-expressing replicon, virus-like particles, and full-length virus for West Nile discovery. *Antimicrob. Agents Chemother.*, **49**, 4980–4988.
2. Puig-Basagoiti, F., Tilgner, M., Forshey, B. M., Philpott, S. M., Espina, N. G., Wentworth, D. E., Goebel, S. J., Masters, P. S., Falgout, B., Ren, P., Ferguson, D. M., and Shi, P.-Y. (2006) Triaryl pyrazoline compound inhibits flavivirus RNA replication, *Antimicrob. Agents Chemother.*, **50**, 1320–1329.
3. Goodell, J. R., Puig-Basagoiti, F., Forshey, B. M., Shi, P.-Y., and Ferguson, D. M. (2006) Identification of compounds with anti-West Nile virus activity, *J. Med. Chem.*, **49**, 2127–2137.
4. Gu, B., Ouzunov, S., Wang, L., Mason, P., Bourne, N., Cuconati, A., and Block, T. M. (2006) Discovery of small molecule inhibitors of West Nile virus using a high-throughput sub-genomic replicon screen, *Antiviral Res.*, **70**(2), 39–50.
5. Kumar, P., Lee, S. K., Shankar, P., and Manjunath, N. (2006) A single siRNA suppresses fatal encephalitis induced by two different flaviviruses, *PLoS Med.*, **3**(4), e96.
6. Lieberman, M. M., Clements, D. E., Ogata, S., Wang, G., Corpuz, G., Wong, T., Martyak, T., Gilson, L., Coller, B. A., Leung, J., Watts, D. M., Tesh, R. B., Siirin, M., Travassos da Rosa, A., Humphreys, T., and Weeks-Levy, C. (2007) Preparation and immunogenic properties of a recombinant West Nile subunit vaccine, *Vaccine*, **25**(3), 414–423.
7. Mateo, R., Xiao, S.-Y., Guzman, H., Lei, H., Travassos da Rosa, A., and Tesh, R. B. (2006) Effects of immunosuppression on West Nile virus infection in hamsters, *Am. J. Trop. Med. Hyg.*, **75**(2), 356-362.

Chapter 17

Herpesviruses

The herpesviruses that infect humans include cytomegalovirus (CMV), herpes simplex virus types 1 and 2 (HSV-1 and HSV-2), varicella-zoster virus (VZV), Epstein-Barr virus (EBV), human herpesviruses 6 and 7 (HHV-6 and HHV-7), and Kaposi's sarcoma–associated herpesvirus (KSHV, or HHV-8) *(1)*. The herpesviruses are known for their ability to remain in the body throughout an infected individual's lifetime and either remaining dormant or producing recurrent disease.

The human herpesviruses are important pathogens responsible for a wide range of diseases. Although they vary greatly in their biological properties and clinical manifestations, the essential processes by which their viral DNA is replicated and the virus particle assembled are very similar and use a significant fraction of the 40 "core" genes conserved in all mammalian and avian herpesviruses. These processes are central to the ability of the virus to pass between individuals and infect them; thus, it is important to understand their nature. Current investigations cover three distinct but interlinked areas: (i) studying the mechanism of herpesvirus DNA replication; (ii) analyzing the structure and assembly pathway of the virus particle; and (iii) determining the mechanism of DNA packaging into a preformed particle known as the procapsid (http://www.mrcvu.gla.ac.uk/research/resgrpc.html).

Genome Replication. The genetic information of HSV-1 is carried by a linear double-stranded DNA molecule. In infected cells, the DNA genome is circularized prior to the initiation of DNA synthesis. DNA replication primarily employs virus-coded proteins, and the products are complex high-molecular-weight concatemers in which multiple copies of the viral genome are linked head-to-tail.

Particle Structure. Assembly of the herpesvirus particle is a complex, multistage process involving numerous viral gene products. The capsid is an icosahedral protein shell, which surrounds and protects the virus genome. It is assembled as a precursor procapsid from hundreds of copies of a small number of different proteins. A specialized channel (the portal) is located at a unique vertex and serves as the entry and exit site for the viral genome. Once the DNA has entered, the capsid undergoes further assembly steps involving the addition of more proteins and a lipid envelope before the mature virus particle is released from the infected cell.

DNA Packaging. DNA packaging involves the site-specific cleavage of concatemeric virus DNA into unit length genomes, a process that is tightly coupled to the injection of the DNA into the procapsid. Seven HSV-1 proteins have been identified that have roles in the DNA packaging process. Among the best understood of these are the portal protein and the terminase complex, which pumps the DNA into the capsid shell and cleaves the replicated DNA to initiate and terminate the packaging process.

Other major challenges of clinical importance include:

- Understanding how herpesviruses interact with the immune system to facilitate the development of new vaccines
- Understanding at the molecular level the mechanism(s) by which herpesviruses maintain latency and how reactivation is controlled
- Development and testing of new prophylactic and therapeutic strategies, including vaccines and antiviral drugs

17.1 Cytomegalovirus

In the United States, approximately 50% of the population is seropositive for CMV, with seropositivity varying with socioeconomic status and geographic location. The outcome of CMV infection is highly dependent on the immune status of the host and although it rarely causes overt disease in healthy individuals, it can become serious, even life-threatening, in immunocompromised patients *(2)*.

Intrauterine transmission of CMV can occur whether a mother has prior immunity or acquires CMV for the first time during pregnancy. The degree of protection afforded an infected infant by the presence of the antibody in the mother before conception has been investigated, and the

V. St. Georgiev, *National Institute of Allergy and Infectious Diseases, NIH: Impact on Global Health*, vol. 2, DOI 10.1007/978-1-60327-297-1_17, © Humana Press, a part of Springer Science+Business Media, LLC 2009

results have shown that the presence of a maternal antibody to CMV before conception provided substantial protection against damaging congenital CMV infection in the newborn. Moreover, primary maternal infection during pregnancy was associated with more severe sequelae of congenital CMV infection (3, 4). Most infants born with symptomatic CMV disease, if they survive, may suffer from profound progressive deafness and/or mental retardation. However, even children who are asymptomatic at birth may also develop serious handicaps (5).

Human CMV (HCMV) infection has long been considered to be an immunosuppressive agent capable of inhibiting the host's immune response and contributing to the persistence of the infection (2). In a symptomatic primary CMV infection, the cell-mediated immunity is depressed, with T-cell abnormalities most readily defined (6).

In renal allograft recipients, the primary CMV infections vary from 25% to 100% (average 53%) and recurrent infections from 46% to 100% (average 85%) (2). Similar rates of infection have been seen among cardiac and bone marrow transplant recipients. In addition, HCMV is the most commonly isolated opportunistic pathogen associated with hepatitis after orthotopic liver transplantation (2).

Because of the high rate of seropositivity (90% to 100%) among HIV-infected patients, HCMV was originally thought by some to be the etiologic agent of AIDS (7). Approximately 40% of AIDS patients present with CMV visceral involvement at an advanced stage of the disease. The most common manifestations are retinitis and gastrointestinal infection and to a lesser extent CNS disorders (2).

Antiviral therapy with ganciclovir appears to be effective in limiting neurodevelopmental injury, particularly hearing loss caused by congenital CMV infection. The patients received 6 weeks of intravenous ganciclovir versus no treatment. Results have shown ganciclovir to be able to prevent hearing deterioration at 6 months and having promising effect on preventing hearing deterioration at ≥ 1 year (2, 8).

17.2 Varicella-Zoster Virus

The varicella-zoster virus is associated with two distinct clinical syndromes: (i) the primary infection of VZV is manifested as chickenpox (varicella) and results in a lifelong latent infection and (ii) upon reactivation of the latent virus leads to shingles (herpes zoster) (1, 9). Whereas varicella is a ubiquitous and highly contagious primary infection affecting the general population (especially in childhood), herpes zoster is a less common endemic clinical condition that usually occurs in older and/or immunocompromised

individuals (9). During varicella infection, a lifelong infection of the sensory nerve ganglion is established (10–12).

Predisposing factors associated with the appearance of herpes zoster are generally linked to compromised immune defenses and include Hodgkin's disease and other lymphomas, immunosuppressive therapy, trauma to the spinal cord and adjacent structures, and heavy-metal poisoning (9). The most common complication of herpes zoster is the postherpetic neuralgia that occurs in nearly 50% of patients 60 years and older (9). Furthermore, patients who have received prior repeated acyclovir treatment have the highest risk of harboring acyclovir-resistant VZV strains (13, 14).

AIDS patients with CD4$^+$ T-cell counts of ≤ 500 T-cells/mm^3 and organ transplant recipients (especially bone marrow allograft recipients) are at significant risk of VZV infections.

17.2.1 Varicella-Zoster Virus Vaccine

In 1992, a live-attenuated VZV vaccine was licensed for use in healthy individuals by the Food and Drug Administration (FDA) and was recommended for universal use in early childhood (15). As of July 2006 in the United States, 46 states and the District of Columbia had implemented a varicella vaccination school-entry requirement. The vaccine appears to be safe, with a single-dose regimen showing efficacy of 88% to 94% in preventing all disease and a complete protection against severe disease (16). Surveillance has showed only minor side effects (17).

The protection provided against severe disease by the current single-dose vaccine appears to be durable. Thus, studies on immunity and efficacy in individuals immunized up to 20 years previously have shown persistence of antibody and protection against serious illness (18).

To provide enhanced protection, a routine second dose of varicella vaccine for children aged 4 to 6 years has recently been recommended (http://www.cdc.gov/od/oc/media/pressrel/r060629-b.htm).

In 2006, a live-attenuated vaccine for herpes zoster was approved by the FDA for use in individuals 60 years and older. The vaccine, which is a high-titer version of the Oka varicella vaccine, markedly reduced morbidity from herpes zoster and post-herpetic neuralgia among older adults (19).

17.3 Herpes Simplex Virus

The herpesviruses (family Herpesviridae) are highly disseminated in nature. Herpesvirus hominis is the etiologic agent of herpes simplex in humans *(20)*. Forty years after the isolation of the herpes simplex viruses (HSVs), Schneweiss *(21)* established the existence of two serotypes, HSV-1 and HSV-2. Type 1 infections are primarily nongenital (e.g., herpes labialis, ocular herpes), whereas type 2 infections are primarily genital (herpes genitalis).

Primary HSV-1 infections typically occur in children under 5 years of age and are usually asymptomatic. Reactivation of latent virus most often manifests as herpes labialis (cold sores). However, there are a number of more severe conditions that may be associated with HSV-1 infections. HSV-1 encephalitis is the most common cause of nonepidemic, sporadic, acute focal encephalitis in United States, especially in AIDS patients *(20)*.

Neonatal HSV infections are classified as (i) disseminated disease, which involves multiple organs (lung, liver, adrenal glands, skin, eye, and the brain); (ii) CNS disease, with or without skin lesions; and (iii) disease limited to the skin, eyes, and/or mouth (SEM). With the use of a high dose of acyclovir, 12-month mortality has been reduced to 29% for disseminated neonatal HSV disease and to 4% for CNS HSV disease *(20)*.

HSV-1 infections of the eye are the second leading cause of corneal blindness (after trauma) *(20)*.

17.3.1 *Herpes Simplex Virus Infections in HIV-Infected Patients*

Prior to the emergence of the AIDS pandemic, chronic mucocutaneous HSV infections were seen predominately in patients with congenital cellular immune deficiencies or acquired immune defects associated most often with lymphoproliferative malignancies and organ transplantations *(20)*. Currently, HIV-infected patients represent the major population affected by persistent active HSV infections *(22)*. Because asymptomatic shedding of HSV can continue despite clinically effective suppression with antiviral chemotherapy, the possibility of person-to-person transmission persists. Chronic perianal HSV lesions causing severe morbidity (pain, itching, and painful defecation) have been considered among the first opportunistic infections associated with AIDS in homosexual men. The clinical manifestations of orolabial and genital HSV disease in HIV-infected patients (mild to severe tissue-destructive lesions) are usually similar to that observed in other immunosuppressed persons. As a result, cases of HSV-associated encephalitis in AIDS patients usually occur as complications of orolabial HSV infection. HSV encephalitis is a life-threatening condition with substantial morbidity and mortality despite the use of antiviral therapy *(23, 24)*.

17.3.2 *Acyclovir-Resistant Herpes Simplex Virus*

The incidence of acyclovir-resistant HSV in immunocompromised patients, though still relatively low [by one estimate only 4.7% *(20)*], appears to be on the rise. Whereas most of acyclovir resistance has been reported among AIDS patients, some cases of lethal disseminated visceral HSV infections caused by acyclovir-resistant mutants have been described in bone marrow transplant recipients and in one case of meningoencephalitis in an AIDS patient *(20)*.

17.4 Epstein-Barr Virus

The Epstein-Barr virus is a lymphotropic virus found ubiquitously worldwide *(25)*. There is no convincing evidence that strain differences among various EBV isolates account for the wide range of clinical conditions associated with EBV infections *(26)*.

Based on serology, approximately 90% of the adult U.S. population has been infected with EBV *(1)*. The impact of acute clinical manifestations induced by EBV in immunocompromised patients is less well understood, although it has been suspected that the virus may be the cause of high morbidity and severe illness in immunocompromised hosts *(26)*. Although EBV can be transmitted through blood transfusion, the main portal of entry is the oropharynx. B cells are the only cells known to have surface receptors for EBV, and replication in the epithelial cells of the oropharynx is thought to provide the source of virus that infects the B lymphoid cells *(27)*.

17.4.1 *Immune Response to Epstein-Barr Virus*

The presence of EBV in epithelial and B cells triggers an intense immune response consisting of antibodies to a large host of virally encoded products, a panoply of cell-mediated responses, as well as secretion of lymphokines *(25)*. Although the exact role of the antibodies in controlling the infection is not known, neutralizing antibodies that appear early after infection will persist for life and may limit the spread of infection. In normal individuals, the control of EBV proliferation in B lymphocytes is carried out by a variety of cell-mediated responses. Reactivation of EBV is facilitated by conditions that interfere with the viability of the cell-mediated responses.

Even though EBV may reactivate frequently in immunocompromised patients, it does not usually cause any severe symptoms. However, the cellular hyporesponsiveness associated with EBV reactivation, though less intense and of shorter duration than that associated with cytomegalovirus infections, may contribute to the morbidity observed in immunocompromised patients *(27)*.

Recent evidence has also suggested that EBV may be associated with Hodgkin's lymphoma *(28)*, T-cell lymphomas, some gastric carcinomas, and breast cancer *(29)*

17.4.2 Pathogenesis of EBV-Associated Diseases in AIDS Patients

Three EBV-associated lesions have been characterized in AIDS patients *(30)*: (i) diffuse polyclonal lymphomas that are frequently localized in extranodal sites, such as the gut and CNS; (ii) lymphocytic interstitial pneumonitis; and (iii) oral "hairy" leukoplakia of the tongue *(31)*.

EBV-induced lymphomas in AIDS patients may sometimes take the form of classic Burkitt's lymphoma with its associated chromosome abnormality *(25)*.

17.5 Human Herpesvirus 6

Primary infection with human herpesvirus 6 (HHV-6) is associated with exanthema subitum (roseola) and most frequently results in a highly febrile illness in young children that last 3 to 7 days and that is sometimes responsible for CNS complications, such as seizures. As with other herpesviruses, HHV-6 persists after infection *(32)*. However, the full spectrum associated with HHV-6 primary, persistent, and recurrent infections has not yet been fully defined.

HHV-6 may be responsible for 20% of emergency room visits for acute febrile illness in infants 6 to 12 months old and for one third of febrile seizures in children less than 3 years of age. Seroprevalence is estimated at 90% *(33)*.

In addition, HHV-6 reactivates in 40% to 50% of patients undergoing hematopoietic stem cell and solid organ transplantation, occurring between 2 and 6 weeks after transplantation *(34, 35)*. In another development, studies incorporating serology, PCR, and assessments of active viral replication have tentatively linked HHV-6 with multiple sclerosis and perhaps other demyelinating diseases as well *(36)*; however, such association still remains controversial *(32)*.

17.5.1 Pathogenesis of Human Herpesvirus 6 in AIDS Patients

The occurrence of three events is relevant to both HHV-6 and HIV: (i) the common isolation of HHV-6 from HIV-infected patients; (ii) the finding that HHV-6 can infect CD4$^+$ T

cells (also the target cells for HIV); and (iii) the observation that human herpesvirus immediate-early proteins can *trans*-activate the HIV long terminal repeat (LTR) *(37, 38)*. The presence of HHV-6 in most patients with AIDS has been ascertained by direct isolation, DNA amplification, and serology. In further studies, there is evidence that both HHV-6 and HIV-1 can productively co-infect individual human CD4$^+$ T-lymphocytes, resulting in accelerated HIV-1 expression and cellular death *(38)*. This finding and the observed *trans*-activation of the HIV-1 LTR by HHV-6 are direct evidence of interaction between HIV-1 and HHV-6.

17.6 Human Herpesvirus 7

The human herpesvirus 7 (HHV-7) shares some genomic homology with HHV-6. Seroprevalence for HHV-7 has been estimated at 90% *(32)*. Seroconversion appears to occur early in life, at 3 to 4 years of age. A roseola-like disease can occur at initial HHV-7 infection.

Although HHV-6 and HHV-7 exhibit similar cytopathic effects and virion structure, there is still insufficient information about the genomic and antigenic properties of HHV-7 and its role as an etiologic agent of infections in immunocompromised patients *(32)*. HHV-7 has been found to reactivate in solid organ transplant recipients, although its clinical significance remains unclear and poorly defined *(39)*.

17.7 Human Herpesvirus 8

Human herpesvirus 8 (HHV-8) has been universally associated with all types of Kaposi's sarcoma, whether AIDS-associated, Mediterranean endemic, or African endemic *(40)*. Thus, the presence of either HHV-8 DNA sequences or HHV-8-specific antibodies in HIV-infected patients was found predictive of the development of Kaposi's sarcoma *(41, 42)*. Furthermore, HHV-8 was present in early clinical lesions and was also localized in specific cells associated with tumor development *(43)*.

17.8 Recent Scientific Advances

- *Crystal Structure of Glycoprotein B from Herpes Simplex Virus 1.* The glycoprotein B (gB) is the most conserved component of the complex cell-entry machinery of the herpesviruses. A crystal structure of the gB ectodomain from HSV-1 reveals a multidomain trimer with unexpected homology to glycoprotein G from the completely unrelated vesicular stomatitis virus (VSV G) *(44)*. The structural similarity of these two viruses will raise the question of how these viruses evolved and the mechanisms of virus evolution in general. The elucidation of the crystal structure of gB will help in developing a more detailed understanding of how HSV enters cells.

- *Maternal Antibodies Enhance or Prevent Cytomegalovirus Infection in the Placenta by Neonatal Fc Receptor–Mediated Transcytosis.* As one of the major viral causes of congenital disease, HCMV infects the uterine-placental interface with varied outcomes depending on the strength of the maternal humoral immunity and gestational age. How HCMV reaches the fetus across the placenta is unknown. However, recent data have suggested that HCMV virions could disseminate to the placenta through the receptor-mediated pathway for IgG; this may also explain the efficacy of hyperimmune IgG for treatment of primary HCMV infections during gestation *(45)*.

- *An siRNA-Based Microbicide Protects Mice from Lethal Herpes Simplex Virus 2 Infection.* A microbicide to prevent sexual transmission of HSV-2 would contribute substantially to controlling the spread of HIV and other infections. Recent research *(46)* has demonstrated that vaginal instillation of small interfering RNAs (siRNAs) targeting HSV-2 protected mice from lethal infection. When mixed with lipid, they were efficiently taken up by epithelial and lamina propria cells and silenced the gene expression in the mouse vagina and ectocervix for at least 9 days.

17.9 Clinical Trials

Several clinical trials supported by the Collaborative Antiviral Study Group (CASG) (http://www.casg.uab.edu/) include:

(i) A Phase III double-blind, placebo-controlled study among patients age 12 and older with herpes simplex encephalitis (HSE) to determine whether treatment with oral valacyclovir, after the patients had completed intravenous acyclovir treatment, will reduce brain swelling and nervous system damage, and whether it can increase survival with or without mild neurophysiologic impairment (*CASG 204*).

(ii) A study to test whether a long-term treatment with oral acyclovir will improve the outcome for infants with HSV infection of the brain or spinal cord (CNS disease) (*CASG 103*). A subcomponent supported by the National Institute of Neurological Disorders and Stroke (NINDS/NIH) is also part of this study.

(iii) A study to test if a long-term treatment with oral acyclovir will improve the outcome for infants with HSV disease of the skin, eyes, and mouth (SEM disease) (*CASG 104*).

(iv) A study of oral valganciclovir syrup in neonates and young infants with symptomatic congenital CMV disease to determine its pharmacokinetics, pharmacodynamics, safety, and tolerability in children has been completed. The study identified the oral dose of valganciclovir that is bioequivalent to intravenous ganciclovir, which was shown in a previous CASG study to lead to improvement or maintenance of hearing in symptomatic infants (*CASG 109*).

References

1. Georgiev, V. St. (1998) Herpesviridae. In: *Infectious Diseases in Immunocompromised Hosts*, CRC Press, Boca Raton, FL, pp. 3–122.
2. Georgiev, V. St. (1998) HCMV Infection in immunocompromised hosts. In: *Infectious Diseases in Immunocompromised Hosts*, CRC Press, Boca Raton, FL, pp. 10–13.
3. Stagno, S., Pass, R. F., Cloud, G., Britt, W. J., Henderson, R. E., Walton, P. D., Veren, D. A., Page, F., and Alford, C. A. (1986) Primary cytomegalovirus infection in pregnancy. Incidence, transmission to fetus, and clinical outcome, *J. Am. Med. Assoc.*, **256**(14), 1904–1908.
4. Jeffries, D. J. (1984) Cytomegalovirus infections in pregnancy, *Br. J. Obstet. Gyneacol.*, **91**(4), 305–306.
5. Fowler, K. B., Stagno, S., Pass, R. F., Britt, W. J., Boll, T. J., and Alford, C. A. (1992) The outcome of congenital cytomegalovirus infection in relation to maternal antibody status, *N. Engl. J. Med.*, **326**(10), 663–667.
6. Rinaldo, C. R., Jr., Black, P. H., and Hirsch, M. S. (1977) Interaction of cytomegalovirus with leukocytes from patients with mononucleosis due to cytomegalovirus, *J. Infect. Dis.*, **136**(5), 667–678.
7. Drew, W. L., Conant, M. A., Miner, R. C., Huang, R. C., Ziegler, J. L., Groundwater, J. R., Gullet, J. H., Volberding, P., Abrams, D. I., and Mintz, L. (1982) Cytomegalovirus and Kaposi's sarcoma in young homosexual men, *Lancet*, **2**, 125–127.
8. Kimberlin, D. W., Lin, C.-Y., Sánchez, P. J., Demmler, G. J., Dankner, W., Shelton, M., Jacobs, R. F., Vaudry, W., Pass, R. F., Kiell, J. M., Soong, S.-J., Whitley, R. J., and the NIAID Collaborative Antiviral Study Group (2003) Effect of ganciclovir therapy on hearing in symptomatic congenital cytomegalovirus disease involving the central nervous system: a randomized, controlled trial, *J. Pediatr.*, **143**(1), 16–25.
9. Georgiev, V. St. (1998) Varicella-zoster virus (herpes zoster) infections. In: *Infectious Diseases in Immunocompromised Hosts*, CRC Press, Boca Raton, FL, pp. 49–92.
10. Gilden, D. H., Vafai, A., Shtram, Y., Becker, Y., Devlin, M., and Wellish, M. (1983) Varicella zoster virus DNA in human sensory ganglia, *Nature*, **306**, 478–480.
11. Mahalingam, R., Wellish, M., Wolf, W., Dueland, A. N., Cohrs, R., Vafai, A., and Gilden, D. (1990) Latent varicella-zoster viral DNA in human trigeminal and thoracic ganglia, *N. Engl. J. Med.*, **323**, 627–631.
12. Hyman, R. W., Ecker, J. R., and Tenser, R. B. (1983) Varicella-zoster virus RNA in human trigeminal ganglia, *Lancet*, **2**(8354), 814–816.
13. Balfour, H. H., Benson, C., Braun, J., Cassens, B., Erice, A., Friedman-Kien, A., Klein, T., Polsky, B., and Safrin, S.

(1994) Management of acyclovir-resistant herpes simplex and varicella-zoster virus infection, *J. Acquir. Immune Defic. Syndr.*, **7**, 254–260.

14. Jacobson, M. A., Berger, T. G., Fikrig, S., Becherer, P., Moohr, J. W., Stanat, S. C., and Biron, K. K. (1990) Acyclovir-resistant varicella-zoster virus infection after chronic oral acyclovir therapy in patients with the acquired immunodeficiency syndrome (AIDS), *Ann. Intern. Med.*, **112**(3), 187–191.

15. Centers for Disease Control (1996) Prevention of varicella: recommendations of the Advisory Committee on Immunization Practices (ACIP), *Morb. Mortal. Wkly Rep.*, **45**(RR-11), 1–36.

16. Vazquez, M., LaRussa, P. S., Gershon, A. A., Steinberg, S. P., Freudigman, K., and Shapiro, E. D. (2001) The effectiveness of the varicella vaccine in clinical practice, *N. Engl. J. Med.*, **344**, 955–960.

17. Wise, R. P., Salive, M. E., Braun, M. M., Mootrey, G. T., Seward, J. F., Rider, L. G., and Krause, P. R. (2000) Postlicensure safety surveillance for varicella vaccine, *J. Am. Med. Assoc.*, **284**(10), 1271–1279.

18. Ampofo, K., Saiman, L., LaRussa, P., Steinberg, S., Annunziato, P., and Gershon, A. (2002) Persistence of immunity to live attenuated varicella vaccine in healthy adults, *Clin. Infect. Dis.*, **34**(6), 774–779.

19. Oxman, M. N., Levin, M. J., Johnson, G. R., Schmader, K. E., Straus, S. E., Gelb, L. D., Arbeit, R. D., Simberkoff, M. S., Gershon, A. A., Davis, L. E., Weinberg, A., Boardman, K. D., Williams, H. M., Zhang, J. H., Peduzzi, P. N., Beisel, C. E., Morrison, V. A., Guatelli, J. C., Brooks, P. A., Kauffman, C. A., Pachucki, C. T., Neuzil, K. M., Betts, R. F., Wright, P. F., Griffin, M. R., Brunell, P., Soto, N. E., Marques, J. W., Keay, S. K., Goodman, R. P., Cotton, D. J., Gnann, J. W., Loutit, J., Holodniy, M., Keitel, W. A., Crawford, G. E., Yeh, S.-S., Lobo, Z., Toney, J. F., Greenberg, R. N., Keller, P. M., Harbecke, R., Hayward, A. R., Irwin, M. R., Kyriakides, T. C., Chan, C. Y., Chan, I. S. F., Wang, W. W. B., Annunziato, P. W., and Silber, J. L., for the Shingles Prevention Study Group. (2005) A vaccine to prevent herpes zoster and postherpetic neuralgia in older adults, *N. Engl. J. Med.*, **352**(22), 2271–2284.

20. Georgiev, V. St. (1998) Herpes simplex virus. In: *Infectious Diseases in Immunocompromised Hosts*, CRC Press, Boca Raton, FL, pp. 92–106.

21. Schneweiss, K. E. (1962) Serologische untersuchungen zur typendifferenzierung des herpesvirus hominis, *Z. Immuno-Forsch. Exp. Ther.*, **124**, 24.

22. Straus, S. E. (1988) Treatment of persistent active herpesvirus infections, *J. Virol. Meth.*, **21**(1–4), 305–313.

23. Whitley, R. J., Alford, C. A., Hirsch, M. S., Schooley, R. T., Luby, J. P., Aoki, F. Y., Hanley, D., Nahmias, A. J., Soong, S.-J., and the NIAID Collaborative Antiviral Study Group (1986) Vidarabine versus acyclovir therapy in herpes simplex encephalitis, *N. Engl. J. Med.*, **314**, 144–149.

24. Sköldenberg, B., Forsgren, M., Alestig, K., Bergström, T., Burman, L., Dahlqvist, E., Forkman, A., Frydén, A., Lövgren, K., Norlin, K., Norrby, R., Olding-Stenkvist, E., Stiernstedt, G., Uhnoo, I., and de Vahl, J. (1984) Acyclovir versus vidarabin in herpes simplex encephalitis: randomized multicentre study in consecutive Swedish patients, *Lancet*, **324**(8405), 707–717.

25. Georgiev, V. St. (1998) Epstein-Barr virus. In: *Infectious Diseases in Immunocompromised Hosts*, CRC Press, Boca Raton, FL, pp. 106–113.

26. Yoser, S. L., Forster, D. J., and Rao, N. A. (1993) Systemic viral infections and their retinal and choroidal manifestations, *Surv. Ophthalmol.*, **37**(5), 313–352.

27. Schooley, R. T. (1991) Epstein-Barr virus infections, including infectious mononucleosis. In *Harrison's Principles of Internal Medicine*, 12th ed. (Wilson, J. D., Braunwald, E., Isselbacher, K.

J., Petersdorf, R. G., Martin, J. B., Fauci, A. S., and Root, R. K., eds.), McGraw-Hill, New York, p. 689.

28. Cartwright, R. A. and Watkins, G. (2004) Epidemiology of Hodgkin's disease: a review, *Hematol. Oncol.*, **22**(1), 11–26.

29. Glaser, S. L., Hsu, J. L., and Gulley, M. L. (2004) Epstein-Barr virus and breast cancer: state of the evidence for viral carcinogenesis, *Cancer Epidemiol. Biomarkers Prev.*, **13**(5), 688–697.

30. Miller, G. (1990) Epstein-Barr virus. In: *Fields Virology*, 2nd ed. (Fields, B. N., Knipe, D. M., Chanock, R. M., Hirsch, M. S., Melnick, J. L., Monath, T. P., and Roizman, B., eds.), Raven Press, New York, p. 1921.

31. Greenspan, J. S., Greenspan, D., Lennette, E. T., Abrams, D. I., Conant, M. A., Petersen, V., and Freese, U. K. (1985) Replication of Epstein-Barr virus within the epithelial cells of oral "hairy" leukoplakia, an AIDS-associated lesion, *N. Engl. J. Med.*, **313**(25), 1564–1571.

32. Georgiev, V. St. (1998) Human herpesvirus-6, human herpesvirus-7, and human herpesvirus-8. In: *Infectious Diseases in Immunocompromised Hosts*, CRC Press, Boca Raton, FL, pp. 114–122.

33. Hall, C. B., Long, C. E., Schnabel, K. C., Caserta, M. T., McIntyre, K. M., Costanzo, M. A., Knott, A., Dewhurst, S., Insel, R. A., and Epstein, L. G. (1994) Human herpes virus-6 infection in children– a prospective study of complications and reactivation, *N. Engl. J. Med.*, **331**(7), 432–438.

34. Zerr, D. M., Corey, L., Kim, H. W., Huang, M.-L., Nguy, L., and Boeckh, M. (2005) Clinical outcomes of human herpesvirus 6 reactivation after hematopoietic stem cell transplantation, *Clin. Infect. Dis.*, **40**, 932–940.

35. Hentrich, M., Oruzio, D., Jäger, G., Schlemmer, M., Schleuning, M., Schiel, X., Hiddemann, W., and Kolb, H.-J. (2005) Impact of human herpesvirus-6 after hematopoietic stem cell transplantation, *Br. J. Haematol.*, **128**(1), 66–72.

36. Derfuss, T., Hohlfeld, R., and Meinl, E. (2005) Intrathecal antibody (IgG) production against human herpesvirus type 6 occurs in about 20% of multiple sclerosis patients and might be linked to a polyspecific B-cell response, *J. Neurol.*, **252**(8), 968–971.

37. Rando, R. F., Pellett, P. E., Luciw, P. A., Bohan, C. A., and Srinivasan, A. (1987) *Trans*-activation of human immunodeficiency virus by herpesviruses, *Oncogene*, **1**(1), 13–18.

38. Lusso, P., Ensoli, B., Markham, P. D., Ablashi, D. V., Salahuddin, S. Z., Tschachler, E., Wong-Staal, F., and Gallo, R. C. (1989) Productive dual infection of human CD4+ T lymphocytes by HIV-1 and HHV-6, *Nature*, **337**, 370–373.

39. Razonable, R. R., Brown, R. A., Humar, A., Covington, E., Alecock, E., Paya, C. V., and the PV16000 Study Group (2005) Herpesvirus infections in solid organ transplant patients at high risk of primary cytomegalovirus disease, *J. Infect. Dis.*, **192**(8), 1331–1339.

40. Huang, Y. Q., Li, J. J., Zhang, W. C., Feiner, D., Friedman-Kien, A. E., Kaplan, M. H., Poiesz, B., and Katabira, K. (1995) Human herpesvirus-like nucleic acid in various forms of Kaposi's sarcoma, *Lancet,* **345**(8952), 759–761.

41. Whitby, D., Boshoff, C., Hatzioannou, T., Weiss, R. A., Schulz, T. F., Howard, M. R., Brink, N. S., Tedder, R. S., Tenant-Flowers, M., Copas, A., Suggett, F. E. A., Aldam, D. M., Denton, A. S., Miller, R. F., and Weller, I. V. D. (1995) Detection of Kaposi's sarcoma associated herpesvirus in peripheral blood of HIV-infected individuals and progression to Kaposi's sarcoma, *Lancet*, **346**(8978), 799.

42. Gao, S.-J., Kingley, L., Hoover, D. R., Spira, T. J., Rinaldo, C. R., Saah, A., Phair, J., Detels, R., Parry, P., Chang, Y., and Moore, P. S. (1996) Seroconversion to antibodies against Kaposi's sarcoma-associated herpesvirus-related latent nuclear antigens before the development of Kaposi's sarcoma, *N. Engl. J. Med.*, **335**(4), 233.

43. Foreman, K. E., Bacon, P. E., His, E. D., and Nickoloff, B. J. (1997) In situ polymerase chain reaction-based localization studies sup-

port role of human herpesvirus-8 as the cause of two AIDS-related neoplasms: Kaposi's sarcoma and body cavity lymphoma, *J. Clin. Immunol.*, **99**(12), 2971–2978.

44. Heldwein, E. E., Lou, H., Bender, F. C., Cohen, G. H., Eisenberg, R. J., and Harrison, S. C., (2006) Crystal structure of glycoprotein B from herpes simplex virus 1, *Science*, **313**(5784), 217–220.

45. Maidji, E., McDonagh, S., Genbacev, O., Tabata, T., and Pereira, L. (2006) Maternal antibodies enhance or prevent cytomegalovirus infection in the placenta by neonatal Fc receptor-mediated transcytosis, *Am. J. Pathol.*, **168**, 1210–1226.

46. Palliser, D., Chowdhury, D., Wang, Q. Y., Lee, S. J., Bronson, R. T., Knipe, D. M., and Lieberman, J. (2006) An siRNA-based microbicide protects mice from lethal herpes simplex virus 2 infection, *Nature*, **432**, 89–94.

Chapter 18

Paramyxoviridae: Nipah Virus and Hendra Virus

The Paramyxoviridae family of lipid-enveloped negative-strand RNA viruses comprises several genera that include such human pathogens as the human parainfluenza virus, the measles and mumps viruses, the Newcastle disease virus (NDV), and the human respiratory syncytial virus, among others.

In September 1994, an outbreak of acute respiratory illness in Hendra, a suburb of Brisbane, Australia, resulted in the deaths of 14 racing horses and a horse trainer. The causative agent of the disease, a new member of the Paramyxoviridae family, was originally called *equine morbillivirus*. Later, the virus was renamed *Hendra virus* after the molecular characterization highlighted differences between it and other members of the Morbillivirus. In 1998, a closely related virus, *Nipah virus*, was isolated in Malaysia from an outbreak that spread rapidly through the pig population and caused severe respiratory disease and fatal encephalitis in humans *(1–3)*. Fruit bat species were found to be the natural reservoir of these viruses, and human encroachment onto their habitat enabled these viruses to come into contact with new host species *(3)*. The pork industry and human handlers who came in contact with infected pigs suffered greatly when more than 100 people died, and 1.2 million pigs had to be sacrificed to contain the outbreak *(1)*. An outbreak of Nipah virus disease in Bangladesh in April 2004 was confirmed or suspected in at least 29 people, and 25 have died.

Extensive serologic studies have identified the natural reservoir of Hendra virus as fruit- and nectar-feeding bats (suborder Megchiroptera), commonly known as flying foxes, such as the gray-headed flying-fox (*Pteropus polocephalus*) and the black flying-fox (*P. alecto*) *(4–6)*. Vertical transmission has been reported for this species.

Spillover of Hendra virus to horses is a rare event. Infected bat urine or an aborted bat fetus may have spread Hendra virus to horses. The Hendra virus can also infect cats and guinea pigs. Infected horses, cats, and guinea pigs excrete the virus in their urine. The virus is also carried through the breath of horses, but it is not highly contagious.

The natural reservoir for Nipah virus is still under investigation, but preliminary data have suggested that bats of the genus *Pteropus* (*P. vampyrus*, *P. hypomelanus*) are also the reservoirs for Nipah virus in Malaysia. How Nipah virus infected pigs is not entirely clear. It is believed that bat wastes or fruit contaminated by bat saliva fell into piggeries and were consumed by pigs, which then became infected. Nipah virus caused a relatively mild disease in pigs in Malaysia and Singapore and was transmitted to humans, cats, and dogs through close contact with infected pigs (http://www.cdc.gov/ncidod/dvrd/spb/mnpages/dispages/nipah.ttm).

18.1 Phylogeny

Although they manifest diverse biological properties, viruses of the families Filoviridae, Rhabdoviridae, Paramyxoviridae, and Bornaviridae all contain a nonsegmented negative-strand RNA genome and share features of genome organization *(7)*. These features, together with similarities in domain structure and sequence of the viral polymerase proteins, suggest a close phylogenetic relationship, which prompted the grouping of these four families taxonomically into the order Mononegavirales, the first taxon above the family level to be recognized in virus taxonomy *(8, 9)*.

The taxonomy within Paramyxoviridae has significantly changed over the past several years, and currently the family is divided into two subfamilies: Paramyxovirinae and Pneumovirinae *(7, 10–12)*. The Paramyxovirinae include three genera, Respirovirus (formerly known as Paramyxovirus), Morbillivirus, and Rubulavirus, whereas Pneumovirinae contains two genera, Pneumovirus and Metapneumovirus.

Two interesting observations can be made from the comparison of the viral genome sizes. First, there is no overlap of genome size between the viral families, and second, the genome size ranges differ significantly between the two families in which multiple genera have been defined, the Rhabdoviridae and Paramyxoviridae *(7)*. Thus, within the Rhabdoviridae, the genome length can vary more than 40%, whereas variation within the Paramyxoviridae is no more than 5%. This difference in variation led the paramyxoviruses, especially those of the subfamily Paramyxovirinae, to be traditionally described as having a "uniform genome size" *(8,10)*. The universality of this feature has recently been challenged with the discovery of a much larger genome for the Hendra virus *(7)*.

The two newly discovered paramyxoviruses, Nipah virus (NiV) and Hendra virus (HeV), prompted the establishment of a new genus, Henipavirus, within the Paramyxoviridae. The large genome size (18,234 nucleotides), the unique complementary genome terminal sequences of HeV, and the limited homology with other members of the Paramyxoviridae suggested that the Hendra virus, together with the Nipah virus, should be classified as a new genus in this family.

The henipaviruses have unique biological characteristics—they are the only *zoonotic* paramyxoviruses and are highly pathogenic. The range of species that are susceptible to these viruses is also remarkable—in addition to at least three pteropid species, NiV infects five terrestrial species in four mammalian orders.

In addition to Henipavirus, several other newly emerged Mononegavirales members of bat origin have been identified. These include the *Australian bat lyssavirus (13)* and the *Menangle virus (14)*. The Australian bat lyssavirus is closely related to the rabies virus and was responsible for the death of a bat handler in 1996 *(15)*. The Menangle virus (MeV) caused fetal death and abortion in pigs and respiratory illness in humans *(14, 16)*. The MeV appears to be a member of the Rubulavirus genus *(7)*. Another, apparently new, member of Paramyxoviridae has recently been isolated from bat urine in Malaysia and has displayed some cross-reactivity with the Menangle virus *(7)*.

Yet another virus, *Tupaia paramyxovirus,* has been isolated and characterized from tree shrews *(17)*, and recently, the *Salem virus*, a novel paramyxovirus, has been isolated from horses *(18)*. These two viruses are phylogenetically related to each other and to the Hendra virus and morbilliviruses *(7)*.

18.2 Molecular Biology of Paramyxoviruses

Morphology. The Henipavirus virion is helical, enveloped with distinct surface projections, 150 to 200 nm in diameter, and 10,000 to 10,040 nm long. It is spherical or filamentous, but pleomorphic forms also occur.

Structure. Like other paramyxoviruses, the henipaviruses contain a linear ribonucleoprotein (RNP) core consisting of a single-stranded genomic RNA molecule of negative polarity to which nucleocapsid proteins (N) are tightly bound in a

ratio of one N for every six nucleotides *(19)*. The RNP also contains smaller numbers of the phosphoprotein (P) and the large (L) polymerase protein, both of which are required to transcribe genomic RNA into mRNA and antigenome RNA. The RNP core is surrounded by an envelope from which two spikes protrude: one is the receptor-binding glycoprotein (G) and the other the fusion (F) protein. The G and F proteins are arranged as homotetramers and homotrimers, respectively. The matrix protein (M), which underlines the viral envelope, is important in determining the virion architecture and is released from the RNP core when it enters the cells *(20)*.

18.2.1 The Genome

The negative-sense genomic RNA is presented in the 3′ to 5′ orientation. The open reading frames (ORFs) encode the nucleocapsid (N), phosphoprotein (P), matrix protein (M), fusion protein (F), glycoprotein or attachment protein (G), and large protein (L) or RNA polymerase in the order 3′-N-P-M-F-G-L-5′. All genes except the P gene are monocistronic. The P gene of henipaviruses encodes not only the P protein but also the V, C, and W proteins. Genomic RNA in RNPs is transcribed by the viral polymerase, which associates with the RNP at the 3′ terminus and sequentially generates discrete mRNAs from each of the viral genes *(6, 20)*.

The successful molecular characterization of the HeV L gene and protein, the genome termini, and the gene boundary sequences completed the sequence of the largest genome in the Paramyxoviridae family *(7)*.

The HeV L gene encodes the RNA polymerase and determines the sequence of the genome termini and gene boundaries. In the highly conserved region of the L protein, the HeV sequence GDNE differed from the GDNQ found in nearly all other nonsegmented negative-strand (NNS) RNA viruses. The Hendra virus possessed an absolutely conserved intergenic trinucleotide sequence, 3′-GAA-5′, and highly conserved transcription initiation and termination sequences similar to those of respiroviruses and morbilliviruses.

The increase in the genome size of HeV was mainly the result of the expansion of the 5′ and 3′ untranslated regions (UTRs), especially at the 3′ end of the mRNA with the exception of the L gene *(7)*.

The data on the L protein sequence, genome end sequences, hexamer-phasing positions, and the gene start and stop signals, together with the sequences and molecular features reported for the other five gene of HeV *(21–24)* have strongly indicated that HeV is a member of the Paramyxovirinae subfamily. These data have also demonstrated the clear need to create a separate genus, Henipavirus, within the subfamily to accommodate the many significant differences between HeV and other members of Paramyxovirinae *(7)*.

Although the complete genome structure of Nipah virus is not yet available, the strong antigenic cross-reactivity between NiV and HeV and the high sequence homology for their N, P, M, F, and G genes *(25)* have indicated that both are very closely related viruses *(7)*.

18.2.2 Host Evasion by Paramyxoviruses: Inhibition of Interferon Signaling

The RNA genome of henipaviruses encodes several proteins necessary for viral replication *(1, 7, 25)*. One feature common to many paramyxoviruses is the presence of a *polycistronic gene*, which encodes two or more different proteins through the use of overlapping ORFs. The genomic transcripts of both HeV and NiV contain three ORFs, the largest of which encodes the P protein *(22)*. Of the remaining two, the +1 ORF encodes the C protein and the V protein *C*-terminal domain (CTD), and the +2 ORF encodes the W protein CTD. Whereas all three P, V, and W proteins are amino co-terminal, they have unique C-termini *(26)*.

The cysteine-rich CTD was found to be highly conservative among all paramyxovirus V proteins. It contains seven invariant cysteine residues, and although it has been shown to bind two atoms of zinc, it is not homologous to any known zinc-binding cellular proteins. Furthermore, even if the paramyxovirus V protein is not required for growth in interferon (IFN)-deficient systems, it was shown to inhibit the IFN signaling, thereby making it essential for avoiding host antiviral responses *(6, 20, 26)*.

Inhibition of the Interferon Response. The interferons (type I, IFN-α/β; and type II, IFN-γ) are innate antiviral cytokines that signal through the JAK-STAT (Janus kinases–signal transducers and activators of transcription) pathway to establish a broadly effective antiviral state in mammalian cells *(6, 27, 28)*. The IFN-α/β initiates a receptor-dependent tyrosine phosphorylation of both STAT1 and STAT2, which together with a DNA-binding subunit, IRF9, will form a heterotrimeric transcription factor complex called ISGF3 *(29, 30)*. The IFN-γ responses are mediated through formation of a transcription factor complex called GAF, which is a STAT1 homodimer *(31)*. These activated STAT transcription factor complexes rapidly translocate to the nucleus and bind to distinct target gene promoter elements to drive the transcription of antiviral gene products *(26)*.

Recent studies have linked the paramyxovirus V protein to inhibition of IFN signaling through a direct targeting of STAT proteins by ubiquitylation and proteozome-dependent degradation of STATs. Whereas both HeV and NiV V proteins inhibited the transcriptional activity in response to IFN-α/β and IFN-γ signaling in human cells similar to their paramyxovirus V proteins *(32, 33)*, the inhi-

bition occurred through a distinct mechanism. Biochemical analysis revealed that although both Henipavirus V proteins bound to both STAT1 and STAT2 and prevented their IFN-induced tyrosine phosphorylation, these V proteins did not cause degradation of either STAT1 or STAT2 by converting them from their latent monomeric state into high-molecular-weight complexes with an average size in the range of 300 to 500 kDa *(26)*.

Furthermore, the Henipavirus V proteins blocked the translocation of STAT1 and STAT2 in response to IFN. In normal cells, prior to IFN stimulation, latent STAT1 is localized in the cytoplasm and nucleus, a result of its basal nuclear-cytoplasmic shuttling *(34)*. However, expression of either Henipavirus V protein caused a dramatic redistribution of the latent STAT1 from the nucleus to the cytoplasm *(26)*.

Based on these and other studies, it has been postulated that a V protein–deficient Henipavirus would be severely attenuated in IFN-competent hosts, and thus a recombinant virus could be used as a potential source of a human and animal vaccine strain against henipaviruses *(26)*.

18.2.3 Viral Fusion and Entry

The identification of ephrin B2 as the cell surface receptor for both HeV and NiV *(35, 36)*, as well as the recent finding that ephrin B3 can serve as an alternate NiV receptor *(37)*, has provided valuable information about the pathogenicity of these two henipaviruses. Endothelial syncytia, composed of multinucleated giant-endothelial cells, are frequently found in NiV and HeV infections and are mediated by the fusion (F) and attachment (G) envelope glycoproteins.

Ephrins are ligands for the Eph family of receptor tyrosine kinases, and the signaling mediated by the Eph receptor-ephrin interaction is critical to a series of developmental pathways, including angiogenesis and axonal guidance, as well as tumorigenesis *(38)*. Although in vertebrates the Eph receptors are regulators of axon pathfinding, neuronal cell migration, and vasculogenesis, the Eph receptors and ephrins have primordial ancestors that predate the appearance of the neural pathways.

Ephrin B2, the membrane-bound cell surface glycoprotein ligand for the EphB class of receptor tyrosine kinases (RTKs), is expressed specifically on endothelial cells, neurons, and the smooth muscle cells surrounding the arterioles, a distribution pattern that parallels the cellular tropism of NiV and HeV diseases *(39, 40)*. The structure of ephrin B2 has been determined by x-ray crystallography *(41)*.

Ephrin B3 is not expressed in the endothelium but rather in the central nervous system, especially in some locations where ephrin B2 is lacking but NiV disease is manifested.

Depending on the biological properties of a virus, the attachment proteins are either the hemagglutinin-neuraminidase, the hemagglutinin, or, as is the case for HeV and NiV, the attachment glycoprotein (G), which lacks both hemagglutinating and neuraminidase activities *(42)*.

The fusion glycoprotein (F) belongs to the family of class I fusion proteins and is characterized by the presence of two heptad repeat (HR) regions, HR1 and HR2. These two regions associate to form a fusion-active hairpin conformation that juxtaposes the viral and cellular membranes to facilitate membrane fusion and enable subsequent viral entry. The Hendra and Nipah virus fusion core proteins have been crystallized and their structures determined to 2.2 Å resolution *(43)*.

Once triggered by the receptor-bound glycoprotein G, the fusion glycoprotein (F), an oligomeric homotrimer, facilitates the fusion of the virion and host cell membranes *(44)* by undergoing multistep conformational changes leading to a six-helix bundle (6HB) structure *(43)* that accomplishes fusion of the viral and cellular membranes. For HeV, once F reaches the cell surface, it is again internalized and then cleaved by cathepsin L, yielding a membrane-distal and membrane-anchored subunit *(45, 46)*. The ectadomain of the paramyxovirus F glycoprotein contains two conserved heptad repeat regions (HRN and HRC) near the fusion peptide and the transmembrane domains, respectively.

The possibility of inhibiting paramyxovirus fusion with HRC peptides has been raised *(47)*, and various peptides have been reported as candidate therapeutic agents. It has been proposed that peptides derived from the HRN and HRC regions of F inhibit fusion by preventing the F protein, after the initial triggering step, from forming the 6HB structure that is required for fusion *(38)*. HRC peptides have generally been the peptides discussed in this context, as they were more potent than HRN peptides because they acquired less coiled-coil structure in solution and therefore will aggregate less *(47)*. In the case of HeV, peptides derived from the HRC region of HPIV3 F were found to be highly effective inhibitors of HeV infection *(38)*.

18.3   Henipavirus Zoonoses

18.3.1   Hendra Virus Infection

Epidemiology and Transmission. The Hendra virus infection (also known as the Australian equine morbillivirus infection, equine morbillivirus pneumonia, and acute equine respiratory syndrome) was initially documented only in Australia. Two outbreaks occurred from 1994 to 1995, and a single horse died of the disease in 1999. However, in March 1999,

Malaysian authorities reported that Hendra virus was isolated from people who had worked closely with pigs *(48)*.

The transmission of HeV occurs from close contact, as the virus is not highly contagious. Aerosol transmission appears to be inefficient, and human-to-human transmission has not been observed. In infected horses and experimentally infected cats, the virus has been isolated from the urine and oral cavities but not from nasal or rectal swabs. In fruit bats, HeV has been isolated from fetal tissues and blood. Furthermore, vertical transmission has been documented in this species. It is assumed that infected bat urine or an aborted bat fetus may have spread the infection to horses.

Clinical Manifestations. In two of three outbreaks of HeV disease in horses, infections were also seen in humans. The incubation period of HeV infection is not known. Two people working at the stable became acutely ill 5 and 6 days after the infected horse had died. The patients developed a serious influenza-like disease with fever, myalgia, and respiratory symptoms. One of them died from septic pneumonia; the other recovered over the next 6 weeks *(49)*.

In the third case, the patient came into contact with sick horses during their illness and at necropsy, and shortly thereafter he developed a mild case of meningoencephalitis. He was successfully treated and became asymptomatic; however, a year later he developed fatal encephalitis *(49)*.

The virus was isolated from the kidneys of one of the dead patients.

There has been no evidence of seroconversion in persons who are often in close contact with fruit bats.

Treatment. A treatment for HeV infection has not been developed. Currently, a vaccine against HeV and NiV is in development in Australia and the United States, using the viral G glycoprotein after removing its membrane to make it soluble in the blood. The experimental vaccine provided complete protection in a feline model (http://www.vetscite.org/publish/items/002767/index.html).

18.3.2   Nipah Virus Infection

Epidemiology and Transmission. During the Nipah virus outbreaks in Malaysia and Singapore in the period 1998 to 1999, there were 105 deaths among 265 reported cases of severe febrile encephalitis, a mortality rate of nearly 40% *(2, 50)*. The outbreak was associated with respiratory illness in pigs and was initially attributed to Japanese encephalitis (JE). JE is a mosquito-borne viral infection that is enzootic in the region, and pigs are among the amplifying hosts. However, because some of the epidemiologic characteristics of the disease in humans were distinct from those of JE, most cases occurred in adult males who worked with pigs, in very few cases patients were young children, and neither mosquito control nor JE vaccination appeared to affect the course of the outbreak—investigators in Malaysia made attempts to isolate the causative agent, which was determined to be a new paramyxovirus, Nipah virus (2, 51).

Fruit bats (flying foxes) are believed to be the natural reservoir for Nipah virus. The ecologic changes associated with land use and animal husbandry practices appeared most likely to be associated with the emergence of the Nipah virus (3). Fruit bats exist in great numbers from India to Australia, and the presence of NiV was also reported between 2001 and 2004 in Thailand, Cambodia, Bangladesh, and India. This has demonstrated that Nipah virus represents a major health problem worldwide that could affect the economies of many countries; the outbreak in Malaysia ceased when more than 1 million pigs were culled from the outbreak area and the immediate surrounding vicinity, representing more than 50% of the number of live herds of swine (2).

The mode of transmission from animal to animal, and from animal to human, is uncertain, but appears to require close contact with contaminated tissue or body fluids from infected animals. Nipah antibodies have been detected in pigs and other domestic and wild animals. The role of species other than pigs in transmitting infection to other animals has not yet been determined. It is unlikely that NiV is easily transmitted to humans, although data from outbreaks seems to suggest that Nipah virus was transmitted from animals to humans more readily than was Hendra virus. Despite frequent contact between fruit bats and humans, there has been no serologic evidence of human infection among bat caretakers (http://www.who.int/mediacentre/factsheets/fs262/en). Pigs were the apparent source of infection in most human cases in Malaysia, but other sources, such as infected dogs and cats, cannot be excluded. Human-to-human transmission of Nipah virus has not been reported.

Serologic studies in which Hendra virus was used to detect the Nipah virus immunoglobulin M (IgM) and IgG confirmed NiV in all cases in Singapore and all but one of the initially identified encephalitis cases from Malaysia (2). Results from a recent study indicated that the NiV nucleocapsid protein (N) was a highly immunogenic protein in human and swine infections and a good target for serodiagnosis in large-scale epidemiologic investigations, especially in developing countries (52).

Pathogenesis. The main histologic findings of NiV disease included a systemic vasculitis with extensive thrombosis and parenchymal necrosis, particularly in the central nervous system. Endothelial damage, necrosis, and syncytial giant cell formation were observed in the affected vessels, with widespread presence of NiV antigens in the endothelial and smooth muscle cells of the blood vessels (51).

Infection of the endothelial cells and neurons (53), as well as vasculitis and thrombosis, seem to be the major pathogenic signs of the NiV disease. Several human neuronal cell proteins that are differently expressed after NiV infection have been associated with various cellular functions, and their abundance reflects their significance in the cytopathologic responses to the infection and the regulation of NiV replication. Thus, data from a study of the SK-N-MC human neuronal cell protein response to NiV infection has shown that the heterogenous nuclear ribonucleoprotein (hnRNP) F, guanine nucleotide binding protein (G protein), voltage-dependent anion channel 2 (VDAC2), and the cytochrome bc1 were abundantly present in the NiV-infected SK-N-MC cells. Conversely, hnRNP H and hnRNP H2 were significantly downregulated. The hnRNPs F, H, and H2 are cellular proteins that could be associated with NiV replication or RNA synthesis. The other two proteins, VDAC2 and cytochrome bc1, are proteins associated with the mitochondria, whereas the G protein is known to be involved with the cell signaling pathways. The abundant presence of the mitochondria-associated proteins, coupled with the ultrastructural changes to the mitochondria in the NiV-infected neuronal cells, raised the possibility of induction of apoptosis in these cells. The number of apoptotic cells steadily increased 24 hours after infection, and at 96 hours after infection the apoptosis of NiV-infected SK-N-MC cells was nearly complete (53).

Clinical Manifestations. The incubation period of Nipah virus disease is between 4 and 18 days. In many cases the infection is mild or unapparent (subclinical). In symptomatic cases, the onset is usually with influenza-like symptoms (lasting 3 to 14 days), including high fever, headache, dizziness, vomiting, and myalgia (54, 55) (http://www.cdc.gov/ncidod/dvrd/spb/mnpages/dispages/nipah.htm). The disease may progress to inflammation of the brain (encephalitis) with drowsiness, disorientation, convulsions, and coma. More than 50% of patients presented with reduced level of consciousness and prominent brain-stem dysfunction. Distinctive clinical signs included segmental myoclonus, areflexia and hypotonia, hypertension, and tachycardia, all suggesting the involvement of the brain stem and the upper cervical spinal cord (54). The initial cerebrospinal fluid findings were abnormal in 75% of patients. Abnormal doll's eye reflex and tachycardia were factors associated with poor prognosis. Death was probably the result of severe brainstem involvement.

Patients who had recovered from clinical illness might have a clinical relapse 13 to 39 days after an initial mild illness (54). These patients presented with either neurologic symptoms after an initial illness without re-exposure to pigs or long latency from an initial exposure to the virus. The onset of symptoms was acute, with fever, headache, focal neurologic signs, seizure, dizziness, reduced consciousness, and myoclonus *(55)*.

Treatment. No drug therapies have yet proved to be effective in treating Nipah infection (http://www.who.int/mediacentre/factsheets/fs262/en). Treatment relies on providing intensive supportive care. There is early evidence that ribavirin can reduce both the duration of feverish illness and the severity of disease. However, the efficacy of this treatment in curing the disease or improving survival is still uncertain.

After the Nipah virus outbreak, ribavirin was used in an open-label trial of acute Nipah encephalitis *(56)*. Oral ribavirin was given to 128 patients, and 12 patients received intravenous ribavirin. There were 45 deaths (32%) in the treated group and 29 (54%) in the controls (51 patients who were previously managed prior to the availability of ribavirin)—the results suggested a 36% reduction in mortality and an increased survival without neurologic deficits, although the latter was not statistically significant.

18.3.2.1 Nipah Virus as a Potential Biological Weapon

The global importance of emerging infectious disease and the discoveries that followed in the field have raised the potential of some of these infectious agents to be used as biological weapons or in bioterrorism.

The Nipah virus, a deadly zoonotic paramyxovirus, has a number of important attributes that puts it in this category *(56)*:

- NiV is extremely pathogenic to humans, and the case-fatality rate may be as high as 50%. Because of that, it has been classified as a Biosafety Level 4 organism. Besides causing acute infection, it can also give rise to clinical relapse months or even years after infection. There is no effective treatment at the present time, and no vaccine may be available for at least several years.
- Diagnostic capability is limited at present to very few laboratories worldwide, although this will improve once a noninfectious, specific test becomes available.
- Nipah virus can be produced in large quantities in cell culture, an important criterion for consideration as a biological weapon.
- Because the complete viral genome has been characterized, genetic manipulations of NiV can be easily achieved if desired.
- It would be possible to stabilize the virus as an aerosol with the capacity of widespread dispersal.
- Besides infecting humans, NiV can also infect livestock, domestic animals, and wildlife. Even small outbreaks like those in Southeast Asia could result in mass culling of affected herds, thereby causing significant economic loss

to the industry or to the national economy of the affected country.

- Because little is known about the Nipah virus, an outbreak in animals or humans could lead to substantial fear, social disruption, or even economic chaos. In a multiracial country such as Malaysia, the handling of the outbreak would be a delicate and sensitive problem that could be turned into a serious political, religious, and racial issue.

Since the discovery of Nipah virus, only a handful of laboratories have access to the virus. However, because its natural reservoir is readily accessible, it will not be difficult to isolate the virus from wildlife, making it readily available to any country. From that perspective (availability, ease of production and dissemination, and high morbidity and mortality rates), the CDC has listed the Nipah virus as a critical Category C biological agent.

References

1. Chua, K. B. (2003) Nipah virus outbreak in Malaysia, *J. Clin. Virol.*, **26**, 265–275.
2. Chua, K. B., Bellini, W. J., Rota, P. A., Harcourt, B. H., Tamin, A., Lam, S. K., Ksiazek, T. G., Rollin, P. E., Zaki, S. R., Shieh, W.-J., Goldsmith, C. S., Gubler, D. J., Roehrig, J. T., Eaton, B., Gould, A. R., Olson, J., Field, H., Daniels, P., Ling, A. E., Peters, C. J., Anderson, L. J., and Mahy, B. W. J. (2000) Nipah virus: a recently emergent deadly paramyxovirus, *Science*, **288**, 1432–1435.
3. Field, H., Young, P., Yob, J. M., Mills, J., Hall, L., and Mackenzie, J. (2001) The natural history of Hendra and Nipah viruses, *Microbes Infect.*, **3**, 307–314.
4. Young, P. L., Halpin, K., Selleck, P. W., Field, H., Gravel, J. L., Kelly, M. A., and Mackenzie, J. S. (1996) Serologic evidence for the presence on Pteropus bats of a paramyxovirus related to equine morbillivirus, *Emerg. Infect. Dis.*, **2**, 239–240.
5. Halpin, K., Young, P. L., Field, H. E., and Mackenzie, J. S. (2000) Isolation of Hendra virus from pteropid bats: a natural reservoir of Hendra virus, *J. Gen. Virol.*, **81**, 1927–1932.
6. Eaton, B. T., Broder, C. C., and Wang, L.-F. (2005) Hendra and Nipah viruses: pathogenesis and therapeutics, *Curr. Mol. Med.*, **5**, 805–816.
7. Wang, L.-F., Yo, M., Hansson, E., Pritchard, L. I., Shiell, B., Michalski, W. P., and Eaton, B. T. (2000) The exceptionally large genome of Hendra virus: support for creation of a new genus within the family *Paramyxoviridae*, *J. Virol.*, **74**(21), 9972–9979.
8. Pringle, C. R. (1991) The order *Mononegavirales*, *Arch. Virol.*, **117**, 137–140.
9. Pringle, C. R. and Easton, A. J. (1997) Monopartite negative strand RNA genomes, *Semin. Virol.*, **8**, 49–57.
10. Rima, B., Alexander, D. J., Billeter, M. A., Collins, P. L., Kingsburry, D. W., Lipkind, M. A., Nagai, Y., Orvell, C., Pringle, C. R., and ter Meulen, V. (1995) Family *Paramyxoviridae*. In: *Virus Taxonomy. Sixth Report of the International Committee on Taxonomy of Viruses* (Murphy, F. A., Fauquet, C. M., Bishop, D. H. L., Ghabrial, S. A., Jarvis, A. W., Martelli, G. P., Mayo, M. A., and Summers, M. D., eds.), Springer-Verlag, Vienna, Austria, pp. 268–274.
11. Mayo, M. A. and Pringle, C. R. (1998) Virus taxonomy – 1997, *J. Gen. Virol.*, **79**, 649–657.

12. Pringle, C. R. (1998) Virus taxonomy – San Diego 1998, *Arch. Virol.*, **143**, 1449–1459.

13. Fraser, G. C., Hooper, P. T., Lunt, R. A., Gould, A. R., Gleeson, L. J., Hyatt, A. D., Russell, G. M., and Kattenbelt, J. A. (1996) Encephalitis caused by a lyssavirus in fruit bats in Australia, *Emerg. Infect. Dis.*, **2**, 327–331.

14. Philbey, A. W., Kirkland, P. D., Ross, A. D., Davis, R., Gleeson, A. B., Love, R. J., Daniels, P. W., Gould, A. R., and Hyatt, A. D. (1998) An apparently new virus (family *Paramyxoviridae*) infectious to pigs, humans, and fruit bats, *Emerg. Infect. Dis.*, **4**, 269–271.

15. Allworth, A., Murray, K., and Morgan, J. (1996) A human case of encephalitis due to a lyssavirus recently identified in fruit bats, *Commun. Dis. Intellig.*, **20**, 504.

16. Chant, K., Chan, R., Smith, M., Dwyer, D. E., and Kirkland, P. (1998) Probable human infection with a newly described virus in the family *Paramyxoviridae*, *Emerg. Infect. Dis.*, **4**, 273–275.

17. Tidona, C. A., Kurz, H. W., Gelderblom, H. R., and Daral, G. (1999) Isolation and molecular characterization of a novel cytopathogenic paramyxovirus from tree shrews, *Virology*, **258**, 425–434.

18. Renshaw, R. W., Glaser, A. L., Van Campen, H., Weiland, F., and Dubovi, E. J. (2000) Identification and phylogenetic comparison of Salem virus, a novel paramyxovirus of horses, *Virology*, **270**, 417–249.

19. Halpine, K., Bankamp, B., Harcourt, B. H., Bellini, W. J., and Rota, P. A. (2004) Nipah virus conforms to the rule of six in a minigenome replication assay, *J. Gen. Virol.*, **85**, 701–707.

20. Eaton, B. T. and Broder, C. C. (2006) Hendra and Nipah viruses: different and dangerous, *Nat. Rev. Microbiol.*, **4**, 23–35.

21. Gould, A. R. (1996) Comparison of the deduced matrix and fusion protein sequences of equine morbillivirus with cognate genes of the *Paramyxoviridae*, *Virus Res.*, **43**, 17–31.

22. Wang, L. F., Michalski, W. P., Yu, M., Pritchard, L. I., Crameri, G., Shiell, B., and Eaton, B. T. (1998) A novel P/V/C gene in a new member of the *Paramyxoviridae* family, which causes lethal infection in humans, horses, and other animals, *J. Virol.*, **72**, 1482–1490.

23. Yu, M., Hansson, E., Langedijk, J. P., Eaton, B. T., and Wang, L. F. (1998) The attachment protein of Hendra virus has high structural similarity but limited primary sequence homology compared with viruses in the genus Paramyxovirus, *Virology*, **251**, 227–233.

24. Yu, M., Hansson, E., Shiell, B., Michalski, W., Eaton, B. T., and Wang, L. F. (1998) Sequence analysis of the Hendra virus nucleoprotein gene: comparison with other members of the subfamily *Paramyxovirinae*, *J. Gen. Virol.*, **79**, 1775–1780.

25. Harcourt, B. H., Tamin, A., Ksiazek, T. G., Rollin, P. E., Anderson, L. J., Bellini, W. J., and Rota, P. A. (2000) Molecular characterization of Nipah virus, a newly emergent paramyxovirus, *Virology*, **271**, 334–349.

26. Rodriguez, J. J. and Horvath, C. M. (2004) Host evasion by emerging paramyxoviruses: Hendra virus and Nipah virus V protein inhibit interferon signaling, *Viral Immun.*, **17**(2), 210–219.

27. Darnell, J. E., Jr. (1997) STATs and gene regulation, *Science*, **277**, 1630–1635.

28. Horvath, C. M. (2000) STAT proteins and transcriptional responses to extracellular signals, *Trends Biochem. Sci.*, **25**, 496–502.

29. Fu, X. Y., Kessler, D. S., Veals, S. A., et al. (1990) ISGF3, the transcriptional activator induced by interferon alpha, consists of multiple interacting polypeptide cells, *Proc. Natl. Acad. Sci. U.S.A.*, **87**, 8555–8559.

30. Levy, D. E. and Darnell, J. E. (2002) STATS: transcriptional control and biological impact, *Nat. Rev. Mol. Cell. Biol.*, **3**, 651–662.

31. Decker, T., Mirkovitch, J., and Darnell, J. E., Jr. (1991) Cytoplasmic activation of GAF, an IFN-gamma-regulated DNA-binding factor, *EMBO J.*, **10**, 927–932.

32. Rodriguez, J. J., Parisien, J. P., and Horvath, C. M. (2002) Nipah virus V protein evades alpha and gamma interferons by preventing STAT1 and STAT2 activation and nuclear accumulation, *J. Virol.*, **76**, 11476–11483.

33. Rodriguez, J. J., Wang, L. F., and Horvath, C. M. (2003) Hendra virus V protein inhibits interferon signaling by preventing STAT1 and STAT2 nuclear accumulation, *J. Virol.*, **77**, 11842–11845.

34. Begitt, A., Meyer, T., van Rossum, M., et al. (2000) Nucleocytoplasmic translocation of Stat1 is regulated by a leucine-rich export signal in the coiled–coil domain, *Proc. Natl. Acad. Sci. U.S.A.*, **97**, 10418–10423.

35. Negrete, O. A., Levroney, E. L., Aguilar, H. C., Bertolotti-Ciarlet, A., Nazarian, R., Tajyar, S., and Lee, B. (2005) EphrinB2 is the entry receptor for Nipah virus, and emergent deadly paramyxovirus, *Nature*, **436**, 401–405.

36. Bonaparte, M. I., Dimitrov, A. S., Bossart, K. N., Cramer, G., Mungall, B. A., Bishop, K. A., Choudhry, V., Dimitrov, D. S., Wang, L.-F., Eaton, B. T., and Broder, C. C. (2005) Ephrin-B2 ligand is a functional receptor for Hendra virus and Nipah virus, *Proc. Natl. Acad. Sci. U.S.A.*, **102**(30), 10652–10657.

37. Negrete, O. A., Wolf, M. C., Aguilar, H. C., Enterlein, S., Wang, W., Muhlberger, E., Su, S. V., Bertolotti-Ciarlet, A., Flick, R., and Lee, B. (2006) Two key residues in Ephrin B3 are critical for its use as an alternative receptor for Nipah virus, *PLoS Pathog.*, **2**, e7.

38. Porotto, M., Doctor, L., Carta, P., Fornabaio, M., Greengard, O., Kellogg, G. E., and Moscona, A. (2006) Inhibition of hendra virus fusion, *J. Virol.*, **80**(19), 9837–9849.

39. Poliakov, A., Cotrina, M., and Wilkinson, D. G. (2004) Diversed roles of eph receptors and ephrins in the regulation of cell migration and tissue assembly, *Dev. Cell*, **7**, 465–480.

40. Drescher, U. (2002) Eph family functions from an evolutionary perspective, *Curr. Opin. Genet. Dev.*, **12**, 397–402.

41. Himanen, J., Rajashankar, K. R., Lackmann, M., Cowan, C. A., Henkemeyer, M., and Nikolov, D. B. (2001) Crystal structure of an Eph receptor-ephrin complex, *Nature*, **414**, 933–938.

42. Eaton, B. T., Wright, P. J., Wang, L. F., Sergeyev, O., Michalski, W. P., Bossart, K. N., and Broder, C. C. (2004) Henipaviruses: recent observations on regulation of transcription and the nature of the cell receptor, *Arch. Virol. Suppl.*, (18), 122–131.

43. Lou, Z., Xu, Y., Xiang, K., Su, N., Qin, L., Li, X., Gao, G. F., Bartlam, M., and Rao, Z. (2006) Crystal structure of Nipah and hendra virus fusion core proteins, *FEBS J.*, **273**, 4538–4547.

44. Baker, K. A., Dutch, R. E., Lamb, R. A., and Jardetzky, T. S. (1999) Structural basis for paramyxovirus-mediated membrane fusion, *Mol. Cell*, **3**, 309–319.

45. Meulendyke, K. A., Wurth, M. A., McCane, R. O., and Dutch, R. E. (2005) Endocytosis plays a critical role in proteolytic processing of the Hendra virus fusion protein, *J. Virol.*, **79**, 12643–12649.

46. Pager, C. T. and Dutch, R. E. (2005) Cathepsin L is involved in proteolytic processing of the hendra virus fusion protein, *J. Virol.*, **79**, 12714–12720.

47. Lambert, D. M., Barney, S., Lambert, A. L., Guthrie, K., Medinas, R., Davis, D. E., Bucy, T., Erickson, J., Merutka, G., and Pettway, S. R. (1996) Peptides from conserved regions of paramyxovirus fusion (F) proteins are potent inhibitors of viral fusion, *Proc. Natl. Acad. Sci. U.S.A.*, **93**, 2186–2191.

48. Centers for Disease Control (1999) Outbreak of Hendra virus – Malaysia and Singapore 1998–1999, *Morb. Mortal. Wkly Rep.*, **48**(3), 265–269.

49. Selvey, L. A., Wells, R. M., McCormack, J. G., Ansford, A. J., Murray, K., Rogers, R. J., Lavercombe, P. S., Selleck, P., and Sheridan, J. W. (1995) Infections of humans and horses by a newly described morbillivirus, *Med. J. Aust.*, **162**, 642–645.

50. Parashar, U. D., Sunn, L. M., Ong, F., Mounts, A. W., Arif, M. T., Ksiazek, T. G., Kamalludin, M. A., Mustafa, A. N., Kaur, H.,

Ding, L. M., Othman, G., Radzi, H. M., Kitsutani, P. T., Stockton, P. C., Arokiasamy, J., Gary, H. E., Jr., and Anderson, L. J. (2000) Case-control study of risk factors for human infection with a new zoonotic paramyxovirus, Nipah virus, during 1998–1999 outbreak of severe encephalitis in Malaysia, *J. Infect. Dis.*, **181**, 1755–1759.

51. Wong, K. T., Shieh, W.-J., Kumar, S., Norain, K., Abdullah, W., Guarner, J., Goldsmith, C. S., Chua, K. B., Lam, S. K., Tan, C. T., Goh, K. J., Chong, H. T., Jusoh, R., Rollin, P. E., Ksiazek, T. G., Zaki, S. R., and the Nipah Virus Pathology Working Group (2002) Nipah virus infection: pathology and pathogenesis of an emerging paramyxoviral zoonosis, *Am. J. Pathol.*, **161**, 2153–2167.

52. Yu, F., Khairullah, S., Inoue, S., Balasubramaniam, V., Berendam, S. J., The, L. K., Ibrahim, N. S. W., Rahman, S. A., Hassan, S. S., Hasabe, F., Sinniah, M., and Morita, K. (2006) Serodiagnosis using recombinant Nipah virus nucleocapsid protein expressed in *Escherichia coli*, *J. Clin. Microbiol.*, **44**(9), 3134–3138.

53. Chang, L.-Y., Ali, A. R. M., Hassan, S. S., and AbuBakar, S. (2007) Human neuronal cell protein responses to Nipah virus infection, *Virol. J.*, **4**, 54.

54. Goh, K. J., Tan, C. T., Chew, N. K., Tan, P. S. K., Kamarulzaman, A., Sarji, S. A., Wong, K. T., Abdullah, B. J. J., Chua, K. B., and Lam, S.-K. (2000) Clinical features of Nipah virus encephalitis among pig farmers in Malaysia, *N. Engl. J. Med.*, **342**(17), 1229–1235.

55. Lam, S.-K. (2003) Nipah virus – a potential agent of bioterrorism? *Antiviral Res.*, **57**, 113–119.

56. Chong, H. T., Kamarulzaman, A., Tan, C. T., Goh, K. J., Thayaparan, T., Kunijapan, S. R., Chew, N. K., Chua, K. B., and Lam, S.-K. (2001) Treatment of acute Nipah encephalitis with ribavirin, *Ann. Neurol.*, **49**, 810–813.

Chapter 19

Arthropod-Borne Viral Encephalitis

Arthropod-borne viruses can be a common cause of sporadic and epidemic encephalitis. These viruses replicate both in vertebrate and nonvertebrate species and include members of many different families, such as Flaviviridae, Bunyaviridae, etc. *(1)*. Typically, these pathogens are transmitted by mosquitoes and ticks; however, there are exceptions like the non-arthropod-borne Arenaviridae, even including—based on morphology—plant viruses [genus Tospovirus in Bunyaviridae (http://edis.ifas.ufl.edu/PP134)].

Among the alphaviruses, major pathogens include the etiologic agents of the eastern, western, and Venezuelan equine encephalitis, as well as the chikungunya virus—a source of human epidemics in Africa and Asia and, recently, in Europe.

The flaviviruses can also cause either mosquito- or tick-borne encephalitis. Examples of the former include Japanese encephalitis, St. Louis encephalitis, Rocio, Murray Valley, and West Nile viruses. Examples of the tick-borne diseases are the Kyasuma Forest and Powassan viruses.

The bunyavirus family includes viruses that are the most common cause of arboviral encephalitic disease in the United States: the La Crosse virus, as well as the Jamestown Canyon and California encephalitis viruses.

"Arboviruses" Classification. The so-called "arboviruses" arthropod-borne viruses) were meant to represent a large (>400) group of enveloped RNA viruses that are transmitted primarily (but not exclusively) by arthropod vectors, such as mosquitoes, sand-flies, fleas, ticks, lice, and so forth. These vector-borne viruses in the past were grouped together under the name *arboviruses*, a term that describes their requirement for a blood-sucking arthropod to complete their life cycle *(2)*. However, more recently, this disordered assemblage has been split into four *bona fide* virus families (Table 19.1).

Since most of the arboviruses are relatively fragile (e.g., not resistant to dessication), they rely on a vector for transmission. With some exceptions (rubella virus, HCV), this dependency tends to limit them to tropical or subtropical regions. Moreover, the rubella virus is also a species that is quite distinct from the other alphaviruses—it is highly contagious but with a limited host range (human mammalian cells only; unknown invertebrate host, if any).

The arboviruses have complex life cycles and replicate in both primary hosts, secondary hosts (which may often be dead-ends), and the arthropod vectors. Therefore, there may be several animal reservoirs for each virus, which would make their eradication practically impossible, unless by blocking transmission through human vaccination and/or eradication of the vector (e.g., mosquitoes).

Arthropod-Borne Viral Encephalitis in the United States. Most of the viruses are transmitted by mosquitoes from a host, such as wild birds, to horses or humans in which clinical symptoms will develop *(1)*. Viral encephalitis outbreaks in the United States have appeared periodically, as with the St. Louis encephalitis in the Ohio and Mississippi River basins in the early 1980s. The St. Louis encephalitis is the second most common arthropod-borne encephalitis in this country. As with other infections of the brain, the ratio of apparent infections is high, varying from 1 in 1,000 to 1 in 100. The mortality rate due to St. Louis encephalitis virus is 10% to 20%, with most deaths occurring in young children and the elderly *(1)*. Other arthropod-transmitted encephalitis infections have either similar mortality rates, such as the Venezuelan equine encephalitis found in the southern United States, or higher mortality rates, such as the eastern equine encephalitis affecting the Gulf and Atlantic coast regions. Western equine encephalitis is associated with a high overall rate of infection but a low incidence of both overt disease and mortality (3% to 7%). The California group of viruses, including the La Crosse virus, are the most significant cause of brain infection in the upper Midwestern United States *(1)*.

19.1 Flaviviruses

The Flavivirus genus contains more than 70 viruses, of which approximately 40 are mosquito-borne, 16 are tick-borne, and 18 have no known vector *(3)*. The type species of the genus is the yellow fever virus, through which the genus and family derive their name. Although all flaviviruses are serologically related, they have been further classified into distinct

V. St. Georgiev, *National Institute of Allergy and Infectious Diseases, NIH: Impact on Global Health*, vol. 2, DOI 10.1007/978-1-60327-297-1_19, © Humana Press, a part of Springer Science+Business Media, LLC 2009

Table 19.1

Family	Genus	Type species	Number of serovars
Togaviridae	Alphaviruses	Sindbis	27
	Rubivirus	Rubella	1
Flaviviridae	Flavivirus	Yellow fever	>70
	Pestivirus	Bovine viral diarrhea	3
	Hepatitis C virus	HCV	1 (variable)
Bunyaviridae	Bunyavirus	Bunyaamwera	168
	Hantavirus	Hantaan	32
	Phlebovirus	Sandfly fever	51
	Nairovirus	Crimean-Congo hemorrhagic fever	35
	Tospovirus	Tomato spotted wilt	2
	Unassigned		42
Arenaviridae	Arenavirus	Lymphocytic choriomeningitis	17

groups *(4, 5)*, the most important of which are the dengue serologic group, the Japanese encephalitis serologic group, and the less serologically cohesive yellow fever virus group (see also Chapter 23).

The flaviviruses are positive-strand RNA viruses with a genome of about 11 kb. The genome's RNA represents the only messenger RNA in infected cells and encodes three structural proteins (C, capsid protein); prM, the membrane precursor protein that is proteolytically cleaved by a cellular protease to form the M protein in mature virions; and E, envelope protein), and seven nonstructural (NS) proteins (NS1, NS2a, NS2b; NS3, NS4a, NS4b, and NS5) *(6, 7)*. The E glycoprotein is the most immunologically important protein.

Phylogeny. The origin, evolution, and spread of the flaviviruses have been studied by extensive analyses of genomic sequence and calculating base substitution rates using sequences from the NS5, NS3, or E genes, or from complete genomic sequences *(8–14)* The obtained data has unambiguously proved that (i) the tick-borne and mosquito-borne viruses represented two distinct and separate evolutionary lineages *(8, 9)*; (ii) most of the viruses with no known vector were also in a distinct lineage; and (iii) the three lineages had diverged early in the evolution of the Flavivirus genus *(13)*. Taking all of the phylogenetic data, together with the biological characteristics of the different flaviviruses, it has been hypothesized that the Flavivirus genus evolved from an ancestral virus in Africa within the past 10,000 years *(9, 12, 14)*. The tick-borne lineage is believed to have diverged approximately 3,000 years ago, followed by the mosquito-borne viruses *(8–13)*.

The most divergent of the mosquito-borne viruses form a clade typified by the yellow fever virus. These viruses are all found in the Old World and are largely associated with *Aedes* mosquitoes, with some of them also being associated with hemorrhagic fever disease in primates and humans (see Chapter 23). A subsequent divergence led to the emergence of new clades containing viruses associated with *Aedes* mosquitoes, including some causing hemorrhagic disease (e.g., members of the dengue virus serologic group); and

clades associated primarily with *Culex* mosquitoes and causing encephalitis, as typified by the Japanese encephalitis virus serologic group *(2, 3, 14)*.

Epidemiology. The flaviviruses are zoonoses that depend on animal species other than humans for their maintenance in nature, with the notable exception of the dengue viruses *(3)*. Humans are usually the incidental and dead-end hosts that do not contribute to the natural transmission cycle. The dengue viruses, however, have adapted completely to humans and are maintained in large urban areas in the tropics in human-mosquito-human transmission cycles that no longer depend on animal reservoirs, although such reservoirs are still maintained in the jungles of Africa and Southeast Asia in mosquito-monkey-mosquito transmission cycles *(3, 15, 16)*.

The changing epidemiology of the flaviviruses is complex and unique to each virus *(16)*, and many factors and properties affect their potential to spread and colonize new areas and to cause an increased incidence of infection *(3)*. Even though complex, these factors are closely associated with certain demographic and societal changes arising from increased and changing human activities, such as urbanization, transportation, and changes in land use. Genetic changes in the virus, host-vector relationships, bird migration and movement, climate, and wind patterns have also contributed to the changing epidemiology of the flaviviruses *(3)*.

19.1.1 Japanese Encephalitis Serologic Group

The Japanese encephalitis serologic group comprises eight species and two subtype viruses with a geographic range encompassing all continents except Antarctica *(3, 17)*.

The major virus species and their geographic range are as follows:

(i) *Japanese encephalitis virus (JEV)* in eastern, southern, and southeastern Asia, Papua New Guinea, and the Torres Strait of Northern Australia. Wind-blown mosquitoes are believed to have been important in the virus's spread in the mid-1990s from Papua New Guinea to the Torres Strait islands and the Australian mainland.

(ii) *West Nile virus (WNV)* in Africa, southern and central Europe, India, the Middle East, and North America, and as the Kunjin virus (a subtype of WNV) in Australia and Papua New Guinea.

(iii) *Murray Valley encephalitis virus (MVEV)* in Australia, Papua New Guinea, and the western Indonesian archipelago.

(iv) *St. Louis encephalitis virus (SLEV)* in North and South America.

Other minor members of the group include the *Usuto (USUV)*, *Koutango,* and *Yaounde* viruses in Africa; *Cacipacore virus* in South America; and the *Alfuy virus,* a subtype of MVEV, in Australia *(3).*

Most members have avian hosts and are vectored primarily by *Culex* spp. mosquitoes.

There are at least four genotypes of JEV distinguished by approximately 10% divergence at the nucleotide level *(18).* For unknown reasons, genotype III has spread most widely.

19.1.1.1 Japanese Encephalitis

The major vector for the Japanese encephalitis virus in humans appears to be the *Culex* mosquito species (*C. tritaeniorhynchus* and *C. vishnui*), which breed in large numbers in rice fields and pig-farming regions. Incubation in the mosquito, known as the gestational incubation period or the interval between ingestion of infected blood and spread from the midgut to the salivary glands, is inoculum and temperature dependent. Once the human is infected, the resultant pathology is similar for mice and humans, with hematogenous spread to the brain that frequently involves the basal ganglia. A predictive factor for the disease outcome is the rapid appearance of antibodies directed against JEV in the cerebrospinal fluid (CSF), which will ameliorate the severity of the disease *(1).*

JEV is transmitted in an enzootic cycle involving birds, particularly wading ardeids, such as herons and egrets. Pigs can become infected and act as amplifying hosts, bringing the virus closer to human habitats, especially when pigs are kept near homes *(18).*

Epidemiology. JEV is the most important cause of viral encephalitis in eastern (China, Japan, Korea) and southern Asia (Thailand, Vietnam, Malaysia, Cambodia) and in India and Pakistan, with 30,000 to 50,000 cases reported annually *(19).* During the second half of 2005, one of the largest outbreaks of JEV in recent years

occurred in northern India, with nearly 5,000 cases and 1,300 deaths *(18).* There have also been rare outbreaks of JEV in U.S. territories in the Western Pacific region (http://cdc/gov/ncidod/dvbid/jencephalitis/facts.htm).

Historically, epidemics of JEV have been recognized in Japan since the 1870s. The virus was first isolated from the brain of a fatal human case in 1935 and was subsequently found throughout most of eastern and southern Asia *(3).*

Most JEV infections are asymptomatic, with estimates *(20)* of the ratio of symptomatic to asymptomatic infections ranging from 1 in 25 to 1 in 1,000. This variation depends on many factors *(19),* including endemicity, exposure to mosquitoes, preexisting antibodies to flaviviruses, and differences among virus strains *(3).*

Pathogenicity and Clinical Manifestations. The incubation period for JEV is 5 to 15 days. Most clinical cases occur in infants and children, although in areas where JEV occurs for the first time or only at rare intervals, clinical disease may affect all age groups *(3).* The clinical disease varies from a nonspecific febrile illness to a severe disease in which patients present with meningoencephalitis, aseptic meningitis, or a polio-like acute flaccid paralysis *(19, 21).*

At the onset of disease, patients typically will present with a nonspecific febrile illness with cough, nausea, vomiting, diarrhea, and photophobia, followed by a reduced level of consciousness. Convulsions occur frequently in children and less commonly in adults. A number of patients will make a rapid, spontaneous recovery *(3).*

The classic description of Japanese encephalitis includes a Parkinsonian syndrome of dull, flat, mask-like facies with wide, unblinking eyes, tremor, generalized hypertonia, cogwheel rigidity, and other abnormalities of movement *(19).*

There may also be upper motor neuron signs, cerebellar signs, and cranial nerve palsies. Paralysis of the upper extremities is more common than that of the legs. About 30% of the survivors will display frank persistent motor deficits and about 20% will have severe cognitive and language impairment *(3).*

Treatment. There is no established treatment for the disease. Typically, 20% to 30% of patients with JEV will die, and approximately 50% of survivors will develop severe neuropsychiatric sequelae *(18, 22).* Treatment efforts are directed at controlling both the immediate complications of infection, including seizures and increased intracranial pressure, and the long-term consequences of neurologic impairment, such as limb contractures and bed sores *(18).*

Japanese Encephalitis Vaccines

Soon after JEV was discovered, crude vaccines were produced, primarily in Japan but in other countries as well, by growing the virus in a mouse brain and inactivating it in formalin. Production was refined, and the vaccine's efficacy was demonstrated in large, placebo-controlled trials in Taiwan in the 1960s and Thailand in the 1980s (18).

A summary Japanese encephalitis vaccine became available in the United States in the 1980s (1983–1987) (http://www.cdc.gov/mmwr/preview/mmwrhtml/00020599.htm). In 1992, an inactivated monovalent Japanese encephalitis (JE) vaccine (JE-VAX; the Biken vaccine) was licensed in the United States. It is prepared with the Nakayama-NIH strain of JEV, originally isolated in 1935 from an infected human. The overall efficacy of the Biken vaccine as determined in clinical trials was 91%. A second, bivalent JE vaccine, prepared from the Beijing strain, was found to be equally effective to JE-VAX. The dosage regimen shown to be effective for primary vaccination in many areas of Asia consists of two doses administered 1 to 4 weeks apart. However, immunogenicity studies conducted in the United States and Britain have indicated that three doses (administered during a 30-day period on days 0, 7, and 30) are needed to provide protective levels of neutralizing antibody in the majority of vaccinees.

Adverse Reactions. JE vaccination is associated with a moderate frequency of local and mild systemic side effects. Local effects include tenderness, redness, and swelling, among others, in approximately 20% of vaccinees. Systemic side effects, including fever, headache, malaise, rash, chills, dizziness, myalgia, nausea, vomiting, and abdominal pain, have been reported in about 10% of vaccinees. Since 1989, an apparently new pattern of adverse reactions has been observed—primarily among travelers vaccinated in Australia, Europe, and North America—characterized by urticaria often in a generalized distribution, and/or angioedema of the extremities, oropharynx and face, especially the lips. Less frequently, respiratory disease and distress or collapse due to hypotension have occurred (http://www.cdc.gov/mmwr/preview/mmwrhtml/00020599.htm). The vaccine constituent or constituents responsible for these adverse events have not been identified.

- *Contraindications.* Individuals with a history of allergic disorders (allergic rash or hives, or wheezing after a wasp sting or taking medications) appear to be at greater risk for developing an adverse reaction to JE vaccine. There are no data supporting the efficacy of prophylactically administered antihistamines or steroids in preventing JE vaccine–related allergic reactions. Furthermore, the vaccine should not be given to a person who has ever had a life-threatening reaction to mouse protein, thimerosal, or a previous dose of JE vaccine.

The vaccine is contraindicated for pregnant or nursing women, as well as for people who will be traveling for fewer than 30 days, especially in major urban areas (http://www.cdc.gov/mmwr/preview/mmwrhtml/00020599.htm).

19.1.1.2 Murray Valley Encephalitis (Australian Encephalitis)

The Murray Valley encephalitis virus (MVEV) is the etiologic agent of the Murray Valley encephalitis, also known as Australian encephalitis (23). It is endemic to the tropical regions of North Australia, particularly Western Australia and the Northern Territory, but can occur in other parts of Australia. Australian encephalitis is the second most serious acute viral encephalitis to be encountered in Australia.

Australian encephalitis is a mosquito-borne infection caused by the MVE virus and, occasionally, by the closely related Kunjin virus (24). These viruses are related antigenically and genomically to the St. Louis encephalitis and West Nile viruses, and together with JEV form the JEV serologic group of the flaviviruses (25, 26). The MVEV is most closely related to the Japanese encephalitis virus. The last epidemic of Murray Valley encephalitis virus occurred in the Murray Valley region of southeastern Australia in 1974 (27). Since then, it has occurred sporadically throughout the tropical north, mostly in the Northern Territory and Western Australia (24, 27). The wading birds act as a natural reservoir (25) and the outbreaks were mostly seasonal, during the monsoon rains (24).

Clinical Manifestations. The onset of clinical disease begins with a prodromal stage characterized by fever, headache, nausea, vomiting, and dizziness (24, 25, 27). This might progress, usually within 5 days, to symptoms such as dysphasia, memory impairment, confusion, tremor, and, in severe cases, to coma, paralysis, respiratory failure, and death (23, 27, 28).

The mortality rate of Australian encephalitis is approximately 20% and a significant residual neurologic deficit of approximately 50% (23, 24, 27, 28).

Computed tomography (CT) seems to be nonspecific in showing neurologic changes for Murray Valley encephalitis (23).CT findings have shown abnormalities in about 34% of patients, including the presence of mild hydrocephalus, flattening of the lateral walls of the right ventricle, cerebral edema, cerebral and cerebellar atrophy, diffuse reduced attenuation extending from the thalami to the brain stem, and a left cerebral infarct (23, 24, 27).

There is no available vaccine against Australian encephalitis (25).

19.1.1.3 St. Louis Encephalitis

The St. Louis encephalitis virus (SLEV) is the etiologic agent of St. Louis encephalitis (SLE), a mosquito-transmitted disease of major medical importance in North America (http://www.cdc/ncidod/dvbid/arbor/sle_qa.htm). First recognized in 1932 in the town of Paris, Illinois, and the following year in St. Louis and Kansas City, Missouri, SLE has been the cause of sporadic and unpredictable epidemics, affecting large numbers of people with serious illness and sometimes even death *(29,30)*. Although rarely, in addition to North America, SLEV has caused human disease in Central and South America and the Caribbean *(31)*.

Mosquitoes become infected with SLEV by feeding on infected birds and then transmit the virus to humans and animals during the feeding process. After inoculation of the virus into the human host via mosquito saliva, replication is initiated in local tissues and regional lymph nodes. Subsequent spread occurs in extraneural tissues through the lymphatics and blood.

Culex pipiens is the mosquito species transmitting SLEV in the Eastern and Central United States. During the 1940s, the disease was recognized in the Pacific Coast states, where the virus was isolated from *C. tarsalis*. In Florida, *Culex nigripalpus* has been linked to recent SLE epidemics *(29)*. The last major SLE epidemic in the United States occurred in the Midwest from 1974 to 1977. During that outbreak, more than 2,500 cases in 35 states were reported to the CDC.

St. Louis encephalitis is not transmitted from person-to-person.

The SLEV has a genome organization similar to all other flaviviruses. Its antigenic and structural properties have been described *(30)*, and its nucleotide sequence was elucidated *(31)*.

Clinical Manifestations. St. Louis encephalitis is an acute viral disease causing meningeal and brain parenchymal inflammation and injury. The incubation period is usually 5 to 15 days.

Mild infections occur without apparent symptoms other than a fever with headache. More severe infections are characterized by generalized malaise marked by headache, high fever, neck stiffness, stupor, and disorientation. In severe cases, the disease is marked by a rapid onset and could further progress to coma, tremors, convulsions (especially in infants), spastic (but rarely flaccid) paralysis, and death *(30)*. The case mortality rates range from 3% to 30% (especially in the elderly) (http://www.cdc/ncidod/dvbid/arbor/sle_qa.htm).

There is no specific treatment or vaccine for St. Louis encephalitis. The care of sick patients is focused on treatment of symptoms and complications. A period of prolonged convalescence occurs in 30% to 50% of cases, characterized by asthenia, irritability, tremulousness, sleeplessness, depression, memory loss, and headaches, lasting up to 3 years. Approximately 20% of these patients have symptoms persisting for longer periods, including gait and speech disturbances, sensorimotor impairment, psychoneurotic complaints, and tremors. Old age and severity of acute illness appear to predispose to these sequelae.

19.2 Alphaviruses

Three Alphavirus species are known as the etiologic agents of equine encephalitis: eastern equine encephalitis (EEE), western equine encephalitis (WEE), and Venezuelan equine encephalitis (VEE). However, they have also shown sufficient potential to invade the central nervous system in humans and to be recognized as causes of encephalitis *(32)*. Of the three infections, the disease pattern of EEE is most dangerous to humans, whereas human infections with WEE and VEE are much less likely to seriously damage the central nervous system unless the host is under 1 year of age.

19.2.1 Eastern Equine Encephalitis Virus

The eastern equine encephalitis virus (EEEV) was known as the cause of epizootics of eastern equine encephalitis in North American horses as far back as 1831 *(33, 34)*. It was during the 1935 outbreak that birds were considered to be a possible reservoir host, but it was not until 1950 that the virus was isolated from a wild bird *(35)*. Subsequent studies have shown that many birds, including virtually all passerine species, are susceptible to EEEV infection *(36, 37)*.

Alphavirus Transmission. Mosquitoes were first implicated as potential vectors of EEEV in 1934. In North America, the predominant vector of EEEV is female *Culiseta melanura*, which feed almost exclusively on passerine birds. The latter serve as the amplifying host for this virus in endemic areas. However, a number of studies have demonstrated that numerous other mosquito species could become infected and then transmit EEEV from one vertebrate to another *(33)*, including different genera: *Aedes* (*A. sollicitans*, *A. canadensis*, *A. atlanticus-tormentor*, *A. cantator*, *A. infirmatus*, *A. vexans*, *A. triseriatus*, *A. mitchellae*), *Culex* (*C. tarsalis*, *C. nigripalpus*, *C. salinarius*, *C. restians*, *C. specias*, *C. territans*, *C. quinquefasciatus*), *Anopheles* (*A. quadrimaculatus*, *A. crucians*, *A. punctipennis*), *Culiseta* (*Cs. morsitans*, *Cs. minnesotae*), *Uranotaenia sapphirrina*, and *Coquillettidia perturbans*.

Mosquitoes carry the virus from their wild bird reservoir to the dead-end hosts, horses and humans. Female mosquitoes acquire the virus by taking a blood meal from an infected host. The virus infects the epithelial cells of the midgut of the mosquito and spreads through the circulation to the salivary glands where it sets up a *persistent* infection. The alphavirus enters a new host when the mosquito regurgitates virus-containing saliva into the victim's bloodstream. Inside the host, the alphaviruses replicate in the capillary endothelial cells, macrophages, monocytes, liver, spleen, or lymphatic tissue.

Epidemiology. The first human cases of eastern equine encephalitis (EEE) were confirmed in 1938 by virus isolation from brain tissue *(38, 39)*. Other vertebrates besides humans that could be infected with EEEV include, in addition to horses and birds, turtles, snakes, swine, bovines, hamsters, and fish. However, none of these are considered to play any role in the epidemiology of the virus.

Outbreaks of EEE are infrequent, and, perhaps because of the lack of sufficient knowledge of how to manage an outbreak when it occurs, the disease might have a significant health, economic, and social impact once an endemic focus has been identified. Hence, the mosquito control for EEE prevention is critical when the potential of the disease is recognized in an area *(33)*.

EEEV is endemic in focal habitats along the East Coast of the United States encompassing a range from southern Canada (Quebec) to the northern areas of South America, including the Caribbean *(40)*.

The strict ornithophilic behavior of *Cs. melanura* restricts the likelihood of this mosquito species playing a major vector role for both equines and humans. The *Culex* mosquito species have been implicated as the enzootic vectors for South American strains of EEEV *(41)*. *Coquillettidia perturbans* is an opportunistic feeder and feeds equally on birds and mammals, especially humans and equines, thus making it an ideal potential vector.

Pathogenesis and Clinical Manifestations. Viremia follows soon after infection with EEEV and may be accompanied by a febrile prodrome.

There are two types of EEE illness: systemic and encephalitic. A systemic infection is abrupt and is characterized by malaise, arthralgia, and myalgia. In a few hours, the patient is chilly and experiences severe muscular shaking, which last for a few days. The temperature reaches 100°F to 104°F. The illness, which lasts for 1 to 2 weeks and without central nervous system (CNS) involvement, usually results in complete recovery *(33, 42)*.

The encephalitic form of EEE is by far the most severe of all arboviral encephalitis, with a mortality between 50% and 75%, and commonly resulting in crippling sequelae *(32, 33, 43)*. Nearly all patients who recover have disabling mental and physical residua, which are progressive *(44)*.

The primary pathologic features of the encephalitic form of EEE are confined to the central nervous system and best visualized by magnetic resonance imaging (MRI) *(43)*. Lesions are scattered throughout the cortex and are particularly severe in the basal ganglia, thalami, and the brain stem; the cerebellum and spinal cord are minimally involved; cortical lesions, meningeal enhancement, and periventricular white-matter changes are less common. Other pathologic features include extensive neuronal necrosis and thrombosis of the arterioles and venules *(32)*. The characteristic early involvement of the basal ganglia and thalami as identified by MRI distinguishes EEE from herpes simplex encephalitis *(43)*.

The encephalitic form of the disease in infants is characterized by an abrupt onset, whereas in older children and adults the onset of active encephalitis typically will occur after a few days of indisposition *(44)*. Clinical manifestations in adults may begin with a febrile prodrome up to 11 days before the onset of disease *(32)*. Regardless of the presence or absence of prodrome, encephalitis begins abruptly with fever, dizziness, decreasing level of consciousness, and nuchal rigidity. Patients become comatose and exhibit tremors, muscular twitching, seizures, loss of abdominal reflexes, and focal signs. The majority of patients will continue with relentless febrile deterioration and die within the first few days of hospitalization. Pediatric patients usually have a more abrupt onset and more serious residual effects, with motor deficiency and serious intellectual and emotional damage in most *(45)*.

Treatment of EEE. Currently, there are no drug options to treat EEE. Medical treatment is symptomatic and may include pain relievers, corticosteroids to reduce brain swelling, antibiotics (for secondary infections), anticonvulsants to treat seizures, and the use of respirator to help with breathing *(32)*.

19.2.2 Western Equine Encephalitis Virus

The western equine encephalitis virus (WEEV) is the arthropod-borne etiologic agent of western equine encephalitis (WEE) spread to horses and humans by infected mosquitoes. Compared with EEEV, WEEV is not as neuroinvasive, and although their transmission and pathogenesis are similar, the encephalitis it causes is not as severe as the diseases inflicted by EEEV *(32)*.

WEE virus, as described in some earlier literature reports, is in fact a WEE complex of serologically related viruses: WEE, Sindbis (SIN), Whataroa, Aura, Highlands (HJ), and Y62-33 *(46, 47)*. Moreover, some of the earlier references to WEEV may be confused with what is now known as the HJ virus. The latter is commonly isolated from the eastern United States and differs from western United States isolations of WEE virus in serology, epidemiology, and presumably virulence *(32)*. WEE and HJ viruses have been molecularly analyzed and demonstrated to be markedly different by oligonucleotide mapping *(48)*.

Culex tarsalis is the most important mosquito vector of WEEV in North America. In addition, this mosquito species is also a vector of Llano Seco, Turlock, Gay Lodge, and Hart Park viruses, and several species of avian malaria *(49)*.

Epidemiology. Western equine encephalitis is found in North, Central, and South America, but most cases have been reported from the plains regions of the western and central United States. Disease range extends from northern Mexico and Baja California north to southern Canada, and from the Pacific east to the southern Atlantic coast.

WEE is a relatively rare disease in humans and can occur in isolated areas or in epidemics.

However, the risk of exposure to WEEV has been increasing in recent years as people move into previously undeveloped areas where the virus lives. Expansion of irrigated agriculture in the North Platte River Valley during the past several decades has created habitats and conditions that favor increases in the number of grain-eating birds and the mosquitoes that feed on them and spread WEEV.

Pathogenesis and Clinical Manifestations. The pathogenesis of WEEV-induced disease in humans, although similar to that of EEE, is clearly less neuroinvasive and neurovirulent *(32)*.

As with EEE, the significant primary findings are in the central nervous system, as presented by multiple foci of necrosis (often without cellular infiltrate) found in the striatum, globus pallidus, cerebral cortex, thalamus, and the pons. There is widespread perivascular cuffing and meningeal reaction.

Symptoms usually appear in 5 to 10 days after the bite from an infected mosquito. Diagnosis is based on tests of blood or spinal fluid. WEE typically will begin suddenly with malaise, fever, and headache, often accompanied by nausea and vomiting *(50)*. Other common symptoms include vertigo, photophobia, sore throat, respiratory abnormalities, abdominal pain, and myalgia. Over a few days, the headache will intensify, and in severe cases, drowsiness and restlessness may merge into stupor or coma *(32)*.

In infants and children, the onset of disease may be more abrupt and is often associated with seizures. Focal or generalized convulsions would occur in nearly all patients under 2 months of age, in 90% of those under 1 year, and with decreasing frequency until they are seen only occasionally in adult patients *(51)*. After about 10 days, patients usually begin a gradual convalescence. Fatal cases (about 3% in patients who develop severe symptoms) generally succumb during the first week. However, many cases of WEE are mild and may present only as aseptic meningitis or an undifferentiated febrile syndrome *(32)*.

There is no specific treatment effective against WEE, and patients' care is mainly supportive, focused on symptoms and complications.

19.2.3 Venezuelan Equine Encephalitis Virus

Venezuelan equine encephalitis (VEE) remains a naturally emerging disease threat as well as a potential biological weapon *(52)*. The Venezuelan equine encephalitis virus (VEEV), like its western (WEEV) and eastern (EEEV) counterparts, is a member of the genus Alphavirus in the family Togaviridae. Similarly, all three viruses contain a single-stranded, message-sense RNA genome of approximately 11,500 kb *(52, 53)*.

First isolated in 1938 as a distinct viral agent from equine epizootics in Venezuela *(54, 55)*, the Venezuelan equine encephalitis virus became the prototype for the VEE complex of related alphaviruses, pathogenic both to equines and humans by causing massive epizootics with extensive human infection *(32)*. The VEE complex encompasses six subtypes (serotypes) (I, VEE; II, Everglades; III, Mucambo; IV, Pixuna; V, Cabassou; and subtype VI) further divided according to different variants (IA–F, IIIA–C).

Viral Genome. The full-length genomes representing the VEEV antigenic subtypes I to VI range in size from 11.3 to 11.5 kb, with 48% to 53% overall G+C contents *(56, 57)*.

The VEEV genomic RNA encodes for nonstructural proteins (nsP1–4) that participate in genome replication and polyprotein processing, and a subgenomic message designated 26S encodes the three main structural proteins: the capsid and the E2 and E1 envelope glycoproteins. The E2 glycoprotein of the alphaviruses forms spikes on the surface of the virion, and the E1 protein lies below the spikes, adjacent to the envelope *(58)*.

The alphavirus replication and propagation depends on the protease activity of the viral nsP2 protein, which cleaves the nsP1–4 polyprotein replication complex into functional components. The recent elucidation of the crystal structure of the VEEV nsP2 protease (nsP2pro) at 2.45Å resolution *(59)* will make the nsP2 protein an attractive target for drug discovery to combat this highly pathogenic alphavirus *(57)*.

Epidemiology. Transmitted between mosquito vectors and vertebrate hosts, the Venezuelan equine encephalitis viruses exist in two epidemiologic forms: (i) enzootic viruses (antigenic subtypes ID, IE, and IF; subtypes II–VI), which are transmitted continuously in sylvanic habitats by *Culex* (*Melanoconion*) spp. mosquitoes among rodent reservoir hosts *(52)*; and (ii) epidemic/epizootic viruses (usually subtypes IAB and IC) *(52, 53)*. The epizootic subtypes IAB and IC viruses use equines as amplification hosts and develop much higher viremia titers in horses than do the enzootic strains, which generally are incapable of sufficient levels of amplification to cause outbreaks (60–62).

An important question pertaining to the natural history of VEEV concerns the source of the equine-virulent epizootic strains. An endemic source of epizootic virus has not been identified, despite intensive surveillance. However, several studies (52, 60, 63, 64) and oligonucleotide fingerprint analyses (65) of South American IC and ID viruses provide the most conclusive evidence suggesting that the VEE equine-virulent strains arise naturally from minor variants present in populations of ID VEE virus maintained in enzootic foci in northern South America. Thus, the equine-avirulent enzootic serotype ID strains appeared to alter their serotype to the equine-virulent IAB and IC strains (as well as their vertebrate and mosquito host range), to mediate repeated VEE emergence via mutations, mainly in the E2 envelope glycoprotein, which represent convergent evolution (52, 64, 66). Reverse genetic studies implicated a Ser→Asn substitution in the E2 envelope glycoprotein as the major determinant of the increased vector infectivity phenotype (60).

Although epizootic VEEV strains are opportunistic in their use of mosquito vectors, the most widespread outbreaks appeared to involve specific adaptation to *Ochlerotatus taeniorhynchus*, the most common vector in many coastal areas of northern South America; this adaptation to an efficient epizootic vector contributed to VEE disease emergence. In contrast, the enzootic VEEV strains are highly specialized and appear to use vectors (*C. spissipes*) exclusively of the *Culex* (*Melanoconion*) subgenus.

Taken together, these findings clearly underscore the capacity of RNA viruses to alter their vector host range through minor genetic changes, resulting in the potential for disease emergence.

19.2.3.1 Clinical Manifestations of VEE

Epizootic Viruses. The majority of VEEV infections are believed to lead to disease. After an incubation period of 24 hours to as long as 4 to 6 days, there will be an abrupt onset of fever and malaise, characterized in most clinical cases by a temperature of 102°F to 105°F, chills, myalgia, headache, and lethargy. Other common symptoms include photophobia, hyperesthesia, prostration, and vomiting. Occasionally, remission of fever and symptoms occur with recrudescence the next day. The usual duration of acute symptoms is 2 to 5 days, with residual asthenia for 1 to 2 weeks (32).

Epizootic virus infection causes encephalitis in a small proportion of cases. However, there is an increased incidence of encephalitis in children. More severe cases of VEE may present with coma and paralysis, and in some cases death may result after a fulminant 48- to 72-hour course as a result

of lymphoid necrosis (67). The case fatality rate may reach 10% to 15% of severe cases during large outbreaks. Only a small number of cases have been followed for a year or more to assess residual effects; however, in patients who survive, the recovery has been virtually complete (68).

Enzootic Viruses. Enzootic VEEV infections present a threat to humans in the warm, moist habitats where it is transmitted. Serum antibody rates show virtually 100% infection in adults in many endemic zones (69). Usually, patients will present with symptoms typical for VEE syndrome (70). Asymptomatic seroconversions have also been documented (32).

The Everglades (VEE subtype II) virus, which has been active in several ecologic zones in Florida, has been implicated in human CNS disease of modest severity (71). All cases occurred in older persons with preexisting hypertension or cerebrovascular disease who recovered without sequelae.

Treatment. Currently, there is no specific and effective treatment or licensed human vaccine for VEEV available. Therapy is primarily supportive and prevention relies on avoidance of mosquitoes.

Epizootic VEE infection should be best controlled by equine vaccination. This will not only protect the veterinary target against disease but also prevent amplification of the VEEV in mosquitoes feeding on viremic horses and mules. The live-attenuated human vaccine TC-83 is safe in equines and is capable of inducing immunity within 3 days of vaccination (72). The formalin inactivation of TC-83 produces a killed immunogen capable of protecting equines. However, inactivated vaccines made from virulent strains should not be used in humans because of the risk of residual live virus, which may initiate epizootics.

A live-attenuated vaccine has been developed to be used in humans (73). The strain, which was developed by passage of the Trinidad donkey strain of IAB virus in cell culture, and designated as TC-83, has been administered to several thousand volunteers. The vaccination led to the development of neutralizing antibodies in more than 90% and provided long-lasting protection against laboratory infections. Nevertheless, about 15% of vaccine recipients developed moderate fever and malaise. Furthermore, there is no convincing evidence that the TC-83 vaccine is safe in pregnant women. Preexisting alphavirus antibodies may also prevent primary immunization, and booster immunization may become difficult (32).

To overcome some of the difficulties inherent in the TC-83 vaccine, an inactivated product was prepared from the attenuated viral strain (74). The vaccine was immunogenic and has been highly useful in boosting waning immunity from TC-83 immunization (75), a particularly important feature for laboratory workers handling enzootic strains (32).

19.3 Bunyaviruses

The California serogroup viruses of the genus *Bunyavirus* includes 14 viruses and subtypes, all of which are transmitted by mosquitoes, and each one has a very narrow range of mosquito and mammalian hosts and a limited geographic distribution *(76)*. A number of the California serogroup viruses can infect humans, and one of them, the La Crosse virus, is an endemic cause of summer encephalitis in the Midwestern United States *(77)*. Extensive studies have identified a number of other California serogroup viruses that are enzootic in North America, and several of these pathogens (the snowshoe hare virus—an antigenic variant of the La Crosse virus, and the Jamestown Canyon virus) have also been implicated in causing sporadic cases of human encephalitis.

19.3.1 La Crosse Encephalitis Virus

In 1963, a pathogenic virus subsequently named La Crosse virus was isolated from a fatal case of encephalitis in La Crosse, Wisconsin *(78)*. It is the most pathogenic member of the California encephalitis serogroup.

La Crosse encephalitis virus (LCEV) was found to be closely related to, but distinct from, the California encephalitis virus. LCEV is the etiologic agent of a relatively rare mosquito-borne disease that has been identified in several Midwestern and Mid-Atlantic states and reaching south to the Florida peninsula *(79)*.

La Crosse virus is transmitted mainly by *Ochlerotatus triseriatus*, a treehole-breeding woodland mosquito that frequently feeds on small mammals, particularly chipmunks and squirrels. These vertebrates develop sufficient viremia to be infectious for mosquitoes that subsequently feed on them. *O. triseriatus* can also breed in water-holding containers (tires, cans, etc.), which can certainly expand the ecologic range of the virus to suburban areas. Recently, eggs of the Asian tiger mosquito, *Aedes albopictus*, infected with the La Cross encephalitis virus were collected in North Carolina and Tennessee. The virus can be maintained during the winter by vertical transmission in mosquito eggs *(79)*. Small infected mammals do not show signs or symptoms of the disease. Humans serve as "dead-end" hosts, meaning that they cannot further transmit the disease, because sufficient amplification of the virus does not occur in humans.

Epidemiologic surveys have indicated that the California serogroup encephalitis is geographically concentrated in the Midwest—Minnesota, Wisconsin, Iowa, Illinois, Indiana, and Ohio—which report more than 90% of all cases in the United States (on average, around 74 annually), as well as in the Appalachian region (West Virginia, North Carolina, Tennessee, and Virginia).

Children and young adults ages 1 to 19, particularly boys, are at greatest risk of exposure to the principal vector during camping and hiking in woodlands. The fatality rate of clinical cases of the disease is 1%.

Clinical Manifestations. The incubation period of the disease is between 5 and 15 days after the mosquito bite. Diagnosis is based on tests of blood and typically cannot be recovered from cerebrospinal fluid. The disease can be mistaken as enteroviral meningitis when mild and as herpes simplex encephalitis when severe *(80, 81)*.

The acute illness lasts for 10 days or fewer in most cases. Typically, the first symptoms are nonspecific, lasting for 1 to 3 days, followed by the appearance of CNS signs and symptoms, such as stiff neck, lethargy, and seizures, which usually abate within 1 week. If cerebrospinal fluid is obtained during the initial presentation, meningitis with both polymorphonuclear neutrophil leukocytes (PMNs) and mononuclear cells is found in about 65% of patients *(76)*.

La Crosse encephalitis virus, which produces classic acute encephalitis in children, is the most prevalent arboviral infection in this population in North America *(82)*. The usual clinical course is the mild form, in which headache, fever, and vomiting frequently occur on days 1 to 3. Lethargy, behavioral changes, and/or brief seizures may occur on days 3 and 4, followed by improvement over a 7- to 8-day period. The less common (10% to 20%), more severe presentations include abrupt fever and headache, disorientation and seizures, occurring within the first 8 to 24 hours of onset. The disease may sometimes progress to deep coma, associated in rare cases with cerebral edema. Overall, symptomatic children present with seizures (in about 50%) and status epilepticus (in about 10% to 15%).

There is no specific treatment currently available for La Crosse encephalitis. The therapy is supportive, directed at relieving the symptoms and preventing complications. Because there is evidence of inhibition of La Crosse virus by ribavirin *(83)*, its intravenous use has been piloted as compassionate therapy in a randomized clinical trial in patients with severe disease *(81)*.

References

1. Whitley, R. J. and Kimberlin, D. W. (1999) Viral encephalitis, *Pediatr. Rev.*, **20**, 192–198.
2. Porterfield, J. S. (1975) The basis of arbovirus classification, *Med. Biol.*, **53**, 400–405.
3. Mackenzie, J. S., Gubler, D. J., and Petersen, L. R. (2004) Emerging flaviviruses: the spread and resurgence of Japanese encephalitis, West Nile and Dengue viruses, *Nat. Med.*, **10**(12), S98–S109.
4. Lindenbach, B. D. and Rice, C. M. (2001) *Flaviviridae*: the viruses and their replication. In: *Fields Virology*, 4th ed. (Knipe, D. M.,

Howley, P. M., Griffin, D. E., Lamb, R. A., Martin, M. A., Roizman, B., and Strauss, S. E., eds.), Lippincott Williams & Wilkins, Philadelphia, pp. 991–1042.

5. Westaway, E. G. and Blok, K. (1997) Taxonomy and evolutionary relationships of flaviviruses. In: *Dengue and Dengue Hemorrhagic Fever* (Gubler, D. J. and Kuno, G., eds.), CAB International, London, pp. 147–173.

6. Marin, M. S., Zanotto, P. M., Gritsun, T. S., and Gould, E. A. (1995) Phylogeny of TYU, SRE, and CFA virus: different evolutionary rates in the genus *Flavivirus*, *Virology*, **206**, 1133–1139.

7. Zanotto, P. M., Gould, E. A., Gao, G. F., Harvey, P. H., and Holmes, E. C. (1996) Population dynamics of flaviviruses revealed by molecular phylogenetics, *Proc. Natl. Acad. Sci. U.S.A.*, **93**, 548–553.

8. Kuno, G., Chang, G. J., Tsuchiya, K. R., Karabatsos, N., and Cropp, C. B. (1998) Phylogeny of the genus *Flavivirus*, *J. Virol.*, **72**, 73–83.

9. Billoir, F., de Chesse, R., Tolou, H., de Micco, P., Gould, E. A., and de Lamballerie, X. (2000) Phylogeny of the genus *Flavivirus* using complete coding sequences of arthropod-borne viruses and viruses with no known vector, *J. Gen. Virol.*, **81**, 781–790.

10. Gould, E. A., de Lamballier, X., Zanotto, P. M. A., and Holmes, E. C. (2001) Evolution, epidemiology, and dispersal of flaviviruses revealed by molecular phylogenies, *Adv. Virus Res.*, **57**, 71–103.

11. Gould, E. A., de Lamballier, X., Zanotto, P. M. A., and Holmes, E. C. (2003) Origins, evolution, and vector/host coadaptations within the genus *Flavivirus*, *Adv. Virus Res.*, **59**, 277–314.

12. Gould, E. A., Moss, S. R., and Turner, S. L. (2004) Evolution and dispersal of encephalitic flaviviruses, *Arch. Virol. Suppl.*, **18**, 65–84.

13. Gould, E. A. (2002) Evolution of Japanese encephalitis serocomplex viruses, *Curr. Top. Microbiol. Immunol.*, **267**, 391–404.

14. Gritsun, T. S., Lashkevich, V. A., and Gould, E. A. (2003) Tick-borne encephalitis, *Antiviral Res.*, **57**, 129–146.

15. Gubler, D. J. (1997) Dengue and dengue haemorrhagic fever: its history and resurgence as a global public health problem. In: *Dengue and Dengue Hemorrhagic Fever* (Gubler, D. J. and Kuno, G., eds.), CAB International, London, pp. 1–22.

16. Gubler, D. J. (2002) The global emergence/resurgence of arboviral diseases as public health problems, *Arch. Med. Res.*, **33**, 330–342.

17. Mackenzie, J. S., Barrett, A. D. T., and Deubel, V. (2002) The Japanese encephalitis serological group of Flaviviruses: a brief introduction to the group, *Curr. Top. Microbiol.*, **267**, 1–10.

18. Solomon, T. (2006) Control of Japanese encephalitis – within our grasp? *N. Engl. J. Med.*, **355**(9), 869–871.

19. Solomon, T. and Vaughn, D. W. (2002) Pathogenesis and clinical features of Japanese encephalitis and West Nile virus infections, *Curr. Top. Microbiol. Immunol.*, **267**, 171–194.

20. Solomon, T. and Winter, P. M. (2004) Neurovirulence and host factors in flavivirus encephalitis – evidence from clinical epidemiology, *Arch. Virol. Suppl.*, **18**, 161–170.

21. Solomon, T., Kneen, R., Dung, N. M., Khanh, V. C., Thuy, T. T., Ha, D. Q., Day, N. P., Nisalak, A., Vaughn, D. W., and White, N. J. (1998) Poliomyelitis-like illness due to Japanese encephalitis virus, *Lancet*, **351**, 1094–1097.

22. Burke, D. S., Lorsomrudee, W., Leake, C. J., Hoke, C. H., Nisalak, A., Chongsvasdi, V., and Laurakpongse, T. (1985) Fatal outcome in Japanese encephalitis, *Am. J. Trop. Med. Hyg.*, **34**(6), 1203–1210.

23. Kienzle, N. and Boyes, L. (2003) Murray Valley encephalitis: case report and review of neurological features, *Australas. Radiol.*, **47**, 61–63.

24. Burrow, J. N., Whelan, P. I., Kilburn, C. J., Fisher, D. A., Currie, B. J., and Smith, D. W. (1998) Australian encephalitis in the Northern territory: clinical and epidemiological features, *Aust. NZ J. Med.*, **28**, 590–596.

25. Russell, R. C. and Dwyer, D. E. (2000) Arboviruses associated with human disease in Australia, *Microbes Infect.*, **2**, 1693–1704.

26. Marshall, I. D. (1998) Murray Valley and Kunjin encephalitis. In: *The Arboviruses: Epidemiology and Ecology* (Monath, T. P., ed.), CRC Press, Boca Raton, FL, pp. 151–190.

27. Mackenzie, J. S., Smith, D. W., Broom, A. K., and Bucens, M. R. (1993) Australian encephalitis in Western Australia, 1978–1991, *Med. J. Aust.*, **158**, 591–595.

28. Bennett, N. M. C. K. (1976) Murray Valley encephalitis 1974. Clinical features, *Med. J. Aust.*, **2**, 446–450.

29. Shroyer, D. A. (2004) Saint Louis encephalitis: a Florida problem. A FMELMG337 document from the Entomology and Nematology Department, Florida Cooperative Extension Service, Institute of Food and Agricultural Sciences, University of Florida, Gainesville (http://edis.ifas.ufl.edu).

30. Monath, T. P. (1990) Flaviviruses. In: *Fields Virology*, 2nd ed. (Fields, B. N., Knipe, D. M., Chanock, R. M., Hirsch, M. S., Melnick, J. L., Monath, T. P., and Roizman, B., eds.), Raven Press, New York, pp. 763–814.

31. Santos, C. L., Sallum, M. A., Franco, H. M., Oshiro, F. M., and Rocco, I. M. (2006) Genetic characterization of St. Louis encephalitis virus in Sao Paulo, Brazil, *Mem. Inst. Oswaldo Cruz*, **101**(1), 57–63.

32. Peters, C. J. and Dalrymple, J. M. (1990) Alphaviruses. In: *Fields Virology*, 2nd ed. (Fields, B. N., Knipe, D. M., Chanock, R. M., Hirsch, M. S., Melnick, J. L., Monath, T. P., and Roizman, B., eds.), Raven Press, New York, pp. 713–761.

33. Morris, C. D. (1992) Eastern equine encephalitis. An ENY-700-6-1 document and part of the Mosquito Control Handbook cooperatively by the Department of Entomology and Nematology, University of Florida and a number of other institutions. The electronic version of the Mosquito Control Handbook is provided by the Florida Cooperatice Extension Service, Institute of Food and Agricultural Sciences, University of Florida, Gainesville (http://hammock.ifas.ufl.edu).

34. Hanson, R. P. (1957) An epizootics of equine encephalomyelitis that occurred in Massachusetts in 1831, *Am. J. Trop. Med. Hyg.*, **6**, 858–862.

35. Kissing, R. E., Rubin, H., Chamberlain, R. W., and Eidson, M. E. (1951) Recovery of virus of eastern encephalomyelitis from blood of a purple grackle, *Proc. Soc. Exp. Biol. Med.*, **77**, 398–399.

36. Kissling, R. E., Chamberlain, R. W., Sikes, R. K., and Eidson, M. E. (1954) Studies on the North American arthropod-borne encephalitides: III. Eastern equine encephalitis in wild birds, *Am. J. Hyg.*, **60**, 251–265.

37. Kissling, R. E., Chamberlain, R. W., Nelson, D. B., and Stamm, D. D. (1955) Studies on the North American arthropod-borne encephalitides. VIII. Equine encephalitis studies in Louisiana, *Am. J. Hyg.*, **62**, 233–254.

38. Howitt, B. (1938) Recovery of the virus of equine encephalomyelitis from a brain of a child, *Science*, **88**, 455–456.

39. Fothergill, L. D., Dingle, J. H., Farber, S., and Connerley, M. L. (1938) Human encephalitis caused by the virus of the eastern variety of equine encephalomyelitis, *N. Engl. J. Med.*, **219**, 411.

40. Monath, T. R. (1979) Arthropod-borne encephalitis in the Americas, *Bull. WHO*, **158**, 513–533.

41. Shope, R. E., de Andrade, A. H. P., Bensabeth, G., Causey, O. R., and Humphrey, P. S. (1966) The epidemiology of EEE, WEE, SLE and Tralock viruses, with special reference to birds, in a

tropical rain forest near Belem, Brazil, *Am. J. Epidemiol.*, **84**, 467–477.

42. Clarke, D. H. (1961) Two nonfatal human infections with virus of eastern encephalitis, *Am. J. Trop. Med. Hyg.*, **10**, 67–70.

43. Deresiewicz, R. L., Thaler, S. J., Hsu, L., and Zamani, A. A. (1997) Clinical and neuroradiographic manifestations of eastern equine encephalitis, *N. Engl. J. Med.*, **336**(26), 1867–1874.

44. Hauser, G. H. (1948) Human equine encephalomyelitis, easter type, in Louisiana, *New Orleans Med. Surg.*, **100**, 551–558.

45. Ayres, J. C. and Feemster, R. F. (1949) The sequelae of eastern equine encephalomyelitis, *N. Engl. J. Med.*, **240**, 960–962.

46. Chanas, A. C., Johnson, B. K., and Simpson, D. I. H. (1976) Antigenic relationships of alphaviruses by a simple microculture cross-neutralization method, *J. Gen. Microbiol.*, **32**, 295–300.

47. Karabatsos, N. (1975) Antigenic relationships of group A arboviruses by plaque reduction neutralization testing, *Am. J. Trop. Med. Hyg.*, **24**, 527–532.

48. Trent, D. W. and Grant, J. A. (1980) A comparison of New World alphaviruses in the western equine encephalomyelitis complex by immunochemical and oligonucleotide fingerprint techniques, *J. Gen. Virol.*, **47**, 261–282.

49. Reisen, W. (1993) The Western encephalitis mosquito, *Culex tarsalis*, *Wing Beats*, **4**(2), 16.

50. Baker, A. B. (1958) Western equine encephalitis. Clinical features, *Neurology*, **8**, 880–881.

51. Finley, K. H. (1959) Postencephalitis manifestations of viral encephalitis. In: *Viral Encephalitis* (Fields, N. S. and Blattner, R. J., eds.), Charles Thomas, Springfield, IL, pp. 69–91.

52. Weaver, S. C., Ferro, C., Barrera, R., Boshell, J., and Navarro, J.-C. (2004) Venezuelan equine encephalitis, *Ann. Rev. Entomol.*, **49**, 141–174.

53. Weaver, S. C., Anischenko, M., Bowen, R., Brault, A. C., Estrada-Franco, J. G., Fernandez, Z., Greene, I., Ortiz, D., Paessler, S., and Powers, A. M. (2004) Genetic determinants of Venezuelan equine virus emergence, *Arch. Virol. Suppl.*, **18**, 43–64.

54. Beck, C. E. and Wyckoff, R. W. G. (1938) Venezuelan equine encephalomyelitis, *Science*, **88**, 530.

55. Kubes, V. and Rios, F. A. (1939) The causative agent of infectious encephalomyelitis in Venezuela, *Science*, **90**, 20–21.

56. Meissner, J. D., Huang, C. Y.-H., Pfeffer, M., and Kinney, R. M. (1999) Sequencing of prototype viruses in the Venezuelan equine encephalitis antigenic complex, *Virus Res.*, **64**, 43–59.

57. Kinney, R. M., Pfeffer, M., Tsuchiya, K. R., Chang, G.-J. J., and Roehrig, J. T. (1998) Nucleotide sequences of the 26S mRNAs of the viruses defining the Venezuelan equine encephalitis antigenic complex, *Am. J. Trop. Med. Hyg.*, **59**, 952–964.

58. Pletnev, S. V., Zhang, W., Mukhopadhyay, S., Fisher, B. R., Hernandez, R., Brown, D. T., Baker, T. S., Rossman, M. G., and Kuhn, R. J. (2001) Locations of carbohydrate sites of alphavirus glycoproteins show E1 forms an eicosahedral scaffold, *Cell*, **105**, 127–136.

59. Russo, A. T., White, M. A., and Watowich, S. J. (2006) The crystal structure of the Venezuelan equine encephalitis alphavirus nsP2 protease, *Structure*, **14**, 1449–1458.

60. Brault, A. C., Powers, A. M., Ortiz, D., Estrada-Franco, J. G., Navarro-Lopez, R., and Weaver, S. C. (2004) Venezuelan equine encephalitis emergence: enhanced vector infection from a single amino acid substitution in the envelope protein, *Proc. Natl. Acad. Sci. U.S.A.*, **101**(31), 11344–11349.

61. Walton, T. E., Alvarez, O., Buckwalter, R. M., and Johnson, K. M. (1973) Experimental infection of horses with an attenuated Venezuelan equine encephalitis vaccine (strain TC-83), *J. Infect. Dis.*, **128**, 271–282.

62. Wang, E., Bowen, R. A., Medina, G., Powers, A. M., Kang, W., Chandler, L. M., Shope, R. E., and Weaver, S. C. (2001) Virulence and viremia characteristics of 1992 epizootic subtype IC Venezuelan equine encephalitis viruses and closely related enzootic subtype ID strains, *Am. J. Trop. Med. Hyg.*, **65**, 64–69.

63. Kinney, R. M., Tsuchiya, K. R., Sneider, J. M., and Trent, D. W. (1992) Genetic evidence that epizootic Venezualan equine encephalitis (VEE) viruses may have evolved from enzootic VEE subtype I-D virus, *Virology*, **191**(2), 569–580.

64. Wang, E., Barrera, R., Boshell, J., Ferro, C., Freier, J. E., Navarro, J. C., Salas, R., Vasquez, C., and Weaver, S. C. (1999) Genetic and phenotypic changes accompanying the emergence of epizootic subtype IC Venezuelan equine encephalitis viruses from an enzootic subtype ID progenitor, *J. Virol.*, **73**(5), 4266–4271.

65. Trent, D. W., Clewley, J. P., France, J. K., and Bishop, D. H. L. (1979) Immunochemical and oligonucleotide fingerprint analyses of Venezuelan equine encephalomyelitis complex viruses, *J. Gen. Virol.*, **43**, 365–381.

66. Kinney, R. M., Chang, G. J., Tsuchiya, K. R., Sneider, J. M., Roehrig, J. T., Woodward, T. M., and Trent, D. W. (1993) Attenuation of Venezuelan equine encephalitis virus strain TC-83 is encoded by the 5′-noncoding region and the E2 envelope glycoprotein, *J. Virol.*, **67**(3), 1269–1277.

67. Avilan Rovira, J. (1972) Discussion. In: *Proceedings of the Workshop-Symposium on Venezuelan Encephalitis Virus*, Sci. Publ. 243, Pan American Health Organization, Washington, DC, pp. 189–195.

68. Bowen, G. S., Fashinell, T. R., Dean, P. B., and Gregg, M. G. (1976) Clinical aspects of human Venezuelan equine encephalitis in Texas, *Bull. Pan Am. Health Organ.*, **10**, 46–57.

69. Johnson, K. M. and Marin, D. H. (1974) Venezuelan equine encephalitis, *Adv. Vet. Sci. Comp. Med.*, **18**, 79–116.

70. Dietz, W. H., Jr., Peralta, P. H., and Johnson, K. M. (1979) The clinical cases of human infection with Venezuelan equine encephalomyelitis virus, subtype I-D, *Am. J. Trop. Med. Hyg.*, **28**, 329–334.

71. Ehrenkranz, N. J. and Ventura, A. K. (1974) Venezuelan equine encephalitis virus infection in man, *Annu. Rev. Med.*, **25**, 9–14.

72. Walton, T. E. and Grayson, M. A. (1988) Venezuelan equine encephalomyelitis. In: *The Arboviruses: Epidemiology and Ecology*, vol. IV, (Monath, T. P., ed.), CRC Press, Boca Raton, FL, pp. 204–231.

73. McKinney, R. M. (1972) Inactivated and live VEE vaccines – a review. In: *Proceedings of the Workshop-Symposium on Venezuelan Encephalitis Virus*, Sci. Publ. 243, Pan American Health Organization, Washington, DC, pp. 369–389.

74. Cole, F. E., Jr., May, S. W., and Eddy, G. A. (1974) Inactivated Venezuelan equine encephalomyelitis vaccine prepared from attenuated (TC-83 strain) virus, *Appl. Microbiol.*, **97**, 150–153.

75. Burke, D. S., Ramsburg, H. H., and Edelman, R. (1977) Persistence in humans of antibody to subtypes of Venezuelan equine encephalomyelitis (VEE) virus after immunization with attenuated (TC-83) VEE virus vaccine, *J. Infect. Dis.*, **136**, 354–359.

76. Gonzales-Scarano, F. and Nathanson, N. (1990) Bunyaviruses. In: *Fields Virology*, 2nd ed. (Fields, B. N., Knipe, D. M., Chanock, R. M., Hirsch, M. S., Melnick, J. L., Monath, T. P., and Roizman, B., eds.), Raven Press, New York, pp. 1195–1228.

77. Kappus, K. D., Monath, T. P., Kaminski, R. M., and Calisher, C. H. (1983) Reported encephalitis associated with California serogroup virus infections in the United States, 1963–1981, *Prog. Clin. Biol. Res.*, **123**, 31–41.

78. Thompson, W. H., Kalfayan, B., and Anslow, R. O. (1965) Isolation of California encephalitis group virus from a fatal human illness, *Am. J. Epidemiol.*, **81**, 245–253.

79. Rey, J. R. (2006) La Crosse encephalitis. An ENY-672 (IN420) document by the Entomology and Nematology Department, Florida Cooperative Extension Service, Institute of Food and Agricultural Sciences, University of Florida, Gainesville (http://edis.ifas.ufl.edu).

80. McJunkin, J. E., Khan, R. R., and Tsai, T. F. (1998) California La Crosse encephalitis, *Infect. Dis. Clin. North Am.*, **12**, 83–93.

81. McJunkin, J. E., Khan, R., de los Reyes, E. C., Parsons, D. L., Minnich, L. L., Ashley, R. G., and Tsai, T. F. (1997) Treatment of a severe case of La Crosse encephalitis with intravenous ribavirin following diagnosis by brain biopsy, *Pediatrics*, **99**(2), 261–267.

82. McJunkin, J. E., de los Reyes, E. C., Irazuzta, J. E., Ceceres, M. J., Khan, R. R., Minnich, L. L., Fu, K. D., Lovett, G. D., Tsai, T., and Thompson, A. (2001) La Crosse encephalitis in children, *N. Engl. J. Med.*, **344**, 801–817.

83. Cassidy, L. F. and Patterson, J. L. (1989) Mechanism of La Crosse virus inhibition by ribavirin, *Antimicrob. Agents Chemother.*, **33**, 2009–2011.

Chapter 20

Malaria

Malaria is an infectious disease caused by parasites of the genus *Plasmodium* that are transmitted by mosquitoes. The illness results in recurrent attacks of chills and fever and is characterized by high morbidity and mortality rates. Of the four known human *Plasmodium* species, *Plasmodium falciparum* is the most lethal. Although malaria has been virtually eradicated in regions with temperate climates, it is still prevalent in the tropical and subtropical countries in Africa, Asia, the Middle East, and Central and South America. Evolving strains of drug-resistant parasites and insecticide-resistant mosquitoes continue to make the threat of malaria a global health peril, especially in children in sub-Saharan Africa. One of the most prevalent diseases worldwide, malaria affects more than 400 million people and causes more than 2.5 million deaths every year *(1)*. Approximately 10,000 to 30,000 travelers from industrialized countries are expected to contract malaria each year *(2)*. The incidence of imported malaria is increasing, and the case fatality rate remains high despite progress in intensive care and anti-malarial treatment.

Without prompt and appropriate treatment, malaria represents a medical emergency because it may rapidly progress to complications and death *(3)*.

These facts have renewed the urgency for the identification of new susceptible drug targets for chemotherapy as well as for the development of vaccines for malaria.

20.1 Life Cycle and Morphology of Plasmodium

The etiologic agent of malaria is a eukaryotic obligate intraerythrocytic protozoa of the genus *Plasmodium*. Humans can be infected with one or more of four species: *P. falciparum*, *P. vivax*, *P. ovale*, and *P. malariae*.

The malaria parasites are members of Apicomplexa, a phylum of the subkingdom Protozoa, which includes the class Sporozoea and the subclasses Coccidia and Piroplasma, and is characterized by the presence of an apical complex. The apical complex represents a set of organelles—collectively known as apical organelles because of their localization at one end of the parasite—that are involved in interactions between the parasite and the host cell (http://www.tulane.edu/~wiser/malaria/cmb.html).

The life cycle of plasmodia consists of three major stages: the mosquito stage, the liver stage, and the intraerythrocyte stage *(4)*. The intraerythrocytic developmental cycle (IDC), or red blood cell stage, is markedly short in length—from 48 hours (*P. ovale*, *P. vivax*, and *P. falciparum*) to 72 hours (*P. malariae*)—among the four human species. During this cycle, plasmodia will undergo an identical series of morphologic changes *(5)* to complete iterative cycles of parasite replication, escape from red blood cells, and re-infection within the host *(4)*. These morphologic transformations imply that a high degree of regulation must exist to ensure that proteins necessary throughout the IDC are present at the appropriate times for precise developmental progression.

When the infected anopheline mosquitoes take a blood meal, parasite sporozoites are inoculated into the bloodstream. Within an hour, sporozoites will enter the hepatocytes and will start to divide into exoerythrocytic merozoites (the so-called *tissue schizogony*). For *P. vivax* and *P. ovale*, dormant forms called *hypnozoites* typically remain quiescent in the liver until a later time; *P. falciparum* does not produce hypnozoites *(3)*. Once merozoites leave the liver, they will invade the erythrocytes and develop into early *trophozoites*, which are ring-shaped, vacuolated, and unnucleated. Once the parasites begin to divide, the trophozoites are called *schizonts*, consisting of many daughter merozoites (*blood schizogony*). Eventually, the infected erythrocytes are lysed by the merozoites, which subsequently will invade other erythrocytes, starting a new cycle of schizogony *(3)*. The duration of each cycle in *P. falciparum* is about 48 hours. In nonimmune humans, the infection is amplified about 20-fold each cycle. After several cycles, some of the merozoites will transform into *gametocytes*, the sexual stage of malaria. Although gametocytes do not generate any significant pathology (except their relation to anemia),

V. St. Georgiev, *National Institute of Allergy and Infectious Diseases, NIH: Impact on Global Health*, vol. 2, DOI 10.1007/978-1-60327-297-1_20, © Humana Press, a part of Springer Science+Business Media, LLC 2009

they are infective for mosquitoes, and from an epidemiologic standpoint they are important by perpetuating the plasmodial cycle *(6, 7)*. Nevertheless, decreased hemoglobin concentrations, hyperparasitemia, and severe malaria have been associated with increased *P. falciparum* gametocyte carriage (see Section 20.5.1) *(7)*.

20.2   Cellular and Molecular Biology of Plasmodium

During their life cycle as eukaryotic intracellular parasites, the *Plasmodium* parasite must enter the host cell and, once inside, they will modify the host cell. Plasmodia are primarily transmitted by the bite of an infected female *Anopheles* mosquito, although infections can also occur through exposure to infected blood products (transfusion malaria) and by congenital transmission *(3)*.

20.2.1   Host Cell/Erythrocyte Invasion

The apical organelles have been implicated in the process of host cell invasion. In the case of *Plasmodium*, three distinct invasive forms have been identified: sporozoite, merozoite, and ookinete (http://www.tulane.edu/~wiser/malaria/cmb.html). The merozoites rapidly (about 20 seconds) and specifically enter the host erythrocytes. The specificity is manifested both for erythrocytes as the preferred host cell type and for a particular host species as well, thus implying receptor-ligand interactions *(8)*. Four distinct steps in the invasion process have been recognized: (i) initial merozoite binding; (ii) reorientation and erythrocyte deformation; (iii) specific interactions and junction formation; and (iv) parasite entry.

Merozoite Surface Proteins and Host-Parasite Interactions. The initial interaction between the merozoite and the erythrocyte is probably a random collision and presumably involves reversible interactions between *merozoite surface proteins (MSPs)* and the host erythrocyte. The best characterized MSP is MSP-1. However, the exact role(s) that MSP-1 and its processing play in the merozoite invasion process is not known *(9)*.

Reorientation and Secondary Organelles. After binding to the erythrocyte, the parasite reorients itself so that its apical end is juxtaposed to the erythrocyte membrane. This process also coincides with a transient erythrocyte deformation. The *apical membrane antigen (AMA-1)* has been implicated in this reorientation *(10)*. AMA-1 is a transmembrane protein located at the apical end of the merozoite that binds to the erythrocyte. Although AMA-1 it is not involved in the merozoite attachment, antibodies against AMA-1 have pre-

vented the reorientation of the merozoite, thereby blocking merozoite invasion.

Three morphologically distinct, specialized secretory organelles (micronemes, rhoptries, and dense granules) are located at the apical end of the invasive stages of the apicomplexan parasites. Of those secretory organelles, the dense granules are not always included with the apical organelles and probably represent a heterogeneous population of secretory vesicles.

The contents of the apical organelles are expelled as the parasite invades, which suggests that these organelles play some role in the invasion. The increase in the cytoplasmic concentration of calcium associated with the macroneme discharge is typical of regulated secretion in other eukaryotes *(11)*. The rhoptries are discharged formation of the parasitophorous vacuole. The contents of the dense granules [the ring-infected erythrocyte surface antigen (RESA) protein, and subtilisin-like proteases] are released after the parasite has completed its entry and, therefore, are usually implicated in the modification of the host cell *(12–14)*.

Specific Interactions and Junction Formation. After the merozoite reorientation and microneme discharge, a junction will form between the parasite and the host cell. Presumably, the microneme proteins [the *erythrocyte-binding antigen (EBA)-175*, the *Duffy-binding protein (DBP)*, the *circumsporozoite-related protein (CTRP)*, and the *thrombospondin-related adhesive protein (TRAP)*] are important for the formation of the junction. Of these proteins, EBA-175 and DBP recognize the sialic acid residues of the glycophorins and the Duffy antigen, respectively, and are probably involved in receptor-ligand interactions with proteins exposed on the erythrocyte surface *(15)*.

The other microneme proteins in the TRAP family have also been implicated in locomotion and/or cell invasion *(16)*.

The junction formation is an important stage in the parasite's invasion of the host cell. It is likely initiated by microneme discharge, which exposes the receptor-binding domains of parasite ligands, and represents a strong connection between the erythrocyte and the merozoite that is mediated by receptor-ligand interactions.

Parasite Entry. Apicomplexan parasites actively invade host cells, and entry is not due to uptake or phagocytosis by the host cell. At the time of junction formation, the erythrocyte membrane proteins are redistributed so that the contact area is free of erythrocyte membrane proteins. A merozoite serine protease that cleaves erythrocyte band 3 has been described *(17)*. Because of the pivotal role band 3 plays in the homeostasis of the submembrane skeleton, its degradation could result in a localized disruption of the cytoskeleton.

An incipient parasitophorous vacuolar membrane (PVM) forms in the junction area, which expands as the parasite enters the erythrocyte. Once the parasite has completed its entry, the tight junction will disappear and the respective

PVM and the host erythrocyte membrane will fuse and separate, thus completing the entry process.

Plasmodium sporozoites and ookinetes, as well as the invasive stages of many other apicomplexan parasites, are motile organisms that crawl along a substratum. This movement along a substratum, or *gliding motility*, is accompanied by the deposition of a trail of TRAP proteins *(16, 18)*. The gliding motility presumably involves attachment of the parasite ligands (i.e., TRAP) to the substratum.

Gene distribution studies have confirmed that TRAP *(19, 20)* and CTRP *(21, 22)* proteins play essential roles in both motility and cell invasion.

20.2.2 Host Erythrocyte Modification

Once inside the erythrocyte, the parasite undergoes a trophic phase followed by a replicative phase. During this intraerythrocytic period, the parasite modifies the host cell to make it a more suitable habitat (http://www.tulane.edu/~wiser/malaria/cmb.html). For example, the erythrocyte membrane becomes more permeable to small-molecular-weight metabolites, presumably reflecting the needs of an actively growing parasite.

Another modification of the host cell concerns the cytoadherence of *P. falciparum*–infected erythrocytes to endothelial cells and the resulting sequestration of the mature parasites in capillaries and postcapillary venules. This sequestration likely leads to microcirculatory alterations and metabolic dysfunctions that could be responsible for many of the manifestations of severe falciparum malaria. The cytoadherence to endothelial cells confers at least two advantages for the parasite: a microaerophilic environment that is better suited for parasite metabolism, and avoidance of the spleen and subsequent destruction.

Knobs and Cytoadherence. Major structural alterations of the host erythrocyte are electron-dense protrusions, or "knobs," on the erythrocyte membrane of *P. falciparum*–infected cells. The knobs are induced by the parasite, and several parasite proteins are associated with the knobs *(23)*. Two proteins that might participate in knob formation or affect the host erythrocyte submembrane cytoskeleton and indirectly induce knob formation are the *knob-associated histidine rich protein (KAHRP)* and the *erythrocyte membrane protein-2 (PfEMP2; MESA)*. Both of these proteins are localized on the cytoplasmic face of the host membrane and not exposed to the outer surface of the erythrocyte. Although their exact role in knob formation is still unknown, they may be involved in reorganizing the submembrane cytoskeleton.

The knobs are believed to play a role in the sequestration of infected erythrocytes, because they are points of contact between the infected erythrocytes and vascular endothelial cells, and parasite species that express knobs exhibit the highest levels of sequestration.

A polymorphic protein known as PfEMP1 has also been localized on the knobs and is exposed to the host erythrocyte surface. PfEMP1 is considered to be a key adhesive ligand mediating sequestration *(24)*. The translocation of PfEMP1 to the erythrocyte surface depends in part on another erythrocyte membrane-associated protein, PfEMP3 *(25)*. PfEMP1 probably functions as a ligand that binds to receptors on host endothelial cells. Other proposed cytoadherence ligands include a modified band 3 (pfalhesin) *(26)*, sequestrin, rifins, and clag9 *(27)*.

Endothelial Cell Receptors. Several possible endothelial receptors have been identified by testing the ability of infected erythrocytes to bind in static adherence *in vitro* assays *(28)*:

(i) CD36.
(ii) Ig superfamily: intercellular cell adhesion molecule-1 (ICAM1), vascular cell adhesion molecule-1 (VCAM1), and platelet endothelial cell adhesion molecule-1 (PECAM1)
(iii) Chondroitin sulfate A, heparin sulfate, hyaluronic acid, E-selectin, and thrombospondin.
(iv) Roseting ligands: CR-1, blood group A antigen, and glycosaminoglycan.

One of the best characterized receptors is CD36, an 88-kDa integral membrane protein found on monocytes, platelets, and endothelial cells. Infected erythrocytes from most parasites bind to CD36, and the binding domain has been mapped to the cysteine interdomain region (CIDR) of PfEMP1.

ICAM1 is a member of the immunoglobulin superfamily and functions in cell-cell adhesion. In addition, sequestration of infected erythrocytes and ICAM1 expression has been co-localized in the brain *(29)*.

Chondroitin sulfate A (CSA) has been implicated in the cytoadherence within the placenta and may contribute to the adverse effects of *P. falciparum* in pregnancy.

The roles of some of the other potential receptors (thrombospondin, VCAM1, PECAM1, and E-selectin) appear unclear, and questions about their constitutive expression on endothelial cells have been raised. However, cytoadherance could involve multiple receptor/ligand interactions.

Roseting is another adhesive phenomenon exhibited by *P. falciparum*–infected erythrocytes, where the binding of infected erythrocytes to multiple uninfected erythrocytes and PfEMP1 appears to have some role in at least some resetting. Possible receptors include complement receptor-1 (CR1), blood group A antigen, or glycosaminoglycan moieties on an unidentified proteoglycan.

The different classes of Duffy-binding-like (DBL) domains (such as Duffy-binding-like (DBL)α) and CIDR may also bind to different endothelial cell receptors *(27, 30)*. The binding of CIDR to CD36 may account for the abundance of this particular binding phenotype among parasite isolates.

Antigenic Variation. In a process known as antigenic variation, clonal *P. falciparum* parasites can vary the type of PfEMP1 molecule they express, so as to avoid antibody-mediated clearance *(24)*. Furthermore, different PfEMP1 ligands mediate adherence to different receptors on endothelial cells, including the scavenger receptor CD36, chondroitin sulfate A, and the intracellular adhesion molecule-1.

In some instances, parasite populations with a predisposition to adhere to certain receptors have been more commonly associated with certain disease outcomes, such as cerebral and placental malaria, although the precise role of parasite-receptor interactions in determining disease severity remains to be understood.

The encoding of the cytoadherence ligand by a highly polymorphic gene family presents a paradox, in that receptor/ligand interactions are generally considered to be highly specific. However, selection for different cytoadherent phenotypes results in a concomitant change in the surface antigenic type *(31)*. Similarly, examination of clonal parasite lines reveals that changes in the surface antigenic type correlate with differences in binding to CD36 and ICAM1. Furthermore, the expression of a particular PfEMP1 will result in a parasite with a distinct cytoadherent and may affect its pathogenesis. Similarly, the association of PfEMP1 with resetting also explains the variability of the resetting phenotype. The parasite counters the host immune response by expressing antigenically distinct PfEMP1 molecules on the erythrocyte surface. This would allow the parasite to avoid clearance by the host immune system and yet maintain the cytoadherent phenotype. The molecular mechanism of this antigenic switching is not known. Preliminary data suggest that expression is controlled by epigenic factors that affect the local chromosomal structure of the expressed gene *(27, 32)* (http://www.tulane.edu/~wiser/malaria/cmb.html).

20.2.3 *P. falciparum Transcription Factors*

During the complex life cycle of *P. falciparum* divided between mosquito and human hosts, the regulation of morphologic changes implies a fine control of transcriptional regulation to correspond precisely with the state of differentiation in the host. The different developmental stages of the parasite would require coordinated modulation of expression of distinct sets of genes, which could be achieved by transcriptional and/or posttranscriptional controls. In *P. falciparum*, as in all eukaryotes, gene expression is controlled by the interaction of elements within promoters acting *in cis* (DNA regulatory elements) and elements acting *in trans*

(transcriptional factors) whose availability is modulated during cellular development.

To elucidate the molecular mechanisms implicated in transcriptional regulation (i.e., the interplay between *cis* and *trans* elements throughout the *P. falciparum* erythrocytic development), studies have been carried out among diverse families of transcription factors, especially Myb-related proteins belonging to the tryptophan cluster family *(33)*. In eukaryotes, the highly conserved Myb proteins have been shown to bind DNA in a sequence-specific manner and to participate in the regulation of expression of genes implicated in growth control and differentiation *(34)*.

One Myb protein, PfMyb1, was the first transcription factor not belonging to general transcription factors to be cloned and analyzed in *P. falciparum (35)*. In that study, it was demonstrated that *pfmyb1* mRNA reached its highest level at the trophozoite stage (at least as regarding the 3D7 clone), and the PfMyb1 protein present in nuclear extracts was able to bind specifically to a prototype *myb*-regulatory element (MRE) from the chicken *mim-1* gene promoter *(36)*, and two putative MRE annotated within the *Plasmodium* promoters *(35)*. These results have strongly suggested that PfMyb1 can be considered to be a genuine Myb transcription factor.

In further studies, by taking advantage of the ability of the long *pfmyb1* double-stranded RNA (dsRNA) to interfere with the cognate messenger expression, the role of PfMyb1 transcription factor was investigated during the *P. falciparum* erythrocytic cycle *(33)*. Using chromatin immunoprecipitation, it was shown that PfMyb1 bound within the parasite nuclei to several promoters, thereby directly participating in the transcriptional regulation of the corresponding genes—the first evidence of a regulation network involving a *P. falciparum* transcription factor during its erythrocytic cycle *(33)*.

20.2.4 *P. falciparum Enzyme Complex: Ribonucleotide Reductase*

Ribonucleotide reductase (RNR) is a key tetrameric enzyme that is responsible for the maintenance of a continuous and balanced supply of deoxynucleotides (dNTPs) by catalyzing the reduction of ribonucleotides. The concentrations of dNTPs (the precursors for DNA synthesis) fluctuate during the eukaryotic cell cycle because of changes in the activity of the ribonucleotide reductase. RNR catalyzes the rate-limiting step in the biosynthesis of all four dNTPs and is regulated by multiple mechanisms. The enzyme's allosteric activity site controls the concentration of dNTP: when the dNTP reaches a certain level, the activity of RNR is downregulated by dATP feedback inhibition *(37, 38)*. Of the three classes of RNR that have been currently identified, class I, which most of the eukaryotic and some of the prokaryotic holoenzymes belong to, is a complex of homodimers of two large (R1) and two small (R2) subunits *(39)*. The R1 subunit accommodates the allosteric regulatory sites and the catalytic sites, and the R2 subunit houses the diferric-tyrosyl radical that is essential for catalysis *(40)*.

A component of the *P. falciparum* enzyme complex, the RNR consists as expected of R1 and R2 subunits. However, a third small subunit, termed R4 (PfR4), has also been identified and characterized *(41)*. RfR4 encodes a 324-amino-acid residue polypeptide that shares only 25% identity with RfR2, another small subunit of *P. falciparum*. RfR4 expression is cell-cycle-regulated, and the profile of the transcript and protein expression corresponds with that of RfR2. Co-immunoprecipitation experiments detected interactions between the RfR1, RfR2, and RfR4 subunits. All three RNR subunits exist in a native enzyme complex of $\alpha_2\beta\beta'$ configuration *(41)*.

20.2.5 Glycosylphosphatidylinositol Protein Anchors and P. falciparum Pathogenicity

Parasite glycosylphosphatidylinositols (GPIs) are a distinct class of glycolipids found ubiquitously in eukaryotic cells and implicated in several biological responses *(42–45)*. GPIs are particularly abundant in parasites, where they are found as free lipids and attached to proteins.

In intraerythrocytic *P. falciparum*, GPIs represent the major glycoconjugates, and their ability to induce proinflammatory cytokine responses in macrophages and endothelial cells is believed to contribute to malaria pathogenesis *(46–49)*. Several functionally important parasite proteins, including the merozoite surface proteins MSP-1, MSP-2, and MSP-4, are anchored to the cell membranes through GPI moieties *(50–52)*.

Parasite fractions enriched with GPIs have induced TNF-α and IL-1 release from macrophages *(42, 46)*. In mice, GPIs have caused transient pyrexia, hypoglycemia, lethal cachexia, and even death in *D*-galactosamine–sensitized animals *(46)*. The *P. falciparum* GPIs exert their toxic effects through the expression of TNF-α, IL-1, inducible nitric oxide synthase (iNOS), and endothelial cell adhesion molecules by activating nuclear factor κB transcription factors *(47–49)*.

As *P. falciparum*–infected erythrocytes are sequestered in specific organs, the local high concentrations of toxic responses to the parasite GPIs can affect vital physiologic functions and cause severe illness. However, antagonists of GPI-mediated signaling and monoclonal antibody against *P. falciparum* GPIs can block the induction of toxic responses *(47–49)*, suggesting that GPI-based therapy is possible. Thus, adults who have shown resistance to clinical malaria presented with high levels of persistent anti-GPI antibodies,

whereas susceptible children lack or have low levels of short-lived antibody response. Individuals who were not exposed to the malaria parasite completely lack anti-GPI antibodies and the absence of a persistent anti-GPI antibody response correlated with malaria-specific anemia and fever, suggesting that anti-GPI antibodies provide protection against clinical malaria. The antibodies were mainly directed against the acylated phosphoinositol portion of GPIs *(42)*.

The elucidation of the complete structures of the *P. falciparum* GPIs has been accomplished using a combination of direct biochemical analysis and mass spectrometry. Two novel structural features were identified: the presence of palmitate and myristate on C-2 of the inositol moiety, and the presence of predominately oleic and minor amounts of *cis*-vaccenic acid and C-18:2 at the *sn*-2 position *(42)*.

20.2.6 P. falciparum Genome Sequence

After an international effort was launched in 1996, the genome sequence of *P. falciparum* clone 3D7 was determined, and all information, including description of chromosome structure, gene content, functional classification of proteins, metabolism and transport, as well as other features of parasite biology, was published in 2002 *(53)*.

The 22.8-megabase nuclear genome, which consists of 14 chromosomes and encodes about 5,300 genes, is the most (A + T)-rich genome sequenced to date—overall at 80.6% and rising to ~90% in introns and intergenic regions. Genes involved in antigenic variation were found to be concentrated in the subtelomeric regions of the chromosomes. When compared with the genomes of free-living eukaryotic microorganisms, the genome of *P. falciparum* encoded fewer enzymes and transporters, but a large number of genes were devoted to immune evasion and host-parasite interactions. Many nuclear-encoded proteins are targeted to the apicoplast, an organelle involved in fatty-acid and isoprenoid metabolism *(4, 53, 54)*.

Unlike many other eukaryotes, the genome of *P. falciparum* did not contain long tandemly repeated arrays of ribosomal RNA (rRNA) genes. Instead, the malaria parasite contained several single 18S-5.8S-28S rRNA distributed on different chromosomes. The two types of rRNA genes were the S-type, expressed primarily in the mosquito vector, and the A-type, expressed primarily in the human host.

Furthermore, the sequence encoded by a rRNA gene in one unit differed from the sequence of the corresponding rRNA in the other units, and the expression of each rRNA unit was developmentally regulated, resulting in the expression of a different set of rRNA at different stages of the parasite life cycle *(53)*.

The parasite chromosomes varied considerably in length, with most of the variations occurring in the subtelomeric regions where the chromosomes displayed a striking degree of conservation—probably due to promiscuous interchromosomal exchange of subtelomeric regions.

20.3 Human Malaria and Inherited Hemoglobin Abnormalities

The progression to disease and sometimes death from malaria is determined by several factors, including the level of host immunity, the innate resistance characteristics of the host, and the virulence of the infected parasites *(55)*. Innate host resistance is manifested, for example, by (i) inherited red blood cell (RBC) characteristics, such as the Duffy blood group determinant Fy^{a}Fy^b that renders the RBCs resistant to invasion by *Plasmodium vivax*; (ii) alterations in the erythrocyte membrane, as in ovalocytosis; (iii) deficiency in glucose-6-phosphate dehydrogenase; or (iv) abnormalities of the hemoglobin composition as in thalassemia or sickle-cell trait. A hypothesis was proposed as far back as the 1940s *(56)* that the high gene frequencies of hemoglobinopathies in malaria-endemic regions may have resulted from protection conferred against malaria; *that is to say that several hereditary factors have been subject to natural selection of the relative resistance they confer against malaria.*

This "malaria hypothesis" has been verified for carriers of the sickle-cell trait (hemoglobin [Hb] type AS), who have been less likely to experience severe, potentially fatal, malaria *(55–59)*.

The overall result has been the establishment of an equilibrium or "balanced polymorphism" in which the homozygote hematologic disadvantage was balanced by the heterozygote advantage of protection from malaria. For example, point mutations in the hemoglobin β chain have been responsible for some of the best known of these polymorphisms, including sickle hemoglobin S (HbS), hemoglobin C (HbC), and hemoglobin E (HbE) *(57)*. Other genetic mutations cause underproduction of the α- and β-chains of hemoglobin and have been responsible for the thalassemias *(60)*.

The geographic distributions of these various hemoglobinopathies generally favor areas where *strong natural selection* has been present from the morbidity and mortality from malaria. Thus, hemoglobin E, resulting from a single point mutation (Glu→Lys) at codon 26 of the β-globin gene, is common in Southeast Asia (Thailand, Laos, Myanmar) *(61–63)*.

It has been suggested that an impaired antioxidant defense may account for the persistence of the hemoglobin E gene in areas where malaria is endemic *(64)*.

Moreover, a high-resolution linkage disequilibrium (LD) map across the human genome can detect recent variants that have been subjected to positive selection. To examine the effects of natural selection on the pattern of linkage disequilibrium and to infer the evolutionary history of the HbE variant, biallelic markers surrounding the HbE variant have been analyzed in a Thai population *(65)*. The results of the study supported the conjecture that the HbE mutation occurred recently, and the allele frequency has increased rapidly.

Early Studies. Although early laboratory studies suggested that hemoglobin E (HbE) retarded the intraerythrocytic growth of *P. falciparum* *(66)*, subsequent investigations have yielded conflicting results *(67)*. Cross-sectional epidemiologic studies have also given contradictory results *(68, 69)*, although these were focused on risk of infection and not on severity of disease. However, in a later hospital-based study in Thailand, the presence of HbE trait (HbAE) was associated with reduced disease severity in acute *P. falciparum* malaria *(70)*.

20.3.1 Mechanisms of Malaria Protection by Hemoglobin Abnormalities

The mechanisms underlying malaria protection by the genetic RBC variants have been studied extensively and can be classified into several broad groups: (i) reduced probability of merozoite invasion into variant RBCs; (ii) impairment of parasite growth within the variant RBCs; (iii) enhanced removal of the parasitized variant RBCs; and (iv) enhanced probability of infection early in life, particularly with *P. vivax*, which protects against subsequent severe *P. falciparum* malaria *(55, 71)*. However, despite considerable research, the relative roles of these processes and the cellular mechanisms that mediate resistance of many of these genetic RBC variants to malaria parasites still remain unclear. Thus, recent results from a study on two hemoglobinopathies frequently occurring in sub-Saharan Africa, sickle hemoglobin (HbS) and α$^+$-thalassemia (a condition characterized by reduced production of the normal α-globin component of hemoglobin), have provided evidence that negative epistasis between them profoundly affected their prevalence. For example, individually each HbS and α$^+$-thalassemia is protective against severe *P. falciparum* malaria; however, malaria protection from these two hemoglobinopathies seemed to be suppressed when they were present (inherited) together, so that children who inherit both of them were at the same risk of malaria as children who inherit neither *(72)*. It is clear that HbS and α$^+$-thalassemia—two of the most common human genetic polymorphisms conferring protection against malaria—when present together may interfere with each other, thus raising questions about their mechanisms of protection.

There have been other examples where it has proved difficult to explain how exactly protective mechanisms operate. For instance:

(i) how erythrocytes containing sickle cell hemoglobin (HbS) retard parasite maturation and thus reduce multiplication *(73–75)*;

(ii) why *P. falciparum* grows slowly in homozygous HbE RBCs, but not in heterozygous RBCs *(66, 76)*;

(iii) why in hereditary ovalocytosis, there is both increased membrane rigidity and a hostile intraerythrocytic milieu *(77)*;

(iv) why the increased amount of hemoglobin F (HbF) present in patients with some hemoglobinopathies is also associated with impaired malaria parasite growth *(78–80)*.

Some studies *(81, 82)*, but not others *(83)*, have shown greatly reduced cytoadherence and rosette formation by α- and β-thalassemic RBCs infected with *P. falciparum*. Other studies *(84, 85)* have demonstrated that α- and β-thalassemic RBCs preferentially bind surface antibody, which would be expected to enhance their clearance. There is also evidence for enhanced immune clearance in sickle cell trait *(86)*. However, epidemiologic studies *(71)* in the South Pacific nation of Vanuatu provided a new twist in this subject—children with α-thalassemia had more malaria in the first years of life compared with children who had normal hemoglobin types. Because infection with *P. vivax* is more common in the region, it has been suggested that co-infection or previous infection with this parasite might have attenuated the severity of the more virulent *P. falciparum*. Thus, it is still uncertain whether α-thalassemic RBCs facilitate or inhibit parasite invasion or multiplication *(55)*.

20.3.2 Hemoglobin Polymorphism: Heterozygous Versus Homozygous State

The HbS mutation (β6 Glu→Val in the gene encoding the β-chain on chromosome 11) was the first point mutation to be associated with malaria protection *(87)*. It is nearly a textbook example of balanced polymorphism, where fatalities from the sickle cell condition in HbS homozygotes have been offset by the survival advantage of HbAS (sickle trait) heterozygotes with malaria over HbAA homozygotes with malaria *(57)*. HbS frequencies of 15% or more occur in regions of India and Africa *(88)*.

The α-thalassemia conditions are the result of genetic mutations that reduce (α^+) or abolish (α^0) the production of α-globin chains from a pair of nearly identical genes on chromosome 16 *(57)*. The most common of these conditions are

forms of α^+-thalassemia that result from a crossover event and loss of one α-chain gene from the chromosome *(60)*. Inherited states of α^+-thalassemia can therefore be "heterozygous" when one parental chromosome is lacking an α gene (-α/αα, a three-gene "silent carrier") or "homozygous" when both parental chromosomes are lacking an α gene (-α/- α, a two-gene "trait" state also known as α-thalassemia minor) *(57)*. Heterozygous α^+-thalassemia lacks clinical features, whereas homozygous α^+-thalassemia results in a mild microcytic anemia. Both states are associated with protection against malaria, with the homozygous state probably offering greater protection than does the heterozygous state *(89–91)*. The α^+-thalassemia deletions are widespread, usually exceeding 10% in regions affected by malaria and approaching fixation in some regions of Nepal, India, and Papua New Guinea *(92)*.

20.3.3 Recent Scientific Advances

● *Hemoglobin E: A Balanced Polymorphism Protective Against Severe P. falciparum.* The malaria protective effects of hemoglobin E (HbE), prevalent in Southeast Asia (Thailand), were studied *in vitro* in a mixed erythrocyte invasion assay *(55)*. Starting at 1% parasitemia, *P. falciparum* invaded preferentially normal (HbAA) compared with abnormal hemoglobin [HbH disease, HbE heterozygote HbE trait (HbAE), HbE homozygote (HbEE), HbHCS (Constant Spring), β-thalassemia E] red blood cells (HRBCs). The heterozygote AE cells differed markedly from all other cells tested. Despite their microcytosis, AE cells were functionally relatively normal in contrast with the RBCs from other hemoglobulinopathies studied. These findings suggested that HbAE erythrocytes have an unidentified membrane abnormality that renders the majority of the RBC population relatively resistant to invasion by *P. falciparum*. Although this would not protect from uncomplicated malaria infections, it would prevent the development of heavy parasite burdens and is consistent with the "Haldane" hypothesis that hemoglobin E provides heterozygote protection against severe malaria *(55, 56)*.

● *Hemoglobin C: Resistance to Severe Malaria in Children.* Although hemoglobin (Hb) C has been reported to protect against severe malaria, it was not clear whether the relative resistance affected infection, disease, or both. As with HbS, an amino acid substitution ($\alpha_2\beta_2$ 6Glu→Lys) in adult HbA forms the underlying disorder of HbC. In a case-controlled study in Ghana of children with severe malaria, asymptomatic parasitemic children, and healthy children, HbAC did not prevent infection but reduced the possibility of developing severe malaria and severe anemia *(58)*. Protection was stronger for carriers of the sickle-cell trait (hemoglobin type AS; HbAS). The frequencies of HbCC and HbSC decreased from healthy children to asymptomatic parasitemic children to children with severe malaria. These data support the notion that natural selection of HbC occurs because of the relative resistance it confers against severe malaria but argues against the notion that HbC offers resistance to infection *(58)*.

- *Hemoglobin C: Reduced P. falciparum Parasitemia and Low Risk of Mild Malaria Attack.* In a longitudinal study of families living in an endemic urban area in Burkina Faso, the association of hemoglobin C (HbC) with reduced *P. falciparum* parasitemia and low risk of mild malaria attack was investigated during a 2-year period *(93)*. HbC carriers had less frequent malaria attacks than did AA individuals within the same age group, as well as HbC-reduced parasitemia.

- *Aberrant Development of P. falciparum in Hemoglobin CC.* Although selection of hemoglobin C (HbC) by malaria was reported long ago, only recently the reduced risk of malaria associated with the homozygous CC state has been attributed to the inability of CC (HbCC-homozygous state) cells to support parasite multiplication *in vitro*. When *P. falciparum* growth in CC cells was investigated *in vitro*, the experimental results have shown that the multiplication rate of several lines of the parasite was measurable in CC cells, but lower than that in AA (HbA-normal) cells *(94)*. A high proportion of rings formed and trophozoites disintegrated within a subset of CC cells—an observation that accounted for the lower replication rate. In addition, knobs present on the surface of infected CC cells were fewer and morphologically aberrant compared with those on AA cells.

- *Hemoglobin E-β-Thalassemia.* Hemoglobin E (HbE)-β-thalassemia is the most common severe form of the disease in many Asian countries. In Thailand, for example, approximately 3,000 children are born with this condition annually, and there are about 100,000 patients in the population carrying this syndrome, with a life expectancy of about 30 years. Other counties in the region (Indonesia, Bangladesh, Vietnam, Cambodia, Laos, and Malaysia) have also been severely afflicted *(92)*. A long-term observational study of hemoglobin E-β-thalassemia in Sri Lanka has begun to define some of the genetic and environmental factors responsible for its remarkable phenotypic variability. Although the frequency of the deletion forms of α^+-thalassemia was too low to assess their contribution to phenotypic modification, a Hardy-Weinberg analysis indicated that α^+-thalassemia was underrepresented in the HbE-β-thalassemia population compared with those with β-thalassemia major or healthy individuals; this finding raised the possibility of a significant

ameliorating effect on the severity of the disease. The overall results have shown a very small difference between the steady-state hemoglobin levels between the mild and severe phenotypes, and it has been possible to stop blood transfusion in many of those who were on long-term treatment of that kind

20.4 Molecular Mechanisms of Virulence

Severe Malaria. At present, it is not clear whether there are polymorphisms that cause some *P. falciparum* parasites to be inherently more virulent than others. It is probable that the most common virulence polymorphisms that can be studied are targets of immunity, as balancing selection from the frequency-dependent acquired immune response would slow down or arrest fixation of optimally fit alleles *(95)*.

There is evidence to suggest differences in the infected erythrocyte *variable surface antigen (VSA)* repertoire expressed by parasites isolated from patients with severe and mild malaria, and also differences between infections from naïve and immune individuals *(96)*. It is proposed that VSA subsets causing most efficient cytoadhesion, rapid parasite replication, and higher virulence will predominate in the naïve host, but immunity to these can be gained after only a few selections (if the host survives), after which the VSAs expressed will be associated with a lower parasite replication rate and thus milder clinical infections.

However, it has not yet been possible to define VSA patterns that are reproducibly associated with severity of disease *(97, 98)*. Although the *var* gene family is very diverse *(99)*, the genes can be clustered into different groups, with one classification system identifying major groups A to E based on the arrangement and number of Duffy binding-like (DBL) domains *(100)* and another based on the comparative sequence analysis of a region of the *N*-terminal DBL domain (DBL-1α) that is contained in most *var* genes *(97)*.

Variation among *P. falciparum* genotypes in intrinsic replication rate in the blood *(101)* is likely to be due in part to efficiency of the erythrocyte invasion mediated by alternative receptor usage *(95)*.

Isolates of *P. falciparum* have shown a broad range of erythrocyte invasion phenotypes (defined as reliance on different erythrocyte receptors that have distinct susceptibility to proteolytic enzymes and neuraminidase) in culture invasion assays, with those samples from single areas of endemicity showing as great a range of phenotypes as those from diverse geographic sources *(102–104)*.

The whole transcript profile of isolates may be assayed using microarray methodology. Technical methods for analysis of clinical isolates have been established that were sensitive enough *(105)*, and a small number of isolates analyzed from patients in Senegal have been compared with cultured isolate 3D7, demonstrating a significant excess in the expression of surface protein gene transcripts in the clinical isolates *(106)*. It may be that a small subset of these surface protein genes are overexpressed in severe malaria isolates compared with mild malaria controls (or in cerebral malaria compared with other presentations such as severe malarial anemia), and that identification of these would define clinically important virulence factors *(95)*.

Placental Malaria. Placental *P. falciparum* infection during pregnancy causes a substantial risk of miscarriage or poor birth outcome. The enhanced infection of the placenta is largely due to a variant ligand on the *P. falciparum*–infected erythrocyte that binds to chondroitin sulfate A on the placental capillary endothelia *(107)*, with some evidence that a secondary ligand may bind to hyaluronic acid *(108)*. There has been substantial evidence to indicate that the product of a particular *P. falciparum var* gene (*var2csa*) that encoded a variant of PfEMP1 was responsible *(109, 110)* and was expressed at high levels in most infections of pregnant women *(111, 112)*, but only occasionally in infections in others *(112)*.

Infected pregnant women can make antibodies against pregnancy-associated malaria (PAM)-specific parasite molecules, of which the response to the *var2csa*-encoded PfEMP1 appeared to be the most important, as it can block adhesion of these parasites to chondroitin sulfate A *(95)*. The presence of such antibodies has been associated with better pregnancy outcome, such as higher birth weight *(113)*. The specificity of the PAM-associated antigenic targets has been emphasized by the observation that the presence of antibodies to other (non–PAM-associated) VSAs did not correlate with improved birth outcome *(113)*.

20.5   Human Malaria: Clinical Manifestations

Diagnosis of Malaria. Light microscopy of thick and thin stained blood smears remains the standard method for diagnosing malaria *(114)*. Thick smears are 20 to 40 times more sensitive than thin smears for screening malarial parasites, with a detection limit of 10 to 50 trophozoites/μL. Thin smears allow for identification of malaria species (including diagnosis of mixed infections), quantifying parasitemia, and assessment for the presence of schizonts, gametocytes, and malarial pigment in neutrophils and monocytes.

However, important advances have been made to allow new diagnostic techniques (fluorescence microscopy of parasite nuclei stained with acridine orange, rapid dipstick immunoassay, and polymerase chain reaction) to be used, with the sensitivity and specificity of some of them approaching or even surpassing the thin and thick smear technique *(115)*.

20.5.1 Plasmodium Gametocyte Pathology

There was a linear relation between the probability of observing gametocytes on the blood smear and the degree of anemia. The peak gametocyte count and the duration of gametocyte carriage were also negatively correlated with hemoglobin concentrations. The relation between anemia and gametocyte carriage has also been observed recently on the western border of Thailand and was construed as a reflection of a longer duration of the malarial episode *(116)*. At comparable hemoglobin concentrations, male mosquitoes are more likely to carry gametocytes, and for longer times. The affinity of hemoglobin for oxygen is lower in female mosquitoes than in males *(117)*, and this may also influence the prevalence of gametocyte carriage in males.

One of the main consequences of acute anemia is reduced oxygenation of tissue. In response to hypoxia, erythropoietin will stimulate erythropoiesis, and the concentration of 2,3-diphosphoglycerate (2,3-DGP) will increase, thus reducing the affinity of hemoglobin for oxygen and facilitating the transfer of oxygen to the tissues *(118)*.

The oxyhemoglobin disassociation curve in patients with chronic anemias will shift to the right, facilitating the release of oxygen in the tissues. However, in cases of acute decrease of hemoglobin concentrations, the adaptive capacity will be reduced *(118, 119)*. During malaria, the reduction in oxygen transport capacity via hypochromia may have overwhelmed the adaptive mechanisms in patients who were likely to have preexisting anemia and major hypoxia. The fact that patients with HbE polymorphism (see Section 20.3) were less likely to carry gametocytes might seem to conflict with this notion. However, differences in affinity of abnormal hemoglobins, such as HbE for oxygen *(118, 119)*, may explain these differences. Moreover, these findings also suggest that reticulocytosis was not the primary reason for gametocytogenesis because HbE patients would be expected to have higher reticulocyte counts than would non-HbE patients with microcytic hypochromic anemia *(118)*.

Increased parasitemia and duration of the malarial episode were associated with an increased frequency of gametocyte carriage *(116)*. The presence of peripheral schizonts, reflecting the sequestration potential and a high parasite biomass *(120)*, was also associated with increased gametocyte carriage.

As the affinity of hemoglobin for oxygen decreases during hypoxia, free nitric oxide (NO) radicals are released *(121, 122)*, thus leading to the notion that stress reticulocytes may be vital for the parasite to continue gametocytogenesis *(118, 123, 124)* because of the increased affinity of hemoglobin for oxygen and greater NO scavenging potential *(121, 122)*. This may then explain the preference of *P. falciparum* for young erythrocytes *(125, 126)*.

These and other studies *(114, 115)* suggested that because of increased gametocyte counts and gametocyte carriage, anemic patients may be greater sources of transmission. The age-structured epidemiology of anemias could partly explain why children are frequent gametocyte carriers.

20.5.2   Signs and Symptoms of Malaria

In nonimmune individuals with *P. falciparum* infection, the median *pre-patent period* (time from sporozoite inoculation to detectable parasitemia) is 5 to 10 days, and the median *incubation period* (time from sporozoite inoculation to development of symptoms) is 6 to 14 days; depending on the level of acquired immunity from previous exposure, antimalarial prophylaxis, or prior partial treatment (which may mitigate but not prevent disease), the incubation period may be prolonged significantly *(3)*.

Most nonimmune travelers will develop symptoms of falciparum malaria within 1 month after departing from a malaria-endemic area (median 10 days); however, there have been reports of falciparum malaria presenting up to 4 years later *(127)*.

For non-falciparum malaria, the inoculation period is usually longer (median 15 to 16 days), and both *P. vivax* and *P. ovale* malaria may relapse months or even years after exposure due to the presence of hypnozoites in the liver. The longest reported incubation period for *P. vivax* was 30 years *(127)*.

The clinical symptoms of malaria are primarily due to schizont rupture and destruction of erythrocytes, and the disease may present either as gradual illness or a fulminant infection with nonspecific symptoms *(3)*.

Generally, a malarial infection is characterized by recurrent attacks of moderate to severe shaking chills, high fever, profuse sweating (diaphoresis) as body temperature falls, and a general feeling of unease and discomfort (malaise). Other symptoms include headache, nausea, vomiting, abdominal pain, myalgia, dizziness, dry cough, and diarrhea *(128)*. Physical signs include tachycardia, jaundice, pallor, orthostatic hypotension, hepatomegaly, and splenomegaly.

Clinical examination in nonimmune persons may be completely unremarkable, even without fever *(3)*.

20.5.3   Severe Malaria

Nearly all severe forms and deaths from malaria are caused by *P. falciparum*. Rarely, *P. vivax* or *P. ovale* may produce serious complications, debilitating relapses, and even death *(128, 129)*. In 1990, the World Health Organization (WHO)

established criteria for severe malaria to assist future clinical and epidemiologic studies *(130)*. In 2000, WHO revised these criteria to include other clinical manifestations and laboratory values that portend a poor prognosis based on clinical experience in semi-immune patients *(130)*.

Severe malaria may develop even after response to initial treatment and complete clearance of parasitemia, due to delayed cytokine release.

Patients who develop severe malaria should be treated aggressively with parenteral antimalarial therapy. Oral medications (quinine, chloroquine, or mefloquine) are not recommended for initial treatment *(130)*.

20.5.3.1   Complications in Severe Malaria

If clinical deterioration to severe malaria occurs, it usually develops in 3 to 7 days after onset of fever, although there have been rare reports of nonimmune patients dying within 24 hours of developing symptoms *(3)*.

Cerebral Malaria. This is the most common clinical presentation and cause of death in adults with severe malaria. The onset of cerebral malaria may be dramatic, with generalized convulsion, or gradual, with initial drowsiness and confusion, followed by coma lasting from several hours to several days. Apart from cerebral malaria, other neurologic sequelae can also occur, including cranial nerve abnormalities, extrapyramidal tremor, and ataxia. The mortality from cerebral malaria ranges from 10% to 50% with treatment *(3)*. Most survivors (>97% adults and >90% children) have shown no neurologic abnormalities after recovery *(131)*.

Pulmonary Complications. Acute lung injury usually occurs a few days into the disease course. It may develop rapidly, even after initial response to antimalarial treatment and clearance of parasitemia. The first indications of impending pulmonary edema include tachypnea and dyspnea, followed by hypoxemia and respiratory failure requiring intubation *(3)*. Noncardiogenic pulmonary edema rarely occurs with *P. vivax* and *P. ovale* malaria.

Renal Complications. Acute renal failure in severe malaria is usually oliguric (<400 mL urine/day) or anuric (<100 mL urine/day), rarely nonoliguric, and may require temporary dialysis. In severe cases, acute tubular necrosis may develop secondary to renal ischemia *(132)*. The term *blackwater fever* refers to passage of dark red, brown, or black urine secondary to massive intravascular hemolysis and resulting hemoglobinuria. Usually, this condition is transient and not accompanied by renal failure *(3)*.

Hypoglycemia. Hypoglycemia is a common feature in patients with severe malaria. This condition may be the result of quinine- or quinidine-induced hyperinsulinemia, but it may be found also in patients with normal insulin levels *(3)*.

Hypotension and Shock. Most patients with shock exhibit a low peripheral vascular resistance and elevated cardiac output. Severe hypotension can develop suddenly, usually with pulmonary edema, metabolic acidosis, sepsis, and/or massive hemorrhage due to rupture of the spleen or from the gastrointestinal tract *(3)*.

Hematologic Abnormalities. Severe anemia is more common in children in highly endemic areas as a result of repeated or chronic *Plasmodium* infections. Thrombocytopenia is common but usually not associated with bleeding *(3)*.

20.6 Treatment of Malaria

Treatment for malaria should not be initiated until the diagnosis has been confirmed by laboratory investigations. Presumptive treatment without the benefit of laboratory confirmation should be reserved for extreme circumstances. Once the diagnosis of malaria is made, the treatment should be guided by three main factors: the infecting *Plasmodium* species, the clinical status of the patient, and the drug susceptibility of the infecting parasites as determined by the geographic area where the infection was acquired (http://www.cdc.gov/malaria/diagnosis/treatment/clinicians2.htm).

Determination of the infecting *Plasmodium* species for treatment purposes is important for three major reasons:

(i)   *P. falciparum* infections can cause rapidly progressive severe illness or death, whereas the non-falciparum (*P. vivax*, *P. ovale*, or *P. malariae*) species rarely cause severe manifestations.

(ii) *P. vivax* and *P. ovale* infections require treatment for the hypnozoite forms that remain dormant in the liver and can cause a relapsing infection.

(iii) *P. falciparum* and *P. vivax* species have different drug resistance patterns in different geographic regions. For *P. falciparum* infections, the urgent initiation of appropriate therapy is especially critical.

The second factor affecting treatment is the clinical status of the patient. Patients diagnosed with malaria are generally categorized as having either uncomplicated or severe malaria. Patients diagnosed with uncomplicated malaria can be effectively treated with oral antimalarial drugs.

The third factor, knowledge of the geographic area where the infection was acquired, provides information on the likelihood of drug resistance of the infecting parasites and enables the treating clinician to choose an appropriate drug or drug combination and treatment course (http://www.cdc.gov/malaria/diagnosis/treatment/clinicians2.htm).

For recent systematic reviews on the treatment of malaria, see Refs. *(133)* and *(134)*, as well as the following Web sites:

- Centers for Disease Control and Prevention (CDC), National Center for Infectious Diseases: http://www.cdc.gov/travel
- World Health Organization (WHO): http://www.who.int/health_topics/malaria
- Health Canada, Population and Public Health Branch: http://www.TravelHealth.gc.ca
- Public Health Laboratory Service, Malaria Reference Laboratory at the London School of Hygiene and Tropical Medicine, UK: http://www.malaria-references.co.uk
- Swiss Tropical Institute, Switzerland: http://www.sti.ch
- Safe Travel: http://www.safe travel.ch
- International Society of Travel Medicine: http://www.istm.org
- Malaria Foundation International: http://www.malaria.org

20.6.1 Antimalarial Chemotherapy

Malaria infections, particularly with *P. falciparum*, require prompt evaluation and treatment. In most cases, the disease is treated effectively with one or more of the following medications:

- Chloroquine (Aralen)
- Quinine sulfate
- Combination of sulfadoxine and pyrimethamine (Fansidar)
- Mefloquine (Lariam)
- Combination of atovaquone and proguanil (Malarone)
- Doxycycline (Doryx, Vibramycin, others)
- Artemisinin and its congeners such as artesunate

In addition, several other drugs have found use as antimalarials, including halofantrine and primaquine.

Halofantrine, which is not marketed in the United States, is contraindicated in patients with heart problems and already on mefloquine medication; the use of halofantrine can cause death.

Primaquine may be given against the dormant liver form of the parasite and prevent relapses. However, the CDC has issued a warning that primaquine not be taken by pregnant women or patients having glucose-6-phosphate dehydrogenase (G6PD) enzyme deficiency.

Quinine and Quinidine. Intravenous quinine (usually as its HCl salt) is currently the most widely used antimalarial agent, especially in the treatment of severe falciparum malaria *(3)*. In the United States, quinidine gluconate (the dextrorotatory optical diastereoisomer of quinine) is the only available intravenous antimalarial and is used instead of quinine *(135)*. Although quinidine is two- to threefold more active than quinine, it is also more cardiotoxic *(136)*. Side effects of both quinine and quinidine include cinchonism (bitter taste, dysphoria, tremor, tinnitus, reversible high-tone hearing loss, headache, nausea, vomiting, and abnormal pain) or pruritus. In addition, both drugs have narrow therapeutic windows. Severe toxicities include cardiac arrhythmias, hypotension, blindness, deafness, and hyperinsulinemic hypoglycemia *(130, 137)*.

Artemisinin Derivatives. Artemisinin is the sweet wormwood extract, initially used as an antimalarial agent in Asia, but now used also in other parts of the world. Although artemisinin and its derivatives clear plasmodia parasites from blood 20% faster than does quinine dihydrochloride, improved survival was observed only in patients in Southeast Asia with recognized quinine resistance *(138)*. Furthermore, recovery from coma may be delayed and the incidence of seizures was higher than that with quinine·2HCl *(130, 139, 140)*.

At present, artemisinin derivatives are recommended for treatment of quinine-resistant falciparum malaria, combined with mefloquine, doxycycline, or clindamycin to prevent recrudescence (see the new WHO Guidelines in Section 20.6.4 and Ref. *(141)*.

There are four artemisinin formulations: dihydroartemisinin, artesunate (a water-soluble compound for intramuscular injection), arteether, and artemether (an oil-soluble compound for intravenous administration). Artesunate and artemether are metabolized to the biologically active metabolite dihydroartemisinin. The artemisinin derivatives are well tolerated. Side effects include nausea, vomiting, pruritus, and fever; bleeding and cardiac arrhythmias rarely occur. Contrary to reports of brain-stem neurotoxicity with high doses in animal studies, this side effect has not been observed in humans to date *(3)*.

Artemisinin acts quickly in the bloodstream by rapidly clearing away parasites and helping to reduce disease transmission by decreasing the number of gametocytes, the infective stage of the parasite.

Chloroquine. Parenteral chloroquine is the drug of choice for severe chloroquine-susceptible falciparum malaria and for those rare cases of life-threatening malaria caused by other plasmodia (*P. vivax, P. ovale,* and *P. malariae*) in some specific regions of the world *(141)*. Chloroquine may be more rapid in lowering parasitemia than either quinine or quinidine, but it also has a more profound hypotensive side effect *(142)*. It has been recommended that it be given by a controlled intravenous infusion with a loading dose of 10 mg/kg base over 8 hours, followed immediately by a maintenance dose of 15 mg/kg base infused over 24 hours *(3)*.

20.6.1.1 Antimalarial Drug Resistance

The history of antimalarial therapy has been marked by constantly evolving drug-resistant parasite strains *(143)*.

In certain regions of the world, for example, the use of chloroquine has been rendered completely ineffective. In another example, increased drug efflux is also a mechanism of chloroquine resistance in *Plasmodium falciparum (144–146)*.

To avoid the development of drug resistance, it is therefore strongly recommended that antimalarial therapies always comprise combinations of artemisinin derivatives with other companion drugs, such as lumefantrine, sulfadoxine-pyrimethamine, amodiaquine (a drug similar ot chloroquine), and mefloquine (see Section 20.6.2). One such drug combination, artesunate-amodiaquine Winthrop (ASAQ), became available in sub-Saharan Africa in 2007.

20.6.2 Uncomplicated Malaria

After initiation of treatment, the patient's clinical response should be monitored, as well as patient's parasitologic status, especially for drug resistance (decrease in parasite density and clearance).

P. falciparum or Species Not Identified. For falciparum infections acquired in areas without chloroquine-resistant strains (Central America west of the Panama Canal, Haiti, the Dominican Republic, and most of the Middle East), patients should be treated with oral chloroquine (http://www.cdc.gov/malaria/diagnosis/treatment/clinicians2.htm).

For falciparum infections acquired from chloroquine-resistant strains, three treatment options are available: (i) quinine sulfate plus doxycycline, tetracycline, or clindamycin; (ii) atovaquone-proguanil (Malarone); and (iii) mefloquine. Mefloquine is, however, associated with higher rate of severe neuropsychiatric reactions and should be used only when the first two options cannot be used. For pediatric patients, the treatment options are the same except at lower doses adjusted by the patient's weight but never exceeding adult doses (http://www.cdc.gov/malaria/ diagnosis/treatment/clinicians2.htm).

If infections initially attributed to "species not identified" are subsequently diagnosed as being due to *P. vivax* or *P. ovale*, additional treatment with primaquine should be administered (see below).

P. malariae. There has been no widespread evidence of chloroquine resistance in *P. malariae* species. Therefore, chloroquine remains the drug of choice for all *P. malariae* infections. As a second-line alternative for treatment, hydroxychloroquine may be given instead (http://www.cdc.gov/malaria/diagnosis/treatment/clinicians2.htm).

P. vivax and *P. ovale*. Chloroquine (or hydroxychloroquine as second-line alternative for treatment) remains the treatment of choice for all *P. vivax* and *P. ovale* infections except for *P. vivax* infections acquired in Papua New Guinea and Indonesia, where there have been published reports of high chloroquine resistance. Rare reports of chloroquine resistance have been reported in Myanmar, India, and South America. Two drug regimens equally effective for chloroquine-resistant *P. vivax* infections are quinine sulfate plus doxycycline or tetracycline, or mefloquine. There are no adequate reports and/or well-controlled studies to support the use of atovaquone-proguanil to treat chloroquine-resistant *P. vivax* infections (http://www. cdc.gov/malaria/diagnosis/treatment/clinicians2.htm).

In addition to requiring blood stage treatment, infections with *P. vivax* and *P. ovale* can relapse due to the presence of hypnozoites that remain dormant in the liver. To eradicate the hypnozoites, patients should be treated with a 14-day course of primaquine phosphate (30 mg base, orally). Accordingly, prior precautions should be taken, because primaquine can cause hemolytic anemia in persons with G6PD deficiency. Furthermore, primaquine must not be used during pregnancy.

For pediatric patients, the treatment options for *P. vivax* and *P. ovale* are the same as in adults except that the drug dose is adjusted by patient weight and must never exceed the adult dose regimens (http://www.cdc.gov/malaria/diagnosis/treatment/clinicians2.htm).

Alternative Treatments During Pregnancy. Malaria infections in pregnant women are associated with high risk of both maternal and perinatal morbidity and mortality likely due to a reduced immune response to malaria infections. Malaria infections during pregnancy can lead to miscarriage, premature delivery, low birth weight, and/or perinatal death (http://www.cdc.gov/malaria/diagnosis/ treatment/clinicians3.htm).

For pregnant women diagnosed with uncomplicated malaria caused by *P. malariae*, *P. vivax*, *P. ovale*, or chloroquine-sensitive falciparum infection, prompt treatment with chloroquine is recommended as scheduled for nonpregnant adult patients. As a second-line alternative for treatment, hydroxychloroquine may be given instead. For pregnant women diagnosed with uncomplicated malaria caused by chloroquine-resistant falciparum infection, prompt treatment with quinine sulfate and clindamycin is recommended (http://www.cdc.gov/malaria/diagnosis/treatment/clinicians3.htm).

Doxycycline and tetracycline are generally not indicated for use in pregnant women. Atovaquone-proguanil and mefloquine (both pregnancy category C medications) are generally not recommended for use in pregnancy unless in uncomplicated cases of chloroquine-resistant falciparum infection, if other options are not available or not tolerated (http://www.cdc.gov/malaria/diagnosis/treatment/clinicians3.htm).

For *P. vivax* or *P. ovale* infections, primaquine phosphate for radical treatment of hypnozoites should not be given during pregnancy.

In general, pregnant patients with *P. vivax* or *P. ovale* infections should be maintained on chloroquine prophylaxis for the duration of their pregnancy; after pregnancy those who do not have G6PD deficiency should be treated with primaquine.

20.6.3   Severe Malaria

Parenteral Antimalarial Therapy. Since 1991, quinidine gluconate has been the only parenterally administered antimalarial drug available in the United States *(147)*. Quinidine levels should be maintained in the range of 3 to 8 mg/L *(*Ref. *136,* and Tables 1 and 2 in Ref. *3)* (http://www.cdc.gov/malaria/diagnosis/treatment/ clinicians3.htm). Parenteral quinidine gluconate is cardiotoxic and should be administered in an intensive care setting with continuous cardiac and blood pressure monitoring *(130, 148)*.

While *exchange blood transfusion (EBT) and erythrocytapheresis (red cell exchange)* have not been adequately proven beneficial in randomized clinical trials, the CDC has recommended that EBT be strongly considered for patients with a parasite density of more than 10% or if complications such as cerebral malaria, non–volume overload pulmonary edema, or renal complications exist. The parasite density should be monitored until it falls below 1%, which usually requires the exchange of 8 to 10 units of blood *(149)* (http://www.cdc.gov/malaria/diagnosis/treatment/clinicians3.htm).

Therapy with monoclonal antibodies against TNF-α has shortened the duration of fever, but had no impact on mortality in patients with severe and/or complicated malaria *(150)*, and may increase morbidity due to neurologic sequelae *(3)*.

Although corticosteroids (dexamethasone) have been used in the past to treat patients with cerebral malaria, a controlled trial has shown that they are harmful by prolonging the duration of coma *(151)*.

Oral Medication. When patients with severe falciparum malaria show significant clinical improvement (after at least 24 hours of parenteral therapy) and can tolerate tablets, they should be switched to oral medication (see Table 3 in Ref. *3*). The choice of oral antimalarial drugs should be guided by the susceptibility pattern of the plasmodia. Combined regimens, such as artemether-lumefantrine or atovaquone-proguanil, are associated with lower risk for the development of drug resistance than are mefloquine or quinine *(3)*.

20.6.4   The New WHO Guidelines for Malaria Treatment

Since April 2001, WHO has recommended the use of artemisinin-based combination therapies (ACTs) in countries where *P. falciparum* malaria is resistant to chloroquine, sulfadoxine-pyrimethamine, and amodiaquine therapies. Although at present 60 countries have adopted ACTs, as recommended by WHO, and 33 are deploying ACTs in the general health services, the private sector markets in endemic countries have recommended the use of artemisinin derivatives—*mainly as monotherapies at lower prices than ACTs.*

The increasing consumption of artemisinin monotherapies in the private sector, if unabated, will produce resistance to artemisinin and compromise the effectiveness of ACTs.

Thus, in April 2006, WHO issued the new guidelines for the treatment of malaria by requesting the pharmaceutical companies to end the marketing and sale of "single-drug" artemisinin malaria medicines in order to prevent malaria parasites from developing resistance to this drug *(141).*

When used correctly in combination with other antimalarial drugs in the so-called ACTs, artemisinin is nearly 95% effective in curing malaria and the parasite is highly unlikely to become resistant.

Currently, the ACTs are the most effective medicines available to treat malaria. According to the new WHO guidelines, uncomplicated falciparum malaria *must* be treated with ACTs rather than by artemisinin alone or any other monotherapy because the use of a "single-drug" artemisinin treatment or monotherapy will hasten the development of resistance by weakening but not killing the parasite.

20.7   Vaccines Against Malaria

Over the past three decades, great strides have been made toward the development of a vaccine against malaria, which now seems to be a distinct possibility—despite the fact that malarial infection does not induce a solid immune protection against future exposure. However, even though natural infection will not produce complete immunity against the plasmodia, long-term exposure to malaria has been shown to induce partially protective immune responses to the disease, as documented by fewer and less dense parasitemias, a reduction in malaria-related illness, and antibody production against erythrocytic stage parasites.

In the early 1970s, the first report of human protection against malaria by vaccination was published *(152).* The vaccination consisted of the bites of about a thousand mosquitoes infected with malaria parasites that had been x-irradiated *(153).* However, the irradiated sporozoites had to be delivered through irradiated, infected mosquitoes, which was impractical and too expensive for widespread use. During the next 20 years, progress toward the development of an antimalarial vaccine occurred mainly in experimental models rather than in human vaccine trials *(154).* Then, much speculation was generated by the SPf66 candidate vaccine, despite the uncertainty of how such a construct could work.

Eventually, Phase III clinical trials showed that Spf66 lacked efficacy *(155–160).* During this past decade, many candidate vaccines are being tested in clinical trials *(161).*

20.7.1   Concepts in Vaccine Development in Malaria

An ideal malaria vaccine will need to incorporate three essential features: (i) multiple components that will induce an effective immune response to the different stages of the malaria infection: sporozoites, infected hepatocytes, and the asexual and sexual erythrocytic stages; (ii) multivalence, containing multiple epitopes restricted by different MHC molecules in order to overcome genetic restriction and allelic and antigenic variations (problems existing in single-antigen-based vaccine); and (iii) multi-immunogenicity, inducing more than one type of immune response, including cell-mediated and humoral. Such a multicomponent vaccine would increase the probability of a more sustainable and effective host response *(162).*

In general, vaccine strategies in malaria may be classified into four major groups: (i) transmission-blocking vaccines; (ii) blood-stage (erythrocytic) vaccines; (iii) liver-stage (pre-erythrocytic) vaccines; and (iv) sexual-stage vaccines *(163).*

Transmission-blocking vaccines would not protect the recipient from contracting malaria, but could be helpful in preventing the spread of disease.

Most blood-stage vaccines are designed to elicit antibodies to merozoites (the blood-cell-infecting stage of plasmodia), because in humans with natural immunity such antibodies will protect from human illness. However, the variability of blood-stage antigens among parasite strains would complicate vaccine development *(163).*

Liver-stage vaccines are designed to prevent malaria but must be 100% effective in order to protect humans with no natural immunity. Such vaccines include those containing whole killed sporozoites and those based on antigenic portions of sporozoite proteins *(163).*

The sexual-stage parasite antigens are complex and have been difficult to produce.

Multistage vaccines are designed to target antigens from multiple stages of the plasmodia life cycle. However, although highly desirable, these vaccines are complicated and expensive to produce.

20.7.2   Definition of Malaria Vaccine Efficacy

With the expanding search for malaria vaccines, a few candidates have already been tested in Phase I/II clinical trials. However, it has been difficult to compare the results of these trials, because even independent trials of the same vaccine candidate will give highly discrepant results. One major obstacle to overcome in evaluating malaria vaccines is the difficulty of diagnosing clinical malaria. In this context, many aspects of vaccine trial design are important in ensuring reliable outcomes, but among the most critical are the choice of primary end points, and thereby, the definition of vaccine efficacy *(164)*. In practice, clinical end points will depend on three equally important components of malaria diagnosis: detection, quantification, and case definition.

Measuring Vaccine Efficacy. The malaria vaccine candidates are categorized by the stage of the parasite life cycle that they target, and that determines the end point that will be used to evaluate its efficacy (see Table 1 in Ref. *(164)*). At present, no currently studied malarial vaccine will induce complete protection against infection or clinical malaria, and the vaccine efficacy will reflect considerable underlying heterogeneity in individual protection and immune response to the vaccine, including the relative frequency of the specified disease event within an individual as well as within the population; and the continued occurrence of infections and symptoms in those successfully vaccinated, albeit less often and/or with less severity *(164)*.

Currently, the vaccine efficacy *is calculated as a ratio*, which leads to the common misconception that *uncertainty* (i.e., false positives or false negatives) *in the numerator and uncertainty in the denominator will cancel or balance*. In fact, however, this assumption will not reflect measurement error or other types of uncertainty that might be introduced during the trial. The effect of the uncertainty of the measurement technique on the reliability of calculations of vaccine efficacy has not been fully evaluated and must be properly incorporated *(164)*.

Detecting Malaria. When making measurements with categorical conclusions, such as the presence or absence of parasites, measurement uncertainty can decrease the sensitivity and specificity of the end point. Low sensitivity results in a misclassification of true positives and may arise as a result of measurement error or a case definition that is too stringent.

Moreover, false positives may be generated by measurement error or a case definition that is too inclusive. Specificity less than 100% can have a dramatic impact on the ability to accurately measure a vaccine's efficacy *(165)*.

In detecting malaria, classification of an individual as parasite-negative or -positive by microscopy is not a true binary measurement, because a parasite-negative slide is one that has a parasite density below the sensitivity, or limit of detection of microscopy *(164)*. The limit of detection (LOD) is operator-dependent but is also correlated with parasite density and has been shown to be highly variable at low densities *(165a)*. This would point to the difficulty of dealing with a source of uncertainty that scales directly with the success of the intervention: if vaccination reduces the parasite density, then the sensitivity will be lower in the vaccinated cohort *(164)*.

To further complicate interpretation of results, the specificity of malaria microscopy is also less than perfect, with rates of false positives reaching 24% *(166, 167)*.

Quantifying Malaria. Quantifying malaria by microscopy is a difficult task *(168)*, but the importance of this well-known fact is often overlooked *(160)*.

When comparing parasite densities in the vaccinated and control groups, uncertainty arising from quantification of the parasite density can be introduced directly into the calculation of the vaccine's efficacy. Thus, at intermediate efficacies (40% to 50%), a 3% to 4% uncertainty could obscure the differences between successive iterations of a vaccine over the course of its development, leading to unwarranted rejection or pursuit of a vaccine candidate *(164)*.

Factors other than measurement error can also contribute to uncertainty in measurements of parasite density, including the method by which parasites are counted using white blood cells as an index *(169)* and temporal fluctuation in parasite density in peripheral blood, which are common and which may have greater consequences for parasite density measurement than does the uncertainty associated with microscopic quantification.

Defining Malaria. In malaria-endemic areas with moderate to high transmission, the presence of parasites alone or parasites with fever are not adequate indicators of a clinical episode of malaria. Therefore, criteria must be chosen to define whether or not a patient is experiencing a clinical malaria episode *(164)*. This uncertainty in definition will undoubtedly lead to misclassification of cases, both false positives and false negatives, resulting in decreased sensitivity and specificity.

The fraction of parasitemic, symptomatic persons whose malaise is caused by plasmodia parasites is referred to as the *attributable fraction*. Most commonly, a logistic regression model is fit to the data *(170)* to describe the probability that a fever can be attributed to malaria at any density. Then, the overall attributable fraction is calculated by averaging this probability over all cases. The logistic regression model for determining the attributable fraction has been used to determine the sensitivity and specificity of case definitions in numerous epidemiologic settings *(164)*.

Once a threshold density has been chosen to define a clinical episode of malaria, the effect of measurement uncertainty inherent in detecting and quantifying the infection can be evaluated. As expected, the vaccine efficacy increases with increasing threshold density and, therefore, increasing specificity of the case definition *(164)*.

20.7.3 Attenuated Sporozoite Vaccines

Although immunization experiments with irradiated sporozoites have consistently provided solid and sterile immunity in experimental animal models *(171)* and human volunteers *(153)*, the development of whole sporozoite vaccines was abandoned because it was impractical and expensive. However, with the advances in recombinant DNA technology, there has been renewed interest in protective recombinant subunit vaccines. Hence, attenuated sporozoites are receiving attention—technological advances in culturing *P. falciparum in vitro* and the transfection have made it possible to produce irradiated or transgenic sporozoites *(172, 173)*.

Radiation-Attenuated Sporozoites (RAS). Sporozoites are irradiated when infected mosquitoes are subjected to irradiation. Like normal sporozoites, after inoculation into a susceptible host, the irradiated sporozoites penetrate the hepatocytes and begin intracellular development *(174)*. However, unlike their normal counterparts, the irradiated sporozoites are not capable of nuclear division and do not develop further, but persist for several weeks or months *(153)*. It is this prolonged stay in the liver and the state of the sporozoites that would result in the stimulation of protective immune responses mediated by cytotoxic CD8$^+$ T-lymphocytes and antibodies, which target infected hepatocytes and sporozoite surface proteins, respectively. Although, on balance, the whole organism sporozoite vaccine looks promising, there are technical and safety concerns that need to be addressed. These include mass production of sterile parasites, proper storage by cryopreservation to maintain low infectivity and high immunogenicity, the correct irradiation dosage, and the safety of a mosquito-derived vaccine with the risk of co-administration of unknown pathogen(s). Another drawback of RAS is that the duration of protection is under 1 year, and this will require boosting doses of RAS vaccines to be administered annually. The latter may not be practical and sustainable in resource-limited endemic countries *(153, 174)*.

Genetically Attenuated Sporozoites (GAS). Genetically attenuated sporozoites, like their RAS counterparts, have low infectivity, undergo arrested development in the liver, and stimulate potent protection against challenge infections in murine models of malaria *(175)*. The difference is that in GAS sporozoite, attenuation is not due to irradiation but to the deletion of specific genes, such as *UIS3*, *UISE4*, and *P36p*, which are essential for the pre-erythrocytic stage of plasmodia *(175–177)*. When these genes are deleted, the sporozoites displayed an arrested development in the liver, did not mature into the blood stages, but were able to induce complete protection against challenge infections in a *P. berghei*–infected mouse model *(176)*. Furthermore, because GAS are produced by double-crossover recombination, they may not pose the safety concerns associated with RAS because the risk of breakthrough infections due to genetic reversion is considerably lower *(176, 177)*. However, the sustainable production of GAS will face similar constraints by the same technical and logistic problems as

those observed for RAS *(174)*. To date, *P. falciparum* GAS have yet to be generated.

20.7.4 Subunit Recombinant Vaccines

One of the most important advances in recombinant DNA technology during the 1980s was the cloning of a malarial vaccine candidate, the circumsporozoite protein of *P. falciparum (178)*. Ever since, the hope has been that cloning and expression of recombinant plasmodia genes will lead to control of malaria by recombinant subunit vaccines. That hope has not materialized. More than 20 years later, despite considerable effort, less than 20 *P. falciparum* antigens are being studied as potential malaria vaccines *(174)*. The current research is focused on four pre-parasitic stage antigens (CSP-1, LSA-1, LSA-3, and TRAP), 13 blood stage antigens (AMA-1, MSP-1, MSP-3, MSP-4, GLURP-1, RESA, SERA5, EBA-175, EBP-2, MAEBL, RAP-2, EMP-1, and DBL-α), and the sexual stage antigen Pf25 of *P. falciparum (179)*.

One serious obstacle to overcome is that malarial proteins vary greatly in their immunogenicity. Moreover, induced antibodies must have the correct avidity to bind, specificity, and biological activity and must be produced in high enough titer to block infection. In addition, recombinant protein subunit vaccines are generally poor at inducing effector T-cell responses, such as CD8$^+$ cytotoxic T-lymphocytes, that are necessary for eliminating intracellular pathogens such as liver-stage malaria parasites *(160)*.

DNA-Based Subunit Vaccines. The newest generation of subunit vaccines are the DNA-based vaccines *(180–183)*.

DNA-based vaccines are taken up by the host cells, then protein is expressed, and the T-cell epitopes bound to HLA molecules and prime naïve T cells to form memory T-cell populations *(184)*. Recombinant viral vaccines work in a similar way but actively infect cells and express the recombinant malaria proteins before aborting infection *(185)*.

Both DNA and recombinant viral subunit vaccines can induce high levels of effector T-cell immune responses, although antibody responses have been poor in clinical trials *(184, 186)*

The assessment of T-cell responses has been significantly advanced by the enzyme-linked immunospot (ELISPOT) and the tetramer assays. ELISPOT is highly sensitive in quantitatively detecting functional antigen-specific T-cells. On the other hand, the tetramer assay will allow for a detailed characterization of antigen-specific T cells. Together, these advances, when coupled with those of subunit vaccination in malaria, will raise the possibility of identifying robust antibody and T-cell immune correlates of protection and increase the level of understanding of vaccine design around immune correlates of protection, to systematically improve vaccine efficacy—a process dubbed *iterative vaccine development (160)*.

20.7.5 Pre-erythrocytic Vaccines

One strategy for developing a malaria vaccine is to target the parasites at the pre-erythrocytic stage during the short period that the sporozoites are in the bloodstream. The aim of this approach is to induce the production of protective antibodies that will block and neutralize the sporozoites from invading the liver cells. The alternative strategy is to target the sporozoites once they are inside the liver cells by inducing potent cytotoxic T-lymphocyte (CTL) immunogenicity that will destroy sporozoite-infected liver cells while not harming the human host *(160)*.

The leading candidate vaccine of this type is RTS,S—a recombinant protein vaccine *(187)*. Hepatitis B surface antigen DNA has been fused to DNA encoding a large part of the best characterized pre-erythrocytic malaria antigen, the circumsporozoite (CS) protein *(188, 189)*. When expressed in yeast, the fusion product (RTS) will bind the hepatitis B surface antigen (S) to form the RTS,S particles. Mixed with an adjuvant (AS02), the RTS,S vaccine induced high titer of antibodies against CS and hepatitis B. After a randomized controlled field trial of three-dose RTS,S/AS02 vaccine in Gambian adults, the vaccine protection was 34% during the 15-week surveillance period, but with 71% efficacy in the first 9 weeks and 0% in the next 6 weeks *(190)*. Protection was not strain-specific. Although the duration of efficacy was short, RTS,S was the first pre-erythrocytic stage vaccine to demonstrate clear protection against natural *P. falciparum* infection. Because RTS,S was not particularly successful at reducing the rate of mild episodes of fever, the finding that it appeared to reduce the rate of severe illness came as a surprise.

Several other pre-erythrocytic vaccine candidates have reached the clinical evaluation stage. Thus, the ICC-1132 vaccine is being tested in the United States, Germany, and the United Kingdom. It represents a hepatitis B core particle that was genetically engineered to include a region of CS for high-titer antibody induction.

Another strategy for vaccine development, the so-called *heterologous prime-boost vaccination*, is to sequentially give two different vaccine vectors encoding the same antigen. The rationale behind the "prime-boost" strategy is that combining malarial antigens with one or more attenuated viruses will stimulate a powerful T-cell response. Viral vectors can be given first (priming) or second (boosting). Whereas DNA vaccines are efficient priming vaccines, they do not boost efficiently *(191)*. Three carriers have been clinically tested: (i) DNA; (ii) modified vaccinia virus

Ankara (MVA); and (iii) attenuated pox virus FP9. The insert included thrombospondin-related adhesive protein (TRAP), a well characterized pre-erythrocytic antigen, and a string of T-cell epitopes (called ME for multiple epitope). These so-called ME-TRAP vaccines have been given in prime-boost sequence—i.e., DNA then MVA, or FP9 then MVA *(192, 193)*. This approach has induced high T-cell responses and some protection, as manifested by a substantial delay to parasitemia in sporozoite challenge studies *(194)*. A randomized controlled trial of the efficacy of DNA and ME-TRAP followed by MVA and ME-TRAP was completed in The Gambia and the United Kingdom *(160, 195)*.

20.7.6 Blood-Stage (Erythrocytic) Vaccines

There are two possible classes of blood-stage vaccines: anti-invasion and anticomplication *(160)*. The guiding principle of the strategy is that if a vaccine could prevent invasion of the red blood cells by the malarial merozoites, it would prevent malarial disease. However, the development of such vaccines has been hampered by the lack of established human challenge, by the limitations of available animal models, and by the unclear immunologic correlates of protection. The merozoite surface protein-1 (MSP-1) is the best-characterized antigen involved in invasion and served as the basis of several vaccine candidates. However, vaccine development has been complicated by the discovery of parallel pathways of invasion and by the demonstration that some antibodies to MSP-1 can block the activity of malaria-protective antibodies *(196)*.

In a small efficacy study conducted in Papua New Guinea, a blood-stage vaccine incorporating the MSP-2 antigen as well as two other blood-stage antigens reduced the parasitic density in the vaccine recipients *(197)*.

A recombinant viral vaccine, NYVAC Pf-7 (*P. falciparum-7*), has been developed that encoded seven antigens from various life-cycle stages *(198)*. Although results of a sporozoite challenge study of NYVAC Pf-7 in rhesus monkeys demonstrated encouraging delays in time to parasitemia and some antibody and cytotoxic T-lymphocyte immunogenicity, this candidate vaccine has not been further developed *(160)*. In human Phase I/II safety, immunogenicity, and efficacy trials, the antibody responses were poor; however, cellular responses were detected in well over 90% of vaccine recipients.

An anti-invasion vaccine based on MSP-1, known as falci-parum malaria protein (FMP-1), is being clinically assessed in a Phase I study in western Kenya *(160)*.

Two blood-stage candidates, glutamate rich protein (GLURP) *(199)* and MSP-3 *(200)*, have been clinically assessed in Europe.

A key issue with all protein-based vaccine candidates is the identification of a safe, immunogenic adjuvant, because the traditional adjuvant, alum, seemed to be insufficiently immunogenic for many malaria proteins. In addition, vaccine with an alum adjuvant would induce a Th2 response rather than the more desirable Th1 response.

Sequestration of *P. falciparum* by adherence to vascular endothelial cells in the brain, kidneys, and placenta is one of the important causes of severe malaria. Hence, the PfEMP-1 antigen (erythrocyte membrane protein-1), the main ligand for such adherence, is being studied as a vaccine candidate.

In this context, PfEMP-1 is also the major ligand for CSA-binding. Placental malaria is caused by chondroitin sulfate A (CSA)-binding parasites that sequester in the placenta, resulting in adverse pregnancy outcomes *(201)*; for this reason, PfEMP-1 is currently targeted for the development of pregnancy-specific malaria vaccine.

Recent studies in a primate model confirmed the usefulness of the PfEMP-1 DBL-1α domain for developing a vaccine for severe malaria *(202)*. However, PfEMP-1 has a high degree of variability, rapid rate of antigenic variation, and high copy number within each parasite, which tend to complicate its vaccine development *(160)*.

20.7.7 Sexual-Stage Vaccines

Induction of antibodies to gametocyte antigens can prevent fertilization in the mosquito; as well as its blood meal, the mosquito ingests antibodies that block fertilization. As a result, it would be possible to assess the efficacy of gametocyte vaccines with a simple *ex vivo* assay *(160)*. Mosquitoes are fed on gametocytes with or without the addition of human serum samples from vaccinated volunteers. The NIAID Malaria Vaccine Development Unit has focused on the clinical assessment of a *P. falciparum* gametocyte candidate vaccine, Pfs25, a recombinant protein.

20.7.8 Reverse Vaccinology and Genome-wide Identification of Vaccine Targets

The reverse vaccinology approach uses the genomic information (genomics, proteomics, and transcriptomics) on pathogens to systematically screen their components for protective efficacy. It is uniquely suited for organisms that are not easy to culture and thus far has yielded promising results for chlamydial infections and some bacterial diseases. The use of genome-wide surveys to search for malaria vaccine targets started in earnest several years ago when the first

extensive microarray and proteomics studies of *P. falciparum* were reported *(203, 204)*.

Results of whole-genome sequencing indicate that there are probably 5,300 *P. falciparum* antigens, and genome databases that can be used to identify hundreds of vaccine candidates. Thus, a recent genome-wide survey for polymorphisms and signatures of selections led to the identification of potential malarial vaccine targets *(205)*. Other developments include a comprehensive proteome analysis of ookinetes, which allowed for a systematic assessment of predicted ookinete surface proteins *(175)*, and the discovery of the vital *P. berghei* pre-erythrocytic stage-specific gene *UIS3* (the genetic target for a novel GAS vaccine), which came as the result of gene-profiling studies *(175)*.

However, the number of possible antigens is not rate-limiting for malaria vaccine development. Moreover, identification of antigens alone will not help to solve some key problems in malaria vaccine development, such as how to induce strong, durable immune responses and how to combine multiple antigens without interference or competition. Nevertheless, the postgenomic antigen identification should generate a wealth of information of long-term value to vaccine development *(160)*.

20.8 NIAID Involvement in Malaria Research

The NIAID has a long-standing interest in and commitment to malaria research, focused on understanding the biology of malaria parasites and their interactions with mosquito vectors and human hosts and developing tools needed for effective and sustainable prevention, treatment, and control of malaria *(206)*.

Despite extraordinary political, economic, social, and medical advances, more than 40% of the world's population lives in areas where people are at risk of contracting malaria. Because of this, NIAID recently announced a new initiative on *NIAID Partnerships with Public-Private Partnerships* designed to strengthen the pipeline for novel products and interventions against malaria and other neglected tropical diseases (http://www3.niaid. nih.gov/about/directors/news/malaria/).

Because of its very high annual mortality rate, malaria continues to be the most important tropical parasitic disease and a research area of high priority to NIAID. Thus, laboratory-based studies on malaria have been funded by NIAID through the traditional investigator-initiated research grant mechanism. In addition, intervention strategies at the preclinical level are being supported through the Tropical Disease Research Units (TDRU) program, and the partnership Program for Development of Novel Vector Control Interventions. NIAID is continuing to pursue the implementation of its *Malaria Vaccine Development Plan* (http://www.niaid.nih.gov/dmid/malaria/malvacdv/toc.htm) designated to accelerate research leading to the development of malaria vaccines. Moreover, field and clinical studies are supported through various solicited research programs, such as the International Collaborations in Infectious Diseases Research, the Tropical Medicine Research Centers, and the Malaria Vaccines: Clinical Research and Trial Sites in Endemic Areas.

According to estimates by WHO, between 300 million and 500 million cases of acute clinical malaria occur annually (WHO: World Malaria Report 2005). Worldwide in 2003, malaria has accounted for an estimated 1.27 million deaths and more than 46 million lost Disability-Adjusted Life Years (DALYs) (WHO: World Health Report 2004). In 2002, 1,252 cases of malaria in the United States were reported to the CDC.

In June 2005, the White House announced the *President's Malaria Initiative (PMI)* to reduce the burden of malaria in Africa by pledging to increase funding of malaria prevention and treatment by more than US$1.2 billion over 5 years. Among the PMI's main objectives is to focus on (i) vector control activities; (ii) procurement and distribution of artemisinin-combination treatment; and (iii) prevention of malaria in pregnant women by intermittent presumptive treatment. The countries included in PMI include Angola, Uganda, Tanzania, Zambia, Equatorial Guinea, Malawi, Mozambique, Rwanda, and Senegal.

Major goals and objectives of NIAID-supported malaria research include:

- *Vaccine Development.* Characterization of the immunologic responses to malaria parasites and their antigenic constituents. Such analysis should lead to the development of vaccine candidates from various life stages, which, when appropriately presented to humans, would protect from infection or disease. Alternative strategies will seek to identify vaccines that will block malaria transmission to the mosquito vector. In addition, efforts to identify, validate, and clinically evaluate candidate vaccines and vaccine strategies will be supported through grants and contracts (http://www.niaid.nih.gov/dmid/malaria/malvacdv/toc.htm).
- *Drug Development.* Design and development of new drugs, and improving of existing drugs, would lead to new chemotherapeutic treatments of malarial infections. In the context of this objective, NIAID efforts will be expanded to search for (i) identification and characterization of unique parasite biochemical pathways that may serve as targets for new drugs; (ii) determination of mode of action of existing and potential antimalarial drugs; and (iii) analysis of mechanisms by which the parasite

has become resistant to existing drugs (http://www.niaid.nih.gov/dmid/malaria/malvacdv/toc.htm).
- *Pathogenesis.* NIAID efforts will be aimed at characterizing the mechanisms by which the parasite survives in the human host and by which infection results in disease. Understanding such mechanisms should lead to new approaches to control and treatment of malaria (http://www.niaid.nih.gov/dmid/malaria/malvacdv/toc.htm).
- *Epidemiology, Vector Biology, and Control.* NIAID will support studies conducted to develop new methods, and improve existing ones, for diagnosing infection, detecting drug-resistant parasites, and vector characterization. Relevant studies will also focus on analyzing the physiologic interactions between the parasite and its mosquito vector, exploring the biology and ecology of vector populations, and devising novel means of interrupting transmission at the level of the arthropod vector. In addition, NIAID will support studies to determine age-specific incidence rates of relevant clinical end-points for clinical trials of interventions aimed at preventing and treating malaria-related morbidity and mortality (http://www.niaid.nih.gov/dmid/malaria/malvacdv/toc.htm).
- *Disease Emergence.* This objective will include research to identify and characterize factors that explain the changes in the distribution of malaria, such as studies aimed at evaluation and spread of drug-resistant parasites, and changing land-use practices associated with the spread of the anopheline vectors (http://www.niaid.nih.gov/dmid/malaria/malvacdv/toc.htm).
- NIAID will also continue to systematically implement its *Research Plan to Accelerate Development of Malaria Vaccines* (http://www.niaid.nih.gov/dmid/malaria/malvacdv/toc.htm).

20.8.1 NIAID Malaria Programmatic Developments: Partners

NIAID is working closely with organizations, such as the U.S. Agency for International Development (USAID), the WHO, the European Commission, the European-Developing Countries Clinical Trials Partnership, the European Malaria Vaccine Initiative, the Wellcome Trust, the Bill & Melinda Gates Foundation, the Malaria Vaccine Initiative, and the Medicines for Malaria Venture. NIAID has also joined with the Fogarty International Center (FIC), the National Library of Medicine, the Special Programme on Research and Training in Tropical Diseases at WHO, and other institutions, to form the *Multilateral Initiative on Malaria.* The mission of this initiative is to increase and enhance research on malaria worldwide by facilitating multinational research cooperation and by supporting the career development and research efforts of African scientists working in malaria endemic areas. In addition, NIAID has developed and is supporting the *Malaria Research and Reference Reagent Resource Center (MR4)* to provide reagents, materials, and protocols necessary for malaria research (http://www3.niaid.nih.gov/about/directors/news/malaria/).

NIAID is participating in many collaborative projects with other U.S. agencies, international organizations, and foreign governments to curb the global impact of malaria (http://www3.niaid.nih.gov/research/topics/malaria/partners. htm). NIAID-supported researchers in Burkina Faso, Mali, Cameroon, The Gambia, Gabon, Ghana, Malawi, Kenya, Mozambique, Tanzania, Uganda, Thailand, Indonesia, Papua New Guinea, and Brazil have been working to strengthen the research capabilities of scientists in their own countries (http://www3.niaid.nih.gov/research/topics/ malaria/research.htm).

Programmatic developments related to international malaria research include:

- Sites in Ghana and Mali, supported by contracts under the *Malaria: Clinical Research and Trial Preparation Sites in Endemic Areas* initiative, have been identified in order to carry out studies characterizing the epidemiology and entomology of malaria in potential clinical trial sites. Over time, NIAID has projected establishing a strong clinical research capacity in Africa. To this end, in collaboration with the U.S. Navy, USAID, and the National Library of Medicine, a satellite Internet connectivity has been established at two research centers in Ghana to facilitate collaborative research (http://www3.niaid.nih.gov/ about/overview/profile/fy2004.pdf/research_malaria.pdf).
- NIAID, in collaboration with Walter Reed Army Institute of Research (WRAIR), GlaxoSmithKline Biologicals, the USAID, the University of Maryland School of Medicine Center for Vaccine Development (Md/CVD), and the University of Bamako, Mali, completed a Phase I adult clinical trial in Mali to evaluate a novel candidate vaccine that targets the blood-stage of malaria parasites. Under the initiative *International Collaborations in Infectious Disease Research*, an award was made to the University of Maryland Center for Vaccine Development and the University of Bamako to carry out additional clinical trials of this promising candidate vaccine in Malian children.
- In an ongoing Cooperative Research and Development Agreement (CRADA) with the Genzyme Transgenics Corp., mice have been genetically engineered to produce malaria vaccine candidate antigen (MSP-1-42) in their milk. Preliminary results from studies on the transgenically produced immunogen provide an indication that it can elicit protective immunity against challenge infection in non-human primates. Transgenic production of candidate malaria vaccines

may offer an *economical alternative* to conventional vaccine production methods (http://www.transgenics. com/pressreleases/pr102298.html).

- In 1999, the Bill & Melinda Gates Foundation awarded US$50 million to the *Program for Appropriate Technology in Health (PATH)* to administer the *Malaria Vaccine Initiative (MVI)* program promoting the development of a vaccine candidate to prevent malaria. PATH, based in Seattle, is an international nonprofit organization whose mission is to improve health, particularly of women and children (http://www.path.org).
- A *Memorandum of Understanding* was established between MVI and NIAID to facilitate collaboration on malaria vaccine development. MVI and NIAID are jointly supporting the development of a promising candidate malaria vaccine and are working together to develop jointly supported product-development efforts for other promising candidates (http://malariavaccine.org).
- *Malaria Vaccine Development Plan.* NIAID continues to pursue the systematic implementation of its Malaria Vaccine Development Plan designed to accelerate research leading to the development of malaria vaccines. Under a contract with SAIC (Science Applications International Corp.), NIAID has completed the required extensive preclinical development activities and has filed new INDs for two new malaria vaccine candidates. These new vaccine candidates include an adjuvanted recombinant protein that targets falciparum malaria blood stages and a recombinant adenovirus serotype 35-vectored circumsporozoite (CS) protein vaccine candidate targeting pre-erythrocytic stages of malaria parasites. In addition, reagents generated under the SAIC contract were also provided to the *Malaria Research and Reference Reagent Resource (MR4)*, which will make them available to the international malaria research community.
- An *Interagency Agreement* is in place between NIAID and the USAID supporting the *Malaria Vaccine Development Program* for collaborative vaccine development.
- In response to the Presidential Millennium Vaccine Initiative (2000), NIAID has launched a new initiative, "Millennium Vaccine Initiative—Novel Vaccines for Tuberculosis and Malaria." Because vaccines for tuberculosis and malaria have not, historically, been high priority areas for private-sector investment, this NIAID initiative seeks *to increase collaboration between the public sector and the pharmaceutical and biotechnology industries,* to identify and actively pursue novel approaches to vaccine development for tuberculosis and malaria (http://www. niaid.nih.gov/publications/jordan/whitehouse.htm).
- Malaria anemia is a leading cause of morbidity and mortality among malaria-infected individuals. To this end, together with NHLBI and FIC, NIAID held an International Malaria Anemia Workshop in 2000. The workshop,

attended by leading scientists from developed and developing countries, produced recommendations and suggestions for future initiatives. Based on these recommendations, NIAID launched a new initiative, "Malaria Vaccine Development: Understanding Malaria Anemia" (NIH Guide: RFA-AI-01-007).

- *The Malaria Research and Reference Reagent Resource Center (MR4)* is continuing to provide expanded access to quality-controlled parasite and vector reagents for the international malaria research community through the MR4 Catalog (http://mr4.org/mr4_catalog).
- NIAID is continuing its support of the "Multilateral Initiative on Malaria (MIM)" through grants to African scientists at African institutions under the MIM/TDR (Tropical Diseases Research) Program. NIAID joined with FIC, WHO, and other institutions to form MIM, whose mission is to increase and enhance worldwide research on malaria by facilitating multinational research cooperation (http://www.who.int/tdr/diseases/malaria/mimprojectsall.htm).
- NIAID continues to participate in the *Federal Malaria Vaccine Coordinating Committee (FMVCC)* and is continuing to provide support to the MIM/TDR Task Force, the WHO Initiative for Vaccine Research (WHO/IVR), and the External Scientific Advisory Committee of the Medicines for Malaria Venture (a public-private partnership that fosters accelerated development of new antimalarial compounds) (http://www3.niaid.nih.gov/research/topics/malaria/partners.htm).
- NIAID has also worked with the European Commission and the European-Developing Countries Clinical Trial Partnership (EDCTP) to coordinate product development and clinical trial activities in vaccines and drugs.
- *Resources for Researchers* (http://www3.niaid.nih.gov/reesrach/topics/malaria/resources/):

  (i) Malaria Research and Reference Reagent Resource Center (MR4).
  (ii) NIAID Microbial Genome Sequencing Centers.
  (iii) The *Plasmodium falciparum* genome Database (PFDB)– J. Craig Venter Institute.
  (iv) The Sanger Institute *Plasmodium falciparum* Genome Projects.
  (v) Stanford Genome Technology Center Malaria Genome Project.

20.8.2   NIAID-Supported Malaria Clinical Trials

NIAID-supported clinical trials can be accessed at http://www.clinicaltrials.gov and http://www3.niaid.nih.gov/research/topics/malaria/clinical.htm. They include:

- Chloroquine alone or in combination for malaria in children in Malawi.
- Rapid diagnostic tests for malaria in Uganda.
- Time to infection with malaria parasites.
- Adenovirus vaccine for malaria.
- Relationship between HIV and malaria in Ugandan children.
- Safety of and immune response to a malaria vaccine (MSP-1 42-C1) with or without CPG 7909 adjuvant.
- Evaluation, treatment, and monitoring of patients with a known or suspected parasitic infection.
- Severe malaria and antimalarial drug resistance in Cambodia.
- Examination of protective factors against severe malaria.
- Randomized, controlled, Phase I study of the safety and immunogenicity of the AMA1-C1/alhydrogel + CPG 7909 vaccine for *Plasmodium falciparum* malaria in semi-immune Malian adults (NCT00114010). This study will examine the safety and immune response of healthy adult volunteers to ANA1-C1, an experimental malaria vaccine developed at NIAID.
- Malaria transmission and immunity in highland Kenya.
- Longitudinal antimalarial combinations in Uganda (NCT00123552). The purpose of the trial is to compare different ways of treating uncomplicated malaria in a group of Ugandan children.
- Malaria prevalence in children.
- Congenital and neonatal malaria in Mali.
- In collaboration with the Walter Reed Army Institute of Research (WRAIR), GlaxoSmithKline Biologicals, the USAID, the University of Maryland, and the University of Bamako, Mali, a Phase I trial was conducted in Mali to evaluate a novel candidate vaccine that targeted the blood-stage of malaria parasites. Additional clinical trials with this promising vaccine candidate will be carried out in Malian children by the University of Maryland Center for Vaccine Development and the University of Bamako.
- Under a contract with Science Application International (SAIC), NIAID has established the capacity to undertake targeted research essential to translating basic research concepts into prototype vaccine products for clinical evaluation. The new vaccine candidates include an adjuvanted recombinant protein targeting falciparum malaria blood stages and a recombinant adenovirus serotype 35-vectored circumsporozoite (CS) protein targeting pre-erythrocyte stages of the malaria parasites (http://www3.niaid.nih.gov/research/topics/malaria/vaccine.htm).
- Through an NIAID-supported contract under the "Malaria Vaccines: Clinical Research and Trial Sites in Endemic Areas" initiative, clinical research capacity has been strengthened in sites in Ghana and Burkina Faso in West Africa. Studies conducted to date or ongoing include (i) cohort studies to determine malaria incidence,

correlates of protective immunity, and drug resistance; (ii) case-control studies identifying potential risk factors for severe malaria; and (iii) molecular epidemiology studies of genetic polymorphisms in *P. falciparum*. In addition, two Phase I clinical trials of novel candidate vaccines targeting the blood-stage of malaria parasites were initiated in U.S. adults in NIAID-sponsored Vaccine and Treatment Evaluation Units (VTEUs). If found to be safe and immunogenic, these two vaccine candidates will be tested under contract in malaria endemic sites in Africa.

20.9 Recent Scientific Advances

- *Elevated Plasma Phenylalanine in Severe Malaria and Implications for Pathophysiology of Neurologic Complications.* The pathophysiology of severe malaria is poorly understood, and once its mechanism is induced, antimalarial treatment alone is not adequate, resulting in severe residual disability or death even if appropriate antimalarial therapy is given. Recent data have indicated that additional amino acid abnormalities have been associated with the severity of malaria *(207)*. Thus, disruption of plasma phenylalanine homeostasis led to significant hyperphenylalaninemia, a likely result of an acquired abnormality in the function of the liver enzyme phenylalanine hydroxylase.

- *Impact of HIV-Associated Immunosuppression on Malaria Infection and Disease.* HIV infection and malaria coexist in much of Africa. Although the prevalence of malaria infection was not associated with lower $CD4^+$ cell counts, the incidence of clinical malaria episodes was higher in patients with $CD4^+$ cell counts of <200 cells/mm^3. Profoundly immunosuppressed adults with HIV infection required more frequent treatment for uncomplicated malaria. However, malaria infection and disease were less strongly associated with HIV-associated immunosuppression than were other opportunistic infections. Therefore, where malaria is common, the high incidence of fever found among immunosuppressed adults may lead to misclassification of illness episodes as malaria *(208)*. This finding underscores the impact that concomitant HIV infection may have on the presumptive diagnosis of malaria and highlights the need for rapid and reliable malaria diagnostics to prevent the inappropriate use of antimalarial drugs

- *A Critical Role for the Mediator Macrophage Migration Inhibitory Factor in the Pathogenesis of Malaria Anemia.* Anemia is a leading cause of morbidity and mortality associated with malaria. The pathogenesis of malarial anemia is multifactorial, and the mechanisms responsible for its high mortality are poorly understood. Recent studies have shown an intrinsic role for the macrophage

migration inhibitory factor (MIF) in the development of the anemic complications and bone marrow suppression associated with malaria *(209)*. Infection of MIF knockout mice with *Plasmodium chabaudi* resulted in less severe anemia, improved erythroid progenitor development, and increased survival compared with wild-type controls. This and other findings suggested that polymorphisms at the MIF locus may influence the levels of MIF produced in the innate response to malaria infection and the likelihood of anemic complications *(209)*.

- *A Mosquito-Specific Protein Family Includes Candidate Receptors for Malaria Sporozoite Invasion of Salivary Glands.* Research has shown the widespread presence of a previously unrecognized protein family (SGS proteins) in *Aedes* and *Anopheles* mosquitoes *(210)*. The *Ae. aegyptii* aaSGS1 mRNA and protein were found to be salivary gland specific, and the protein was localized in the basal lamina covering the anatomic regions that are preferably invaded by the malaria sporozoites. Furthermore, anti-aaSGS1 antibodies inhibited sporozoite invasion into the salivary glands *in vivo*, confirming aaSGS1 as a candidate sporozoite receptor. By homology to aaSGS1, the complete complement of four SGS genes were also identified in *An. gambiae*. It has been postulated that sporozoite invasion of the mosquito salivary glands and subsequently the vertebrate liver may share similar sulfation-based mechanisms *(210)*.

- *Structural Basis for Unique Mechanisms of Folding and Hemoglobin Binding by a Malarial Protease.* Falciparin-2 (FP2), the major cysteine protease of the human malarial parasite, *Plasmodium falciparum*, is a hemoglobinase and a promising drug target. The crystal structure of FP2, which has been recently elucidated as a complex with a protease inhibitor, cystatin, has shown two previously unknown cysteine protease structural motifs, $FR2_{nose}$ and $FP2_{arm}$, in addition to details of the active site that would help focus a potential drug-inhibitor design *(211)*. Furthermore, unlike most cysteine proteases, FR2 will not require a prodomain but only the short $FR2_{nose}$ motif to correctly fold and gain catalytic activity. The $FP2_{arm}$ motif will be required for hemoglobinase activity. The latter and other topographic features suggested that $FP2_{arm}$ may serve as an exo-site for hemoglobin binding. Motifs similar to $FP2_{nose}$ and $FP2_{arm}$ have been found only in related plasmodial proteases, suggesting that they confer malaria-specific functions and may serve as potential targets for antimalarial drug design.

References

1. Sachs, J. and Malaney, P. (2002) The economic and social burden of malaria, *Nature*, **415**, 680–685.

2. Kain, K. C. and Keystone, J. S. (1998) Malaria in travelers. Epidemiology, disease, and prevention, *Infect. Dis. Clin. North Am.*, **12**, 267–284.

3. Trampuz, A., Jereb, M., Muzlovic, I., and Prabhu, R. M. (2003) Clinical review: severe malaria, *Crit. Care*, **7**, 315–323.

4. Llinás, M. and DeRisi, J. L. (2004) Pernicious plans revelead: *Plasmodium falciparum* genome wide expression analysis, *Curr. Opin. Microbiol.*, **7**, 382–387.

5. Bannister, L. H., Hopkins, J. M., Fowler, R. E., Krishna, S., and Mitchell, G. H. (2000) A brief illustrated guide to the ultrastructure of *Plasmodium falciparum* asexual blood stages, *Parasitol. Today*, **16**, 427–433.

6. Garcia, L. S. (2001) Malaria and babesiosis. In: *Diagnostic Medical Parasitology* (Garcia, L. S., ed.), American Society of Microbiology, Washington, DC, pp. 159–204.

7. Nacher, M., Singhasivanon, P., Silachamroon, U., Treeprasertsuk, S., Tosukhowong, T., Vannaphan, S., Gay, F., Mazier, D., and Looareesuwan, S. (2002) Decreased hemoglobin concentrations, hyperparasitemia, and severe malaria are associated with increased *Plasmodium falciparum* gametocyte carriage, *J. Parasitol.*, **88**(1), 97–101.

8. Gratzer, W. B. and Dluzewski, A. R. (1993) The red blood cell and malaria parasite invasion, *Semin. Hematol.*, **30**, 232–247.

9. Aubouy, A., Migot-Nabias, F., and Derolon, P. (2003) Polymorphism in two merozoite surface proteins of *Plasmodium falciparum* from Gabon, *Malar. J.*, **2**, 12 (http://www.malariajournal.com/content/2/1/12).

10. Mitchell, G. H., Thomas, A. W., Margos, G., Dluzewski, A. R., and Banister, L. H. (2004) Apical membrane antigen 1, a major malaria vaccine candidate, mediates the close attachment of invasive merozoites to host red blood cells, *Infect. Immun.*, **72**, 154–158.

11. Carruthers, V. B. and Sibley, L. D. (1999) Mobilization of intracellular calcium stimulates microneme discharge in *Toxoplasma gondii*, *Mol. Microbiol.*, **31**, 421–428.

12. Culvenor, J. G., Day, K. P., and Anders, R. F (1991) *P. falciparum* ring-infected erythrocyte surface antigen is released from merozoite dense granules after erythrocyte invasion, *Infect. Immun.*, **59**, 1183–1187.

13. Blackman, M. J., Fujioka, H., Stafford, W. L., Sajid, M., Clough, B., Fleck, S. L., Aikawa, M., Grainger, M., and Hackett, F. (1998) A subtilisin-like protein in secretory organelles of *Plasmodium falciparum* merozoites, *J. Biol. Chem.*, **273**, 23398–23409.

14. Barale, J. C., Blisnick, T., Fujioka, H., Alzari, H., Aikawa, M., Braun-Breton, C., and Langsley, G. (1999) *Plasmodium falciparum* subtilisin-like protease 2, a merozoite candidate for the merozoite surface protein 1–42 maturase, *Proc. Natl. Acad. Sci. U.S.A.*, **96**, 6445–6450.

15. Reed, M. B., Caruana, S. R., Batchelor, A. H., Thompson, J. K., Crabb, B. S., and Cowman, A. F. (2000) Targeted disruption of an erythrocyte binding antigen in *Plasmodium falciparum* is associated with a switch toward a sialic acid-independent pathway of invasion, *Proc. Natl. Acad. Sci. U.S.A.*, **97**, 7509–7514.

16. Tomley, F. M. and Soldati, D. S. (2001) Mix and match modules: structure and function of microneme proteins in apicomplexan parasites, *Trends Parasitol.*, **17**, 81–88.

17. Braun-Breton, C. and Pereira da Silva, L. H. (1993) Malaria proteases and red blood cells, *Parasitol. Today*, **9**, 92–96.

18. Sibley, L. D., Hakansson, S., and Carruthers, V. B. (1998) Gliding motility: an efficient mechanism for cell penetration, *Curr. Biol.*, **8**, R12–R14.

19. Sultan, A., Thathy, V., Frevert, U., Robson, K., Crisanti, A., Nussenzweig, V., Nussenzweig, R., and Menard, R. (1997) TRAP is necessary for gliding motility and infectivity of *Plasmodium falciparum*, *Cell*, **90**, 511–522.

20. Wengelnik, K., Spaccapelo, R., Naitza, S., Robson, K. J. H., Janse, C. J., Bisoni, F., Waters, A. P., and Crisanti, A. (1999) The A-domain and the thrombospondin-related motif of *Plasmodium falciparum* TRAP are implicated in the invasion process of mosquito salivary glands, *EMBO J.*, **18**, 5195–5204.

21. Yuda, M., Sakaida, H., and Chinzei, Y. (1999) Targeted disruption of the *Plasmodium berghei* CTRP gene reveals its essential role in malaria infection of the vector mosquito, *J. Exp. Med.*, **190**, 1711–1716.

22. Dessens, J. T., Beetsma, A. L., Dimopoulos, G., Wengelnik, K., Crisanti, A., Kafatos, F. C., and Sinden, R. E. (1999) CTRP is essential for mosquito infection by malaria ookinetes, *EMBO J.*, **18**, 6221–6227.

23. Deitsch, K. W. and Wellems, T. E. (1996) Membrane modifications in erythrocytes parasitized by *Plasmodium falciparum*, *Mol. Biochem. Parasitol.*, **76**, 1–10.

24. Crabb. B. S. and Cowman, A. F. (2002) *Plasmodium falciparum* virulence determinants unveiled, *Genome Biol.*, **3**(11), 1031.1–1031.4.

25. Waterkeyn, J. G., Wickham, M. E., Davern, K. M., Cooke, B. M., Coppel, R. L., Reeder, J. C., Culvenor, J. G., Waller, R. F., and Cowman, A. F. (2000) Targeted mutagenesis of *Plasmodium falciparum* erythrocyte membrane protein 3 (PfEMP3) disrupts cytoadherence of malaria-infected red blood cells, *EMBO J.*, **19**, 2813–2823.

26. Sherman, I. W., Crandall, I. E., Guthrie, N., and Land, K. M. (1995) The sticky secrets of sequestration, *Parasitol. Today*, **11**, 378–384.

27. Craig, A. and Scherf, A. (2001) Molecules on the surface of the *Plasmodium falciparum*-infected erythrocyte and their role in malaria pathogenesis and immune evasion, *Mol. Biochem. Parasitol.*, **115**, 129–143.

28. Beeson, J. G. and Brown, G. V. (2002) Pathogenesis of *Plasmodium falciparum* malaria: the roles of parasite adhesion and antigenic variation, *Cell. Mol. Life Sci.*, **59**, 258–271.

29. Turner, G. D. H., Morrison, H., Jones, M., Davis, T. M.E., Looareesuwan, S., Buley, I. D., Gatter, K. C., Newbold, C. I., Pukritayakamee, S., Nagachinta, B., White, N. J., and Berendt, A. R. (1994) An immunohistochemical study of the pathology of fatal malaria – evidence for widespread endothelial activation and a potential role for intercellular adhesion molecule-1 in cerebral sequestration, *Am. J. Pathol.*, **145**, 1057–1069.

30. Smith, J. D., Gamain, B., Baruch, D. I., and Kyes, S. (2001) Decoding the language of *var* genes and *Plasmodium falciparum* sequestration, *Trends Parasitol.*, **17**, 538–545.

31. Biggs, B. A., Anders, R. F., Dillon, H. E., Davern, K. M., Martin, M., Petersen, C., and Brown, G. V. (1992) Adherence of infected erythrocytes to venular endothelium selects for antigenic variants of *Plasmodium falciparum*, *J. Immunol.*, **149**, 2047–2054.

32. Deitsch, K. W., del Pinal, A., and Wellems, T. E. (1999) Intracluster recombination and var transcription switches in the antigenic variation of *Plasmodium falciparum*, *Mol. Biochem. Parasitol.*, **101**, 107–116.

33. Gissot, M., Briquet, S., Refour, P., Boschet, C., and Vaquero, C. (2005) PfMyb1, *Plasmodium falciparum* transcription factor, is required for intra-erythrocytic growth and controls key genes for cell cycle regulation, *J. Mol. Biol.*, **346**, 29–42.

34. Lipsick, J. S. (1996) One billion years of Myb, *Oncology*, **13**, 223–235.

35. Boschet, C., Gissot, M., Briquet, S., Hamid, Z., Claudel-Renard, C., and Vaquero, C. (2004) Characterization of PfMyb1 transcription factor during erythrocyte development of 3D7 and F12 *Plasmodium falciparum* clones, *Mol. Biochem. Parasitol.*, **138**, 159–163.

36. Ness, S. A., Marknell, A., and Graf, T. (1989) The v-myb onco-gene product binds to and activates the promyelocyte-specific mim-1 gene, *Cell*, **59**, 1115–1125.

37. Reichard, P. (2002) Ribonucleotide reductase: the evolution of allosteric regulation, *Arch. Biochem.*, **397**, 149–155.

38. Chabes, A. and Stillman, B. (2007) Constitutively high dNTP concentration inhibits cell cycle progression and the DNA damage checkpoint in yeast *Saccharomyces cerevisiae*, *Proc. Natl. Acad. Sci. U.S.A.*, **104**, 1183–1188.

39. Jordan, A. and Reichard, P. (1998) Ribonucleotide reductases, *Annu. Rev. Biochem.*, **67**, 71–98.

40. Eklund, H., Uhlin, U., Farnegardh, M., Logan, D. T., and Nordlund, P. (2000) Structure and function of the radical enzyme ribonucleotide reductase, *Prog. Biophys. Mol. Biol.*, **77**, 177–268.

41. Bracchi-Ricard, V., Moe, D., and Chakrabarti, D. (2005) Two *Plasmodium falciparum* ribonucleotide reductase small subunits, RfR2 and RfR4, interact with each other and are components of the *in vivo* enzyme complex, *J. Mol. Biol.*, **347**, 749–758.

42. Naik, R. S., Branch, O. H., Woods, A. S., Vijaykumar, M., Perkins, D. J., Nahlen, B. L., Lal, A. A., Cotter, R. J., Costello, B. L., Ockenhouse, C. F., Davidson, E. A., and Gowda, D. C. (2000) Glycosylphosphatidylinositol anchors of *Plasmodium falciparum*: molecular characterization and naturally elicited antibody response that may provide immunity to malaria pathogenesis, *J. Exp. Med.*, **192**(11), 1563–1575.

43. McConville, M. J. and Ferguson, M. A. J. (1993) The structure, biosynthesis, and functions of glycosylated phosphatidylinositols in the parasite protozoa and higher eukaryotes, *Biochem. J.*, **294**, 305–324.

44. Englund, P. T. (1993) The structure and biosynthesis of glycosylphosphatidylinositol protein anchors, *Annu. Rev. Biochem.*, **62**, 121–138.

45. Ferguson, M. A. J., Brimacombe, J. S., Brown, J. R., Crossman, A., Dix, A., Field, R. A., Guther, M. L., Milne, K. G., Sharma, D. K., and Smith, T. K. (1999) The GPI biosynthetic pathway as a therapeutic target for African sleeping sickness, *Biochim. Biophys. Acta*, **1455**, 327–340.

46. Schofield, L. and Hackett, F. (1993) Signal transduction in host cells by a glycosylphosphatidylinositol toxin of malaria parasites, *J. Exp. Med.*, **177**, 145–153.

47. Schofield, L., Vivas, L., Hackett, F., Gerold, P., Schwartz, R. T., and Tachado, S. (1993) Neutralizing monoclonal antibodies to glycosylphosphatidylinositol, the dominant TNF-α-inducing toxin of *Plasmodium falciparum*: prospects for the immunotherapy of severe malaria, *Ann. Trop. Med. Parasitol.*, **87**, 617–626.

48. Schofield, L., Novakovic, S., Gerold, P., Schwartz, R. T., McConville, M. J., and Tachado, S. D. (1996) Glycosylphosphatidylinositol toxin of *Plasmodium* up-regulates intercellular adhesion molecule-1, vascular cell adhesion molecule-1, and E-selectin expression in vascular endothelial cells and increases leukocyte and parasite cytoadherence via tyrosine kinase-dependent signal transduction, *J. Immunol.*, **156**, 1886–1896.

49. Tachado, S. D., Gerold, P., Schwartz, R., Novakovic, S., McConville, M., and Schofield, L. (1997) Signal transduction in macrophages by glycosylphosphatidylinositols of *Plasmodium*, *Trypanosoma*, and *Leishmania*: activation of protein tyrosine kinases and protein kinase C by inositolglycan and diacylglycerol moieties, *Proc. Natl. Acad. Sci. U.S.A.*, **94**, 4022–4027.

50. Miller, L. H., Roberts, T., Shahabuddin, M., and McCutchan, T. F. (1993) Analysis of sequence diversity in the *Plasmodium falciparum* merozoite surface protein-1 (MSP-1), *Mol. Biochem. Parasitol.*, **59**, 1–14.

51. Marshall, V. M., Silva, A., Foley, M., Cranmer, S., Wang, L., McColl, D. J., Kemp, D. J., and Coppel, R. L. (1997) A second merozoite surface protein (MSP-4) of *Plasmodium falciparum* that contains an epidermal growth factor-like domain, *Infect. Immun.*, **65**, 4460–4467.

52. Braun-Breton, C., Rosenberry, T. L., and Pereira da Silva, L. H. (1990) Glycolipid anchorage of *Plasmodium falciparum* surface antigens, *Res. Immunol.*, **141**, 743–755.

53. Gardner, M. J., Hall, N., Fung, E., White, O., Berriman, M., Hyman, R. W., Carlton, J. M., Pain, A., Nelson, K. E., Bowman, S., Paulsen, I. T., James, K., Eisen, J. A., Rutherford, K., Salzberg, S. L., Craig, A., Kyes, S., Chan, M.-S., Nene, V., Shallom, S. J., Suh, B., Peterson, J., Angiouli, S., Pertea, M., Allen, J., Selengut, J., Haft, D., Mather, M. W., Vaidya, A. B., Martin, D. M. A., Fairlamb, A. H., Fraunholz, M. J., Roos, D. S., Ralph, S. A., McFadden, G. I., Cummings, L. M., Subramanian, G. M., Mungall, C., Venter, J. C., Carucci, D. J., Hoffman, S. L., Newbold, C., Davis, R. W., Fraser, C. M., and Barrell, B. (2002) Genome sequence of the human malaria parasite *Plasmodium falciparum*, *Nature*, **419**, 498–511.

54. Berry, A. E., Gardner, M. J., Caspers, G.-J., Roos, D. S., and Berriman, M. (2004) Curation of the *Plasmodium falciparum* genome, *Trends Parasitol.*, **20**(12), 548–552.

55. Chotivanich, K., Udomsangpetch, R., Pattanapanyasat, K., Chierakul, W., Simpson, J., Looaraasuwan, S., and White, N. (2002) Hemoglobin E: a balanced polymorphism protective against high parasitemias and thus severe *P. falciparum* malaria, *Blood*, **100**(4), 1172–1176.

56. Haldan, J. B. S. (1949) The rate of mutation of human genes, *Hereditas*, **35**, 267–272.

57. Wellems, T. E. and Fairhurst, R. M. (2005) Malaria-protective traits at odds in Africa? *Nature*, **37**(11), 1160–1162.

58. Aidoo, M., Terlouw, D. J., Kolczak, M. S., McElroy, P., ter Kuile, F., Kariuki, S., Nahlen, B., Lal, A., and Udhayakumar, V. (2002) Protective effects of the sickle cell gene against malaria morbidity and mortality, *Lancet*, **359**, 1311–1312.

59. Mockenhaupt, F. P., Ehrhardt, S., Cramer, J. P., Otchwemah, R. N., Anemana, S. D., Goltz, K., Mylius, F., Dietz, E., Eggelte, T. A., and Bienzle, U. (2004) Hemoglobin C and resistance to severe malaria in Ghanaian children, *J. Infect. Dis.*, **190**, 1006–1009.

60. Flint, J., Harding, R. M., Boyce, A. J., and Clegg, J. B. (1998) The population genetics of the haemoglobinopathies, *Baillieres Clin. Haematol.*, **11**, 1–51.

61. Looareesuwan, S., Tokunaga, K., Ohashi, J., Clark, A. G., Naka, I., Patarapotikul, J., Hananatachai, H., and Brittenham, G. (2004) Extended linkage disequilibrium surrounding the hemoglobin E variant due to malarial selection, *Am. J. Hum. Genet.*, **74**(6), 1198–1208.

62. Flatz, G., Sanguansermsri, T., Sengchanh, S., Horst, D., and Horst, J. (2004) The "hot spot" of Hb E [β26(B8)Glu→Lys] in Southeast Asia: β-globin anomalies in the Lao Theung population of Southern Laos, *Hemoglobin*, **28**(3), 197–204.

63. Win, N, Lwin, A. A., Oo, M. M., Aye, K. S., Soe-Soe, and Okada, S. (2005) Hemoglobin E prevalence in malaria-endemic villages in Myanmar, *Acta Med. Okayama*, **59**(2), 63–66.

64. Lachant, N. A. and Tanaka, K. R. (2006) Impaired antioxidant defense in hemoglobin E-containing eruthrocytes: a mechanism protective against malaria? *Am. J. Hematol.*, **26**(3), 211–219.

65. Ohashi, J., Naka, I., Patarapotikul, J., Hananantachai, H., Brittenham, G., Looareesuwan, S., Clark, A. G., and Tokunaga, K. (2004) Extended linkage disequilibrium surrounding the hemoglobin E variant due to malarial selection, *Am. J. Hum. Genet.*, **74**, 1198–1208.

66. Nagel, R. L., Raventos-Suarez, C., Febby, M. E., Tonowitz, H., Sicard, D., and Labie, D. ((1981) Impairment of the growth of *P. falciparum* in HbEE erythrocytes, *J. Clin. Invest.*, **68**, 303–305.

67. Santiyanont, R. and Wilairat, P. (1981) Red cells containing hemoglobin E do not inhibit malaria parasite development *in vitro*, *Am. J. Trop. Med. Hyg.*, **30**, 541–543.

68. Kruatrachue, M., Bhaibulaya, M., Klongkamnaunkam, K., and Harinasula, C. (1969) Haemoglobinopathies and malaria in Thailand, *Bull. World Health Organ.*, **40**, 459–463.

69. Flatz, G., Pik, C. and Sundharagiati, B. (1964) Malaria and haemoglobin E in Thailand, *Lancet*, *ii*, 385–387.

70. Hutagalung, R., Wilairatana, P., Looareesuwan, S., Brittenham, G. M., Aikawa, M., and Gordeuk, V. R. (1999) Influence of hemoglobin E trait on the severity of falciparum malaria, *J. Infect. Dis.*, **179**, 283–286.

71. Williams, T. N., Maitland, K., Bennett, S., Ganczakowski, M., Peto, T. E. A., Newbold, C. I., Bowden, D. K., Weatherall, D. J., and Clegg, J. B. (1996) High incidence of malaria in α-thalassaemic children, *Nature*, **383**, 522–525.

72. Williams, T. N., Mwangi, T. W., Wambua, S., Peto, T. E. A., Weatherall, D. J., Gupta, S., Recker, M., Penman, B. S., Uyoga, S., Macharia, A., Mwacharo, J. K., Snow, R. W., and Marsh, K. (2005) Negative epistasis between the malaria-protective effects of α⁺-thalassemia and the sickle cell trait, *Nat. Genet.*, **37**(11), 1253–1257.

73. Friedman, M. J. (1978) Erythrocytic mechanism of sickle cell resistance to malaria, *Proc. Natl. Acad. Sci. U.S.A.*, **75**, 1994–1997.

74. Friedman, M. J., Roth, E. F., Nagel, R. L., and Trager, W. (1979) The role of hemoglobin C, S and NBatl in the inhibition of malaria parasite development in vitro, *Am. J. Trop. Med. Hyg.*, **28**, 777–780.

75. Pasvol, G. (1980) The interaction between sickle haemoglobin and the malaria parasite *Plasmodium falciparum*, *Trans. R. Soc. Trop. Med. Hyg.*, **74**, 701–705.

76. Vernes, A. J.-M., Heynes, J. D., Tang, D. B., Dutoit, E., and Diggs, C. L. (1986) Decreased growth of *Plasmodium falciparum* in red cells contain haemoglobin E, a role for oxidative stress, and a sero-epidemiological correlation, *Trans. R. Soc. Trop. Med. Hyg.*, **80**, 642–648.

77. Bunyaratvej, A., Butthep, P., Kaewkettong, P., and Yuthavong, Y. (1997) Malaria protection in hereditary ovalocytosis: relation to red cell deformability, red cell parameters and degree of ovalocytosis, Southeast Asia, *Southeast Asian J. Trop. Med. Publ. Health*, **28**, 38–42.

78. Pasvol, G., Weatherall, D. J., Wilson, R. J., Smith, D. H., and Giles, H. M. (1976) Fetal hemoglobin and malaria, *Nature*, **1**(7972), 1269–1270.

79. Pasvol, G., Weatherall, D. J., and Wilson, R. J. (1977) Effects of fetal hemoglobin on susceptibility of red cell to *Plasmodium falciparum*, *Nature*, **270**, 171–173.

80. Bunyaratvej, A., Butthep, P., Sae-Ung, N., Fuchareon, S., and Yuthavong, Y. (1992) Reduced deformability of thalassemic erythrocytes and erythrocytes with abnormal hemoglobins and relation with susceptibility to *Plasmodium falciparum* invasion, *Blood*, **79**, 2460–2463.

81. Udomsangpetch, R., Sueblinvong, T., Pattanapanyasat, K., Dharmkrong-al, A., and Webster, H. K. (1993) Alteration in cytoadherance and resetting of *Plasmodium falciparum*-infected thalassemic red blood cells, *Blood*, **82**, 3752–3759.

82. Carlson, J., Nash, G. B., Gabutti, V., Al Yaman, F., and Wahlgren, M. (1994) Natural protection against severe *Plasmodium falciparum* malaria due to impaired rosette formation, *Blood*, **84**, 3909–3914.

83. Luzzi, G. A. and Pasvol, G. (1990) Cytoadherence of *Plasmodium falciparum*-infected α-thalassemic red cells, *Ann. Trop. Med. Parasitol.*, **84**, 413–414.

84. Bayoumi, R. A., Abu-Zeid, Y. A., Abdulhadi, N. H., Saeed, B. O., Theander, T. G., Hviid, L., Ghalib, H. V., Nugud, A.

H., Jepsen, S., and Jensen, J. B. (1990) Cell-mediated immune responses to *Plasmodium falciparum* purified soluble antigens in sickle-cell trait subjects, *Immunol. Lett.*, **25**, 243–249.

85. Luzzi, G. A., Merry, A. H., Newbold, C. I., Marsh, K., Pasvol, G., and Weatherall, D. J. (1991) Surface antigen expression on *Plasmodium falciparum*-infected erythrocytes is modified in α- and β-thalassemia, *J. Exp. Med.*, **173**, 785–791.

86. Abu-Zeid, Y. A., Theander, T. G., Abdulhadi, N.H., Hviid, L., Saeed, B. O., Jepsen, S., Jepsen, J. B., and Bayoumi, R. A. (1992) Modulation of the cellular immune response during *Plasmodium falciparum* infections in sickle cell trait individuals, *Clin. Exp. Immunol.*, **88**, 112–118.

87. Allison, A. C. (1964) Polymorphism and natural selection in human populations, *Cold Spring Harb. Symp. Quant. Biol.*, **29**, 137–149.

88. Nagel, R. L. and Fleming, A. F. (1992) Genetic epidemiology of the beta S gene, *Baillieres Clin. Haematol.*, **5**, 331–365.

89. Williams, T. N., Wambua, S., Uyoga, S., Macharia, A., Mwacharo, J. K., Newton, C. R. J. C., and Maitland, K. (2005) Both heterozygous and homozygous alpha⁺ thalassemias protect against severe and fatal *Plasmodium falciparum* malaria on the coast of Kenya, *Blood*, **106**, 368–371.

90. Mockenhaupt, F. P., Ehrhardt, S., Gellet, S., Otchwemah, R., N., Dietz, E., Anemana, S. D., and Bienzle, U. (2004) α⁺ Thalasemia protects African children from malaria, *Blood*, **104**, 2003–2006.

91. Allen, S. J., O'Donnell, A., Alexander, N. D. E., Alpers, M. P., Peto, T. E. A., Clegg, J. B., and Weatherall, D. G. (1997) α⁺-Thalasemia protects children caused by other infections as well as malaria, *Proc. Natl. Acad. Sci. U.S.A.*, **94**, 14736–14741.

92. Weatherall, D. J. and Clegg, J. B. (2001) Inherited haemoglobin disorders: an increasing global health problem, *Bull. World Health Organ.*, **79**, 704–712.

93. Rihet, P., Flori, L., Tall, F., Traore, A. S., and Fumoux, F. (2004) Hemoglobin C is associated with reduced *Plasmodium falciparum* parasitemia and low risk of mild malaria attack, *Hum. Mol. Genet.*, **13**(1), 1–6.

94. Fairhurst, R. M., Fujioka, H., Hayton, K., Collins, K. F., and Wellems, T. E. (2003) Aberrant development of *Plasmodium falciparum* in hemoglobin CC red cells: implications for the malaria protective effect of the homozygous state, *Blood*, **101**(8), 3309–3315.

95. Conway, D. J. (2007) Molecular epidemiology of malaria, *Clin. Microbiol. Rev.*, **20**(1), 188–204.

96. Nielsen, M. A., Staalsoe, T., Kurtzhals, J. A. L., Goka, B. Q., Dodoo, D., Alifrangis, M., Theander, T. G., Akanmori, B. D., and Hviid, L. (2002) *Plasmodium falciparum* variant surface antigen expression varies between isolates causing severe and nonsevere malaria and is modified by host immunity, *J. Immunol.*, **168**, 3444–3450.

97. Bull, P. C., Berriman, M., Kyes, S., Quail, M. A., Hall, N., Kortok, M. M., Marsh, K., and Newbold, C. I. (2005) *Plasmodium falciparum* variant surface antigen expression patterns during malaria, *PLoS Pathol.*, **1**, e26.

98. Bull, P. C., Pain, A., Ndungu, F. M., Kinyanjui, S. M., Roberts, D. J., Newbold, C. I., and Marsh, K. (2005) *Plasmodium falciparum* antigenic variation: relationships between in vivo selection, acquired antibody response, and disease severity, *J. Infect. Dis.*, **192**, 1119–1126.

99. Gardner, M. J., Hall, N., Fung, E., White, O., Berriman, M., Hyman, R. W., Carlton, J. M., and Pain, A. (2002) Genome sequence of the human malaria parasite *Plasmodium falciparum*, *Nature*, **419**, 498–511.

100. Lavstsen, T., Salanti, A., Jensen, A. T. R., Arnot, D. E., and Theander, T. G. (2003) Sub-grouping of *Plasmodium falciparum*

3D7 var genes based on sequence analysis of coding and non-coding regions, *Malar. J.*, **2**, 27.

101. Simpson, J. A., Aarons, L., Collins, W. E., Jeffery, G. M., and White, N. J. (2002) Population dynamics of untreated *Plasmodium falciparum* malaria within the adult human host during the expansion phase of the infection, *Parasitology*, **124**, 247–263.

102. Baum, J., Pinder, M., and Conway, D. J. (2003) Erythrocyte invasion phenotypes of *Plasmodium falciparum* in The Gambia, *Infect. Immun.*, **71**, 1856–1863.

103. Lobo, C. A., de Frazao, K., Rodriguez, M., Reid, M., Zalis, M., and Lustigman, S. (2004) Invasion profiles of Brasilian field isolates of *Plasmodium falciparum*: phenotypic and genotypic analyses, *Infect. Immun.*, **72**, 5886–5891.

104. Okoyeh, J. N., Pillai, C. R., and Chitnis, C. E. (1999) *Plasmodium falciparum* field isolates commonly use erythrocyte invasion pathways that are independent of sialic acid residues of glycophorin A, *Infect. Immun.*, **67**, 5784–5791.

105. Daily, J. P., Le Roch, K. G., Sarr, O., Fang, X., Zhou, Y., Ndir, O., Mboup, S., Sultan, A., Winzeler, E. A., and Wirth, D. F. (2004) In vivo transcriptional profiling of *Plasmodium falciparum*, *Malar. J.*, **3**, 30.

106. Daily, J. P., Le Roch, K. G., Sarr, O., Ndiaye, D., Lukens, A., Zhou, Y., Ndir, O., Mboup, S., Sultan, A., Winzeler, E. A., and Wirth, D. F. (2005) *In vivo* transcriptome of *Plasmodium falciparum* reveals overexpression of transcripts that encode surface proteins, *J. Infect. Dis.*, **191**, 1196–1203.

107. Hviid, L. (2004) The immuno-epidemiology of pregnancy-associated *Plasmodium falciparum* malaria: a variant surface antigen-specific perspective, *Parasite Immunol.*, **26**, 477–486.

108. Beeson, J. G. and Brown, G. V. (2004) *Plasmodium falciparum*-infected erythrocyte demonstrate dual specificity for adhesion to hyaluronic acid and chondroitin sulfate A and have distinct adhesive properties, *J. Infect. Dis.*, **189**, 169–179.

109. Salanti, A., Dahlback, M., Turner, L., Nielsen, M. A., Barfod, L., Magistrado, P., Jensen, A. T., Lavstsen, T., Ofori, M. F., Marsh, K., Hviid, L., and Theander, T. G. (2004) Evidence for the involvement of VAR2CSA in pregnancy-associated malaria, *J. Exp. Med.*, **200**, 1197–1203.

110. Viebig, N. K., Gamain, B., Scheidig, C., Lepolard, C., Przyborski, J., Lanzer, M., Gysin, J., and Scherf, A. (2005) A single member of the *Plasmodium falciparum* var multigene family determines cytoadhesion to the placental receptor chondroitin sulphate A, *EMBO J.*, **6**, 775–781.

111. Duffy, M. F., Caragounis, A., Noviyanti, R., Kyriacou, H. M., Choong, E. K., Boysen, K., Healer, J., Rowe, J. A., Molyneux, M. E., Brown, G. V., and Rogerson, S. J. (2006) Transcribed *var* genes associated with placental malaria in Malawian women, *Infect. Immun.*, **74**, 4875–4883.

112. Tuikue Ndam, N. G., Salanti, A., Bertin, G., Dahlback, Fievet, N., Turner, L., Gaye, A., Theander, T., and Deloron, P. (2005) High level of *var2csa* transcription by *Plasmodium falciparum* isolated from the placenta, *J. Infect. Dis.*, **102**, 331–335.

113. Staalsoe, T., Shulman, C. E., Bulmer, J. N., Kawuondo, K., Marsh, K., and Hviid, L. (2004) Variant surface antigen-specific IgG and protection against clinical consequences of pregnancy-associated *Plasmodium falciparum* malaria, *Lancet*, **363**, 283–289.

114. Moody, A. H. and Chiodini, P. L. (2000) Methods for the detection of blood parasites, *Clin. Lab. Haematol.*, **22**, 189–201.

115. Lee, S. H., Kara, U. A., Koay, E., Lee, M. A., Lam, S., and Teo, D. (2002) New strategies for the diagnosis and screening of malaria, *Int. J. Hematol.*, **76**(Suppl. 1), 291–293.

116. Nacher, M., Singhasivanon, P., Silachamroon, U., Treeprasertsuk, S., Tosukhowong, T., Vannaphan, S., Gay, F., Mazier, D., and Looareesuwan, S. (2002) Decreased hemoglobin concentra-

tions, hyperparasitemia, and severe malaria are associated with increased *Plasmodium falciparum* gametocyte carriage, *J. Parasitol.*, **88**(1), 97–101.

117. Samaja, M., Rovida, E., Motterlini, R., Tarantola, M., Rubinacci, A., and di Prampero, P. E. (1990) Human red cell age, oxygen affinity and oxygen transport, *Respir. Physiol.*, **79**, 69–79.

118. Hoffman, R. E., Benz, J., Shattil, S. J., Furie, B., and Cohen, H. (1991) *Hematology: Basic Principles and Practice*, Churchill Livingstone, Edinburgh, Scotland, pp.458–468.

119. Robert, V., Tchuinkam, T., Mulder, B., Bodo, J. M., Verhave, J. P., Carnevale, P., and Nagel, R. L. (1996) Effect of the sickle cell trait status of gametocyte carriers of *Plasmodium falcipare* on infectivity to anophelines, *Am. J. Trop. Med. Hyg.*, **54**, 111–113.

120. Silamut, K. and White, N. J. (1993) Relation of the stage of parasite development in the peripheral blood to prognosis in severe falciparum malaria, *Trans. R. Soc. Trop. Med. Hyg.*, **87**, 436–443.

121. Hsia, C. C. (1998) Respiratory function of hemoglobin, *N. Engl. J. Med.*, **338**, 239–247.

122. Taylor-Robinson, A. (2000) The sequestration hypothesis: an explanation for the sensitivity of malaria parasites to nitric oxide-mediated immune effector function in vivo, *Med. Hypothesis*, **54**, 638–641.

123. Jarra, W. and Brown, K. N. (1989) Invasion of mature and immature erythrocytes of CBA/Ca mice by a cloned line of *Plasmodium chabaudi*, *Parasitology*, **99**, 157–163.

124. Gautret, P., Miltgen, F., Gantier, J. C., Chabaud, A. G., and Landau, I. (1996) Enhanced gametocyte formation by *Plasmodium chabaudi* in immature erythrocytes: pattern of production, sequestration, and infectivity to mosquitoes, *J. Parasitol.*, **82**, 900–906.

125. Trager, W. and Gill, G. S. (1992) Enhanced gametocyte formation in young erythrocytes by *Plasmodium falciparum* in vitro, *J. Protozool.*, **39**, 429–432.

126. Trager, W., Gill, G. S., Lawrence, C., and Nagel, R. L. (1999) *Plasmodium falciparum*: enhanced gametocyte formation in vitro in reticulocyte-rich blood, *Exp. Parasitol.*, **91**, 115–118.

127. White, N. J. (2003) Malaria. In: *Manson's Tropical Diseases* (Cook, G. C., Zumla, A. I., and Weir, J., eds.), W. B. Saunders, Philadelphia, pp. 1205–1295.

128. Genton, B. and D'Acremont, V. (2001) Clinical features of malaria in returning travelers and migrants. In: *Travelers' Malaria* (Schlagenhauf, P., ed.), Hamilton, Ontario, Canada, B. C. Decker, pp. 371–392.

129. Swenson, J. E., MacLean, J. D., Gyorkos, T. W., and Keystone, J. (1995) Imported malaria. Clinical presentation and examination of symptomatic travelers, *Arch. Intern. Med.*, **155**, 861–868.

130. World Health Organization (1990) Severe and complicated malaria, *Trans. R. Soc. Trop. Hyg.*, **84**(Suppl. 2), S1–S65.

131. Brewster, D. R., Kwiatkowski, D., and White, N. J. (1990) Neurological sequelae of cerebral malaria in children, *Lancet*, **336**, 1039–1043.

132. Mehta, K. S., Halankar, A. R., Makwana, P. D., Torane, P. P., Satija, P. S., and Shah, V. B. (2001) Severe acute renal failure in malaria, *J. Postgrad. Med.*, 47, 24–26.

133. Griffith, K. S., Lewis, L. S., Mali, S., and Parise, M. E. (2007) Treatment of malaria in the United States. A systematic review, *J. Am. Med. Assoc.*, **297**(20), 2264–2277.

134. Lalloo, D. G., Shingadia, D., Pasvol, G., Chiodini, P. L., Whitty, C. J., Beeching, N. J., Hill, D. R., Warrell, D. A., and Bannister, B. A., for the HPA Advisory Committee on Malaria Prevention in UK Travelers (2007) UK malaria treatment guidelines, *J. Infect., Dis.*, **54**, 111–121.

135. Centers for Disease Control (2000) Availability and use of parenteral quinidine gluconate for severe or complicated malaria, *Morb. Mortal. Wkly Rep.*, **49**, 1138–1140.

136. White, N. J. (1996) The treatment of malaria, *N. Engl. J. Med.*, **335**, 800–806.

137. Bonington, A., Davidson, R. N., Winstanley, P. A., and Pasvol, G. (1996) Fatal quinine cardiotoxicity in the treatment of falciparum malaria, *Trans. R. Soc. Trop. Med. Hyg.*, **90**, 305–307.

138. Pittler, M. H. and Ernest, E. (1999) Artemether for severe malaria: a meta-analysis of randomized clinical trials, *Clin. Infect. Dis.*, **28**, 597–601.

139. Tran, T. H., Day, N. P., Nguyen, H. P., Nguyen, T. H., Tran, T. H., Pham, P. L., Dinh, X. S., Ly, V. C., Ha, V., Waller, D., Peto, T. E., and White, N. J. (1996) A controlled trial of artemether or quinine in Vietnamese adults with severe falciparum malaria, *N. Engl. J. Med.*, **335**, 76–83.

140. Murphy, S., English, M., Waruiru, C., Mwangi, I., Amukoye, E., Crawley, J., Newton, C., Winstanley, P., Peshu, N., and Marsh, K. (1996) An open randomized trial of artemether versus quinine in the treatment of cerebral malaria in African children, *Trans. R. Soc. Trop. Med. Hyg.*, **90**, 298–301.

141. World Health Organization (WHO) (2006) *Guidelines for Treatment of Malaria*, NLM classification: WC 770, ISBN 978 92 4 154694 2.

142. Hatz, C. F. (2001) Clinical treatment of malaria in returned travelers. In: *Traveler's Malaria* (Schlagenhauf, P., ed.), Hamilton, Ontario, Canada, B. C. Decker, pp. 431–445.

143. Gold, H. S. and Moellering, R. C. (1996) Antimalarial-drug resistance, *N. Engl. J. Med.*, **335**, 1445–1453.

144. Barat, L. M. and Bloland, P. B. (1997) Drug resistance among malaria and other parasites, *Infect. Dis. Clin. North Am.*, **11**, 969–987.

145. Krogstad, D. J. (1996) Malaria as a reemerging disease, *Epidemiol. Rev.*, **18**, 77–89.

146. White, N. J. (1992) Antimalarial drug resistance: the pace quickens, *J. Antimicrob. Chemother.*, **30**, 571–585.

147. Centers for Disease Control (2000) Availability and use of parenteral quinidine gluconate for severe or complicated malaria, *Morb. Mortal. Wkly Rep.*, **49**(50), 1138–1140.

148. Miller, K. D., Greenberg, A. E., and Campbell, C. C. (1989) Treatment of severe malaria in the United States with a continuous infusion of quinidine gluconate and exchange transfusion, *N. Engl. J. Med.*, **321**(2), 65–70.

149. Powell, V. I. and Grima, K. (2002) Exchange transfusion for malaria and *Babesia* infection, *Transfus. Med. Rev.*, **16**(3), 239–250.

150. Kwiatkowski, D., Molyneux, M. E., Stephens, S., Curtis, N., Klein, N., Pointaire, P., Smit, M., Allan, R., Brewster, D. R., and Grau, G. E. (1993) Anti-TNF therapy inhibits fever in cerebral malaria, *Q. J. Med.*, **86**, 91–98.

151. Warrell, D. A., Looareesuwan, S., Warrell, M. J., Kasemsarn, P., Intaraprasert, R., Bunnag, D., and Harinasuta, T. (1982) Dexamethazone proves deleterious in cerebral malaria. A double-blind trial in 100 comatose patients, *N. Engl. J. Med.*, **306**, 313–319.

152. Clyde, D. F., Most, H., McCarthy, V. C., and Vanderberg, J. P. (1973) Immunization of man against sporozoite-induced falciparum malaria, *Am. J. Med. Sci.*, **266**, 169–177.

153. Hoffman, S. L., Goh, L. M., Luke, T. C., Schneider, I., Le, T. P., Doolan, D. L., Sacci, J., de la Vega, P., Dowler, M., Paul, C., Gordon, D. M., Stoute, J. A., Church, L. W. P., Sedegah, M., Heppner, D. G., Ballou, W. R., and Richie, T. L. (2002) Protection of humans against malaria by immunization with radiation-attenuated *Plasmodium falciparum* sporozoites, *J. Infect. Dis.*, **185**, 1155–1164.

154. Kwiatkowski D. and Marsh, K. (1997) Vaccine series: development of a malaria vaccine, *Lancet*, **350**, 1696–1701.

155. Patarrouo, G., Franco, L., Amador, R., Murillo, L. A., Rocha, C. L., Rojas, M., and Patarroyo, M. E. (1992) Study of the safety and immunogenicity of the synthetic malaria SPf66 vaccine in children aged 1–14 years, *Vaccine*, **10**, 175–178.

156. Alonso, P. L., Smith, T., Schellenberg, J. R., et al. (1994) Randomized trial of efficacy of SPf66 vaccine against *Plasmodium falciparum* malaria in children in Tanzania, *Lancet*, **344**, 1175–1181.

157. D'Allesandro, U., Leach, A., Drakely, C. J., et al. (1995) Efficacy trial of malaria vaccine SPf66 in Gambian infants, *Lancet*, **346**, 462–467.

158. Nosten, F., Luxemburger, C., Kyle, D. E., et al. (1996) Randomized double-blind placebo-controlled trial of SPf66 malaria vaccine in children in northwestern Thailand. Shoklo SPf66 Malaria Vaccine Trial Group, *Lancet*, **348**, 701–707.

159. Acosta, C. J., Galindo, C. M., Schellenberg, D., et al. (1999) Evaluation of the SPf66 vaccine for malaria control when delivered through the EPI scheme in Tanzania, *Trop. Med. Int. Health*, **4**, 368–376.

160. Moorthy, V. S., Good, M. F., and Hill, A. V. S. (2004) Malaria vaccine developments, *Lancet*, **363**, 150–156.

161. Moorthy, V. and Hill, A. V. (2002) Malaria vaccines, *Br. Med. Bull.*, **62**, 59–72.

162. Shi, Y. P., Hasnain, S. E., Sacci, J. B., Holloway, B. P., Fujioka, H., Kumar, N., Wohlhueter, R., Hoffman, S. L., Collins, W. L., and Lal, A. A. (1999) Immunogenicity and in vitro protective efficacy of a recombinant multistage *Plasmodium falciparum* candidate vaccine, *Proc. Natl. Acad. Sci. U.S.A.*, **96**, 1615–1620.

163. Okie, S. (2005) Betting on a malaria vaccine, *N. Engl. J. Med.*, **353**, 1877–1881.

164. Prudhomme O'Meara, W., Hall, B. F., and McKenzie, F. E. (2007) Malaria vaccine efficacy: the difficulty of detecting and diagnosing malaria, *Malar. J.*, **6**, 36.

165. Lachenbruch, P. A. (1998) Sensitivity, specificity, and vaccine efficacy, *Control Clin. Trials*, **19**(6), 569–574.

165a. Prudhomme O'Meara, W., Barkus, M., Wongsrichamalai, et al. (2006) Reader technique as a source of variability in determining malaria parasite density by microscopy, *Malaria J.*, **5**, 118.

166. McKenzie, F. E., Sirichaisinthrop, J., Miller, R. S., Gasser, R. A., and Wongsrichanalai, C. (2003) Dependence of malaria detection and species diagnosis by microscopy on parasite density, *Am. J. Trop. Med. Hyg.*, **69**(4), 372–376.

167. Ohrt, C., Purnomo, Sutamihardja, M. A., Tang, D., and Kain, K. C. (2002) Impact of microscopy error on estimates of protective efficacy in malaria-prevention trials, *J. Infect. Dis.*, **186**(4), 540–546.

168. Prudhomme O'Meara, W., McKenzie, F. E., Magill, A. J., Forney, J. R., Permpanich, B., Lucas, C., Gasser, R. A., and Wongsrichanai, C. (2005) Sources of variability in determining malaria parasite density by microscopy, *Am. J. Trop. Med. Hyg.*, **73**(3), 593–598.

169. Deley, V., Bouvier, P., Breslow, N., Doumbo, O., Sagara, I., Diakite, M., Mauris, A., Dolo, A., and Rougemont, A. (2000) What does a single determination of malaria parasite density mean? A longitudinal survey in Mali, *Trop. Med. Int. Health*, **5**(6), 404–412.

170. Alonso, P. L., Sacarlal, J., Aponte, J. J., Leach, A., Macete, E., Milman, J., Mandomando, I., Spiessens, B., Guinovart, C., Espasa, M., Bassat, Q., Aide, P., Ofori-Anyinam, O., Navia, M. M., Corachan, S., Ceuppens, M., Dubois, M. C., Demoitie, M. A., Dubovsky, F., Menendez, C., Tornieporth, N., Ballou, W. R., Thompson, R., and Cohen, J. (2004) Efficacy of the RTS,S/AS02A vaccine against *Plasmodium falciparum* infection and disease in young African children: randomized controlled trial, *Lancet*, **364**(9443), 1411–1420.

171. Nussenzweigg, R., Vanderberg, J., Most, H., and Orton, C. (1967) Protective immunity produced by the injection of

X-irradiated sporozoites of *Plasmodium berghei*, *Nature*, **216**, 160–162.

172. Srivastava, K., Singh, S., Singh, P., and Puri, S. K. (2007) *In vitro* cultivation of *Plasmodium falciparum*: studies with modified medium supplemental with ALBUMAX II and various animal sera, *Exp. Parasitol.*, **116**(2), 171–174.

173. Balu, B. and Adams, J. H. (2007) Advancement in transfection technologies for plasmodium, *Int. J. Parasitol.*, **37**, 1–10.

174. Kanoi, B. N. and Egwang, T. G. (2007) New concepts in vaccine development in malaria, *Curr. Opin. Infect. Dis.*, **20**, 311–316.

175. Mueller, A.-K., Labaied, M., Kappe, S. H. I., and Matuschewski, K. (2005) Genetically modified *Plasmodium* parasites as a protective experimental malaria vaccine, *Nature*, **433**, 164–167.

176. Mueller, A.-K., Camargo, N., Kaiser, K., Andorfer, C., Frevert, U., Matuschewski, K., and Kappe, S. H. I. (2005) *Plasmodium* liver stage developmental arrest by depletion of a protein at the parasite-host interface, *Proc. Natl. Acad. Sci. U.S.A.*, **102**, 3022–3027.

177. Van Dijk, M. R., Douradinha, B., Franke-Fayard, B., Heussler, V., van Dooren, M. W., van Schaijk, B., van Gemert, G.-J., Sauerwein, R. W., Mota, M. M., Waters, A. P., and Janse, C. J. (2005) Genetically attenuated, P36p-deficient malarial sporozoites induce protective immunity and apoptosis of infected liver cells, *Proc. Natl. Acad. Sci. U.S.A.*, **102**, 12194–12199.

178. Enea, V., Ellis, J., Zavala, F., (1984) DNA cloning of *Plasmodium falciparum* circumsporozoite gene: amino acid sequence of repetitive epitope, *Science*, **225**, 628–630.

179. Girard, M. P., Reed, Z. H., Friede, M., and Kieny, M. P. (2007) A review of human vaccine research and development: malaria, *Vaccine*, **25**, 1567–1580.

180. Ulmer, J. B., Donnelly, J. J., Parker, S. E., Rhodes, G. H., Felgner, P. L., Dwarki, V. J., Gromkowski, S. H., Deck, R. R., DeWitt, C. M., Friedman, A., et al. (1993) Heterologous protection against influenza by injection of DNA encoding a viral protein, *Science*, **259**, 1745–1749.

181. Li, S., Rodrigues, M., Rodriguez, D., Esteban, M., Palese, P., Nussenzweig, R. S., and Zavala, F. (1993) Priming with recombinant influenza virus followed by administration of recombinant vaccinia virus induces CD8+ T-cell-mediated protective immunity against malaria, *Proc. Natl. Acad. Sci. U.S.A.*, **90**, 5214–5218.

182. Wang, R., Doolan, D. L., Le, T. P., et al. (1998) Induction of antigen-specific cytotoxic T lymphocytes in humans by a malaria DNA vaccine, *Science*, **282**, 476–480.

183. Schneider, J., Gilbert, S. C., Blanchard, T. J., et al. (1998) Enhanced immunogenicity for CD8+ T cell induction and complete protective efficacy of malaria DNA vaccination by boosting with modified vaccinia virus Ankara, *Nat. Med.*, **4**, 397–402.

184. Gurunathan, S., Klinman, D. M., and Seder, R. A. (2000) DNA vaccines: immunology, application, and optimization, *Annu. Rev. Immunol.*, **18**, 927–974.

185. Miyahira, Y., Garcia-Sastre, A., Rodriguez, D., et al. (1998) Recombinant viruses expressing a human malaria antigen can elicit potentially protective immune CD8(+) responses in mice, *Proc. Natl. Acad. Sci. U.S.A.*, **95**, 3954–3959.

186. Paoletti, E. (1996) Application of pox virus vectors to vaccination: an update, *Proc. Natl. Acad. Sci. U.S.A.*, **93**, 11349–11353.

187. Stoute, J. A., Slaoui, M., Heppner, D. G., et al. (1997) A preliminary evaluation of a recombinant circumsporozoite protein vaccine against *Plasmodium falciparum* malaria. RTS,S Malaria Vaccine Evaluation Group, *N. Engl. J. Med.*, **336**, 86–91.

188. Potocnjak, P., Yoshida, N., Nussenzweig, R. S., and Nussenzweig, V. (1980) Monovalent fragments (Fab) of monoclonal antibodies to a sporozoite surface antigen (Pb44) protect mice against malarial infection, *J. Exp. Med.*, **151**, 1504–1513.

189. Nardin, E. H., Nussenzweig, V., Nussenzweig, R. S., et al. (1982) Circumsporozoite proteins of human malaria parasites *Plasmodium falciparum* and *Plasmodium vivax*, *J. Exp. Med.*, **156**, 20–30.

190. Bojang, K. A., Milligan, P. J., Pinder, M., et al. (2001) Efficacy of RTS,S/AS02 malaria vaccine against *Plasmodium falciparum* infection in semi-immune adult men in The Gambia: a randomized trial, *Lancet*, **358**, 1927–1934.

191. Schneider, J., Gilbert, S. C., Hannan, C. M., et al. (1999) Induction of CD8+ T cells using heterologous prime-boost immunization strategies, *Immunol. Rev.*, **170**, 29–38.

192. Moorthy, V. S., McConkey, S., Roberts, M., et al. (2003) Safety of DNA and modified vaccinia virus Ankara vaccines against liver-stage *P. falciparum* malaria in non-immune volunteers, *Vaccine*, **21**, 2004–2011.

193. Moorthy, V. S., Pinder, M., Reece, W. H. H., et al. (2003) Safety and immunogenicity of DNA/modified vaccinia virus Ankara malaria vaccination in African adults, *J. Infect. Dis.*, **188**, 1239–1244.

194. McConkey, S., Reece, W. H. H., Moorthy, V. S., et al. (2003) Enhanced T-cell immunogenicity in humans of plasmid DNA vaccines boosted by recombinant modified vaccinia virus Ankara, *Nat. Med.*, **9**, 729–735.

195. Moorthy, V. S., Imoukhuede, E. B., Milligan, P., et al. (2004) A randomized, double-blind, controlled vaccine efficacy trial of DNA/MVA ME-TRAP against malaria infection in Gambian adults, *PLoS Med.*, **1**(2), e33.

196. Holder, A. A., Guevara Patino, J. A., Uthaipibull, C., et al. (1999) Merozoite surface protein 1, immune evasion, and vaccines against asexual blood stage malaria, *Parasitologia*, **41**, 409–414.

197. Genton, B., Betuela, I., Felger, I., et al. (2002) A recombinant blood-stage malaria vaccine reduces *Plasmodium falciparum* density and exerts selective pressure on parasite populations in a phase 1–2b trial in Papua New Guinea, *J. Infect. Dis.*, **185**, 820–827.

198. Ockenhouse, C. F., Sun, P. F., Lanar, D. E., et al. (1998) Phase I/II safety, immunogenicity, and efficacy trial of NYVAC-Pf7, a pox-vectored, multiantigen, multistage vaccine candidate for *Plasmodium falciparum* malaria, *J. Infect. Dis.*, **177**, 1664–1673.

199. Oeuvray, C., Theisen, M., Rogier, C., Trape, J. F., Jepsen, S., and Druilhe, P. (2000) Cytophilic immunoglobulin responses to *Plasmodium falciparum* glutamate-rich protein are correlated with protection against clinical malaria in Dielmo, Senegal, *Infect. Immun.*, **68**, 2617–2620.

200. Oeuvray, C., Bouharoun-Tayoun, H., Gras-Masse, H., et al. (1994) Merozoite surface protein-3: a malaria protein inducing antibodies that promote *Plasmodium falciparum* killing by cooperation with blood monocytes, *Blood*, **84**, 1594–1602.

201. Fried, M., Domingo, G. J., and Gowda, C. D., et al. (2006) *Plasmodium falciparum*: chondroitin sulfate A is the major receptor for adhesion of parasitized erythrocytes in the placenta, *Exp. Parasitol.*, **113**, 36–42.

202. Moll, K., Pettersson, F., Vogt, A. M., et al. (2007) Generation of cross-protective antibodies against *Plasmodium falciparum* sequestration by immunization with an erythrocyte membrane protein 1-Duffy binding-like1α domain, *Infect. Immun.*, **75**, 211–219.

203. Hall, N., Karras, M., Raine, J. D., et al. (2005) A comprehensive survey of the *Plasmodium* life cycle by genomic, transcriptomic, and proteomic analyses, *Science*, **307**, 82–86.

204. Daily, J. P., Le Roch, K. G., Sarr, O., et al. (2005) In vivo transcriptome of *Plasmodium falciparum* reveals overexpression of transcripts that encode surface proteins, *J. Infect. Dis.*, **191**, 1196–1203.

205. Mu, J., Awadalla, P., Duan, J., McGee, K. M., Keebler, J., Seydel, K., McVean, G. A. T., and Su, X.-Z. (2007) Genome-wide variation and identification of vaccine targets in *Plasmodium falciparum* genome, *Nat. Med.*, **39**, 126–130.

206. Hall, B. F. (Lee) and Fauci, A. S. (2007) Africa Malaria Day and Malaria Awareness Day, April 25, 2007 (http://www3.niaid.nih.gov/about/directors/news/malaria_07.htm).

207. Lopansri, B. K., Anstey, N. M., Stoddard, G. J., Mwaikambo, E. D., Bouitlis, C. S., Tjitra, E., Maniboey, H., Hobbs, M. R., Levesque, M. C., Weinberg, J. B., and Granger, D. L. (2006) Elevated plasma phenylalanine in severe malaria and implications for pathophysiology of neurological complications, *Infect. Immun.*, **74**(6), 3355–3359.

208. Laufer, M. K., van Oosterhout, J. J. G., Thesing, P. C., Thumba, F., Zijlstra, E. E., Graham, S. M., Taylor, T. E., and Plowe, C. V. (2006) Impact of HIV-associated immunosuppression on malaria infection and disease in Malawi, *J. Infect. Dis.*, **193**, 872–878.

209. McDevitt, M. A., Xie, J., Shanmugasundaram, G., Griffith, J., Liu, A., McDonald, C., Thuma, P., Gordeuk, V. R., Metz, C. N., Mitchell, R., Keefer, J., David, J., and Bucala, R. (2006) A critical role for the host mediator macrophage migration inhibitory factor in the pathogenesis of malarial anemia, *J. Exp. Med.*, **203**(5), 1185–1196.

210. Korochkina, S., Barreau, C., Pradel, G., Jeffery, E., Li, J., Natarajan, R., Shabanowitz, J., Hunt, D., Frevert, U., and Vernick K. D. (2006) A mosquito-specific protein family includes candidate receptor for malaria sporozoite invasion of salivary glands, *Cell. Microbiol.*, **8**, 163–175.

211. Wang, S. X., Oandey, K. C., Somoza, J. R., Sijwali, P. S., Korteme, T., Brinen, L. S., Fletterick, R. J., Rosenthal, P. J., and McKerrow, J. H. (2006) Structural basis for unique mechanisms of folding and hemoglobin binding by a malarial protease, *Proc. Natl. Acad. Sci. U.S.A.*, **103**(31), 11503–11508.

Chapter 21

Rickettsia: The Typhus Group

The phylogenetic position of *Rickettsia*, as inferred from rRNA sequence data, is within the α-proteobacteria group *(1)*. The genus *Rickettsia* comprises two main groups: the typhus group *Rickettsia* and the spotted fever group *Rickettsia*. However, several species, such as *Rickettsia bellii* and *Rickettsia canada*, although phylogenetically close, have been shown to be distinct from the two main groups *(2, 3)*.

Rickettsia prowazekii and *Rickettsia typhi* are the only two members of the typhus group. Both species are pathogenic to humans *(4)*. The Latin name of the typhus pathogen, *Rickettsia prowazekii*, was given to honor the scientists who in 1909 first described this organism, H. T. Ricketts and S. J. M. Prowazek. Unfortunately, both scientists contracted typhus and died during their studies of the pathogen.

For hundreds of years, epidemics of typhus have taken the lives of tens of millions of people, making this pathogen one of the main sources of human disasters. The discovery in 1909 by Charles Nicolle of the Pasteur Institute that typhus is transmitted by the human body louse, *Pediculus humanus corporis (5)*, is considered to have had immeasurable importance when simple hygienic measures saved the lives of thousands of soldiers and civilians throughout World Wars I and II.

According to the World Health Organization (WHO), even though epidemics of typhus are now very rare, the disease is still a major health problem in some countries in Africa, where, as recently as 1995, there had been an outbreak of louse-borne epidemic typhus in Burundi *(6)*.

21.1 Rickettsia prowazekii Genome

The genome of *R. prowazekii* is very small, only 1.11 Mb *(4, 7)*. It is remarkable that as much as 24% of its genome consists of noncoding DNA. It has been convincingly demonstrated that the intergenic sequences in *R. prowazekii* comprise decayed genes that are no longer active but have not yet been completely eliminated *(8–10)*. The lack of coding potential in these regions was first established by comparative analyses of closely related strains and species, which revealed sequence similarities between genes in one species and pseudogenes or noncoding DNA in another species *(8–10)*.

As seen from the genome sequence data, as much as one third of the coding capacity of the ancestral *R. prowazekii* genome has been lost since its divergence from *Rickettsia conorii* (see Chapter 22). From a human perspective, it is remarkable that the genome of the highly pathogenic *R. prowazekii* is essentially only a degraded version of its close relative, *R. conorii*, which is a less-pathogenic species *(4)*.

The first information about the detailed pattern of degradation of single-gene sequences in *Rickettsia* was obtained from the *metK* gene, which codes for *S*-adenosylmethionine synthetase, an essential enzyme required for the biosynthesis of the essential cofactor *S*-adenosylmethionine (SAM) *(8)*. This gene contains a single termination codon in the Madrid E strain of *R. prowazekii*, but the reading frame is open in the Brein1 strain of *R. prowazekii* as well as in *R. typhi*. In all other *Rickettsia* species, this gene seems to have accumulated mutations in a random manner. It has been shown that there is a transport system for SAM in *Rickettsia* that presumably has rendered this gene nonessential *(11)*.

The mutations in the *metK* gene, which are supposed to represent neutral mutations, involved mainly deletions of one or a few bases *(8)*. The strong bias for deletion mutations has indicated that a gene inactivated by the accumulation of internal stop codons or frameshift mutations will eventually be eliminated solely as a function of the rate at which mutations are produced by the replication-repair machinery *(4)*.

As suggested by sequence data analyses (including genes, pseudogenes, noncoding DNA, and repeated sequences), compared with the spotted fever group (SFG) *Rickettsia*, the process of sequence elimination has occurred more rapidly in the typhus group *Rickettsia*. That is to say, genes that evolve within the SFG seemed to have higher probability

V. St. Georgiev, *National Institute of Allergy and Infectious Diseases, NIH: Impact on Global Health*, vol. 2, DOI 10.1007/978-1-60327-297-1_21, © Humana Press, a part of Springer Science+Business Media, LLC 2009

of survival than those that evolve within the typhus group *Rickettsia*.

Thus, it has been suggested that the difference in size and rate of genome degradation may be related to some intrinsic mechanisms by which deletion mutations are produced, or it may be related to the different population structures of the various species *(4)*. For example, there is a striking difference between the ticks that transmit *R. conorii* and the lice that transmit *R. prowazekii*. Whereas a tick has a life span of 5 to 6 years, mates once per year, and takes a blood meal only twice in its lifetime, a louse has a life span of only 1 month, mates once per day, and takes a blood meal 5 times daily. It then becomes apparent that the bacterial population will expand much more frequently in lice than in ticks. Hence, if deletion mutations arise primarily during the replication phase of the parasite lifestyle, the pathogen using a vector with a shorter life span (the louse) is expected to go through more generations per year, thereby increasing the probabilities for all types of deletion mutations to accumulate in the population *(4)*.

Taken together, the data obtained to date have demonstrated that both *R. conorii* and *R. prowazekii* are exposed to similar evolutionary pressures, but the difference in their lifestyles will make these processes operate at different rates. This suggests that *R. conorii* is slowly on its way to becoming a copy of the modern *R. prowazekii* genome, which will by then be even smaller. Eventually, all repeats will be consumed, and gene degradation will occur by infinitesimally small steps *(4)*.

21.2 Epidemiology and Clinical Manifestations of Typhus

Humans are the main host and currently the only known natural reservoir for *R. prowazekii*, which uses the human body louse as its vector of transmission *(12)*. Lice are strictly blood-sucking insects that excrete feces containing millions of infected bacterial cells at the skin bite lesion. If rubbed or scratched into the skin, the pathogen will enter the human body *(4)*. In an unusual twist, infection with the pathogen is also fatal to the vector transmitting the disease because *R. prowazekii* multiplies intensively inside the midgut epithelial cells of the louse, inducing cell lysis.

Rickettsia may enter the host cells by induced phagocytosis, with phagocytic vesicles formed simultaneously with the binding of the bacterium to the receptors of the host cells. The primary target of the pathogen is the epithelium, which *Rickettsia* enters by an actin-dependent process *(13)*.

The incubation period for typhus is typically 10 to 14 days. At the onset of illness, the clinical symptoms include high fever, headache, and the development of rash on the trunk, limbs, and the axillar areas after 5 to 7 days. The central nervous system is invaded and neurologic disorders are common. Patients may fall into a coma during which body temperature is high and blood pressure is low. The mortality rate of typhus is between 10% and 30%.

Patients who have contracted typhus may retain *Rickettsia* in a chronic form, known as *Brill-Zinsser disease*, which may be activated under stressful conditions *(14)*. In turn, a single case of Brill-Zinsser disease may initiate a new outbreak of epidemic typhus if lice infestations are high in the population.

Murine typhus, a milder form of human disease, is caused by *R. typhi*. Rats are the main reservoir for this species, which is transferred to humans by rats or rat fleas.

Treatment. Typhus can still be cured by use of antibiotics, and natural antibiotic resistance has not yet been observed in rickettsial populations. Because epidemic outbreaks are strictly dependent on lice infestations, improved hygienic measures have significantly limited the spread of the disease in the past 100 years.

References

1. Olsen, G. J., Woese, C. R., and Overbeek, R. (1994) The winds of (evolutionary) change, breathing new life into microbiology, *J. Bacteriol.*, **176**, 1–6.
2. Roux, V., Ridkina, E., Eremeeva, M., and Raoult, D. (1997) Citrate synthase gene comparison, a new tool for phylogenetic analysis, and its application for Rickettsiae, *Int. J. Syst. Bacteriol.*, **47**, 252–261.
3. Andersson, S. G. E., Stothard, D. R., Fuerst, P., and Kurland, C. G. (1999) Molecular phylogeny and rearrangement of rRNA genes in *Rickettsia* species, *Mol. Biol. Evol.*, **47**, 252–261.
4. Andersson, S. G. E. (2004) Obligate intracellular pathogens. In: *Microbial Genomes* (Fraser, C. M., Read, T. D., and Nelson, K. E., eds.), Humana Press, Totowa, NJ, pp. 291–308.
5. Gross, L. (1996) How Charles Nicolle of the Pasteur Institute discovered that epidemic typhus is transmitted by lice: reminiscences from my years at the Pasteur Institute in Paris, *Proc. Natl. Acad. Sci. U.S.A.*, **93**, 10539–10540.
6. Raoult, D., Ndihokubwayo, J. B., Tissot-Dupont, H., et al. (1998) Outbreak of epidemic typhus associated with trench fever in Burundi, *Lancet*, **352**, 353–358.
7. Andersson, S. G. E., Zomorodipour, A., Andersson, J. O., et al. (1998) The genome sequence of *Rickettsia prowazekii* and the origin of mitochondria, *Nature*, **296**, 133–140.
8. Andersson, J. O. and Andersson, S. G. E. (1999) Genome degradation is an ongoing process in *Rickettsia*, *Mol. Biol. Evol.*, **16**, 1178–1191.
9. Andersson, J. O. and Andersson, S. G. E. (1999) Insights into the evolutionary process of genome degradation, *Curr. Opin. Genet. Dev.*, **9**, 664–671.
10. Andersson, J. O. and Andersson, S. G. E. (2001) Pseudogenes, junk DNA and the dynamics of *Rickettsia* genomes, *Mol. Biol. Evol.*, **18**, 829–839.
11. Tucker, A., Winkler, H. H., Driskell, L. O., and Wood, D. O. (2003) *S*-adenosylmethionine transport in *Rickettsia prowazekii*, *J. Bacteriol.*, **185**, 3031–3035.

12. Hackstadt, T. (1996) The biology of Rickettsiae, *Inf. Agents Dis.*, **5**, 127–143.

13. Walkers, T. S. (1984) Rickettsial interactions with human endothelial cells in vitro: adherence and entry, *Infect. Immun.*, **44**, 205–210.

14. Raoult, D. and Roux, V. (1997) Rickettsioses as paradigms of new or emerging infectious diseases, *Clin. Microbiol. Rev.*, **19**, 694–719.

Chapter 22

Tick-Borne Bacterial, Rickettsial, Spirochetal, and Protozoal Diseases

Approximately 900 tick species exist worldwide, parasitizing a broad array of mammals, including humans, and thereby playing a significant role in the transmission of infectious diseases (1). In the United States, tick-borne diseases are generally seasonal and geographically distributed. They occur mostly during the spring and summer but can occur throughout the year.

These blood-feeding arthropods that parasitize all vertebrates can be classified into three families: (i) Ixodidae (hard ticks) comprising approximately 700 species and 13 genera; (ii) Argasidae (soft ticks), which consists of approximately 180 species and 5 genera; and (iii) Nuttaliellidae, which is composed of only one species and is found only in Africa (1, 2).

Ticks are major vectors of arthropod-borne infections and not only can transmit a wide variety of pathogens, such as rickettsia and other bacteria, viruses, and protozoa, but also may carry more than one infectious agent and thus transmit one or more infections to humans at the same time (1).

Infections transmitted by the Ixodidae family (hard ticks) include (i) Lyme disease (borreliosis); (ii) human ehrlichiosis; (iii) Rocky Mountain spotted fever; (iv) tularemia; (v) southern tick-associated rash illness; and (vi) babesiosis. Infections transmitted by the Argasidae family (soft ticks) include the tick-borne relapsing fever (1).

Ticks of the Ixodidae family that transmit infections to humans are most often associated with the genera *Amblyomma*, *Ixodes*, *Dermacentor*, and *Rhicephalus*. They live in diverse but relatively humid habitats, and the infections they transmit are usually seasonal and geographically distributed. The hard ticks can attach securely to their hosts and feed slowly for prolonged periods, which will facilitate the transmission of infectious pathogens (1). In contrast, the only important disease-transmitting soft ticks belonging to the Argasidae family are those of the genus *Ornithodoros*, and they transmit spirochetes throughout their life cycle. *Ornithodoros* feed rapidly, typically at night, and may transmit disease in as little as 30 seconds (2).

In the United States, ticks have been found in all regions of the country, and the incidence rates of tick-borne diseases have increased steadily over the past decade or so (http://www3.niaid.nih.gov/research/topics/lyme/introduction/htm). Although Lyme disease and Rocky Mountain spotted fever are well known to the general public, recently emerging infections, such as ehrlichiosis and anaplasmosis (formerly known as human granulocytic ehrlichiosis), have now also been firmly established in the country. The increasing reports of tick-borne diseases likely reflect improved awareness, surveillance and diagnosis, but the growing U.S. population and the spread of human communities into previously undeveloped environments also increase the regions of tick-human contact.

Since the identification of *Borrelia burgdorferi* as the causative agent of Lyme disease in 1982, 11 tick-borne human bacterial pathogens have now been described throughout Europe. These include five spotted fever rickettsiae, the etiologic agent of human granulocytic anaplasmosis (HGA), four species of *B. burgdorferi* complex, and a new relapsing fever–causing *Borellia* (3).

If left untreated, the tick-borne infections can be associated with significant morbidity and even mortality.

22.1 Lyme Disease (Lyme Borreliosis, Lyme Arthritis)

Lyme disease (borreliosis) is the most prevalent tick-borne infectious disease in the United States. The disease is caused by a spiral-shaped bacterium *Borrelia burgdorferi* and is spread by the deer tick *Ixodes scapularis*. The likelihood for a person to be bitten by a deer tick is greater during the times of the year when ticks are most active. Young deer ticks, called *nymphs*, are active from mid-May to mid-August and are approximately the size of poppy seeds. Adult ticks, which are approximately the size of sesame seeds, are most active from March to mid-May and from mid-August to November. Both nymphs and adult ticks can transmit Lyme disease at any time when the temperatures are above freezing.

V. St. Georgiev, *National Institute of Allergy and Infectious Diseases, NIH: Impact on Global Health*, vol. 2,
DOI 10.1007/978-1-60327-297-1_22, © Humana Press, a part of Springer Science+Business Media, LLC 2009

During 2003–2005, CDC received reports of 64,382 Lyme disease cases from 46 states and the District of Columbia *(4)*; 93% of cases occurred among residents of the 10 *Healthy People 2010* reference states (see Table and Fig. 1 in Ref. *4*). The average annual rate in these 10 reference states for the 3-year period was 29.2 cases per 100,000 population: 29.1 in 2003, 26.8 in 2004, and 31.6 in 2005 *(4)*.

Not all deer ticks are infected with Lyme disease. Ticks can become infected only if they feed on small animals that are infected. In most cases, the tick must stay attached to humans for 36 hours or more before the bacteria can be transmitted. There is no person-to-person spread of Lyme disease. In extremely rare cases reported, the bacteria may be transferred from an infected pregnant woman to the fetus. Even if successfully treated, a person may become re-infected if bitten later by another infected tick.

22.1.1 Pathophysiology of Lyme Borreliosis

The complex life cycle of *B. burgdorferi*, which passes through ticks and various intermediate hosts (mice and deer) before infecting humans, is still not completely understood *(5,6)* (http://www3.niaid.nih.gov/research/topics/lyme). The outer surface protein A (OspA) of *B. burgdorferi* has been extensively studied, leading to a number of hypotheses regarding its role in conjunction with other cell surface proteins (OspB and OspC) in transmission of Lyme disease *(5)*.

Although *B. burgdorferi* depends on *Ixodes* ticks and mammalian hosts for its life cycle, the search for the borrelial genes responsible for its parasitic dependence on these diverse hosts has been hindered by the difficulties in genetically manipulating virulent strains of the pathogen. Nevertheless, there is strong evidence indicating that the inactivation and complementation of a linear plasmid-25-encoded gene, *bptA* (formerly known as *bbe16*), is essential for the persistence of *B. burgdorferi* in *I. scapularis* ticks, and therefore, it must be considered to be a major virulence factor that is critical for *B. burgdorferi*'s overall parasitic strategy *(7)*.

22.1.2 Symptoms of Lyme Disease

Early symptoms of Lyme disease usually appear within 3 to 30 days after the bite of an infected tick. In 60% to 80% of cases, a rash resembling a bull's eye or solid patch (about 2 inches in diameter) will appear and expand around or near the site of the bite. Occasionally, multiple rash sites may also appear. In the early stage of the Lyme disease, one or more of the following symptoms will appear: chills and fever, headache, fatigue, stiff neck, muscle and/or joint pain, and

swollen glands. If not recognized or left untreated, symptoms become more severe, and include fatigue, a stiff aching neck, and tingling or numbness in the arms and legs, or facial paralysis.

The most severe symptoms can occur even weeks, months, or years after the tick bite and include severe headache, painful arthritis, swelling of the joints, and heart and central nervous system problems. Some evidence points to an autoimmune disease, perhaps triggered by the initial infection *(8, 9)* (http://www3.niaid.nih.gov/topics/lymeDisease/research/autoimmune.htm).

Early treatment of Lyme disease involves the use of antibiotics, which in nearly all cases results in a complete cure. However, the likelihood of a full cure will decrease if treatment is delayed. And whereas in most infected individuals Lyme disease can be easily treated with antibiotics, in a small percentage of patients it may lead to debilitating symptoms that may continue for years after treatment.

22.1.3 Neuropsychiatric Lyme Disease

As a result of dissemination through the bloodstream, *B. burgdorferi* can invade the central nervous system within days to a week after the initial skin infection. Once in the central nervous system, the spirochete may affect the brain, most commonly causing a disturbance in thinking (cognition), known as Lyme encephalopathy. Other symptoms may include headache, mood swings, irritability, depression, and a high degree of fatigue. These symptoms comprise the typical features of neuropsychiatric Lyme disease in adults (http://www.columbia-lyme.org/flatp/lymeoverview.html). Many of these symptoms are common manifestations in other disorders, such as mood or anxiety disorders, collagen vascular or autoimmune diseases, spinal cord compression, multiple sclerosis, metastatic diseases, endocrinologic disorders, fibromyalgia, chronic fatigue syndrome, and residual damage from past brain trauma or toxin exposure. Nevertheless, knowing the typical cluster of symptoms can be helpful in diagnosing this condition. The majority of patients with Lyme encephalopathy will not present with joint problems at the time that their cognitive symptoms have been recognized.

It is important to emphasize that bedside neurologic examination does not usually disclose neurologic findings, and standard office-based cognitive screening test may not detect cognitive impairment. To detect cognitive disturbance, a more comprehensive neuropsychological examination would be needed. In addition, lumbar puncture, even though important in the differential diagnosis, should not be used to exclude neurologic Lyme disease, as approximately 20% to 40% of patients with confirmed neurologic Lyme disease may test negative in routine cerebrospinal fluid (CSF) assays (http://www.columbia-lyme.org/flatp/lymeoverview.html).

In general, the majority of patients who undergo early antibiotic therapy will not incur long-term central nervous system problems.

22.1.3.1 Time Course of Manifestations of Chronic Cognitive Disorders in Lyme Encephalopathy

The typical time course of the manifestations of Lyme encephalopathy (http://www.columbia-lyme.org/flatp/lymeoverview.html) is as follows:

(i) Very early: erythema migrans (a red, round, expanding rash).
(ii) One to 2 months after infection: cardiac or early neurologic involvement (meningitis, encephalitis, cranial neuropathies) with mild to marked neuropsychiatric symptoms.
(iii) Six to 10 months after infection: arthritis of multiple joints.
(iv) Two to 8 years after infection: chronic cognitive problems.

22.1.3.2 Symptoms of Neuropsychiatric Lyme Disease

Typical symptoms among adult patients with neuropsychiatric Lyme disease (http://www.columbia-lyme.org/flatp/lymeoverview.html) include:

(i) Mild to severe fatigue (a need for prolonged sleep), low-grade fevers, night sweats, migrating arthralgias (joint pains) or arthritis (joint inflammation or swelling), muscle pains, sleep disturbances, and frequent and severe headaches.
(ii) Cranial nerve disturbance. Though either facial nerve palsy or optic neuritis is not frequently manifested, patients may more commonly present with facial numbness and/or tingling.
(iii) Sharp, stabbing, deep/boring, burning, or lancinating (shooting) pains, as well as signs of peripheral neuropathy (multifocal numbness or tingling in hands or feet).
(iv) Cognitive problems may include problems of attention, memory, verbal fluency, and thinking speed. Some patients may experience what is otherwise a normal environmental stimulation to be excessive, resulting in a cognitive "short-circuiting" (cognitive overload) where patients may start to feel confused, lose focus, stutter, or panic.
(v) "Brain fog," a term frequently used by patients with Lyme disease to describe a syndrome characterized by

lack of clarity in their cognitive processes similar to "depersonalization or derealization" in which the person's sense of self and place are altered.
(vi) Sensory hyperacuities characterized by heightened sensitivity to sound or to light, particularly in the early stages of neurologic Lyme disease.
(vii) Spatial or geographic orientation problems where a patient may bump into the door jambs; try to place an object on a table only to have it fall to the floor due to a misjudgment of spatial distance; or get lost in a familiar place.
(viii) Less common neurologic syndromes include partial or complex seizures, multiple sclerosis–like illness, dementia-like illness, Guillain-Barré syndrome, strokes, and Tullio phenomenon.

Symptoms of Neuropsychiatric Disorders in Children

Most common symptoms of neuropsychiatric disorders in children suffering from Lyme disease include headaches, disturbances of behavior or mood, fatigue (falling asleep in class), and problems with auditory and visual attention (*some children could be mistakenly diagnosed as having attention deficit disorder*).

They may have fluctuating symptoms: worse on some days, remarkably better on others, without a clear cause (http://www.columbia-lyme.org/flatp/lymeoverview.html).

As noted among adults, when Lyme disease is treated early, few children will develop long-term cognitive or neuropsychiatric problems.

22.1.4 Treatment of Lyme Borreliosis

Prior vaccination with the licensed recombinant outer surface protein A (OspA) vaccine reduces the risk of developing Lyme disease associated with tick bites *(10)*.

22.1.4.1 Early Lyme Disease

Administration of doxycycline (100 mg, twice daily) or amoxicillin (500 mg, 3 times daily) for 14 to 21 days is recommended for the treatment of early localized or early disseminated Lyme disease associated with erythema migrans, in the absence of neurologic involvement or third-degree atrioventricular heart block *(9)*. In prospective studies, these two drugs have been shown to be effective in treating erythema migrans and associated symptoms. Doxycycline has the advantage of being effective also for treating human granulocytic anaplasmosis (HGA), another tick-borne infection that may occur simultaneously with Lyme disease. However, doxycycline may be relatively contraindicated for pregnant women, during lactation, and for children aged 8 years or younger (see also Section 22.2.2.2).

Because of its higher cost, cefuroxime axetil (500 mg orally, twice daily), which is as effective as doxycycline in the treatment of erythema migrans, should be reserved as an alternative agent for those patients who can take neither doxycycline nor amoxicillin *(9)*.

For children, the recommended dose of amoxicillin is $50 \, \text{mg} \, \text{kg}^{-1} \, \text{day}^{-1}$, divided into 3 doses per day (maximum, 500 mg/dose). Cefuroxime axetil is an acceptable alternative given at a dose of $30 \, \text{mg} \, \text{kg}^{-1} \, \text{day}^{-1}$, divided into 2 doses daily (maximum, 500 mg/dose).

Macrolide antibiotics (azithromycin, erythromycin, and clarithromycin) are not recommended as first-line therapy for early Lyme disease; when used they should be reserved for patients who are intolerant of amoxicillin, doxycycline, and cefuroxime axetil *(9)*.

Intravenous ceftriaxone (2.0 g daily), although effective, is not superior to oral agents and is not recommended as a first-line agent for treatment of Lyme disease in the absence of neurologic involvement or third-degree atrioventricular heart block. However, ceftriaxone is recommended for acute neurologic disease manifested by meningitis or radiculopathy *(9)*. For children, the recommended dose of ceftriaxone is 75 to $100 \, \text{mg} \, \text{kg}^{-1} \, \text{day}^{-1}$, in a single daily intravenous dose (maximum, 2.0 g), or cefotaxime (150 to $200 \, \text{mg} \, \text{kg}^{-1} \, \text{day}^{-1}$) divided into 3 or 4 doses (maximum, 6.0 g/daily) for 14 to 28 days *(9)*.

Patients with first- or second-degree atrioventricular heart block associated with early Lyme disease should be treated with the same antimicrobial regimens as patients with erythema migrans without carditis. The recommended treatment for patients with a third-degree atrioventricular heart block is parenteral antibiotics such as ceftriaxone in a hospital setting *(9)*.

Although antibiotic treatment does not hasten resolution of seventh cranial nerve palsy associated with *B. burgdorferi* infection, antibiotics should be used to prevent further sequelae *(9)*.

22.1.4.2 Lyme Arthritis

Lyme arthritis usually can be treated successfully with antimicrobial agents administered orally or intravenously. Thus, administration of oral doxycycline (100 mg, twice daily) or amoxicillin (500 mg, 3 times daily), in each instance for 28 days, is recommended for patients without clinically evident neurologic disease *(9)*. For children, the recommended dose of doxycycline (1.0 to 2.0 mg/kg, twice daily; maximum, 100 mg/dose) could be given to children age 8

and older, or amoxicillin ($50 \, \text{mg} \, \text{kg}^{-1} \, \text{day}^{-1}$, divided into 3 doses per day; maximum, 500 mg/dose) for 28 days *(9)*.

Whereas oral therapy is easier to administer than intravenous antibiotics, is associated with fewer adverse effects, and is significantly less expensive, its disadvantage is that some patients treated with oral antimicrobials have subsequently developed overt neuroborreliosis, which may require intravenous therapy for successful resolution *(9)*.

22.1.4.3 Late Neuroborreliosis

The recommended therapy for patients with late neuroborreliosis affecting the central or peripheral nervous system is treatment with intravenous ceftriaxone (2.0 g, once daily for 2 to 4 weeks) *(9)*. Response to treatment is usually slow and may be incomplete. However, unless relapse is shown by reliable objective means, repeat treatment is not recommended *(9)*. For children, the recommended treatment is a 14- to 28-day course of ceftriaxone (75 to $100 \, \text{mg} \, \text{kg}^{-1} \, \text{day}^{-1}$, in a single daily intravenous dose; maximum, 2.0 g) *(9)*.

22.1.4.4 Chronic Lyme Disease or Post–Lyme Disease Syndrome

After an episode of Lyme disease that is treated appropriately, some patients have a variety of subjective complaints, such as myalgia, arthralgia, or fatigue. Such patients may then be classified as having either *chronic Lyme disease* or *post–Lyme disease syndrome*. However, both conditions are poorly defined because these patients represent a heterogenous group. Because there have not been any randomized, controlled studies of patients who remain unwell after standard courses of antibiotic therapy for Lyme disease, there are no convincing published data demonstrating that repeated or prolonged courses of either oral or intravenous antimicrobial therapy are effective for such patients *(9)*.

22.1.5 NIAID Research Agenda in Lyme Disease

22.1.5.1 Background and Goals

The NIAID has had a long-standing commitment to conduct research on Lyme borreliosis, or Lyme disease, beginning more than 20 years ago when the cause of the disease was not yet known (http://www3.niaid.nih.gov/research/topics/lyme/research/). In 1981, NIAID-funded research efforts resulted in identifying *Borrelia burgdorferi*, a spiral-shaped bacterium, or spirochete, as the causative agent of Lyme disease *(11)*. Since then, basic and clinical research efforts have been expanded in scope to address many different aspects of this infectious disease (http://www3.niaid.nih.gov/research/topics/lyme/research/). They include systematic studies of:

- Animal models of disease.
- Microbial physiology.
- Molecular, genetic, and cellular mechanisms of pathogenesis.
- Mechanisms of protective immunity.
- Vectors, as well as vector competency and their influence on transmission of the disease.
- Efficacy of different modes of antibiotic therapy.
- Development of more sensitive and reliable diagnostic tests for both early (acute) and late (chronic) Lyme disease.
- Diagnosis, including the development and application of new technologies for rapid and sensitive diagnostic assays, as well as assessment, refinement, and standardization of improved diagnostic procedures.
- Treatment and prevention, including the development, application, and evaluation of novel and safe therapeutic approaches, as well as identification and characterization of candidate vaccines.
- Immune mechanisms, including understanding the development of protective immunity, characterizing the immunomodulatory properties of microbial antigens and evaluating their role in the pathogenesis, and characterizing the response of the host's immune system both during infection and after deliberate immunization.
- Pathogenesis, including the identification and characterization of virulence factors and the molecular basis for damage to host tissues during infection, and defining the role of cytokines and other immunomodulatory agents in the expression of disease.
- Epizootiology/ecology, including defining potential and established vectors and reservoirs, assessing the role of ticks and other vectors in transmitting the disease and maintaining virulence, relating the role of genetic variation in the incidence of disease in endemic areas, and defining effective measures for significantly reducing or eliminating populations of infected ticks in endemic areas.

Other developments of NIAID-supported Lyme borreliosis and tick-borne rickettsial disease research include:

(i) The sequencing of the *B. burgdorferi* genome, including the DNA within plasmids—small segments of DNA that reside outside the *B. burgdorferi* chromosome and can be exchanged among bacteria. Microarray technology is now being applied to identify genes involved in pathogenesis and adaptation to various host environments, as

well as to evaluate the utility of this approach for the early diagnosis of infection.

(ii) The development of tick salivary protein-based, transmission blocking vaccines to interfere with the ability of infected ticks to feed on intermediary mammalian hosts.

(iii) Research is continuing to sequence multiple *Rickettsia* species, including the spotted fever group bacteria *R. rickettsii* and *R. akari*, and the typhus-group pathogen *R. canada*. In addition, the genome sequence of *R. bellii*, which represents a third group of *Rickettsia* species, is also under way.

22.1.5.2 Ongoing Research

NIAID's current Lyme disease research portfolio is extensive and diverse (http://www3.niaid.nih.gov/research/topics/lyme/research/). It encompasses basic and clinical research studies conducted by extramural and intramural investigators, including intramural scientists at NIAID's Rocky Mountain Laboratories (RML) in Hamilton, Montana, as well as at NIAID intramural laboratories in Bethesda, Maryland.

Specific NIAID-supported activities on Lyme disease include extramural research on:

- The transmission of Lyme disease
- Diagnostic procedures
- Co-infection
- Antibiotic therapy
- The role of autoimmune reactivity
- Vaccine production

Lack of Evidence of Borrelia Involvement in Alzheimer's Disease. Because various published reports have suggested the possibility that *B. burgdorferi* may play a role in the etiology of Alzheimer's disease, NIAID intramural scientists have examined this issue in greater detail. The results of these studies, using a very sensitive polymerase chain reaction (PCR) assay capable of amplifying a *Borrelia*-specific DNA target sequence from all strains of *B. burgdorferi sensu lato* species known to cause disease in humans, have provided *no evidence* to indicate the presence of *B. burgdorferi* in the brains of patients with Alzheimer's disease *(12)*.

22.1.5.3 Antibiotic Therapy and Animal Models

Whereas early acute Lyme borreliosis is easily cured by conventional antibiotic therapy, some patients who have been correctly diagnosed initially as having Lyme disease may experience serious neurologic and musculoskeletal symptoms several months after receiving what appeared to have been successful antibiotic therapy. Because it is unclear whether such symptoms are due to long-term persistent infections or other causes, the term *posttreatment chronic Lyme disease (PTCLD)* is often used to describe this condition, so as not to impose any judgment on the actual mechanism(s) that might be involved (see also Section 22.1.4.4).

Over the years, NIAID has supported research regarding PTCLD as well as other clinical issues (http://www3. niaid.nih.gov/research/topics/lyme), including:

- *New England Medical Center (NEMC) Clinical Study.* This study, which was carried out in NEMC in Boston and completed in 2000, was aimed at studying the clinical efficacy of antibiotic therapy for treating PTCLD. It involved randomized, double-blind, placebo-controlled, multicenter trials to examine the safety and efficacy of ceftriaxone and doxycycline in patients with either seropositive or seronegative chronic Lyme disease. The trials compared treatment with 30 days of intravenous ceftriaxone followed by 60 days of oral doxycycline to treatment with intravenous placebo followed by oral placebo for the same duration in patients who were either seropositive or seronegative at the time of enrollment. Preliminary results from the trials showed that after 90 days of continuous antibiotic therapy, there were no significant differences in the percentage of patients who felt that their symptoms had improved, gotten worse, or stayed the same between the antibiotic treatment and placebo groups in either trial *(13)*. Other results from the trials indicated that patients with PTCLD did not show objective evidence of cognitive impairment and that 90 days of continuous antibiotic therapy was not more beneficial for these patients than was administering a placebo *(14)*.
- *State University of New York (SUNY) Clinical Study.* In another placebo-controlled study conducted at SUNY at Stony Brook, patients with PCTLD were treated with either intravenous ceftriaxone or a placebo for 28 days. They were then evaluated to determine whether there was significant improvement with respect to fatigue, cognitive function, and the clearance of OspA antigen that was present in the spinal fluid of only 16% of all enrolled patients. The results of the trial have shown that ceftriaxone therapy was associated with improvement in fatigue but not with the other primary outcome markers considered *(15)*. Because fatigue, which is a nonspecific symptom, was the only primary outcome measure affected and because the treatment examined was associated with adverse events, the results of the SUNY study do not support the use of additional antibiotic therapy with parenteral ceftriaxone in posttreatment, persistently fatigued PTCLD patients (http://www3.niaid.nih.gov/research/topics/lyme).
- *Animal Models.* Appropriate animal models also have provided considerable information on the transmission

and pathogenesis of Lyme borreliosis, as well as on the mechanisms involved in the development of protective immunity. NIAID, in collaboration with the National Institute of Neurological Disorders and Stroke (NINDS), has broadened these efforts to include comprehensive studies on non-human primate animal models for experimental research on the neuropathology associated with chronic Lyme borreliosis *(16)*. A major goal of these studies is to optimize the rhesus model of Lyme borreliosis as well as to determine the pathogenesis of the disease with a focus on the neurologic manifestations. It is anticipated that these studies will expand the knowledge of those factors that contribute to the pathology associated with persistent infection of the central nervous system by *B. burgdorferi* and ultimately will enable scientists to devise more effective clinical approaches for treating chronic Lyme borreliosis in humans. These studies will also supplement and enhance the results of current clinical research on the efficacy of antibiotic therapies for treating chronic Lyme disease and provide precedents for use in designing future clinical studies and will ultimately enhance the results of current clinical studies on chronic Lyme disease.

Inflammation of skeletal muscle is a consistent feature of Lyme borreliosis, both in humans and in experimental animal models of infection. Although several cytokines are expressed in muscle tissue, proinflammatory cytokines commonly associated with inflammation are not upregulated in *Borrelia*-infected muscle. However, the expression of *B-lymphocyte chemoattractant (BLC)*, a chemokine implicated in the trafficking of B cells to tissues, is increased in *Borrelia*-infected muscles of non-human primates *(17)*. Using protein expression profiling, it has been shown that BLC is upregulated in the spinal fluid of patients with neuroborreliosis but not in patients with noninflammatory and various other inflammatory neurologic diseases *(18)*. Because the upregulation of BLC was found in every neuroborreliosis patient examined, it may be a valuable diagnostic marker for neuroborreliosis.

Other studies have shown that *B. burgdorferi* can be detected in mice for at least 3 months after treatment with therapeutic doses of various antibiotics (ceftriaxone, doxycycline, or azithromycin). These surviving spirochetes could not be transmitted to healthy mice and some lacked plasmid genes associated with infectivity. By 6 months, antibiotic-treated mice no longer tested positive for the presence of *B. burgdorferi*, and even cortisone immunosuppression failed to alter this result; that is, it failed to activate infection. Nine months after antibiotic treatment, low levels of *Borrelia* DNA still could be detected in some, but not all of the mice. These findings *(19)* have indicated that noninfectious *B. burgdorferi* can persist for a limited time after antibiotic therapy. The implications of these findings to persistent infection and the nature of chronic Lyme disease in humans remain to be assessed.

22.1.5.4 The Role of Autoimmune Reactivity in Lyme Disease

Results from recent studies have indicated that T cells from patients with chronic Lyme disease were reactive not only against *B. burgdorferi*–specific antigens but also against various host (self) antigens *(20)*. Such antigenic mimicry might generate autoimmune inflammatory reactions that could be responsible for arthritic as well as neurologic symptoms associated with chronic Lyme disease (http://www3.niaid.nih.gov/research/topics/lyme/research/autoimmune/).

In other studies, antibodies against the OspA epitopes of *B. burgdorferi* have also been shown to cross-react with neural tissue *(21)* as well as myocin *(22)*. Such antigenic mimicry may have the potential to generate autoimmune inflammatory reactions that could be responsible for the neurologic symptoms associated with chronic Lyme disease. In this context, it is interesting to note that homologies between proteins of *B. burgdorferi* and thyroid antigens have also been reported *(23)*.

In NIAID-supported clinical studies, case subject patients with PTCLD were compared with control subjects without such symptoms for the presence of several human leukocyte antigen (HLA) class II (DRB1 and DQB1) genetic markers, some of which are known to be associated with the expression of autoimmune reactivity. The results obtained did not support the involvement of an autoimmune mechanism in PTCLD *(24)*. However, because not all autoimmune diseases are associated with specific HLA haplotypes, these findings do not necessarily exclude that possibility. Definitive proof would clearly involve demonstrating the presence of significant levels of relevant autoimmune antibodies and/or autoreactive T cells in patients with PTCLD but not in treated control subjects without such symptoms. A greater frequency of DRB1*0401, which has been reported to be associated with antibiotic-treatment-resistant arthritis, was noted in the case subject patients; although this finding appeared to be nominally significant (p < 0.05), its biological significance is ambiguous because none of the case subjects considered had symptoms of inflammatory arthritis (http://www3.niaid.nih.gov/research/topics/lyme/research/autoimmune/).

22.1.5.5 Co-infections

Co-infection could represent a major potential problem, mainly because the *Ixodes* ticks that transmit *B. burgdorferi* often carry—and simultaneously transmit—other emerging pathogens, such as *Anaplasma (Ehrlichia)* species, the causative agent of human granulocytic ehrlichiosis (HGE), and *Babesia microti*, which causes babesiosis (http://www3.niaid.nih.gov/research/topics/lyme/research/co-infection/). In Europe and Asia, *Ixodes* ticks also are known to transmit tick-borne encephalitis viruses. Fortunately, this tick-borne viral infection has not yet been reported in the United States, although co-infections with Powasan virus and deer tick virus have been reported.

Co-infection by some or all of these other infectious agents may interfere with the clinical diagnosis of Lyme borreliosis and/or adversely influence host defense mechanisms, thereby altering landmark characteristics of the disease and the severity of infection *(25)*. NIAID-supported studies have indicated that co-infection with HGE increases the severity of Lyme borreliosis *(26)*. By contrast, when mice were co-infected with *B. microti* and *B. burgdorferi*, neither agent influenced the course of infection induced by the other as evidenced by the percentage of parasitemia, spleen weights, and hematologic and clinical chemistry parameters *(27)*.

In NIAID-supported clinical studies on chronic Lyme disease, patients with persisting symptoms were examined to determine if they might have been co-infected with other tick-borne infectious diseases at the time of their acute episode of Lyme disease. Among the tick-borne infectious diseases considered were babesiosis (*Babesia microti*), granulocytic ehrlichiosis (*Anaplasma phagocytophilum*), and tick-borne encephalitis virus infection. The seroprevalence rates for *B. microti* and *A. phagocytophilum* were found to be 2.5% and 8.6%, respectively, and no patient examined was found to be positive for tick-borne encephalitis viruses *(27)*. Thus, the persistence of symptoms in patients with "post–Lyme syndrome" could not be attributed to co-infection with one of these pathogens.

An examination of pathogen distributions in the tissues of mice infected with both *B. burgdorferi* and *A. phagocytophilum*, the bacterium that causes HGE in humans, showed an increase in the numbers of *B. burgdorferi* in the ears, heart base, and skin of co-infected mice; however, the numbers of *A. phagocytophilum* remained relatively constant. The serum antibody response to *A. phagocytophilum* (but not to *B. burgdorferi*) decreased as a result of co-infection. These findings suggest that co-infection can influence not only pathogen burden but also host antibody responses *(28)*. NIAID intramural and extramural research programs have initiated clinical studies on chronic Lyme disease. The intramural research program is conducting a comprehensive clinical, microbiologic, and immunologic assessment of patients with Lyme disease. This involves multiple lines of investigation with emphasis on (i) defining various biological markers of infection; (ii) assessing clinical course and outcomes of patients with Lyme borreliosis; and (iii) characterizing the immune response generated in response to *B. burgdorferi* (http://www3.niaid.nih.gov/research/topics/lyme/research/co-infection/).

22.1.5.6   Diagnostic Procedures

NIAID is supporting various efforts to evaluate and improve existing diagnostic procedures. Approximately 20% of its extramural Lyme disease research portfolio is devoted to developing novel and more sensitive diagnostic procedures (http://www3.niaid.nih.gov/ research/ topics/ lyme/ research/ diagnostics/). In 1998, the FDA granted approval to Chembio Diagnostic Systems to market the Wampole *PreVue Borrelia burgdorferi* Antibody Detection Assay. The assay is a single-use, unitized immunochromatographic test that uses recombinant *B. burgdorferi* antigens for the qualitative presumptive (first step) detection of IgG and IgM antibodies to *B. burgdorferi* in human serum or whole blood. This test is to be used only in patients with history, signs, and symptoms that are consistent with Lyme disease. It is intended for use in clinical and physicians' office laboratories.

In collaboration with CDC, NIAID is also playing a major role in encouraging the development of novel approaches to improve the diagnosis of Lyme borreliosis in humans with various co-infections (e.g., ehrlichiosis or babesiosis), as well as in immunized people (http://www3.niaid.nih.gov/research/topics/lyme/research/diagnostics/). For example, it has been shown in NIAID-supported research that a synthetic peptide composed of 26 amino acid residues (C6) derived from a variable surface antigen (VlsE) of *B. burgdorferi* can be used in a new, rapid, and extremely sensitive ELISA test (the C6 ELISA) for diagnosing Lyme disease. Because this diagnostic test for Lyme disease, which has been approved by FDA, does not detect antibodies specific for recombinant OspA, it can be used even for those who have been immunized with the licensed OspA-based LYMErix vaccine *(29)*.

Although the *Lyme Urinary Antigen Test (LUAT)* is one of several diagnostic tests used routinely in NIAID's clinical studies on chronic Lyme disease, the results of independent quality control assessments of tests conducted by extramural and intramural scientists showed the LUAT to be unreliable because it yields an unacceptably high percentage of false-positive reactions *(30)*. A critical evaluation of urine-based PCR assays for the diagnosis of Lyme borreliosis likewise affirmed that urine is not a suitable material for the diagnosis of Lyme borreliosis *(31)*. By contrast, the similar assessments confirmed a high degree of reproducibility and concordance (virtually 100%) for the results obtained using ELISA and Western blot assays *(30)*.

Of great importance is the fact that decreases in the titer of antibodies against C6 can be used as an indicator of the efficacy of antibiotic therapy for patients with localized or disseminated Lyme disease, but not for chronic Lyme disease *(32)*. This is indeed a major advancement, because no other laboratory test enables one to obtain such information *(29)*. The results obtained with the C6 ELISA assay are consistent with those obtained with other diagnostic tests and may eliminate the time and expense of conducting additional laboratory tests to confirm the diagnosis of Lyme disease *(33)*. NIAID-supported investigators are now working closely with the CDC to determine if the C6 ELISA can eventually replace the traditional two-tiered conventional ELISA and Western blot assays. The results of other studies confirmed that a decline in the anti-C6 antibody titer coincides with the efficacy of antimicrobial therapy in patients with early localized or early disseminated Lyme borreliosis *(34)* (see also *22.1.6*).

The *B. burgdorferi*–specific immune complex (IC) test in which polyethylene glycol (PEG) is used to isolate ICs from serum has been advocated by some investigators as an approach for the early diagnosis of active borreliosis. However, recent findings indicate that it may not be more effective in detecting early and active infections than other conventional tests in which unprocessed serum specimens are used *(35)*.

There is a great need to develop additional simple, sensitive, and rapid procedures to distinguish those persons who are actively infected with *B. burgdorferi* from those who have either recovered from a previous infection or have been immunized previously. Because the genome of *B. burgdorferi* has now been completely sequenced, greater advances toward this goal are anticipated as this information is used in conjunction with microarray technology and proteomics to improve diagnosis, as well as to provide new insights on the pathogenesis of this disease and pathogen-specific host response mechanisms (http://www3.niaid.nih.gov/research/topics/lyme/research/diagnostics/).

22.1.5.7   Transmission of Lyme Disease

There is no clear understanding about the molecular basis of how *B. burgdorferi* maintains itself in nature via a complex life cycle that involves passage through ticks and various intermediate hosts, such as mice and deer, before infecting humans. The outer surface protein A (OspA) of *B. burgdorferi* has been well studied, and there is much speculation about its role—in conjunction with other cell surface proteins (OspB and OspC)—in transmitting Lyme disease *(5)*.

Although *B. burgdorferi* depends on *Ixodes* ticks and mammalian (rodent) hosts for its persistence in nature *(6)*, the search for borrelial genes responsible for its parasitic dependence on these types of diverse hosts has been hampered by limitations in the ability to genetically manipulate virulent strains of *Borrelia*. Despite this constraint, there is evidence to indicate that the inactivation and complementation of a gene (*bbe16*) encoded by a linear plasmid (lp25) plays a major role in the virulence, pathogenesis, and survival of *B. burgdorferi* during its natural life cycle *(36)*. This gene, which has been renamed BptA (for borrelial persistence in ticks-gene A), potentiates virulence in mice and is essential for the persistence of *B. burgdorferi* in *Ixodes scapularis* ticks. Although BptA appears to be a lipoprotein expressed on the outer surface membrane of *B. burgdorferi*, the molecular mechanism(s) by which BptA promotes persistence within its tick vector remains to be elucidated. Because BptA appears to be highly conserved (>88% similarity and >74% identity in amino acid sequence) in all *B. burgdorferi sensu lato* strains examined, it may be widely used to promote persistence in nature. Given the absolute dependence on—and intimate association with—its tick and rodent hosts, BptA must be considered to be a major virulence factor that is critical for *B. burgdorferi's* overall infectious strategy *(7)*. Strategies designed to block the synthesis or expression of BptA could be of great value in preventing the transmission of Lyme disease.

The potential role that differentially upregulated surface proteins play in the transmission of borreliosis and Lyme disease pathogenesis have prompted investigators to conduct a comprehensive gene expression profiling analysis of temperature-shifted and mammalian host–adapted *B. burgdorferi*. The combined microarray analyses revealed that many genes encoding known and putative outer surface proteins are downregulated in mammalian host–adapted *B. burgdorferi*. However, at the same time, several different genes encoding at least seven putative outer surface proteins were found to be upregulated during the transmission and infection process. All seven proteins are immunogenic and generate the production of bactericidal antibodies in infected baboons *(37)*. This suggests that these outer surface proteins might be excellent second-generation vaccine candidates.

The above findings have been consistent with the results of published studies *(19)* in which a novel experimental technique (*xenodiagnosis by ticks*) was used to determine whether *B. burgdorferi* can persist in mice long after antibiotic therapy. In these studies, an immunofluorescence assay and the PCR assay were used to demonstrate that *B. burgdorferi* could be detected in doxycycline- and ceftriaxone-treated mice for at least 3 months (if not longer) after antibiotic therapy. However, the resulting surviving spirochetes were unable to infect other naïve mice because they lacked those linear plasmids (lp25 and lp28) that are essential for their ability to transmit infection *(19)*. It is noteworthy that lp25 also encodes for a gene product (PncA or BBE22) that is essential for the survival of *B. burgdorferi* in a mammalian host *(36)*.

NIAID-supported investigators have now been able to create various mutant strains of *B. burgdorferi* and have shown that although OspA and OspB are not required for infection of mice, they were essential for the colonization and survival of *B. burgdorferi* in ticks (http://www3.niaid.nih.gov/research/topics/lyme/research/transmission/). *Ixodes scapularis* ticks have a receptor on the inner wall of their intestines to which *B. burgdorferi* is able to bind tenaciously by means of OspA, a cell surface protein. This receptor is called the *tick receptor for OspA (TROSPA)*. Attachment to TROSPA will enable *B. burgdorferi* to persist in the gut from the time they were ingested by ticks through a subsequent molt, thereby avoiding elimination; this would allow *Borrelia* to be injected into a new host when the ticks take their next blood meal *(38)*. When ticks take a blood meal, the production of OspA is downregulated in favor of the increased production of OspC. This results in gut-bound spirochetes becoming detached, which enables them to migrate to the salivary glands, where they can be injected into mammalian hosts. Thus, TROSPA, in addition to other bacterial cell surface components, such as OspA, appears to play a key role in the transmission of Lyme disease to humans. Other studies have shown that if ticks are permitted to feed on mice that have been immunized previously with OspA, or have been treated with the antibody specific for OspA, the attachment and subsequent colonization of ticks by *B. burgdorferi* would be significantly impaired, if not prevented. This suggests the feasibility of developing oral- or vector-expressed transmission-blocking vaccines that involve the immunization of the intermediate hosts upon which ticks feed *(39)*. Several NIAID-supported investigators are now examining and testing this approach under controlled laboratory conditions (http://www3.niaid.nih.gov/research/topics/lyme/research/transmission/).

Results from other studies conducted by NIAID-supported investigators *(40)* have demonstrated that *B. burgdorferi* uses an immunosuppressive *tick salivary protein (Salp 15)* to facilitate the transmission of infection to mammalian hosts. This finding is based on observations that (i) the level of Salp 15 expression is enhanced by the presence of *B. burgdorferi* in infected ticks; (ii) Salp 15 adheres specifically to spirochete surface OspC both *in vivo* and *in vitro*, thereby increasing the ability of *B. burgdorferi* to infect mice; and (iii) the binding of Salp 15 protects *B. burgdorferi* from antibody-mediated killing *in vitro*, a factor that confers marked survival advantage. All of these observations suggest that Salp 15 and/or other tick salivary proteins might be excellent candidates for vaccines to block the transmission of Lyme disease *(41)*. In this context, prior and repeated exposure of experimental animals to uninfected ticks—and presumably their salivary proteins—has been shown to limit the capacity of infected ticks to transmit Lyme disease *(42)*.

22.1.5.8 Vaccine Production

Two large pharmaceutical companies [GlaxoSmithKline (SKB) and Pasteur Merieux Connaught (PMC)] have devoted considerable effort to developing a vaccine for Lyme disease. Double-blind, randomized, placebo-controlled clinical trials, involving more than 10,000 volunteers from areas of the United States where Lyme disease is highly endemic, have been completed for each of two *B. burgdorferi* recombinant OspA vaccines manufactured by SKB and PMC. These vaccines were found to be 49% to 68% effective in preventing Lyme disease after two injections and 68% to 92% effective in preventing Lyme disease after three injections. The duration of the protective immunity generated in response to the SKB vaccine (LYMErix), which was licensed by the FDA in December 1998, is not known. Consequently, the need for yearly booster injections remains to be established. Researchers and health experts anticipate that the use of these vaccines in endemic areas would likely result in a significant reduction in the incidence of Lyme disease in the future.

NIAID was not directly involved in the design and implementation of these particular vaccine trials; however, patents for cloning the genes used for the expression of recombinant OspA, as well as knowledge of the role of antibodies against OspA in the development of protective immunity, were derived from basic research funded by NIAID (http://www3. niaid.nih.gov/research/topics/lyme/research/vaccine/).

In April 2002, GlaxoSmithKline announced that even with the incidence of Lyme disease continuing to increase, sales for LYMErix declined from about 1.5 million doses in 1999 to a projected 10,000 doses in 2002. Although studies conducted by FDA failed to reveal that any reported adverse events were vaccine-associated, GlaxoSmithKline has discontinued manufacturing the vaccine for economic reasons *(43)*.

NIAID-funded investigators have developed an experimental bait delivery system for an OspA-based vaccine against *B. burgdorferi* in which mice were immunized orally (via gavage or bait feeding) with a strain of *Escherichia coli* expressing the gene for OspA, which resulted in the appearance of serum antibody specific for OspA. When mice were exposed to *Ixodes* nymphs carrying multiple strains of *B. burgdorferi*, oral vaccination was found to protect 89% of the mice from infection, and the resultant serum antibody response confirmed the presence of IgG2a/2b antibody specific for OspA (http://www3.niaid.nih. gov/topics/lymeDisease/research/vaccine.htm). This vaccination approach is able to generate a significant protective immune response against a variety of infectious strains of *B. burgdorferi*, thereby indicating that it can eliminate *B. burgdorferi* from a major host reservoir. It suggests that the broad delivery of an oral vaccine to wildlife reservoirs in an endemic area is likely to disrupt the transmission of Lyme disease *(44)*. These findings are consistent with the results reported by other investigators *(39)*, thus affirming the utility of this approach.

In other NIAID-supported studies, scientists have developed a murine-targeted OspA vaccine using the vaccinia virus to interrupt the transmission of disease in reservoir hosts, thereby having the potential to reduce the incidence of human disease. Oral vaccination of mice with a single dose of vaccinia virus expressing OspA resulted in high antibody titers to OspA, 100% protection of vaccinated mice from infection by *B. burgdorferi*, and a significant clearance of *B. burgdorferi* from infected ticks fed on vaccinated animals *(44)*. These findings indicate that such a vaccine may effectively reduce the incidence of Lyme disease in endemic areas.

NIAID is also funding preclinical studies to develop and test other candidate vaccines (e.g., decorin-binding protein A, or DbpA) for Lyme disease. Thus, MedImmune, Inc., and Sanofi-Aventis Pharmaceuticals have reported that a combination vaccine composed of the DbpA and OspA of *B. burgdorferi* was more effective than either one given alone in preventing the development of borreliosis in experimental animals. On the basis of these encouraging findings, both companies have entered into an agreement to develop a new, more effective second-generation vaccine to prevent Lyme disease in humans. Although the results of previous studies indicate that DbpA induces the development of protective immunity in a murine model of Lyme borreliosis when mice have been challenged (needle-inoculated) intradermally with *in vitro*–cultivated *B. burgdorferi*, such mice were not protected from infection transmitted by ticks carrying virulent *B. burgdorferi*.

22.1.5.9 Other NIH Institutes and Centers Working on Lyme Disease

The principal mission of NIAID is to study infectious diseases and host immune defense mechanisms; therefore, the institute conducts and supports most of the basic and clinical research on Lyme disease funded by the National Institutes of Health (NIH). However, because Lyme disease affects different tissue and organ systems of the body, it is also a matter of great concern to other NIH institutes and centers (http://www3.niaid.nih.gov/research/topics/lyme/centers/).

The *National Institute of Arthritis and Musculoskeletal and Skin Diseases (NIAMS)* is funding research on chronic Lyme-induced arthritis, including the role of the immune system and genetic factors in contributing to its development.

The *National Institute of Neurological Disorders and Stroke (NINDS)* is funding research to characterize the neurologic, neuropsychological, and psychosocial manifestations of early and late Lyme disease in both adults and children, as well as to characterize pathogenic mechanisms associated with the neurologic symptoms of chronic Lyme disease.

The *National Center for Research Resources (NCRR)* provides resource support (non-human primates) for basic and clinical studies on both acute and chronic infection, as well as support for testing and developing candidate vaccines for Lyme disease.

In addition, the *Fogarty International Center (FIC)* is funding research on Lyme disease abroad, and the *National Institute on Aging (NIA)* and the *National Institute of Mental Health (NIMH)* have focused on those aspects of Lyme disease that relate to their specific missions.

To facilitate cooperative interactions as well as to ensure that the research activities of all NIH components are complementary, an *NIH Lyme Disease Coordinating Committee (LDCC)* was established in 1992. LDCC meets annually to review the results of current studies and recent advances in research on Lyme disease. Because the FDA is responsible for evaluating the efficacy and safety of vaccines against Lyme disease (e.g., the LYMErix vaccine) and the CDC is especially interested in developing new and improved diagnostic procedures, representatives from FDA and CDC have been invited to serve on the LDCC and to provide updates on their activities related to Lyme disease.

22.1.6 Recent Scientific Advances

- *C6 ELISA Diagnostic Procedure.* It has been shown that a synthetic peptide comprising 26 amino acid residues (C6) derived from a variable surface antigen (V1sE) of *B. burgdorferi* can be used in a new, rapid, and extremely sensitive ELISA test (the C6 ELISA) for diagnosing Lyme disease *(29)*. The C6 ELISA test is sensitive only to antibodies generated during an active infection (both early and late stages of Lyme disease). Another advantage of the test is its ability to detect antibodies specific for both North American and European strains of *Borrelia*. Of great importance is the fact that decreases in the titer of antibodies against C6 can be used as an indicator of the efficacy of antibiotic therapy for patients with localized or disseminated Lyme disease, but not for chronic Lyme disease. Because the C6 ELISA test would not detect antibodies specific for recombinant OspA, it can be used even for those patients who have been immunized with the licensed OspA-based LYMErix vaccine *(29)*. This is a major advance, because except for the C6 ELISA no other laboratory test is capable of obtaining such information *(32)*.
- *An Ecologic Approach to Preventing Lyme Disease.* In a recently developed, ecologic approach to Lyme disease prevention, researchers have intervened in the natural life cycle of *B. burgdorferi* by immunizing the wild white-footed mouse (*Peromyscus leucopus*), a reservoir host species, with either a recombinant antigen (OspA) of the spirochete or a negative control antigen in a repeated field experiment with paired experimental and control grids stratified by site *(39)*. OspA vaccination significantly reduced the prevalence of *B. burgdorferi* in nymphal black-legged ticks (*I. scapularis*) collected at the sites the following year in both experiments. The magnitude of the vaccine's effect at a given site correlated with the prevalence of tick infection found on the control grid, which in turn correlated with mouse density. These data, as well as differences in the population structure of *B. burgdorferi* in sympatric ticks and mice, indicated that non-mouse hosts contributed more toward infecting ticks than previously expected. Thus, where non-mouse hosts play a large role in the infection dynamics, vaccination should be directed at additional species *(39)*.

- *Variable Nature of Antibodies Specific for OspC Influence Virulence.* The outer surface protein C (OspC) of *B. burgdorferi*, the spirochete that causes Lyme disease, has been studied for its potential in the development of a vaccine *(45)*. Of the 21 OspC types currently identified, a surprisingly large number (types A, B, C, D, K, N, and 1) are associated with invasive disease. Because a detailed knowledge of the antigenic structure of OspC would be essential for vaccine development, the antibody response against several different recombinant OspC proteins was examined in detail. The results have revealed a high degree of specificity, indicating that the immunodominant epitopes of OspC reside in the variable regions of the protein. To localize these epitopes, OspC fragments were generated and screened against serum collected from infected mice, thus allowing the identification of previously uncharacterized epitopes that define the type specificity of the OspC antibody response. The reported findings have provided valuable insights into the antigenic structure of OspC, as well as a basis for understanding the variable nature of the antibody response to this important virulence factor.
- *B. burgdorferi Uses an Immunosuppressive I. scapularis Salivary Protein to Infect the Mammalian Host.* The Lyme disease spirochete, *B. burgdorferi*, is maintained in a tick-mouse cycle. Evidence has demonstrated that the spirochete usurps a tick (*I. scapularis*) salivary protein, Salp15, to facilitate the infection of mice *(40)*. The level of *salp15* expression was selectively elevated by the presence of *B. burgdorferi* in *I. scapularis*. The salivary protein was shown to adhere to the spirochete and to specifically interact with *B. burgdorferi*'s outer surface protein C. The binding of Salp15 protected *B. burgdorferi* from antibody-mediated killing, thereby providing the spirochetes with a marked advantage when

they were inoculated into naïve mice or mammals previously infected with *B. burgdorferi*.

- *Development of a New Transmission Blocking Vaccine for Lyme Disease.* It has long been known that immunization of mice with outer surface protein A (OspA) will protect against transmission of *B. burgdorferi* infection and will reduce the carriage of this pathogen in feeding ticks. In a recent study, the development of a murine-targeted OspA vaccine using vaccinia virus to interrupt the transmission of disease in reservoir hosts has been reported *(44)*. Thus, oral vaccination with a single dose of the OspA-expressing vaccinia virus construct resulted in high antibody titers against OspA, 100% protection against infection by *B. burgdorferi*, and a significant clearance of *B. burgdorferi* from infected ticks that fed on immunized mice. The reported findings indicated that such a vaccine was effective and may provide a means to lower the incidence of human disease in endemic areas.

- *Identification of a Genetic Deficiency That Enhances Acquisition and Transmission of Lyme Disease by Ticks.* *B. burgdorferi* strains exhibit various degrees of infectivity and pathogenicity in mammals, which may be due to their relative ability to evade initial host immunity. Innate immune cells recognize *B. burgdorferi* by Toll-like receptors (TLRs) that use the intracellular molecule myeloid differentiation factor-88 (MyD88) to mediate effector functions *(46)*. In a mouse model of Lyme disease using mutant strains of mice, the absence of MyD88 was found to facilitate tick-transmission of strains of *B. burgdorferi* of both low and high infectivity *(47)*. The reported data will broaden the understanding of factors that contribute the degree of pathogenicity observed between different clinical isolates of *B. burgdorferi*, as well as the genetic basis for host resistance or susceptibility to infection.

22.2 Tick-Borne Rickettsial Diseases

Tick-borne rickettsial diseases (TBRDs) are caused by pathogens of the second main group (the *spotted fever group*) of the genus *Rickettsia* (the other being the *typhus group*; see Chapter 21). TBRDs continue to cause severe illness and death in otherwise healthy adults and children despite the availability of low-cost, effective antimicrobial therapy, and the reported incidence of TBRDs has increased during the previous decade. The greatest challenge to clinicians is the difficulty of diagnosing these illnesses early in their clinical course when antibiotic therapy is most effective—early signs and symptoms are often nonspecific or mimic benign viral diseases, making diagnosis difficult *(48)*.

Although clinically similar, the TBRDs are epidemiologically and etiologically distinct diseases. In the United States,

they include (i) human monocytotropic (or monocytic) ehrlichiosis (HME); (ii) human granulocytotropic (or granulocytic) anaplasmosis (HGA; formerly known as human granulocytotropic ehrlichiosis or HE); (iii) Rocky Mountain spotted fever (RMSF); (iv) *Ehrlichia ewingii* infection; and (v) other emerging TBRDs *(48)*.

Additional diseases caused by the pathogenic members of the spotted fever group of *Rickettsia* are the African tick typhus and rickettsial pox. It is interesting to note that the pathogenic tick-borne *R. rickettsii*, *R. parkeri*, and *R. sibirica* are phylogenetically distinct from the nonpathogenic species *R. rhipicephali* and *R. montana*. Other species, such as *R. felis* and *R. helvetica*, are early diverging within the spotted fever group. The difference at the molecular level between the pathogenic and nonpathogenic species has not yet been completely elucidated.

Genome Sequence of Rickettsia conorii. Complete genome sequence data has been generated for only one species of the spotted fever group, *R. conorii (49)*. The genome of *R. conorii* is very small, only 1.29 Mb, and similar to that of *R. prowazekii* (see Chapter 21). The overall architecture of these two rickettsial genomes is essentially the same, with the exception of a few rearrangements near the terminus of replication. Symmetric DNA inversions at the regions surrounding the origins of replication and termination have been observed also in *Chlamydia (50)*. The symmetric nature of these rearrangements is thought to be the outcome of recombination events at the open replication forks. Such translocation and inversion events have since been identified in a variety of genomes, suggesting that the replicating DNA at the open replication fork is particularly vulnerable to recombination events *(49)*.

22.2.1 Treatment and Management of TBRDs: General Comments

Appropriate antibiotic treatment should be initiated immediately after diagnosis is made based on clinical, laboratory, or epidemiologic findings *(48)*. Any delay in treatment may lead to severe disease and even a fatal outcome.

Because any of the TBRD pathogens is susceptible to tetracycline antibiotics (especially doxycycline), these drugs are considered the therapy of choice in nearly all clinical situations. Fever typically subsides within 24 to 48 hours after doxycycline treatment is initiated during the first 4 to 5 days of illness *(48)*.

Doxycycline is bacteriostatic against rickettsiae and is active in both children and adults. The recommended dose for adults is 100 mg, twice daily (orally or intravenously). For children weighing less than 100 lb (45.5 kg), the recommended dose is 2.2 mg/kg body weight, twice daily (orally or intravenously). Intravenous administration is frequently indicated for hospitalized patients. The length of antibiotic therapy would be at least 3 days after the fever subsides and until evidence of clinical improvement is noted (typically 5 to 7 days) *(48)*.

The tetracycline antibiotics are generally *contraindicated for use in pregnant women* because of risks associated with malformation of teeth and bones in the fetus and hepatotoxicity and pancreatitis in the mother *(48, 51)*. However, tetracycline has been used successfully to treat HME in pregnant women *(52)*, and its use may be warranted during pregnancy in life-threatening situations where clinical suspicion of TBRD is high. Nevertheless, therapeutic choices for pregnant women with ehrlichiosis should be weighed cautiously, even when the benefits of doxycycline therapy generally outweigh its risks *(1)*.

Chloramphenicol (no longer available as an oral formulation) is an alternative drug that has been used to treat TBRDs such as Rocky Mountain spotted fever (RMSF) *(53)*. However, the drug is associated with various side effects and may need monitoring of the patient's blood indices. Moreover, epidemiologic studies using CDC case report data have suggested that patients with RMSF treated with chloramphenicol have a higher risk of dying than do patients who receive tetracycline *(48, 54)*. Whereas chloramphenicol is typically the preferred treatment for RMSF during pregnancy, care *must be used* especially when administering the drug late in the third trimester of pregnancy because of the risk of gray baby syndrome *(51)*.

22.2.1.1   Drug Resistance

Only the tetracycline antibiotics have demonstrated *in vitro* susceptibility and *in vivo* activity toward *Ehrlichia* species. In spite of *in vitro* susceptibility against *Ehrlichia*, the clinical effectiveness of rifampin is unknown *(55)*.

Ehrlichia chaffeensis has demonstrated resistance to gentamicin, ciprofloxacin, penicillin, macrolides, and sulfa-containing drugs *(56)*.

22.2.1.2   Severe Manifestations of TBRDs

A substantial number of patients with TBRDs may require hospitalization because of severe manifestations, including prolonged fever, renal failure, disseminated intravascular coagulopathy (DIC), hemophagocytic syndrome, meningoencephalitis, and acute respiratory distress syndrome (ARDS) *(48)*. A notable exception is anaplasmosis (HGA), which has not been associated with meningoencephalitis.

Rocky Mountain spotted fever frequently presents as a severe illness, during which patients commonly require hos-

pitalization. Up to 20% of untreated cases and 5% of treated cases have a fatal outcome, *making RMSF the most often fatal rickettsial disease in the United States (57)*. Host factors associated with severe or fatal RMSF include advanced age, male gender, black race, chronic alcohol abuse, and *glucose-6-phosphate dehydrogenase (G6PD)* deficiency *(53)*. Deficiency of G6PD is a sex-linked genetic condition affecting approximately 12% of the U.S. black male population *(48)*. Deficiency of G6PD is associated with a high proportion of fulminant cases of RMSF *(53)*. Fulminant cases follow a clinical course that is fatal within 5 days of the onset of infection. Long-term health effects of severe, life-threatening RMSF that may persist for more than 1 year include partial paralysis of the lower extremities, gangrene requiring amputation (fingers, toes, arms, or legs), hearing loss, blindness, loss of bowel or bladder control, movement disorders, and speech disorders *(58)*.

Similarly to RMSF, HME and HGA can also cause serious or fatal illness, although at a lower frequency than that observed with RMSF. Clinical conditions that may require hospitalization may include immunocompromised state, pain (headache, myalgia), mental confusion, cough, infiltrate in chest radiograph, abnormal spinal fluid findings, or specific acute organ failure *(48)*.

22.2.1.3   TBRDs Overlapping with Invasive Meningococcal Infection

It must be emphasized that during diagnosis, clinicians should be aware of the overlap of early symptoms of invasive meningococcal infection and TBRDs. These conditions are difficult to distinguish early in the course of the illness. In patients for whom both conditions are included in the initial differential diagnoses, after performing blood cultures and lumbar puncture, empirical treatment for both diseases *would be appropriate*. Such treatment could be accomplished by adding an appropriate parenteral penicillin (or cephalosporin) that has activity against *Neisseria meningitides* to doxycycline therapy *(48)*.

22.2.1.4   Pathogen Tropism

R. rickettsii, E. chaffeensis, E. ewingii, and *A. phagocytophilum* have specific and distinct cell tropism *(48)*.

R. rickettsii infects endothelial cells and, more rarely, underlying smooth muscle cells, where it multiplies freely in the cytoplasm. The rickettsiae cause a small-vessel vasculitis resulting in a maculopapular or petechial rash in the majority of patients. Vasculitis, when occurring in organs (brain or lungs), could cause life-threatening complications *(48)*.

Rickettsiae are not evident in blood smears and do not stain with the majority of conventional stains.

Ehrlichiosis and anaplasmosis are characterized by infection of leukocytes where the causative pathogens multiply in cytoplasmic membrane-bound vacuoles to form microcolonies known as *morulae*. *E. chaffeensis* most frequently infect monocytes, whereas *A. phagocytophilum* and *E. ewingii* demonstrate a predilection for granulocytes *(48)*. Morulae can be stained with conventional Wright or Giemsa stains and are occasionally observed in leukocytes in smears of peripheral blood, buffy coat preparations, or cerebrospinal fluid. Although a routine blood smear can provide a presumptive clue *for early diagnosis* because of the visualization of morulae, still a confirmatory testing for *Ehrlichia* or *Anaplasma* species *is required* by serology, PCR, or immunostaining methods. Also important to note is that the available methodology to demonstrate morulae in blood smears is not very sensitive, and a case of ehrlichiosis or anaplasmosis might be missed if the diagnosis relies solely on detecting morulae on blood smears. Although the diagnostic sensitivity of blood smears is greater for HGA than for HME, blood smears might only be positive in up to 60% of patients with HGA *(59)*.

22.2.2 Human Ehrlichiosis

Since 2000, the CDC has been tracking reported cases of several diseases collectively called human ehrlichiosis. However, the term "ehrlichiosis" is somewhat misleading, because when studied in detail it became clear that the etiologic agents of these emerging tick-borne infections are two different bacterial genera, *Ehrlichia* and *Anaplasma*. Geographically, they have occurred primarily east of the Rocky Mountains *(8, 48)*.

In the United States, infections caused by *Ehrlichia* spp. are typically transmitted by tick species of the genera *Amblyomma* (*A. americanum*) and *Ixodes* (*I. scapularis* and *I. pacificus*). Both genera use small mammals and birds as their primary reservoirs *(1)*. Morphologically, *Ehrlichia* spp. are small intracellular Gram-negative cocci that infect different hematopoietic cells, causing two etiologically and epidemiologically distinct forms of ehrlichiosis: *human monocytic ehrlichiosis (HME)* and *human granulocytic anaplasmosis (HGA)*. In the United States, most cases of both HME and HGA occur in the spring and summer (April to September for HME, and May to August for HGA), when ticks are at their peak *(1)*.

Recently, the CDC has described a new group of diseases called "other and unspecified" human ehrlichiosis. These infections include diseases caused by a second *Ehrlichia* species as well cases of previously mentioned illnesses that

could not be definitely diagnosed as either HME or anaplasmosis *(8, 48)*.

22.2.2.1 Human Monocytic Ehrlichiosis

The etiologic agent of human monocytic ehrlichiosis (HME) is *Ehrlichia chaffeensis* (Lone Star tick), which infects the macrophages and monocytes. The pathogen is transmitted primarily by *Amblyomma americanum*, but *Dermacentor variabilis* (American dog tick) can also transmit the disease. The major reservoir for *E. chaffeensis* is the white-tailed deer, with most cases being reported in the south central and southeastern regions of the United States. HME has been mainly associated with males (3 times more often than females), the elderly (over 65 years of age), and immunocompromised hosts (HIV/AIDS patients, and those with asplenia or Down's syndrome, and patients receiving immunosuppressive therapy) *(48, 60, 61)*.

Clinical manifestations of HME include fever, headache, and rash presented as part of a prodrome consisting of abrupt, high-grade fever (>95% of patients) often with an associated headache (60% to 80%), malaise (30% to 80%), nausea (40% to 50%), myalgia (40% to 60%), arthralgia (30% to 35%), lower back pain (30% to 40%), and gastrointestinal disorders (20% to 25%). The rash (on the trunk, extremities, and face, but rarely on the sole and palms) may be petechial, macular, maculopapular, or erythematous *(60)*. The prodrome typically manifests itself 7 to 14 days (median 9 days) after exposure to a tick. Neurologic manifestations (symptoms of meningitis and encephalopathy) have been observed in approximately 20% of patients.

Laboratory findings of HME are characterized by reduction in the multiple hematopoietic cell lines (occurring early in the course of the disease), thrombocytopenia, and leukopenia. A large decline in the total lymphocyte count is often seen in the early stage of the disease, whereas lymphocytosis occurs later, during the recovery phase of HME. Elevated liver enzyme levels (aspartate aminotransferase and alanine aminotransferase) are another characteristic laboratory finding of the disease and occur in 80% to 90% of patients *(1)*.

The manifestations of HME are typically moderate to severe and would require hospitalization of at least 50% of infected patients. If left untreated, HME may be fatal within the first 2 weeks, especially in men, the immunocompromised, and the elderly *(1)*.

22.2.2.2 Human Granulocytic Anaplasmosis

The black-legged tick (*Ixodes scapularis*) is the vector for *Anaplasma phagocytophilum* in the New England and north central regions of the United States, whereas the western black-legged tick (*Ixodes pacificus*) is the principal vector in northern California. Because these *Ixodes* species also transmit *Borrelia burgdorferi* (the causative agent of Lyme disease) and various *Babesia* species, the preponderance of cases of HGA occur in the same states that usually report high incidence of Lyme disease and human babesiosis *(48)*. Simultaneous infection with *A. phagocytophilum* and *B. burgdorferi* has been reported *(55, 62)*, and discerning such a mixed infection is vital because it *might affect the choice of antimicrobial medication*; whereas amoxicillin can be used to treat early stage of Lyme disease, it is not effective against HGA *(48)*.

In the absence of tick exposure, other modes of HGA transmission have also been reported—butchers cutting fresh deer carcasses had contracted the disease *(63)*. This suggests blood as a potential source of transmission and represents a risk of occupational exposure.

At-risk populations include the elderly, patients with chronic diseases (e.g., diabetes, collagen-vascular diseases), and patients on immunosuppressive therapy.

HGA is manifested as a constellation of nonspecific symptoms that occur after an incubation period of 7 to 10 days after tick exposure; generally 4 to 8 days elapse before a patient will seek medical care *(55)*.

The disease is commonly characterized by high-grade fever (over 39°C), rigors, nonspecific myalgia, severe headache, and malaise *(1)*. Other symptoms may include nausea, nonproductive cough, arthralgia, and anorexia. Although less common, 11% of patients with HGA will present with rash *(55)*, which is thought to be due to co-infection with Lyme borreliosis *(62)*. Though associated with less morbidity and mortality than is HME, 50% of patients with HGA will require hospitalization *(1)*.

Unlike patients with HME, those with HGA may have normal blood cell counts *(1)*. Nevertheless, approximately 70% of patients will have leukopenia and thrombocytopenia. Increased levels of liver enzymes, in particular, hepatic transaminases and C-reactive protein, are also commonly observed. In general, laboratory abnormalities will reach their peaks within 1 week after the onset of symptoms.

During acute HGA, morulae can be visualized (with microscopy) in the cytoplasm of leukocytes. This finding, if present, is diagnostic of HGA. However, the absence of morulae does not exclude the diagnosis of HGA *(55)*.

Typically, the nonspecific disease presentation, lack of morulae, and the transient nature of the blood cell counts *would make the diagnosis of HGA difficult*. As a result, the Consensus Approach for Ehrlichiosis (CAFE) Society has developed a set of definitions to help clinicians with the diagnosis of HGA *(1, 64)*.

Although HME and HGA are two distinct forms of human ehrlichiosis, the treatment is the same for both infections *(1)*. Doxycycline is the primary agent recommended for treat-

ment of HGA. However, similarly to HME, doxycycline is *contraindicated for pregnant women and children younger than age 9*, posing a dilemma for clinicians treating these patients. Data demonstrating the efficacy of rifampin in the treatment of ehrlichiosis in pregnant women are limited to just case reports *(56)*. Therapeutic choices for pregnant women with ehrlichiosis should be weighed cautiously, but the benefit of doxycycline therapy generally outweigh its risks *(1)*, and according to recommendations by the American Academy of Pediatrics and the CDC, doxycycline should be used in the treatment of children *(65)* and neonates *(66)*. It is recommended for children to start with oral doxycycline (4.4 mg/kg in 2 divided doses) on day 1, followed by a single dose of 2.2 mg kg^{-1} day^{-1}; the CDC is recommending the use of doxycycline 4.0 mg/kg in divided doses for children weighing less than 45 kg, and 100 mg twice daily (adult dose) for children weighing 45 kg or more (http://www.cdc.gov/ncidod/dvrd/rmsf/treatment).

22.2.2.3 Rocky Mountain Spotted Fever

In 1916, *Rickettsia rickettsii* was described in the blood vessels of infected patients and later identified as the etiologic agent of the Rocky Mountain spotted fever (RMSF).

The Rocky Mountain spotted fever has long been established in the United States. In spite of its common name, it is relatively rare in the Rocky Mountain region but far more prevalent in the southeastern regions of the United States.

Most often the infection is transmitted by ticks of the genus *Dermacentor*, which include the American dog tick (*D. variabilis*) in the eastern, central, and Pacific coastal United States, and by the Rocky Mountain wood tick (*D. andersoni*) in the western United States. In 2005, the common brown dog tick (*Rhipicephalus sanguineus*), a vector in Mexico, was also implicated in an Arizona outbreak *(8)*. The cayenne tick (*Amblyomma cajennense*) is a common vector of RMSF in Central and South America, and its range has extended into the United States in Texas *(48)*.

A case report of *Rickettsia parkeri* infection was recently published *(67)*. The organism was first discovered in Texas in *Amblyomma maculatum* (Gulf Coast tick); before that, the disease had not been reported in humans.

The main reservoirs for *D. variabilis* are small animals, such as mice and voles, and dogs and other large animals; and for *D. andersoni*, both small and large animals, typically wild rodents *(1)*. Ticks become infected by feeding on infected animals, by transtadial and transovarian passage. Humans are not a primary reservoir for *R. rickettsii* but are merely secondary hosts that enter the organism's life cycle tangentially through contact with arthropods. For humans to become infected with rickettsiosis, a tick may need to be attached for as little as 6 to 8 hours. However, attachment of 24 hours or more is generally needed for transfer of the disease *(1)*. Human infection may also result from contact with contaminated tick fluid and tissues during tick removal or from laboratory contact during culture and isolation.

In cases reported to the CDC, approximately 90% occurred from April to September and 40% during the May to June period, although infections have occurred in every month *(57)*.

Today, if left untreated, RMSF is the most fatal tick-borne infection in the United States, with an overall mortality of 25% *(68)*. However, treatment with antibiotics has reduced the mortality rates to 3% to 4%, and this, in most cases, may be due to delay in the diagnosis of the disease. The causative agent of RMSF, *R. rickettsii*, has been included as a NIAID Category C biodefense priority pathogen.

Dogs are susceptible to RMSF, and they frequently develop the disease concurrently with other household members in an endemic area *(48)*.

The clinical and laboratory manifestations of RMSF are similar to those of HME and HGA and generally appear within 2 to 14 days after a tick bite *(1, 48)*. In RMSF, a rash typically appears 2 to 4 days after the onset of fever and will occur earlier in children than in adults; it is eventually observed in approximately 90% of children. The exanthema typically will begin with the appearance of small, blanching, pink macules on the ankles, wrists, or forearms that evolve to maculopapules. The classic centripetal spread of rash is typically not noticed by the patient and might be difficult to elicit from the clinical history *(48)*. Although the rash may expand to involve the entire body, its presence on the face is usually limited. Patients with petechial rash are often severely ill, and although fever and organ dysfunction may resolve quickly with treatment, complete recovery can take longer.

The rash progression of RMSF includes several critical exceptions and considerations as follows *(48)*:

(i) A rash on the palms and soles is not pathognomonic and may occur in illnesses caused by drug hypersensitivity reactions, infective endocarditis, and a diverse group of other pathogens, including *Treponema pallidum, Streptobacillus moniliformis, E. chaffeensis*, and especially *Neisseria meningitides*, as well as certain enteroviruses.
(ii) The rash might be evanescent or localized to a particular region of the body.
(iii) A rash might be completely absent or atypical in up to 20% of patients with RMSF.

In certain cases, patients with RMSF (or ehrlichiosis) may seek medical attention for a febrile illness that mimics viral meningoencephalitis. Focal neurologic deficits, including cranial or peripheral motor nerve paralysis or sudden transient deafness, may also be observed *(48)*.

Laboratory findings, especially the complete blood cell count (CBC), are essential for the diagnosis of RMSF *(48)*.

The total white blood cell (WBC) count is typically normal in patients with RMSF, but increased numbers of immature bands are generally observed. Thrombocytopenia, mild elevation in hepatic transaminases, and hyponatremia may be observed with RMSF. By comparison, leukopenia (up to 53% of patients), thrombocytopenia (up to 94% of patients), and modest elevation of liver transaminase levels are particularly suggestive for HME and HGA *(48)*.

Patients with RMSF may have various signs and symptoms that differ in degree of severity *(1, 48)*. Orally given antibiotics are adequate in cases of mild illness, whereas severely ill patients should be hospitalized and treated with intravenous antibiotics. In a retrospective study, information based on multivariate analysis has shown that only increased serum creatinine levels and neurologic symptoms were associated with mortality *(69)*. The clinical outcome of RMSF is apparently strongly dependent on the time span between the patient's first visit and the start of therapy; if therapy had begun more than 5 days after the first visit, the outcome is significantly poorer than if treatment had been initiated earlier.

The tetracyclines are the cornerstone of therapy for RMSF, with doxycycline being the drug of choice *(1, 48)*. However, as with ehrlichiosis, the use of doxycycline in pediatric and pregnant patients again poses a problem. Generally, short courses of doxycycline may be administered in children younger than 9 years of age. However, according to the guidelines of the American Academy of Pediatrics and the CDC, the *empiric use* of doxycycline in children and pregnant women, although possible, should be applied with caution and with careful consideration for maternal hepatotoxicity and permanent tooth discoloration. Chloramphenicol has long been recommended as an alternative therapy for RMSF and is considered a suitable choice for patients who are pregnant or allergic to tetracyclines *(1)*. However, the adverse effects of chloramphenicol are well known: aplastic anemia, reversible bone marrow suppression, and gray baby syndrome *(70)*. Moreover, the chloramphenicol concentrations and reticulocyte counts should be monitored when the treatment exceeds 3 days.

Clearly, the administration of either doxycycline or chloramphenicol in pregnant women is not without risks.

22.2.2.4 Ehrlichia ewinglii Infection

Amblyomma americanum is also the principal vector of the ehrlichial pathogen *Ehrlichia ewinglii (48)*. The ecologic features of *E. ewinglii* are not completely known. However, dogs and deer have been naturally infected. Cases of granulocytotropic ehrlichiosis caused by *E. ewinglii* have been reported primarily in immunocompromised hosts. Human infections with this pathogen have been reported throughout the range of the Lone Star tick *(48)*.

Early clinical presentations in patients with *E. ewinglii* include fever, headache, myalgia, and malaise, and they are difficult to distinguish from other TBRDs and noninfectious diseases *(48)*.

As in patients with HGA, rash is rare in patients with *E. ewinglii* infection, and blood smears are useful for identifying patients with *E. ewinglii*. Furthermore, evaluation of CSF in patients with *E. ewinglii* has shown neutrophilic pleocytosis *(71)*.

Appropriate antibiotic treatment should be initiated immediately when a diagnosis of *E. ewinglii* is made. Doxycycline is the drug of choice for both children and adults, and as with the treatment of other TBRDs, caution must be applied when doxycycline is used for the treatment of *E. ewinglii (48)*.

22.3 Tularemia

The first report of tularemia in the United States occurred in 1911, in Tulare County, California *(72)*. One year later, the pathogen responsible for this outbreak was isolated and named *Bacterium tularense (72)*. The first report of tularemia in humans occurred in 1914 in two patients bitten by deerfly *(72)*. The infection is transmitted by ticks and is passed transovarially among ticks. In 1959, the organism was renamed *Francisella tularensis*.

F. tularensis is a highly contagious organism, which, in the context of biological weapons defense, is considered to be a potential threat. In fact, a tularemia outbreak in 1942 before the Battle of Stalingrad was the result of weaponized *F. tularensis*. There is no person-to-person transmission, but tularemia delivered as an aerosol could infect a large number of people.

Ecologically, tularemia is a disease of the northern hemisphere (North America, Northern Asia, Scandinavia, Europe, Japan, and Russia).

In addition to transmission by ticks and other arthropods, *F. tularensis* can be transmitted by inhalation, ingestion of contaminated food or drinking water supplies, and animal bites *(1)*. More than 250 animal species are implicated as carriers of *F. tularensis*. Consequently, in different regions of the world the disease is known by different names (rabbit fever, hare fever, deerfly fever, and lemming fever).

In the United States, when transmitted by ticks, *F. tularensis* is primarily transmitted by *A. americanum, D. andersoni*, and *D. variabilis (72)*. Except for Hawaii, all states have reported cases of tularemia, with the highest rates coming from Arkansas, Missouri, South Dakota, and Oklahoma.

The disease has a predilection for males, especially Native Americans and Alaskan Natives, and children age 5 to 9 and adults age 75 or older. Most human outbreaks occur in spring and summer, which correlates with arthropod transmission *(1, 72)*.

22.3.1 Bacteriology and Taxonomy of F. tularensis

The bacteriology and taxonomy of *F. tularensis* is complex *(1)*. It is a small, pleomorphic, aerobic, Gram-negative coccobacillus that can be found both inside and outside of cells.

The genus *Francisella* is divided into three major biovars. Biovar A (biogroup tularensis) predominates in North America and is the most virulent. Biovar B (biogroup holarica) is found primarily in Europe and Asia, but also exists in North America. Biovar C (biogroup novicida; formerly known as *F. novicida*) is found in parts of North America and has very low virulence *(73)*.

22.3.2 Clinical Manifestations and Laboratory Findings

The clinical course of tularemia is quite diverse, ranging from asymptomatic disease to septic shock and death *(1)*. Typically, tularemia is divided into six forms, reflecting the mode of transmission: (i) ulceroglandular; (ii) glandular; (iii) oculoglandular; (iv) oropharyngeal; (v) pneumonic (pleuritic); and (vi) typhoidal.

Tularemia is characterized by abrupt but nonspecific symptoms, such as fever, chills, headache, vomiting, fatigue, and anorexia, which make the disease difficult to diagnose. Pulse-temperature disparity in which the patients may exhibit a high temperature without reflexive increase in pulse is a *hallmark manifestation of the disease (73)*.

Ulceroglandular tularemia is the most common syndrome, accounting for 70% to 80% of *F. tularensis* infections. The pathogen enters through a scratch, abrasion, or tick and spreads via the proximal lymphatic system. As few as 10 organisms can cause disease. This syndrome usually appears as a papule at the tick-bite site and progresses to a pustular, ulcerated lesion called an inoculation eschar *(73)*.

Glandular tularemia is a relatively rare syndrome (15% of patients) with no ulcer present. The organism causes regional lymphadenopathy and is presumed to have gained access to the host through clinically unapparent abrasion *(74)*. Diagnosis may be difficult because the patient presents one or several enlarged lymph nodes with no skin lesion.

Oculoglandular tularemia occurs in approximately 1% of patients and results from inoculation of the eye by tularemia-contaminated fluids or fingers, perhaps after removal of the tick *(1)*. The clinical manifestations of oculoglandular tularemia are conjunctivitis with adjacent lymph node involvement, periorbital edema, and erythema.

Oropharyngeal tularemia accounts for less than 5% of all cases. This syndrome is not acquired by contact with ticks but results from ingestion of infected raw meats or contaminated water supplies *(1)*. Symptoms include fever, exudative pharyngitis, or oropharyngeal ulcerations. Because the manifestations mimic those of other upper respiratory infections, the diagnosis of oropharyngeal tularemia is based on exclusion from lack of response to antibiotics given for bacterial pharyngitis.

Pneumonic tularemia, the most severe form of the infection, may not be directly associated with tick exposure, but rather can develop through inhalation or secondarily by hematogenous spread *(1)*. Disease mortality is estimated to be around 7% *(72)*.

Typhoidal tularemia is a rare syndrome *(72)* manifested by fever, chills, and local findings to culture-negative septic shock. The syndrome may also be accompanied by pneumonia, elevated transaminase levels, and rhabdomyolysis, which leads to renal failure *(75)*.

The diagnosis of tularemia is confirmed when an antibody response occurs approximately 2 weeks after the onset of disease. The preferred serologic methods are agglutination (latex or tube agglutination tests) or PCR. The latter is highly sensitive and safer, but its specificity is dependent on the DNA sample and its purity *(1)*.

22.3.3 *Antibiotic Therapy of Tularemia*

Treatment of tularemia is based solely on case reports and anecdotal experience. Based on the latter, aminoglycosides, especially streptomycin and gentamicin, are regarded as the cornerstone of therapy *(1)*. A meta-analysis found that streptomycin was successful in 97% of patients, whereas gentamicin was successful in 86% *(76)*. In addition, gentamicin was associated with a 6% relapse rate and an 8% failure rate. However, despite these drawbacks of gentamicin, its cure rate was equal to or greater than that of other classes of antimicrobials, thus making it an acceptable alternative to streptomycin.

Results from tetracycline therapy of tularemia have shown 88% success and no treatment failures; however, it was associated with 12% relapse rate *(76)*. The high relapse rate of tetracycline may be the result of its bacteriostatic mode of action. In addition, tetracycline can be given only orally, which limits its use in patients with severe tularemia—the

drug levels achieved with oral administration only minimally exceeded the minimum inhibitory concentration (MIC) for *F. tularensis*.

In patients treated with chloramphenicol, the success rate was 77% with a 21% relapse rate *(76)*. Like tetracycline, chloramphenicol is bacteriostatic. However, when compared with aminoglycosides and tetracycline, one advantage of chloramphenicol is its enhanced penetration into the central nervous system. This feature makes chloramphenicol a *therapeutic option for treatment of meningeal tularemia*.

The fluoroquinolones are another therapeutic option for treating tularemia. Ciprofloxacin and levofloxacin have been used in the treatment of pneumonic tularemia, with the former showing a low failure rate and fewer adverse effects *(77)*, and no relapses (levofloxacin) 1 year later. Although data describing the efficacy of fluoroquinolones in the treatment of tularemia are still evolving, these agents have been as successful as other treatments of the disease *(1)*.

In vitro data demonstrated that *F. tularensis* isolates have shown resistance to β-lactams and therefore they should not be recommended for treatment of tularemia *(1)*.

22.4 Southern Tick-Associated Rash Illness

Erythema migrans, the characteristic rash associated with Lyme disease, has been reported in patients living in the south central and southeastern United States. Typically, it is associated with the bite of *Amblyomma americanum*. However, the spirochete that causes Lyme disease in North America, *Borrelia burgdorferi* sensu stricto, has not been confirmed in these regions of the United States by culture from clinical specimens, and serum antibodies rarely indicate exposure *(1)*. Although *Amblyomma americanum* is apparently not a vector for *B. burgdorferi sensu stricto*, the same ticks carry another spirochete, *Borrelia lonestari*. In a case report *(78)*, a patient was described with erythema migrans and *Amblyomma americanum* attachment. Importantly, *Borrelia lonestari* was identified both in the patient and the tick, and serology for *B. burgdorferi sensu stricto was negative*. Therefore, this observation strongly suggested that *Amblyomma americanum* can transmit the spirochete to humans, and the resulting rash, which resembled that seen with Lyme disease, has become known as southern tick-associated rash illness (STARI).

Borrelia lonestari (family Treponemataceae) is a spirochete that has been detected in *Amblyomma americanum* by DNA analysis. Unlike *Ixodes scapularis*, a vector for Lyme disease, *Amblyomma americanum* is less likely to be infected with a spirochete, with only 1% to 3% of *Amblyomma americanum* infected *(79)*. In contrast, 10% to 20% of nymph stage ticks and 30% to 40% of the adult-stage ticks of *I. scapularis* are infected with a spirochete.

The natural reservoir for *B. lonestari* has not been identified even though it was detected in white-tailed deer.

22.4.1 Clinical Manifestations, Laboratory Findings, and Treatment

In the only published case report of STARI, the patient showed only mild symptoms, such as fatigue, cough, and right shoulder discomfort *(78)*. Fever and headache were absent, and results of musculoskeletal, neurologic, pulmonary, and cardiac examinations were normal. Two erythematous lesions were also noted. The only abnormal laboratory finding was a slightly elevated serum alkaline phosphatase level.

There is no specific serologic test for exposure to *B. lonestari (1)*.

In the only case reported, the patient underwent antibiotic therapy with doxycycline for 2 weeks *(78)*; the skin lesions resolved in 11 days, and the patient returned to health about 24 days after therapy was initiated.

22.5 Babesiosis

Babesiosis, a malaria-like disease caused by intraerythrocyte protozoa named *Babesia bigemina*, was first described in 1888 *(80)*. The parasite is also the cause of the Texas cattle fever *(1)*. The first case of babesiosis in humans was reported in the former Republic of Yugoslavia in 1957 and in the United States in the late 1960s *(1)*.

The *Babesia* protozoa may vary in size (1 to 5 μm) and can be oval, round, or pear shaped *(81)*. More than 100 different species have been identified, but only four have been reported to be pathogenic in humans. In the United States, infection is caused primarily by *B. microti*, and two new strains of *Babesia* that can cause infection are designated as WA-1 and MO-1. Although human infections in the United States caused by *B. divergens* have not been reported, this protozoa is the primary cause of babesiosis in Europe *(1)*.

In the northeastern United States, the primary vector for *B. microti* is *Ixodes scapularis*, and the primary reservoir is the white-footed mouse. Although all stages of *I. scapularis* feed on humans, the nymph-stage tick is typically responsible for transmission of *B. microti* in humans. Vectors and reservoirs for WA-1 and MO-1 have not been identified *(1)*.

While babesiosis infections have been observed in patients of all ages, it appears that the occurrence is higher in men, and persons older than 40 years are prone to more severe infection. The infection is contracted most commonly during the summer (June to August) *(1)*.

22.5.1 Clinical Manifestations and Laboratory Findings of Babesiosis

Like malaria, the *Babesia* species reproduce within the red blood cells and produce hemolysis, which is responsible for the clinical presentation of babesiosis *(82)*. Manifestations of the disease are diverse and may range from asymptomatic to fulminant, leading to prolonged illness and even death. Although in the United States most cases of babesiosis are subclinical, when patients become symptomatic, manifestations usually appear after an incubation period of 1 to 6 weeks. The most common symptoms include fever (85% of patients), fatigue (79%), chills (63%), and headache (39%). Less often, myalgia, anorexia, cough, nausea, vomiting, arthralgia, emotional liability, depression, sore throat, abdominal pain, conjunctival injection, photophobia, and weight loss have been reported *(82)*. Physical findings are generally nonspecific (high fever, mild splenomegaly, and hepatomegaly). Unlike other tick-borne infections, rash is not common in babesiosis.

The most common complications in patients with severe babesiosis are acute respiratory failure (21% of patients), disseminated intravascular coagulation (18%), heart failure (12%), coma (9%), and renal failure (6%). Babesiosis is fatal in 5% to 9% of cases *(83)*.

Laboratory findings may include a decreased hematocrit value, thrombocytopenia, and a normal or decreased white blood cell count. Elevated levels of hepatic transaminases, bilirubin, and lactate dehydrogenase have also been observed. Urinalysis may reveal proteinuria and hemoglobinuria *(81)*.

22.5.2 Treatment of Babesiosis

Most cases of human babesiosis in the United States are mild and may resolve without treatment *(1)*. However, therapy is required in those patients who have undergone splenectomy, are immunosuppressed, are elderly, or have significant symptoms.

Historically, the cornerstone of babesiosis therapy is a combination of clindamycin and quinine given for period of 7 to 10 days *(82)*. However, even though effective, the combination clindamycin-quinine has been associated with significant drug-related toxicities, such as hearing loss, tinnitus, vertigo, and diarrhea.

Atovaquone, an antiprotozoal drug, has been studied in combination with azithromycin for the treatment of *B. microti* infections *(83)*. The atovaquone-azithromycin combination was compared with a 7-day oral treatment with clindamycin-quinine in immunocompetent adults with non–life-threatening babesiosis *(84)*. Resolution of parasitemia and symptoms was similar in both groups; however, the adverse reactions were significantly less in patients receiving atovaquone-azithromycin (15%) than in those receiving clindamycin-quinine (72%).

Another drug combination found effective in the treatment of babesiosis was clindamycin-doxycycline-azithromycin in an AIDS patient who developed an allergy to quinine *(81)*.

The combination of sulfamethoxazole-trimethoprim-pentamidine has been used successfully in the treatment of *B. divergens (84)*.

Exchange transfusions, administered concurrently with antibiotic therapy, may be necessary for patients with severe babesiosis showing significant parasitemia (more than 5%), coma, hypotension, heart failure, pulmonary edema, or renal failure *(82)*. Exchange transfusions reduce parasitemia and will facilitate the removal of *Babesia*-, erythrocyte-, and macrophage-produced by-products *(85)*.

22.6 Tick-Borne Relapsing Fever

In 1905, tick-borne relapsing fever (TBRF) was first described in West Africa where it was transmitted by *Ornithodoros moubata* soft ticks *(86)*. Tick-borne relapsing fever (TBRF) is a systemic *Borrelia* infection caused by a group of closely related species of spirochetes: *B. hermsii*, *B. turicatae*, and *B. parkeri*.

22.6.1 Pathophysiology of TBRF

The *Ornithodoros* species are soft ticks belonging to the Argasidae family. In the United States, two of these species, *O. hermsii* and *O. turicata*, cause most cases of TBRF *(1)*. *O. hermsii* transmits *Borrelia hermsii*, *O. turicata* transmits *B. turicatae*, and *O. parkeri* transmits *B. parkeri (86)*.

TBRF is endemic in the western United States. It occurs sporadically, but several common source epidemics have been reported. As with other tick-borne diseases, TBRF is a seasonal illness; 71% of reported cases have occurred during the June to September period. However, in Texas most episodes occur during the late autumn and early winter, with 50% reported from November to January *(1)*. This difference in seasonality may be related to differences in both organisms and habitats; in Texas, cases typically represent

B. turicatae infections acquired in caves, whereas in the northwestern United States, cases are generally *B. hermsii* infections acquired in mountainous regions *(1)*.

These spirochetes possess the unique ability to change outer surface proteins under pressure from the host immune system in a process known as *antigenic variation*, a phenomenon responsible for the recurring nature of the disease *(87)*. Thus, borreliae will sequester themselves in internal organs during afebrile periods and then will reappear with modified surface antigens to evade eradication.

As *Borrelia* organisms invade the endothelium, this can produce a low-grade, disseminated intravascular coagulation and thrombocytopenia. The relapse phenomenon occurs because of the antigenic variation—a genetically programmed shifting of outer surface proteins of *Borrelia* that allows a new clone to avoid destruction by antibodies directed initially against the majority of the original infecting organisms. As a result, the patient will improve clinically until the new clone multiplies sufficiently to cause another relapse. The tick-borne illness tends to have more relapses (average of 3) than does the louse-borne variety (often just one relapse).

22.6.1.1 Louse-Borne Relapsing Fever

Relapsing fever (RF) is an infectious disease transmitted to humans by two vectors, ticks and lice. The human body louse, *Pediculus humanus*, is the specific vector for borreliae. *Pediculus pubis* is not a vector. Louse-borne relapsing fever is a more severe form than the tick-borne variety. Regardless of the mode of transmission, a spirochetemia will develop.

The louse-borne relapsing fever is caused by *Borrelia recurrentis*. No animal reservoir exists. The lice that feed on infected humans acquire the *Borrelia* organisms, which then multiply in the gut of the louse. When an infected louse feeds on an uninfected human, the organism gains access when the victim crushes the louse or scratches the area where the louse is feeding. *B. recurrentis* infects the person through either abraded or intact skin (or mucous membranes) and then invades the bloodstream.

22.6.2 Clinical Manifestations and Laboratory Findings of TBRF

Because *Ornithodoros* ticks feed so rapidly, patients with TBRF are often unaware of the tick bite. A pruritic eschar may develop at the soft tick attachment site *(1)*.

Symptoms will appear abruptly on average 7 days after tick exposure *(88)*. Common manifestations include fever, headache, myalgia, arthralgia, nausea, and vomiting. The primary febrile period when the temperature can rise as high as 104°F (or even higher) lasts about 3 days (range, 12 hours to 17 days). Patients then experience an afebrile period lasting about 1 week, during which time they may experience malaise before symptoms suddenly recur. Without treatment, several (three to five) relapses can be expected. However, the length and severity of the illness will typically decrease with each relapse *(88)*.

Less common symptoms of TBRF include abdominal pain, confusion, dry cough, eye pain, diarrhea, dizziness, photophobia, and neck pain. Rash (petechial, macular, or popular) occurs in about 18% of patients and develops as the fever subsides. Other physical findings can be splenomegaly and hepatomegaly *(1)*.

Neurologic complications (neuroborreliosis) will occur predominately in patients infected with *B. turicatae* (27% to 80%), but much less in patients infected with *B. hermsii* (5%). The most common manifestations of neuroborreliosis are cranial nerve palsies and meningism *(89)*. Rare complications of TBRF are ocular disorders, myocarditis, and ruptured spleen *(86)*.

The most common hematologic abnormalities are thrombocytopenia (32% of patients), proteinuria (46%), and hematuria (30%). Most patients with TBRF have a normal white blood cell count.

22.6.3 Treatment of TBRF

No controlled studies have been published regarding treatment of TBRF. Based on clinical experience, the tetracycline antibiotics have been the treatment of choice *((90, 91)*. Oral doxycycline, 100 mg every 12 hours for 7 to 10 days, is the typical treatment. In addition, penicillin, chloramphenicol, and erythromycin have all been used successfully to treat TBRF. Tetracycline, erythromycin, and chloramphenicol are usually administered at dosages of 500 mg every 6 hours *(90)*. Patients with meningitis should receive intravenous therapy with penicillin G, cefotaxime, or ceftriaxone for 14 days or more *(91)*.

22.6.3.1 Jarisch-Herxheimer Reaction

The Jarisch-Herxheimer reaction is a serious consequence of TBRF treatment. It is manifested as an acute exacerbation of the patient's symptoms that can occur with the start of the antibiotic treatment. It has been reported in more than 50% of patients treated for TBRF *(89)*.

The pathophysiology of the Jarisch-Herxheimer reaction has been studied most extensively in patients with louse-borne relapsing fever. The reaction is associated with transient increases in plasma concentrations of tumor necrosis factor-α (TFN-α), interleukin-6, and interleukin-8 *(92)*. Anti-TNF-α antibodies prevented this reaction in patients with louse-borne relapsing fever *(93)*. Furthermore, meptazinol, an opioid partial agonist, reduced the severity of symptoms, whereas naloxone was ineffective *(94)*.

References

1. Amsden, J. R., Warmack, S., and Gubbins, P. O. (2005) Tick-borne bacterial, rickettsial, spirochetal, and protozoal infectious diseases in the United States: a comprehensive review, *Pharmacotherapy*, **25**(2), 191–210.
2. Parola, P. and Raoult, D. (2001) Ticks and tickborne bacterial diseases in humans: an emerging infectious threat, *Clin. Infect. Dis.*, **32**, 897–928.
3. Parola, P. and Raoult, D. (2001) Tick-borne bacterial diseases emerging in Europe, *Clin. Microbiol. Infect.*, **7**(2), 80–83.
4. Centers for Disease Control (2007) Lyme disease—United States, 2003–2005, *Morb. Mortal. Wkly Rep.*, **55**(23), 573–576.
5. Steere, A. C., Coburn, J., and Glickstein, L. (2004) The emergence of Lyme disease, *J. Clin. Invest.*, **113**(4), 1093–1101.
6. Schwan, T. G. and Piesman, J. (2000) Temporal changes in outer surface proteins A and C of the Lyme disease-associated spirochete *Borrelia burgdorferi*, during the chain of infections in ticks and mice, *J. Clin. Microbiol.*, **38**(1), 382–388.
7. Revel, A. T., Blevins, J. S., Almazán, C., Neil, L., Kocan, K. M., de la Fuente, J., Hagman, K. E., and Norgard, M. V. (2005) bptA (bbe16) is essential for the persistence of the Lyme disease spirochete, *Borrelia burgdorferi*, in its natural tick vector, *Proc. Natl. Acad. Sci. U.S.A.*, **102**(19), 6972–6977.
8. Latov, N., Wu, A. T., Chin, R. L., Sander, H. W., Alaedini, A., and Brannagan, T. H., III (2004) Neuropathy and cognitive impairment following vaccination with the OspA protein of *Borrelia burgdorferi*, *J. Peripheral Nervous System*, **9**, 165–167.
9. Wormser, G. P., Nadelman, R. B., Dattwyler, R. J., Dennis, D. T., Shapiro, E. D., Steer, A. C., Rush, T. J., Rahn, D. W., Coyle, P. K., Persing, D. H., Fish, D., and Luft, B. J. (2000) Practice guidelines for the treatment of Lyme disease, *Clin. Infect. Dis.*, **31**(Suppl. 1), S1–S14.
10. Marques, A. R., Martin, D. S., and Phillipp, M. T. (2002) Evaluation of the C6 peptide enzyme-linked immunosorbent assay for individuals vaccinated with the recombinant OspA vaccine, *J. Clin. Microbiol.*, **40**(7), 2591–2593.
11. Burgdorfer, W., Barbour, A. G., Hayes, S. F., Benach, J. L., Grunwaldt, E., and Davis, J. P. (1982) Lyme disease—a tick-borne spirochete? *Science*, **216**, 1317–1319.
12. Marques, A. R., Weir, S. C., Fahle, G. A., and Fischer, S. H. (2000) Lack of evidence of *Borrelia* involvement in Alzheimer's disease, *J. Infect. Dis.*, **182**, 1006–1007.
13. Klempner, M. S., Hu, L. T., Evans, J., Schmid, C. H., Johnson, G. M., Trevino, R. P., Norton, D., Levy, L., Wall, D., McCall, J., Kosinski, M., and Weinstein, A. (2001) Two controlled trials of antibiotic treatment in patients with persistent symptoms and a history of Lyme disease, *N. Engl. J. Med.*, **354**(2), 85–92.
14. Kaplan, R. F., Trevino, R. B., Johnson, G. M., Levy, L., Dornbush, R., Hu, L. T., Evans, J., Weinstein, A., Schmid, C. H., and Klempner, S. S. (2003) Cognitive function in post-treatment Lyme disease: do additional antibiotics help? *Neurology*, **60**(12), 1916–1922.
15. Krupp, L. B., Hyman, L. G., Grimson, R., Coyle, P. K., Melville, P., Ahnn, S., Dattwyler, R., and Chandler, B. (2003) Study and

treatment of post Lyme disease (STOP-LD): a randomized double masked clinical trial, *Neurology*, **60**(12), 1923–1930.

16. Pachner, A. R., Dail, D., Bai, Y., Sondey, M., Pak, L., Narayan, K., and Cadavid, D. (2004) Genotypes determine phenotype in experimental Lyme disease, *Ann. Neurol.*, **56**(3), 361–370.

17. Pachner, A. R., Dail, D., Narayan, K., Dutta, K., and Cadavid, D. (2002) Increased expression of B-lymphocyte chemoattractant but not pro-inflammatory cytokines, in muscle tissue in rhesus chronic Lyme borreliosis, *Cytokine*, **19**(6), 297–307.

18. Rupprecht, T. A., Pfister, H. W., Angele, B., Kastenbauer, S., Wilske, B., and Koedel, U. (2005) The chemokine CXCL13 (BLC): a putative diagnostic marker for neuroborreliosis, *Neurology*, **65**(3), 448–450.

19. Bockenstedt, L. K., Mao, J., Hodzic, E., Barthold, S. W., and Fish, D. (2002) Detection of attenuated, noninfectious spirochetes of *Borrelia burgdorferi*-infected mice after antibiotic treatment, *J. Infect. Dis.*, **186**(6), 1430–1437.

20. Hemmer, B., Gran, B., Zhao, Y., Marques, A., Pascal, J., Tzou, A., Kondo, T., Cortese, I., Bielekova, B., Straus, S. E., McFarland, H. F., Houghten, R., Simon, R., Pinilla, C., and Martin, R. (1999) Identification of candidate T-cell epitopes and molecular mimics in chronic Lyme disease, *Nat. Med.*, **5**, 1375–1382.

21. Alaedini, A. and Latov, N. (2005) Antibodies against OspA epitopes of *Borrelia burgdorferi* cross-react with neural tissue, *J. Neuroimmunol.*, **159**(1–2), 192–195.

22. Raveche, E. S., Schutzer, S. E., Fernandes, H., Bateman, H., McCarthy, B. A., Nickell, S. P., and Cunningham, M. W. (2005) Evidence of *Borrelia* autoimmunity-induced component of Lyme carditis and arthritis, *J. Clin. Microbiol.*, **43**, 850–856.

23. Benvenga, S., Guarniei, F., Vaccaro, M., Santarpia, L., and Trimarchi, F. (2004) Homologies betwen proteins of *Borrelia burgdorferi* and thyroid autoantigens, *Thyroid*, **14**(11), 964–966.

24. Klempner, M. S., Wormser, G. H., Wade, K., Trevino, R. P., Tang, K., Kaslow, R., and Schmid, C. (2005) A case-control study to examine HLA haplotype associations in patients with posttreatment chronic Lyme disease, *J. Infect. Dis.*, **192**(6), 1010–1013.

25. Moro, M. H., Zegara-Moro, O. L., Bjornsson, J., Hofmeister, E. K., Bruinsma, E., Germer, J. J., and Persing, D. H. (2002) Increased arthritis severity in mice coinfected with *Borrelia burgdorferi* and *Babesia microti*, *J. Infect. Dis.*, **186**(3), 428–431.

26. Thomas, V., Anguita, J., Barthold, S. W., and Fikrig, E. (2001) Co-infection with *Borrelia burgdorferi* and the agent of human granulocytic ehrlichiosis alters the murine immune responses, pathogen burden, and severity of Lyme arthritis, *Infect. Immun.*, **69**(5), 3359–3371.

27. Klempner, M. S. (2002) Controlled trials of antibiotic treatment in patients with post-treatment chronic Lyme disease, *Vector Borne Zoonotic Dis.*, **2**, 255–263.

28. Ge, Z., Feng, Y., Whary, M. T., Nambiar, P. R., Xu, S., Ng, V., Taylor, N. S., and Fox, J. G. (2005) Cytolethal distending toxin is essential for colonization of *Helicobacter hepaticus* in outbread Swiss Webster mice, *Infect. Immun.*, **73**(6), 3440–3467.

29. Liang, F. T., Jacobson, R. H., Straubinger, R. K., Grooters, A., and Philipp, M. T. (2000) Characterization of a *Borrelia burgdorferi* VlsE invariable region useful in canine Lyme disease serodiagnosis by enzyme-linked immunosorbent assay, *J. Clin. Microbiol.*, **38**(11), 4160–4166.

30. Klempner, M. S., Schmid, C. H., Hu, L., Steere, A. C., Johnson, G., McCloud, B., Noring, R., and Weinstein, A. (2001) Intralaboratory reliability of serologic and urine testing for Lime disease, *Am. J. Med.*, **110**(3), 217–219.

31. Rauter, C., Mueller, M., Diterich, I., Zeller, S., Hassler, D., Meergans, T., and Hartung, T. (2005) Critical evaluation of urine-based PCR assay for diagnosis of Lyme borreliosis, *Clin. Diag. Lab. Immunol.*, **12**(8), 910–917.

32. Fleming, R. V., Marques, A. R., Klempner, M. S., Schmid, C. H., Dally, L. G., Martin, D. S., and Phillipp, M. T. (2004) Pretreatment and post-treatment assessment of the C6 test in patients with persistent symptoms and a history of Lyme borreliosis, *Eur. J. Clin. Microbiol. Infect. Dis.*, **23**(6), 615–618.

33. Mogilyansky, E., Loa, C. C., Adelson, M. E., Mordechai, E., and Tilton, R. C. (2004) Comparison of Western immunoblotting and the C_6 Lyme antibody test for laboratory detection of Lyme disease, *Clin. Diag. Lab. Immunol.*, **11**(5), 924–929.

34. Philipp, M. T., Wormser, G. P., Marques, A. R., Bittker, S., Martin, D. S., Nowakowski, J., and Dally, L. G. (2005) A decline in C_6 antibody titer occurs in successfully treated patients with culture-controlled early localized or early disseminated Lyme borreliosis, *Clin. Diag. Lab. Immunol.*, **12**(9), 1069–1074.

35. Marques, A. R., Hornung, R. L., Dally, L., and Philipp, M. T. (2005) Detection of immune complexes is not independent of detection of antibodies in Lyme disease patients and does not confirm active infection with *Borrelia burgdorferi*, *Clin. Diag. Lab. Immunol.*, **12**(9), 1036–1040.

36. Purcer, J. E., Lawrenz, M. B., Caimano, M. J., Howell, J. K., Radolf, J. D., and Norris, S. J. (2003) A plasmid-encoded nicotinamidase (PncA) is essential for infectivity of *Borrelia burgdorferi* in a mammalian host, *Mol. Microbiol.*, **48**(3), 753–764.

37. Brooks, C. S., Vuppala, S. R., Jett, A. M., and Akins, D. R. (2006) Identification of *Borrelia burgdorferi* outer surface protein, *Infect. Immun.*, **74**(1), 296–304.

38. Pal, U., Xin, L., Wang, T., Montgomery, R. R., Ramamoorthi, N., deSilva, A. M., Bao, F., Yang, X., Pypaert, M., Pradham, D., Kantor, F. S., Telford, S., Anderson, J. F., and Fikrig, E. (2004) TROSPA, and *Ixodes scapularis* receptor for *Borrelia burgdorferi*, *Cell*, **119**(4), 457–468.

39. Tsao, J. I., Wootton, J. T., Binikis, J., Luna, M. G., Fish, D., and Barbour, A. G. (2004) An ecological approach to preventing human infection: vaccinating wild mouse reservoirs intervenes in the Lyme disease cycle, *Proc. Natl. Acad. Sci. U.S.A.*, **101**(52), 18159–18164.

40. Ramamoorthy, N., Narasimhan, S., Pal, U., Yang, X. F., Fish, D., Anguita, J., Norgard, M. V., Kantor, F. S., Anderson, J. F., Koski, R. A., and Fikrig, E. (2005) The Lyme disease agent exploits a tick protein to infect the mammalian host, *Nature*, **436**, 573–577.

41. Brossard, M. and Wikel, S. K. (2004) Tick immunobiology, *Parasitology*, **129** (Suppl.), S161–S176.

42. Burke, G., Wikel, S. K., Spielman, A., Telford, S. R., McKay, K., Krause, P. Y., and the Tick-borne Infection Study Group (2005) Hypersensitivity to ticks and Lyme disease risk, *Emerg. Infect. Dis.*, **11**(1), 36–41.

43. Lathrop, S. L., Ball, R., Haber, P., Mootrey, G. T., Braun, M. M., Shadomy, S. V., Elllenberg, S. S., Chen, R. T., and Hayes, E. B. (2002) Adverse event reports following vaccination against Lyme disease: December 1998–July 2000, *Vaccine*, **20**(11–12), 1603–1608.

44. Schekelhoff, M. R., Telford, S. R., and Hu, L. T. (2006) Protective efficacy of an oral vaccine to reduce carriage of *Borrelia burgdorferi* (strain N40) in mouse and tick reservoirs, *Vaccine*, **24**(11), 1949–1957.

45. Earnhart, C. G., Buckles, E. L., Dumler, J. S., and Marconi, R. T. (2005) Demonstration of OspC type diversity in invasive human Lyme disease isolates and identification of previously uncharacterized epitopes that define the specificity of the OspC murine antibody response, *Infect. Immun.*, **73**(12), 7869–7877.

46. Velegraki, M., Samonis, G., Eliopoulos, G. D., and Papadaki, H. (2007) Toll like receptors: molecular structure and functional role in innate and adaptive immunity, *Haema*, **10**(1), 18–26.

47. Bockenstedt, L. K., Liu, N., Schwartz, I., and Fish, D. (2006) MyD88 deficiency enhances acquisition and transmission of

Borrelia burgdorferi by *Ixodes scapularis* ticks, *Infect. Immun.*, **74**(4), 2154–2160.

48. Centers for Disease Control (2006) Diagnosis and management of tickborne rickettsial diseases: Rocky Mountain spoted fever, ehrlichioses, and anaplasmosis—United States, (2006), *Morb. Mortal. Wkly Rep.*, **55**(RR-4), 1–27.

49. Andersson, S. G. E. (2004) Obligate intracellular pathogens. In: *Microbial Genomes* (Fraser, C. M., Read, T. D., and Nelson, K. E., eds.), Humana Press, Totowa, NJ, pp. 291–308.

50. Tillier, E. R. M. and Collins, R. A. (2000) Genome rearrangement by replication-directed translocation, *Nature*, **26**, 195–197.

51. Walker, D. H. and Sexton, D. J. (1999) *Rickettsia rickettsii*. In: *Antimicrobial Therapy and Vaccines* (Yu, V. L., Merigan, T. C., Jr., and Barriere, S. L., eds.), Williams & Wilkins, Baltimore, pp. 562–568.

52. Smith Sendev, A. E., Sehdev, P. S., Jacobs, R., and Dumler, J. S. (2002) Human monocytic ehrlichiosis presenting as acute appendicitis during pregnancy, *Clin. Infect. Dis.*, **35**, e99–e102.

53. Walker, D. H. and Raoult, D. (2005) *Rickettsia rickettsii* and other spotted fever group Rickettsiae (Rocky Mountain spotted fever and other spotted fevers). In: *Mandell, Douglas, and Bennett's Principles and Practice of Infectious Disease*, 6th ed., Churchill Livingstone, Philadelphia, pp. 2287–2295.

54. Holman, R. C., Paddock, C. D., Curns, A. T., Krebs, J. W., McQuiston, J. H., and Childs, J. E. (2001) Analysis of risk factors for fatal Rocky Mountain spotted fever: evidence for superiority of tetracyclines for therapy, *J. Infect. Dis.*, **184**, 1437–1444.

55. Bakken, J. S., Krueth, J., Wilson-Nordskog, C., Tilden, R. L., Asanovich, K., and Dumler, J. S. (1996) Clinical and laboratory characteristics of human granulocytic ehrlichiosis, *J. Am. Med. Assoc.*, **275**, 199–205.

56. Brouqui, P. and Raoult, D. (1992) In vitro antibiotic susceptibility of the newly recognized agent of ehrlichiosis in humans, *Ehrlichia chaffeensis, Antimicrob. Agents Chemother.*, **36**, 2799–2803.

57. Treadwell, T. A., Holman, R. C., Clarke, M. J., Krebs, J. W., Paddock, C. D., and Childs, J. E. (2000) Rocky Mountain spotted fever in the United States, 1993–1996, *Am. J. Trop. Med.*, **63**, 21–26.

58. Archibald, L. K. and Sexton, D. J. (1995) Long-term sequelae of Rocky Mountain spotted fever, *Clin. Infect. Dis.*, **20**, 1122–1125.

59. Bakken, J. S. and Dumler, J. S. (2000) Human granulocytic ehrlichiosis, *Clin. Infect. Dis.*, **31**, 554–560.

60. Fishbein, D. B., Dawson, J. E., and Robinson, L. E. (1994) Human ehrlichiosis in the United States, 1985 to 1990, *Ann. Intern. Med.*, **120**, 736–743.

61. Paddock, C. D. and Childs, J. E. (2003) *Ehrlichia chaffeensis*: a prototypical emerging pathogen, *Clin. Microbiol. Rev.*, **16**, 37–64.

62. Nadelman, R. B., Horowitz, H. W., Hsieh, T.-C., Wu, J. M., Aguero-Rosenfeld, M. E., Schwartz, I., Nowakowski, J., Varde, S., and Wormser, G. P. (1997) Simultaneous human granulocytic ehrlichiosis and Lyme borreliosis, *N. Engl. J. Med.*, **337**(1), 27–30.

63. Bakken, J. S., Krueth, J. K., Lund, T., Malkovitch, D., Asanovich, K., and Dumler, J. S. (1996) Exposure to deer blood may be the cause of human granulocytic ehrlichiosis [letter], *Clin. Infect. Dis.*, **23**, 198.

64. Walker, D. H. (2000) Diagnosing human ehrlichiosis: current status and recommendations, *Am. Soc. Microbiol. News*, **66**, 287–291.

65. Masters, E. J., Olson, G. S., Weiner, S. J., and Paddock, C. D. (2003) Rocky Mountain spotted fever: a clinician's dilemma, *Arch. Intern. Med.*, **163**, 769–774.

66. Horowitz, H. W., Kilchevsky, E., Haber, S., Aguero-Rosenfeld, M., Kranwinkel, R., James, E. K., Wong, S. J., Chu, F., Liveris, D., and Schwartz, I. (1998) Perinatal transmission of the agent of human granulocytic ehrlichiosis, *N. Engl. J. Med.*, **339**(6), 375–378.

67. Paddock, C. D., Sumner, J. W., Comer, J. A., Zaki, S. R., Goldsmith, C. S., Goddard, J., McLellan, S. L. F., Tamminga, C. L., and Ohl, C. A. (2004) *Rickettsia parkeri*: a newly recognized cause of

spotted fever rickettsiosis in the United States, *Clin. Infect. Dis.*, **38**, 805–811.

68. Jones, T. E., Craig, A. S., Paddock, C. D., McKechnie, D. B., Childs, J. E., Zaki, S. R., and Schaffner, W. (1999) Family cluster of Rocky Mountain spotted fever, *Clin. Infect. Dis.*, **28**, 853–859.

69. Conlon, P. J., Procop, G. W., Fowler, V., Eloubeidi, M. A., Smith, S. R., and Sexton, D. J. (1996) Predictors of prognosis and risk of acute renal failure in patients with Rocky Mountain spotted fever, *Am. J. Med.*, **101**, 621–626.

70. Stallings, S. P. (2001) Rocky Mountain spotted fever and pregnancy: a case report and review of the literature, *Obstet. Gynecol. Surv.*, **56**, 37–42.

71. Buller, R. S., Arens, M., Hmiel, S. P., Paddock, C. D., Sumner, J. W., Rikihisa, Y., Univer, A., Gaudreault-Keener, M., Manian, F. A., Liddell, A. M., Schmulewitz, N., and Storch, G. A. (1999) *Ehrlichia ewingii*, a newly recognized agent of human ehrlichiosis, *N. Engl. J. Med.*, **341**(3), 148–155.

72. Evans, M. E., Gregory, D. W., Schaffner, W., and McGee, Z. A. (1985) Tularemia: a 30-year experience with 88 cases, *Medicine*, **64**, 251–269.

73. Cassady, K. A., Dalzell, A., Guffey, M. B., and Kelly, D. R. (2007) Ulceroglandular tularemia in a nonendemia area. (Disease/Disorder overview), *South. Med. J.*, **100**(3), 304–308.

74. Choi, E. (2002) Tularemia and Q fever, *Med. Clin. North Am.*, **86**, 393–416.

75. Hayes, E., Marshall, S., and Dennis, D. (2002) Tularemia: United States, 1990–2000, *Morb. Mortal. Wkly Rep.*, **51**, 182–184.

76. Enderlin, G., Morales, L., Jacobs, R. F., and Cross, J. T. (1994) Streptomycin and alternative agents for the treatment of tularemia: review of the literature, *Clin. Infect. Dis.*, **19**, 42–47.

77. Perez-Castrillon, J. L., Bachiller-Lique, P., Martin-Luquero, M., Mena-Martin, F. J., and Herreros, V. (2001) Tularemia epidemic in northwestern Spain: clinical description and therapeutic response, *Clin. Infect. Dis.*, **33**, 573–576.

78. James, A. M., Liveris, D., Wormser, G. P., Schwartz, I., Montecalvo, M. A., and Johnson, B. J. (2001) *Borrelia lonestari* infection after a bite by an *Amblyomma americanum* tick, *J. Infect. Dis.*, **183**, 1810–1814.

79. Burkot, T. R., Mullen, G. R., Anderson, R., Schneider, B. S., Happ, C. M., and Zeidner, N. S. (2001) *Borrelia lonestari* DNA in adult *Amblyomma americanum* ticks, Alabama, *Emerg. Infect. Dis.*, **7**, 471–473.

80. Homer, M. J., Aguilar-Delfin, I., Telford, S. R., Krause, P. J., and Persing, D. H., (2000) Babesiosis, *Clin. Microbiol. Rev.*, **13**, 451–469.

81. Boustani, M. R. and Gelfand, J. A. (1996) Babesiosis, *Clin. Infect. Dis.*, **22**, 611–615.

82. Krause, P. J. (2002) Babesiosis, *Med. Clin. North Am.*, **86**, 361–373.

83. Hatcher, J. C., Greenberg, P. D., Antique, J., and Jimenez-Lucho, V. E. (2001) Severe babesiosis in Long Island: review of 34 cases and their complications, *Clin. Infect. Dis.*, **32**, 1117–1125.

84. Krause, P. J., Lepore, T., Sikand, V. K., Gadbaw, J., Jr., Burke, G., Telford, S. R., 3rd, Brassard, P., Pearl, D., Azlanzadeh, J., Christianson, D., McGrath, D., and Spielman, A. (2000) Atovaquone and azithromycin for the treatment of babesiosis, *N. Engl. J. Med.*, **343**(20), 1454–1458.

85. Jacoby, G. A., Hunt, J. V., Kosinski, K. S., Demirjian, Z. N., Huggins, C., Etkind, P., Marcus, L. C., and Spielman, A. (1980) Treatment of transfusion-transmitted babesiosis by exchange transfusion, *N. Engl. J. Med.*, **303**(19), 1098–1100.

86. Dworkin, M. S., Schwan, T. G., and Anderson, D. E., Jr. (2002) Tick-borne relapsing fever in North America, *Med. Clin. North Am.*, **86**, 417–433.

87. Barbour, A. (1990) Antigenic variation of a relapsing fever *Borrelia* species, *Annu. Rev. Microbiol.*, **44**, 155–171.

88. Southern, P. M. and Sanford, J. P. (1969) Relapsing fever: a clinical and microbiological review, *Medicine*, **48**, 129–149.

89. Dworkin, M. S., Anderson, D. E., Jr., Schwan, T. G., Schoemaker, P. C., Banerjee, S. N., Kassen, B. O., and Burgdorfer, W. (1998) Tick-borne relapsing fever in the northwestern United States and southwestern Canada, *Clin. Infect. Dis.*, **26**(1), 122–131.

90. Horton, J. M. and Blaser, M. J. (1985) The spectrum of relapsing fever in the Rocky Mountains, *Arch. Intern. Med.*, **145**, 871–875.

91. Cadavid, D. and Barbour, A. G. (1998) Neuroborreliosis during relapsing fever: review of the clinical manifestations, pathology, and treatment of infections in humans and experimental animals, *Clin. Infect. Dis.*, **26**, 151–164.

92. Negussie, Y., Remick, D. G., DeForge, L. E., Kunkel, S. L., Eynon, A., and Griffin, G. E., (1992) Detection of plasma tumor necrosis factor, interleukins 6 and 8, during the Jarisch-Herxheimer reaction of relapsing fever, *J. Exp. Med.*, **175**, 1207–1212.

93. Fekade, D., Knox, K., Hussein, K., Melka, A., Lalloo, D. G., Coxon, R. E., and Warrell, D. A. (1996) Prevention of Jarisch-Herxheimer reactions by treatment with antibodies against tumor necrosis factor, *N. Engl. J. Med.*, **335**(5), 311–315.

94. Teklu, B., Habte-Michael, A., Warrell, D. A., White, N. J., and Wright, D. J. (1983) Meptazinol diminishes the Jarisch-Herxheimer reaction of relapsing fever, *Lancet*, **1**, 835–839.

Chapter 23

Defense Against Biological Weapons (Biodefense)

Biological warfare (germ warfare) is defined as the use of any disease-causing organism or toxin(s) found in nature as weapons of war with the intent to destroy an adversary. Though rare, the use of biological weapons has occurred throughout the centuries.

The ban on the use of biological weapons was enacted as an international law by the Geneva Protocol of 1925. Subsequently, because a successful biological attack could conceivably result in thousands, even millions, of casualties, causing severe disruptions to societies and economies, the creation and stockpiling of biological weapons were banned in 1972 by the Geneva Biological and Toxin Weapons Convention, which was signed by more than 100 states. The convention extended the ban to almost all production, storage, and transport of biological weapons. *However, oddly enough, the convention did not prohibit the use of biological weapons.* The consensus among military experts is that, except in the context of bioterrorism, biological warfare is militarily of little use (http://www.biocrawler.com/encyclopedia/biological_warfare). It is believed that since the signing of the convention, the number of countries capable of producing such weapons has increased.

For the military, the main problem with use of biological weapons is that a biological attack would take some time to have an effect and, therefore, unlike a nuclear or chemical attack, would not necessarily stop an advancing army. As a strategic weapon, biological warfare would again be militarily problematic, because unless it is used to poison the enemy's civilian population, it would be difficult to prevent the biological attack from spreading, either to allies or to the attacker. Besides, a biological attack would almost certainly invite immediate massive retaliation, usually in the same form (http://www.biocrawler.com/encyclopedia/biological_warfare).

On the other hand, a terrorist attack using biological agents, once thought to be a remote possibility, occurred in autumn 2001 when *B. anthracis* spores were sent through the U.S. mail, causing 18 confirmed cases of anthrax (11 inhalation, 7 cutaneous). Recent events have raised awareness of both the possibility of a bioterrorist attack and the vulnerability of the U.S. population to such an event. In 2003 and 2004, ricin was found in an envelope at a postal facility in South Carolina and in a U.S. Senate office building in Washington, DC, and was used to contaminate several jars of baby food in California. Although the U.S. Department of Defense (DoD) has developed defenses for biological warfare, there are additional concerns that need to be addressed to provide an adequate civilian defense from a bioterrorist attack. The potential list of microbial pathogens that threaten civilian populations is larger than the list of classic biological warfare threats. The list of biodefense priority pathogens targeted by NIAID research can be found at http://www3.niaid.nih.gov/Biodefense/bandc_priority.htm. In addition, the populations to be protected are different, because civilians include people of all ages and physical conditions.

Diseases considered for weaponization, or known to be weaponized, include anthrax, Ebola, bubonic plague, cholera, tularemia, brucellosis, Q fever, Machupo, Venezuelan equine encephalomyelitis (VEE), and smallpox. Naturally occurring toxins that can be used as weapons include ricin, staphylococcal enterotoxin B (SEB), the botulism toxin, and many mycotoxins.

Instead of targeting humans, biological weapons could be designed to target food crops. Such bioweapons are known as bioherbicides, or mycoherbicides if the agent is a fungus.

23.1 History of Biological Warfare

The use of biological agents in military confrontations is not new and before the 20th century occurred in three main forms:

- *Deliberate poisoning of food and water with infectious material.* For example, in the 6th century BC, the Assyrians poisoned enemy wells with a fungus that would make the enemy delusional. During the U.S. Civil War, General George Sherman reported that Confederate forces shot farm animals in ponds upon which the Union forces depended for drinking water, thus effectively poisoning the water (http://www.biocrawler.com/encyclopedia/biological_warfare).

- *Use of microorganisms, toxins, or animals, living or dead, in a weapons system.* During the Middle Ages, victims of bubonic plague were used for biological attacks, often by flinging their corpses and excrement over castle walls using catapults *(1)*. In medieval medical theory, the stench of rotting organic material was believed to be a potent cause of disease. Thus, in 1340, the enemy hurled dead horses and other animals by catapult at the castle of Thun L'Eveque in Hainault (now in Northern France). At Caffa in the Crimea in 1346, it was human plague cadavers, and in Karlstein in Bohemia in 1422, it was human battle casualties and waste of some kind—probably human and animal manure. The purpose was almost certainly to transmit disease, and at least in 1346 at Caffa it succeeded: after the battle a large number of the defenders came down with plague, and by fleeing Caffa they helped transmit the disease around the Mediterranean basin, initiating the Black Death *(1)*.

The last known incident of using plague corpses for biological warfare occurred in 1710, when Russian forces attacked the Swedes by flinging plague-infected corpses over the city walls of Reval.

- *Use of biologically inoculated humans and fabrics.* Much of the Native American population suffered after contact with the Old World as a result of the introduction of many different diseases. The British army at least once used smallpox as a weapon. In 1763, at Fort Pitt on the Pennsylvania frontier during the parlay, the British gave as gifts to the Indians blankets and handkerchiefs that were taken from smallpox patients in the infirmary *(1)*.

During the American Revolutionary War, Britain apparently used smallpox as a biological weapon, possibly on several occasions *(1, 2)*. In the northern colonies they were suspected on several occasions of inoculating civilians with smallpox with the intent that they would transmit the disease to the Continental Army *(1)*. Deliberate inoculation with material from a small pustule was a well-known protective measure: it gave the recipient a mild case of smallpox, with lower chance of death than that with natural transmission and led to lifelong immunity. However, the induced disease was as contagious as natural smallpox, and the inoculated persons were commonly quarantined until their symptoms abated.

23.1.1 German Biological Sabotage in World War I

From 1915 through 1918, Germany waged a campaign of covert biological attack on animals (horses, mules, sheep, and cattle) being shipped from neutral countries to the Allies *(3)*. For biological weapons, the program used glanders and anthrax and employed secret agents to administer the bacterial cultures to animals penned for shipment from Romania, the United States, Spain, Argentina, and perhaps Norway. It is not clear how effective these programs of biological sabotage were.

23.1.2 Japanese Biological Warfare in World War II

Contrary to expectations, in fact only Japan made significant use of biological weapons during World War II *(4, 5)*. During 1939, the Japanese carried out biological attacks on military and civilian targets. The methods were primitive, and all efforts to develop reliable and effective biological munitions failed. Most attacks relied on saboteurs contaminating wells with intestinal pathogens and on distribution of microbe-laced foods, air drops of plague-infected fleas, and probably aerial spraying of microbial cultures. Their effectiveness is hard to evaluate.

23.1.3 Terrorist Use of Biological Weapons

In 1984, followers of the Bagwan Shree Rajneesh (the Rajneeshee cult) living in a ranch in rural Oregon tested a crude biological weapon in the small town of The Dulles *(6)*. Cultures of *Salmonella typhimurium* were grown in the infirmary of the ranch and then sprinkled on food in restaurants, in particular at salad bars. The result was more than 750 cases of salmonellosis, 45 of which required hospitalization. The intent of the attack, which was apparently successful, was to determine the feasibility of keeping voters from the polls in an upcoming election, with the hope that the Rajneeshees could win a majority in the county government, allowing them to make changes in the zoning and land-use policies that the existing government had turned down *(1)*.

During September and October 2001, several letters (probably five to six) containing *Bacillus anthracis* spores were mailed from Trenton, New Jersey, to several media representatives and to two offices at the U.S. Senate *(1)*. As these envelopes were processed through automatic sorting machines, they contaminated a great number of postal workers, and upon being opened, they contaminated hundreds more people in the receiving premises. A total of 22 cases of anthrax are thought to have resulted (a few more are possible). Eleven of the episodes were cutaneous, none of which was fatal. The other cases were pulmonary, and five of them were fatal. The widespread and extensive use of prophylactic antibiotic treatment undoubtedly prevented many additional cases of infection.

23.2 Biological and Toxin Weapons Factors

Delivery of biological weapons through food or water is of concern. However, it is restricted by the quantity of biological agent required, which limits use to objectives where less than mass morbidity is intended (e.g., psychological impact on civilian populations) *(7)*. Contrary to popular perception, dilution factors and modern technology for refining the food supply, including water purification, will significantly limit the efficient use of biological weapons by the oral use of exposure *(8)*. By comparison, in the context of biological warfare and/or terrorist action, biological weapons are most likely to be delivered covertly and by aerosol, with the intention of causing mass casualties *(7)*.

Potential biological weapons are usually designated as either lethal or incapacitating, although these terms are not absolute but imply statistical probability of response.

In April 1997, the U.S. Department of Health and Human Services (DHHS) and the Centers for Disease Control and Prevention (CDC) set forth a set of regulations governing hazardous biological agents (Tables 23.1 and 23.2) *(9)*.

23.2.1 Aerosol Delivery: Biological/Toxin Agent Factors

Biological weapons can be disseminated most effectively in an aerosol form through the use of either conventional delivery systems, such as bombs and missiles, or by unconventional systems, such as agricultural sprayers. Either way, respirable aerosols represent the most serious threat of effectively exposing large numbers of people *(7)*.

Factors that can influence the effectiveness of aerosol delivery of potential biological/toxin agents include infectivity, virulence, toxicity, pathogenicity, incubation period, transmissibility, lethality, and stability *(7, 10)*.

Infectivity. The capability of microorganisms to establish themselves in the host environment differs. Whereas pathogens with high infectivity cause disease with relatively few organisms, those with low infectivity will require a larger number. To this end, high infectivity does not necessarily imply that the symptoms of disease will appear more quickly or that the disease will be more severe *(7)*.

Virulence. The propensity of an agent for causing severe disease is dependent on a diverse combination of agent and host factors. These factors are dynamic and malleable, leading often different strains of the same microorganisms to cause diseases with different severity *(7)*.

Toxicity. The toxicity relates to the severity of the illness (toxicosis) elicited by the toxin *(7)*.

Pathogenicity. Pathogenicity is defined as the ability of an agent to initiate a set of events (e.g., propagate attachment and penetration) that will culminate in a disease or abnormality. In this regard, a sufficient number of microorganisms or quantity of toxin must penetrate the host to initiate an infection (the infective dose) or intoxication (the intoxicating

Table 23.1 The CDC list of restricted agents, 1997

Viral	Bacterial	Toxins	Rickettsial	Fungal
Crimean-Congo hemorrhagic fever	*Bacillus anthracis*[1]	Abrin	*Coxiella burnetii*[1]	*Coccidioides*
Eastern equine encephalitis virus	*Brucella abortus, melitensis,*	Aflatoxins	*Rickettsia prowazekii*	*immitis*
Ebola virus[1]	and *suis*[1]	Botulinum neurotoxins[1]	*Rickettsia rickettsii*	
Equine morbillivirus	*Burkholderia (Pseudomonas*	*Clostridium perfringens*		
Lassa fever virus	*mallei)*[1]	epsilon toxin[1]		
Marburg virus[1]	*Burkholderia (Pseudomonas*	Conotoxins		
Rift Valley fever virus	*pseudomallei)*[1]	Diacetoxyscirpenol		
South American hemorrhagic fever	*Clostridium botulinum*	Ricin[1]		
viruses	*Francisella tularensis*[1]	Saxitoxin		
Tick-borne encephalitis complex viruses	*Yersinia pestis*[1]	Shigatoxin		
Variola major virus (smallpox virus)[1]		*Staphylococcus enterotoxins*[1]		
Venezuelan equine encephalitis virus[1]		Tetradotoxin		
Hantavirus pulmonary syndrome		T-2 toxin (trichothecene)[1]		
Yellow fever virus				

[1]Based on various assumptions and estimations as discussed in Section 23.2.1, these agents possess the attributes that make them candidates for biological aerosol weapons affecting large populations [with permission *(7)*].

Table 23.2 Emergency preparedness and response: Bioterrorism agents/diseases by categories

Category A[1]	Category B[2]	Category C[3]
Anthrax (*Bacillus anthracis*)	Brucellosis (*Brucella* spp.)	Nipah virus
Botulism (*Clostridium botulinum* toxin)	Epsilon toxin (*Clostridium perfringens*)	Hantavirus
Plague (*Yersinia pestis*)	Food safety threats (e.g., *Salmonella* spp., *Escherichia coli*	
Smallpox (variola major)	0157:H7, *Shigella*)	
Tularemia (*Francisella tularensis*)	Glanders (*Burkholderia mallei*)	
Viral hemorrhagic fevers [filoviruses (e.g., Ebola,	Melioidosis (*Burkholderia pseudomallei*)	
Marburg) and arenaviruses (e.g., Lassa, Machupo)]	Psittacosis (*Chlamydia psittaci*)	
	Q fever (*Coxiella burnetii*)	
	Ricin toxin from *Ricinus communis* (castor beans)	
	Staphylococcal enterotoxin B	
	Typhus fever (*Rickettsia prowazekii*)	
	Viral encephalitis [alphaviruses (e.g., Venezuelan equine encephalitis,	
	eastern equine encephalitis, western equine encephalitis)]	
	Water safety threats (e.g., *Vibrio cholerae, Cryptosporidium parvum*)	

[1]High-priority agents because they (i) can be easily disseminated or transmitted from person to person; (ii) result in high mortality rates and have the potential for major public health impact; (iii) might cause public panic and social disruption; and (iv) require special action for public health preparedness.
[2]Second highest priority agents/toxins, including those that (i) are moderately easy to disseminate; (ii) result in moderate morbidity rates and low mortality rates; and (iii) require specific enhancements of CDC's diagnostic capacity and enhanced disease surveillance.
[3]Third highest priority agents, including emergency pathogens that could be engineered for mass dissemination in the future because of (i) availability; (ii) ease of production and dissemination; and (iii) potential for high morbidity and mortality rates and major health impact.

dose). Infectious agents must then multiply (replicate) to produce disease *(7)*.

Incubation Period. Incubation period is the time between exposure and the appearance of symptoms of disease. This period depends on many variables, including the initial dose, virulence, route of entry, rate of replication, and host immunologic factors *(7)*.

Transmissibility. Some biological agents can be transmitted from person-to-person directly. However, indirect transmission such as by arthropod vectors may also be a significant means of transmission and spread of disease to humans. With regard to managing casualties in biological warfare, the relative ease with which an agent is passed from person to person (i.e., its transmissibility) constitutes the principal concern *(7)*.

Lethality. Lethality reflects the relative ease with which an agent causes death in a susceptible population.

Stability. The viability of an agent is affected by various environmental factors, including temperature, relative humidity, atmospheric pollution, and sunlight. A quantitative measure of stability is an agent's decay rate (e.g., "aerosol decay rate") *(7)*.

bioterrorism *(11, 12)*. From 1979 to 1985, a large outbreak (about 10,000 cases) occurred in Zimbabwe—at that time, a civil war caused the interruption of veterinary and public health services in the country, which contributed significantly to the magnitude of the outbreak *(11)*. This, and the accidental release of spores into the air in Sverdlovsk (in the former Soviet Union), and the recent mail attacks in the United States in 2001 that led to human casualties, became a stark reminder of the pathogenic potential of *B. anthracis* as a biological weapon. Furthermore, for some time, *B. anthracis* has been the subject of intense research and genetic manipulation with the intent of generating pathogen variants with increased virulence or with resistance to medical therapies and vaccine prevention strategies *(4, 11–13)*.

B. anthracis can be obtained from infected animals or soil, and spores from the pathogen can be easily prepared. The anthrax spores usually display very low visibility when delivered as an aerosol spray or powder. The lethal dose (LD_{50}) after human inhalation of the spores is not known, but when estimated from animal studies it is of the order 10,000 spores, corresponding to approximately 0.01 μg *(14)*.

23.3 Anthrax (Bacillus anthracis)

Anthrax is caused by *Bacillus anthracis*. A disease in animals, anthrax can be transmitted to humans. Because *B. anthracis* forms spores that can be aerosolized and sprayed with the intent to kill, this pathogen represents a very serious threat as an agent of biological warfare and

23.3.1 Bacteriology of B. anthracis

B. anthracis was shown to be the etiologic agent of anthrax by Robert Koch *(15)*. Its name derived from the Greek word for *coal* (*anthracis*), because of the black skin lesions that arise during the course of cutaneous infections.

B. anthracis is a Gram-positive, aerobic, spore-forming bacillus *(15)*. The vegetative cell is rather large (1 to 8 μm long, and 1.0 to 1.5 μm wide), whereas the spore size is approximately 1.0 μm. The bacilli are nonmotile and form large colonies with irregularly tapered outgrowths.

When ingested by herbivores, *B. anthracis* germinate within the host as they enter an environment rich in amino acids, nucleosides, and glucose. The vegetative bacilli multiply rapidly in the host and express virulence factors that kill the host. Then they sporulate in the cadaver once in contact with air and then contaminate the soil, anticipating another host. Vegetative bacilli have poor survival outside of an animal or human host. For example, when inoculated into water, colony counts will decline rapidly within 24 hours *(11)*.

23.3.2 Pathogenesis of B. anthracis

The vegetative form of *B. anthracis* elaborates a capsule that confers an antiphagocytic property on the bacilli *(16, 17)* and secretes the three-component protein toxin, PA (*pagA* encoded), LF (*lef* encoded), and EF (*cya* encoded) *(18)*. The combined action of the protein toxins is believed to kill infected animals by triggering the release of interleukin (IL-1) and tumor necrosis factor-α from the intoxicated macrophages *(19)*. The two binary exotoxins are referred to as LeTx when comprising PA and LF and as EdTx when encompassing PA and EF *(11)*.

LeTx has been implicated in both macrophage and host death *(20, 21)*. It acts as a zinc protease and cleaves the mitogen-activated protease kinase kinase (MAPKK), presumably interfering with signal transduction events of the p38 pathway and causing apoptosis of activated macrophages and release of IL-1 cytokine *(20, 22)*.

EdTx is thought to be involved in phagocyte inhibition and the massive edema occurring during anthrax infection *(23)*. EF is an adenylate cyclase *(24)*. After binding to calmodulin, EdTx cleaves the adenosine triphosphate (ATF) to generate the second messenger cyclic adenosine monophosphate (cAMP), thereby presumably interfering with the normal immune function of the macrophages *(24)*. At this stage, *B. anthracis* will multiply in the lymph system and in the blood but not within the macrophages *(11)*.

23.3.2.1 Virulence Plasmids

The virulence of all *B. anthracis* strains requires two large plasmids, pXO1 and pXO2 *(25,26)*. pXO1 carries the genetic determinants responsible for the synthesis of the anthrax exo-

toxin complexes PA, LF, and EF *(27)*, whereas pXO2 is involved in the capsule production *(28)*.

23.3.3 Human Disease

Humans are accidental hosts of *B. anthracis*. Infection is initiated with the introduction of spores into skin lesions, or entry through the intestinal or respiratory mucosa. Depending on the route of entry, anthrax could be classified as either cutaneous, gastrointestinal, or inhalational *(11, 29)*.

Humans acquire anthrax infections from contact with infected animals or contaminated animal products (e.g., hides, wool, hair, ivory tusks). Ingestion of poorly cooked infected meat may lead to gastrointestinal anthrax. Cases of inhalational anthrax have been observed in individuals who process animal products, and where aerosolized spores may be inhaled *(11)*.

23.3.3.1 Inhalational Anthrax

Inhalation of spores by humans will cause bacterial germination in the hilar and mediastinal lymph nodes *(29)*. The classic clinical description of inhalational anthrax is that of a biphasic illness. After an incubation period of 1 to 6 days, mild fever, malaise, myalgia, nonproductive cough, and some chest and abdominal pain may be observed *(11)*. As the disease develops further, fever, acute dyspnea, diaphoresis, and cyanosis will occur. The entry of the pathogen into the bloodstream will lead to systemic spread to the intestines and the meninges. During the meningitis, the cerebrospinal fluid is hemorrhagic with polymorphonuclear pleocytosis *(11)*.

23.3.3.2 Cutaneous Anthrax

In cases of cutaneous anthrax, spores of *B. anthracis* will enter through a small abrasion or wound in the human skin, typically in the face, hands, or neck *(29)*. Cutaneous anthrax represents 95% of all naturally occurring anthrax. The primary lesion, a pruritic papule, appears within a few days (1 to 7 days). Then, it develops into an ulcer with surrounding vesicles; occasionally, a single larger vesicle will form (1 to 2 cm in diameter) *(29)*. The vesicle is filled with clear or serosanguineous fluid containing occasional leukocytes and numerous large bacilli. After 2 days, the vesicle will rupture and will undergo necrosis, and a painless characteristic black eschar with a surrounding edema can be observed. After 1 to 2 weeks, the lesion will dry and the eschar separates, revealing an underlying scar. Systemic infections are almost always lethal if left untreated *(11)*. Antibiotic therapy will not prevent the progression of skin lesions but will abbreviate or prevent systemic infection.

23.3.3.3 Gastrointestinal Anthrax

Consumption of food that is contaminated with *B. anthracis* spores will lead to gastrointestinal anthrax *(29)*. The characteristic skin lesion is not present, and the establishment of a definitive diagnosis outside of an epidemic is difficult *(11)*. The incubation period of gastrointestinal anthrax is only 3 to 7 days. Abnormal symptoms with nausea, vomiting, anorexia, and fever may develop. The disease manifestations will progress rapidly, and patients will present with severe, bloody diarrhea. The primary intestinal lesions are ulcerative and occur mainly in the terminal ileum or cecum. Hemorrhagic mesenteric lymphadenitis is also a feature of gastrointestinal anthrax, and marked ascites may occur. The mortality associated with gastrointestinal anthrax is greater than 50%, and death can occur within 2 to 5 days after the onset of symptoms *(11)*.

23.3.3.4 Treatment of Anthrax

With the availability of antibiotics, these agents became the preferred drugs of treatment *(30)*. Successful therapy usually relies on the prompt uptake of antibiotics. Chemotherapy is rarely effective in cases of inhalational anthrax because the exposure to spores may not be recognized for some time. In this regard, the first stages of the illness are often mistaken for bronchitis and the second stage for cardiac failure or cerebrospinal accidents. Spores engulfed by alveolar macrophages are carried to local lymph nodes, germinate, and will rapidly multiply in the bloodstream *(11)*.

During the anthrax attack in the United States in 2001, the antimicrobial susceptibility patterns of all *B. anthracis* isolates displayed susceptibility to ciprofloxacin, doxycycline, chloramphenicol, clindamycin, tetracycline, rifampin, vancomycin, penicillin, and amoxicillin *(31)*. Because of the mortality associated with inhalational anthrax, CDC-issued guidelines recommended that two or more antimicrobial agents be used for effective treatment and that ciprofloxacin or doxycycline be used in an initial intravenous therapy. The duration of the therapy should be prolonged over 60 days *(31)*. Treatment of systemic anthrax using penicillin alone is no longer recommended, because *B. anthracis* genome encodes for at least two β-lactamases: a penicillinase and a cephalosporinase *(31)*.

However, whereas the currently available antibiotic treatments are capable of killing multiplying bacteria, they are unable to interfere with the toxin-mediated killing of the host. Another avenue to be explored is the possibility of combining passive immunization of infected patients with aggressive antibiotic treatment. Most attempts described to date have been directed at interfering with the correct functioning of the PA exotoxin subunit. However, no matter how effective a vaccine may be, multiple immunizations would be required for protection to build up *(11)*.

Studies on the *anthrax toxin receptor (ATR)*, a recently discovered membrane protein on the surface of macrophages *(32)*, have demonstrated that the soluble region of ATR can block the killing by PA, suggesting that the design of a receptor decoy may represent a new therapeutic strategy. However, because the physiologic function of ATR (TEM8) is not known, it is unclear whether such a therapeutic agent (a receptor decoy) will also affect the host *(11)*.

Another strategy for blocking the function of PA is to take advantage of mutant PA exhibiting a dominant negative phenotype. Such mutant PAs when co-assembled with the wild-type protein in a test tube prevented pore formation and translocation of EF and LF into cultured cells. Injection of the mutant PA in rats challenged with anthrax conferred protection from disease *(33)*. It is conceivable that administration of mutant PA into individuals infected with anthrax may block the progression of the disease at even more advanced stages of the disease *(11)*.

Recently, in a new therapeutic approach, the inherent binding specificity and lytic action of the bacteriophage enzymes, *lysins*, has been explored *(34)*. As a normal part of their life cycle, bacteriophages multiply in host cells and their progeny are released upon lysis of the cell wall. Purified PlyG, an enzyme synthesized by bacteriophage-γ, was found to destroy the cell wall of both vegetative cells and germinating spores of *B. anthracis (34)*. PlyG is a specific lysine for *B. anthracis* and other members of the *B. anthracis* "cluster" of bacilli and may well be exploited as a tool for treating and detecting anthrax.

The *Anthrax Vaccine Absorbed (AVA)* is an adjuvant absorbed preparation of the culture supernatant of vaccine strains and has been licensed by the Food and Drug Administration (FDA) for the prevention of anthrax in humans *(35)*. The AVA vaccine has been successfully used to prevent laboratory infections in the United States, and its effectiveness in preventing anthrax after a respiratory challenge has been demonstrated in rodents and non-human primates *(36)*. The active component of the AVA vaccine, anti-PA IgG, is believed to exert sporicidal effect. However, the effectiveness of the AVA vaccine in preventing human anthrax after a bioterrorist attack or biological warfare use of *B. anthracis* is hitherto unknown *(11)*.

23.4 Variola Major Virus (Smallpox)

The month of October 1977 will be remembered as the time when the world's last acquired case of smallpox occurred in Somalia, Africa (37). The last case of smallpox (a laboratory-associated infection) occurred in England in September of 1978. After a worldwide program to verify the eradication of smallpox in May 1980, the 33rd World Health Assembly accepted the report of the Global Commission for the Certification of Smallpox Eradication that smallpox had been eradicated (38). However, even though smallpox had been eliminated as a threat to humanity as the result of worldwide efforts involving intensive planning, geopolitical cooperation, and effective vaccination, it still remains a great public health concern. Although two WHO-approved repositories of variola virus remain at the CDC in Atlanta, Georgia, and at "Vector" in Novosibirsk, Russia, the extent of concealed stockpiles in other parts of the world is unknown. The former Soviet Union has admitted to weaponizing variola major (39).

Until its eradication in 1980, smallpox was one of the most dangerous infectious diseases, responsible over the centuries for more deaths and disabilities than any other pathogen (37). Those fortunate to survive the infection often faced lifelong complications and sequelae such as blindness, arthritis, encephalitis, permanent osteoarticular anomalies, and severely scarred complexion (40).

It is thought that the variola virus evolved as a human pathogen from an Orthopoxvirus of animals in the Central African rainforests and established itself in the valley of the Nile and the Fertile Crescent of Egypt thousands of years ago (37). Examination of Egyptian mummified remains demonstrated the presence of typical pustular eruptions of smallpox (41).

Before the development of the cowpox vaccine by Dr. Edward Jenner in 1796, there was no safe and consistently effective prevention method for smallpox (42).

Global terrorism, the continued research and development of biological weapons, and other geopolitical events have generated a concern that smallpox could be directed at susceptible populations (38). Even if the legally sanctioned repositories of smallpox in the United States and Russia were to be destroyed, other potential sources of smallpox could exist, including clandestine stockpiles, cadavers in permafrost, and strains reverse-engineered by scientists using data obtained from genetically sequenced strains. In fact, it is generally agreed that the likelihood of smallpox virus existing outside WHO-sanctioned laboratories is high (38).

These and other findings have led the U.S. federal authorities to conclude that the threat of smallpox as a biological weapon is significant enough to warrant reinstituting a vaccination program for selected members of the U.S. population, including the military, health care workers, and certain emergency responders, as well as the possibility of making the vaccine available to the general population on a volunteer basis in the future (43).

23.4.1 Variola Virus

The variola virus is a member of the family Poxviridae, subfamily Chordopoxvirinae, genus Orthopoxvirus. The genus Orthopoxvirus comprises many related viruses and includes, in addition to variola major, vaccinia virus, cowpox, monkeypox, ectromelia (mousepox), camelpox, taterapox (gerbilpox), Uasin Gishu disease, and racoonpox (38). The variola virus is exclusively a human disease, with no known animal reservoir. Other members of the genus produce disease primarily in their respective animal hosts. However, because of the close relationships between the orthopoxviruses, species jumping can occur, as evidenced by cowpox and monkeypox; monkeypox is capable of producing large outbreaks of human disease (44, 45), with clinical manifestations very similar to those of variola major and a mortality rate of 10% to 15% (44).

23.4.1.1 Morphology and Antigenic Structure of Orthopoxviruses

Poxviruses are the largest of all viruses, with a genome consisting of a single molecule of double-stranded DNA cross-linked with a hairpin loop at the ends (38). Their genomes vary in size from 130 to 300 kbp (46). The physical properties of the poxviruses are very similar in that they are "brick-shaped" or ovoid, and are 200 to 400 nm long. The external surface of the virus contains an envelope consisting of host cell membrane protein plus virus-specific polypeptides such as hemagglutinin. Based on studies of vaccinia virus, the presence or absence of an outer envelope defines two major infectious forms of the virus: the intracellular mature virion (IMF) and the extracellular enveloped protein (EEV) (47). The IMF form is stable in the environment and plays a predominant role in the host-to-host transmission. The EEV form plays an important role in dissemination within the host. Below the envelope is the outer membrane, consisting of a complex of surface tubules and globular proteins and enclosing large lateral bodies. The viral core consists of double-stranded DNA that is unique to each virus as shown by restricted fragment length polymorphism (RFLP) analysis; the genomes of the orthopoxviruses have a very well-preserved central region, allowing classification within the genus, whereas heterology in the terminal regions can be used to differentiate species (38).

The antigenic structure of the orthopoxviruses is characterized by large number of polypeptides that define cellular receptors and antigenic sites for protective immunity. The close relations of these viruses (e.g., vaccinia virus and variola virus) and serologic cross-reactivity help to explain the importance of the type of antigen required for protective immunogenicity. Thus, mice vaccinated with VACV L1R (IMV immunogen) and A33R (EEV immunogen) were protected from a lethal poxvirus challenge *(47)*. Both antigens induced greater protection than did either antigen alone, suggesting that for complete protective immunity, both IMF and EEV antigens are required *(38)*.

23.4.1.2 Replication and Virulence of Variola Virus

The orthopoxviruses, like all viruses, depend on host cellular mechanisms for DNA replication, protein synthesis, and viral assembly and release *(38)*. The viral attachment to the host cell is carried out through specific cellular receptors on the outer surface of the virus. Although both IMF and EEV forms are infectious, they differ in the way they attach to and enter the host cells. Whereas the EEV form has a more rapid cellular entry and requires uncoating of the virus in the cellular cytoplasm, the IMF form can enter either through the host-cell outer membrane or within a vacuole formed by the invagination of the plasma membrane releasing its core directly into the cytoplasm *(38)*. Once the core enters the host cytoplasm, there is an immediate transcription of viral enzymes that leads to viral uncoating and the release of DNA into the cytoplasm. Next, DNA replication occurs, followed by translation of both structural and nonstructural polyproteins, resulting in viral assembly first as IMF, which is then wrapped in modified Golgi membranes and transported to the periphery of the cell, with subsequent release of the EEV form of the mature virion *(46)*.

The variola virus represents a collection of many distinct strains, which, although difficult to differentiate antigenically or serologically, is suggested by clinical evidence indicating wide variation in mortality caused by different strains during outbreaks in various parts of the world—mortality rates between 5% and 40% in some regions compared with mortality of only 0.1% to 2% in other areas *(38)*. This distinct difference in virulence led to classification of the variola virus as variola major and variola minor. The genetic differences between the variola major and minor strains have been analyzed by RFLP mapping *(48, 49)*. The observed genetic difference between the variola strains most likely reflects differences in their replication and host-cell assembly, leading to greater or lesser virulence. Thus, a variant of variola virus has been described that produced a unique late polypeptide of different size and endonuclease site *(50)*. This marker was demonstrated to be genetically independent, expressed by 14

of the 48 variola strains examined and correlated with variola major and not variola minor.

23.4.1.3 Immune Evasion Strategies

The observed pathogenesis and virulence among the poxviruses is directly related to the ability of different strains to manipulate the immune response mechanisms of the host in which they replicate, such as the ability to produce many proteins that react with the host at both the cellular and systemic levels *(51, 52)*. Thus, a direct inhibition of the host's cellular immune response by the orthopoxviruses has been demonstrated through the production of soluble receptors for interferon-γ (IFN-γ), which prevented the host-produced IFN-γ from binding to its receptor *(53)*.

The potential of genetic manipulation of the orthopoxviruses, leading to expression of novel proteins and evasion of the host immune responses, introduces the potential to engineer a variola virus that may be used as a biological weapon *(38)*. Thus, recombinant vaccinia viruses that have been engineered to express genes encoding cytokines and chemokines were studied extensively to understand the pathogenesis of the orthopoxviruses *(54)*. The introduction of the interleukin (IL)-4 gene, a human interleukin involved in the type-2 immune response, significantly increased viral virulence by downregulating the cellular, type-1 immune responses. Similarly, IL-4–expressing engineered ectromelia virus was found to overcome genetic resistance to this virus in mice and produced an infection characterized by high mortality similar to the disease seen when genetically sensitive mice have been infected with the wild-type virus *(55)*.

23.4.2 Smallpox: Clinical Manifestations

The morbidity and mortality of smallpox depend on various factors, including the type of the smallpox virus (variola major or variola minor), clinical manifestations, previous smallpox vaccination, age, geography, urban or rural setting, underlying immune status, and, for women, pregnancy *(38)*.

The variola virus gains entry into its human hosts through the oropharynx or respiratory tract. Direct inoculation through the skin can also occur as demonstrated by the practice of variolation. The infectious 50% dose of variola virus is not known. From the time of inoculation with the virus, there is an incubation period of 10 to 14 days *(56)*. During this period, the virus replicates in the respiratory tract and disseminates throughout the body during viremia. Transmission of variola virus from infected patients rarely occurs during the incubation period. However, with the onset of rash, the period of maximum infectivity begins, then gradually subsides until the rash evolves to the point where all scabs have separated. Because the variola virus is present in the scabs, isolation of patients is necessary until the last scab has become separated *(38)*.

23.4.2.1   Ordinary or Classic Smallpox

As noted above, two distinct types of smallpox have come to be recognized over time: major and minor. The prototypical disease, variola major, or ordinary smallpox, usually results in 30% mortality in unvaccinated patients. However, other clinical forms associated with variola major, such as flat-type and hemorrhagic-type smallpox, have been known for severe mortality *(38)*.

Ordinary smallpox can be classified into three distinct clinical presentations or types: (i) *discrete*, in which individual lesions are separated by normal-appearing skin; (ii) *confluent*, in which lesions on any part of the body coalesce; (iii) *semiconfluent*, in which lesions on the face are confluent but are discrete on the rest of the body. Those patients manifesting discrete lesions tended to have a significantly lower mortality rate than did those with confluent lesions (9% vs. 62% in unvaccinated cases in Rao's clinical series) *(38)*.

Disease manifestations begin acutely, with malaise, fever, rigors, vomiting, headache, and backache, and as many as 15% of patients develop delirium. Two to 3 days after the initial symptoms, an enanthem (rash in the oropharynx) appears concomitantly with a cutaneous rash (exanthem) that covers the face, hands, and the forearms. The exanthema will then spread to the lower extremities and subsequently to the trunk. The lesions will quickly progress from macules to papules to vesicles, and eventually to pustular vesicles. Lesions are more abundant on the extremities and the face, and this centrifugal distribution is an *important diagnostic feature*.

It should be emphasized that in distinct contrast with varicella (chickenpox), lesions on the various segments of the body remain generally synchronous in their stages of development. From 8 to 14 days after the onset of the exanthema, the pustules will scab, leaving depressed depigmented scars upon healing. The major sequela of smallpox is the presence of permanent pockmarks, often leading to an extremely disfigured complexion. Corneal scarring resulting in blindness occurs in 1% to 4% of patients *(38)*.

Smallpox in Children

Smallpox in children is clinically similar to that seen in adults, with several notable exceptions *(38)*. Thus, in infants the overall mortality rate often exceeds 40% *(57)*, and in one report *(58)* it reached 85%. In addition, children have a higher incidence of vomiting, conjunctivitis, seizures, and cough *(59)*. Infections during pregnancy were associated with uterine hemorrhage, premature labor, and fetal demise, although no distinct congenital syndrome has been associated with smallpox infection *in utero (57)*.

23.4.2.2   Hemorrhagic Smallpox

This form of smallpox accounts for about 2% to 3% of all cases. Hemorrhagic smallpox can be subdivided into early and late hemorrhagic smallpox.

Early hemorrhagic smallpox is manifested with a different clinical presentation than is ordinary smallpox and would often kill patients before they exhibited the focal rash *(38)*. Patients develop a toxic clinical picture resembling disseminated intravascular coagulation and in most cases rapidly succumb to the disease. Death occurs in excess of 95% in unvaccinated patients with hemorrhagic smallpox.

In late hemorrhagic smallpox, the focal rash appears but hemorrhages occur between the pustules. In general, hemorrhagic smallpox is more common in adults, and pregnant women would appear to be at greatest risk.

Host factors, such as some form of immune system deficiency, rather than a unique variola strain, are believed to be responsible for the development of hemorrhagic smallpox; however, immunologic data are generally lacking *(60)*.

23.4.2.3   Flat-Type or Malignant Smallpox

The flat-type smallpox accounted for about 6% of all cases in the pre-eradication era and occurred most often in children *(38)*. The disease has a mortality rate of more than 95% in unvaccinated patients. The rash characteristically involves flattened, confluent lesions rather than the characteristic firm pustules observed in ordinary smallpox. As with hemorrhagic smallpox, the flat-type illness has been associated with deficient cellular immune responses to the virus.

23.4.2.4   Modified Smallpox

Modified smallpox for the most part has been associated with persons who had been previously vaccinated but whose immunity had waned with time. According to the WHO definition of modified smallpox, the observed difference is related to the character and development of the focal eruption, with crusting being completed within 10 days. The prodrome may or may not be shortened or lessened in severity, but the secondary fever is typically absent *(57)*. Typically, there are fewer skin lesions, and the lesions tend to be more superficial. In addition, the lesions evolve more rapidly and do not show the typical uniformity observed in ordinary smallpox. Diagnosis of modified smallpox is more difficult, and patients are still contagious, although often ambulatory *(38)*.

23.4.2.5 Variola Sine Eruptione

Variola sine eruptione occurs in previously vaccinated for smallpox after exposure to smallpox and is characterized by sudden onset of fever, headache, and backache, but *no rash followed the prodrome*. The illness usually is short lived and resolves in 1 to 2 days. However, patients can still transmit the virus to others for a short period of time *(38)*.

23.4.2.6 Variola Minor

The second form of smallpox, variola minor, is distinguished by milder systemic toxicity, a lesser degree of pox lesions, and a mortality rate of 1% in unvaccinated persons. Although the viral exanthema is the most prominent feature of both forms of smallpox, when patients with variola major and variola minor were matched for the same extent of exanthema, mortality rates differed substantially. Patients with variola minor illness can be confused with those presenting with modified smallpox *(38)*.

23.4.3 Treatment of Smallpox

In the pre-eradication era and through the last human case of smallpox infection in 1978, the standard treatment consisted of supportive measures such as hydration, fever and pain control, and meticulous care for the skin to prevent bacterial superinfection *(38)*.

Although drug research has found a new momentum as the threat of biological weapons attack has been fully appreciated, very few drugs against orthopoxviruses have advanced to the stage of human trials and, if they did, the results were disappointing *(61, 62)*. Among the first antiviral drugs tested for anti-orthopoxvirus activity were cytosine arabinoside and adenine arabinoside, and the thiosemicarbazones (methisazone, M&B 7714). The latter showed excellent activity in mouse models of vaccinia and variola *(61, 62)*. However, randomized, placebo-controlled human trials for treating smallpox infection yielded disappointing results *(63,64)*. In addition, the adverse side effects (gastrointestinal, nausea, vomiting) were severe, and the expense of the thiosemicarbazones is prohibitive *(61, 62)*.

Other antiviral compounds that have shown *in vitro* activity against orthopoxviruses included inosine monophosphate (IMP), dehydrogenase inhibitors, *S*-adenosylhomocysteine hydrolase inhibitors, orotidine monophosphate decarboxy-

lase inhibitors, cytosine triphosphate synthetase inhibitors, thymidylate synthetase inhibitors, nucleoside analogues, thiosemicarbazones, acyclic nucleoside phosphonates, and carbocyclic imidodisulfamide analogues *(61, 62, 65–68)*. Most of the *in vitro* activity has been determined against orthopoxviruses other than variola, but several classes of the available antiviral drugs were found to be specifically active against the variola virus in addition to other orthopoxviruses *(66–68)*.

Of the current commercially available drugs, HPMPC (cidofovir), *bis*-POM PMEA (adefovir dipivoxil), and ribavirin have been shown to have an IC_{59} in cell culture assays well below the levels associated with cytotoxicity *(61,62,65)*. Both cidofovir and adefovir dipivoxil have been associated with severe nephrotoxicity.

Whereas no human data exist for cidofovir for treating smallpox, there were case reports documenting success in its use against other poxvirus infections. In addition, topical and parenteral cidofovir have been used to effectively treat patients with severe immunodeficiency disorders (AIDS and Wiskott-Aldrich syndrome) and disfiguring molluscum contagiosum *(69, 70)*.

An orally bioavailable anti-poxvirus compound (ST-246) was found to inhibit extracellular virus formation and protected mice from lethal orthopoxvirus challenge. ST-246 has been shown to be highly active against a number of orthopoxviruses both *in vitro* and in animal models. These results, coupled with its lack of toxicity, make ST-246 a very promising candidate for further development to prevent or treat smallpox infection in humans *(71)*.

23.4.4 Smallpox Vaccines

Several different vaccinia strains have been used in the production of vaccines against smallpox *(38)*. Currently in the United States, the Dryvax vaccine (Wyeth) is the only licensed vaccinia-based vaccine. It consists of a lyophilized (freeze-dried) preparation of live vaccinia virus obtained from New York City calf lymph, which is derived from a seed virus of the New York City Board of Health (NYCBH) strain. Other strains used in preparing smallpox vaccines also include the New York City chorioallantoic membrane (also derived from the NYCBH strain), EM-63 (former Soviet Union), the temple of heaven strain (China), and the Lister or Elestree strain (United Kingdom). Whereas all strains seemed to be equally effective in preventing smallpox, a difference existed in the adverse reactions *(38)*.

A vaccinia strain referred to as *modified vaccinia Ankara (MVA)* was successfully used in Europe throughout the 1970s. The attenuated vaccinia virus in MVA appeared to have less virulence than did the other vaccinia strains, especially with regard to postvaccination encephalitis *(38)*.

23.5 Yersinia pestis: Plague

Plague has been associated with three pandemics—in the 6th, 14th, and 20th centuries. During World War II, the Japanese Army apparently used plague as a biological weapon in China.

The causative agent of plague is *Yersinia pestis*, a Gram-negative, nonacid-fast, nonmotile, nonsporulating, nonlactose-fermenting, bipolar coccobacillus. The genus *Yersinia* (family Enterobacteriaceae) consists of 11 species, of which three are human pathogens (*Y. pestis*, *Y. pseudotuberculosis*, and *Y. enterocolitica*). In common with other enteric bacteria, *Y. pestis* has typical cell wall and whole-cell lipid composition and an enterobacterial antigen *(72)*. A facultative intracellular pathogen, *Y. pestis*, is now thought to maintain intracellular residence only during the early stages of infection, with extracellular growth being predominant at later stages.

All three human pathogens (*Y. pestis*, *Y. pseudotuberculosis*, and *Y. enterocolitica*) have a nearly identical siderophore-dependent iron transport system. The majority of *Y. pestis* strains, regardless of biotype or origin, contain three plasmids termed pPCP1 (pesticin, coagulase, plasminogen activator), pCD1 (calcium dependence), and pMT1 (murin toxin). A low-calcium response stimulon (LCRS) is encoded on pCD1 and includes regulatory genes controlling the expression of secreted virulence proteins and a dedicated multiprotein secretory system. The LCRS region is highly conserved, and the LCRS plasmids are necessary for virulence in all three human pathogenic *Yersinia* species *(72)*.

The naturally occurring disease is transmitted to humans from rodents by fleas. The most common form of plague is the *bubonic plague* (about 90%). Secondary *septicemic plague* occurs in about one fifth of patients and secondary *pneumonic plague* in about 10%. If *Y. pestis* were used as a biological weapon, the primary manifestation would be epidemic pneumonia. The transmission of pneumonic plague from person to person is extremely high *(7, 72)*.

Among the numerous animal models used over the years, those that exhibit the closest relationship to pathology in humans include the mouse and non-human primate (NHP) models *(73–77)*. The pathology of plague infection in humans and NHPs is strikingly similar.

23.5.1 Epidemiology of Y. pestis

Plague is a zoonotic disease primarily affecting rodents; humans play no role in the long-term survival of *Y. pestis*. Transmission between rodents is accomplished by their associated fleas. Whereas infection can occur by direct contact or ingestion, these routes normally do not play a role in the

maintenance of *Y. pestis* in an animal reservoir. Fleas will acquire the pathogen from an infected blood meal—the oriental rat flea (*Xenopsylla cheopis*) is the classic vector for plague. Another flea, *Xenopsylla astia*, is also a known vector of *Y. pestis (72)*. Currently, only a small number (around 31) of flea species were proven as vectors of plague. The cat flea (*Ctenocephalides felis*) and the so-called human flea (*Pulex irritans*) were found to be very poor vectors.

Y. pestis has also been isolated from lice and ticks. However, there is no evidence yet for transmission of plague by ticks to mammals.

Through the start of the third pandemic, transmission from urban rodents (especially rats) was most common. Currently, most human plague cases in the world and all cases in the United States are classified as sylvatic plague, contracted from rural wild animals, such as squirrels, chipmunks, marmots, voles, gerbils, mice, and rabbits *(72)*. In the United States, transmission to humans occurs primarily via the bites of fleas from infected rodents.

It is accepted that the pathogen spreads from the site of the flea bite to the regional lymph nodes and grows to high numbers, causing the formation of a *bubo* (swollen lymph node). Then, the infection spreads into the bloodstream, where the bacilli are preferentially removed in the spleen and liver but also colonize other internal organs.

23.5.2 Bubonic Plague

Human epidemics generally start as bubonic plague, which is the classic form of the disease. When a bubonic plague victim develops secondary pneumonic plague, the potential for respiratory droplets spreads, and a primary pneumonic plague epidemic occurs. However, this type of epidemic is currently uncommon because of the advent of effective antibiotics and modern public health measures *(72)*.

Patients with bubonic plague usually develop symptoms of fever, headache, chills, and swollen, extremely tender lymph nodes (buboes) within 2 to 6 days after contact with the pathogen. In addition, gastrointestinal complaints, such as nausea, vomiting, and diarrhea, are common. Depending on the duration of the infection, symptoms of disseminated intravascular coagulation (DIC) can also develop. Skin lesions infrequently develop at the initial site of the infection. Buboes are typically found in the inguinal and femoral regions but can also occur in other nodes *(78)*. Bacteremia or secondary plague septicemia is frequently seen in patients with bubonic plague *(72)*.

Intracellular *Y. pestis* survive by an undefined mechanism, but most eventually escape their intracellular captivity within the lymph node *(77)*. Within hours of the infection, extracellular bacteria in the lymph nodes express a range of anti-host proteins, including the proteinaceous Fraction One (F1) capsule *(72)*.

23.5.3 Septicemic Plague

Primary septicemic plague is generally defined as occurring in patients with positive blood cultures but no palpable lymphadenopathy. Clinically, septicemic plague resembles septicemia caused by other Gram-negative bacteria, during which patients present with chills, headache, malaise, and gastrointestinal disturbances. Compared with patients with bubonic plague, patients with septicemic disease have a higher incidence of abdominal pain. The mortality rate of patients with septicemic plague is fairly high, ranging from 30% to 50%, probably because the antibiotics generally used to treat undifferentiated sepsis are not effective against *Y. pestis (72, 79)*.

During the development of septicemic plague, it is not clear if the invading bacteria actually avoid the regional lymph nodes or, if infection of the nodes does occur, the invading bacteria fail to induce gross pathologic or physiologic changes *(80)*.

23.5.4 Pneumonic Plague

Pneumonic plague is a rare form of the disease with a very high mortality rate *(72)*. It is spread through respiratory droplets by close contact (2 to 5 ft) with an infected person. It progresses rapidly from a febrile flu-like illness to an overwhelming pneumonia, manifested by coughing and the production of bloody sputum. The incubation period of pneumonic plague is between 1 and 3 days. In the United States, the vast majority of cases were contracted from infected cats; during the period 1970–1993, 12% of the U.S. plague patients developed pneumonia secondary to either the bubonic or septicemic form of plague *(81)*.

Clinical disease after exposure to "intentionally" aerosolized plague is markedly different *(77)*. Primary pneumonic plague occurs after inhaling plague bacilli dispersed in a size that can reach the deep lungs (1 to 10 μm in diameter). Deposited bacilli may be unencapsulated and phenotypically negative for the virulence-associated *Yersinia* outer proteins (Yops) or, if transmitted from an infected person, may be expressing both. The effect of expressing or not expressing capsule and/or Yop proteins in the lungs at the time of infection is still not clear *(77)*.

An asymptomatic infection in some humans and nonhuman primates (NHPs) presumably exposed to aerosolized plague is *pharyngeal plague (82, 83)*. Pharyngeal carriage is thought to eventually resolve asymptomatically or progress after an extended time to fulminate into plague pneumonia *(77)*.

23.5.5 Treatment of Plague

All patients suspected of having bubonic plague should be placed in isolation until 2 days after starting antibiotic treatment to prevent the potential spread of the disease should the patient develop secondary plague pneumonia *(72)*.

Numerous antibiotics have been used to treat *Y. pestis* infections or as prophylaxis. Streptomycin has for many years remained the drug of choice. It is given intramuscularly to adults at a daily dose of 2.0 g, twice daily (at 12-hour intervals); the dose in children is 30 mg/kg, 2 to 3 times daily. Because streptomycin is bacteriolytic, it should be administered with care to prevent the development of endotoxic shock. Because of its toxicity, patients are not usually maintained on streptomycin for the full 10-day treatment regimen but are gradually switched to one of the other antibiotics, usually tetracycline.

The tetracyclines are commonly used for prophylactic therapy. In adults, tetracycline is administered at an oral daily dose of 2.0 g (4 times daily at 6-hour intervals); the oral daily dose for children ($\geq$ 9 years) is 25 to 50 mg/kg (4 times daily at 6-hour intervals). Chloramphenicol is typically used to treat plague meningitis.

Whereas *Y. pestis* is susceptible to penicillin *in vitro*, the antibiotic is considered to be ineffective against plague. Antibiotic-resistant strains of *Y. pestis* are rare and are not increasing in frequency *(72)*.

23.5.5.1 Killed Whole-Cell Plague Vaccines

Historically, whole-cell plague vaccines are effective in preventing bubonic plague in humans. The basis for their inability to protect against pneumonic plague is not well understood; it may be caused by alteration in the quality or quantity of the F1 antigen and the limited presence of other important proteins. A major criticism of the whole-cell plague vaccines is the predicted duration of "immunity" and the inability to induce a mucosal immune response *(77)*.

The Haffkine Vaccines. First developed in India in the 1890s by W. M. W. Haffkine *(84, 85)*, the original vaccine was a whole-cell killed vaccine made from stationary-phase broth cultures of the virulent Indian strain of *Y. pestis* 195/P. An improved Haffkine vaccine was subsequently produced using log-phase broth cultures grown at 37°C. A retrospective comparison of the old and new Haffkine vaccines revealed that the latter contained 4 times the amount of F1 antigen, which had been directly linked to its greater efficacy. Although the Haffkine vaccine was reported to be relatively effective, its drawbacks included severe side effects, a high number of vaccine failures, and contamination of some of the vaccine preparations. It was ultimately abandoned in favor of the development of the new live-attenuated plague vaccines *(77)*. In addition, there has been no evidence that the Haffkine-type vaccines were effective against aerosol challenge by *Y. pestis*.

The "Army" Vaccine. In 1941, the U.S. National Research Council recommended the use of a new "Army" whole-cell killed plague vaccine for deploying U.S. troops. The decision to use this vaccine was based on its less severe vaccine reactions in humans compared with that of the Haffkine vaccine, and it was credited for reducing bubonic plague morbidity and mortality of U.S. soldiers during World War II *(77)*. Later, with minor modifications, the Army vaccine became the Plague Vaccine USP. As with the Haffkine vaccine, there is no evidence that the Army vaccine protected against pneumonic plague.

The Cutter/Greer Vaccines. The first U.S. licensed vaccine was manufactured by Cutter Co. and was an adaptation of the Army product *(77)*. The Cutter vaccine underwent several modifications, with a final formulation developed in 1967 and its subsequent manufacture by Greer Laboratories. The Greer vaccine was prepared from fully virulent *Y. pestis* 195/P. The principal protective antigen in the Cutter/Greer vaccines is the capsular antigen F1 because the induction of antibodies to F1 was considered essential for the development of a protective immune response.

23.5.5.2 Live-Attenuated Plague Vaccines

The first live-attenuated plague vaccines were tested for efficacy in large-scale trials in the 1930s using the Tjiwidej and EV strains. Of the two vaccines, the EV-type vaccine was more extensively used and reported to be more effective *(86)*. Whereas the Tjiwidej strain was reported negative for the production of V antigen (VW-), the EV-type vaccine did produce V antigen *(77)*. Trials in NHPs indicated that the EV-type vaccines exhibited significant protection from bubonic plague after parenteral challenge. There is also evidence that the live-attenuated plague vaccines were effective in reducing the incidence of bubonic plague in humans *(87)*.

A potential problem with the EV-type vaccines has been the maintenance of seed cultures, as the EV-76 strain has undergone several changes after its original isolation, and these cultures are known to change phenotypes *(88)*. On average, only about 30% of a delivered dose of EV-type vaccines is viable. Currently, there is no methodology to control for this fluctuation in viability. This aspect of the EV-type vaccine has significant implications for vaccinating elderly, young, and immunocompromised populations *(77)*.

Very little is known concerning protection from pneumonic plague with live-attenuated plague vaccines. There is one published report of EV-76–dependent protection in rhesus monkeys intratracheally challenged *(89)*. Resistance in

vaccinated monkeys was related to circulating levels of anti-F1 antibody.

Serious side effects caused by live-attenuated plague vaccines were first reported in Africa (Senegal) then in the former Soviet Union and included fever, lymphadenopathy, malaise, headache, and sloughing of skin at the inoculation side *(90)*. These and other reports of adverse side effects raised serious questions about the acceptability of the EV-type live-attenuated plague vaccines, especially for mass vaccination. In addition, the induction of long-term immunity may also be a problem with the EV-type vaccines—as determined from intradermal inoculation of pestin, immunity may wane in 60% of vaccinees between 6 months and 1 year *(91)*. It was noted that in general, prior vaccination with a killed plague vaccine had an ameliorating effect on subjects given the live vaccine *(77)*.

23.5.5.3 Subunit Plague Vaccines

The subunit vaccines are essentially acellular preparations that contain one or a number of bacterial antigens, proteins, and/or carbohydrates, formulated with a characterized adjuvant *(77)*. Because the basis for selecting purified plague antigens is their immunogenicity in the host during infection, it should be noted that not all plague immunogens by any means induce a protective response in the host.

Capsular F1 Antigen. *Y. pestis* has long been known to produce a highly immunogenic, proteinaceous capsular antigen F1 that is actively synthesized both *in vitro* and *in vivo* *(92)*. The F1 antigen, regardless of the source and whether cell-associated or cell-free, provides a high degree of protection against either lethal parenteral (SC) or aerosolized plague infection. However, because the capsular F1 antigen may not be the only determinant of virulence that induces protective immunity in the host *(93)*, additional protective components may also be included in the vaccine preparation, giving an added advantage to the protected host.

Lipopolysaccharide (LPS). In addition to large amounts of F1 capsule, Plague Vaccine UPS also contains very high levels of LPS, which may be a contributing factor to the reactogenicity of this product observed in many recipients of the vaccine *(94)*. Like most Gram-negative bacteria, the *Y. pestis* LPS contains 2-keto-3-deoxyoctulosonic acid but is lacking a true *O*-side-chain antigen, probably as the result of mutations in existing genes required for the biosynthesis of the *O*-antigen. Even though the immunomodulatory effects of LPS are unquestionable, in light of experimental evidence that purified LPS failed to protect mice *(95)*, the contribution of *Y. pestis* LPS in the development of a protective immune response in the host remains tenuous *(77)*.

pH 6.0 Antigen. The pH 6.0 antigen is a fibrillar-like protein polymer. Like the F1 capsule, the pH 6.0 antigen is a protein structure that appears across the surface of the pathogen as filamentous strands only at 37°C *(96)*. However, unlike the F1 antigen, a low pH is required for the expression of pH 6.0 antigen. This phenomenon is highly suggestive for the selective expression of the antigen in acidified host cell compartments such as the phagolysosome of a macrophage *(97)*. Nonetheless, purified preparations of recombinant pH 6.0 antigen protein failed to protect inoculated mice against parenteral plague challenge—although the protein induced very high levels of circulating antibody *(77)*.

Plasminogen Activator (Pla). The plasminogen activator is a protein encoded by the small virulence plasmid unique to *Y. pestis (77)*. It possesses an enzymatic activity that leads to clot lysis by converting plasminogen to the plasmin protease *(98)*. The bacterial plasminogen activator activity is not unique to *Y. pestis* and is associated with the virulence of many bacterial species *(99)*. It has been hypothesized that Pla has a dual enzymatic function: as a dissemination factor in the mammal, and as a clotting factor in the flea. However, as with the pH 6.0 antigen, preliminary studies evaluating the efficacy of recombinant Pla in mice yielded inconclusive results *(77)*.

V Antigen. The virulence determinant known as the V antigen present in *Yersinia* species is required for full virulence of these bacteria *(100)*. This polypeptide is encoded by the medium-molecular-weight virulence plasmid pLCR and is temperature-regulated (expressed only at 37°C). It is induced *in vitro* only in the absence of calcium cations, hence the term *low calcium response*. It is thought that the function of the V antigen is regulatory and associated with secretions of other virulence proteins *(101, 102)*. In addition, there has been experimental evidence suggesting host immunomodulatory effects *(103, 104)*.

The use of the V antigen as a protective immunogen was documented several decades ago *(105)*. In a recent study, purified recombinant V antigen demonstrated excellent efficacy against high-level parenteral and aerosol challenges *(106)*. These and other results have strongly suggested using the V antigen as at least one of the components in a new acellular vaccine *(77)*.

Other pLCR-Encoded Proteins. Additional antigenic proteins identified on pLCR that could be used as subunit vaccine candidates include a group of effector proteins (known as the *Yersinia* outer proteins, or Yops) that are translocated intracellularly by a type-III secretion apparatus *(77)*. Various biochemical functions have been defined for these proteins, including apoptosis (YopJ), cytolysis (YopB/D), dephosphorylation of host cell proteins (YopH), serine/threonine kinase activity (YpkA), actin microfilament disruption (YopE), and inhibition of platelet aggregation (YopM). Studies have shown that at least some Yops are immunogenic, as antibodies to these proteins have been detected in human convalescent sera *(107)*.

Multiple Subunit Vaccines. The preponderance of experimental evidence collected to date strongly suggests that a rational approach for new cell-free plague vaccine would consist of both the F1 capsule and V antigens *(77)*. In this regard, a unique recombinant hybrid protein, consisting of a gene fusion between the F1 structural gene *caf1* and *lcrV* encoding V antigen, has been generated *(108)*. The gene product was then expressed in *E. coli* to reasonably high levels and purified by standard chromatographic techniques. In a single-dose vaccination study, the F1-V fusion protein has shown a synergistic effect as demonstrated by its ability to protect against very high doses of virulent plague organisms *(109)*.

One great advantage of the F1-V fusion protein is its easy manufacturing, as the components of an F1 plus V mixture would be considered as separate products.

Another approach to a multiple subunit vaccine would be to use a "complex" of antigens *(77)*. In the case of *Yersinia*, the most likely vaccine candidate would be the YopB/D cytolytic porin. This bipartite complex will attach to the target host cell to form a "portal of entry" for the pathogen's effector proteins *(110)*. It is hypothesized that when the YopB/D complex is used, an improved and potentially synergistic immune response may be developed, with the caveat of potential toxicity to the host *(77)*.

23.6 Brucellosis

Brucellosis is a chronic, systemic, febrile, granulomatous infection caused by at least four different *Brucella* species *(111, 112)*. The latter are Gram-negative, aerobic, nonmotile, nonspore-forming intracellular coccobacilli. As intracellular bacteria of mononuclear phagocytes, the *Brucella* species successfully evade many host immune responses and resist easy eradication by antimicrobial agents. Because of its great infectivity, ability to incapacitate infected individuals, and the persistent nature of human disease, brucellosis has long been considered a prime biowarfare threat. Both the United States and the former Soviet Union weaponized *Brucella* in the 1940s *(111)*.

The traditional classification of *Brucella* species is largely based on their preferred hosts. There are six classic pathogens—*Brucella melitensis*, *B. abortus*, *B. suis*, *B. canis*, *B. ovis*, and *B. neotomae*—of which the first four are recognized human zoonoses. The presence of rough or smooth lipopolysaccharide (LPS) correlates with the virulence of the disease in humans. New *Brucella* species, provisionally called *B. pinnipediae* and *B. cetaceae*, were recently isolated from marine mammals and found to be pathogenic to humans *(111, 112)*. *Brucella ovis* and *B. neotomae* are not known to cause human disease.

Taxonomically, *Brucella* is a monospecific genus that should be termed *B. melitensis*, and all other species are subtypes with an interspecies homology above 87%. The phenotypic difference and host preference may be attributed to various proteomes, as exemplified by specific outer-membrane markers *(112, 113)*.

The complete sequencing of the *B. melitensis* genome was determined in 2002 *(114)*. The complete genome sequencing of two other *Brucella* species, *B. abortus (115)* and *B. suis (116)*, have also been accomplished. The genome of *Brucella melitensis* reveals the presence of two circular replicons of 1.1 and 2.2 Mb, respectively, with a 57% CG content and no plasmids. The *B. abortus* biovars 1 and 4 and *B. suis* biotype 1 were found to be remarkably similar to *B. melitensis*. In contrast, *B. suis* biotypes 2 and 4 are composed of two replicons of 1.35 and 1.85 Mb, respectively, and *B. suis* biotype 3 is composed of a single circular replicon of 3.3 Mb *(112)*.

23.6.1 Pathogenesis of Brucella Species

The *Brucella* species do not produce exotoxins and do not naturally harbor plasmids or phages. Their most remarkable virulence factor is the outer membrane LPS *(111)*. At least two features contribute to the ability of LPS to enhance bacterial survival in the host, namely (i) the endotoxic activity (ability to trigger a systemic inflammatory response) of LPS is much less than that of typical enteric Gram-negative organisms, so innate immune responses are poorly activated by encounters with the bacterium; and (ii) smooth strains of *Brucella*, which have long chains of *O*-polysaccharide (OPS) on their LPS, fix small amount of serum complement to their surface but are resistant to complement-mediated lysis *(117)*. Moreover, smooth strains have a reduced ability to induce cytokine responses from the monocytes, most likely because of steric interference by their surface OPS with the binding of the lipid A endotoxic component of LPS to mononuclear phagocyte surface receptors *(111)*. Furthermore, smooth, virulent brucellae that have been coated with complement are readily phagocytosed by mononuclear phagocytes. Inside these cells, brucellae foster phagosomal acidification, inhibit the fusion of phagosomes with lysosomes, remain in the phagosomes, and replicate to an enormous number inside their host cells *(111)*.

Brucellae are resistant to damage from polymorphonuclear cells due to the suppression of the myeloperoxidase–hydrogen peroxide–halide system and copper-zinc superoxide dismutase, and the production of inhibitors of adenylate monophosphate and guanyl monophosphate *(112)*. Impaired activity of the natural killer cells and impaired macrophage generation of reactive oxygen intermediates and interferon regulatory factors have also been documented *(118–120)*.

Interferon-γ has a central role in the pathogenesis of brucellosis *(121, 122)* by activating macrophages, producing reactive oxygen species and nitrogen intermediates; by inducing apoptosis, enhancing cell differentiation and cytokine production; by converting immunoglobulin G to immunoglobulin G2a; and by increasing the expression of antigen-presenting molecules *(112)*.

After the lysis of infected cells, the bacteria are ingested by other mononuclear phagocytes, and the cycle of bacterial proliferation will continue. However, with the development of an effective host response, the bacterial proliferation is controlled and brucellae are gradually eliminated. Nevertheless, the bacteria may persist in their host cells for months or even years and recommence replication if the activity of immunologic control mechanisms declines *(111)*. In addition to mononuclear phagocytes, placental trophoblasts are also highly susceptible to infection with brucellae and support rampant intracellular proliferation of the bacteria. In this location, brucellae associate with the rough endoplasmic reticulum *(123)*, where they may have access to more nutrients than are available in the macrophage phagosome.

23.6.2 Clinical Manifestations of Brucellosis

In humans, *B. melitensis* is the most virulent species, followed by *B. abortus* and *B. suis*. *Brucella canis* and *B. maris* (isolated from marine mammals) appear to be approximately as virulent as *B. abortus*.

Transmission of brucellosis to humans occurs through the consumption of infected, unpasteurized animal milk products (raw milk, soft cheese, butter, and ice cream), through direct contact with infected animal parts (such as placenta by inoculation through ruptures of skin and mucous membranes), and through the inhalation of infected aerosolized particles *(112)*. Airborne transmission of brucellosis has been studied in the context of using brucellae as a biological weapon *(111)*.

After brucellae encounter a susceptible host, the bacteria enter across the mucous membranes and are ingested by mononuclear phagocytes, then travel to local lymph nodes, and disseminate via the thoracic duct and blood throughout the mononuclear phagocyte system *(111)*. At the time of dissemination, humans typically present with fever, chills, and malaise. In addition, neuropsychiatric abnormalities, including depression and inability to concentrate on task performance, are common *(124)*.

Focal disease may occur in almost any organ but more often tend to develop in sites where blood supply is particularly rich. Osteoarticular disease, which is universally the most common complication of brucellosis, is manifested in three distinct forms: peripheral arthritis, sacroiliitis, and spondylitis. Approximately one third of patients will have disease in vertebrae or in one or more joints (knees, hips, ankles, wrists, and especially the sacroiliacs). *Brucella* vertebral osteomyelitis, which may be clinically indistinguishable from tuberculosis, tends to develop in older patients. Spondylitis remains very difficult to treat and often seems to result in residual damage *(125)*.

The reproductive system is the second most common site of focal brucellosis. Epididymitis or epididymoorchitis occur in about 2% to 10% of male patients. Brucellosis in pregnancy poses a serious risk of spontaneous abortion *(126)*.

Endocarditis and CNS disease occur in 2% to 5% of patients; meningitis, encephalitis, meningoencephalitis, meningovascular disease, brain abscesses, and demyelinating syndromes have all been reported *(127)*. However, endocarditis remains the principal cause of morbidity in brucellosis and the major cause of death. It usually involves the aortic valve and typically requires immediate surgical valve replacement *(111, 112)*.

The blood count is often characterized by mild leukopenia and relative lymphocytosis, along with mild anemia and thrombocytopenia. The thrombocytopenia may be severe *(111)*.

Relapses, which are rare (about 10% of cases), usually occur in the first year after infection and are often milder in severity than is the initial disease.

In contrast with humans, livestock do not show systemic signs of disease during the dissemination phase. Brucellae have also been found in milk macrophages, leading to infection in young animals and providing a source of human infection.

Diagnosis of brucellosis is usually made serologically based on the detection of antibody directed against OPS.

23.6.3 Treatment of Brucellosis

Treatment of human brucellosis should involve antibiotics that can penetrate macrophages and can act in the acidic intracellular environment. There is a general need for antibiotic combination treatment because all monotherapies are characterized by unacceptably high relapse rates *(111, 112)*. In addition, the general discrepancy between *in vitro* activity and *in vivo* observations will preclude the study of resistance patterns of brucellae or *in vitro* evaluation of the efficacy of individual antibiotics.

In 1986, WHO issued guidelines for the treatment of human brucellosis. The guidelines discussed two regimens, both using doxycycline (100 mg, twice daily) for a period of 6 weeks, in combination with either streptomycin (15 mg/kg, intramuscularly) for 2 to 3 weeks or rifampin (600 to 1,200 mg daily) for 6 weeks *(112)*.

Alternative drug combinations have also been used, including aminoglycosides such as gentamicin (5.0 mg/kg daily in 3 divided intravenous doses for 5 to 7 days) and netilmicin. The trimethoprim-sulfamethoxazole combination (960 mg, twice daily for 6 weeks) is usually used in triple regimens. Various combinations that incorporate ciprofloxacin (500 mg, twice daily for 6 weeks) and ofloxacin (400 mg, twice daily for 6 weeks) have been tried clinically and found to have similar efficacy as those of the classic regimens *(112)*.

In various combinations, rifampin is the drug of choice in the treatment of brucellosis in pregnancy. Brucellosis in children has been treated with a combination based on rifampin and trimethoprim-sulfamethoxazole *(112)*.

23.6.3.1 Human Brucellosis Vaccines

It is likely that a human vaccine against brucellosis will elicit both humoral and cellular immune responses. However, although several vaccines have been tested in the past, none was completely satisfactory *(128)*. Vaccines from *B. abortus* strain 19 were used in the former Soviet Union, and strains of *B. abortus* 104M have been used in China. A phenol-insoluble peptidoglycan fraction of *B. melitensis* strain M15 was used in France *(111, 112)*.

Theoretical vaccine targets for use in future vaccine development may include the *rfbK* mutations of *B. melitensis*, the outer-membrane protein 25, and the cytoplasmic protein BP26 *(129)*.

23.7 Coxiella burnetii: Q Fever

Q fever was first discovered in Australia as an occupational disease and was found in the United States just before the outbreak of World War II. Currently, this zoonotic disease caused by *Coxiella burnetii* has nearly worldwide distribution *(130, 131)*. Cattle, sheep, and goats are the primary reservoirs of *C. burnetii*. Organisms are excreted in the milk, urine, and feces of infected animals. However, *C. burnetii* infection has been noted in a wide variety of other animals, including other species of livestock and domesticated pets, as well as arthropods. *C. burnetii* does not usually cause clinical disease in these animals, although abortion in goats and sheep has been linked to *C. burnetii* infection. Humans are the only hosts identified that normally would experience an illness as a result of infection (http://cdc.gov/ncidod/dvrd/qfever). *C. burnetii* is resistant to heat, drying, and many common disinfectants, which enables the bacteria to survive in the environment for long periods.

Infections in humans usually occur from inhaling these organisms from air that contains airborne barnyard dust contaminated with dried placental material, birth fluids, and excreta of infected herd animals. Ingestion of contaminated milk, followed by regurgitation and inspiration of the contaminated food, is a less common mode of transmission. Other modes of transmission to humans, including tick bites and human-to-human transmission, are rare.

Humans are often very susceptible to the disease, and very few organisms may be required to cause infection. Because of its infectivity, *C. burnetii* could be developed for use in biological warfare and is considered a potential terrorist threat.

Coxiella burnetii is an obligated intracellular organism that grows as a small coccobacillus, approximately 0.8 to 1.0 μm in length by 0.3 to 0.5 μm in width, and may occur either singly or in short chains. It is classified in the family Rickettsiaceae but is not included in the genus, and therefore is not a true rickettsia. Moreover, it was not found to be closely related to any other bacterial species when comparative 16s ribosomal ribonucleic acid analysis was performed. Thus, the genus *Coxiella* has only one species. Its closest relative, according to 16s ribosomal RNA analysis, is *Legionella (132,133)*, even though *Legionella* has different growth characteristics—the ability to survive and multiply extracellularly and causing a different clinical syndrome *(131)*. In contrast, *C. burnetii* cannot have sustained growth and replication outside a host cell.

C. burnetii replicates only within the phagolysosomal vacuoles of animal cells, primarily macrophages. The replication occurs by binary fission.

The most important biological feature of the organism is the existence of small, compacted cell types within mature populations growing in animal hosts. These forms, called small-cell variants (SCVs), are absolutely distinct from the large-cell variants (LCVs) in the population. The latter are likely the metabolizing stage in what is obviously a developmental life cycle in *C. burnetii (130)*. It is thought that the SCVs of the developmental cycle of the organism are mainly linked to the unusual resistance characteristics of *C. burnetii*, as well as its long-term durability within different environments.

The virulent *C. burnetii*, which is usually linked to natural infection and a smooth LPS, is designated as phase I. This phase is resistant to complement and is a potent immunogen. Serial passage of *C. burnetii* in eggs eventually results in the bacterium's conversion to phase II, which has a rough LPS and is much less virulent than phase I. Phase II is sensitive to complement and is a poor immunogen. The conversion of phase I to phase II is irreversible and is the result of a mutation caused by a chromosomal deletion *(131)*.

C. burnetii also contains several plasmids, and dissimilar plasmid types may be associated with different manifestations of disease *(134)*. In addition, the cell wall of a phase I *C. burnetii* organism contains, in association with the LPS,

an immunomodulatory complex *(135)* that produces toxic reactions in mice (e.g., hepatomegaly, splenomegaly, liver necrosis) and lymphocyte hyporesponsiveness *in vitro (131)*.

23.7.1 Q Fever: Clinical Manifestations

C. burnetii is extremely infectious; under experimental conditions, a *single organism* is capable of producing infection and disease in humans *(136)*. Human infection is usually the results of inhalation of infected aerosols. The incubation period varies from 10 to 40 days, with its duration being inversely correlated with the magnitude of the inoculum— a higher inoculum also increases the severity of the disease *(131)*.

Q fever in humans may be manifested as asymptomatic seroconversion, acute illness, or chronic disease. Infection with *C. burnetii* has been reported to persist in humans (as it does in animals) in an asymptomatic state. Although possible, infection with Q fever may adversely affect the outcome of pregnancy.

Q fever is usually diagnosed by serologic testing because culture of *C. burnetii* is potentially dangerous to laboratory personnel and requires animal inoculation or cell culture. A number of serologic methods have been used, including complement fixation, indirect fluorescent antibody, macroagglutination and microagglutination, and the enzyme-linked immunosorbent assay (ELISA). Of the methods currently used for serologic testing of Q fever, ELISA is the most sensitive (80% to 84% in early convalescence, and 100% in intermediate and late convalescence) *(137)* and easiest to perform. In general, antibodies to the rough phase II organism are identified earlier in the illness, during the first few months after infection, followed by a decline in antibody to phase II organisms and a rise in antibody to the smooth, virulent phase I organism *(131)*.

23.7.1.1 Acute Q Fever

There is no characteristic illness for acute Q fever, and manifestations may vary considerably among locations where the disease is acquired *(131)*.

When symptomatic, the onset of Q fever may be abrupt or insidious, with fever, chills (including frank rigors), and headache (usually severe, throbbing, and frontal or retro-orbital in location) being the most common. Diaphoresis, malaise, fatigue, and anorexia are also very common. Relatively infrequent symptoms include sore throat, gastrointestinal upset, and neck stiffness; the last symptom may be severe enough to require a lumbar puncture to exclude bacterial meningitis *(131)*.

A common clinical manifestation of Q fever is pneumonia *(138)*. Atypical pneumonia is most frequent, and asymptomatic patients can also exhibit radiologic changes (usually nonspecific, but also rounded opacities and hilar adenopathy).

Neurologic complications were observed in up to 23% of acute cases, including encephalopathic symptoms, hallucinations (visual and auditory), expressive dysplasia, hemifacial pain resembling trigeminal neuralgia, diplopia, and dysarthria. Other symptoms involving the CNS, such as encephalitis, encephalomyelitis, optic neuritis, or myelopathy, may also occur, particularly late in acute illness *(131)*.

23.7.1.2 Chronic Q Fever

Chronic infection with *C. burnetii* is usually rare but, unlike acute illness, is often fatal *(130)*. Chronic disease occurs almost exclusively in patients with prior coronary illness or in immunocompromised patients with AIDS or cancer or transplant recipients.

Chronic Q fever is manifested mainly by infective endocarditis, which also is the most severe complication of Q fever. Other syndromes, such as chronic hepatitis and infection of surgical lesions, have also been observed *(130, 131)*. In Q fever endocarditis, fever has been recorded in 85% of patients, along with other systemic symptoms such as chills, headache, myalgias, and weight loss. Other complications resulting from Q fever endocarditis include congestive heart failure (76%), splenomegaly (42%), hepatomegaly (41%), clubbing (21%), and cutaneous signs, often the result of a leukocytoclastic vasculitis (22%).

23.7.2 Treatment of Q Fever

In the treatment of Q fever, the use of tetracyclines has been the preferred therapy. When initiated within the first 3 days of illness, treatment with tetracyclines shortens the duration of disease. Doxycycline has been the treatment of choice for acute Q fever—a dose of 100 mg of oral doxycycline twice daily for 15 to 21 days is the most frequently prescribed therapy.

Macrolide antibiotics, such as erythromycin, have also proved effective for the treatment of acute Q fever *(139)*.

Chronic Q fever endocarditis is much more difficult to treat effectively and often requires the use of multiple drugs. Two different treatments protocols have been evaluated: (i) doxycycline in combination with quinolones for at least 4 years; and (ii) doxycycline in combination with hydroxychloroquine for 1.5 to 3 years. The second regimen leads to fewer relapses but requires routine eye examinations to detect accumulation of chloroquine. Surgery to remove damaged valves may be required in some cases of *C. burnetii* endocarditis (http://cdc.gov/ncidod/dvrd/qfever).

23.7.2.1 Vaccines

An effective Q fever vaccine was developed in 1948. This preparation, consisting of formalin-killed and ether-extracted *C. burnetii* containing 10% yolk sac, was effective in protecting human volunteers from aerosol challenge *(140)*.

Vaccines prepared from phase I microorganisms, which were found to be 100 to 300 times more potent than phase II vaccines, form the basis for most current Q fever vaccines *(130)*. Purification methods have been improved over the years to better separate bacterial cells from egg proteins and lipids. However, use of the early phase I cellular vaccines has frequently been accompanied by adverse reactions, including induration of the vaccination site or the formation of sterile abscesses or granulomas. In addition, administration of a cellular vaccine to persons previously infected may result in severe and persistent local reactions *(130)*.

Attempts to maintain the vaccine's efficacy while decreasing the potential for adverse reactions led to testing cell extract as vaccines. Although such extracted cellular antigens were less reactive than were the intact microorganisms after injection, they were also less effective as vaccines *(130)*.

For the most part, attenuated Q fever vaccines are not used. However, a phase II attenuated strain, designated M-44, was developed in the former Soviet Union and has been used since 1960. This vaccine was shown to cause myocarditis, hepatitis, liver necrosis, granuloma formation, and splenitis in guinea pigs *(141)*.

In the late 1970s, a new CMR (chloroform-methanol residue) Q fever vaccine was developed. Initial testing has shown that the CMR vaccine did not cause adverse reactions in mice at doses several times larger than doses of phase I cellular vaccine. In addition, CMR vaccine did reduce the shedding of *C. burnetii* when used to vaccinate sheep *(130)*.

The most thoroughly tested Q fever vaccine in use today is Q-Vax. This is a formalin-killed, Henzerling strain, phase I cellular vaccine produced and licensed for use in Australia *(142)*. Q-Vax has been used successfully to prevent clinical Q fever in occupationally at-risk individuals. Thus, when a single subcutaneous dose (30 µg) of this vaccine was given to more than 2,000 abattoir workers screened for prior immunity, the protective efficacy was 100% *(142)*. The duration of protection was more than 5 years. The currently available Q fever vaccines would be of benefit to those occupationally at risk for Q fever, to those in areas endemic for Q fever, as well as to military and civilian populations who might be exposed as a result of a bioterrorist or biowarfare attack *(130)*.

23.8 Glanders

The causative agents of glanders and melioidosis are the non-fermenting Gram-negative bacilli *Burkholderia mallei* and *Burkholderia pseudomallei*, respectively.

Glanders is a disease of antiquity that has followed human civilization and has been described in writings by ancient Greek and Roman writers. The disease symptoms were recorded by Hippocrates around the year 425 BC, and the disease was given the name *melis* by Aristotle in approximately 350 BC.

Glanders (also known as equine, farcy, malleus, and droes) is naturally found in equines (horses, mules, and donkeys), and could occasionally be transmitted to humans *(143, 144)*. In addition, glanders can also be naturally contracted by goats, dogs, lions, and cats.

Through much of recorded history, glanders has been a world problem because horses and mules were vital means of transportation. The military also used them for moving supplies and troops and in battles among cavalries.

Only when horses were replaced by motorized transport in the early 20th century did the incidence of glanders decrease. Critical factors in reducing glanders in the Western world were the development of an effective skin test, a process of identification, and slaughter of infected animals. In the United States, glanders was eradicated in 1934 and has not been seen since 1945 *(143)*. Although developed nations have essentially been free of glanders, the disease is still commonly seen among domestic animals in Africa, Asia, the Middle East, and Central and South America (http://cdc.gov/ncidod/dbmd/diseaseinfo/glandrs_g.htm).

In World War I, *B. mallei* was used as biological weapon for the first time. The Central Powers infected Russian equines, causing disruption of supply lines and associated human deaths. Later, the Japanese used *B. mallei* against the Chinese, and there is anecdotal evidence that the former Soviet Union attempted to weaponize the pathogen and use it in Afghanistan (http://pathema.tigr.org/pathema/b_mallei.shtml).

The ease of transmission and severity of the disease have made *B. mallei* an obvious choice as an agent for biowarfare and bioterrorism, leading NIAID to categorize *B. mallei* as a category B Biological Disease *(145)*.

23.8.1 *Burkholderia mallei*

Burkholderia mallei (also previously known as *Pseudomonal mallei*, *Bacillus mallei*, *Pfeifferella mallei*, *Acinetobacter mallei*, *Loefferella mallei*, *Malleomyces mallei*, and *Acinetobacter mallei*) is a rod-shaped, nonmotile, obligate, Gram-negative bacillus that is an obligate animal pathogen, unlike the closely related *Burkholderia pseudomallei*, which can be found in tropical soil *(143)*. *Burkholderia mallei* was incorporated in its current genus in 1992 *(146)*. It produces an extracellular capsule that is an important virulence determinant and can survive drying for 2 to 3 weeks but is susceptible to heat (55°C for 10 minutes) and ultraviolet light.

In addition, *B. mallei* is susceptible to numerous disinfectants, including benzalkonium chloride, iodine, mercuric chloride in alcohol, potassium permanganate, 1% sodium hypochlorite, 70% ethanol, and 2% glutaraldehyde. It is less susceptible to phenolic disinfectants.

23.8.1.1 Genome Sequence of Burkholderia mallei

The complete genome sequence of *B. mallei* ATCC 23344, a highly pathogenic clinical isolate, has provided valuable insights into a number of putative virulence factors whose function was supported by comparative genome hybridization and expression profiling of the bacterium in hamster liver *in vivo* *(147)*. The genome consists of two chromosomes comprising approximately 5.7 million base pairs and an average G+C content of 68%. Its sequence is riddled with insertion sequences that have had a dramatic effect on its chromosomal structure.

The bioinformatics and laboratory analysis of the genome also provides further insight into the pathogenesis and biology of *B. mallei* and its relationship to the pathogenic *Burkholderia pseudomallei* and the nonpathogenic *B. thailandensis*.

The *B. mallei* genome was found to contain numerous insertion elements that have mediated extensive deletions and rearrangements of the genome relative to *B. pseudomallei*. The genome also contains a vast number of simple sequence repeats (more than 12,000). Furthermore, the observed variation in simple sequence repeats in key genes can provide a mechanism for generating antigenic variation, which may account for the mammalian host's inability to mount a durable adaptive response to a *B. mallei* infection *(147)*.

The location of the only virulence factors definitely shown to be essential for the pathogenicity of *B. mallei*, an extracellular capsule *(148)*, and a *Salmonella typhimurium*–like type III secretion system *(149)*, have been determined in the chromosome *(147)*.

In evolving from a metabolically versatile soil organism to a highly specialized obligate mammalian pathogen, structural flexibility appeared to be a major adaptive feature of the *B. mallei* genome.

23.8.1.2 Virulence of Burkholderia spp.

Better understanding of the *B. mallei* virulence determinants and pathogenesis will be critical for the development of suitable vaccine candidates *(143)*. Some virulence factors of this pathogen have been characterized *(148, 149)*, and the recently completed genome of *B. mallei* ATCC 23344 (see Section 23.8.1.1) revealed putative gene products that were similar to virulence factors in other Gram-negative bacteria, including a type II secretion system, a type III secretion system, type IV pili, autotransporter proteins, iron acquisition proteins, fimbriae, quorum-sensing systems, and various transcriptional regulators *(150–152)*.

Capsule. Polysaccharide capsules represent highly hydrated polymers that mediate the interaction of bacteria with their immediate surroundings and often play integral roles in the interaction of pathogens with their hosts. A number of studies have provided clear evidence that *B. mallei* does form a capsule and that it is important for the pathogen's virulence *(143)*. Taken together, these studies have indicated that the *B. mallei* capsule may prevent phagocytosis early in the infection and may block the microbicidal action of the phagocytes after internalization. It is also possible that the capsule will confer resistance of the bacteria to lysosomal enzymes and will allow *B. mallei* to persist long enough to escape from the phagosome and/or phagolysosome, albeit by unknown mechanism. However, as of yet the chemical structure of the *B. mallei* capsule is unknown.

Subtractive hybridization has been used to identify genetic determinants present in *B. mallei (148)* and *B. pseudomallei (153)*. In both species, subtractive hybridization products have been mapped to a genetic locus encoding proteins involved in the biosynthesis, export, and translocation of a capsular polysaccharide *(148, 153)*. Furthermore, the *B. mallei* capsule gene cluster exhibited 99% nucleotide identity to a *B. pseudomallei* capsule gene cluster that encodes a homopolymeric surface polysaccharide *(148)*, and based on genetic and biochemical criteria, both *B. mallei* and *B. pseudomallei* gene clusters most closely resemble group 3 gene clusters because of their gene arrangement and because they lack the *kpsF* and *kpsU* homologues that are present in group 2 gene clusters *(148, 153)*. As shown in an immunogold electron micrograph study, *B. mallei* ATCC 23344 reacted with polyclonal capsular antibodies by forming a thick (approximately 200 nm) and evenly distributed surface layer around the bacteria.

Antigen 8. In several studies, an extracellular capsule-like substance called antigen 8 (Ag8) has been identified on the surface of both *B. mallei* and *B. pseudomallei* and is thought to be a pathogenicity factor because of its antiphagocytic and immunosuppressive properties *(154,154a,155)*. Ag8 is a glycoprotein composed of 10% protein and 90% carbohydrate and has a molecular mass of approximately 88 kDa *(154)*. In *B. mallei* cultures, Ag8 production was not detected until the second half of the exponential growth phase, and production was maximal during the stationary phase

(154). Because the carbohydrate moiety of Ag8, a homogeneous polymer of 6-d-*D*-mannoheptose *(155)*, was found to be identical in structure to the capsular polysaccharide of *B. pseudomallei* and *B. mallei*, further studies will be necessary to determine whether Ag8 and the capsule (see the preceding paragraph) are the same molecule or are distinct molecular moieties *(143)*.

Lipopolysaccharide (143). Similar to *Burkholderia pseudomallei (156)*, *B. mallei* strains deficient in LPS *O*-antigen are sensitive to killing by 30% normal human serum (NHS) and are less virulent than the wild-type strains *(157)*. Previous studies have revealed that *B. mallei* LPS *O*-antigens cross-react with polyclonal antibodies raised against *B. pseudomallei* LPS *O*-antigens *(48, 157, 158)*, and that the LPS *O*-antigen gene clusters of these species are 99% identical at the nucleotide level *(156, 157)*. In fact, the *B. mallei* LPS *O*-antigen was found to be similar to the previously described *B. pseudomallei* LPS *O*-antigen, a heteropolymer of repeating *D*-glucose and *L*-talose *(157, 159, 160)*. However, changes are apparent in the *O*-acetylation pattern of the *B. mallei* *L*-talose residue compared with the pattern in *B. pseudomallei*. Similar to the *B. pseudomallei* LPS *O*-antigen, the *B. mallei* LPS *O*-antigen contained an *O*-acetyl or *O*-methyl substitution at the 2′-position of the talose residue. On the other hand, the *B. mallei* LPS *O*-antigen is devoid of an *O*-acetyl group at the 4′-position of the talose residue *(157)*. Thus, the structure of *B. mallei* LPS *O*-antigen is best described as "3-β-*D*-glucopyranose-(1,3)-6-deoxy-α-*L*-talopyranose-(1-" in which the talose residue contains 2-*O*-methyl or 2-*O*-acetyl substituents *(157)*.

Pathoadaptive Mutations (143). Comparative genomic analysis of closely related bacteria has demonstrated that gene loss and gene inactivation are common themes in host-adapted pathogens *(161)*. These mutations, called pathoadaptive mutations, will improve fitness/virulence by modifying traits that interfere with survival in host tissues *(161)*. *B. mallei* is a host-adapted parasite of equines whereas *B. pseudomallei* is an opportunistic parasite of numerous hosts. The genomic sequences of *B. mallei* ATCC 23344 *(147)* and *B. pseudomallei (162)* have been completed and can be directly compared (see also Section 23.8.1.1). Although the genes conserved between these species were approximately 99% identical, *B. pseudomallei* contained approximately 1 megabase (Mb) of DNA that was not present in *B. mallei*. It is plausible that *B. pseudomallei* may have acquired this DNA through lateral transfer after the divergence of these two species from a common progenitor *(163)*. Alternatively, this DNA was present in the common progenitor and was subsequently deleted in *B. mallei (164)*. In addition, *B. mallei* has numerous insertion sequences, and several of these are present within genes (gene inactivation). Gene loss and gene inactivation probably played important roles in the evolution of *B. mallei* by eliminating factors that were not required (or were inhibitory) for a successful host-pathogen interaction. Thus, it appears that pathoadaptive mutations have played an important role in the evolutionary adaptation of *B. mallei* to a parasitic mode of existence *(143)*.

Exopolysaccharide. A survey of the phenotypic traits that are present in *B. mallei* and *B. pseudomallei* (but absent in the nonpathogenic *B. thailandensis*) may allow for the identification of new virulence determinants *(143)*. One virulence factor that fits these criteria is a capsule-like exopolysaccharide *(165)*. This exopolysaccharide is a linear tetrasaccharide repeating unit consisting of three galactose residues, one bearing a 2-linked *O*-acetyl group and a 3-deoxy-*D*-manno-2-octulosonic acid residue *(166)*. However, the genes encoding the exopolysaccharide have not been identified in *B. mallei* and *B. thailandensis*, and its role in the pathogenesis is currently unknown.

23.8.2 Clinical Manifestations of Glanders in Humans

Humans can become infected with *B. mallei* after contact with sick animals or infectious materials. Transmission is typically through small wounds and abrasions in the skin. Ingestion or inhalation with invasion through the mucous membranes (nasal, oral, and conjunctival), eyes, and by inhalation into the lungs is also possible. Cases are usually seen in people who handle laboratory samples *(167)* or who have frequent close contact with equines.

Case fatality rate is 95% for untreated septicemic infections and more than 50% with traditional antibiotic treatment, although susceptibility data suggest that newer antibiotics should be effective.

In natural infections, the incubation period is 1 to 14 days. Infections from aerosolized forms in biological weapons are expected to have an incubation period of 10 to 14 days.

In humans, the clinical symptoms of glanders depend on the route of infection with the organism. The types of infection include localized, pus-forming cutaneous infections, pulmonary infections, bloodstream (septicemic) infections, and chronic suppurative infections of the skin. *Combinations of syndromes can occur.* Generalized symptoms of glanders include fever, muscle pain, chest pain, muscle tightness, and headache. Additional symptoms have included excessive tearing of the eyes, light sensitivity, and diarrhea (http://cdc.gov/ncidod/dbmd/diseaseinfo/glandrs_g.htm).

Localized Infections. If there is a cut or scratch in the skin, a localized infection with ulceration will develop within 1 to 5 days at the site where the bacteria entered the body. Swollen lymph nodes may also be present. Infections (ulcers) involving the mucous membranes in the eyes, nose, and respiratory tract will cause increased mucus production and blood-tinged discharge from the affected sites. Mucosal or skin infections can disseminate; symptoms of disseminated infections include a popular or pustular rash, abscesses in the internal organs (particularly the liver and spleen), and pulmonary lesions. Disseminated infections are associated with septic shock and high mortality.

Pulmonary Infections. In pulmonary infections, pneumonia, pulmonary abscesses, and pleural effusion can also occur. Chest x-rays will show localized infection in the lobes of the lungs. Symptoms include cough, fever, dyspnea, and mucopurulent discharge. Skin abscesses sometimes develop after several months.

Bloodstream (Septicemic) Infections. Glanders bloodstream infections are usually fatal within 7 to 10 days. In the septicemic form, fever, chills, myalgia, and pleuritic pain develop acutely. Other symptoms may include generalized erythroderma, jaundice, photophobia, lacrimation, diarrhea, and granulomatous or necrotizing lesions. Tachycardia, cervical adenopathy, and mild hepatomegaly or splenomegaly may also be observed.

In the septicemic form, blood cultures of *B. mallei* may be negative just before death.

Chronic Infections. The chronic form of glanders involves multiple abscesses within the muscles of the arms and legs or in the spleen or liver.

23.8.3 Treatment of Glanders

Because *B. mallei* is considered a potential biological weapon and its intentional release has already been documented *(143, 168)*, there is a clear need for effective treatment strategies of human glanders as well as postexposure prophylaxis.

Because *B. mallei* is variably susceptible to antibiotics *(169, 171)*, long-term treatment or multiple drugs may be necessary. However, treatment may be ineffective, especially in septicemia, because of the pathogen's *intrinsic resistance* to a wide range of antimicrobial agents including β-lactam antibiotics, aminoglycosides, and macrolides *(170, 171)*.

The antibiotic susceptibility pattern profile of *B. mallei* has shown *in vitro* susceptibility to ceftazidime, imipenem, meropenem, and doxycycline. Although initial treatment with imipenem or meropenem, or with ceftazidime for 2 to 3 weeks has been recommended, there is little experience in treating glanders in humans. In severe cases, a combination therapy with doxycycline or co-trimoxazole may be considered *(172, 173)*. In mild cases, initial oral therapy with an antimicrobial agent (doxycycline, co-amoxiclav, fluoroquinolones, TMP-SMZ) may be sufficient *(174)*.

Dose Regimens (www.emea.eu.int/pdfs/human/bioterror/10.glandersmelioidosis.pdf)

(i) *Imipenem*. In adults: 50 mg/kg daily, up to 1.0 g, 4 times daily. In children over 3 years of age: 15 mg/kg, 4 times daily (up to maximum of 2.0 g daily); over 40 kg, use adult dose. In children between 3 months and 3 years: 15 to 25 mg/kg, 4 times daily. In pregnancy, same regimens as in nonpregnant adults should be considered; it is recommended when possible to cease breastfeeding *(174)*.

(ii) *Meropenem*. In adults: 500 to 1,000 mg, intravenously, 3 times daily. In children over 3 months: 10 to 20 mg/kg, 3 times daily; adult dose for 50 kg and over. In pregnancy, same regimens as in nonpregnant adults should be considered; it is recommended when possible to cease breastfeeding *(174)*.

(iii) *Ceftazidime*. In adults: 2.0 g, intravenously, 3 times daily. In children over 2 months: 100 mg/kg daily in 3 divided doses (maximum dose is 6.0 g). In children younger than 2 months: 60 mg/kg daily in 2 divided doses. In pregnancy, same regimens as in nonpregnant adults should be considered; it is recommended when possible to cease breastfeeding *(174)*.

(iv) *Doxycycline*. In adults: 100 mg, intravenously, twice daily. In children over age 8 and over 45 kg weight: use the adult dose. In children over 8 years and less than 45 kg weight: 2.2 mg/kg, intravenously, twice daily. In children younger than 8: 2.2 mg/kg, intravenously, twice daily. Maximum dose 200 mg per day. In pregnancy, same regimens as in nonpregnant adults should be considered; it is recommended when possible to cease breastfeeding *(174)*.

(v) *TMP-SMX (trimethoprim-sulfamethoxazole)*. In adults: TMP: 6 to 8 mg/kg daily and SMX: 40 mg/kg daily, intravenously, in 1 or 2 divided doses, followed by TMP: 6 to 8 mg/kg daily and SMX: 40 mg/kg daily orally in 1 or 2 divided doses. Maximum total dose is 1,440 mg, twice daily. Consideration could be given to reducing the dose after 2 weeks *(174)*.

In children younger than 8: TMP: 6 to 8 mg/kg daily and SMX: 30 to 40 mg/kg daily, intravenously in 2 divided doses, followed by TMP: 6 to 8 mg/kg daily and SMX: 30 to 40 mg/kg daily, orally in 1 or 2 divided doses. Consideration could be given to reducing the dose after 2 weeks. In pregnancy, same regimens as in nonpregnant adults should be considered; it is recommended when possible to cease breastfeeding *(174)*.

23.8.3.1 Vaccines

Currently, there is no evidence for immunity against glanders by virtue of previous infection or vaccination *(143, 175)*. Infections in horses that seemed to recover symptomatically from glanders would recrudesce when the animals were challenged with *B. mallei*. Numerous attempts to vaccinate horses and laboratory animals against glanders were unsuccessful during the period 1895–1928 *(143)*. Even though vaccination resulted in some resistance to infection, the animals still contracted glanders.

23.9 Melioidosis

Melioidosis, also called *Whitmore's disease*, is an infection caused by *Burkholderia pseudomallei*, a Gram-negative bacterium closely related to *B. mallei*, the etiologic agent of glanders (see Section 23.8). Melioidosis is clinically and pathologically similar to glanders, but the ecology and the epidemiology of melioidosis are different from those of glanders. Melioidosis is predominately a disease of tropical climates, and the bacterium that causes melioidosis is found in contaminated water and soil. It is spread to humans and animals through direct contact with the contaminated source. Glanders is contracted by humans from infected domestic animals or by inhalation *(176)* (http://www.cdc.gov/ncidod/dbmd/diseaseinfo/melioidosis_g.htm).

B. pseudomallei is an organism that has been considered as a potential agent for biological warfare and bioterrorism. Melioidosis is endemic to Southeast Asia, with the highest concentration of cases in Vietnam, Cambodia, Laos, Thailand, Malaysia, Myanmar (Burma), and northern Australia. In addition, it is also seen in the South Pacific, Africa, India, and the Middle East. The bacterium is so prevalent that it has been isolated from troops of all nationalities that have served in areas of endemic disease. A few isolated cases of melioidosis have occurred in the Western Hemisphere, in Mexico, Panama, Ecuador, Haiti, Peru, Guyana, and in the states of Hawaii and Georgia. In the United States, confirmed cases range from none to five each year and occur among travelers and immigrants. Since the infamous "Affaire du Jardin des Plantes," in which a panda donated by Mao Ze Dong to French President Pompidou was the index case in an epidemic of melioidosis that decimated the large animals of the Paris zoological gardens *(176, 177)*, *B. pseudomallei* has also emerged as a major veterinary pathogen. Animals susceptible to melioidosis include sheep, goats, horses, swine, cattle, dogs, and cats. Transmission occurs by direct contact with contaminated soil and surface waters. In Southeast Asia, the pathogen has been repeatedly isolated from agricultural fields, with infection occurring primarily during the rainy season. Humans and animals are believed to acquire the infection by inhaling dust, ingesting contaminated water, and having contact with contaminated soil, especially through skin abrasions, and for military troops by contamination of war wounds. Person-to-person transmission can also occur. Two cases of sexual transmission have been reported—the transmission in both cases was preceded by a clinical history of chronic prostatitis in the source patient (http://www.cdc.gov/ncidod/dbmd/diseaseinfo/melioidosis_g.htm).

In endemic areas, melioidosis is a disease of the rainy season and affects mainly people with underlying predisposition to infection, such as those with diabetes, renal disease, cirrhosis, thalassemia, or alcoholism, as well as those who are immunosuppressed (176). However, melioidosis seems not to be associated with HIV infection. In addition, melioidosis has been recognized as a possible cause of chronic infection in patients with cystic fibrosis (178, 179).

23.9.1 Burkholderia pseudomallei

Burkholderia pseudomallei, the etiologic agent of melioidosis, is a motile, aerobic, nonspore-forming, Gram-negative bacterium. It is a soil saprophyte and can be recovered readily from water and wet soils in rice paddies in endemic areas (176).

The genome of B. pseudomallei was recently sequenced and found to be relatively large, 7.24 megabase (Mb) pairs (161). It is unequally divided between two chromosomes (4.07 and 3.17 Mb) with a G+C content of 68%, and a significant functional partitioning between them. The larger chromosome encodes many of the core functions associated with central metabolism and cell growth, whereas the smaller chromosome carries more accessory functions associated with adaptation and survival in different niches. Genomic comparisons with closely (see Section 23.8.1.1) and more distantly related bacteria revealed a greater level of gene order conservation and a greater number of orthologous genes on the large chromosome, suggesting that the two replicons have distinct evolutionary origins (161).

One striking feature of the B. pseudomallei genome was the presence of 16 genomic islands that together made up 6.1% of the genome. Further analysis revealed that these islands were variably present in a collection of invasive and soil isolates but entirely absent from the clonally related organism B. mallei; it has been hypothesized that variable horizontal gene acquisition by B. pseudomallei is an important feature of recent genetic evolution and that this has resulted in a genetically diverse pathogenic species (161).

23.9.2 Pathogenesis and Virulence Determinants of Burkholderia pseudomallei

B. pseudomallei, like many soil bacteria, is difficult to kill. It can survive in triple-distilled water for years (143). It is resistant to complement, lysosomal defensins, and cationic peptides, and it produces proteases, lipase, lecithinase, catalase,

peroxidase, superoxide dismutase, hemolysins, a cytotoxic exolipid, and at least one siderophore (180–183). Furthermore, the pathogen can survive inside several eukaryotic cell lines and is seen within phagocytic cells in pathologic specimens (183–185). After internalization, the pathogen escapes from the endocytic vacuoles into the infected cell cytoplasm and then forms membrane protrusions by inducing actin polymerization at one pole. The actin protrusions from the infected cell membrane mediate spread of the organism from cell to cell (186). B. pseudomallei contains several type III secretion systems that play an important role both in its spread and in intracellular survival (185, 186).

The role of the exotoxins in the pathogenesis of melioidosis is still unresolved (176). The high mortality of melioidosis is related to an increased propensity to develop high bacteremias (> 1 CFU/mL), but the relation between bacterial counts in blood and mortality is similar to that of other Gram-negative bacteria (187). This finding suggests that exotoxins do not contribute directly to the outcome.

The cell wall LPS, which is the immunodominant antigen, is highly conserved. In addition, B. pseudomallei produces a highly hydrated glycocalyx polysaccharide capsule (188), an important virulence determinant (189) that helps to form slime. This capsule facilitates the formation of microcolonies in which the organism is both protected from antibiotic penetration and phenotypically altered, resulting in reduced susceptibility to antibiotics (small colony variants) (190). Passive immunization with antibody to this exopolysaccharide reduced the lethality in mice (191). To date, the organisms that cause invasive disease are indistinguishable from those found in the environment (176).

The position-308 promoter region of the TNF-α gene has been associated with polymorphism (TNF2 allele) that is related to acquisition of melioidosis and disease severity (192). Furthermore, melioidosis has been positively associated with HLA class II DRB1*1602 in Thailand (193, 193a). This allele was associated significantly with septicemic melioidosis, whereas DQA1*03 was negatively associated; this association was independent of confounders such as diabetes mellitus (193).

23.9.3 Clinical Manifestations of Melioidosis

Generally, melioidosis presents as a febrile illness ranging from an acute fulminant septicemia to a chronic debilitating localized infection. The majority of patients are septicemic (176) (http://www.cdc.gov/ncidod/dgmd/diseaseinfo/melioidosis_g.htm). The disease can be categorized as acute or localized infection, acute pulmonary infection, acute bloodstream (septicemic) infection, and chronic suppurative infection. Asymptomatic infection is also possible.

Melioidosis can spread from person to person by contact with the blood and body fluids of an infected person. Two documented cases of male-to-female sexual transmission have involved males with chronic prostatic infection due to melioidosis. The incubation period of melioidosis is not clearly defined but may range between 2 days and many years (http://www.cdc.gov/ncidod/dgmd/diseaseinfo/melioidosis_g.htm).

Acute Localized Infection. This form is generally localized as a nodule and results from inoculation through a break in the skin. Symptoms include fever, general muscle pain, and may progress rapidly to infection of the bloodstream.

Pulmonary Infection. The lung is the most commonly affected organ, either presenting with cough and fever resulting from a primary lung abscess or pneumonia, or secondary to septicemic spread (blood-borne pneumonia). The clinical picture of the disease may be characterized from mild to severe pneumonia. The onset is typically accompanied by high fever, headache, anorexia, and general muscle soreness. Chest pain is common, but a nonproductive or productive cough with normal sputum is the hallmark of pulmonary melioidosis. However, sputum may also be purulent but rarely blood-stained. Large or peripheral lung abscesses may rupture into the pleural space to cause empyema *(176)*.

Acute Bloodstream Infection. Patients with underlying disease such as diabetes, HIV infection, and renal failure are affected by this form of melioidosis, which usually will result in septic shock. The symptoms of the bloodstream infection vary depending on the site of the original infection, but in general, they will include respiratory distress, severe headache, fever, diarrhea, development of pus-filled lesions on the skin, muscle tenderness, and disorientation. This is typically an infection of short duration, and abscesses will be found throughout the body.

Chronic Suppurative Infection. Chronic melioidosis is an infection that involves the organs of the body. Seeding and abscess formation may arise in any organ, although the joints, viscera, lymph nodes, skin, brain, liver, spleen, skeletal muscle, and the prostate are common sites. Renal abscesses are often associated with calculi and urinary infection. Corneal ulcers secondary to trauma and then exposure to contaminated water can be rapidly destructive *(193a)*.

23.9.4 Treatment of Melioidosis

Melioidosis is difficult to treat, and the initial intensive care management of severe illness includes resuscitation of patients with adequate intravenous fluids, because hypovolemia is common in the acute phase, as well as administration of high doses of parenteral antibiotics *(176)*. The antibiotic of choice is ceftazidime *(194, 195)*. Other third-generation cephalosporins were less effective.

Carbapenems kill *B. pseudomallei* more rapidly than do cephalosporins *(196)*, and in a large randomized trial imipenem proved equivalent to ceftazidime *(197)*.

Antibiotic combinations have also been used as empirical treatment of melioidosis including parenteral amoxicillin-clavulanate and cefoperazone-sulbactam; however, such treatment should be changed to ceftazidime or a carbapenem once the diagnosis of melioidosis has been confirmed *(176)*.

The risk of relapse has been related to the adherence to treatment and the initial extent of the disease, but not to the underlying condition *(176)*. The prognosis of melioidosis has been much better in children than in adults, and relapse was rarely observed. Adult patients require follow-up observation throughout their lives *(176)*.

Parenteral Treatment. Because the therapeutic response is very slow, parenteral treatment should be given for at least 10 days and should continue until improvement is noted and the patient can take oral drugs. Dose regimens often need to be adjusted for renal failure *(176)*.

Ceftazidime is usually given intravenously at 40 mg/kg every 8 h for a total of 120 mg/kg daily, or at 19 mg/kg intravenously immediately followed by a continuous infusion of 3 to 5 $mg\,kg^{-1}\,h^{-1}$. Other third-generation cephalosporins (e.g., cefotaxime, ceftriaxone) should not be used, because these antibiotics have been associated with increased mortality despite evidence of acceptable *in vitro* susceptibility *(176)*.

Imipenem is administered intravenously at 20 mg/kg every 8 hours for a total of 60 mg/kg daily *(176)*.

Intravenous amoxicillin-clavulanate is effective as empirical treatment of suspected septicemia at doses of 27 mg/kg given every 4 h *(not every* 8 h) for a total of 162 mg/kg daily *(176)*.

Oral Treatment. Oral treatment should be administered to complete a full 20 weeks of treatment. In adults, the oral treatment of choice is a four-drug combination of chloramphenicol (40 mg/kg daily in 4 divided doses), doxycycline (4 mg/kg daily in 2 divided doses), and trimethoprim-sulfamethoxazole (10 mg and 50 mg/kg daily, respectively, in 2 divided doses). *Note: chloramphenicol should be given only for the first 8 weeks.*

In children (8 years of age) and pregnant women, the recommended drug regimen comprises amoxicillin-clavulanate (amoxicillin 30 mg/kg daily; clavulanic acid 15 mg/kg daily) plus amoxicillin (30 mg/kg daily) *(176)*.

23.9.5 Melioidosis Acute Suppurative Parotitis

Melioidosis acute suppurative parotitis is a unique syndrome that occurs mainly in children in Southeast Asia without any other evidence of an underlying predisposing condition

(198). The syndrome is unusual in Australia. Patients present with fever, pain, and swelling over the parotid gland. In about 10% of cases, parotitis is bilateral. In advanced cases, rupture can arise, either to the skin or through the external ear *(198)*.

This condition has been managed with antibiotics (initially ceftazidime, followed by oral amoxicillin-clavulanate) and with incision and drainage, with great care applied not to damage the facial nerve. Delay in drainage can result in permanent Bell's palsy. The syndrome is usually managed with 8 weeks of treatment *(176)*.

23.9.6 Brain-Stem Encephalitis

In about 4% of cases from Australia and rarely elsewhere, melioidosis presents as brain-stem encephalitis with peripheral motor weakness of flaccid paraparesis *(199–201)*. Prominent features of this neurologic syndrome include unilateral limb weakness, cerebellar signs, and cranial nerve palsies. The pathogenesis of this condition has been uncertain, but new evidence has suggested that multiple focal microabscesses in the brain stem and spinal cord have been the cause. Antibiotic treatment has been similar to that given for other forms of melioidosis *(176)*.

23.10 Viral Hemorrhagic Fever: Filoviruses

The filoviruses are enveloped particles classified in the family Filoviridae, and together with two other families (Paramyxoviridae and Rhabdoviridae) they belong in the order Mononegavirales. Within the family Filoviridae, there is a single genus, Filovirus, that is separated into two sero-/genotypes, Marburg (MARV) and Ebola (EBOV). Ebola is further subdivided into four subtypes: Zaire, Sudan, Reston, and Ivory Coast (http://www.cdc.ncidod/dvrd/spb/mnpages/dispages/filoviruses.htm).

Structurally, Filovirus virions (complete viral particles) may appear in several shapes, a biological feature known as pleomorphism. These shapes include long, sometimes branched filaments, as well as shorter filaments shaped like a "6," or "U," or a circle. Viral filaments may measure up to 14,000 nm in length, have a uniform diameter of 80 nm, and are enveloped in a lipid membrane. Each virion contains one molecule of single-stranded, negative-sense RNA, approximately 19 kb long. New viral particles are created by budding from the surface of their host's cells. However, the Filovirus replication pathways are not well understood.

The first Filovirus was recognized in 1967 when a number of laboratory workers in Germany and the former Republic of Yugoslavia, who were handling tissues of green monkeys (*Cercopithecus aethiops*), developed hemorrhagic fever. A total of 31 cases and seven deaths were associated with these outbreaks. The virus was named for the city of Marburg, Germany, the site of one of the outbreaks. After the initial outbreaks, the virus disappeared. It did not re-emerge until 1975, when a traveler, most likely exposed in Zimbabwe, became ill. A few sporadic cases of Marburg hemorrhagic fever have been identified since that time.

The Ebola virus was first identified in 1976 when two outbreaks of Ebola hemorrhagic fever (Ebola HF) occurred in northern Zaire (Democratic Republic of Congo) and southern Sudan *(202–207)*. These two outbreaks eventually involved two different species of Ebola virus; both were named after the nations in which they were first discovered. Both the Zaire and Sudan subtypes proved to be highly lethal, as 90% of the Zairian cases and 50% of the Sudanese cases resulted in death. Since 1976, the Ebola virus has sporadically appeared in Africa, with small to midsize outbreaks confirmed between 1976 and 1979. Large epidemics of Ebola HF occurred in Kikwit, Zaire, in 1995 and in Gulu, Uganda, in 2000. Smaller outbreaks were identified in Gabon between 1994 and 1996 (http://www.cdc.ncidod/dvrd/spb/mnpages/dispages/filoviruses.htm). The Ebola-Reston subtype was isolated from cynomolgus monkeys (*Macaca fascicularis*) imported from the Philippines into the United States in 1989 and into Italy in 1992. The Ebola–Ivory Coast subtype emerged on the Ivory Coast in 1994 *(208, 209)*.

Epidemiology. It appears that the filoviruses are zoonotic because they are transmitted to humans from ongoing life cycles in animals other than humans. The Ebola-Reston subtype is the only known Filovirus that does not cause severe disease in humans; however, it can be fatal to monkeys *(210, 211)*. In spite of numerous attempts to locate the natural reservoir(s) of Ebola and Marburg viruses, their origins remain undetermined. However, because the virus can be replicated in some species of bats, some bat species native to the areas where the viruses are found may prove to be their carriers (http://www.cdc.ncidod/dvrd/spb/mnpages/dispages/filoviruses.htm).

Just how the virus is transmitted to humans is not known. However, once a human is infected, person-to-person transmission is the means by which further infections occur. Usually, transmission involves close contact between an infected individual or his or her body fluids and another person. During recorded outbreaks of hemorrhagic fever caused by Filovirus infection, persons who cared for or worked very closely with infected patients were especially at risk of becoming infected themselves *(212)*. Nosocomial transmission through contact with infected body fluids (reuse of unsterilized syringes, needles, or other contaminated material) has also been an important factor in spreading the disease. Although the viruses display some capability of infection through small-particle aerosols, airborne spread among humans has not been clearly demonstrated (http://www.cdc.ncidod/dvrd/spb/mnpages/dispages/filoviruses.htm).

In conjunction with the WHO, the CDC has developed practical, hospital-based guidelines, titled *Infection Control for Viral Haemorrhagic Fevers in the African Health Care Setting* (available at the CDC Web site under Ebola Hemorrhagic Fever) to help health care facilities recognize cases and prevent further hospital-based transmission of disease, using locally available materials and few financial resources.

23.10.1 Genome Structure of Filoviruses

The genomes of Ebola and Marburg consist of a single, negative-stranded, RNA linear molecule and are approximately 19 kb long (Marburg, 19.1 kb; Ebola, 18.9 kb) *(213)* (see also http://www.gsbs.utmb.edu/microbook/ch072.htm). The RNA is noninfectious, not polyadenylated, and complementary to polyadenylated viral subgenomic RNA species. The genes have been defined by highly conserved transcriptional start and termination signals at their 3′ and 5′ ends. Some genes overlap, but the positions and numbers of overlaps differ between the two types of viruses. The length of the overlaps is limited to five highly conserved nucleotides within the transcriptional signals. Most genes tended to possess long noncoding sequences at their 3′ and/or 5′ ends, which have contributed to the increased length of the genome. The genomes were complementary at the very extreme ends.

The filoviruses' nucleoprotein (NP) is the major structural phosphoprotein, and only the phosphorylated form is incorporated into the virions, as demonstrated for Marburg. The NP is the major component of the ribonucleoprotein complex (RNP). The RNP consists of the nonsegmented negative-stranded RNA genome and four of the structural proteins: nucleoprotein (NP); virion structural protein (VP) 30; VP35; and L (large or polymerase) protein. Two other virion proteins, VP24 and VP40, are membrane-associated, and the spikes are formed by the glycoprotein (GP).

23.10.2 Pathogenesis of Filoviruses

The fatal outcome in filoviral infection is associated with an early reduction in the number of circulating T cells, the host's failure to develop specific humoral immunity, and the release of proinflammatory cytokines *(214–217)*.

The lack of evidence for massive direct vascular involvement in infected hosts supports the role of active mediator molecules in the pathogenesis of the disease. Although the source of these mediators during Filovirus infections is still unknown, candidate cells exist. Besides the endothelium, the common denominator remains the macrophage, which is known as a pivotal source of a different protease, H_2O_2, and mediators such as tumor necrosis factor (TNF)-α. The latter finding supports the concept of a mediator-induced vascular instability, thus suggesting that increased permeability may be a key mechanism for the development of the shock syndrome in severe and fatal cases. The tendency toward bleeding could be the result of endothelial damage caused directly by virus replication, as well as indirectly by cytokine-mediated processes. Furthermore, the combination of viral replication in endothelial cells and the virus-induced cytokine release from macrophages may also promote a distinct proinflammatory endothelial phenotype that can trigger the coagulation cascade (http://www.gsbs.utmb.edu/microbook/ch072.htm).

Clinical and biochemical findings have supported the anatomic observations of extensive liver involvement, renal damage, changes in vascular permeability, and activation of the clotting cascade (http://www.gsbs.utmb.edu/microbook/ch072.htm). Necrosis of visceral organs is the consequence of virus replication in parenchymal cells. However, no organ is sufficiently damaged to cause death. Fluid distribution problems and platelet abnormalities indicate dysfunction of endothelial cells and platelets. The shock syndrome in severe and fatal cases seems to be mediated by virus-induced release of humoral factors such as cytokines. The Filovirus glucoprotein is believed to carry an immunosuppressive domain, and immunosuppression has been observed in monkeys (http://www.gsbs.utmb.edu/microbook/ch072.htm).

Recent experimental data have shown that some of the antibodies produced during Ebola virus infection have enhanced its infectivity, and this enhancement was mediated by antibodies to the viral glycoprotein and by complement component C1q. This finding suggested a novel mechanism of antibody-dependent enhancement (ADE) of virus infection. Cross-links between virus and cell, via antibodies, C1q, and C1q ligands at the cell surface may promote either binding of the virus to Ebola virus–specific receptors or endocytosis of the target cells, suggesting that ADE of infectivity may account for the extreme virulence of Ebola virus. Furthermore, the human macrophage galactose- and N-acetyl galactosamine-specific C-type lectins enhanced the infectivity of the filoviruses. Interestingly, these C-type lectins are present on cells known to be major Filovirus targets (e.g., macrophage hepatocytes and dendritic cells), suggesting a role for these C-type lectins in viral tissue tropism *in vivo*. The overall results led to a hypothesis suggesting that the filoviruses may use antibodies, complement components, and C-type lectins to gain cellular entry, depending on the cell type, and promote efficient viral replication (http://www.czc.hokudai.ac.jp/epidemiol/research_e.html).

23.10.2.1 Filoviral Glycoprotein

The membrane-anchored Filovirus glycoprotein (GP) is attached on the surface of virions and infected cells. It mediates receptor binding and fusion. The Filovirus glycoproteins are considered to be major determinants of viral pathogenicity and contribute to both immunosuppression and vascular dysregulation (214, 218–221).

The transmembrane glycoproteins of many animal and human retroviruses share structural features, including a conserved region that has strong immunosuppressive properties (222, 223). As a result, CKS17, a synthetic peptide corresponding with the conserved region in oncogenic retroviruses, has been used to study the pathophysiology of immunosuppression (224, 225). In particular, CKS17 causes an imbalance of human type-1 and type-2 cytokine production, suppresses the cell-mediated immunity (226), and blocks the activity of protein kinase C, a cellular messenger involved in T-cell activation (227, 228). Furthermore, it has been determined that there is a region of strong secondary structure conservation between the *C*-terminal domain of the envelope glycoprotein of the filoviruses and CKS17 (214). Thus, a 17-amino-acid domain in the filoviral glycoproteins was shown to resemble an immunosuppressive motif in the retroviral envelope proteins; that is, dysregulating the Th-1 and Th2 responses and depleting CD4$^+$ and CD8$^+$ T-cells through apoptosis. Moreover, an alignment of the filoviral glycoprotein and the retroviral immunosuppressive domains illustrated primary sequence similarity between a wide range of retroviruses and filoviruses. Three cysteine residues implicated in disulfide bonding were also conserved, reinforcing similarities in secondary structure. Functional analysis of the putative immunosuppressive domains in various species of Ebola and Marburg has demonstrated that the immunosuppressive effect of different species of the GP peptides was consistent with the pathogenicity observed in different animal hosts (214). These and other findings have also been consistent with a previous observation that the Ebola-Reston subtype was not pathogenic in humans (221) and may enable the development of specific strategies to reduce the extreme morbidity and mortality associated with hemorrhagic fever due to the Ebola and Marburg filoviruses (214).

23.10.2.2 Filovirus Replication

It is thought that the cell entry of the filoviruses is mediated by the GP as the only surface protein of virion particles.

Studies on Marburg (strain Musoke) infection of hepatocytes have identified the asialoglycoprotein receptor as a receptor candidate (229). It is not known if the next step in the virus entry involves a fusion process at the plasma membrane or fusion after endocytosis of virus particles. Neither has the uncoating mechanism been studied. The Filovirus transcription and replication take place in the cytoplasm of the infected cells. The role of gene overlaps in regulating transcription is not known, but transcription may be re-initiated by repositioning of the polymerase at the downstream start site (back-up mechanism). Alternatively, the polymerase may occasionally terminate transcription at the overlap and initiate transcription of the downstream gene without polyadenylation of the upstream gene. The switch mechanism between transcription and replication has not been studied. Virions usually bud at the plasma membrane. Mature particles usually exit preferentially in a vertical mode, but budding via the longitudinal axis has also been observed (229).

With the Ebola GP gene, the transcription occurs from two open reading frames (229). The primary gene product is a small nonstructural glycoprotein that is secreted from the infected cells. To express the full-length GP, two independent mechanisms are possible: transcriptional editing of a single nucleotide at a run of uridine residues; or translational frame shifting (−1) at or just past the editing site of unedited transcripts. The Marburg GP, however, is expressed in a single frame, and the gene does not contain sequences favoring mechanisms such as editing or frame shifting (229).

23.10.3 Hemorrhagic Fever: Clinical Manifestations

The filoviruses cause a severe hemorrhagic fever in humans and non-human primates (229). The onset of disease is very sudden, with fever, chills, headache, myalgia, and anorexia. These symptoms may be followed by abdominal pain, sore throat, nausea, vomiting, cough, arthralgia, diarrhea, and pharyngeal and conjunctival vasodilation. Patients are dehydrated, apathetic, and disoriented. Further symptoms include the development of characteristic, nonpruritic, maculopapular centripetal rash associated with varying degree of erythema, which desquamates by day 5 or 7 of the illness (229).

Hemorrhagic manifestations will develop at the peak of the illness and are of prognostic value. Bleeding into the gastrointestinal tract is the most prominent, in addition to petechia and hemorrhages from puncture wounds and mucous membranes. The laboratory parameters, although less characteristic, include leukopenia (as low as $1,000/\mu$L); left shift with atypical lymphocytes; thrombocytopenia (50,000 to $100,000/\mu$L); markedly elevated serum transaminase levels (typically aspartate aminotransferase exceeding alanine aminotransferase); hyperproteinemia; and proteinuria.

There is a fever in patients who eventually recover in about 5 to 9 days. In cases ending in death, clinical signs will occur at an early stage, and the patient will die between days 6 and 16 from hemorrhage and hypovolemic shock. The mortality rate is between 30% and 90% depending on the virus, with the highest rate reported for the Ebola-Zaire subtype. The Ebola-Reston subtype seems to possess a very low pathogenicity for humans or may be even apathogenic. Convalescence is prolonged and sometimes associated with myelitis, recurrent hepatitis, psychosis, or uveitis. An increased risk of abortion exists for pregnant women, and clinical observations indicate a high death rate for children of infected mothers (229).

23.10.3.1 Treatment of Filovirus Hemorrhagic Fever

A filovirus-specific treatment does not exist (229). Supportive therapy should be directed toward maintaining effective blood volume and electrolyte balance. The management of shock, cerebral edema, renal failure, coagulation disorders, and secondary bacterial infection is of ultimate importance for the survival of patients. Heparin treatment should only be considered when there is clear evidence of disseminated intravascular coagulopathy (DIC). Although human interferon and human reconvalescence plasma have been used in the past, there is a lack of experimental data showing efficacy. On the contrary, the filoviruses are resistant to the antiviral effects of interferon, and administering interferon to monkeys failed to increase the survival rate or to reduce the virus titer. Ribavirin is of no clinical value either.

Isolation of patients is strongly recommended, and the protection of medical and nursing staff is required.

23.10.3.2 Vaccines

Cross-protection among different Ebola subtypes in experimental animal models has been reported, thus suggesting a general value of vaccines. Inactivated vaccines have been developed by treating cell culture–propagated Marburg and Ebola, subtypes Sudan and Zaire, with formalin or heat. Protection, however, has only been achieved by careful balancing of the challenge dose and virulence. Immunizing monkeys with purified NP and GP has demonstrated the induction of the humoral and cellular immune responses and protection of animals against challenge with lethal doses (229).

In a highly effective vaccine strategy for Ebola virus infection in cynomolgus macaques, a combination of DNA immunization and boosting with adenoviral vectors that encoded viral proteins generated cellular and humoral immunity (230). Challenge with a lethal dose of the highly pathogenic, wild-type, 1976 Mayinga strain of Ebola-Zaire virus resulted in uniform infection in controls, who progressed to a moribund state and death in less than 1 week. In contrast, all vaccinated animals were asymptomatic for more than 6 months with no detectable virus after the initial challenge. These findings have demonstrated that it would be possible to develop a preventive vaccine against Ebola virus infection in non-human primates if the proposed vaccine strategy is proven effective against a more substantial viral challenge (231–233).

In another study, monkeys have been protected against high doses of Marburg virus by a vaccine based on a modified Alphavirus construct (234). The construct was an RNA replicon, based on the Venezuelan equine encephalitis (VEE) virus, which was used as a vaccine vector. The VEE structural genes were replaced by genes for the Marburg NP, GP, VP40, VP35, VP30, and VP24. Guinea pigs were vaccinated with recombinant VEE replicons (packaged into VEE-like particles) inoculated with the Marburg virus and evaluated for viremia and survival. The results indicated that either NP or GP were protective antigens, whereas VP35 afforded incomplete protection. In further evaluation of the vaccine's efficacy, cynomolgus macaques were inoculated with VEE replicons expressing the Marburg GP and/or NP. The results showed that the NP afforded incomplete protection, sufficient to prevent death but not disease in two of three macaques. Three monkeys vaccinated with replicons that expressed Marburg GP, and three others vaccinated with both replicons that expressed GP or NP, remained aviremic and were completely protected from disease (234).

23.11 Viral Hemorrhagic Fever: Bunyaviridae

The family Bunyaviridae is one of the largest groupings of animal viruses comprising more than 300 species classified into five genera: Orthobunyavirus, Hantavirus, Phlebovirus, Nairovirus, and Tospovirus (235). The Bunyaviridae have the capacity for sudden dramatic variation comparable with the antigenic shift associated with the influenza viruses, and this warrants continuing surveillance (236). Several members of the Bunyaviridae family are the causative agents of the often lethal hemorrhagic fevers, most notably the Crimean-Congo hemorrhagic virus (Nairovirus), Rift Valley fever virus (Phlebovirus), Hantaan, Sin Nombre, and related viruses (Hantavirus).

Recently, another bunyavirus, Garissa (Orthobunyavirus) was found to be the cause of hemorrhagic fever (237). The Garissa virus is now identified as an isolate of Ngari virus, which, in turn, is a Bunyamwera virus reassortant, which acquired the L and S segments (near complete identity) of Bunyamwera virus *(238)*.

The Bunyaviridae virus particles are spherical, 90 to 100 nm in diameter and enveloped with glycoprotein surface projections. The virions contain three unique segments of negative-sense, single-stranded RNA in the form of circular ribonucleoprotein complexes (nucleocapsids) and a transcriptase enzyme. The nucleotide stretches are highly conserved at the segment ends *(236, 239–241)*. The 3'-terminal nucleotide sequences of the three genomic RNA segments are conserved within each genus.

Intrastrand base pair interaction between these terminal nucleotides leads to noncovalently closed, circular RNAs providing the functional promoter region for the interaction of the viral polymerase with the genome segments *(241)*.

The viruses replicate in the cytoplasm of the infected cell and mature by budding into smooth-surface vesicles in or near the Golgi region *(242)*. The budding site seems to be defined by the retention of the glycoproteins G_N and G_C at that particular site *(239, 242)*.

The Bunyaviridae viruses have the ability to interact genetically with certain other closely related viruses by *genome segment reassortment (238)*.

23.11.1 Crimean-Congo Hemorrhagic Fever Virus

Crimean-Congo hemorrhagic fever virus (CCHFV) is the causative agent of the Crimean-Congo hemorrhagic fever (CCHF). It is a member of the genus Nairovirus of the family Bunyaviridae *(239)*. The genus Nairovirus includes 34 identified viruses and is divided into seven different serogroups. Only three are known to be pathogenic to humans (CCHF, Dugbe, and the Nairobi sheep disease viruses) *(239)*.

23.11.1.1 CCHFV Structural Proteins

The three genome segments of the bunyaviruses encode four structural proteins: the RNA-dependent RNA polymerase (L protein) is encoded by the large (L) segment, which has recently been sequenced *(243, 244)*; the glycoproteins (G_N and G_C) are encoded by the medium (M) segment; and the nucleoprotein (N) is encoded by the small (S) segment *(239)*. Together with hantaviruses, the nairoviruses seem to possess the simplest genome expression strategy among the Bunyaviridae.

Structurally, CCHF virions represent spherical particles approximately 90 nm in diameter. The two glycoproteins G_N and G_C, which are inserted into the lipid envelope as spike-like structures, are responsible for the virion's attachment to

receptors on the host cells and for the induction of neutralizing antibodies *(239)*.

The CCHFV glycoproteins are likely to play an important role in the natural tick-vertebrate cycle of the virus, as well as for the high pathogenicity in humans. Indeed, a highly variable mucin-like region at the amino terminus of the CCHFV glycoprotein precursor has been identified, a unique feature of nairoviruses within the family Bunyaviridae *(245)*. A similar serine-threonine–rich domain has been associated with increased vascular permeability and the development of hemorrhages in Ebola hemorrhagic fever *(218, 246)*.

The mature viral proteins, G_N and G_C, are generated by proteolytic cleavage from precursor proteins *(247)*. The amino termini of G_N and G_C are immediately preceded by the tetrapeptides RRLL and RKPL, respectively, leading to the hypothesis that SKI-1 or related proteases may be involved *(245)*. *In vitro* peptide cleavage data have shown that an RRLL tetrapeptide representing G_N processing site was efficiently cleaved by SKI-1 protease, whereas an RKPL tetrapeptide representing the G_C processing site was cleaved at negligible levels. The efficient cleavage of RRLL tetrapeptide is consistent with the known recognition sequences of SKI-1, including the sequence determinants involved in the cleavage of the Lassa virus (family Arenaviridae) glycoprotein precursor. Comparison of the SKI-1 cleavage efficiency between peptides representing Lassa virus GP2 and CCHFV G_N cleavage sites suggested that amino acids flanking the RRLL may modulate the efficiency. The apparent lack of SKI-1 cleavage of the CCHFV G_C RKPL site has indicated that related proteases other than SKI-1 are likely to be involved in the processing at this site and identical or similar sites used in several New World arenaviruses *(247)*.

After the complete genome sequence of the CCHFV reference strain IbAr10200 was determined, several expression plasmids were generated for the individual expression of the glycoproteins G_N and G_C, using CMV- and chicken β-actin-driven promoters *(248)*. The results of the study showed that the *N*-terminal glycoprotein G_N is localized in the Golgi complex, a process mediated by retention/targeting signal(s) in the cytoplasmic domain and ectodomain of this protein. In contrast, the *C*-terminal glycoprotein G_C remained in the endoplasmic reticulum but could be rescued into the Golgi complex by coexpression of G_N *(248)*.

23.11.1.2 Reverse Genetics

A thorough molecular analysis of CCHFV transcription/replication, protein biosynthesis, and processing would provide basic information to better understand the pathogenesis of the disease and to formulate concepts for antiviral treatment and vaccine development *(239)*. To this end, the generation of recombinant CCHFV particles based on DNA transfection (infectious clone system) would greatly promote these studies.

As of recently, a new methodology, commonly referred to as *reverse genetics*, became available and allowed the genomes of negative-stranded viruses to be genetically manipulated and infectious viruses to be rescued entirely from cloned cDNAs. Application of reverse genetics has revolutionized the analysis of viral gene expression and has enabled the dissection of regulatory sequences important for replication and transcription *(249)*. The ability to rescue infectious viruses from cloned cDNAs has by now been well established for nonsegmented, negative-strand viruses, such as members of the families Rhabdoviridae *(250, 251)*, Paramyxoviridae *(252, 253)*, and Filoviridae *(254)*. However, the development of similar methodology for manipulating the genomes and generating viruses from cloned cDNAs of segmented, negative-strand viruses, such as members of the families Bunyaviridae, Orthomyxoviridae, and Arenaviridae, have turned out to be much more difficult *(249, 255)*.

Recently, a reverse genetics technology for CCHF virus was developed *(256)* using the RNA polymerase I system *(257, 258)*. Artificial viral RNA genome segments (minigenomes) were generated that contained different reporter genes in antisense (VRNA) or sense (cRNA) orientation flanked by the noncoding regions (NCR) of the CCHFV S segment. Reporter gene expression was observed in different eukaryotic cell lines after transfection and subsequent superinfection with CCHFV confirming encapsulation, transcription, and replication of the pol I–derived minigenomes. The successful transfer of reporter gene activity to secondary uninfected cells has demonstrated the generation of recombinant CCHFV and confirmed the packaging of the pol I–derived minigenomes into progeny viruses *(256)*. The system will offer a unique opportunity to study the biology of nairoviruses and to develop therapeutic and prophylactic measures against CCHFV infections *(239)*.

23.11.1.3 Genome Reassortment

One problem common to all segmented genome viruses is the production of virus particles that package the correct genetic complement *(236)*. In the Bunyaviridae viruses, the RNAs extracted from purified virus preparations are rarely equimolecular, and the S segment usually predominates. Although it is not clear how much of the deviation from an equimolar ratio is the result of degradation of the larger RNAs during the sample preparation, it does appear that virions containing different numbers of genome segments are produced *(259)*. A potential advantage of a segmented genome is the possibility for RNA segment reassortment to occur, which could confer new and desirable genetic traits on the progeny reassortants *(236)*.

In Bunyaviridae, reassortment has been demonstrated in the laboratory between certain related viruses, but not between viruses in different genera, nor between viruses in different serogroups in the same genus. There are further restrictions on reassortment, as seen by the difficulty in obtaining reassortants with a certain genotype (e.g., Batai, Bunyamwera, and Maguari bunyaviruses) where the L and S segments appeared to cosegregate in heterologous crosses, but this linkage could be broken when heterologous reassortants were used as parental viruses *(260)*. Genome segment reassortment has also been demonstrated experimentally in dually infected mosquitoes *(261–263)*, and evidence that reassortment also occurs in nature has been obtained *(237, 238, 264, 264a)*.

To assess the genetic reassortment of Rift Valley fever virus in nature, several isolates from diverse localities in Africa were studied by reverse transcription–PCR, followed by direct sequencing of a region of the small (S), medium (M), and large (L) genomic segments *(264b)*. The phylogenetic analysis showed the existence of three major lineages corresponding with geographic variants from West Africa, Egypt, and Central-East Africa. However, incongruences detected between the L, M, and S phylogenies suggested that genetic exchange through reassortment occurred between strains from different lineages. This hypothesis depicted by parallel phylogenies was further confirmed by statistical tests. The results of the study have strongly suggested that exchanges between strains from areas of endemicity in West and East Africa strengthen the potential existence of a sylvatic cycle in the tropical rainforest and also emphasize the risk of generating uncontrolled chimeric viruses by using live-attenuated vaccines in areas of endemicity *(264b)*.

23.11.2 Epidemiology of the Crimean-Congo Hemorrhagic Fever

The Crimean-Congo hemorrhagic fever is believed to be a very old disease, described as early as the 12th century, from southeastern Russia in the region that is currently Tadzhikistan *(264c)*. The first well-documented report of CCHF was from an epidemic in the western Crimea region of Russia (currently in Ukraine) *(264d)*. Later, a similar disease was observed in Africa in 1956 *(265)*; the virus was subsequently isolated and found to be antigenically indistinguishable from the Crimean hemorrhagic fever virus *(266)*. The name Crimean-Congo hemorrhagic fever virus was suggested and commonly accepted to designate the disease *(267)*.

The known distribution of the CCHFV covers the greatest geographic range of any tick-borne virus, with reports of virus isolation and/or disease from more than 30 countries in Africa, Asia, southeastern Europe, and the Middle East *(239)*.

In general, the known occurrence of CCHFV in Europe, Asia, and Africa coincides with the world distribution of ticks of the genus *Hyalomma* (e.g., *Hyalomma marginatum*) of the Ixodidae family *(264c)*, followed by members of the genera *Rhipicephalus* and *Dermacentor*. Altogether, the virus has been isolated from at least 31 species of ticks and one species of biting midge (*Culicoides* spp.).

The natural cycle of CCHFV includes transovarial (i.e., passed through the eggs) and transstadial (i.e., passed directly from immature ticks to subsequent life stages) transmission among ticks in a tick-vertebrate-tick cycle involving a variety of wild and domestic animals. *Hyalomma* ticks normally feed on livestock (sheep, goats, and cattle), large wild herbivores, hares, and hedgehogs, which become infected with CCHFV *(264c)*. Infection in these animals generally results in an unapparent or subclinical disease but generates viremia levels capable of supporting virus transmission to uninfected ticks *(264c)*. Regarding the role of birds in the epidemiology of CCHF, it appears that birds (with the exception of ostriches) are refractory to CCHFV infection, even though they can support large numbers of CCHFV-infected ticks.

Transmission to humans can occur either through tick bites or possibly by crushing engorged infected ticks. Direct contact with virus-contaminated blood or tissues from infected animals or humans is another source of virus transmission and is generally characterized by more severe clinical symptoms and high mortality *(239, 268)*.

23.11.3 *Crimean-Congo Hemorrhagic Fever: Clinical Manifestations*

The family Bunyaviridae contains at least 41 tropical viruses that cause fever *(239)*. Some of these viruses also cause meningoencephalitis, hemorrhage, arthritis, or retinitis.

The CCHFV is associated with hemorrhages and is often fatal *(239,264c,269)*. Outbreaks of CCHF are focal in nature, and clinically they present with fever, malaise, and prostration, to severe and fatal hemorrhagic disease. The fatality rate varies from 25% to more than 75%, with most deaths occurring 5 to 14 days after the onset of illness.

Four different phases of the disease are recognized: incubation; prehemorrhagic; hemorrhagic; and convalescence.

The incubation period of the CCHFV is between 3 and 6 days in nosocomial outbreaks and 2 to 12 days in other situations *(264c)*.

The prehemorrhagic phase is characterized by a sudden onset of flu-like symptoms, including dizziness, neck pain and stiffness, myalgia, back and abdominal pain, severe headache, eye pain and photophobia, arthralgias, chills,

anorexia, sore throat, nausea, and vomiting. Neuropsychiatric changes have also been reported—patients have developed altered consciousness progressing to aggressive behavior and unconsciousness *(270)*. About 50% of the patients will develop hepatomegaly.

In moderate to severe illness, fever will last between 5 and 20 days (average, 9 days). The disease may be biphasic, with fever followed by two afebrile days, then a return of fever associated with epistaxis, petechiae, purpura, and thrombocytopenia *(239)*.

Hemorrhage often begins with blood leakage at sites of needlesticks and may become quite profuse. Shock ensues in severe cases and may be accompanied by liver failure, cerebral hemorrhage, anemia, dehydration, diarrhea, myocardial infarction, pulmonary edema, and pleural effusions *(239)*.

The convalescence phase starts 15 to 20 days after the onset of illness and is characterized by weakness, weak pulse, confusion, asthenia, alopecia, and neuralgias for 2 to 4 months *(264c)*.

Factors contributing to a fatal outcome include hemorrhage, severe dehydration, severe anemia, and shock associated with prolonged diarrhea, lung edema, myocardial infarction, and pleural effusion. Multiple organ failure is common, and liver lesions may vary from disseminated necrotic foci to massive necrosis *(218)*.

23.11.3.1 CCHF: Diagnosis, Treatment, and Prognosis

Bunyaviral fevers are commonly encountered in the tropics. Even though an early diagnosis of CCHF is very important for the disease outcome in the patient, the cause is usually left undetermined because laboratory diagnostic capabilities are lacking *(239)*. The differential diagnosis should include borreliosis, leptospirosis, and rickettsiosis. Usually the first indicators of CCHF are the clinical symptoms combined with the patient's history (e.g., tick bites, travel to endemic areas, and exposure to blood or tissue of livestock or human patients).

From the available classic and modern techniques that can be used to diagnose CCHF, the antigen capture enzyme-linked immunoassay (ELISA) seems to be the most efficient, allowing viral antigen in the patient's serum to be detected in 5 to 6 hours; however, this assay is less sensitive *(239)*. Nevertheless, ELISA is of value for the more severe CCHF cases because of higher viral titer and prolonged viremia. Recently, new immunologic assays have been reported using recombinant CCHFV nucleoprotein in an indirect fluorescent-antibody (IFA) assay as well as an ELISA assay *(271, 272)*.

Treatment options for CCHF are very limited. Currently, there is no antiviral therapy available for use in humans with CCHF. Supportive therapy still remains the major means of controlling hematologic and fluid imbalances *(239)*.

Ribavirin, an antiviral nucleoside analogue, has been found effective for inhibiting CCHFV replication *in vitro (273)* and in animal models *(274)*. Case reports have suggested that oral or intravenous administration of ribavirin has been helpful in treating human CCHF *(275–278)*. However, there are no randomized, controlled clinical studies to confirm these reports. Suggested doses for intravenous ribavirin are 30 mg/kg for one dose, then 16 mg/kg every 6 hours for 4 days; then 8 mg/kg every 8 hours for 6 days *(279)*.

Immunotherapy using passive transfer of CCHF survivor plasma (hyperimmune serum) has also been used *(280)*. Although limited in scope, these studies have suggested that the CCHF immune serum may be beneficial when administered intravenously at a dose of 250 mL over 1 to 2 hours on successive days and when given early in the infection *(280, 281)*. The beneficial effect of this treatment has been based on observed clinical improvement, but the study did not include placebo control patients.

A vaccine for CCHF derived from inactivated mouse brain has been in use in Bulgaria *(282, 283)* but is not available outside of the country. It is not clear whether the efficacy of this vaccine has been well quantified.

23.11.4 Rift Valley Fever Virus

Rift Valley fever is considered to be one of the most important viral zoonoses in Africa, and the causative viral agent was first isolated in 1931 after an outbreak with large number of aborting sheep and lamb deaths near Naivasha in the Rift Valley of Kenya. At the same time, it was noticed that people attending to the sheep simultaneously suffered from a febrile illness *(284)*. The Rift Valley fever virus (RVFV) was classified later as member of the Bunyaviridae family, genus Phlebovirus. Initially, the virus was endemic to the region, but later spread to West, Central, and southern Africa and Madagascar. In 1997, RVFV provoked a sudden and dramatic outbreak in Egypt, then in 2000 RVFV spread outside Africa to the Arabian Peninsula and caused two simultaneous outbreaks, in Yemen and Saudi Arabia *(284)*. Phylogenetic analysis indicated three major lineages for RVFV: Western Africa, Eastern/Central Africa, and Egypt. All of the strains isolated from the Arabian Peninsula and Madagascar were closely related to each other and mapped together with the Kenyan isolate. The phylogenetic studies also revealed the ability of this segmented RNA virus to exchange genetic material between isolates from different geographic areas *(264b)* (see Section 23.11.1.3).

RVHV is transmitted to ruminants and humans by the bite of infected mosquitoes. Occasionally, humans may be infected by contact with infected tissues or aerosols. Circumstantial evidence exists that infection can occur through contact with raw milk, although very rarely *(285)*.

In Africa, 23 species of mosquitoes from the genera *Aedes*, *Culex*, *Anopheles*, *Eretmapodites*, and *Mansonia* have been found to be involved in RVFV transmission. In addition, numerous strains of RVFV have been isolated from various species of biting midges (*Culicoides*), black flies (*Simuli*), and occasionally from ticks (*Rhipicephalus*). In some cases, the virus can also be transmitted mechanically *(284)*.

23.11.4.1 RVFV: Molecular Biology

Like all of the Bunyaviridae, RFFV has a tripartite single-stranded RNA genome consisting of L (large), M (medium), and S (small) segments *(284)*. The L and M segments are of negative polarity and express, respectively, the RNA-dependent RNA polymerase L and the precursor to the glycoproteins G_N and G_C. Posttranslational cleavage of this precursor protein also generates a nonstructural protein (MSm) of yet undetermined role.

The S segment of RVFV (like all other phleboviruses) uses an ambisense strategy and encodes for the nucleoprotein N in antisense and for the nonstructural protein NSs in sense orientation.

The viral genes are flanked by noncoding regions containing important *cis*-acting elements for the regulation of viral genome transcription, replication, encapsulation, and packaging into progeny virions *(284)*.

A highly efficient reverse genetics system was developed that allowed generation of recombinant RVFVs to assess the role of NSm protein in virulence in a rat model in which wild-type RVFV strain ZH501 (wt-ZH501) resulted in 100% lethal hepatic disease 2 to 3 days after infection *(286)*.

Minigenome Systems

Recently, it has become possible to genetically manipulate the genomes of negative-stranded viruses and to generate infectious virions entirely from cloned cDNAs. By using *minigenome rescue systems*, this reverse genetics technique has revolutionized the study of viral gene expression and has enabled regulatory elements required for viral transcription and replication steps to be dissected, as well identifying viral components interacting with the host cells *(249–255)* (see Section 23.11.1.2).

In a typical minigenome system, virus-like RNA (minigenome) transcripts contain an internal open reading frame (ORF) of a reporter gene in place of a viral ORF sandwiched by untranslated regions (UTRs) of viral RNA termini. The expressed minigenome RNA transcripts undergo RNA replication and transcription in the presence of coexpressed viral proteins or co-infected helper virus; the levels of reporter expression are a measure of the efficiency of minigenome RNA replication and transcription. Minigenome transcripts are expressed by either host RNA polymerase I or T7 RNA polymerase, the latter of which is often provided by vaccinia virus or Sindbis virus *(287)*.

However, in the case of RVFV, the reverse genetics system was relatively inefficient and it was not possible to clearly demonstrate whether replication did occur. For this reason, an RNA polymerase I (pol I)-driven system *(287, 288)* has been developed and found to be more efficient and functional for transcription and replication *(284, 289)*. A minigenome rescue system expressing a CAT reporter has been established to investigate the role of the noncoding regions in this process. The results of the study have shown that the L, M, and S segment-based minigenomes have driven *bona fide* transcription and replication and have expressed variable levels of CAT reporter, indicating differential promoter activities within the noncoding sequences. In addition, there was a good correlation between the relative promoter strength and the abundance of viral RNA species in RVFV-infected cells *(290)*.

The coexpression of NSs protein with L and N proteins substantially enhanced minigenome replication and transcription, suggesting that RVFV NSs protein played a critical role in the RVFV RNA synthesis *(287)*. The enhancement of the minigenome RNA synthesis by the NSs protein occurred in cells lacking α/β interferon (IFN-α/β) genes, indicating that the effect of NSs protein on minigenome RNA replication was unrelated to a putative NSs protein–induced inhibition of IFN-α/β production *(287)*. Unlike other viral IFN antagonists, NSs did not inhibit IFN-specific transcription factors but blocked the IFN gene expression at a subsequent step *(291)*.

The Interferon Response Circuit

The type I interferons (IFN-α/β) are potent antiviral cytokines and modulators of the adaptive immune system. They are induced by viral infection or by double-stranded RNA (dsRNA), a by-product of viral replication, and lead to the production of a broad range of antiviral proteins and immunoactive cytokines. However, viruses, in turn, have evolved multiple strategies or mechanisms to counter the IFN system, which would otherwise stop the virus growth early in infection, leading to a complicated balancing act between the virus-induced IFN responses and the viral escape countermeasures by suppressing IFN production, down-modulating IFN signaling, and blocking the action of antiviral effector proteins *(292)*.

Induction of type I (α/β) IFN gene expression is tightly regulated. Recent findings suggested that the cells make use of two major but distinct cellular signal transduction pathways to sense viruses and activate their type I IFN genes. Most cells in the body, including fibroblasts, hepatocytes, and conventional dendritic cells, use the *classic pathway*. Using their intracellular sensors, upon infection these cells will detect viral components in the cytoplasm and then activate the main IFN regulatory transcription factors IRF-3 and NF-κB, which in turn will transactivate the IFN-β gene expression. Infected cells secrete mainly IFN-β as an initial response to infection but would switch to IFN-α during the subsequent amplification phase of the IFN response *(293)*. In contrast, plasmacytoid dendritic cells use Toll-like receptors expressed on the cell surface or in endosomes to sense extracellular or engulfed viral material.

The IFN receptor signaling pathway is now firmly established, and IFN-β and multiple IFN-α subspecies activate a common type I IFN receptor (IFNAR), which sends a signal to the nucleus through the so-called JAK-STAT pathway *(292, 294)*.

Type I IFNs activate the expression of several hundred IFN-stimulated genes *(295)*, some of which code for antiviral proteins via three antiviral pathways: the protein kinase R, the 2,5-OAS/RNasel system, and the Mx proteins *(292)*.

23.11.4.2   Pathogenesis and Immune Response

The RVFV affects primarily the liver, with rapid hepatocellular changes progressing to massive necrosis. Hepatic necrosis and vasculitis are the most characteristic microscopic lesions of RVFV in domestic animals and humans *(284)*. A profound leukopenia, elevated serum enzymes associated with severe liver damage, and thrombocytopenia are strongly associated with the development of the hemorrhagic state *(296)*. It is likely that the virus is transported from the inoculation site to the lymph nodes by lymphatic drainage. Once in the lymph nodes, the virus replicates and is spread into the circulation to produce primary viremia, leading to infection of the target organs *(284)*. In addition, RVFV replicates in hepatocytes in the liver and in the walls of small vessels (adrenocortical cell and glomeruli of the kidney).

As with most viral infections, RVFV is expected to induce both adaptive and innate immune responses *(284)*. It is a common feature of bunyavirus infections that the antibody response plays an important role in protection. Antibodies are raised against the internal nucleoprotein (the major immunogen) and the surface glucoproteins G_N and G_C, which carry neutralizing epitopes *(297)*.

With respect to innate immunity, major studies have been carried out on the virulence of the nonstructural protein NSs, which antagonizes the antiviral response by blocking type I interferon production *(298)*. As a general inhibitor of transcription, NSs must have a wide range of action on cellular transcription by not only inhibiting the antiviral response and preventing the synthesis of IFN-β but also by affecting the transcriptional activity in response to hormonal stimuli *(284)*.

Infection with RVFV leads to a rapid and drastic suppression of host cellular RNA synthesis that parallels a decrease in the transcription factor II H (TFIIH) cellular concentration *(299)*. It was further found that the nonstructural viral protein NSs interacts with the p44 component of TFIIH to form nuclear filamentous structures that also contain the XPB subunit of TFIIH. By competing with XPD (the natural partner of p44 within TFIIH), and sequestering the p44 and XPB subunits, NSs prevented the assembly of the TFIIH subunits, thus destabilizing the normal host cell life *(299)*. These observations shed light on the mechanism used by the RVFV to evade the host response.

23.11.4.3 Clinical Manifestations

The incubation period of the disease varies from 2 to 6 days. The symptoms include an influenza-like illness, headache, myalgia, and backache. Some patients will present with neck stiffness, photophobia, and vomiting. The symptoms of Rift Valley fever (RVF) usually last from 4 to 7 days, after which time the immune response becomes detectable with the appearance of IgM and IgG antibodies, and the disappearance of circulating virus from the bloodstream (http://www.who.int/mediacente/factsheets/fs207/en).

Whereas most human cases are relatively mild, a small proportion of patients (0.5% to 2%) may develop a much more severe illness characterized with several recognizable syndromes: eye disease (retinal lesions), meningoencephalitis, or hemorrhagic fever (severe liver disease, jaundice, vomiting blood, passing blood in the feces, purpuric rash, and bleeding from the gums). The case-fatality rate from hemorrhagic disease is about 50% (http://www.who.int/mediacente/factsheets/fs207/en).

23.11.4.4 Treatment

Because most human cases of RVF are relatively mild and of short duration, they will not require any specific treatment.

Concerning treatment, it has been shown that administrations of antibodies, interferon, interferon inducer, or ribavirin in experimentally RVFV-infected mice, rats, and monkeys have exerted protective effects against the disease *(300)*. However, these treatments have never been tested to treat RVFV infection in humans.

An inactivated vaccine has been developed for human use. Although the vaccine has been used to protect veterinary and laboratory personnel at high risk of exposure to RVF, it is not licensed and not available commercially. Other candidate vaccines are under investigation.

23.11.5 Hantaviruses

Hantaviruses are trisegmented, negative-strand RNA viruses that belong to the family Bunyaviridae *(301)*. Unlike other viruses of the same family, in nature, the hantaviruses do not have an arthropod vector but are exclusively maintained in the population of their specific rodent hosts *(302)*. In their natural host species, hantaviruses usually develop a persistent infection with prolonged virus shedding in excreta. Humans become infected by inhaling virus-contaminated aerosol, but unlike the asymptomatic infection in rodents, in humans the hantaviruses are the etiologic agents of two acute febrile diseases: hemorrhagic fever with renal syndrome (HFRS) and hantavirus pulmonary syndrome (HPS) *(303, 304)*. The mortality rate varies from 0.1% to 40% depending on the virus involved.

Both HFRS and HPS appear to be immunopathologic, and inflammatory mediators are important in causing the clinical manifestations. In HPS, T cells act on heavily infected pulmonary endothelium, and both IFN-γ and TFN-α are major agents of a reversible increase in vascular permeability that leads to severe, noncardiogenic pulmonary edema. HFRS has prominent systemic manifestations in which the retroperitoneum is a major site of vascular leak and the kidneys suffer tubular necrosis. Both syndromes are accompanied by myocardial depression and hypotension or shock *(304)*.

While HFRS is primarily a Eurasian disease, HPS appears to be confined to the Americas. These geographic distinctions correlate with the phylogenies of the rodent hosts and the viruses that co-evolved with them.

23.11.5.1 Hantavirus Genome

The Hantavirus genome consists of large (L), medium (M), and small (S) segments that code for the viral RNA-dependent RNA polymerase (RdRp), the glycoprotein precursor (GPC) of two envelope glycoproteins (G1 and G2), and the nucleocapsid protein (N), respectively. In the virion, the viral RNA is complexed with the multiple N protein molecules to form individual L, M, and S ribonucleocapsid structures. Furthermore, the nucleocapsids and RdRp are packaged within a lipid envelope that is embedded with viral glycoproteins. Each virion usually contains equimolar amounts of the three genomic viral RNAs *(305)*.

Nucleocapsid Protein

The nucleocapsid (N) protein is the most abundant Hantavirus protein synthesized early after infection, and similarly to other Bunyaviridae viruses, it is central to virus replication. It may also protect newly synthesized viral RNA (vRNA) from nuclease degradation as well as play a role in preventing intrastrand base pairing within the vRNA template *(301)*. The N protein binds to membranes and vRNAs, associates with transcription and replication complexes, and oligomerizes during the process of virus assembly. The pathway of Hantavirus nucleocapsid oligomerization involves helix bundling or alternative amino-terminal coiled-coil conformation *(306)*.

In addition, recent studies provided evidence that the N protein can interact with host cell proteins. Although the nature of this interaction is unclear, it may be hypothesized that it is important for virus replication by blocking the inhibitory action of the host cell antiviral proteins and preventing infected cell apoptosis *(301)*.

Glycoproteins

The Hantavirus glycoproteins precursor (GPC) is synthesized in the ribosomes bound to the endoplasmic reticulum (ER) *(307)*. The GPC is then translocated into the ER lumen and is co-translationally cleaved. Two glycoproteins (G1 and G2) are generated by posttranslational cleavage of GPC at the conserved amino acid sequence WAASA *(308)*, and G1 and G2 are glycosylated to form heterodimers that constitute a Golgi retention signal. However, for Golgi translocation of the glycoproteins, they have to be coexpressed *(308)*, resulting in the formation of a G1/G2 complex. In the Golgi, G1/G2 complexes complete maturation and become ready for virus assembly *(309)*.

The G1 and G2 glycoproteins are known to mediate cell attachment and fusion *(310–312)*. It has been demonstrated that the hantaviruses use integrin receptors for cell attachment. Thus, β_3 integrins, which regulate vascular permeability and platelet function and are present on the surfaces of platelets, endothelial cells, and macrophages, facilitate the cellular entry of HFRS-associated hantaviruses *(313)*.

Viral RNA–Dependent RNA Polymerase (RdRp)

Hantavirus RNA-dependent RNA polymerase (RdRp) mediates transcription and replication. Therefore, it has been suggested that RdRp should have endonuclease, transcriptase, replicase, and possibly RNA-helicase activities *(301)*. Shortly after virion entry, RdRp initiates transcription and uncoating *(314)*.

23.11.5.2   Hantaviruses and Their Diseases

It is well known that, in general, the geographic distribution and epidemiology of hantaviruses reflect the distribution and natural history of their primary rodent hosts. To this end, there are several distinct, regional hantaviruses:

(i)   Hantaan virus or Korean hemorrhagic virus (also known as epidemic hemorrhagic fever), found in Asia; etiologic agent of HFRS.

(ii) Seoul virus, associated with domestic rats, and causing HFRS.

(iii) Sin Nombre virus (previously known as Muerto canyon virus and Four Corners virus), found in the United States, and causing Hantavirus-associated respiratory/pulmonary syndrome (HARDS).

(iv) Puumala virus, found in Scandinavia, Europe, and western Russia.

(v)   Dobrava or Belgrade virus, found in Eastern Europe; etiologic agent of HPS.

(vi) Baltimore rat virus or New York virus, a fairly unrecognized form that is suspected of causing chronic renal disease and/or hypertension, as well as HPS.

In addition, other serologically distinct viruses causing human disease have been identified, including [*Note: human disease and geographic distribution given in parenthesis*]: Amur virus (HFRS; Siberia, Far East, Russia), Dobrava-like virus (HFRS; Europe, Northern Caucasus), Andes virus (HPS; South America: Argentina and Chile), Lechiguanas virus (HPS; South America: Argentina), Oran virus or "Andes-Nort" virus (HPS; South America), Laguna Negra virus (HPS; South America), Choclo virus (HPS; South America), and Araucaria virus (HPS; South America: Brazil).

Although hantavirus diseases are associated with seasonal changes that coincide with the life cycle of the host rodents, the greater incidence of HFRS cases occur in rural areas among farmers, forest workers, military personnel, and so forth, and always coincides with increased human agricultural activities in spring and autumn.

No vectors have been shown to be involved in the Hantavirus transmission cycle. It is believed that infection is spread horizontally by inhaling virus-contaminated aerosol, and very rarely through bites. Infectious virus is shed in the rodent's saliva, urine, and feces, possibly throughout the rest of its life.

With the exception of the Andes virus, there is no evidence of human-to-human transmission of Hantavirus. In fact, human-to-human transmission has not been confirmed with the Andes virus, but the pattern of infection implied a human vector (http://www.cdc.gov/ncidod/EID/vol11no12/05-0501.htm).

Some of the known rodent vectors associated with human disease include *Apodemus agrarius*—Asian subspecies (Hantaan virus), *A. flavicollis* and *A. agrarius* (Dobrava virus), *A. ponticus* (Dobrava-like virus), *Rattus norvegicus* (Seoul virus), *Clethrionomys glareolus* (Puumala virus), *Peromyscus maniculatus*—grassland subspecies (Sin Nombre virus), *P. maniculatus*—forest species (Monongahela virus), *Oligoryzomys longicaudatus* (Argentina), and *Calomys laucha* (Choclo virus).

Genome segment reassortment is one of the important ways used by segmented viruses to achieve high infectivity and adaptation to new animal species *(315–317)*. Thus, preferential reassortment with homologous L-M and L-S segments has been described for many viruses of the Bunyaviridae family *(318–320)*.

23.11.5.3 Pathogenesis and Immune Responses to Hantavirus Diseases

Currently, there is no single factor identified to explain the complexity of the pathogenesis of HFRS and HPS *(301)*. Most likely, the Hantavirus pathogenesis is a multifunctional process involving mainly endothelial cell damage, immune effectors, cytokines, and chemokines *(321, 322)*.

Immune complexes (ICs) were found in the HFRS serum before Hantavirus-specific antibodies could be detected. The levels of ICs gradually increase during the febrile, oliguric, and polyuric phases of HFRS, and then usually decline during the convalescent phase of the disease. However, it is still not clear whether the levels of serum ICs correlate with the severity of clinical manifestations *(323, 324)*. Furthermore, electron microscopic studies of kidney biopsies collected 3 days after the onset of HFRS revealed C3 complement component and IgM deposits along the basal capillary membrane of the glomeruli, and in the interstitial tissue of kidney later during HFRS *(325, 326)*. The morphologic hallmarks of ICs-mediated tissue injury are necrosis and predominately neutrophil-composed cellular infiltrates.

Classic and alternative pathways of complement activation are induced in HFRS patients, and the severity of the disease correlates with the degree of complement activation *(301)*. Increased serum levels of activated C1 complement component were found in HFRS patients 5 to 6 days after the onset of disease, and its presence coincides with manifestations of the hemorrhagic syndrome, proteinuria, and shock *(327)*. A number of studies have suggested that the nature of ICs formed during HFRS (in particular, ICs containing IgG1 and IgG3 subclass antibody) may contribute to complement activation and prolonged ICs circulation in the blood *(301)*.

B-Cell Immune Responses

HFRS and HPS patients have manifested with high levels of Hantavirus IgM detected simultaneously with the onset of clinical symptoms. The IgM antibodies were directed against all three of the structural proteins of Hantavirus *(328)*. The IgM levels declined during the convalescent stage of the

disease, which usually coincides with the rise of Hantavirus IgG *(301)*.

In general, the IgG subclass responses are comparable for both HFRS and HPS patients. The Hantavirus induces an early IgG1 response that increases with the progression of the disease, with antibody titers higher against the G1 and G2 glycoproteins than against the N protein *(301)*.

The neutralizing IgA response is most important in the development of mucosal immunity, especially in recovery from acute infection and long-term immunity. The mechanism of antiviral IgA protection remains unclear, although some evidence suggests that it may interfere with the replication of the virus by binding to newly synthesized viral proteins within infected cells and neutralizing the virus intracellularly *(329)*.

Hantavirus infection has been shown to significantly increase the serum levels of IgE compared with that of other viral diseases, such as influenza, cytomegalovirus, and Epstein-Barr virus *(330)*.

T-Cell Responses

Detection of virus strain–specific cytotoxic T-lymphocytes (CTL) in the blood of convalescent donors suggests that CTL plays an important role in the pathogenesis of hantaviruses. The Hantavirus N protein is believed to be the major antigen activating the CTL response *(331, 332)*. Although the importance of virus-specific CD8$^+$ CTL for clearance of the virus and recovery is well recognized, virus clearance by the CD8$^+$ CTL has often been associated with apoptosis of infected cells and tissue damage. In fact, viral clearance and tissue injury (destruction of infected endothelial cells) are believed to be two interrelated consequences of the cellular immune response *(332, 333)*.

CTL can control virus infections and induce disease pathogenesis by secreting cytokines such as IFN-γ and TFN-α *(334, 335)*. Cytokines play a major role in facilitating the CD8$^+$ CTL cytotoxic activity, and the cytokine profile [as a function of the particular viral epitope *(336)*] may contribute to the lung injury. Furthermore, proinflammatory cytokines secreted by activated CD8$^+$ T-cells can attract inflammatory cells to the site of infection and activate parenchymal cells to release more chemokines, such as IP-10 and Mig *(337)*, and monocyte chemotactic protein-1 (MCP-1) and the macrophage inflammatory protein-2 *(338)*.

23.11.5.4 Hantavirus Hemorrhagic Fever with Renal Syndrome

Epidemiology

HFRS (also known as the *Korean hemorrhagic fever*, epidemic nephrosonephritis, nephropathica epidemica, Hantaan fever, Hantaan hemorrhagic fever, and Songo fever) caused by the hantaviruses is a major public health problem, with hundred of thousands of cases annually in Asia (China, Korea, and eastern Russia) and Europe (Scandinavia, western Europe, the Balkans, and western Russia).

The Korean hemorrhagic fever, caused by a Hantavirus infection, first attracted attention during and after the Korean War (1951–1953), when more than 3,000 U.S. and Korean soldiers fell severely ill with an infectious disease characterized by renal failure, generalized hemorrhage, and shock, and with a mortality rate over 10%. The causative agent was first isolated in 1976 from the lungs of the striped field mouse, *Apodemus agrarius*, and designated as the Hantaan virus *(339, 340)*.

The incidence of HFRS in the United States is not very well known. The most likely etiologic agent is the Seoul virus (vector: *Rattus norvegicus*), which causes mild to moderately severe HFRS in Asia and is the only Hantavirus associated with urban disease *(303, 304)*. The rodent and its virus have been spread around the world by maritime commerce. The prevalence of antibodies in inner city residences in the United States has been estimated to be about 1% or less, with only several acute cases suggestive of Seoul virus being reported *(341)*. Other North American hantaviruses from voles (e.g., *Microtus pennsylvanicus*) have not yet been implicated as causes of HFRS *(303, 304)*.

Clinical Manifestations of HFRS

Symptoms of HFRS usually occur between 1 and 6 weeks after exposure to the virus. The initial onset is marked by nonspecific flu-like symptoms: fever, myalgia, headache, abdominal pain, nausea, and vomiting. There is a characteristic facial flushing, and usually a petechial rash (mainly limited to the axilla or the armpits). Sudden and extreme albuminuria will occur about day 4; this is characteristic of severe HFRS. Ecchymosis also occurs, and commonly, scleral injection and bloodshot eyes. Additional symptoms may include hypotension, shock, respiratory distress and/or failure, and renal impairment and/or failure. *Damage to the renal medulla is characteristic and unique for the hantaviruses.*

There are five phases of HFRS, although any one or more of these stages may not be apparent *(304)*:

(i) *Febrile*—lasting 3 to 5 days; it may often include the initial symptoms of the disease: thirst, nausea and vomiting, abdominal pain, blurred vision and photophobia, characteristic flushing of the face and the V-area of the neck and thorax, conjunctival suffusion, and periorbital edema.

(ii) *Hypotensive*—lasting for a few hours to 2 days; nausea and vomiting are common, thrombocytopenia

is almost universal, and laboratory evidence of disseminated intravascular coagulation is common. The blood pressure then falls, perhaps with severe or fatal shock. One-third of the deaths will occur at this stage.

(iii) *Oliguric*—lasting from few days to 2 weeks; marked polymorphonuclear leukocytosis with a left shift is typically present, and $CD8^+$-activated T cells appear on the peripheral blood smear as atypical lymphocytes. Proteinuria is marked and the urine-specific gravity falls to 1.010, followed by oliguria. CNS manifestations (obtundation or coma) may be present either from the disease process or from metabolic disturbances. Hemorrhagic tendencies continue, including ecchymoses and mucous membrane hemorrhages. Half of all deaths occur during this stage.

(iv) *Polyuric/diuretic*—renal function returns within a few days to 2 weeks but the subsequent polyuria and hyposthenuria pose new problems in fluid and electrolyte management. Death can still occur from shock or pulmonary complications.

(v) *Convalescent*—fluid and electrolyte imbalance still exist and can last weeks or months.

The more severe cases of HFRS are usually caused by the Hantaan virus infections in Asia or Dobrava virus infection in the Balkans *(341a, 341b)*, both of which have a case fatality rate of 5–15%. The milder cases of HFRS (caused generally by the Seoul or Puumala viruses) usually do not display the full spectrum of clinical manifestations and have a case fatality of less than 1% *(304)*.

Management of HFRS

Successful treatment of HFRS begins with prompt diagnosis. Shock is usually managed with the administration of pressors and judicious administration of fluids—1 to 2 fluid units of human serum albumin is thought to be a useful adjunct *(304)*. Dialysis reduces the mortality rate from 5% to 15% to less than 5% and should begin promptly to treat hyperkalemia, volume overexpression, or uremia. Furthermore, volume adjustment is particularly important because pulmonary edema and intracerebral hemorrhage are two major causes of death in the oliguric phase of the disease. Later, diuresis of large volumes of isosthenuric urine will lead to potentially fatal volume and electrolyte abnormalities *(304)*.

Intravenous ribavirin, when given within the first 4 days of onset, has been shown to lessen renal failure, decrease the bleeding manifestations, and decrease the case fatality rate in a Chinese setting in which dialysis and other supportive measures were less available *(342, 343)*.

The classic Salk-type Hantavirus vaccines have been widely and successfully used for a number of years in Korea and China. Meanwhile, more sophisticated recombinant and DNA vaccines are being developed in Europe and North America, but none has entered the market *(344)*. In addition to cloning sequences for Hantavirus genomes for diagnostic purposes, researchers at the U.S. Army Medical Research Institute of Infectious Diseases (USAMRIID) have constructed and engineered a vaccine for Hantaan virus that expresses the virus M gene products, G1 and G2 *(344a)*. Other vaccine developments include testing of suckling mouse and suckling rat brain vaccines in North and South Korea *(345)*, as well as other inactivated vaccines *(346)*.

23.11.5.5 Hantavirus Pulmonary Syndrome

Epidemiology

The initial association of HPS was with the Sin Nombre virus and its rodent reservoir, the deer mouse (*Peromyscus maniculatus*). Later, HPS cases were identified outside the range of the deer mouse, and the Bayou, Black Creek Canal, and the New York viruses have been implicated as the etiologic agents of HPS; each apparently infects a distinctive species of rodents *(304)*. Although the number of these recognized HPS cases is small, there may be more prominent component of renal failure in the Bayou and Black Creek Canal infections *(347–350)*.

Studies in South America have also identified an increasing number of viruses that cause HPS in humans, but only chronic asymptomatic infections in rodents of the Sigmodontinae subfamily of the family Muridae *(351)*. The actual incidence of HPS in South America is not known, but local epidemics and sporadic cases have been reported in several countries *(304)*.

Human-to-human transmission has not been recognized in any Hantavirus disease, with exception of a single HPS epidemic caused by the Andes virus in Argentina in 1996 *(352, 353)*. A combination of human epidemiology, rodent studies, and molecular genetics of the virus has established the transmission.

Clinical Manifestations of HPS

The HPS is primarily a lung infection, with the kidneys largely unaffected. The initial manifestations of HPS include mainly flu-like symptoms: fever, myalgia, headache, and cough; other symptoms can include chills, abdominal pain, diarrhea, and malaise. However, cardiopulmonary dysfunction, ranging from mild hypoxemia with stable hemodynamics to rapidly progressive respiratory failure with cardiogenic

shock, is the hallmark of patients with fully developed HPS *(304, 351)*. The disease progresses rapidly. Eventually, the patients experience thrombocytopenia, hypoxemia, and interstitial pulmonary edema concurrently with hypotension, shock, and respiratory distress followed by respiratory failure. Most patients infected with Sin Nombre virus will die within few days of onset of symptoms.

Patients with severe pulmonary edema have copious, amber-colored, nonpurulent pulmonary secretions associated with diffuse pulmonary infiltrates on chest radiograph.

The average duration of HPS prior to hospitalization is 3 to 4 days, and in those patients who deteriorated, the usual time until death was an additional 1 to 3 days, although patients can die within hours of admission. Severe cardiopulmonary dysfunction predicts a poor prognosis in HPS, with myocardial depression leading to shock and severe oxygen deficiency dominating the hemodynamic picture *(304)*.

There has been a general absence of associated multiple organ failure, renal failure, or hepatic failure in Sin Nombre virus infections.

Management of HPS

During diagnosis, HPS is commonly confused with acute respiratory distress syndrome from other infectious pathogens, pyelonephritis, intra-abdominal processes, pneumonias, and systemic infections such as rickettsial disease or plague. Therefore, early diagnosis for optimal management is paramount.

No instance of person-to-person transmission of HPS has been reported in the United States. Respiratory isolation of suspected cases is well warranted, because pneumonic plague is in the differential diagnosis of HPS.

In general, the Sin Nombre and Black Creek Canal viruses were found to be sensitive *in vitro* to ribavirin. However, its efficacy in HPS cases is uncertain. Thus, a small number of patients with HPS has been treated with intravenous ribavirin in open-label protocol. Although the results of the trial showed 47% mortality rate in the ribavirin recipients compared with 50% in nontreated patients *(304)*, data should be interpreted with caution because most of the untreated patients were either ill during the early phase of the epidemic or presented in nonepidemic areas where the diagnosis may have been delayed.

Placement of a flow-directed pulmonary artery catheter for continuous measurement of cardiac output may be beneficial early in the clinical course. In addition, maintenance of low-normal pulmonary wedge pressures, compatible with satisfactory cardiac indices, is recommended because of the extreme capillary leak. Inotropic agents such as dobutamine, dopamine, and noradrenaline should be used earlier in the treatment of shock in HPS patients than in patients with bacterial sepsis, together with judicious intravascular volume expansion with packed red blood cells to maintain delivery of oxygen if hemoglobin concentration falls *(304)*.

23.11.5.6 Baltimore Rat Virus

Disease caused by the Baltimore rat virus is characterized by acute onset of nausea, vomiting, fever, upper abdominal pain, protein in the urine, and hypertension. In some cases, liver and renal involvement occurs. Patients suffer fever, then 1 to 2 days of hypotension, followed by renal failure with liver enzyme derangements. Survivors can experience chronic renal impairment and disease.

23.12 Viral Hemorrhagic Fever: Arenaviruses

The Arenaviridae is a family of viruses whose members are generally associated with rodent-transmitted disease in humans. Each Arenavirus is usually associated with a particular rodent host species in which it is maintained. Arenavirus infections are relatively common in humans in some regions of the world and can cause severe illness (http://www.cdc.gov/ncidod/dvrd/spb/mnpages/dispages/arena.htm).

The family Arenaviridae consists of a single genus, Arenavirus, in which two serotypes are recognized: *LCM/Lassa complex (Old World arenaviruses)*, and *Tacaribe complex (New World arenaviruses)* (Table 23.3).

The first Arenavirus, the lymphocytic choriomeningitis virus (LCMV), was isolated in 1933 during a study of an epidemic of St. Louis encephalitis. By the 1960s, several similar viruses had been discovered and were all classified into a new family, Arenaviridae. Since Tacaribe virus was found in 1956, new arenaviruses have been identified every 1 to 3 years, on average. A number of these viruses are pathogenic to humans, causing hemorrhagic disease. The Junin virus, isolated in 1958, was the first of these to be recognized; it causes the Argentine hemorrhagic fever. In 1963, the Machupo virus, which causes the Bolivian hemorrhagic fever, was isolated, followed in 1969 by the Lassa virus in Africa. Most recently, the Guanarito and Sabia viruses, which cause the Venezuelan and Brazilian hemorrhagic fevers, respectively, were added to the family (http://www.cdc.gov/ncidod/dvrd/spb/mnpages/dispages/arena.htm).

The Junin, Machupo, Guanarito, and Sabia viruses, known to cause severe hemorrhagic fever, are included in the Category A Pathogen List as defined by the CDC and are listed as Biosafety Level 4 (BSL-4) agents *(279)*.

The hosts of arenaviruses are rodents: *Mastomys natalensis* for Lassa virus; *Mus musculus* for LCMV; *Calomys musculinus* for the Junin virus; *C. callosus* for the Machupo virus; *Zygodontomys brevicauda* and *Sigmodon alstoni* for the Guanarito virus, and *Neotoma* rodents for the Whitewater Arroyo virus. Transfer to humans occurs via contact with infected rodents or inhalation of infectious rodent excreta or secreta. The arenaviruses do not require arthropods for spread and do not infect insect cells. Hence, the human infection is *zoonotic*; that is, transmission is from animals to humans.

The Arenavirus particles are spherical to pleomorphic with a diameter ranging from 50 to 300 nm (average, 120 nm) *(354)*. They possess a dense lipid-containing envelope with 8- to 10-nm-long, club-shaped projections. When viewed in

Table 23.3 Arenaviruses (region of isolation is listed in parenthesis)

LCM/Lassa complex (Old World arenaviruses)	Tacaribe complex (New World arenaviruses)
Ippy virus (Central African Republic)	Amapari virus (Brazil)
Lassa virus (Lassa, Nigeria)[1]	Flexal virus (Brazil)
Lymphocytic choriomeningitis virus; LCMV (Missouri)[2]	Guanarito virus (Venezuela)[3]
Mobala virus (Central African Republic)	Junin virus (Argentina)[4]
Mopeia virus (Mozambique)	Machupo virus (Bolivia-Beni region)[5]
SPH 114202 virus	Parana virus (Paraguay)
	Pichinde virus (Colombia)
	Tacaribe virus (Trinidad)
	Sabia virus (Brazil)[6]
	Latino virus (Bolivia)
	Oliveros virus (Argentina)
	Pirital virus (Venezuela)
	Whitewater Arroyo virus (New Mexico)
	Tamiami virus (Florida)

[1]Pathogenic to humans: Lassa fever.
[2]Pathogenic to humans: lymphocytic choriomeningitis/aseptic (nonbacterial) meningitis.
[3]Pathogenic to humans: Venezuelan hemorrhagic fever.
[4]Pathogenic to humans: Argentine hemorrhagic fever.
[5]Pathogenic to humans: Bolivian hemorrhagic fever.
[6]Pathogenic to humans: Brazilian hemorrhagic fever.

cross section, the arenaviruses show grainy particles, which are ribosomes (20 to 25 nm) acquired from their host cells during the budding process (their function is still not yet understood). It is this characteristic that gave them their name (from the Latin *arenosus* meaning *sandy*).

The viruses are quickly inactivated at 56°C, at pH below 5.5 or above 8.5, or by exposure to UV and/or gamma irradiation.

23.12.1 Genome Structure of Arenaviruses

The arenaviruses possess a single-stranded RNA genome consisting of two segments: L (large, ∼ 5.7 kb) and S (small, ∼ 2.8 kb). Each segment forms a circle by hydrogen bonding of its ends. The naked genome is noninfectious. The negative-sense RNA is neither capped nor polyadenylated and is contained in a helical nucleocapsid that comprises two proteins: nucleocapsid (N) and RNA polymerase (L). The L segment encodes the L and Z proteins. The S segment's 5′ part is (+) sense and encodes the N protein; its 3′ part is (−) sense and encodes the G protein.

The envelope contains two glycoprotein spikes: GP1 and GP2. One unique property of the genomes of arenaviruses is their *ambisense* organization.

The most important viral antigens are the nucleoproteins and the glycoproteins, with the nucleoprotein antigens being the most conserved among the arenaviruses.

The replication of the arenaviruses involves two rounds of transcription—one before and one after the formation of the "reverse-sense" RNA intermediate, to cope with the ambisense coding strategy.

Ambisense Organization. Historically, the RNA viruses are classified based on the ability of their naked nucleic acid (RNA separated from the other viral components) to induce a lytic action. The procedure of transforming cells with viral nucleic acid is known as *transfection*. Eventually, it has been demonstrated that the ability to productively transfect a cell corresponded to the "sense" or polarity of the RNA. Viruses (such as the polio virus) whose genomes consist of message-sense (+, or positive sense) single-stranded RNA were the only ones found to be able to productively transfect permissive cells. The other viruses (such as influenza) were shown to have genomes that contained the complement to mRNA. In most cases, the missing factor was the absence of the viral polymerase that allowed the complementary RNA to be transcribed into message (http://virus.stanford.edu/arena/ambisense.htm).

Several complications with this classification system have arisen: (i) the retroviruses have been shown to contain a genome with single-stranded message-sense RNA that was not infectious. They require reverse transcriptase in order to

carry out their complicated replication cycle. (ii) An analogous complication is the sense of the reoviruses, which contain message-sense RNA as part of their double-stranded genome. Enzymatic separation of the strands using a viral protein may be essential for translation. (iii) Some negative ssRNAs (the ssRNA is not infectious) were shown to display *ambisense*. Ambisense is a situation in which both the genome and its complement contain some coding information. Because translation *always* occurs in the 5′–3′ direction, the two strands are being translated in opposite directions, and because each strand has regions of + and − polarity, the viral organization/capability is defined as ambisense. Nevertheless, even though ambisense organization is seen in the arenaviruses (and also in the Bunyaviridae family's phleboviruses and tospoviruses), it is still convenient to classify the arenaviruses with the negative ssRNA viruses because they resemble them in both virion structure and infectivity (http://virus.stanford.edu/arena/ambisense.htm).

23.12.2 Human Significance of Arenaviruses

All South American arenaviruses were identified during the second half of the 20th century. However the arenaviruses seem to be quite ancient and have existed in nature for years as silent zoonotic foci *(354)*.

There have never been any reports of human-to-human transmission of LCMV. However, Machupo virus has clearly been responsible for severe nosocomial outbreaks, in which all cases were associated with a single index case that had returned from an endemic region *(354, 355)*. The common features of the reported nosocomial outbreaks include (i) the index case was critically ill and died; (ii) aerosol spread was the most likely explanation for the route of infection of at least some of the secondary cases; (iii) lethality was high; and (iv) transmission ceased after the secondary or tertiary cases *(354)*.

The case-fatality rate of the *Argentine hemorrhagic fever (AHF)* is approximately 20% in the absence of specific therapy. AHF is typically a seasonal disease with a peak of frequency occurring during the corn harvest (March to June). However, since the late 1980s, the epidemiology of AHF has been dramatically modified by the development of live-attenuated vaccine *(354)*.

The *Bolivian hemorrhagic fever (BHF)* was responsible for a large outbreak with a case-fatality rate of about 20% *(355)*. Most of the recorded infections were acquired by direct contact with rodents or by aerosol through infected excreta *(354)*.

The *Venezuelan hemorrhagic fever (VHF)* was recognized in 1989 and currently about 200 cases have been confirmed *(356)*. The number of reported human cases dropped between 1992 and 2002 despite the continuous circulation of the virus in the rodent population during this period. However, a new outbreak was observed in 2002. The reason(s) for this hiatus and the secondary re-emergence of the disease are unknown *(354)*.

Very little is known about the health consequences of human infections with arenaviruses other than Junin, Machupo, Guanarito, Sabia, and LCMV *(354)*.

Pichinde virus has resulted in numerous seroconversions without any notable clinical significance *(357)*.

The Flexal and Tacaribe viruses have caused febrile illnesses in laboratory workers *(357–359)*. The Flexal virus has caused two symptomatic laboratory infections and should be considered as potentially dangerous *(358, 359)*.

Tacaribe virus has resulted in a single case of febrile illness with mild central nervous system symptoms *(358)*.

In 1999 and 2000, three fatal cases of illness were reported in California, and their association with the Whitewater Arroyo virus was based on PCR and sequencing results *(360)*. The patients infected with the Whitewater Arroyo virus were healthy prior to the viral infection and there was no history of travel outside California during the 4 weeks preceding the illness. In one of the cases, the virus was probably acquired via the aerosol pathway during the removal of rodent droppings from the home.

23.12.3   Transferrin Receptor 1

At least five arenaviruses cause viral hemorrhagic fever in humans. One of these pathogens, the Lassa virus (an Old World Arenavirus), together with the lymphocytic choriomeningitis virus (LCMV) use the cellular receptor α-dystroglycan as the host cellular receptor to infect cells *(361)*. The South American hemorrhagic fever viruses (New World arenaviruses), the Machupo, Guanarito, Junin, and Sabia viruses, do not use the α-dystroglycan receptor. Instead, a specific, high-affinity association between the transferring receptor 1 (TfR1) and the entry glycoprotein (GP) of the Machupo virus has recently been established, demonstrating that TfR1 is the host cellular receptor of the four South American arenaviruses *(362)*. In addition, it has also been shown that expression of TfR1 in hamster cell lines efficiently enhanced the entry of retroviruses expressing the GP of the Machupo virus. Expression of transferring receptor 2 (TfR2) in the same cell lines did not promote Arenavirus infection. This confirmed that TfR1 is a necessary cellular receptor for all New World arenaviruses, and anti-TfR1 antibody was shown to efficiently inhibit infection in all cases *(362)*.

As TfR1 is normally involved in the cellular iron transport, further experiments have been directed at studying the effect of iron on the Arenavirus infection process. When the cell culture medium was depleted of iron, which is known to upregulate the expression of TfR1, there has been a significant enhancement in the efficiency of infection by both the Junin and Machupo viruses. Conversely, supplementation of the medium with iron (and the subsequent downregulation of TfR1 expression) inhibited the Junin and Machupo virus infection *(362)*.

Several properties of TfR1 indicated its possible role in arenaviral replication and disease. Thus, TfR1 was rapidly and constitutively endocytosed to an acidic compartment, which is consistent with the pH dependence of Arenavirus entry *(363)*. Further, it is expressed ubiquitously and at high levels on activated or rapidly dividing cells, including macrophages and activated lymphocytes, major targets of arenaviral infection *(364, 365)*. TfR1 has also been highly expressed on endothelial cells *(366, 367)*, which are thought to be central to the pathogenesis of hemorrhagic fever *(368)*.

TfR1 is a homodimeric type II transmembrane protein comprising a small cytoplasmic domain, a single-pass transmembrane region, and a large extracellular domain. The crystal structure of the butterfly-shaped dimeric TfR1 ectodomain showed that each monomer has three structurally distinct domains: a protease-like domain proximal to the membrane, a helical domain accounting for all the dimer contacts, and a membrane-distal apical domain *(369)*.

Although much is understood of the transferring endocytotic cycle, little has been uncovered of the molecular details underlying the formation of the TfR1 receptor-transferrin complex. Using cryoelectron microscopy, a density map of the TfR1-transferrin complex at subnanometer resolution has recently been produced *(370)*.

The role of iron in this process, the possible consequences of iron deficiency, and the therapeutic potential of a humanized anti-TfR1 antibody remain important directions for future research *(362)*. To this end, several anti-human TfR1 antibodies have already been developed and are currently being investigated as antitumor therapeutics *(365)*. Some of these antibodies, including the anti-TfR1 antibody, did not compete with transferrin, indicating that an anti-TfR1 antibody can limit arenaviral replication in an infected individual without interfering with iron metabolism *(362)*.

23.12.4   Arenaviruses Hemorrhagic Fever: Clinical Manifestations

The clinical manifestations of the South American hemorrhagic fevers are nearly identical regardless of the virus responsible for the disease *(356, 358, 371)*.

The incubation period is typically from 7 to 14 days, with extreme cases extending from 5 to 21 days. Secondary infection to very high-load inoculum may result in the reduction of the incubation period to 2 days.

The onset is gradual, with fever and malaise, followed by myalgia, back pain, headache, and dizziness. Hyperesthesia of the skin is common. However, the most important clinical features of the disease are hemorrhagic and neurologic. They can present separately or combined *(354)*.

The hemorrhagic manifestations, which include petechiae of the skin and hemorrhaging from the gums, vagina, and the gastrointestinal tract, and will typically start around the fourth day of illness, indicate the advent of hypovolemic clinical shock. The blood loss is usually minor, so the hematocrit generally will increase as the capillary leak syndrome, the hallmark of the disease, becomes more severe. Bleeding and prothrombin time may be prolonged, and reduction of factors II and VII of the coagulation cascade have been observed. The renal function is generally delayed until shock occurs, but the urinary protein may be high. Pronounced thrombocytopenia may also occur *(354)*.

Neurologic manifestations, presenting as tremor of the hands and an inability to swallow or to speak clearly, may develop, and these can progress to grand mal convulsions, coma, and death in the absence of significant capillary leak or hemorrhagic signs. Death usually occurs between 7 and 12 days after the onset.

Symptoms that appear to be more specifically associated with one or another of the viruses have been reported *(372)*. For example, while frequency of clinical and laboratory findings were identical for Junin and Machupo virus infections, there have been clear differences with the Guanarito infections: pharyngitis, vomiting, and diarrhea were more frequently observed with the Guanarito virus; in contrast, petechiae, erythema, facial edema, hyperesthesia of the skin, and shock were frequently observed in the case of Junin or Machupo infections. A fatal outcome of Junin virus infection has been more frequently observed in pregnant women in the last trimester, and a high fetal mortality rate was associated with both Junin and Machupo virus infections *(373)*.

In the three fatal cases associated with the Whitewater Arroyo virus, the onset was characterized by nonspecific febrile symptoms including fever, headache, and myalgia *(360)*. All patients presented with acute respiratory distress syndrome, and two developed liver failure and hemorrhagic manifestations. Death occurred within 8 weeks after the onset. The direct implication of the Whitewater Arroyo virus in the pathophysiology of these clinical cases remains to be formally established *(354)*.

23.12.4.1 Diagnosis and Treatment

Arenaviruses can be isolated by propagating in cell cultures (particularly in Vero cells). However, because the cytopathic effect is inconsistent, virus-infected cells are usually detected by direct immunofluorescent tests *(354)*.

Arenaviruses can be isolated from serum and throat washings collected 3 to 10 days after onset; less frequently from urine. Specifically, the Machupo virus is recovered from only 20% of acute-phase sera and even less frequently from throat washings or urine *(354)*. With regard to the Junin virus, reverse transcriptase–polymerase chain reaction (RT-PCR) is to date the only method available for rapid diagnosis.

It should be emphasized that arenaviruses are not recovered from the cerebrospinal fluid (CSF) of patients presenting with CNS symptoms when infected with the South American viruses. Viral RNA can be detected by RT-PCR from serum, plasma, urine, throat washings, and various tissues, and the sequencing of the amplified region can be used to identify the implicated virus. The RT-PCR diagnosis offers the advantage of reducing the delay to response and demonstrates a greater sensitivity compared with that of cell culture. Additional techniques for direct detection of viral presence in tissues include *in situ* nucleic acid hybridization and antigen detection ELISA *(354)*.

Indirect serologic diagnosis is based on the detection of antibodies to the nucleoprotein and/or the envelope glycoproteins. Immunofluorescence (IF) tests and ELISA methods using lysates of infected cells would permit the detection of antibodies to the nucleoprotein. However, because this antigen is the most conserved among the arenaviruses, cross-reactions are frequent. Nevertheless, together with ELISA, the indirect IF tests remain simple, inexpensive, rapid, and sensitive assays for detecting Arenavirus infection. The precise identification of the viral species involved should be based on neutralization tests *(354)*.

For the South American viruses causing hemorrhagic fever, the differential diagnosis principally includes yellow fever, dengue hemorrhagic fever, viral hepatitis, leptospirosis, hemorrhagic fever with renal syndrome caused by hantaviruses, rickettsial diseases, sepsis with disseminated intravascular coagulation, and, in the case of CNS involvement, viral encephalitis *(354)*.

Nonspecific treatment of Arenavirus hemorrhagic fever has been based on monitoring and correcting fluid, electrolyte, and osmotic balance. Hemorrhaging can be treated with clotting factor and/or platelet replacement; however, the most serious symptoms usually are caused by capillary leakage *(354)*.

Immune Therapy

The case-fatality ratio of the Argentine hemorrhagic fever, which is about 20% without specific treatment, has been decreased to less than 1% when patients were treated with convalescent serum *(371)*, especially when the immune serum therapy was given within the first 8 days of illness

(374, 375). There is experimental evidence suggesting that the immune plasma may work through viral neutralization.

In the case of Machupo viral hemorrhagic fever, in spite of the recognized efficacy of the convalescent plasma, the low number of cases since its initial outbreak and the absence of a program for collecting and storing of Bolivian immune plasma creates the possibility of future shortages of plasma *(354)*. Hence, antiviral-based approaches may hold a better promise for Bolivian hemorrhagic fever (BHF) treatment.

Ribavirin

The primary target of ribavirin is thought to be the IMP dehydrogenase, an enzyme that converts inosine 5′-monophosphate (IMP) into xanthosine-5′-monophosphate (XMP) *(376)*. The viral RNA synthesis is reduced by ribavirin through a marked decrease in the levels of guanosine-5′-monophosphate (GMP), guanosine diphosphate (GDP), and guanosine-5′-triphosphate (GTP). The reduction of the GTP pool level is the result of a decrease in the 3′,5′-monophosphate (ATP) pool level, because GTP acts as a cofactor for the conversion of IMP into succinyl AMP by the adenylsuccinate synthethase. Typically, the ribavirin treatment will lead to the rise of the intracellular pool level by (i) directly inhibiting the IMP dehydrogenase; (ii) indirectly inhibiting the adenosuccinyl synthetase subsequent to the reduced GTP pool levels; (iii) directly interfering with viral RNA synthesis *(377)*; (iv) directly interfering with the viral mRNA capping the guanylation process; and *(v)* by directly interfering with the generation and elongation of the primer during the viral RNA transcription *(354)*.

The main side effects of ribavirin include thrombocytosis and severe anemia, which resolve after the administration has been stopped.

In 1994, two patients infected with the Machupo virus were treated with ribavirin *(378)*; both patients recovered without sequelae. In 1995, a case of a laboratory-acquired Sabia virus infection occurred in the United States. The patient was treated intravenously with ribavirin 3 days after the infection and recovered without any sequelae *(379)*. These and other (mainly *in vitro*) studies against arenaviruses have shown them to be susceptible to ribavirin *(354)*.

The protocols for ribavirin administration were defined for Lassa virus infections. With regard to its therapeutic use, ribavirin is usually given intravenously at a loading dose of 30 mg/kg, then 16 mg/kg every 6 hours for 4 days, and then 8 mg/kg every 8 hours for 6 days *(279)*. Concerning its prophylactic use for at-risk populations, the recommended dose regimen is oral administration of 500 mg every 6 hours for 7 days *(279)*. Although there is no specific information for South American hemorrhagic fever arenaviruses, the rib-

avirin dose regimens recommended for Lassa fever may still apply *(354)*.

Hemorrhagic Fever Vaccines

The Argentine hemorrhagic fever is the only South American Arenavirus hemorrhagic fever for which extensive studies have been conducted to develop and evaluate a candidate vaccine *(354)*. Early attempts were based on the Tacaribe virus to elicit protection against a lethal challenge with the Junin virus *(380, 381)*.

Recently, a new vaccine, known as Candid 1, has been developed based on live-attenuated Junin virus *(382)*. Studies in non-human primates (*Macacus rhesus*) have shown full protection against a virulent strain of the Junin virus, most likely by inducing a neutralizing antibody response *(383)* coupled with the development of a virus-specific antibody-dependent cellular cytotoxicity *(384)*. The immunogenicity and safety of Candid 1 have been tested in rhesus macaques by subcutaneous administration at increasing doses. The results have shown no clinical and/or biological adverse reaction, and the Candid 1 is being considered for evaluation in Phase I/II human trials *(385)*.

The neutralizing antibody titers to Candid 1 vaccine against Argentine hemorrhagic fever (AHF) were studied for 2 years after vaccination in volunteers to assess whether the kinetics and/or magnitude of this immune response had been modified by previous infection with the Junin virus and lymphocytic choriomeningitis (LCM). The overall results of this study indicated that the immune response to Candid 1 boosted preexisting immunity to Junin virus but was not changed by previous experience with the LCM virus *(386)*.

Whether Candid 1 vaccine may prove useful to cross-protect populations against the Bolivian hemorrhagic fever infection—and possibly against the Venezuelan hemorrhagic fever—needs to be further explored. Cross-reactivity of Junin virus with other arenaviruses was found to be restricted to nucleoprotein-specific monoclonal antibodies and occurred only with New World arenaviruses *(387)*. Cross-reactivity also showed that the Junin virus was most closely related to the Machupo and Tacaribe viruses.

23.12.5 Lassa Fever

Lassa fever has been found predominately in West Africa, especially in Nigeria, Sierra Leone, and Liberia but was also reported in other West African countries. The actual number of cases must run into the thousands, and the impact of the disease must be considerable. Thus, a study carried out in Sierra Leone from 1977 until 1979 reported that 12% of all hospital admissions to just two hospitals were Lassa fever. Furthermore, deaths due to Lassa fever represented 30% of all hospital deaths. Seroprevalence to Lassa fever was found in 7% of all febrile episodes studied. The multimammate rat (*Mastomys natalensis*) appears to be the natural reservoir, and these rodents sustain chronic viremia and virus shedding in the absence of histologic lesions. Human-to-human transmission has been extensively documented. Lassa fever is also a well-recognized nosocomial infection (http://virology-online.com/viruses/haemorrhagicfever.htm).

The Lassa virus is typically spread through aerosolized particles, via either infected rodents or close contact with infected individuals. Additional contact with infected bodily fluids, including blood, urine, and vomit, has been known to spread the virus.

23.12.5.1 The α-Dystroglycan Receptor

α-Dystroglycan (α-DG), a peripheral membrane protein, has been identified as the receptor of both the Lassa fever virus and the lymphocytic choriomeningitis virus (LCMV) *(361)*.

The α-dystroglycan, which was found to be interactive with LCMV, has been purified from cells permissive to infection. Tryptic peptides from this protein were determined to be α-dystroglycan. Several strains of LCMV and Lassa fever virus (LFV) bound to α-dystroglycan, and soluble α-DG blocked both LCMV and LFV infection. Cells bearing a null mutation of the gene encoding α-DG were resistant to LCMV and LFV infections, and reconstitution of α-DG expression in null mutant cells restored the susceptibility to LCMV and LFV infections, thus demonstrating that α-DG is the cellular receptor for both viruses *(388)*.

23.12.5.2 Lassa Fever: Diagnosis and Clinical Manifestations

The incubation period of Lassa virus is between 5 and 21 days, with symptoms usually appearing 10 days after infection.

Traditional laboratory tests provide little help in the way of diagnosis. Leukocyte levels and platelet counts are not useful means of diagnosis. Albuminuria is common. The aspartate aminotransferase (AST) levels parallel the amount of virus in the blood, which is a useful factor in determining the prognosis: the greater the amount of virus in the blood, the more likely the associated disease will be fatal. The Lassa virus is easily isolated from the blood during the febrile stage of the illness, and complement fixation (CF), immunofluorescent antibody assay (IFA), and ELISA may all be useful for detecting viral antibodies (http:// stanford.edu/group/virus/arena/2005/lassavirus.htm). The antigen-capture ELISA test detects virus antigen or

virus-specific antibodies (either IgM or IgG). Using a combination of antigen and IgM antibody tests will allow virtually all Lassa virus infections to be diagnosed early.

Lassa fever typically begins with sore throat, fever, chills, headache, myalgia, and malaise, which may be followed by anorexia, vomiting, and chest pains. Severe abdominal pain and swelling of the neck and face are common. Hemorrhages develop in about 15% to 20% of patients, predominately in the mucous membranes, and are associated with significant rise in mortality. Other symptoms may also include maculopapular rash, cough, diarrhea, conjunctivitis, tremors, dizziness, or signs of hepatitis.

Neurologic phenomena are less common but are nevertheless important. Aseptic meningitis, encephalitis, and global encephalopathy with seizures have all been documented in cases of Lassa virus infection.

Although unusual, deafness is a common feature during late-stage illness or early convalescence and may be either ephemeral or permanent.

When treated in a hospital setting, the mortality rate of Lassa fever is between 15% and 20%. However, it increases dramatically (up to 60%) in areas where appropriate medical care is unavailable. Fatal cases of Lassa fever rarely show any signs of remission, progressing from fever to shock to death in an unrelenting slide. Survivors remain symptomatic for approximately 2 to 3 weeks after the onset of symptoms.

Lassa fever infections in pregnant women are generally more serious—mortality rates range from 30% to 50%, and 95% of the pregnancies end in abortion.

23.12.5.3 Treatment of Lassa Fever

Treatment of Lassa fever is largely symptomatic. Good supportive care is required in the case of severe illness, and shock must be managed very carefully. Management of bleeding and hydration is critical.

Ribavirin has been shown to be effective against Lassa fever, with a two- to threefold decrease in mortality in high-risk patients. Treatment with intravenous ribavirin should commence as soon as possible. Protocols for ribavirin administration were defined for Lassa virus infections. In regard to its therapeutic use, ribavirin is usually given intravenously at a loading dose of 30 mg/kg, then 16 mg/kg every 6 hours for 4 days, and then at 8 mg/kg every 8 hours for 6 days *(279)*. Concerning its prophylactic use for at-risk populations, the recommended dose regimen is oral administration of 500 mg every 6 hours for 7 days *(279)*. However, the drug was shown to be embryotoxic in animal models, and its use in pregnant women is contraindicated.

Postexposure prophylaxis against Lassa fever may be desirable. However, there is no established safe prophylaxis against the disease. Various combinations of hyperimmune convalescent immunoglobulin and/or oral ribavirin may be considered.

At present, there is no effective vaccine available. The development of inactivated vaccines has been hampered by the inability to obtain large quantities of virus from cell cultures. This problem has redirected research interest toward live-attenuated vaccines.

23.12.6 Lymphocytic Choriomeningitis Virus

The LCMV is the prototype member of the Arenaviridae. The LCMV rarely infects humans and when it does, it is usually under conditions when the indigenously infected mouse populations are extremely dense or from contact with infected animals. Individuals become infected with LCMV after exposure to fresh urine, droppings, saliva, or nesting materials. Transmission may also occur when these materials are directly introduced into broken skin, the nose, eyes, or the mouth, or presumably via the bite of an infected rodent. Person-to-person transmission has not been reported with the exception of vertical transmission from an infected mother to the fetus (http://www.cdc.gov/ncidod/dvrd/spb/mnpages/dispages/lcmv/qa.htm). Recent investigations have indicated that organ transplantation may also be a means of transmission (389).

In spite of an apparent decrease in occurrence, the LCMV continues to circulate in rodents and to infect humans as established by seroepidemiologic studies (390–392).

Based on available data for LCMV infections, immunofluorescence (IF) assays appear to be best suited for making a rapid diagnosis soon after infection (354). Neutralizing antibodies appear relatively late after infection and therefore cannot be recommended for detection of seroconversion early in convalescence. However, because the neutralizing antibodies persist for many years (presumably lifelong), they seem to be well suited for confirmation of unexpected results and for detection of infection from distant past. The complement fixation (CF) tests have been considered of little value for the serologic diagnosis of LCMV (392a).

LCM disease is typically mild and is usually manifested as a form of aseptic meningitis (lymphocytic meningitis) or an influenza-like illness. During the first phase of the disease, the most common laboratory abnormalities are a low white blood cell count (leukopenia) and a low platelet count (thrombocytopenia). After the onset of the neurologic disease during the second phase, an increase of the protein levels, an increase in the number of white blood cells, or a decrease in the glucose levels in the CSF have been observed. CNS complications beyond aseptic meningitis include encephalitis and may involve cranial nerve palsies and/or damage to the autonomic nervous system. Non-CNS complications

include orchitis, myocarditis, and small-joint arthritis—these symptoms developed, if at all, in the late stage of the disease during the recurrence of fever.

Intrauterine infection with LCMV may affect the fetus leading to hydrocephalus and chorioretinitis with persistent spastic pareses and death within several years.

On very rare occasions, severe or fatal LCM disease is seen with hemorrhagic manifestations.

The LCMV may also be pathogenic to the fetus leading to abortion or resulting in delivery of babies with hydrocephalus (increased fluid in the brain), chorioretinitis, and mental retardation.

A peripheral membrane protein, α-dystroglycan (α-DG), has been identified as the cellular receptor for both the lymphocytic choriomeningitis and Lassa fever viruses (see Section 23.12.5.1) (361).

LCM disease requires no more than symptomatic treatment.

23.13   Viral Hemorrhagic Fever: Flaviviruses

The Flaviviridae is a family of more than 66 viruses, with nearly 30 of these viruses associated with human disease. Flaviviruses associated primarily with hemorrhagic fever include the yellow fever virus, dengue hemorrhagic fever virus, Kyasanur Forest virus, and the Omsk hemorrhagic fever virus.

The flaviruses represent single-strand, (+)-sense RNA, enveloped, spherical viruses, 40 to 60 nm in diameter. Their genome has a $5'$ cap but is not polyadenylated at the $3'$ end. The entire Flavivirus genome is translated as a single polyprotein, which is then cleaved into the mature proteins. Complementary ($-$)-strand RNA is synthesized by NS proteins and used as a template for genomic progeny RNA synthesis. The first mechanism for ($-$)-strand RNA synthesis described in Flavivirus has been proposed, in which the promoter element functions from the $5'$ end of a circular viral genome. Because similar $5' - 3'$ long-range interactions were observed in many viral RNA genomes, the proposed mechanism for dengue virus may represent a wide-spread strategy for viral RNA replication (393).

Although the mechanisms of RNA replication of (+)-strand RNA viruses is still unclear, in a recent study, the first promoter element for Flavivirus RNA synthesis has been identified using dengue virus as a model (393).

Flavivirus assembly occurs during budding, characteristically into cytoplasmic vacuoles rather than at the cell surface. Release occurs when the cell lyses.

Many Flavivirus species can replicate in both mammalian and insect cells and survive for long periods in their hosts, such as ticks, by replicating in the insect without causing damage.

23.13.1 *Yellow Fever*

Yellow fever is a viral disease of short duration and varying degree of severity that is transmitted primarily by mosquitoes. The infection caused by the yellow fever Flavivirus is so named because of the yellow skin color (jaundice) observed in persons with serious illness. The disease has been associated with tropical climates (reported in 33 countries worldwide) and caused large epidemics in Africa (90% of all cases) and the Americas (10%). To date, yellow fever has not been reported in Asia and Australia, where very strict quarantine regulations exist as well as a requirement of a valid vaccination certificate for people traveling from areas in Africa and South America where yellow fever occurs (the disease is covered by the International Quarantine Regulations). Although an effective vaccine has been available for 60 years, the number of people infected over the past two decades has increased, and yellow fever is again recognized as a serious public health threat (http://www.who.int/mediacentre/factsheets/fs100/en).

In Africa, there are two distinct genetic types (known as topotypes) associated with East and West Africa. In South America, two different types have been defined, but since 1974 only one has been identified as the cause of disease outbreaks.

Transmission. Humans and monkeys are the principal species to be infected. The virus is transmitted by a biting mosquito (horizontal transmission). The mosquito can also pass the virus via infected eggs to its offspring (vertical transmission). The eggs are resistant to drying and lie dormant through dry conditions, hatching when the rainy season begins, thus making the mosquito the true reservoir of the virus, ensuring transmission from one year to the next.

Female mosquitoes transmit the virus because they take blood from the bitten victim. Male mosquitoes do not take blood from the victim. After the mosquito ingests the virus, it takes about a week to 10 days or so for that mosquito to become infective.

Several different species of the *Aedes* (*Ae. africanus* in Africa) and *Haemagogus* (in South America only) mosquitoes transmit the yellow fever virus. These mosquitoes are either domestic (i.e., they breed around houses), wild (they breed in the jungle), or semidomestic (they display mixture of habits). Any region populated with these mosquitoes can potentially harbor the disease.

23.13.1.1 Yellow Fever: Infections to Humans

There are three types of transmission cycles for the yellow fever: sylvatic, intermediate, and urban. All three cycles exist in Africa, but in South America, only the sylvatic and urban cycles occur (http://www.who.int/mediacentre/factsheets/fs100/en):

(i) *Sylvatic (or Jungle) Yellow Fever.* In the tropical rainforest, yellow fever occurs in monkeys that are infected by wild mosquitoes. The infected animals can pass the virus to other mosquitoes that feed on them. The infected wild mosquitoes can then bite humans, causing sporadic cases of yellow fever. On occasion, the virus spreads beyond the infected individual.

(ii) *Intermediate Yellow Fever.* In the humid or semihumid savannahs of Africa, small-scale epidemics occur. These epidemics behave differently than do the urban epidemics, in that many separate villages in an area suffer cases simultaneously, but fewer people die from infection. The semidomestic mosquitoes infect both monkeys and human hosts. Such areas are often called the *zone of emergence*, where increased contact between humans and infected mosquitoes leads to disease. The intermediate yellow fever is the most common type of outbreak seen in recent decades in Africa. It can shift to a more severe urban-type epidemic if the infection is carried into a suitable environment populated with domestic mosquitoes and unvaccinated humans.

(iii) *Urban Yellow Fever.* This type of disease, causing large epidemics of yellow fever, occurs only in humans. Large epidemics can take place when migrants introduce the virus into areas with high human density. Domestic mosquitoes (*Aedes aegyptii*) feed on humans and carry the virus from person to person, with no monkeys involved in the transmission. These outbreaks tend to spread outwards from one source to cover a wide area.

The disease is diagnosed by a blood serum or tissue tests, antigen detection by immunofluorescence or immunochemistry, RNA detection by RT-PCR, or by specific antibody detection.

23.13.1.2 Yellow Fever: Clinical Manifestations

After an incubation period of 3 to 6 days, 5% to 50% of infected people will develop the disease. The signs and symptoms of yellow fever can be divided into three stages. The early stage is characterized by headache, muscle pain, fever, loss of appetite, vomiting, and jaundice. Transient viremia and primary multiplication in lymph nodes takes place. The second stage is a period of remission where fever and other symptoms resolve—most individuals recover at this stage. However, up to 50% of infected individuals may move onto the third, most dangerous, stage, which is characterized by a multiorgan dysfunction, especially liver and kidney failure, epistaxis, other bleeding disorders such as hemorrhage, disseminated intravascular coagulation, and brain dysfunction including delirium, seizures, coma, and shock; up to 30% of patients will die. Overall, the mortality rate of yellow fever is 40% in severe cases. Genetic variations between different human populations result in different severity of disease; however, the genes involved are still not known (http://microbiologybytes.com/virology/flsaviviruses.html).

23.13.1.3 Yellow Fever: Treatment

At present, there are no antiviral drugs effective against yellow fever. Serious cases of yellow fever *always* need hospital treatment, which is symptomatic—mainly intravenous rehydration with fluids and salts to restore the electrolyte balance. Paracetamol should be avoided if there is already evidence of liver damage. In mild cases, the pain may be relieved with painkiller (analgesic) drugs and high temperature with antipyretics.

23.13.1.4 Yellow Fever Vaccines

Vaccination against yellow fever is the best way of avoiding the disease and doing so is *absolutely recommended*. The vaccine is almost 100% effective against yellow fever, and its tolerance is excellent. It provides protection against the disease for at least 10 years beginning 10 days after its administration.

The yellow fever *17D vaccines* are based on a live-attenuated strain, first developed in 1937 from a parent Asibi strain *(394)* and manufactured with the approval of WHO in 11 countries after standards for its production had been approved, including the adoption of a seed lot system *(395)*. Mass vaccination was conducted in the late 1930s and early 1940s in Brazil, various countries in Africa, and the armed forces of the United States and its allies.

Vaccines currently in use are derived from two distinct substrains (17DD at the 284th to 286th passage level; and 17D-204 at the 233rd to 237th passage level), which represent independently maintained series of passages from the original 17D virus developed in 1937 *(396)*.

The 17D vaccine is administered at 0.5 mL subcutaneously and requires a booster every 10 years.

Adverse reactions include hypersensitivity to eggs, encephalitis in the very young, hepatic failure, as well as rare reports of deaths from massive organ failure. In June 2001, seven cases of yellow fever vaccine–associated viscerotropic disease (YEL-AVD; previously known as multiple organ system failure) were reported as the result of vaccination with 17D-derived yellow fever vaccine *(338–340,397,400)*. These and other reports on two suspected cases of YEL-AVD, and four cases of suspected YEL-associated neurotropic disease

(YEL-AND; previously called postvaccinal encephalitis), prompted the Advisory Committee on Immunization Practices (ACIP) at the CDC to recommend enhanced surveillance for adverse effects after vaccination with the 17D vaccine *(401)*.

However, the risk to unimmunized individuals either living in or traveling to areas where there is known yellow fever transmission is far greater than the risk of having a vaccine-related adverse event, and WHO policy on yellow fever vaccination remains unchanged, strongly recommending vaccination against yellow fever.

Contraindications. Administration of yellow fever vaccines has been contraindicated for certain populations, as follows (http://www.cdc.gov/ncidod/dvbid/yelloefever.html):

(i) The vaccine should never be given to infants under 6 months of age because of a risk of viral encephalitis. Most vaccinations should be deferred until the child is 9 to 12 months of age.

(ii) Pregnant women should not be vaccinated because of the potential risk that the developing fetus may become infected from the vaccine.

(iii) Individuals hypersensitive to eggs should not receive the vaccine because it is prepared in embryonated eggs. In case of questionable history of egg hypersensitivity, an intradermal test dose may be administered under medical supervision.

(iv) Individuals with immunosuppression associated with HIV infection or malignancies or those who are receiving immunosuppressive therapy and/or radiation should not receive the vaccine. Patients with asymptomatic HIV infection may be vaccinated if exposure to yellow fever cannot be avoided.

23.13.2 Dengue Fever

Dengue fever was first described in 1779–1780, and the virus was isolated in 1944 *(402)*. The disease pattern associated with dengue-like illness from 1780 to 1940 was characterized by relatively infrequent but often large epidemics. However, during that time, the dengue viruses seemed to become endemic in many tropical urban centers *(403)*.

The ecologic disruption in the Southeast Asia and the Pacific regions during and after World War II created optimal conditions for increased transmission of mosquito-borne disease and the beginning of a global pandemic of dengue, followed in 1953–1954 by an epidemic of the newly identified dengue hemorrhagic fever (DHF) in the Philippines *(404, 405)*. In Asia, epidemic dengue hemorrhagic fever expanded geographically from Southeast Asian countries west to India, Sri Lanka, the Maldives, and Pakistan, and east to China *(406)* and the Pacific *(407)*. The dengue hemorrhagic fever has emerged as the leading cause of hospitalization and death among children in many Southeast Asian countries *(403)*.

After the eradication of the dengue virus mosquito-vector *Aedes aegyptii*, epidemics of the disease abated. However, after the discontinuation of the eradication program in the early 1970s, this species started to reinvade the countries from which it had been eradicated, and epidemics of dengue invariably followed the re-infestation of a country by *Ae. aegyptii (405, 408)*.

Before the 1980s, there was little information about the distribution of dengue viruses in Africa. Since then, however, major epidemics caused by all four serotypes have occurred in both East and West Africa *(407)*.

Each year, cases of dengue disease are imported to the continental United States and documented by the CDC. These cases represent the introductions of all four serotypes from all tropical regions of the world reflecting the increased number of people traveling from and to those areas, thereby making the potential for epidemic dengue transmission in the United States a possibility. After an absence of more than 40 years, autochthonous transmission, secondary to importation of the virus in humans, occurred on several occasions during the 1980–1997 period *(403, 409)*. Although small, these outbreaks still underscore the potential for dengue transmission in the United States where two competent mosquito vectors (*Ae. aegyptii* and *Ae. albopictus*) exist and can transmit dengue to humans, thereby increasing the risk of autochthonous dengue transmission, secondary to imported cases *(405, 410)*.

The dengue fever virus belongs to the genus Flavivirus of the family Flaviviridae, which contains approximately 70 species *(411)*. It comprises four serotypes, known as DEN-1, DEN-2, DEN-3, and DEN-4. Infection with one dengue serotype provides lifelong immunity to that virus, but since there is no cross-protective immunity to the other serotypes, persons living in an area of endemic dengue can be infected with all four dengue serotypes during their lifetimes *(405)*.

Transmission Cycles. The primitive enzootic transmission cycle of the dengue viruses involves canopy-dwelling *Aedes* mosquitoes and lower primates in the rainforests of Asia and Africa *(405)*. Current evidence suggests that these viruses do not regularly move out of the forests to urban areas *(412)*. The most important transmission cycle from a public health standpoint is the urban endemic/epidemic cycle in large urban centers of the tropical regions. The viruses are maintained in an *Ae. aegyptii*-to-human-to-*Ae. aegyptii* cycle with periodic epidemics. Often, multiple virus serotypes cocirculate in the same urban area (hyperendemicity) *(403)*.

Humans are infected with dengue viruses by the bite of an infected female mosquito. The principal vector, *Aedes aegyptii*, is a small, black-and-white, highly domes-

ticated tropical insect that prefers to lay its eggs in artificial containers in immediate proximity to homes. The adult mosquitoes usually rest indoors, are unobtrusive, and prefer to feed on humans during the daylight hours; they infect several persons in one single blood meal. This feeding pattern makes *Ae. aegyptii* an efficient epidemic vector *(403)*.

23.13.2.1　Dengue Fever Virus Infections: Diagnosis and Clinical Manifestations

Primary infection may be asymptomatic or may result in dengue fever. The incubation period after a bite by an infected mosquito is 3 to 14 days (average, 4 to 7 days) *(403)*.

During the acute initial febrile period, which may be as short as 2 days and as long as 10 days, dengue viruses may circulate in the peripheral blood. If other *Ae. aegyptii* mosquitoes bite the already ill person during this febrile viremic stage, those mosquitoes may become infected and subsequently transmit the virus to other uninfected persons, after an extrinsic period of 8 to 12 days *(405, 413)*.

Dengue virus infection in humans causes a spectrum of illnesses ranging from asymptomatic or mild febrile illness to severe and fatal hemorrhagic disease *(403)*. Infection with any of the four dengue serotypes will elicit a similar clinical presentation, which may vary in severity depending on a host of risk factors, such as the strain and serotype of the infecting virus and the person's immune status, age, and genetic background *(405, 414–416)*.

Dengue Fever

The classic dengue fever is primarily a disease of older children and adults and may vary with age. Infants and young children develop rash and flu-like symptoms, whereas older children and adults may present with high fever and more severe symptoms.

After the end of the incubation period, the person may experience acute onset of fever accompanied by a variety of nonspecific signs and symptoms, such as headache and body aches, retro-orbital pain, nausea and vomiting, arthralgia (pain in the joints) that can progress to arthritis (inflammation of the joints), myositis (inflammation of muscle tissue), and a discrete macular or maculopapular rash. Patients may be anorexic, have an altered taste sensation, and have mild sore throat *(405, 417, 418)*. In this situation, clinical differentiation from other viral diseases may not be possible.

The initial temperature may rise to 102°F to 105°F, and fever may last for 2 to 7 days. The fever may drop after a few days, only to rebound 12 to 24 hours later (saddleback). Lymphadenopathy is common. A second rash may appear between days 2 and 6 of illness.

Hemorrhagic manifestations in dengue fever are not uncommon and range from mild to severe. Hematuria occurs infrequently, and jaundice is rare *(403)*.

Dengue fever is generally self-limiting and is rarely fatal. Whereas the acute phase lasts between 3 and 7 days, the convalescence phase may be prolonged for weeks and may be associated with weakness and depression, especially in adults.

Dengue Hemorrhagic Fever

Dengue hemorrhagic fever (DHF) is primarily a disease in children under 15 years of age, although it may also occur in adults *(419)*. It is characterized by sudden onset of fever, which usually lasts for 2 to 7 days, and a variety of non-specific signs and symptoms. During the acute phase of the illness, it is difficult to differentiate between DHF and dengue fever, as well as other diseases found in tropical settings. However, as fever remits, characteristic manifestations of plasma leakage appear, making accurate clinical diagnosis possible in many cases *(403)*.

The critical stage of DHF is at the time of defervescence, but signs of circulatory failure or hemorrhagic manifestations may occur from about 24 hours before to 24 hours after the temperature falls to normal or below. There is evidence of vascular leak syndrome, and common hemorrhagic manifestations include skin hemorrhages (petechiae, purpuric lesions, and ecchymoses). Epistaxis, bleeding gums, gastrointestinal hemorrhages, and hematuria occur less frequently.

Dengue Shock Syndrome

Dengue shock syndrome (DSS) is usually a progression of dengue hemorrhagic fever and is often fatal. The primary pathophysiologic abnormality seen in DHF and DSS is an acute increase in vascular permeability that leads to leakage of plasma into the extravascular compartment, resulting in hemoconcentration, hypoproteinemia, and decreased blood pressure *(420)*. Plasma volume studies have shown a reduction of more than 20% in severe cases.

One theory explaining the pathogenic changes that take place in DHF and DSS is known as the secondary-infection or immune-enhancement hypothesis *(404, 416, 417)*. Upon infection, the host immune response will produce specific antibodies against the particular serotype's surface proteins that prevent the virus from binding to the macrophages (the target cell that dengue viruses infect) and gaining entry. However, if another dengue serotype infects the same individual, the virus will activate the immune system to respond to the attack as if it had been provoked by the first serotype; the

host antibodies will bind to the viral surface proteins but will not inactivate the virus. Moreover, the immune response will attract numerous macrophages, which the new dengue serotype will proceed to infect because it has not been inactivated. The body will also release cytokines that cause the endothelial tissue to become permeable, resulting in hemorrhagic fever and fluid loss from the blood vessels. Thus, it is hypothesized that prior infection, through a process known as antibody-dependent enhancement (ADE), enhances the infection and replication of dengue virus in cells of the mononuclear cell lineage *(417, 421–423)*. As a result, the patient's condition progresses to dengue shock syndrome.

Another hypothesis assumes that dengue viruses, like all animal viruses, vary and change genetically as a result of selection pressures as they replicate in humans and or mosquitoes and that there are some virus strains that have greater epidemic potential *(405, 424, 425)*. Phenotypic expression of genetic changes in the virus genome may include increased virus replication and viremia, severity of disease (virulence), and epidemic potential *(403)*.

Immunopathogenesis of DHF/DSS

During the past four decades, seroepidemiologic studies in areas endemic for DHF/DSS have provided growing evidence that the risk of severe disease has been significantly higher in secondary dengue infections and suggest that DHF and DSS have an immunologic basis *(426)*. After re-infection with a dengue virus of different serotype, severe disease is linked to high levels of antibody-enhanced viral replication early in the illness, which is followed by a cascade of memory T-cell activation and a host of inflammatory cytokines and other chemical mediators. These compounds are released primarily from T-cells, monocytes/macrophages, and endothelial cells to ultimately cause an increase in vascular permeability. These immunologic events have underscored the fact that the DHF/DSS pathogenesis is a complex, multifactorial process involving cocirculation of various dengue serotypes and the interplay of host and viral factors that influence the disease severity *(426)*.

23.13.3 Omsk Hemorrhagic Fever

The Omsk hemorrhagic fever virus (OHFV) is a member of the tick-borne encephalitis (TBE) antigenic complex of the genus Flavivirus of the family Flaviviridae. The enveloped virions are spherical, about 45 nm in diameter, with a single-stranded, positive-sense RNA genome.

OHFV is native to the western regions of Siberia and was first isolated in 1947 from the blood of a patient with hemorrhagic fever during an epidemic in Omsk and the regions of Novosibirsk, Kurgan, and Tyumen. The virus is carried by ticks of the genera *Dermacentor* (*D. reticulates* and *D. marginatus*) and *Ixodes* (*I. persulcatus*) that remain infective for life. The animal hosts are rodents and the muskrat (*Ondatra zibethica*), and the narrow-skulled (*Microtus gregalis*) and water (*Arvicola terestris*) voles *(427)*.

The virus is susceptible to drying and heating (56°C for 30 minutes) but can survive in water and may be transmitted to humans through contaminated water. In addition to physical inactivation, OHFV is also sensitive to 70% ethanol, 1% sodium hypochlorite, and 2% glutaraldehyde.

Transmission. OHFV is transmitted to humans by the bite of an infected tick or can be caught from infected muskrats and voles (blood, feces, or urine). Rodents are infected with OHFV from the bite of an infected tick. Data suggest direct transmission (zoonosis) from both muskrats and voles. There is no human-to-human transmission reported. Aerosol infections have occurred in the laboratory. OHFV can also be transmitted through the milk of infected goats or sheep and has been isolated from aquatic animals.

All ages and both genders are susceptible to infection, and seasonal occurrence in each area coincides with vector activity.

23.13.3.1 Sequence of the Envelope Glycoprotein of the OHFV

The OHFV is of particular interest because, in contrast with most of other TBE viruses, it produces a hemorrhagic disease closely resembling but milder than that caused by the Kyasanur Forest disease virus, another highly pathogenic member of the group I serocomplex (see Section 23.13.3.2).

To shed light on this intriguing phenomenon, the gene encoding the envelope glycoprotein of the OHFV was cloned and sequenced *(428)*. A freeze-dried preparation of infected suckling mouse brain suspension was used as the source material for the viral RNA. The derived cDNA was amplified using PCR, and the cloned DNA was sequenced by dideoxynucleotide sequencing. Alignment of the OHFV sequence with those of other known tick-borne flaviviruses showed that they shared *N*-glycosylation sites, cysteine residues, the fusion peptide, and the hexapeptide (EHLPTA; amino acids 207 to 212) that identifies tick-borne flaviviruses. Though OHFV was distinguishable from the other viruses, it shared the closest amino acid identity (93%) with the TBE viruses. A sequence of three amino acids (AQN; amino acids 232 to 234), which had previously been known to be specific for the TBE viruses, was altered to MVG (amino acids 232 to 234).

In addition to the amino acid substitutions described above, the OHFV also showed several other unique amino acid substitutions in positions that may have significance for its pathogenesis. For example, the substitution of an amino acid in OHFV at position 67 exactly coincided with that of an escape mutant of TBE virus *(429)* and this is the position of the *N*-glycosylation site in the dengue virus. Furthermore, the amino acids 271 to 282 encompassed a cluster of amino acid changes in OHFV, and an amino acid codon change within this region has been identified in a Japanese encephalitis virus neutralization-resistant mutant *(430)*. Moreover, the vaccine strain of yellow fever virus also showed two amino acid codon substitutions in this region *(431)* compared with the similar regions in most other flaviviruses. These and other observations have strongly implied that changes in several domains within the viral envelope glycoprotein may be required for altering the pathogenic characteristics of the OHFV—that is, there is no single motif that will determine its hemorrhagic pathogenicity, but rather a combination of substitutions of the types described above may be required for stabilizing attenuation *(428)*.

23.13.3.2 Omsk Hemorrhagic Fever: Human Disease

The incubation period after initial infection is usually between 3 and 8 days. The illness begins with a sudden onset of fever, chills, headache, pain in both the lower and upper extremities, and severe prostration. A papulovascular rash on the soft palate, cervical lymphadenopathy, and conjunctival suffusion are usually present. Patients may also experience abnormally low blood pressure. CNS abnormalities (signs of encephalitis) typically develop 1 to 2 weeks after the onset of disease.

Severe cases of illness present with hemorrhages but no cutaneous rash. Other forms of hemorrhages include epistaxis (nosebleed), and gastrointestinal and uterine bleeding. The lungs may also be affected.

The Omsk hemorrhagic fever is a biphasic illness (i.e., after the initial appearance of symptoms, there may be a brief period of recovery before new symptoms appear). The second phase usually will develop after 1 to 2 weeks and will affect the central nervous system.

Laboratory findings including leukopenia and thrombocytopenia are indicative of viral hemorrhagic fever. Other diagnostic tests include detection of antigens or antibody to the virus in the blood—immunoassays distinguishing OHFV from related viruses (which are available in Russia), and ELISA (enzyme-linked immunosorbent serologic assay).

Complications after recovery frequently include hearing loss, hair loss, and behavioral or psychological difficulties associated with neurologic conditions.

Previous infection leads to immunity.

The mortality rate of Omsk hemorrhagic fever is estimated to be between 1% and 10%.

Treatment. There is no specific treatment (e.g., antiviral drugs) for Omsk hemorrhagic fever. A formalized mouse-brain vaccine is in use but is not available commercially. Supportive therapy is important. Replacement therapy should be considered only in severe cases of hemorrhages, and usual precautions should be taken for patients with bleeding disorders. Fluid infusion to deal with dehydration is often counterproductive but can be supportive if accompanied by careful monitoring of serum electrolytes.

23.13.4 Kyasanur Forest Disease

The Kyasanur Forest disease (KFD) virus was first recognized in 1957 as a febrile illness in the Shimoga district of Karnataka State in India *(432)*. Preceding the human epidemic, a large number of sick and dead monkeys had been noticed in the nearby forest area. The virus has been isolated from dead monkeys, sick patients, and the vector tick species *Haemaphysalis spinigera*. Since the first case, there has been a centripetal expansion of the affected area, presumably from an altered ecosystem resulting from deforestation and changing agricultural practices *(433)*. Recently, a virus very similar to KFD virus (KFDV) was discovered in Saudi Arabia.

The KFDV is susceptible to disinfectants (70% ethanol, 1% sodium hypochlorite, and 2% glutaraldehyde), as well as to heating at 56°C for 30 minutes, and to freezing.

The main hosts of KFDV are small rodents, but shrews, bats, and monkeys may also carry the virus (http://www.cdc.gov/ncidod/dvrd/spb/mnpages/dispages/kyasanur.htm).

Transmission. KFDV is transmitted by the bite of an infected tick (*H. spinigera*), especially nymphal ticks. Humans can get the disease from a tick bite or by contact with an infected animal (zoonosis), such as sick or recently dead monkey. Larger animals such as goats, cows, and sheep may become infected with KFDV, but they do not have a role in the transmission of the disease. Furthermore, there is no evidence that the infection is transmitted through unpasteurized milk of any of these animals.

23.13.4.1 KFDV: Structural Protein Gene Sequence

KFDVs have been isolated from monkeys, humans, and ticks from different areas and at different times, and they were found to be antigenically identical *(434)*. Although antigenic relationships have been demonstrated between the KFDV and other tick-borne flaviviruses, significant differences have been found in the neutralization indices between KFD, European tick-borne encephalitis (TBE), and the Russian TBE (formerly known as the Russian spring-summer encephalitis virus) viruses *(435)*. The antigenic discreteness of KFDV was further demonstrated when it was observed

that mice immunized with inactivated KFDV showed no resistance to challenge with the Russian TBE *(436)*.

However, the relationships of KFDV with other members of the tick-borne flaviviruses at molecular level is less clear. The sequence of the structural protein genes of the KFDV has been defined using conserved primers in a PCR assay *(437)*. Data have shown that the KFDV is a distinct member of the tick-borne antigenic complex with characteristic protease cleavage sites, fusion peptides, signal sequences, and hydrophobic transmembrane domains. Among its structural proteins, the KFDV E glycoprotein exhibited maximum similarity (77.4% to 81.3%) to tick-borne flaviviruses.

The C protein was highly basic (21.5% lysine and arginine residues) and similar to other flaviviruses. The C protein is believed to be important in the interaction with RNA during the formation of viral nucleocapsids. Furthermore, the KFDV showed the sequence AKG after the first M (membrane protein), which was unique among all tick-borne flavivirus sequences *(437)*.

The E glycoprotein represents the most important functional component of the KFDV by inducing inhibition of hemagglutination and by neutralizing protective antibodies during the course of natural infection or immunization. It is thought to be one of the major determinants of virulence or attenuation of the virus.

Although the tick-borne flavivirus-specific hexapeptide genetic marker EHLPTA showed a T $\rightarrow$ K substitution (at residues 207 to 212) unique to the KFDV, the alignment of its amino acid sequence with those of other known tick-borne flaviviruses revealed many conserved regions confirming its identity as a member of the TBE antigenic complex *(437)*.

The previous belief that the KFDV was a variant of the Omsk hemorrhagic fever virus (see Section 23.13.3) introduced from Siberia is questionable because the sequence homology of the E glycoprotein of the two viruses was no greater than that of other members of the group 1 serocomplex *(437)*.

23.13.4.2 KFD: Human Disease

After an incubation period of 3 to 8 days, the symptoms of the KFD begin suddenly with fever, headache, severe muscle pain, cough, dehydration, gastrointestinal symptoms, and bleeding abnormalities. Patients may also experience abnormally low blood pressure and low platelet, red blood cell, and white blood cell counts. Relative bradycardia is frequently present, along with inflammation of the conjunctivae (http://www.cdc.gov/ncidod/dvrd/spb/mnpages/dispages/kyasanur.htm) *(438)*. After 1 to 2 weeks of symptoms, some patients recover without complication.

However, in most patients the illness is biphasic, and at the end of the second week, patients begin to experience a second wave of symptoms, including fever and signs of CNS disorders (encephalitis).

It is estimated that there are approximately 400 to 500 cases of KFD annually in India with a mortality rate ranging between 3% and 5%. The hemorrhagic fatality rate is 2% to 50%. A small number of patients will develop coma or bronchopneumonia before death.

Diagnosis of the disease is made by isolating the virus from blood or by serologic testing using the ELISA assay.

Treatment. There is no specific treatment for KFD, but supportive therapy is highly important, including hydration and treatment for bleeding disorders.

23.14 Protein Toxin Weapons

The term *toxin weapon* has been used to describe poisons typically of natural origin and easily accessible by modern chemical synthetic methods. When used in the battlefield or as bioterrorist agents, they cause death or severe incapacitation at relatively low concentrations *(439, 440)*.

Recently, several factors have increased the importance of these agents as biological weapons, namely *(439)*:

(i) The progress in biotechnology that made the large-scale production and purification of protein toxins more feasible.

(ii) New molecular biology techniques such as polymerase chain reaction (PCR) that enable the identification, isolation, and comparison of extended families of previously less well known natural toxins.

(iii) New developments in gene manipulation and microbiology that have significantly expanded the accessible delivery vehicles for proteins to include, for example, natural or genetically modified bacteria and engineered viruses as sources for novel protein toxins.

(iv) The ability for aggressors to use toxins as a tactical weapon to strike at the enemy in a controlled manner that is difficult or impossible with infectious agents, for example by selective contamination of key terrain or high-value targets. Aerosolized protein toxins can be used both as lethal or severe incapacitating agents, greatly complicating medical care and logistical systems.

However, the absence of replicating biological delivery systems will markedly reduce the usefulness of protein toxins as direct mass-casualty biological weapons. Further drawbacks include the facts that:

(i) Proteins are not volatile and generally do not persist long in the environment.

(ii) Simple, physical protection offers an effective natural defense against foreign proteins.

(iii) Relatively sophisticated research, development, testing, and evaluation is required to establish conclusively that each specific protein toxin is a viable open-air aerosol weapon.

23.14.1 *Clostridium botulinum Neurotoxins*

Botulism is caused by a family of potent neurotoxins (*Clostridium botulinum* neurotoxins; BoNTs) produced by *Clostridium botulinum* bacteria from one of at least seven different serotypes designated as BoNT/A through/G *(441)*. Four of these serotypes (BoNT/A,/B,/E, and to a lesser degree/F) are significant as human poisons through contaminated food, wound infection, or infant botulism *(440)*. Although rare, the extreme toxicity of BoNT qualifies it as a potent biological weapon. Thus, after internalized, BoNT may cause fatal paralysis in animals at nonagram/kilogram levels *(442)*.

During the past decade, the three-dimensional structures of holotoxins or isolated toxin domains of *Clostridium* bacteria have been solved, rendering a clearer picture of their functions and toxicities *(443–446)*. Like the closely related tetanus neurotoxin (TeNT) *(443)*, the BoNT proteins are disulfide-bonded heterodimers consisting of an approximately 50-kDa zinc metalloproteinase "light chain" and an approximately 100-kDa receptor-binding "heavy chain" (Hc). The Hc has been subdivided structurally and functionally into a *C*-terminal domain that binds the toxin to gangliosides and other receptors on the surface of the peripheral cholinergic neurons (so-called Hc domain), and the *N*-terminal domain, which is believed to enhance cell binding and translocation of the catalytic light chain across the vascular membrane. In addition, the BoNT naturally is associated with a number of nontoxic "accessory proteins," some of which may stabilize the toxins *in vivo (439)*.

The mechanism by which BoNT traverses the neuron cell membranes is not completely understood, but once inside the neuron, the catalytic light chain subunit of BoNT acts as a selective zinc metalloproteinase to cleave essential polypeptide components of the so-called *SNARE complex* required for normal neurotransmitter release or membrane fusion. The exact mechanism by which the soluble *N*-ethyl maleimide–sensitive factor attachment protein receptors (SNARE) complex mediates vesicle fusion or release of neurotransmitter acetylcholine (ACh) into the synaptic cleft remains controversial; however, it is clear that the integrity of the complex is critical for normal cholinergic nerve transmission *(447, 448)*.

Clinical Manifestations of BoNT Intoxication. By disrupting ACh exocytosis at the peripheral neuromuscular junction,

BoNT causes cholinergic autonomic nervous system dysfunction in affected patients. The signs and symptoms of BoNT intoxication, which typically manifest 12 to 36 hours after toxin exposure, include generalized weakness, lassitude, and dizziness. There may be decreased salivation and dry mouth or sore throat. Furthermore, motor symptoms will reflect cranial nerve dysfunction, including dysarthria, dysphonia, and dysphagia, followed by symmetric descending and progressive muscle paralysis (449). Without adequate supportive care, death may occur abruptly as a result of respiratory failure (439).

Current medical treatment for BoNT intoxication is likely to involve prolonged life-support for incapacitated survivors, including the continual use of mechanical ventilation (450).

23.14.1.1 BoNT Vaccines

It is known that the tetanus neurotoxin (TeNT) Hc fragments could compete for neuron binding and thereby antagonize the neuromuscular blocking properties of native TeNT and, to a lesser degree, BoNT (451, 452). These observation led to the development of a vaccine candidate for BoNT/A based on the recombinant Hc once the BoNT gene was cloned and expressed. Subsequent epitope mapping of BoNT/A identified two specific polypeptides, both from Hc ($H_{455-661}$ and $H_{1150-1289}$), which were capable of protecting mice from supralethal challenge with the botulinum neurotoxin (453).

Further studies at the U.S. Army Medical Research Institute of Infectious Diseases (USAMRIID) have led to the development of recombinant BoNT Hc vaccine candidates for BoNT/A,/B, and/F, which conferred protection in mice against supralethal challenge with the botulinum neurotoxin (454–458). This approach was recently extended to include BoNT Hc fragments from BoNT/C and/D (459).

Unlike the BoNT toxoids, the recombinant Hc vaccine candidates did not require treatment with denaturants and were not susceptible to reversion of catalytic activity (439).

Although apparently safe and effective, the inherent limitation of the recombinant Hc fragment vaccines has been their lack of cross-reactivity among the BoNT serotypes; a separate Hc fragment immunogen would be required for each BoNT serotype and perhaps for some different strains of each BoNT serotype.

Alternative Delivery of BoNT Vaccines. Several alternative vaccine-delivery systems for recombinant BoNT Hc immunogens have been explored recently in animal models, including inhalation and oral vaccine delivery, as well as the use of self-replicating RNA virus or DNA-based vectors (460–463). Proof of concept for the use of inactivated holotoxin as an oral immunogen has also been reported (464, 465). However, it remains unproven whether these experimental delivery approaches offer any practical advantage compared with traditional intramuscular vaccination (439).

23.14.1.2 Immunotherapeutics

The potential of BoNT as a mass casualty biological weapon, coupled with the high cost and logistical burden of symptomatic medical treatment, has prompted an increased effort to develop selective and cost-effective BoNT therapeutics (439).

Animal and human studies have suggested that the presence of preformed, neutralizing antibodies in the serum to bind and eliminate the BoNT before it reaches the target cells can prevent and/or reduce intoxication. Thus, several antitoxin preparations for human use have been developed, including a "trivalent" (serotypes/A,/B, and/E) equine antitoxin product, as well as a monovalent BoNT/E antitoxin (439). In addition, an experimental despeciated equine heptavalent (serotypes/A to/G) product has been developed at USAMRIID and currently is administered under Investigational New Drug (IND) protocol for limited use (439).

Several studies resulted in the production of a human *botulism immune globulin (BIG)* antiserum from different pools of plasma obtained from human donors who had been previously vaccinated with the pentavalent toxoid (PBT) vaccine. Subsequently, a human antitoxin (BIG-IV) was developed and distributed for treating infant botulism under FDA-authorized IND protocol (466). Intravenous administration of BIG significantly reduced the hospital stay of infants diagnosed with botulism. However, it is still not clear to what extent the success of BIG with infant botulism will also apply to treating patients exposed to BoNT by aerosol (439).

23.14.2 *Staphylococcus aureus Enterotoxins*

Whereas BoNT achieves its potency by dampening an amplified extracellular signal of nerve cells via enzymatic catalysis, the *Staphylococcus aureus* enterotoxins (SEs) act by inappropriately amplifying an extracellular signal of key immune cells (439).

The SE belong to an extended family of stable 23- to 29-kDa protein toxins that includes SE serotypes/A,/B,/C1,/C2,/C3,/D,/E, and/H, and streptococcal pyrogenic exotoxin serotypes/A to/C,/F to/H, and/J, as well as toxic shock syndrome toxin (TSST-1) (467). Based on their common ability to cause severe illness in animals by inducing a physiologic overreaction of the host-immune response, these toxins have been categorized collectively as *superantigens (SAgs) (439)*. SAgs are a major cause of human poisoning and contribute significantly to opportunistic bacterial infections in hospital patients.

In the context of biological weapons, the most important SAg is SE serotype/B (SE/B). SE/B is a two-domain, α/β-protein that contains discrete binding sites for the major histocompatibility complex (MHC) class II molecule and the Vβ regions of T-cell antigen receptors (TCRs) *(468–470)*. By binding to these two receptor molecules, and perhaps through other cell-surface interactions, SE/B is able to activate both antigen-presenting cells and a relatively large number of T lymphocytes to cause the release of pyrogenic cytokines, chemokines, and other proinflammatory molecules *(439)*.

Whereas the more common forms of SAg food poisoning can be managed with routine supportive care, SE/B is a formidable aerosol threat because of its high potency and stability. It is estimated that SE/B may produce human incapacitation and death at levels as low as 0.03 and 1.5 μg, respectively *(439)*.

23.14.2.1 SE Vaccines

SE Toxoid Vaccines. During the mid-1960s, it was shown that SE/B can be isolated from bacterial culture supernatants in highly purified form and then inactivated with neutral formaldehyde solution to produce an effective toxoid vaccine *(471)*. However, the requirement of active toxin production as starting material, the possibility of toxoid reversion to yield active SE/B toxin, as well as minor reactogenicity associated with formaldehyde-inactivated vaccines, has prompted research studies directed at the development of improved SE/B vaccines.

Engineered SE Vaccines. Comparative structural and biochemical studies have focused on the development of nontoxic, recombinant immunogens capable of eliciting a protective immune response against multiple SAg toxins. One such initiative was to inactivate SE by modifying three structural regions of the toxin that were involved in HLA-DR1 binding: (i) a polar pocket created by three β-strand elements of the β-barrel domain of the toxin; (ii) a hydrophobic reverse turn; and (iii) a disulfide-bonded loop *(468,472–474)*. By combining substitutions in each of these three structural regions of SE/B (Tyr89Ala, Leu45Arg, and Tyr94Ala) within a single immunogen, a recombinant candidate (rSE/Bv) was produced that was lacking detectable SAg activity. An analogous recombinant immunogen was subsequently developed for SE type A (SE/A) by introducing comparable substitutions (Asp70Arg, Leu48Arg, and Tyr92Ala) *(439)*.

The rSE/Bv vaccine candidate was tested in mouse and non-human primate models and was found to elicit high antibody titers, and the vaccinated mice survived supralethal challenges with SE/B toxin. In contrast with the natural toxin, rSE/Bv showed no evidence of toxic SAg activity *(439)*.

23.14.3 Clostridium perfringens

Clostridium perfringens is an anaerobic Gram-positive spore-forming bacillus that produces at least 15 toxins *(475)*. The toxins of this microorganism are highly toxic phospholipases.

The spores germinate after warming slowly at ambient temperature. The natural reservoir of the microorganism is soil and the gastrointestinal tract of healthy persons and animals.

The virulence factor of *C. perfringens* is responsible for various disease, including gas gangrene, food poisoning, necrotic enteritis, and enterotoxemia *(476)*. Gas gangrene is typically the result of contamination of a wound by spores of *C. perfringens*. Unlike *B. anthracis* spores, there is no apparent disease after inhalation of *C. perfringens* spores. There have been rare case reports of pulmonary infections associated with *C. perfringens (477, 478)*.

Whereas aerosol challenges with *C. perfringens* toxin have been reported to produce lethal pulmonary disease in laboratory animals, there is no established threat from aerosol exposure and inhalation of these toxins in healthy individuals *(475)*.

23.14.4 Ricin Toxin

Ricin is a disulfide-bonded heterodimeric toxin found in the seeds of the castor bean plant (*Ricinus communis*). It has been recognized as a potential toxin weapon since World War I *(439)*. Although less lethal than BoNT and SE, at sublethal doses it can cause incapacitation by pulmonary damage. Moreover, ricin is readily available because the castor bean plant is cultivated worldwide, and the toxin is easily extracted from common by-products of the seeds *(479, 480)*.

The name *ricin* was given to the toxin by R. Stillmark in 1888 when he tested the beans' extract on red blood cells and saw them agglutinate *(481)*. Now it is known that the agglutination was caused by another toxin also present in the extract, called RCA (*Ricinus communis* agglutinin). The difference between these two toxins is that ricin is a potent cytotoxin but a weak hemagglutinin, whereas RCA is a weak cytotoxin but a powerful hemagglutinin. Poisoning by ingestion of the castor bean is due to ricin, not RCA, because the latter does not penetrate the intestinal wall and does not affect the red blood cells unless given intravenously. If injected into the blood, RCA will cause the red blood cells to agglutinate and burst by hemolysis.

History and Military and Medical Significance. In ancient Egypt, *Ricinus communis* was cultivated for its oil's lubricating and laxative effects. Both castor bean oil and whole seeds have also been used in various regions of the world in the treatment of other diseases. During World Wars I and II, the lubricating oil was used in the aircraft industry until synthetic oils replaced the castor oil.

During the Cold War, ricin was used in the highly publicized assassination of the Bulgarian dissident Georgi Markov in 1978. He was killed with ricin contained in a pellet placed in an umbrella tip. Mr. Markov was stabbed with the umbrella while waiting for a bus on a London street *(479)*.

Any attack using ricin is likely to be on a small scale. Experts have estimated that 4 tons would be needed to affect $100\,km^2$, which would make ricin more a tool for assassination than a weapon of mass destruction. Ricin could also be used to contaminate food or water or by leaving it on door handles in busy buildings, with the aim of poisoning and spreading panic.

Recently, with the advent of new immunotherapeutic approaches, ricin has been studied as a component of anti-tumor regimens known as immunotoxins, specifically in chimeric toxins. For example, the native ricin or just its A-chain is conjugated to tumor cell–specific monoclonal antibodies (technically, to other ligands that target the active component of the toxin to tumor cells for selective killing). Some of these conjugates have undergone Phases I and II clinical trials as anticancer agents *(482, 483)*. Although the results have shown promise, two factors appear to limit ricin's immunoefficacy: the lack of specificity of the antibody, and the significant immunogenicity of the toxin moiety, which would result in relatively rapid onset of refractory immunity to the therapeutic agent *(484, 485)*.

When ingested, one to three ricin seeds may be fatal to a child; two to four may be poisonous to an adult, and eight may be fatal. A fatal ingested dose is about 1 mg/kg. Because the alimentary tract will destroy a significant amount of ricin because of its poor oral absorption from the gastrointestinal tract, it is much more potent when administered parenterally—a dose of 2 millionth of the body weight may prove fatal *(486)*.

Molecular Structure. Ricin is a heterodimeric ribosome-inhibiting protein. The ribosome-inactivating 32-kDa protein called A-chain (RTA) is linked by a disulfide bond to a 34-kDa B-chain (RTB), which is a specific galactose/*N*-acetylgalactosamine-binding lectin. Both chains are glycoproteins containing mannose-rich carbohydrate groups; the reticuloendothelial cells have mannose receptors. To confer toxicity, the A- and B-chains must be associated.

The ricin toxin has been crystallized, and its crystal structure was determined by x-ray crystallography to 2.5 Å *(487)*.

Ricin Uptake. Having bound diffusely to the cell membrane, ricin is internalized. The part of ricin bound to the cell surface undergoes receptor-mediated endocytosis. The ricin is taken up in uncoated pits, and pits and vesicles showing the characteristic clathrin coat. Smooth pits and/or large smooth invaginations may also play a part in the ricin uptake. The latter is not nearly as fast as the uptake of molecules such as LDL and transferrin, which use similar mechanisms, and thus there is a lag time between the administration of toxin and development of toxic effect.

The toxin molecule is then internalized to the vacuolar and tubo-vesicular portions of the endosomal system, where most of it remains bound to the plasma membrane, despite the prevailing acidic conditions.

Ricin is transported retrograde via the Golgi apparatus to the *endoplasmic reticulum (ER)*. For the A-chain subunit to reach its target ribosome site and cause toxic effects in the cell, it must first enter the cytosol, which it does through the ER using the so-called *ERAD (ER-associated protein degradation) pathway*. The ERAD pathway is associated with transportation of misfolded proteins to the proteosome. Ubiquitination is an important part of ERAD and may also be important in the ricin retrograde translocation. Once in the cytosol, at least some of the ricin must avoid proteasome degradation so that it can kill the cell. It is possible that ricin may be inefficiently ubiquitinylated due to a low lysine content of its A-chain. It may also be possible that the A-chain has learned to "look" like a misfolded protein in the ER, and once it is exported to the cytosol it will appear as a properly folded protein, thereby avoiding proteasome degradation.

Some ricin may reach the cytosol directly from the endosomes through endosome degradation.

Mechanism of Action. Like many other structurally and functionally related cytotoxic proteins from a variety of plants, ricin inhibits the protein synthesis by specifically and irreversibly inactivating the eukaryotic ribosomes. Typically, these ribosome-inactivating proteins (RIPs) are *N*-glycosylated *(488)*.

Ribosomes are complex structures, consisting of protein and nucleic acid (rRNA) components. Structurally, they have two subunits, a large subunit that contains an rRNA fragment (known as the 60S fragment), and a smaller subunit. The 60S fragment is made of several pieces of RNA, one of which is the 28S rRNA. It is believed that the RNA components are most important in the protein chain elongation catalysis. The ribosomes are responsible for protein synthesis from mRNA and amino acid subunits linked to tRNA.

The ricin A-chain catalytically and irreversibly inactivates the 60S large ribosomal subunit by binding and depurinating a specific adenine (at base A_{4324}) of the 28S rRNA fragment of the 60S RNA chain. The target adenine is a specific RNA sequence that contains the unusual tetranucleotide loop, GAGA. Depurination occurs at base A_{4324}, which is part of the GAGA loop.

The adenine ring of the ribosome becomes sandwiched between two tyrosine rings in the catalytic cleft of the enzyme (A-chain) and is hydrolyzed by the enzyme's N-glycosidase action. This change does not directly cause the hydrolysis of the RNA chain but renders the phosphodiester bonds surrounding the altered base highly susceptible to hydrolysis. This affects the binding of elongation factors to the ribosome and thus halts the protein synthesis; it requires no energy or cofactors.

Inactivation/Decontamination. Ricin can be inactivated by heat: 80°C for 10 minutes or 50°C for approximately 1 hour at pH 7.8. An 0.1% sodium hypochlorite solution is thought to be effective, although some have recommended using a stronger 0.5% sodium hypochlorite solution.

23.14.4.1   Clinical Manifestations of Ricin Intoxication

After ingestion, the incubation period is a few hours to a few days. After inhalation, the incubation period appears to be less than 8 hours. Humans who were accidentally exposed to sublethal doses of ricin would develop symptoms in 4 to 8 hours *(488)*.

Diagnosis. The diagnosis of ricin poisoning is usually based on clinical signs. Ricin can sometimes be detected in serum or respiratory secretions by ELISA and in tissues by immunohistochemistry. PCR assays can often find castor bean DNA in ricin preparations.

Ricin is very immunogenic, and serology can be useful for a retrospective diagnosis. ELISA and chemiluminescence tests are available.

Clinical Symptoms After Ingestion. Natural infections typically occur after ingestion. Onset of symptoms is usually within 4 to 6 hours but may be as late as 10 hours. The initial signs are nonspecific and may include colicky abdominal pain *(488)*. The ingested toxin usually manifests with severe gastrointestinal symptoms, including abdominal pain, diarrhea, fever, nausea, vomiting, incoordination, drowsiness, and hematuria. The fluid loss can lead to dehydration, particularly in children. Vascular collapse and death occur quickly, but most patients who survive for 3 to 5 days will recover.

Clinical Symptoms After Aerosol Inhalation. After aerosol exposure, the symptoms appear acutely with clinical signs that include fever, tightness of the chest, cough, dyspnea, nausea, and arthralgia. In sublethal doses, profuse sweating will occur several hours later, followed by recovery. Lethal human exposures by aerosol have not been reported. Based on studies in laboratory animals, airway necrosis and pulmonary edema would probably develop within 24 hours. Severe respiratory distress and death from respiratory complications and circulatory collapse would be expected to occur within 36 to 72 hours. The symptoms would likely include dyspnea, cyanosis, and hypotension.

Clinical Symptoms After Parenteral Intoxication: The Case of Georgi Markov. In the assassination of Georgi Markov in 1978, the ricin was placed in a pellet hidden in an umbrella tip *(480)*. The pellet, containing about 500 µg ricin, when injected into his body during the attack resulted in almost immediate local pain, then a feeling of weakness within 5 hours. Fifteen to 24 hours later, the victim had a high temperature, nausea, and vomiting. Thirty-six hours after the attack, he was admitted to the hospital feeling very ill, presenting with fever and tachycardia, but normal blood pressure. The lymph nodes of the affected groin were swollen and a 6-cm-diameter area of induration and inflammation was observed at the injection site on his thigh. Just over 2 days after the attack, Mr. Markov became suddenly hypotensive and tachycardic; his pulse rate was 160. The white blood count was $26,300/\text{mm}^3$. Early on the third day after the attack, the victim became anuric and began vomiting blood. An electrocardiogram demonstrated a complete atrioventricular conduction block. Mr. Markov died shortly thereafter; at the time of his death, his white blood cell count was $33,200/\text{mm}^3$ *(480)*.

Intramuscular or subcutaneous injection of toxin doses, as in the case of Mr. Markov, would result in severe local lymphoid necrosis, gastrointestinal hemorrhage, liver necrosis, diffuse nephritis, and diffuse splenitis. In the case of Mr. Markov, a mild pulmonary edema was thought to be secondary to cardiac failure *(480)*. Similar data have been collected after experimental animal studies.

23.14.4.2   Treatment of Ricin Intoxication

Because no antidote exists for ricin poisoning, the most important factor is to get the ricin off or out of the body as quickly as possible and to give the victim supportive medical care to minimize the effects of the poisoning.

For oral intoxication, supportive therapy includes administering activated charcoal and intravenous fluid and replacing electrolytes. For inhalational intoxication, supportive therapy is aimed at counteracting acute pulmonary edema and respiratory distress. Symptomatic care is the only intervention currently available for the treatment of incapacitating or lethal doses of inhaled ricin *(480)*.

Animal studies have shown that either active immunization or passive prophylaxis or therapy (if the therapy is given within a few hours) is extremely effective against intravenous or intraperitoneal intoxication with ricin. On the other hand, inhalational exposure is best countered with active immunization or prophylactic administration of aerosolized specific antiricin antibody *(480)*.

Ricin Vaccines

Ricin Toxoid Vaccines. A toxoid vaccine prepared from formalin-inactivated ricin holotoxin was developed during World War II and was shown to enhance survival significantly in animals exposed to ricin *(489)*.

An improved ricin toxoid vaccine based on denatured toxin adsorbed to Alhydrogel adjuvant was developed at USAMRIID in the 1990s and has been shown to be effective at protecting rhesus monkeys against ricin toxin aerosol exposure *(439)*. However, as with earlier studies, the vaccine did not protect completely against short-term (up to 14 days postexposure) bronchiolar and interstitial pulmonary inflammation.

The general failure of toxoid vaccines to protect the respiratory tract of exposed animals from the cytotoxic effects of ricin underscores the need to develop effective recombinant vaccines and alternative vaccine-delivery systems that can elicit and enhance mucosal immune response *(490, 491)*.

Deglycosylated Ricin A-Chain Vaccine. The ricin A-chain (RTA) conjugated with tumor-specific antibodies has been used clinically in animal and human studies to target and kill tumors *(483, 484)*. These and other studies *(492)* have contributed to the development of a recombinant ricin vaccine by demonstrating convincingly that the ricin A-chain in the absence of the B-chain is much less toxic than is the whole toxin when administered parenterally to animals *(493, 494)*.

Some technical limitations have arisen regarding the use of RTA or dgRTA (chemically deglycosylated RTA) as candidates for human vaccines. Both immunogens have retained residual *N*-glycosidase activity and have shown significant aggregation during expression and purification or upon prolonged storage in solution *(439)*. To this end, recombinant vaccine candidates with active-site–specific substitutions designed to reduce the *N*-glycosidase activity of RTA without disrupting the antigenic properties of the molecule have been proposed as vaccine candidates *(492, 495–498)*. Active-site substitutions in RTA essentially eliminated the problem of residual toxicity but did not address the important manufacturing problem regarding RTA instability and aggregation *(439)*.

Engineered Ricin Vaccines. It is thought that the tendency of subunit-based RTA vaccines to self-aggregate under physiologic conditions is related to the hydrophobic domains being exposed by the absence of the natural B-chain (RTB) subunit. Starting from a theoretical analysis of the functional architecture of the toxin compared with the related single-chain ribosome-inactivating proteins (RIPs) *(498–500)*, it was hypothesized that reducing the hydrophobic surface of RTA by large-scale deletions might result in a better structural platform for presenting the neutralizing epitope than that of the parent molecule.

Furthermore, along with reduced hydrophobic surface, recombinant vaccine candidates would have to retain the surface loop which is thought to serve as a neutralizing immunologic epitope for the ricin toxin (i.e., RTA residues 97 to 106; Ref. *493*). In addition, candidates would also have to lack key amino acid residues of the RNA binding site that is essential for *N*-glycosidase toxicity. Based on experimental trials with an array of recombinant RTA candidates, it was found that immunogens based approximately on the *N*-terminal domain of RTA (residues 1 to 198) best satisfied these design criteria *(439)*.

Under physiologic conditions, polypeptides based on RTA residues 1 to 198 remained folded as seen by circular dichroism and infrared spectroscopy, were more stable thermodynamically than was RTA, and exhibited dynamic light scattering, indicating monodisperse monomers without significant aggregation. Moreover, the single-domain immunogens showed no detectable toxin activity and protected mice against supralethal exposure to ricin toxin by injection or by aerosol *(439)*. In this case, protein engineering based partly on a functional analysis of protein domains has yielded ricin vaccine candidates that were superior to traditional approaches, including inactivated holotoxin or toxin subunit vaccines containing active-site mutations *(439)*.

23.14.5 Abrin Toxin

Abrin is a potent plant toxin that has been isolated from the seeds of *Abrus precatorius* (the rosary pea). Its cell agglutinating activity was first described in 1972 *(501)*, and its biological activity is very similar to that of ricin: the A-chain of abrin inhibits protein synthesis, whereas its B-chain binds to the cell surface receptors containing terminal galactose and acts as an immunotoxin. The A-chain is not active until it is internalized by the cell.

As with ricin, the extreme toxicity of abrin and its relatively easy manner of production makes it a potential biological weapon.

Molecular Structure and Mechanism of Action. Like ricin, abrin structurally represents a heterodimer consisting of two peptide moieties (A-chain and B-chain) linked by a disulfide bridge. Ricin and abrin have a large-scale molecular similarity, with the A-chains of both toxins having a 102 conserved amino acid homology.

Abrin exists in two forms, abrin-a and abrin-b, with both containing the A- and B-chains. A disulfide bond between Cys247 of the A-chain and Cys8 of the B-chain connects the two chains.

The A-chain comprises 251 residues and is divided into three folding domains. The A-chain catalytically inactivates 60S ribosomal subunits by removing adenine from positions

4 and 324 of 28S rRNA, resulting in the inhibition of the protein synthesis.

The B-chain represents a galactose-specific lectin that facilitates the binding of abrin to the cell membranes *(502, 503)*. The B-chain of both forms of abrin consists of 268 amino acid residues and shares 256 identical residues *(504)*. A comparison of the B-chains of abrin-a and abrin-b with that of ricin has shown that 60% of the residues of abrin's B-chain were identical to those of the B-chain of ricin. In addition, two saccharide-binding sites in the ricin B-chain identified by crystallographic studies were highly conserved in the abrin B-chain *(504)*.

The mechanism of action of abrin is identical to that of ricin, but the toxicity of abrin in mice was 75 times that of ricin (0.04 µg/kg for abrin compared with 3.0 µg/kg for ricin).

The diagnosis, clinical features, treatment, protection, and prophylaxis of abrin intoxication are the same as those of ricin *(505)*.

23.14.6 Trichothecene

Trichothecene (T-2 toxin) is a mycotoxin antibiotic produced by the fungus *Trichothecium roseum*. Though its acute toxicity by inhalation is similar to that of the poison blister gas lewisite [dichloro(2-chlorovinyl)arsine] (ca. 10^3 mg- min /m^3), the T-2 toxin is about 10 times more potent than liquid mustard [bis-(2-chloroethyl)sulfide] with dermal exposure *(506)*.

The trichothecenes are considered primarily blister agents that cause severe skin and eye irritation at low exposure doses. Subacute exposure reduces the host's resistance to bacterial or parasitic infections.

In general, the mycotoxins are not considered to be an established threat by aerosol exposure *(507)*.

23.15 Arthropod-Borne Viral Fever and Arthropathy

The arthropod-borne alphaviruses constitute an important genus of the Togaviridae family. Their ecologic maintenance is passage from mosquito to vertebrate to mosquito. The great majority of the Alphavirus-associated human infections are either subclinical or would result in a transient and only temporarily incapacitating febrile illness *(508)*. However, a small but important fraction of these infections will proceed with either viral entry into the central nervous system causing viral encephalitis or viral-associated fever and acute arthropathy, which is caused mainly by the chikungunya virus. Other togaviruses, including the O'nyong-

nyong (ONN), Igbo Ora, Mayaro, and Ross River viruses, as well as some strains of Sindbis (SIN) virus, have been associated with a similar syndrome. The togavirus rubella is also arthritogenic.

23.15.1 Chikungunya Virus

Originally, the chikungunya virus (CHIKV) (also known as the Buggy Creek virus) was probably an infection of primates in the forests and savannahs of Africa, maintained by the sylvatic *Aedes* mosquito, as it continues to be today in transmission mainly between mosquitoes and monkeys *(508)*. However, today the chikungunya virus is also the etiologic agent of *Ae. aegyptii*–transmitted urban epidemics in Africa, the Indian Ocean islands, and Asia, causing crippling arthralgia and arthritis accompanied by fever and other systemic symptoms of clinically distinctive chikungunya infection. The illness is rarely life-threatening. Nevertheless, a re-emerging disease in Africa and Asia that sometimes is clinically indistinguishable from dengue fever, chikungunya epidemics cause substantial morbidity and economic loss *(509)* (http://www.cdc.gov/travel; http://www.cdc.gov/ncidod/dvbid/Chikungunya/chikvfact.htm). In a very recent development, in September 2007 an outbreak of about 160 cases was reported in the Ravenna region of northern Italy (http://news.bbc.co.uk/2/hi/health/6981476.stm).

The word *chikungunya* is thought to be derived from the word *kungunyala* in the Swahili/Makonde language of southeastern Tanzania and northern Mozambique. It is used for both the virus and the disease and means "to walk bent over" or "to dry up or become contorted" referring to the effect of the joint pains that characterize this illness.

Genomic Studies. The complete genomic sequence of chikungunya virus (strain S27 African prototype) has been determined and the presence of an internal polyadenylation [I-poly(A)] site was confirmed within the 3′ nontranslated region (NTR) of this strain *(510)*. The complete genome was 11,805 nucleotides in length, excluding the 5′ cap nucleotide, an I-poly(A) tract and the 3′ poly(A) tail. It comprised two long open reading frames that encoded the nonstructural (2,474 amino acids) and structural proteins (1,244 amino acids). In addition, predicted secondary structures were identified within the 5′ NTR and repeated sequence elements (RSEs) within the 3′ NTR.

Amino acid sequence homologies, phylogenetic analysis of nonstructural and structural proteins, and characteristic RSEs revealed that although CHIKV is closely related to the O'nyong-nyong (ONN) virus, the chikungunya virus is in fact a distinct entity.

In another study *(511)*, the genomic sequence of a sole isolate obtained from the cerebrospinal fluid of a patient from the Indian Ocean islands showed unique changes in nsP1 (T3011), nsP2 (Y622N), and nsP3 (E460 deletion) nonstructural proteins, not obtained from isolates from sera. In the structural protein region, two noteworthy changes (A226V and D284E) were observed in the membrane fusion glycoprotein E1. Homology three-dimensional modeling allowed mapping of these two changes to regions that are important for membrane fusion and virion assembly. Change E1-A226V was absent in the initial strains but observed in more than 90% of subsequent viral sequences from a Réunion Island strain, denoting evolutionary success—possibly due to adaptation to the mosquito *(511)*.

Epidemiology. Epidemics of fever, rash, and arthritis resembling chikungunya fever were recorded as early as 1824 in India. However, the virus was first isolated in 1952–1953 from both humans and mosquitoes during an epidemic of fever in Tanzania.

Chikungunya fever (also known as "chicken guinea") displays interesting epidemiologic profiles: major epidemics appear and disappear in a cyclical manner, usually with an interepidemic period of 7 to 8 years and sometimes as long as 20 years. Between 1960 and 1982, outbreaks of chikungunya fever were reported in Africa and Asia (Thailand, 1960s; India, 1964; Sri Lanka, 1969; Vietnam, 1975; Myanmar, 1975; and Indonesia, 1982). Recently, after an interval of more than 20 years, outbreaks of chikungunya fever have been reported in India and various Indian Ocean islands (Comoros, Mayotte, Mauritius, Réunion, Seychelles, and the Nicobar and Andaman Islands) *(512–517)* (http://www.searo. who.int/en/Section10/Section2246.htm). In some regions of India, the attack rates have reached as high as 45%, with more than 1.25 million cases reported in 2006.

Chikungunya fever, although considered to be rarely life threatening, has been shown to cause fatalities: during the 2005–2006 epidemic in Réunion Island, the number of deaths rose by 34% in February 2006 and by 25% in March 2006, compared with the same months in 2005. These increases represent a total of 170 to 180 additional deaths just for these 2 months, with many of them in patients older than 75 years of age *(518)*. A total excess of 260 deaths was reported by the French National Institute for Public Health Surveillance *(518)* for the outbreak. This would correspond with roughly a 1% case fatality ratio for estimated cases of chikungunya based on seroprevalence studies *(513)*.

The suggestion *(512)* that the recent outbreak of chikungunya fever in India *(516)* could have been caused by the same viral strain that caused the Indian Ocean islands outbreak *(517)* has been challenged, based on comparison of the E1 sequences of both strains *(511, 519)*; microheterogeneity studies have shown the presence of a single nucleotide change (T321C) found in all Indian Ocean isolates, whereas isolates from India retained the ancestral T321 nucleotide present in all other African and Asian strains *(519)*.

The clinical manifestations of chikungunya fever have to be distinguished from dengue fever, especially when co-occurrence of both fevers is observed, as was recently the case in the Maharashtra State in India. Such cases highlight the importance of strong clinical suspicion and efficient laboratory diagnosis support.

The chikungunya virus is killed by common disinfectants, moist heat, and drying.

23.15.1.1 Clinical Manifestations

The incubation period can be 3 to 12 days but is usually 3 to 7 days. There is a sudden onset of flu-like symptoms including severe headache, chills, fever ($> 40°C$, $104°F$), joint pain, nausea, and vomiting. The joints of the extremities in particular become swollen and painful to the touch; most frequently affected joints are fingers, wrists, toes, and ankles. At the early acute stage of the disease (within 10 days of disease onset), rash may also occur *(514)*. However, "silent" CHIKV infections (with no illness) do occur, but how commonly this happens is still not known.

Typically, the clinical course of chikungunya fever involves two stages: an initial severe febrile and eruptive polyarthritis, followed by disabling peripheral rheumatism that can persist for months. Also, during the second stage there is the possibility of transitory peripheral vascular disorders. Besides the arthralgic syndrome, some patients, especially children, may present with neurologic disorders or fulminant hepatitis *(511)*.

All patients suffer from arthritis. Note: The prolonged joint pain with CHIKV is not typical of dengue fever (http://www.cdc.gov/ncidod/dvbid/Chikungunya/chikvfact.htm).

Treatment

No specific therapies are currently available. Symptomatic treatment for mitigating pain and fever using anti-inflammatory drugs along with rest usually is sufficient. While recovery from chikungunya fever is the expected outcome, convalescence is prolonged (up to a year or more), and persistent join pain may require analgesic and long-term anti-inflammatory therapy.

Vaccine. After several successful trials, a vaccine against CHIKV, a potential bioterrorist agent, was developed by the U.S. military after interest in chikungunya was aroused in the 1960s, when Thailand was overrun by simultaneous outbreaks of cholera, dengue, and chikungunya. The vaccine source was a weakened version of the Thailand CHIKV strain 15561 and was labeled TSI-GSD-218. In volunteers, it was safe, well tolerated, and highly immunogenic—8% of vaccine recipients developed chikungunya antibodies by day

28, and 85% of the recipients remained seropositive after 1 year. In 1969, an experimental vaccine using the killed chikungunya virus underwent testing in the Walter Reed Army Institute of Research (WRAIR).

23.15.2   O'nyong-nyong Virus

The O'nyong-nyong (ONN) virus is considered antigenically as a subtype of the chikungunya virus. Although similar in many other respects as well, there are highly significant differences. However, recently published data have shown that chikungunya virus and ONN virus are two distinct viruses after phylogenetic analysis (E1 protein) and serologic studies *(520)*.

The ONN virus was identified as the causative agent of a major East African epidemic in 1959 *(521, 522)*. The disease, which was referred to by the Acholi word meaning "weakening of the joints," had affected at least 2 million people. After the epidemic, ONN virus was not encountered again until its isolation from *Anopheles funestus* in 1978 *(523)*. Another *Anopheles* species, *An. gambiae*, has also been implicated as a vector of ONN.

Clinical Manifestations. ONN and CHIK viral infections result in a similar clinical syndrome *(522)*. After an incubation period thought to be at least 8 days, a sudden onset of joint manifestations occur. Rash occurred in 60% to 70% of patients an average of 4 days later, often accompanied by an improvement in symptoms *(508)*. The morbilliform eruption last for 4 to 7 days before subsiding. Fever was less common than in CHIKV infections, exceeding 101°F in only about one third of outpatients. In contrast with chikungunya disease, ONN illness is characterized by the development of markedly enlarged lymph nodes of a firm, rubbery consistency *(508)*. There are no known drugs against ONN virus, and symptomatic treatment is the therapy of choice.

23.16   NIAID Research Agenda in Biodefense

Improving the United States' defenses against bioterrorism is a key part of the U.S. government's homeland security effort. The Department of Health and Human Services (DHHS) supports activities to improve local and state public health systems, to expand existing biosurveillance efforts, and to fund research on medical countermeasures against potential bioterror agents.

NIAID is committed to accelerating development of medical tools to detect and counter the effects of a bioterrorist attack (http://www3.niaid.nih.gov/topics/Biodefense Related/Biodefense/about/niaidRole.htm), including:

- Vaccines to immunize the public against diseases caused by bioterrorism agents
- Diagnostic tests to help first responders and other medical personnel rapidly detect exposure and provide treatment
- Therapies to help patients exposed to bioterrorism agents regain their health

The capability to detect and counter bioterrorism depends to a substantial degree on the state of the relevant medical science, and basic research provides the essential underpinning. The National Institutes of Health (NIH) biodefense program, spearheaded by NIAID, includes both short- and long-term research targeted at the design, development, and evaluation of the specific public health tools (diagnostics, therapies, and vaccines) needed to control a bioterrorist-caused outbreak. The generation of genome sequence information on potential bioterrorism agents is also an important component of this program.

Since 2001, NIAID has greatly accelerated its biodefense research program, launching several new initiatives to catalyze development of vaccines, therapies, and diagnostic tests. For example, in December 2004, an NIAID-funded clinical trial aimed at boosting the nation's flu vaccine supply began enrolling volunteers at four U.S. sites. In October 2004, NIAID announced $232 million in biodefense contracts for vaccine development against three potential bioterror agents: smallpox, plague, and tularemia. Also, an NIAID-funded study shed new light on how the smallpox virus attacks its victims.

Identifying Research Priorities. NIAID has set research priorities and goals for each microorganism that might be used as an agent of bioterrorism, with particular emphasis on Category A agents—those considered by the CDC to be the worst bioterror threats. NIAID's research agenda and strategic plan cover the following categories (http://www3.niaid.nih.gov/topics/BiodefenseRelated/Biodefense/about/niaidRole.htm):

- *Basic Biology*—understanding how microorganisms and their toxic products function and cause disease
- *Immunology and Host Response*—understanding how the human immune system interacts with and defends the body against potential agents of bioterrorism
- *Design/Development/Clinical Evaluation of Therapies*
- *Vaccines*—working closely with industry to create new and improved vaccines
- *Drugs*—working closely with industry to develop and test drugs to treat diseases that may result from a biological attack
- *Genomics, Basic Research, and Infrastructure*
- *Diagnostics*—developing devices or methods to quickly and accurately diagnose diseases caused by bioterrorism agents

- *Research Resources*—establishing biosafety laboratories, databases, and other resources to help scientists conduct safe and effective biodefense research

23.16.1 Major NIAID Programs in Biodefense Research

- *Modified Vaccinia Ankara Smallpox Vaccine.* NIAID continues to support advanced development and manufacture of a modified vaccinia Ankara (MVA) vaccine for smallpox, with the intention of targeting MVA vaccine candidates that can be produced on a scale to support commercial manufacturing. Two pharmaceutical companies, Bavarian Nordic and Acambis, Inc., have played a key role in the development of MVA vaccine candidates under contracts awarded by NIAID. Clinical trials are under way in the United States to evaluate the safety and immunogenicity of MVA in healthy adults, and in the United States and Europe to determine the safety and immunogenicity of MVA in adults with atopic dermatitis and HIV. A study is under way in the United States to compare routes of administration (intradermal, intramuscular, and subcutaneous) of MVA in healthy individuals (http://www3.niaid.nih.gov/Biodefense/ Public/PDF/spox_niaid_invest.pdf).
- *Smallpox Vaccines.* In addition to work to advance MVA, NIAID continues to support the development of additional smallpox vaccines (http://www3.niaid.nih.gov/ Biodefense/Public/PDF/spox_niaid_invest.pdf).   Three new vaccines are currently supported: (i) a live-attenuated vaccinia virus vaccine that is attenuated by a different mechanism than that of MVA; (ii) a protein subunit vaccine that comprises four variola virus proteins that are known to be largely responsible for stimulating the protective immune response that occurs when the live virus vaccine is used, thereby limiting the adverse reactions that are usually caused by other components of the virus; and (iii) a subunit vaccine in which the homologous immunity-stimulating proteins from vaccinia are expressed in a disabled, nonreplicating Venezuelan equine encephalitis (VEE) vector.

NIAID's Vaccine Research Center (VRC) has tested MVA as an attenuated poxvirus with the potential to protect against vaccinia (the virus used to vaccinate against smallpox) or variola (the virus that causes smallpox). The vaccine has been provided by Therion Biologics Corporation as part of a collaboration agreement with the Vaccine Research Center. Two Phase I clinical trials testing MVA as a component of a safer smallpox vaccine in both vaccinia- naïve and vaccinia-immune populations have concluded.

- *Compound ST-246.* Through a SBIR grant to SIGA Technologies, Inc., NIAID is continuing to support an orally bioavailable anti-poxvirus compound (ST-246) that inhibits extracellular virus formation and protects rodents from lethal Orthopoxvirus challenge. ST-246 has been shown to be highly active against a number of orthopoxviruses both *in vitro* and in animal models. NIAID has supported the preclinical development of ST-246 and recently awarded a contract for advanced manufacturing and clinical studies *(524)*
- *Cidofovir.* Clinical protocols to assess activity of cidofovir as a treatment for complications related to smallpox vaccine have been developed in the Vaccine Treatment and Evaluation Units (VTEUs) as backup therapy after vaccine immune globulin (VIG) has been indicated. To date, no one has needed to be enrolled in this protocol.
- *Recombinant Protective Antigen Anthrax Vaccine.* NIAID is continuing its support of advanced development and production of a recombinant protective antigen (rPA) vaccine for anthrax (http://www3.niaid.nih.gov/topics/ Biodefense/BiodefenseRelated/Biodefense/research/ anthrax.htm).

In 2004, new contracts were awarded to two pharmaceutical companies, Vaxgen and Avecia, to build upon the companies' achievements, supporting production, testing, and evaluation of rPA vaccine; this includes two Phase II clinical trials per contract. Proof-of-concept aerosol challenge efficacy studies in rabbits and non-human primates were successfully completed for both rPA vaccine candidates, as have postexposure efficacy rabbit studies that combined antibiotic and vaccine treatments. Avecia's Phase II clinical trials were completed by the end of 2006. Both companies have validated new facilities and completed validation of processes for large-scale current Good Manufacturing Practice (cGMP) manufacturing of rPA vaccine by the end of 2006.

- *Ebola Vaccine.* Building on their previous results that showed that the prime-boost vaccination strategy produced a strong, long-lasting immune response in vaccinated non-human primates, scientists at the VRC, in collaboration with researchers at the U.S. Army Medical Research Institute for Infectious Disease (USAMRIID), have developed an Ebola vaccine. Testing was conducted to determine whether the immune response mounted against the boost component alone would be sufficient to protect monkeys against Ebola infection. Results have shown that monkeys vaccinated with only the boost survived, even those who received high doses of Ebola virus. In 2005, the VRC completed a 2-year study of the first human trial of a DNA vaccine designed to prevent the Ebola infection. The trial consisted of three vaccinations given over 3 months, and study participants were followed for 1 year. Results have demonstrated that this DNA vaccine was safe and well tolerated with no significant adverse events, and it was capable of inducing an immune response. In another project, VRC scientists have developed a fast-acting, single-shot experimental Ebola vaccine for humans based on previous studies showing protection in monkeys. A Phase I vaccine trial in humans began in autumn 2006 (http://www3.niaid.nih.gov/news/newsreleases/2003/ebolahumantrial.htm).

Vaccines against Ebola and Marburg viruses are also under development by extramural scientists with NIAID support. A partnership grant was awarded in 2002 to develop a vaccine against Marburg virus, using an Alphavirus replicon particle technology. This vaccine is effective in protecting small animals and non-human primates against Marburg virus infection and is in advanced stages of preclinical development. Vaccines against Ebola virus are under early stages of development using a variety of approaches, which include replicon particle vaccines, virus-like particle vaccines, and recombinant protein subunit vaccines.

- *Dengue Fever*. NIAID is funding research to develop countermeasures against Dengue fever (http://www3. niaid.nih.gov/healthscience/healthtopics/dengue/). One direction is to develop a validated, fully automated, portable, point-of-care nucleic acid detection system for the rapid diagnosis of *hemorrhagic fever* syndromes caused by Category A–C biodefense viruses, including dengue. Another direction is to develop a live-attenuated tetravalent dengue (DEN) vaccine. This experimental vaccine is a mixture of the established attenuated DEN-2 vaccine strain, which has been shown to be safe and effective in human clinical trials, and chimeric viruses that express the structural genes of the other three DEN serotypes in the attenuated DEN-2 background.
- *Arenaviruses*. NIAID is supporting efforts to develop and validate new ELISA diagnostic tests to be used in clinics for the rapid detection of arenaviruses that cause viral hemorrhagic fevers in humans. These include the highly pathogenic Lassa virus in Africa, as well as Junin, Machupo, Guanarito, and Sabiá viruses in South America (http://www3.niaid.nih.gov/Biodefense/Research/biotresearchagenda.pdf).
- *Rift Valley Fever*. NIAID is also supporting efforts to develop vaccines against Rift Valley fever virus, a Category A pathogen of both human and veterinary importance. Vaccine candidates are being developed using a variety of approaches, including live-attenuated viruses, virus-like particles, and Sindbis virus replicon-particle-based vaccine.
- The *Food and Waterborne Diseases Integrated Research Network (FWD IRN)*. FWD IRN is supporting multidisciplinary research and the development of products to

rapidly identify, prevent, and treat food- and water-borne diseases. The network currently funds:

- ○ Research and development of improved diagnostics for enteric pathogens.
- ○ Vaccine research on tularemia vaccine strain LVS, *Shigella*, and *S. typhi*. A clinical study to improve response to *S. typhi* vaccination.
- ○ Research on the molecular evolution and transmission of antibiotic-resistant genes in enteric pathogens.
- ○ Development of animal models for botulinum neurotoxins, Shiga toxin–producing *E. coli* (STEC)-mediated hemolytic uremic syndrome (HUS), *Campylobacter*-mediated enteritis, shigellosis, and Crohn's disease.
- ○ Strain repository for STEC.
- ○ Development of high-throughput screening assays for small-molecule drugs against BoNT and Shiga toxin.
- ○ Basic and applied research on *Clostridium difficile*, a pathogen emerging with increased virulence.

- *Botulism*. NIAID is funding research focused on the discovery and development of botulism therapeutics that would be effective in a postexposure scenario; there are two categories of potential postexposure treatments.

NIAID is also funding research to develop protective vaccines against botulism serotypes C, D, E, F, and G and to successfully formulate vaccines that protect against multiple serotypes, including serotypes A and B. Approaches that are being funded include (i) the traditional approach of a vaccine derived from recombinant protein fragments of the neurotoxin; and (ii) novel approaches such as constructing Alphavirus replicon particles that express protective, nontoxic fragments of the neurotoxin or immune enhancing entities *in vivo*. NIAID has also used the simplified acquisition process authority provided by *Project BioShield* to contract for the further development of a serotype E–specific vaccine candidate.

- *Neurotoxin Research*. With regard to inhibitors that prevent the neurotoxins from entering neuronal cells (their site of action), NIAID is funding the discovery and development of human-compatible monoclonal antibody inhibitors. NIAID is also supporting work on human-compatible polyclonal antibodies produced in transgenic animals. NIAID has also used the simplified acquisition process authority provided by *Project BioShield* to contract for the further development of serotype A–specific monoclonal antibodies.

With regard to inhibitors that block the activity of neurotoxin after they have entered the neuronal cell (which would provide the greatest therapeutic value), NIAID is funding, through grants and the FWD IRN contract, research on identifying inhibitors of protease activity, and the development of novel drug carrier systems to deliver inhibitors to the interior of peripheral cholinergic nerve cells.

- *Tularemia*. NIAID is extensively supporting basic research and product development in tularemia. Thus, a Phase I clinical trial is under way using the Army's Live Vaccine Strain (LVS) tularemia vaccine through collaboration with the Department of Defense. NIAID also has a contract with DynPort Co. to support the current clinical trial and the manufacture of an additional clinical batch of LVS for possible future trials, including testing the vaccine's stability. NIAID-supported researchers have discovered critical host-defense mechanisms against tularemia in a mouse model. In research jointly supported with the Department of Defense, a real-time PCR test to simultaneously detect the bacteria that cause tularemia, plague, anthrax, and *Burkholderia* has been developed. In 2006, NIAID awarded two contracts (University of New Mexico and Dynport Co.) for the development of new tularemia vaccine candidates and the assays and animal models with which to evaluate them.

- *Plague*. NIAID is supporting a robust portfolio of basic research and product development for basic research and product development for plague. In 2006, NIAID exercised an option on its contract with Avecia, Inc., for the further development, testing, and evaluation of a plague vaccine, to include additional manufacture of GMP material for Phase II clinical trials. Together with USAMRIID and FDA, NIAID is evaluating licensed antibiotic therapies in a monkey model of pneumonic plague. Studies on gentamicin and ciprofloxacin have been completed and task orders recently given for studies on levofloxacin and doxycycline.

- *Category B and C Agents*

  o *Severe Acute Respiratory Syndrome (SARS) Coronavirus*. The Vaccine Research Center contracted with Vical, Inc., to manufacture a single, closed, circular DNA plasmid–based vaccine encoding the S protein of the SARS coronavirus. Mouse studies conducted at VRC have demonstrated that this vaccine induces T-cell and neutralizing antibody responses, as well as protective immunity. A Phase I open-label clinical study to evaluate safety, tolerability, and immune response was completed in 2006 *(387)*. In the study, healthy 18- to 50-year-old subjects received 4.0-mg DNA vaccinations at three 1-month intervals. Interim study results indicated that the vaccine is well tolerated; immunogenicity analysis of the stored samples is ongoing.

  o *West Nile Virus*. The VRC is currently developing a DNA-based vaccine against West Nile virus (WNV) in collaboration with Vical, Inc. The vaccine is based on an existing codon-modified gene-based DNA plas-

mid vaccine platform designed to express WNV proteins. In 2005, following preclinical safety studies and viral challenge studies, the Vaccine Research Center initiated a Phase I clinical trial to evaluate safety, tolerability, and immune responses of this recombinant DNA vaccine in human volunteers. Also in collaboration with Vical, Inc., the VRC has developed a second-generation DNA vaccine using an improved expression vector expressing the same WNV proteins.

  o *Japanese Encephalitis Virus (JEV)*. NIAID is supporting the development of a novel inactivated vaccine against Japanese encephalitis virus, using promising vaccine and adjuvant technologies. The Japanese encephalitis virus is the leading cause of encephalitis worldwide, and new vaccines against this disease are sorely needed.

  o *Influenza Therapeutics*. In 2006, NIAID made grant awards using authorities granted by the *Project BioShield Act* of 2004 for the development of high-throughput assays to screen influenza therapeutics.

- *Immunity and Biodefense*

  o *Immune Epitope Discovery*. Several of the Immune Epitope Discovery contracts made significant progress in 2004–2005 in identifying antibody and T-cell epitopes to such pathogens as influenza, vaccinia virus, and *Clostridium botulinum* neurotoxins. Investigators at Scripps Research Institute identified three candidate neutralizing antibody Fab fragments with specificity toward *Clostridium botulinum* neurotoxin A. Further characterization of these antibodies and the epitopes recognized is ongoing. Researchers at the Benaroya Research Institute at Virginia Mason characterized 18 MHC class II epitopes recognized by human CD4$^+$ T-cells. Finally, investigators at the La Jolla Institute of Allergy and Immunology identified 49 MHC class I epitopes recognized by CD8$^+$ T-cells from individuals receiving Dryvax vaccine; nine of these epitopes were recognized by T-cells from several donors and may represent common epitopes for monitoring host responses to vaccination or for developing subunit vaccines.

  o *Atopic Dermatitis and Vaccinia Immunization Network (ADVN)*. In 2004, NIAID established the Atopic Dermatitis and Vaccinia Immunization Network (ADVN) to develop short- and long-term approaches to reduce the incidence and severity of eczema vaccinatum and protect individuals with atopic dermatitis from the adverse consequences of vaccinia exposure. The ADVN consists of (i) Clinical Studies Consortium; (ii) Animal Studies Consortium; and (iii) Statistical and Data Coordinating Center.

○ *Systems Approach to Innate Immunity and Inflammation.* The NIAID-supported cooperative agreement Systems Approach to Innate Immunity and Inflammation, which uses systems biology approaches to produce a detailed map of innate immune responses to infection, generated an additional 25 monoclonal antibodies to human and mouse innate immune response genes, thus bringing the total to more than 60. Many of these antibodies are being submitted to the NIAID's Biodefense Research Resource Repository for public distribution. The researchers also produced a total of 69 mutant mouse lines, using random mutagenesis techniques, with defects in immune response genes. Thirty-two of these mutations affect the immune system, 27 of the genes were identified, and 13 were shown to be involved in Toll-like receptors (TLR) signaling pathways of the innate immune responses to viral and bacterial infections. Many of the mutant mice have been deposited in existing mouse repositories (i.e., Jax, NCRR Mutant Mouse Regional Resource Centers) for public distribution.

• *Research Resources*
NAIAD has made available a number of research resources (http://www3.niaid.nih.gov/topics/Biodefense Related/Biodefense/research/resources/default.htm) available as follows:

○ *National Biocontainment Laboratories and Regional Biocontainment Laboratories.* NIAID is continuing to support its network of National Biocontainment Laboratories (NBLs) and Regional Biocontainment Laboratories (RBLs) by providing funds for the maintenance and operation of the NBLs.

○ *The C. W. Bill Young Center for Biodefense and Emerging Infectious Diseases* opened on the NIH campus in Bethesda, Maryland, in May 2006. The center contains BSL-2/3 laboratory space *(387)*. In addition, NIAID is constructing two other intramural BSL-3/4 laboratories, one in collaboration with USAMRIID in Frederick, Maryland, and the other at the Rocky Mountain Laboratory in Hamilton, Montana, as well as funding the upgrade to BSL-3+ of one of its *in vivo* screening contract laboratories at Utah State University to allow the study of pathogenic strains of influenza in a mouse model.

○ *NIAID Vaccine Immune T-Cell and Antibody Laboratory.* The VRC completed the development of the NIAID Vaccine Immune T-Cell and Antibody Laboratory (NVITAL) in collaboration with DAIDS and the Henry Jackson Foundation to create added immune assay capacity and to accelerate the immunologic testing of candidate vaccines, including those for Category A agents such as Ebola, Lassa, and Marburg viruses. Located in Gaithersburg, Maryland, the facility provides state-of-the-art immunogenicity testing to support NIAID vaccine trials that are multinational in scope and that generate thousands of samples. High-throughput immunology assay capabilities are developed and implemented by conforming to the highest scientific standards and goals, while complying with all appropriate quality guidelines. At the start of 2006, NVITAL began its initial experiments and began sample processing. In May 2006, NVITAL completed assay validation and began clinical trials end-point testing.

○ *The Immune Epitope Database and Analysis Resource (IEDB)* became publicly available in February 2005 (www.immuneepitope.org). The IEDB contains extensively curated antibody and T-cell epitope information from the published literature, as well as tools to predict antibody and T-cell epitopes or visualization/mapping of epitopes onto known protein structures. There are currently 17,868 unique epitopes within the database, including all published influenza antibody and T-cell epitopes and approximately 90% of the published epitopes for NIAID Category A, B, and C Priority Pathogens. This program is supported by a DAIT contract to the La Jolla Institute of Allergy and Immunology.

○ *In Vitro and Animal Models for Emerging Infectious Diseases and Biodefense Program.* This program provides a wide range of resources for *in vitro* and *in vivo* nonclinical testing of new therapies and vaccines. These contracts provide resources for development and validation of small laboratory animal and non-human primate infection models for licensure of vaccines and therapeutics by the Food and Drug Administration (FDA). Specific projects include the *in vitro* assays and animal models for anthrax, plague, tularemia, smallpox, ricin, botulinum neurotoxin, SARS, and avian influenza, as well as other antimicrobials.

More information on the numerous NIAID resources available to biodefense researchers is provided at http://www2.niaid.nih.gov/biodefense/research/resources.htm.

23.16.2 Genomics and Proteomics

NIAID has made a significant investment in the genomic sequencing of microorganisms considered agents of bioterrorism. Knowledge of the genomes of these organisms will aid researchers in discovering new targets for therapeutics, vaccines, and diagnostics. To this end, NIAID is currently supporting sequencing efforts of multiple NIAID Category A, B, and C potential agents of bioterrorism. As of September 2006, NIAID-supported investigators completed

131 genome sequencing projects for 105 bacteria, 8 fungi, 15 parasitic protozoans, 2 invertebrate vectors of infectious diseases, and 1 plant. In addition, NIAID completed the sequence for 1,467 influenza genomes.

In 2006, genome sequencing projects (see also Section 25.4.2.1 in Chapter 25) were completed for the following organisms:

Burkholderia mallei (3 strains)
Burkholderia pseudomallei (3 strains)
Burkholderia cenocepacia
Burkholderia dolosa
Campylobacter (9 strains)
Coxiella burnetii (2 strains)
Escherichia coli (1 strain)
Listeria monocytogenes (2 strains)
Mycobacterium tuberculosis (2 strains)
Pseudomonas aeruginosa (3 strains)
Rickettsiella grylli (1 strain)
Shigella dysenteriae
Yersinia pestis (1 strain)
Influenza viruses (1,134 additional isolates)
Aspergillus fischerianus
Aspergillus clavatus
Entamoeba invadens
Entamoeba dispans
Plasmodium falciparum (2 strains)
Toxoplasma gondii (1 strain)
Trichomonas vaginalis
Ricin communis

Ongoing Sequencing Projects. In 2006, NIAID supported approximately 40 large-scale genome sequencing projects for additional strains of viruses, bacteria, fungi, parasites, viruses and invertebrate vectors, and new projects include additional strains of *Borrelia, Clostridium, E. coli, Salmonella, Streptococcus pneumonia, Ureaplasma, Coccidioides, Penicillium marneffei, Talaromyces stipitatus, Lacazia loboi, Histoplasma capsulatum, Blastomyces dermatitidis, Cryptosporidium muris,* dengue viruses, and additional sequencing and annotation of *Aedes aegyptii.*

For more information on the NIAID's genomic program, including resources available to researchers, see Section 25.4.2 in Chapter 25.

23.16.3 Recent NIAID Research Initiatives

Numerous NIAID initiatives resulted in 2006 biodefense awards in the areas of basic research, product development, clinical research, and research resources. For a comprehensive list of awards, see the 2006 Biodefense Awards page at http://www3.niaid.nih.gov/Biodefense/Research/2006awards/default.htm.

● *Basic Research*

○ *Biodefense and Emerging Infectious Diseases Research Opportunities.* Objective: To encourage the submission of investigator-initiated research grant applications in biodefense and select emerging infectious diseases. The goal is to expedite research leading to the diagnosis, prevention, and treatment of diseases caused by potential bioterrorism agents.

○ *Innate Immunity to NIAID Category B Protozoa.* Objective: To discover the cellular/molecular/ biochemical mechanisms by which the mammalian innate immune system responds to NIAID Category B Priority Pathogens.

○ *Training and Career Development for Biodefense and Emerging Diseases.* Objective: To ensure that an adequate cadre of well-trained and motivated investigators are available to pursue research and development objectives in biodefense and emerging diseases.

● *Product Development*

○ *Assays for Influenza Therapeutics: Project BioShield.* Objective: To develop high-throughput *in vitro* screening assays for influenza antiviral therapeutics incorporating validated, high-priority biochemical targets.

○ *Development of Therapeutic Agents for Selected Viral Diseases.* Objective: To develop new, safe, and effective therapeutics for variola major and viral hemorrhagic fevers, viral encephalitis, and influenza.

○ *NIAID Small Business Biodefense Program.* Objective: To encourage SBIR/STTR applications to develop therapeutics, vaccines, adjuvants/immunostimulants, diagnostics, and selected resources for biodefense.

○ *Cooperative Research Partnerships for Biodefense.* Objective: To support the discovery, design, and development of vaccines, therapeutics, adjuvants, and diagnostics for NIAID Category A, B, and C priority pathogens and toxins.

● *Research Resources*

○ *NBL Operations Cooperative Agreements.* Objective: To support operations of NIAID National Biocontainment Laboratories (NBLs).

○ *Services for Pre-Clinical Development of Therapeutic Agents.* Objective: To establish a resource to facilitate preclinical development of therapeutic agents (drugs or biological products) including activities required for Investigational New Drug applications.

23.17 Recent Scientific Advances

- *An Orally Bioavailable Antipoxvirus Compound (ST-246) Inhibits Extracellular Virus Formation and Protects Mice from Lethal Orthopoxvirus Challenge.* Concern over the use of smallpox (variola virus) as a biological weapon has prompted interest in the development of small-molecule therapeutics against the disease. Smallpox is highly transmissible and causes severe disease with high mortality rates. ST-246 has been shown to be highly active against a number of orthopoxviruses both *in vitro* and in animal models. Cowpox virus variants selected in cell culture for resistance to ST-246 were found to have a single amino acid change in the V061 gene. Re-engineering this change back into the wild-type cowpox virus genome conferred resistance to ST-246, suggesting that V061 is the target of ST-246 antiviral activity. The cowpox virus V061 gene is homologous to vaccinia virus F13L gene, which encodes a major envelope protein (p37) required for production of extracellular virus. In cell culture, ST-246 inhibited plaque formation and virus-induced cytopathic effects. In single-cycle growth assays, ST-246 reduced extracellular virus formation 10-fold relative to untreated controls, while having little effect on the production of intracellular virus. *In vivo*, oral administration of ST-246 protected BALB/c mice from lethal injection, after intranasal administration of $10 \times 50\%$ lethal dose (LD_{50}) of vaccinia virus strain IHD-J. ST-246-treated mice that survived infection acquired protective immunity and were resistant to subsequent challenge with lethal dose ($10 \times LD_{50}$) of vaccinia virus. Furthermore, orally administered ST-246 also protected A/NCr mice from lethal infection, after intranasal inoculation with $40,000 \times LD_{50}$ of ectromelia virus. These and other results, coupled with its lack of toxicity, make ST-246 a superb candidate for further development and eventual licensure by the FDA to prevent or treat smallpox infection in humans *(524)*.

- *Activity and Mechanism of Action of N-Methanocarbathymidine Against Herpesvirus and Orthopoxvirus Infections.* N-Methanocarbathymidine [(N)-MCT] is a new conformationally locked analogue that was found to exert *in vitro* activity active against some herpesviruses and orthopoxviruses *(525)*. The antiviral activity of (N)-MCT was dependent on the type I thymidine kinase (TK) in herpes simplex virus and also appeared to be dependent on the type II TK expressed by cowpox and vaccinia viruses, suggesting that it is a substrate for both of these divergent forms of the enzyme. Furthermore, (N)-MCT was also found to exhibit good activity inhibiting viral DNA polymerase once it is activated by the viral TK homologs. This mechanism of action has explained the rather unusual spectrum of activity, which was limited to only orthopoxviruses, alphaherpesviruses, and the Epstein-Barr virus, as all of these viruses express molecules with TK activity that can phosphorylate and thus activate (N)-MCT.

- *Conserved Receptor-Binding Domains of Lake Victoria Marburg Virus and Zaire Ebola Virus Bind a Common Receptor.* The $GP_{1,2}$ envelope glycoproteins (GPs) of the filoviruses (Marburg and Ebola viruses) mediate cell-surface attachment, membrane fusion, and entry into permissive cells. It has been reported that a 151-amino-acid fragment of the Lake Victoria Marburg virus GP_1 subunit bound Filovirus-permissive cell lines more efficiently than did a full-length GP_1 *(526)*. Furthermore, a homologous 148-amino-acid fragment of the Zaire Ebola virus GP_1 subunit similarly bound the same cell lines more efficiently than did a series of longer GP_1 truncation variants. Neither the Marburg virus GP_1 fragment nor that of Ebola virus bound a nonpermissive lymphocyte cell line. Both fragments specifically inhibited the replication of infectious Zaire Ebola virus, as well as the entry of retroviruses pseudotyped with either Lake Victoria Marburg virus or Zaire Ebola virus $GP_{1,2}$. These studies have identified the receptor-binding domains of both viruses, indicating that these viruses use a common receptor, and suggested that a single small molecule or vaccine can be developed to inhibit infection by all filoviruses *(526)*.

- *SV2 is the Protein Receptor for Botulinum Neurotoxin A.* The botulinum toxins (BoNTs) rank among the most toxic substances known and are responsible for food poisoning cases with high morbidity and mortality. These toxins are also potential weapons for bioterrorism, and are currently being used to treat a variety of medical conditions. How the widely used BoNT/A recognizes and enters neurons is poorly understood. A group of researchers at the University of Wisconsin found that BoNT/A enters neurons by binding to the synaptic vesicle protein SV2 (isoforms A, B, and C) *(527)*. Synaptic vesicles served the role of transporting neural cell signaling molecules (transmitters) from the neural cell to the muscle cell to mediate movement. When these vesicles reach the junction between neural cells and muscle cells to release the transmitters, the toxin, which has been absorbed to the bloodstream, takes advantage of the temporary exposure of SV2 to the circulation by binding to SV2. As result, the toxin enters into the neural cell when the vesicle returns to the interior of the cell. Once within the neural cell, the toxin will act as an enzyme to disrupt further transport of transmitters by the vesicles. By dissecting the mechanism by which these toxins gain entry into target cells, new strategies for prophylaxes and therapeutics can be developed. This new information may enable more effective use of the toxins for treatment of conditions such as dystonia, strabismus, and migraine headache.

- *Identification and Characterization of Potent Small-Molecule Inhibitor of Hemorrhagic Fever New World Arenaviruses.* Currently, there are no virus-specific treatments approved for use against Arenavirus hemorrhagic fevers. Ribavirin is the only compound that has shown partial efficacy against some Arenavirus infections, but with a high level of undesirable secondary reactions. ST-294 was discovered via *in vitro* screening and was optimized through iterative chemistry, resulting in a specific small-molecule inhibitor with selective activity against human pathogenic New World arenaviruses (Junín, Machupo, Guanarito, and Sabiá) *(528)*. ST-294 demonstrated favorable pharmacodynamic properties that permitted the demonstration of *in vivo* anti-Arenavirus activity in a newborn mouse model. ST-294 and its related compounds represent a new class of inhibitors that may warrant further development for potential inclusion in a strategic stockpile.

- *Development of High-Throughput Assays for Drug Discovery Against West Nile Virus (WNV).* Although genetic systems have been developed for many flaviviruses, their use in antiviral high-throughput screening (HTS) assays has not been well explored. In this regard, three cell-based assays for WNV have been compared, namely (i) an assay that uses a cell line harboring a persistently replicating subgenomic replicon (containing a deletion of viral structural genes); (ii) an assay that uses packaged virus-like particles containing replicon RNA; and (iii) an assay that uses a full-length reporting virus *(529)*. A *Renilla* luciferase gene was engineered into the replicon or into the full-length viral genome to monitor viral replication. Potential inhibitors could be identified through suppression of luciferase signals upon compound incubation *(530–532)*.

- *Genomic Sequence and Analysis of a Vaccinia Virus Isolate.* In a recent study, the genomic sequence of a vaccinia virus isolate (VACV-DUKE) from a patient diagnosed with progressive vaccinia was determined, and its availability for the first time allowed a genomic sequence of vaccinia virus isolate associated with a smallpox vaccine complication (necrosum) to be analyzed and compared with the genomic sequence of culture-derived clonal isolates of the Dryvax vaccine *(533)*. The study showed that both sequences were overall very similar and that virus in lesions that resulted from progressive vaccinia after vaccination with Dryvax are likely clonal in origin. Although other clones derived from Dryvax vaccine have been sequenced, VACV-Duke was unique in being the only completely sequenced Dryvax isolate obtained from a human source. Detailed analysis of its nucleotide sequence and gene content will allow for better understanding of the population diversity of Dryvax, and the lack of sequence heterogeneity is suggestive of a single clonal lesion source.

- *A Novel Cell Culture–Derived Smallpox Vaccine in Vaccinia-Naïve Adults.* In the context of the potential use of smallpox as a biological weapon, the development of a new generation of smallpox vaccines represents an important part of a viable and efficient biodefense strategy. A Phase II randomized, double-blind, controlled trial was conducted to determine whether a clonal smallpox vaccine, ACAM2000, manufactured in cell culture, was equivalent to the standard calf-lymph vaccine, Dryvax, in terms of cutaneous response rate, antibody responses, and safety *(534)*. All subjects in the highest ACAM2000 dose group and the Dryvax group experienced a successful vaccination. Dilution doses of ACAM2000 were associated with success rates below the 90% threshold established for efficacy. There were no differences in the proportion of subjects who developed neutralizing antibody: 94% in the highest ACAM2000 dose group (95% CI, 84 to 99) and 96% in the Dryvax group (95% CI, 86 to 100). In addition, no significant differences were seen between the effective ACAM2000 and Dryvax groups regarding the occurrence of adverse effects.

- *Safety and Immunogenicity of IMVAMUNE as a Third Generation of Smallpox Vaccine.* A Phase I trial was performed to investigate the safety and immunogenicity of a third-generation of smallpox vaccine MVA-BN (IMVAMUNE), a highly attenuated clone derived from the modified vaccinia Ankara (MVA) virus strain 571, in naïve and pre-immunized subjects *(535)*. The vaccine was administered to healthy subjects in five different doses and routes of administration. All vaccinations were well tolerated, with the most frequent symptom being mild to moderate pain at the injection site. The IMVAMUNE vaccine has the potential to be developed as an efficient and safe alternative to the conventional smallpox vaccine such as Lister-Elstree or Dryvax. Unique attributes render it a promising candidate for prophylactic mass immunization even in subjects for whom conventional smallpox vaccines are contraindicated.

- *Modified Vaccinia Ankara Virus Protects Macaques Against Respiratory Challenge with Monkeypox Virus.* The use of classic smallpox vaccines based on vaccinia virus has been associated with severe complications in both naïve and immune individuals. The modified vaccinia Ankara (MVA) vaccine, a highly attenuated replication-deficient strain of vaccinia virus, has been proven to be safe in humans and immunocompromised animals. In a recent study, the efficacies of MVA alone and in combination with classic vaccinia virus–based vaccines were compared in a cynomolgus macaque monkeypox model *(536)*. The MVA-based smallpox vaccine protected macaques against lethal respiratory challenge with monkeypox virus and should therefore be considered an important candidate for protecting humans against smallpox.

- *Effective Antimicrobial Regimens for Use in Humans for Therapy of Bacillus anthracis Infections and Post-Exposure Prophylaxis.* The objective of this study was to identify a levofloxacin treatment regimen that would serve as an effective therapy for *Bacillus anthracis* infections and as a postexposure prophylaxis *(537)*. An *in vitro* hollow-fiber infection model that replicates the pharmacokinetic profile of levofloxacin observed in humans [half-life $(t_{1/2})$, 7.5 hours] or in animals, such as the mouse or the rhesus monkey $(t_{1/2}, \sim 2$ hours), was used to evaluate a proposed indication for levofloxacin (500 mg, once daily) for treating *Bacillus anthracis* infections. The results obtained with the *in vitro* model served as the basis for the doses and the dose schedules that were evaluated in the mouse inhalational anthrax model. The effects of levofloxacin and ciprofloxacin treatment were compared with those of no treatment (untreated controls). The main outcome measure in the *in vitro* hollow-fiber infection model was a persistent reduction of culture density ($\geq 4 \log_{10}$ reduction) and prevention of the emergence of levofloxacin-resistant organisms. In the mouse inhalational anthrax model, the main outcome measure was survival. The results indicated that levofloxacin given once daily with simulated human pharmacokinetics effectively sterilized *Bacillus anthracis* cultures. By using a simulated animal pharmacokinetic profile, a once-daily dosing regimen that provided a human-equivalent exposure failed to sterilize the cultures. Dosing regimens that "partially humanized" levofloxacin exposures within the constraints of animal pharmacokinetics reproduced the antimicrobial efficacy seen with human pharmacokinetics. In a mouse inhalational anthrax model, once-daily dosing was significantly inferior (survival end point) to regimens of dosing every 12 hours or every 6 hours with identical total daily levofloxacin doses. These results demonstrate the predictive value of the *in vitro* hollow-fiber infection model with respect to the success or the failure of treatment regimens in animals. Furthermore, the model permits the evaluation of treatment regimens that "humanize" antibiotic exposures in animal models, enhancing the confidence with which animal models may be used to reliably predict the efficacies of proposed antibiotic treatments in humans in situations (e.g., the release of pathogens as agents of bioterrorism or emerging infectious diseases) where human trials cannot be performed. A treatment regimen effective in rhesus monkeys was identified *(537)*. This study demonstrated the combinational use of *in vitro* hollow-fiber and animal models to evaluate the effectiveness of certain antibiotics for treating human infections for diseases where human trials

cannot be performed, such as anthrax and plague. Such systemic pharmacokinetic and pharmacodynamic characterization of existing antibiotics will allow scientists to identify agents and to design effective treatment regimens. The findings gained from this study will provide the public with options of more than one antibiotic if there is an urgent need to counteract a bioterror attack or other unexpected outbreak of an emerging infectious disease.

- *Mutual Enhancement of Virulence by Enterotoxigenic and Enteropathogenic Escherichia coli.* Enterotoxigenic and enteropathogenic *Escherichia coli* (ETEC and EPEC, respectively) are common causes of diarrhea in children, especially in developing countries. Dual infections by both pathogens have been noted fairly frequently. It has been previously shown that cholera toxin and forskolin markedly potentiated EPEC-induced ATP (adenosine 5′-triphosphate) release from the host cells, and this potentiated release was found to be mediated by the cystic fibrosis transmembrane conductance regulator. A follow-up study *(538)* examined whether the ETEC heat-labile toxin (LT) or the heat-stable toxin (STa, also known as ST) potentiated the EPEC-induced ATP release. The results showed that crude ETEC culture filtrates, as well as purified ETEC toxins, did potentiate EPEC-induced ATP released in cultured T84 cells. Co-infection of T84 cells with live ETEC plus EPEC bacteria also resulted in enhanced ATP release compared with that of EPEC alone. These and other studies have demonstrated that ETEC toxins and EPEC-induced damage to the host cells both enhanced the virulence of the other type of *E. coli (538)*.

- *Peptidoglycan Recognition Proteins as a New Class of Human Bactericidal Proteins.* Skin and mucous membranes come into contact with the external environment and protect tissues from infections. As one of the components of the innate immune system, the skin and mucous membranes produce antimicrobial peptides, such as defensins. These antimicrobial peptides damage the bacterial cell membrane, thereby protecting the host from infection. The existence of a novel class of human bactericidal and bacteriostatic proteins that are present in the skin, eyes, salivary glands, throat, tongue, esophagus, stomach, and intestine has been recently discovered *(539)*. Thus, the peptidoglycan recognition proteins 3 and 4 (PGLYRP3 and PGLYRP4) are secreted as 89- to 115-kDa disulfide-linked homo- and heterodimers and are bactericidal against several pathogenic and nonpathogenic transient but not normal flora, Gram-positive bacteria. Furthermore, PGLYRP3 and PGLYRP4 were bacteriostatic toward all other tested bacteria, which included Gram-negative bacteria. PGLYRP3 and PGLYRP4 have shown a mechanism of action distinct from their antimicrobial peptide counterparts, as well as different structures and expression patterns. These novel proteins interact with the bacterial cell wall peptidoglycan as a means of killing. *Listeria monocytogenes* was highly sensitive to killing by both PGLYRP3 and PGLYRP4. Furthermore, both were active *in vivo*, protecting mice in a *S. aureus* lung infection model. This novel discovery could ultimately have implications for the development of broad-spectrum vaccines and immunotherapeutics.

- *The Unc93b1 Mutation Is Affecting Both Innate and Adaptive Immune Responses.* By using *N*-ethyl-*N*-nitrosourea (ENU) mutagenesis in mice, researchers have identified a recessive mutant that is a single-base transversion of an allele of UNC-93B (3d) *(540)*. In addition, by positional identification it was found that the 3d mutant was a missense allele of *Unc93b1*, which encodes the 12-membrane-spanning protein UNC-93B, a highly conserved molecule found in the plasma reticulum with multiple paralogs in mammals. The 3d mutant is defective in its response to foreign nucleic acids and cannot signal through the Toll-like receptors (TLR) 3, 7, and 9 of the innate immune system. Using mice with the 3d mutation, an additional function of this protein was discovered that affects the adaptive immune response, independent of TLR signaling. The 3d mutation led to defective presentation of exogenous antigen, abolished cross-priming for CD8$^+$ T-cells, and inhibited CD4$^+$ T-cell priming. Innate responses to nucleic acids and exogenous antigen presentation, both of which begin in the endosomes, seemed to depend on an endoplasmic reticulum–resident protein, which is suggestive of communication between these organellar systems. Hence, the protein has two seemingly unrelated functions, which affect both the innate immune system and the adaptive immune response *(540)*.

- *Systems Biology Revealed a Novel Function of the Transcription Factor ATF3.* Although the innate immune system is absolutely required for host defenses, when uncontrolled it leads to inflammatory disease. This control is mediated, in part, by cytokines that are secreted by macrophages. Because the immune regulation is extraordinarily complex, it can be best investigated with systems approaches—that is, using computational tools to predict regulatory networks arising from global, high-throughput data sets. Using cluster analysis of a comprehensive set of transcriptomic data derived from Toll-like receptor (TLR)-activated macrophages, researchers have identified a prominent group of genes that appeared to be regulated by activating transcription factor 3 (ATF3), a member of the CREB/ATF family of transcription factors *(541)*. Network analysis predicted that ATF3 would be part of a transcriptional complex that also contained members of the nuclear factor NF-κB family of transcription factors. Furthermore, promoter analysis of the putative ATF3-regulated gene cluster demonstrated an over-representation of closely apposed ATF3 and NF-κB binding sites, which was verified by chromatin immunoprecipitation and hybridization to a DNA microarray. In other studies, microarray analysis was used to identify gene transcription factors affected in macrophages at different time points after LPS activation through Toll-like receptor 4. Predictions resulting from the analysis were validated in a number of biochemical assays using LPS-activated macrophages. For example, at early time points, activating transcription factor 3 (ATF3) was found to be a negative regulator of LPS-induced gene expression for IL-6 and IL-12 cytokine production. An *in vivo* model confirmed these findings, as mice deficient in ATF3 were much more susceptible to septic shock. A potential mechanism was described that involves ATF3 binding to histone deacetylase (HDAC) to alter chromatin structure, resulting in inhibition of IL-6 and IL-12 gene transcription. In addition, several useful software tools were developed by this group to predict which regulatory circuits operate under particular activation conditions.

- *Cytokine Milieu of Atopic Dermatitis Skin Subverts the Innate Immune Response to Vaccinia Virus.* Atopic dermatitis (AD) is associated with eczema vaccinatum (EV), a disseminated viral skin infection that follows inoculation with vaccinia virus (VV). A recent study *(542)* examined whether atopic dermatitis skin can control the replication of vaccinia virus, as well as the role of IL-4 and IL-13 in modulating the human cathelicidin LL-37, an antimicrobial peptide that kills vaccinia virus. The results showed that AD skin exhibited increased VV replication and decreased LL-37 expression compared with that of normal or psoriatic skin. Furthermore, IL4/IL-13 enhanced VV replication while downregulating LL-37 in VV-stimulated keratinocytes. Neutralizing IL-4/IL-13 in AD skin augmented LL-37 and inhibited VV replication. Cathelicidins were induced via Toll-like receptor 3 and were inhibited by IL-4/IL-13 through STAT-6. Skin from cathelicidin-deficient mice exhibited reduced ability to control VV replication. Exogenous LL-37 controlled replication of vaccinia virus in infected keratinocytes and atopic dermatitis skin explants. The overall results from the study demonstrated that Th2 cytokines enhanced VV replication in AD skin by subverting the innate immune response against vaccinia virus in a STAT-6-dependent manner *(542)*.

- *Immune Protection of Non-Human Primates Against Ebola Virus with Single Low-Dose Adenovirus Vectors Encoding Modified Glycoproteins.* Ebola virus causes a hemorrhagic fever syndrome that is associated with high mortality in humans. In the absence of effective therapies for Ebola virus infection, the development of a vaccine becomes an important strategy to contain outbreaks. Immunization with DNA and/or replication-defective adenoviral vectors (rAd) encoding the Ebola glycoprotein (GP) and nucleoprotein (NP) has been previously shown to confer specific protective immunity in non-human primates. Furthermore, GP can exert cytopathic effects on transfected cells *in vitro*, and multiple GP forms have been identified in nature, raising the question of which would be optimal for a human vaccine. To address this question, VRC-led researchers have explored the efficacy of mutant GPs from multiple Ebola virus strains with reduced *in vitro* cytopathicity and analyzed their protective effects in the primate challenge model, with or without NP *(543)*. Deletion of the GP transmembrane domain eliminated *in vitro* cytopathicity but reduced its protective efficacy by at least one order of magnitude. In contrast, a point mutation was identified that abolished this cytopathicity but retained immunogenicity and conferred immune protection in the absence of NP. The minimal effective rAd dose was established at 10^{10} particles, two logs lower than that used previously. Expression of specific GPs alone vectored by rAd were found sufficient to confer protection against lethal challenge in a relevant non-human primate model. Elimination of NP from the vaccine and dose reductions to 10^{10} rAd particles did not diminish protection and simplify the vaccine, providing the basis for selecting a human vaccine candidate *(543)*.

- *Protection Against Multiple Influenza A Subtypes by Vaccination with Highly Conserved Nucleoprotein.* Current influenza vaccines elicit antibodies effective against specific strains of the virus, but new strategies are urgently needed for protection against unexpected strains. DNA vaccines have been shown to provide protection in animals against diverse virus strains, but the potency of the vaccines needs improvement. Scientists at the Vaccine Research Center tested a DNA prime-recombinant adenoviral boost vaccine targeted at one of the influenza viral proteins, nucleoprotein (NP). Strong antibody and T-cell responses were induced. Protection against viral challenge was substantially more potent than was DNA vaccination alone. Equally importantly, vaccination protected against lethal challenge with highly pathogenic H5N1 virus. Thus, gene-based vaccination with NP may contribute to protective immunity against diverse influenza viruses through its ability to stimulate cellular immunity *(544)*.

References

1. Wheelis, M. (2003) A short history of biological warfare and weapons, In: *The Implementation of Legally Binding Measures to Strenghten the Biological and Toxin Weapons Convention* (Chevrier, M. I., Chomiczewski, K., Dando, M. R., Garrigue, H., Granaztoi, G., and Pearson, G. S., eds.), ISO Press, Amsterdam, pp. 15–31.

2. Fenn, E. A. (2000) Biological warfare in eighteen-century North America: beyond Jeffery Amherst, *J. Am. History*, **86**(3), 1552–1580.

3. Wheelis, M. (1999) Biological sabotage in World War I. In: *Biological and Toxin Weapons: Research, Development and Use from the Middle Ages to 1945* (Geissler, E. and Moon, J. E. V. C., eds.), Oxford University Press, Oxford, pp. 35–62.

4. Harris, S. H. (1994) *Factories of Death: Japanese Biological Warfare 1932–45 and the American Cover-Up*, Routledge, London.

5. Williams, P. and Wallace, D. (1989) *Unit 731: The Japanese Army's Secret of Secrets*, Hodder & Stoughton, London.

6. Carus, W. S. (2000) The Rajneeshees (1984). In: *Toxic Terror: Assessing Terrorist Use of Chemical and Biological Weapons*, MIT Press, Cambridge, pp. 115–137.

7. LeClaire, R. D. and Pitt, M. L. M. (2005) Biological weapons defense. In: *Biological Weaponse Defense: Infectious Diseases and Counterterrorism* (Lindler, L. E., Lebeda, F. J., and Korch, G. W., eds.), Humana Press, Totowa, NJ, pp. 41–61.

8. Burrows, W. D. and Renner, S. E. (1999) Biological warfare agents as threats to potable water, *Environ. Health Perspect.*, **107**, 975–984.

9. Ferguson, J. R. (1997) Biological weapons and U.S. law, *J. Am. Med. Assoc.*, **278**, 357–360.

10. FM 8–9, (1996) *NATO Handbook on the Medical Aspects of NBC Defensive Operations AMedP-6(B)*, Part II Biological. Department of the Army, Washington, DC, 1996.

11. Missiakas, D. M. and Schneewind, O. (2005) *Bacillus anthracis* and the pathogenesis of anthrax. In: *Biological Weaponse Defense: Infectious Diseases and Counterterrorism* (Lindler, L. E., Lebeda, F. J., and Korch, G. W., eds.), Humana Press, Totowa, NJ, pp. 79–97.

12. Meselson, M. (1999) The challenge of biological and chemical weapons, *Bull. World Health Organ.*, **77**, 102–103.

13. Edsall, J. T. and Meselson, M. (1967) Proliferation of CB warfare, *Science*, **156**, 1029–1030.

14. Enserink, M. (2001) This time it was real: knowledge of anthrax put to the test, *Science*, **294**, 490–491.

15. Koch, R. (1876) Die aetiologie der milzbrand-krankheit, begruendet auf die entwicklungsgeschichte des *Bacillus anthracis*, *Beiträ Biol Pflanzen*, **2**, 277–310.

16. Zwartouw, H. T. and Smith, H. (1956) Polyglutamic acid from *Bacillus anthracis* grown in vivo: structure and aggressin activity, *Biochem. J.*, **63**, 437–454.

17. Preisz, H. (1991) Experimentelle studien ueber virulenz, empfaenglichkeit und immunitaet beim milzbrand, *Zeitschr. Immunitä.-Forsch.*, **5**, 341–452.

18. Leppla, S. H. (1991) The anthrax toxin complex. In: *Sourcebook of Bacterial Protein Toxins* (Alouf, J. and Freer, J. H., eds.), Academic Press, London, pp. 277–302.

19. Hanna, P. C., Acosta, D., and Collier, R. J. (1993) On the role of macrophages in anthrax, *Proc. Natl. Acad. Sci. U.S.A.*, **90**, 10198–10201.

20. Duesbery, N. S., Webb, C. P., Leppla, S. H., Gordon, V. M., Klimpel, K. R., Copeland, T. D., Ahn, N. G., Oskarsson, M. K., Fukusawa, K., Pauli, K. D., and Vande Woude, G. F. (1998) Proteolytic inactivation of map-kinase-kinase by anthrax lethal factor, *Science*, **280**, 734–737.

21. Vitale, G., Pellizzari, R., Recchi, C., Napolitani, G., Mock, M., and Montecucco, C. (1998) Anthrax lethal factor cleaves the N-terminus of MAPKKs and induces tyrosine/threonine phosphorylation of MAPKKs in cultured macrophages, *Biochem. Biophys. Res. Commun.*, **248**, 706–711.

22. Park, J. M., Greten, F. R., Li, Z. W., and Karin, M. (2002) Macrophage apoptosis by anthrax lethal factor through p38 MAP kinase inhibition, *Science*, **297**, 2048–2051.

23. Leppla, S. H. (1984) *Bacillus anthracis* calmodulin-dependent adenylate cyclase: chemical and enzymatic properties and interactions with eukariotic cells, *Adv. Cyc. Nuc. Prot. Phos. Res.*, **17**, 189–198.

24. Leppla, S. H. (1982) Anthrax toxin edema factor: a bacterial adenylate cyclase that increases cyclin AMP concentrations in eukariotic cells, *Proc. Natl. Acad. Sci. U.S.A.*, **79**, 3162–3166.

25. Green, B. D., Battisti, L., Koehler, T. M., Thorne, C. B., and Ivins, B. E. (1985) Demonstration of a capsule plasmid in *Bacillus anthracis, Infect. Immun.*, **49**, 291–297.

26. Mikesell, P., Ivins, B. E., Ristroph, J. D., and Dreier, T. M. (1983) Evidence for plasmid-mediated toxin production in *Bacillus anthracis, Infect. Immun.*, **39**, 371–376.

27. Smith, H., Keppie, H. S., and Stanley, J. I. (1953) The chemical basis of the virulence of *Bacillus anthracis*. I. Properties of bacteria grown in vivo and preparation of extracts, *Br. J. Exp. Pathol.*, **34**, 477–485.

28. Keppie, J., Smith, H., and Harris-Smith, P. W. (1963) The chemical basis of the virulence of *Bacillus anthracis*. II. Some biological properties of bacterial products, *Br. J. Exp. Pathol.*, **34**, 486–496.

29. Dixon, T. C., Meselson, M., Guillemin, J., and Hanna, P. C. (1999) Anthrax, *N. Engl. J. Med.*, **341**, 815–826.

30. Lightfood, N. F., Scott, R. J. D., and Turnbull, P. C. B. (1989) Antimicrobial susceptibility of *Bacillus anthracis*. In: *Proc. Int. Workshop on Anthrax*, Salisbury Medical Bulletin, Winchester, UK, pp. 95–98.

31. Centers for Disease Control (2001) Update: investigation of bioterrorism-related anthrax and interim guidelines for exposure management and antimicrobial therapy, October 2001, *Morb. Mortal. Wkly Rep.*, **50**, 909–919.

32. Bradley, K. A., Modridge, J., Mourez, M., Collier, R. J., and Young, J. A. (2001) Identification of the cellular receptor for anthrax toxin, *Nature*, **414**, 225–229.

33. Sellman, B. R., Mourez, M., and Collier, R. J. (2001) Dominant-negative mutants of a toxin subunit: an approach to therapy of anthrax, *Science*, **292**, 695–697.

34. Schuch, R., Nelson, D., and Fischetti, V. A. (2002) A bacteriolytic agent that detects and kills *Bacillus anthracis, Nature*, **418**, 884–889.

35. Pittman, P. R., Kim-Ahn, G., Pifat, D. Y., Coonan, K., Gibbs, P., Little, S., Pace-Templeton, J. G., Myers, R., Parker, G. W., and Friedlander, A. M. (2002) Anthrax vaccine: immunogenicity and safety of a dose-reduction, route-change comparison study in humans, *Vaccine*, **20**, 1412–1420.

36. Friedlander, A. M. (2001) Tackling anthrax, *Nature*, **414**, 160–161.

37. Fenner, F. (1993) Smallpox: emergence. Global spread, and eradication, *Hist. Philos. Life Sci.*, **15**, 397–420.

38. Darling, R. G., Burgess, T. H., Lawler, J. V., and Endy, T. P. (2005) Virologic and pathogenic aspects of the *Variola* virus (smallpox) as a bioweapon, In: *Biological Weapons Defense: Infectious Diseases and Counterbioterrorism* (Linder, L. E., Lebeda, F. J., and Korch, G. W., eds.), Humana Press, Inc., Totowa, NJ, pp. 99–120.

39. Tucker, J. B. (1999) Historical trends related to bioterrorism: an empirical analysis, *Emerg. Infect. Dis.*, **5**, 498–504.

40. Albert, M., Ostheimer, K., Liewehr, D., Steinberg, S., and Breman, J. (2002) Smallpox manifestations and survival during the Boston epidemic of 1901 to 1903, *Ann. Intern. Med.*, **137**, 993–1000.

41. Smallpox and its eradication (1988) In: *The History of Smallpox and Its Spread Around the World*, World Health Organization, Geneva.

42. Baxby, D. (1996) The Jenner bicentenary: the introduction and early distribution of smallpox vaccine, *FEMS Immunol. Med. Microbiol.*, **16**, 1–10.

43. Bucknell, W. J. (2002) The case of voluntary smallpox vaccination, *N. Engl. J. Med.*, **346**, 1323–1325.

44. Human monkeypox in Kasai Oriental, Zaire (1996–1997) (1997) *Wkly Epidemiol. Rec.*, **72**, 101–104.

45. Centers for Disease Control and Prevention (2003) Multistate outbreak of monkeypox – Illinois, Indiana, and Wisconsin, 2003, *Morb. Mortal. Wkly Rep.*, **52**, 537–540.

46. Moss, B. (2001) Poxviridae: the viruses and their replication. In: *Fields Virology*, 4th ed. (Knipe, D. M. and Howley, P. M., eds.), Lippincott Williams & Wilkins, Philadelphia, pp. 2849–2883.

47. Hooper, J., Custer, D., and Thompson, E. (2003) Four-gene-combination DNA vaccine protects mice against a lethal vaccinia virus challenge and elicits appropriate antibody responses in nonhuman primates, *Virology*, **306**, 181–195.

48. Esposito, J., Obijeski, J., and Nakano, J. (1978) Orthopoxvirus DNA: strain differentiation by electrophoresis of restriction endonuclease fragmented virion DNA, *Virology*, **89**, 53–66.

49. Esposito, J. and Knight, J. (1985) Orthopoxvirus DNA: a comparison of restriction profiles and maps, *Virology*, **143**, 230–251.

50. Dumbell, K., Harper, L., Buchan, A., Douglass, N., and Bedson, H. (1999) A variant of variola virus, characterized by changes in polypeptide and endonuclease profiles, *Epidemiol. Infect.*, **122**, 287–290.

51. Smith, V. and Alcami, A. (2000) Expression of secreted cytokine and chemokine inhibitors by ectromelia virus, *J. Virol.*, **74**, 8460–8471.

52. Buller, R. and Palumbo, G. (1991) Poxvirus pathogenesis, *Microbiol. Rev.*, **55**, 80–122.

53. Alcami, A. and Smith, G. (1995) Vaccinia, cowpox, and camelpox viruses encode soluble gamma interferon receptors with novel broad species specificity, *J. Virol.*, **69**, 4633–4639.

54. Ramshaw, I., Ramsay, A., Karupiah, G., Rolph, M., Mahalingam, S., and Ruby, J. (1997) Cytokines and immunity to infection, *Immunol. Rev.*, **159**, 119–135.

55. Jackson, R., Ramsay, A., Christensen, C., Beaton, S., Hall, D., and Ramshaw, I. (2001) Expression of mouse interleukin 4 by a recombinant ectromelia virus suppresses cytolytic lymphocyte responses and overcomes genetic resistance to mousepox, *J. Virol.*, **75**, 1205–1210.

56. Mack, T. M. (1972) Smallpox in Europe, 1950–1971, *J. Infect. Dis.*, **125**, 161–169.

57. Fenner, F., Henderson, D. A., Arita, I., Jezek, Z., and Ladnyi, I. D. (1988) *Smallpox and Its Eradication*, World Health Organization, Geneva.

58. Mazumder, D. N., Mitra, A. C., and Mukherjee, M. K. (1975) Clinical observations on smallpox: a study of 1233 patients admitted to the Infectious Disease Hospital, Calcutta during 1973, *Bull. World Health Organ.*, **52**, 301–306.

59. Sheth, S. C., Maruthi, V., Tibrewalla, N. S., and Pai, P. M. (1971) Smallpox in children. A clinical study of 100 cases, *Indian J. Pediatr.*, **38**, 128–131.

60. Henderson, D., Inglesby, T., Bartlett, J., Ascher, M. S., Eitzen, E., Jahrling, P. B., Hawer, J., Layton, M., McDade, J., Osterholm, M. T., O'Toole, T., Parker, G., Perl, T., Russell, P. K., Tonat, K., for the Working Group on Civilian Biodefense (1999) Smallpox as a biological weapon: medical and public health management, *J. Am. Med. Assoc.*, **281**, 2127–2137.

61. De Clercq, E. (2002) Cidofovir in the treatment of poxvirus infections, *Antiviral Res.*, **55**(1), 1–13.

62. De Clercq, E., Luczak, M., Shugar, D., Torrence, P. F., Waters, J. A., and Witkop, B. (1976) Effect of cytosine, arabinoside, iododeoxyuridine, ethyldeoxyuridine, thiocyanatodeoxyuridine, and ribavirine on tail lesion formation in mice infected with vaccinia virus, *Proc. Soc. Exp. Biol. Med.*, **151**, 487–490.

63. Rao, A. R., McFadzean, J. A., and Kamalakshi, K. (1966) An isothiazole thiosemicarbazone in the treatment of *Variola major*

in man. A controlled clinical trial and laboratory investigations, *Lancet*, **1**, 1068–1072.

64. Rao, A. R., Jacobs, E. S., Kamalakshi, S., Bradbuty, and Swamy, A. (1969) Chemoprophylaxis and chemotherapy in *Variola major*. II. Therapeutic assessment of CG662 and marboran in treatment of *Variola major* in man, *Indian J. Med. Res.*, **57**, 484–494.

65. Jahrling, P. B., Zaucha, G. M., and Huggins, J. W. (2000) Countermeasures to the reemergence of smallpox virus as an agent of bioterrorism. In: *Emerging Infections 4* (Scheld, W. M., Craig, W. A., and Hughes, J. M., eds.), ASM, Washington, DC.

66. Georgiev, V. St. Drugs for Treating Viral Infections, *U.S. Patent 6,433,016 B1*, 2002.

67. Georgiev, V. St. Drugs for Treating Viral Infections, *U.S. Patent 6,596,771 B2*, 2003.

68. Georgiev, V. St. Drugs for Treating Viral Infections, *U.S. Patent 6,7,192,606 B1*, 2007.

69. Meadows, K. P., Tyring, S. K., Pavia, A. T., and Rallis, T. M. (1997) Resolution of recalcitrant molluscum contagiosum virus lesions in human immunodeficiency virus-infected patients treated with cidofovir, *Arch. Dermatol.*, **133**, 987–990.

70. Davies, E. G., Thrasher, A., Lacey, K., and Harper, J. (1999) Topical cidofovir for severe molluscum contagiosum, *Lancet*, **353**, 2042.

71. Buller, M., Handley, L., Parker, S. (2008) Development of prophylactics and therapeutics against smallpox and monkeypox biothreat agents. In: National Institute of Allergy and Infections Diseases, NIH, vol. 1 Fiontiers Research (Georgiev, V. St., Western, K. A., and McGowan. J. J., eds.), Humana Press, Springer, New York, pp. 145–161.

72. Perry, R. D. and Fetherstone, J. D. (1997) *Yersinia pestis* – etiologic agent of plague, *Clin. Microbiol. Rev.*, **10**(1), 35–66.

73. Smith, P. N. (1959) Pneumonic plague in mice: gross and histopathology in untreated and passively immunized animals, *J. Infect. Dis.*, **104**, 78–84.

74. Chen, T. H. and Mayer, K. F. (1965) Susceptibility of the Langur monkey (*Semnopithesus entellus*) to experimental plague: pathology and immunity, *J. Infect. Dis.*, **115**, 456–464.

75. Smith, J. H. (1976) Plague. In: *Pathology of Tropical and Extraordinary Diseases. An Atlas*, vol. 1 (Binford, C. H. and Connor, D. H., eds.), Armed Forces Institute of Pathology, Washington, DC, pp. 130–134.

76. Davies, K. J., Fritz, D. L., Pitt, M. L., Welkos, S. L., Worsham, P. L., and Friedlander, A. M. (1996) Pathology of experimental pneumonic plague produced by fraction 1-positive and fraction 1-negative *Yersinia pestis* in African green monkeys (*Cercopithecus aetiops*), *Arch. Pathol. Lab. Med.*, **120**, 156–163.

77. Adamovitz, J. J. and Andrews, G. P. (2005) Plague vaccines. Retrospective analysis and future developments. In: *Biological Weapons Defense: Infectious Diseases and Counterterrorism* (Lindler, L. E., Lebeda, F. J., and Korch, G. W., eds.), Humana Press, Totowa, NJ, pp. 121–153.

78. Butler, T. (1989) The Black Death past and present. 1. Plague in the 1980s, *Trans. R. Soc. Trop. Med.*, **83**, 458–460.

79. Crook, L. D. and Tempest, B. (1992) Plague: a clinical review of 27 cases, *Arch. Intern. Med.*, **152**, 1253–1256.

80. Butler, T. (1985) Plague and other *Yersinia* infections. In: *Current Topics in Infectious Disease* (Greenough, W. B. and Marigan, T. C., eds.), Plenum Press, New York, pp. 73–108.

81. Doll, J. M., Zeitz, P. S., Ettestad, P., Bucholtz, A. L., Davis, T., and Gage, K. (1994) Cat-transmitted fatal pneumonic plague in a person who traveled from Colorado to Arizona, *Am. J. Trop. Med. Hyg.*, **51**, 109–114.

82. Ransom, J. P. and Krueger, A. P. (1954) Chronic pneumonic plague in *Macacca mulatta*, *Am. J. Trop. Med. Hyg.*, **3**, 1040–1054.

83. Marshall. J. D., Quy, D. V., and Gibson, F. L. (1967) Asymptomatic pharyngeal plague in Vietnamese, *Am. J. Trop. Med.*, **16**, 175–177.

84. Haffkine, W. M. (1897) Remarks on the plague prophylactic fluid, *Br. Med. J.*, **1**, 1461.

85. Taylor, J. (1933) Haffkine's plague vaccine, *Indian Med. Res. Memoirs*, **27**, 3–125.

86. Grasset, E. (1942) Plague immunization with live vaccine in South Africa, *Trans. R. Soc. Trop. Med. Hyg.*, **35**, 203–211.

87. Grasset, E. (1946) Control of plague by means of live avirulent plague vaccine in Southern Africa (1941–44), *Trans. R. Soc. Trop. Med. Hyg.*, **40**, 275–294.

88. Meyer, K. F., Cavanaugh, D. C., Bartelloni, P. J., and Marshall, J. D., Jr., (1974) Plague immunization I. Past and present trends, *J. Infect. Dis.*, **129**(Suppl.), S13–S17.

89. Chen, T. H., Elberg, S. S., and Eisler, D. M. (1977) Immunity in plague: protection of the vervet (*Cercopithecus aethiops*) against pneumonic plague by the oral administration of live attenuated *Yersinia pestis*, *J. Infect. Dis.*, **135**, 289–293.

90. Alexandrov, N. L., Gefen, N. E., Gapochko, K. G., Grain, N. S., Sergeyev, V. M., and Lasareva, E. S. (1961) Aerosol immunization with dry living vaccines and toxoids. Report VI. A study of postvaccinal reaction and immunological efficacy of aerosol immunization with pulverized vaccines (brucellosis, tularemia, anthrax and plague) in man, *J. Microbiol. Epidemiol. Immunobiol.*, **32**, 1245–1252.

91. Anisimov, A. P., Nikiforov, A. K., Yeremin, S. A., and Drozdov, I. G. (1995) Design of the strain *Yersinia pestis* with improved level of protection, *Bull. Exp. Biol. Med.*, **120**, 532–534.

92. Meyer, K. F., Hightower, J. A., and McCrumb, F. R. (1974) Plague immunization. VI. Vaccination with the fraction 1 antigen of *Yersinia pestis*, *J. Infect. Dis.*, **129**(Suppl.), S41–S45.

93. Du, Y., Rosqvist, R., and Forsberg, A. (2002) Role of fraction 1 antigen of *Yersinia pestis* in inhibition of phagocytosis, *Infect. Immun.*, **70**, 1453–1460.

94. Marshall, J. D., Jr., Bartelloni, P. J., Cavanaugh, D. C., Kadull, P. J., and Meyer, K. F. (1974) Plague immunization II. Relation of adverse clinical reactions to multiple immunizations with killed vaccine, *J. Infect. Dis.*, **129**(Suppl.), S19–S25.

95. Ben-Efraim, S., Aronson, M., and Bichowsky-Slomnicki, L. (1961) New antigenic component of *Pasteurella pestis* formed under specific conditions of pH and temperature, *J. Bacteriol.*, **81**, 704–714.

96. Lindler, L. E. and Tall, B. D. (1993) *Yersinia pestis* pH 6 antigen forms fimbriae and is induced by intracellular association with macrophages, *Mol. Microbiol.*, **8**, 311–324.

97. Lindner, L. E., Klempner, M. S., and Straley, S. C. (1990) *Yersinia pestis* pH 6 antigen: genetic, biochemical, and virulence characterization of a protein involved in the pathogenesis of bubonic plague, *Infect. Immun.*, **58**, 2569–2577.

98. Lahteenmaki, K., Kukkonen, M., and Korhonen, T. K. (2001) The Pla surface protease/adhesin of *Yersinia pestis* mediates bacterial invasion into human endothelial cells, *FEBS Lett.*, **504**, 69–72.

99. Lahteenmaki, K., Kuusela, P., and Kornhonen, T. K. (2001) Bacterial plasminogen activators and receptors, *FEMS Microbiol. Rev.*, **25**, 531–552.

100. Burrows, T. W. (1957) Virulence of *Pasteurella pestis*, *Nature*, **179**, 1246–1247.

101. Price, S. B., Cowan, C., Perry, R. D., and Straley, S. C. (1991) The *Yersinia pestis* V antigen is a regulatory protein necessary for Ca^{2+}-dependent growth and maximal expression of low-Ca^{2+} response virulence genes, *J. Bacteriol.*, **173**, 2649–2657.

102. Nakajima, R. and Brubacker, R. R. (1993) Association between virulence of *Yersinia pestis* and suppression of gamma interferon and tumor necrosis factor alpha, *Infect. Immun.*, **61**, 23–31.

103. Sing, A., Roggenkamp, A., Geiger, A. M., and Heeseman, J. (2002) Yersinia enterocolitica evasion of the host innate immune response by V antigen-induced IL-10 production of macrophages is abrogated in IL-10-deficient mice, *J. Immunol.*, **168**, 1315–1321.

104. Sing, A., Rost, D., Tvardovskaia, N., Roggenkamp, A., Wiedemann, A., Kirschning, C. J., Aepfelbacher, M., and Heeseman, J. (2002) *Yersinia* V antigen exploits Toll-like receptor 2 and CD14 for interleukin 10-mediated immunosuppression, *J. Exp. Med.*, **196**, 1017–1024.

105. Lawton, W. D., Fukui, G. M., and Surgalla, M. J. (1960) Studies on antigens of *Pasteurella pestis* and *Pasteurella pseudotuberculosis, J. Immunol.*, **84**, 475–479.

106. Orth, K. (2002) Functions of the *Yersinia* effector YopJ, *Curr. Opin. Microbiol.*, **5**(1), 38–43.

107. Mazza, G., Karu, A. E., and Kingsbury, D. T. (1985) Immune responses to plasmid- and chromosome-encoded *Yersinia* antigens, *Infect. Immun.*, **48**, 676–685.

108. Heath, D. G., Anderson, G. W., Jr., Welkos, S. L., Andrews, G. P., Friedlander, A. M., and Mauro, J. M. (1997) A recombinant capsular F1-V antigen fusion protein vaccine protects against experimental bubonic and pneumonic plague. In: *Vaccines 97* (Brown, F., Burton, D., Doherty, P., Mekelanos, J., and Norrby, E., eds.), Cold Spring Harbor Laboratory Press, Cold Spring Harbor, NY, pp. 197–200.

109. Anderson, G. W., Jr., Heath, D. G., Bolt, C. R., Welkos, S. L., and Friedlander, A. M. (1998) Short- and long-term efficacy of single-dose subunit vaccines against *Yersinia pestis* in mice, *Am. J. Trop. Med. Hyg.*, **58**, 793–799.

110. Persson, C., Nordfelth, R., Holmstrom, A., Hakansson, S., Rosqvist, R., and Wolf-Watz, H. (1995) Cell-surface bound *Yersinia* translocate the protein tyrosine phosphatase YopH by a polarized mechanism into the target cell, *Mol. Microbiol.*, **18**, 135–150.

111. Hoover, D. L. and Borschel, R. H. (2005) Medical protection against brucellosis. In: *Biological Weapons Defense: Infectious Diseases and Counterterrorism* (Lindner, L. E., Lebeda, F. J., and Korch, G. W., eds.), Humana Press, Totowa, NJ, pp. 155–184.

112. Pappas, G., Akritidis, N., Bosilkovski, M., and Tsianos, E. (2005) Brucellosis, *N. Engl. J. Med.*, **352**(22), 2325–2336.

113. Cloeckaert, A., Vizcaino, N., Paquet, J. Y., Bowden, R. A., and Elzer, P. H. (2002) Major outer membrane proteins of *Brucella* spp.: past, present and future, *Vet. Microbiol.*, **90**, 229–247.

114. DelVecchio, V. G., Kapatral, V., Redkar, R. J., Patra, G., Mujer, C., Los, T., Ivanova, N., Anderson, I., Bhattacharyya, A., Lykidis, A., Reznik, G., Jablonski, L., Larsen, N., D'Souza, M., Bernal, A., Mazur, M., Goltsman, E., Selkov, E., Elzer, P. H., Hagius, S., O'Callaghan, D., Letesson, J.-J., Haselkorn, R., Kyprides, N., and Overbeek, R. (2002) The genome sequence of the facultative intracellular pathogen *Bricella melitensis, Proc. Natl. Acad. Sci. U.S.A.*, **99**, 443–448.

115. Sanchez, D. O., Zandomeni, R. O., Cravero, S., Verdún, R. E., Pierrou, E., Faccio, P., Diaz, G., Lanzavecchia, S., Agüero, F., Frasch, A. C. C., Andersson, S. G. E., Rossetti, O. L., Grau, O., and Ugalde, R. A. (2001) Gene discovery through genomic sequencing of *Brucella abortus, Infect. Immun.*, **69**, 865–868.

116. Paulsen, I. T., Seshadri, R., Nelson, K. E., Eisen, J. A., Heidelberg, J. F., Read, T. D., Dodson, R. J., Umayam, L., Brinkac, L. M., Beanan, M. J., Daugherty, S. C., Deboy, R. T., Durkin, A. S., Kolonay, J. F., Madupu, R., Nelson, W. C., Ayodeji, B., Kraul, M., Shetty, J., Malek, J., Van Aken, S. E., Riedmuller, S., Tettelin, H., Gill, S. R., White, O., Salzberg, S. L., Hoover, D. L., Lindler, L. E., Halling, S. M., Boyle, S. M., and Fraser, C. M. (2002) The *Brucella suis* genome reveals fundamental similarities between animal and plant pathogens and symbionts, *Proc. Natl. Acad. Sci. U.S.A.*, **99**, 13148–13153.

117. Fernandez-Prada, C. M., Nikolich, M., Vemulapalli, R., Sriranganathan, N., Boyle, S. M., Schurig, G. G., Hadfield, T. L., and Hoover, D. L. (2001) Deletion of *wboA* enhances activation of the lectin pathway of complement in *Brucella abortus* and *Brucella melitensis, Infect. Immun.*, **69**(7), 4407–4416.

118. Salmeron, I., Rodriguez-Zapata, M., Salmeron, O., Manzano, L., Vaquer, S., and Alvarez-Mon, M. (1992) Impaired activity of natural killer cells in patients with active brucellosis, *Clin. Infect. Dis.*, **15**, 746–770.

119. Rodriguez-Zapata, M., Reyes, E., Sanchez, L., Espinosa, A., Solera, J., and Alvarez-Mon, M. (1997) Defective reactive oxygen metabolite generation by macrophages from acute brucellosis patients, *Infection*, **25**, 187–188.

120. Ko, J., Gendron-Fitzpatrick, and A. Splitter, G. A. (2002) Susceptibility of IFN regulatory factor-1 and IFN consensus sequence binding protein-deficient mice to brucellosis, *J. Immunol.*, **168**, 2433–2440.

121. Yingst, S. and Hoover, D. L. (2003) T cell immunity to brucellosis, *Crit. Rev. Microbiol.*, **29**, 313–331.

122. Zhan, Y. and Cheers, C. (1993) Endogenous gamma interferon mediates resistance to *Brucella abortus* infection, *Infect. Immun.*, **61**, 4899–4901.

123. Anderson, T. D., Cheville, N. F., and Meador, V. P. (1986) Pathogenesis of placentitis in the goat inoculated with *Brucella abortus*. II. Ultrastructural studies, *Vet. Pathol.*, **23**(3), 227–239.

124. Spink, W. W. (1950) Clinical aspects of human brucellosis. In: *Brucellosis* (Larson, C. H. and Soule, M. H., eds.), Waverly, Baltimore, pp. 1–8.

125. Solera, J., Lozano, E., Martinez-Alfaro, E., Espinosa, A., Castillejos, M. L., and Abad, L. (1999) Brucellar spondylitis: review of 35 cases and literature survey, *Clin. Infect. Dis.*, **29**, 1440–1449.

126. Khan, M. Y., Mah, M. W., and Memish, Z. A. (2001) Brucellosis in pregnant women, *Clin. Infect. Dis.*, **32**, 1172–1177.

127. Shakir, R. A., Al-Din, A. S., Araj, G. F., Lulu, A. R., Mousa, A. R., and Saadah, M. A. (1987) Clinical categories of neurobrucellosis: a report on 19 cases, *Brain*, **110**, 213–223.

128. Schurig, G. G., Sriranganathan, N., and Corbel, M. J. (2002) Brucellosis vaccines: past, present and future, *Vet. Microbiol.*, **90**, 479–496.

129. Ko, J. and Spliter, G. A. (2003) Molecular host-pathogen interaction in brucellosis: current understanding and future approaches to vaccine development for mice and humans, *Clin. Microbiol. Rev.*, **16**, 65–78.

130. Waag, D. M. and Thompson, H. A. (2005) Pathogenesis of and immunity to *Coxiella burnetii*. In: *Bilogical Weapons Defense: Infectious Diseases and Counterterrorism* (Lindner, L. E., Lebeda, F. J., and Korch, G. W., eds.), Humana Press, Totowa, NJ, pp. 185–207.

131. Byrne, W. P. (1997) Q fever. In: *Medical Aspects of Chemical and Biological Warfare* (Zajtchuk, R. and Belamy, R. F., eds.), Office of the Surgeon General, U.S. Department of the Army, pp. 523–537.

132. Weisburg, W. G., Dobson, M. E., Samuel, J. E., Dasch, G. A., Mallavia, L. P., Baca, O., Mandelco, L., Sechrest, J. E., Weiss, E., and Woese, C. R. (1989) Phylogenetic diversity of the Rickettsiae, *J. Bacteriol.*, **171**, 4202–4206.

133. Tzianabos, T., Moss, C. W., and McDade, J. E. (1981) Fatty acid composition of rickettsiae, *J. Clin. Microbiol.*, **13**, 603–605.

134. Samuel, J. E., Frazier, M. E., and Mallavia, L. P. (1985) Correlation of plasmid type and disease caused by *Coxiella burnetii, Infect. Immun.*, **49**, 775–777.

135. Waag, D. M. and Williams, J. C. (1988) Immune modulation by *Coxiella burnetii*: characterization of a Phase I immunosup-

pressive complex expressed among strains, *Immunopharmacol. Immunotoxicol.*, **10**, 231–260.

136. Tigertt, W. D. and Benenson, A. S. (1956) Studies on Q fever in man, *Trans. Assoc. Am. Phys.*, **69**, 98–104.

137. Waag, D., Chulay, J., Marrie, T., England, M., and Williams, J. (1995) Validation of an enzyme immunoassay for serodiagnosis of acute Q fever, *Eur. J. Clin. Microbiol. Infect. Dis.*, **14**(5), 421–427.

138. Fournier, P.-E., Marrie, T. J., and Raoult, D. (1998) Minireview: diagnosis of Q fever, *J. Clin. Microbiol.*, **36**, 1823–1834.

139. Sobradillo, V., Zalacain, R., Capelastegui, A., Uresandi, F., and Corral, J. (1992) Antibiotic treatment in pneumonia due to Q fever, *Thorax*, **47**, 276–278.

140. Smadel, J. E., Snyder, M. J., and Robbins, F. C. (1948) Vaccination against Q fever, *Am. J. Hyg.*, **47**, 71–78.

141. Johnson, J. W., McLeod, C. G., Stookey, J. L., Higbee, G. A., and Pedersen, C. E., Jr. (1977) Lesions in guinea pigs infected with *Coxiella burnetii* strain M-44, *J. Infect. Dis.*, **135**, 995–998.

142. Ackland, J. R., Worswick, D. A., and Marmion, B. P. (1994) Vaccine prophylaxis of Q fever. A follow-up study of the efficacy of Q-Vax (CSL) 1985–1990, *Med. J. Aust.*, **160**, 704–708.

143. Waag, D. M. and DeShazer, D. (2005) Glanders. In: *Biological Weapons Defense: Infectious Diseases and Counterterrorism* (Lindler, L. E., Lebeda, F. J., and Korch, G. W., eds.), Humana Press, Totowa, NJ, pp. 209–237.

144. Miller, W. R., Pannell, L., Cravitz, L., Tanner, W. A., and Rosebury, T. (1948) Studies on certain biological characteristics of *Malleomyces mallei* and *Malleomyces pseudomallei*. II. Virulence and infectivity for animals, *J. Bacteriol.*, **55**, 127–135.

145. Centers for Disease Control (2000) Biological and chemical terrorism: strategic plan for preparedness and response, *Morb. Mortal. Wkly Rep.*, **49**(RR-4), 1–14.

146. Yabuuchi, E., Kosako, Y., Oyaizy, H., Yano, I., Hotta, H., Hashimoto, Y., Ezaki, T., and Arakawa, M. (1992) Proposal of *Burkholderia* gen. nov. and transfer of seven species of the genus *Pseudomonas* homology group II to a new genus, with the type species *Burkholderia cepacia* (Palleroni and Holmes 1981) comb.nov., *Microbiol. Immunol.*, **36**, 1251–1275.

147. Nierman, W. C., DeShazer, D., Kim, H. S., Tettelin, H., Nelson, K. E., Feldblyum, T., Ulrich, R. L., Ronning, C. M., Brinkac, L. M., Daugherty, S. C., Davidsen, T. D., Deboy, R. T., Dimitrov, G., Dodson, R. J., Durkin, A. S., Gwinn, M. L., Haft, D. H., Khouri, H., Kolonay, J. F., Madupu, R., Mohammoud, Y., Nelson, W. C., Radune, D., Romero, C. M., Sarria, S., Selengut, J., Shamblin, C., Sullivan, S. A., White, O., Yu, Y., Zafar, N., Zhou, L., and Fraser, C. M. (2004) Structural flexibility in the *Burkholderia mallei* genome, *Proc. Natl. Acad. Sci. U.S.A.*, **101**(39), 14246–14251.

148. DeShazer, D., Waag, D. M., Fritz, D. L., and Woods, D. E. (2001) Identification of a *Burkholderia mallei* polysaccharide gene cluster by subtractive hybridization and demonstration that the encoded capsule is an essential virulence determinant, *Microb. Pathogen.*, **30**, 253–269.

149. Ulrich, R. L. and DeShazer, D. (2004) Type III secretion: a virulence factor delivery system essential for the pathogenicity of *Burkholderia mallei*, *Infect. Immun.*, **72**, 1150–1154.

150. Finley, B. B. and Falkow, S. (1997) Common themes in microbial pathogenesis revisited, *Microbiol. Mol. Biol. Rev.*, **61**, 136–169.

151. Henderson, I. R. and Nataro, J. P. (2001) Virulence functions of autotransporter proteins, *Infect. Immun.*, **69**, 1231–1243.

152. Zhu, J., Miller, M. B., Vance, R. E., Dziejman, M., Bassler, B. l., and Mekelanos, J. J., Quorum-sensing regulators control virulence gene expression in *Vibrio cholerae*, *Proc. Natl. Acad. Sci. U.S.A.*, **99**, 3129–3134.

153. Reckseidler, S. L., DeShazer, D., Sokol, P. A., and Woods, D. E. (2001) Detection of bacterial virulence genes by subtrac-

tive hybridization: identification of capsular polysaccharide of *Burkholderia pseudomallei* as a major virulence determinant, *Infect. Immun.*, **69**, 34–44.

154. Khrapova, N. P., Tikhonov, N. G., and Prokhvatilova, Y. V. (1998) Detection of glycoprotein of *Bukholderia pseudomallei*, *Emerg. Infect. Dis.*, **4**, 336–337.

154a. Samygin, V.M., Khrapova, N.P., Spiridonov, V.A., and Stepin, A. A. (2001) Antigen 8 biosynthesis during cultivation of *Burkholderia pseudomallei and B. mallei*, *Zh. Mikrobiol. Epidemiol. Immunobiol.*, **4**, 50–52.

155. Piven, N. N., Smirnova, V. L., Viktorov, D. V., Kovalenko, A. A., Farber, S. M., Iarulin, R. G., and Podzolkova, G. G. (1996) Immunogenicity and heterogenicity of *Pseudomona pseudomallei* surface antigen 8, *Zh. Mikrobiol. (Moscow)*, (4), 75–78.

156. DeShazer, D., Brett, P. J., and Woods, D. E. (1998) The type II O-antigenic polysaccharide moiety of *Burkholderia pseudomallei* lipopolysaccharide is required for serum resistance and virulence, *Mol. Microbiol.*, **30**, 1081–1100.

157. Burtnick, M. N., Brett, P. J., and Woods, D. E. (2002) Molecular and physical characterization of *Burkholderia mallei* O antigens, *J. Bacteriol.*, **184**, 849–852.

158. Pitt, T. L., Aucken, H., and Dance, D. A. (1992) Homogeneity of lipopolysaccharide antigens of *Pseudomonas pseudomallei*, *J. Infect.*, **25**, 139–146.

159. Knirel, Y. A., Paramonov, N. A., Shashkov, A. S., Kochetkov, N. K., Yarullin, R. G., Farber, S. M., and Efremenko, V. I. (1992) Structure of the polysaccharide chains of *Pseudomonas pseudomallei* lipopolysaccharides, *Carbohydr. Res.*, **233**, 185–193.

160. Perry, M. B., MacLean, L. L., Schollaardt, T., Bryan, L. E., and Ho, M. (1995) Structural characterization of the polysaccharide O antigens of *Burkholderia pseudomallei*, *Infect. Immun.*, **63**, 3348–3352.

161. Day, W. A. J., Fernandez, R. E., and Maurelli, A. T. (2001) Pathoadaptive mutations that enhance virulence: genetic organization of the *cadA* regions of *Shigella* spp., *Infect. Immun.*, **69**, 7471–7480.

162. Holden, M. T. G., Titball, R. W., Peacock, S. J., Cerdeño-Tárraga, A. M., Atkins, T., Crossman, L. C., Pitt, T., Churcher, C., Mungall, K., Bentley, S. D., Sebaihia, M., Thomson, N. R., Bason, N., Beacham, I. R., Brooks, K., Brown, K. A., Brown, N. F., Challis, G. L., Cherevach, I., Chillingworth, T., Cronin, A., Crossett, B., Davis, P., DeShazar, D., Feltwell, T., Fraser, A., Hance, Z., Hauser, H., Holroyd, S., Jagels, K., Keith, K. E., Maddison, M., Moule, S., Price, C., Quail, M. A., Rabbinowitsch, E., Rutherford, K., Sanders, M., Simmonds, M., Songsivilai, S., Stevens, K., Tumapa, S., Vesaratchavest, M., Whitehead, S., Yeats, C., Barrell, B. G., Oyston, P. C. F., and Parkhill, J. (2004) Genomic plasticity of the causative agent of melioidosis, *Burkholderia pseudomallei*, *Proc. Natl. Acad. Sci. U.S.A.*, **101**(39), 14240–14245.

163. Ochman, H., Lawrence, J. G., and Groisman, E. A. (2000) Lateral gene transfer and the nature of bacterial innovation, *Nature*, **405**, 299–304.

164. Mira, A., Ochman, H., and Moran, N. A. (2001) Deletional bias and the evolution of bacterial genomes, *Trends Genet.*, **17**, 589–596.

165. Steinmetz, I., Rohde, M., and Brenneke, B. (1995) Purification and characterization of an exopolysaccharide of *Burkholderia (Pseudomonas) pseudomallei*, *Infect. Immun.*, **63**, 3959–3965.

166. Nimtz, M., Wray, V., Domke, T., Brenneke, B., Haussler, S., and Steinmetz, I. (1997) Structure of an acidic exopolysaccharide of *Burkholderia pseudomallei*, *Eur. J. Biochem.*, **250**, 608–616.

167. Srinivasan, A., Kraus, C. N., DeShazer, D., Becker, P. M., Dick, J. D., Soacek, L., Bartlett, J. G., Byrne, W. R., and Thomas, D. L. (2001) Glanders in a military research microbiologist, *N. Engl. J. Med.*, **345**(4), 256–258.

168. Neubauer, H., Meyer, H., and Finke, E. J. (1997) Human glanders, *Int. Rev. Armed Forces Med. Serv.*, **70**, 258–265.

169. Thibault, F. M., Hernandez, E., Vidal, D. R., Girardet, M., and Cavallo, J.-D. (2004) Antibiotic susceptibility of 65 isolates of *Burkholderia pseudomallei* and *Burkholderia mallei* to 35 antimicrobial agents, *J. Antimicrob. Chemother.*, **54**, 1134–1138.

170. Heine, H. S., England, M. J., Waag, D. M., and Byrne, R. (2001) In vitro antibiotic susceptibilities of *Burkholderia mallei* (causative agent of glanders) determined by broth microdilution and E-test, *Antimicrob. Agents Chemother.*, **45**(7), 2119–2121.

171. Dance, D., Wuthiekanun, V., Chaowagul, W., and White, N. J. (1989) The antimicrobial susceptibility of *Pseudomonas pseudomallei*. Emergence of resistance in vitro and during treatment, *J. Antimicrob. Chemother.*, **24**, 295–309.

172. Centers for Disease Control (2000) Laboratory-acquired human glanders – Maryland, *Morb. Mortal. Wkly Rep.*, **49**(RR-24), 532–535.

173. Chetchotisakd, P., Porramatikul, S., Mootsikapun, P., Anunnatsiri, S., and Thinkhamrop, E. (2001) Randomized, double-blind, controlled study of cefoperazone-sulbactam plus cotrimazole for the treatment of severe melioidosis, *Clin. Infect. Dis.*, **33**, 29–34.

174. The European Agency for the Evaluation of Medicinal Products (2002) EMEA/CPMP Guidance document on use of medicinal products for treatment and prophylaxis of biological agents that might be used as weapons of bioterrorism. 10. Glanders and melioidosis, European Agency for the Evaluation of Medicinal Products, London.

175. Mohler, J. R. and Eichhorn, A. (1914) Immunization test with glanders vaccine, *J. Comp. Pathol.*, **27**, 183–185.

176. White, N. J. (2003) Melioidosis, *Lancet*, **361**(9370), 1715–1722.

177. Dance, D. A. B. and White, N. J. (1996) Melioidosis. In: *The Wellcome Trust Illustrated History of Tropical Diseases* (Cox, F. E. G., ed.), The Wellcome Trust, London, pp. 72–81.

178. Visca, P., Cazzola, G., Petrucca, A., and Braggion, C. (2001) Travel-associated *Burkholderia pseudomallei* infection (melioidosis) in a patient with cystic fibrosis: a case report, *Clin. Infect. Dis.*, **32**, E15–E16.

179. Holland, D. J., Wesley, A., Drinkovic, D., and Currie, B. J. (2002) Cystic fibrosis and *Burkholderia pseudomallei* infection: an emerging problem, *Clin. Infect. Dis.*, **35**, 138–140.

180. Woods, D. E., DeShazer, D., Moore, R. A., Brett, P. J., Burtnick, M. N., Reckseidler, S. L., and Senkiw, M. D. (1999) Current studies on the pathogenesis of melioidosis, *Microbes Infect.*, **1**(2), 157–162.

181. Sexton, M. M., Jones, A. L., Chaowagul, W., and Woods, D. E. (1994) Purification and characterization of protease from *Pseudomonas pseudomallei*, *Can. J. Microbiol.*, **40**, 903–910.

182. Haussler, S., Nimtz, M., Domke, T., Wray, V., and Steinmetz, I. (1996) Purification and characterization of a cytotoxic exolipid of *Burkholderia pseudomallei*, *Infect. Immun.*, **66**, 1588–1593.

183. Egan, A. M. and Gordon, D. L. (1996) *Burkholderia pseudomallei* activates complement and is ingested but not killed by polymorphonuclear leukocytes, *Infect. Immun.*, **64**, 4952–4959.

184. Wong, K. T., Puthucheary, S. D., and Vadivelu, J. (1995) The histopathology of human melioidosis, *Histopathology*, **26**, 51–55.

185. Kespichayawattana, W., Rattanachetkul, S., Wanun, T., Utaisincharoen, P., and Sirisinha, S. (2000) *Burkholderia pseudomallei* induces cell fusion and actin-associated membrane protrusion: a possible mechanism for cell-to-cell spreading, *Infect. Immun.*, **68**, 5377–5384.

186. Stevens, M. P., Wood, M. W., Taylor, L. A., Monaghan, P., Hawes, P., Jones, P. W., Wallis, T. S., and Galyov, E. E. (2002) An Inv/Mxi-Spa-like type III protein secretion system in *Burkholderia pseudomallei* modulates intracellular behaviour of the pathogen, *Mol. Microbiol.*, **46**, 649–659.

187. Walsh, A. L., Smith, M. D., Wuthiekanun, V., Suputtamongkol, S., Chaowagul, W., Dance, D. A., Angus, B., and White, N. J. (1995) Prognostic significance of quantitative bacteremia in septicemic melioidosis, *Clin. Infect. Dis.*, **21**(6), 1498–1500.

188. Steinmetz, I., Rohde, M., and Brenneke, B. (1995) Purification and characterization of an exopolysaccharide of *Burkholderia* (*Pseudomonas*) *pseudomallei*, *Infect. Immun.*, **63**, 3959–3965.

189. Reckseidler, S. L., DeShazer, D., Sokol, P. A., and Woods, D. E. (2001) Detection of bacterial virulence genes by subtractive hybridization: identification of capsular polysaccharide of *Burkholderia pseudomallei* as a major virulence determinant, *Infect. Immun.*, **69**, 34–44.

190. Haussler, S., Rohde, M., and Steinmetz, I. (1999) Highly resistant *Burkholderia pseudomallei* small colony variants isolated in vitro and in experimental melioidosis, *Med. Microbiol. Immunol. (Berl)*, **188**, 91–97.

191. Jones, S. M., Ellis, J. F., Russell, P., Griffin, K. F., and Oyston, P. C. (2002) Passive protection against *Burkholderia pseudomallei* infection in mice by monoclonal antibodies against capsular polysaccharide, lipopolysaccharide or proteins, *J. Med. Microbiol.*, **51**, 1055–1062.

192. Nuntayanuwat, S., Dharakul, T., Chaowagul, W., and Songsivilai, S. (1999) Polymorphism in the promoter region of tumor necrosis factor-alpha gene is associated with severe melioidosis, *Hum. Immunol.*, **60**, 979–983.

193. Dharakul, T., Vejbaesya, S., Chaowagul, W., Luangtrakool, P., Stephens, H. A., and Songsivilai, S. (1998) HLA-DR and -DQ associations with melioidosis, *Hum. Immunol.*, **59**, 580–586.

193a. Viriyasithavat, P., Chaowagul, W., Dance, D. A., and White, N. J. (1991) Corneal ulcer caused by *Pseudomonas pseudomallei*: report of three cases, *Rev. Infect. Dis.*, **13**(3), 335–337.

194. White, N. J., Dance, D. A., Chaowagul, W., Wattanagoon, Y., Wuthiekanun, V., and Pitakwatchara, N. (1989) Halving of mortality of severe melioidosis by ceftazidime, *Lancet*, **2**, 697–701.

195. Sookpranee, M., Boonma, P., Susaengrat, W., Bhuripanyo, K., and Punyagupta, S. (1992) Multicenter prospective randomized trial comparing ceftazidime plus co-trimozaxole with chloramphenicol plus doxycycline and co-trimoxazole for treatment of severe melioidosis, *Antimicrob. Agents Chemother.*, **36**, 158–162.

196. Smith, M. D., Wuthiekanun, V., Walsh, A. L., and White, N. J. (1994) Susceptibility of *Pseudomonas pseudomallei* to some newer β-lactam antibiotics and antibiotic combination using time-kill studies, *J. Antimicrob. Chemother.*, **33**, 145–149.

197. Simpson, A. J. H., Suputtamongkol, Y., Smith, M. D., Angus, B. J., Rajanuwong, A., Wuthiekanun, V., Howe, P. A., Walsh, A. L., Chaowagul, W., and White, N. J. (1999) Comparison of imipenem and ceftazidime as therapy for severe melioidosis, *Clin. Infect. Dis.*, **29**(2), 381–387.

198. Dance, D. A. B., Davis, T. M. E., Wattanagoon, Y., Chaowagul, W., Saiphan, P., Looareesuwan, S., Wuthiekanun, V., and White, N. J. (1989) Acute suppurative parotitis caused by *Pseudomonas pseudomallei* in children, *J. Infect. Dis.*, **159**(4), 654–660.

199. Currie, B. J., Fisher, D. A., Howard, D. M., Burrow, J. N. C., Lo, D., Selva-nayagam, S., Anstey, N. M., Huffman, S. E., Snelling, P. L., Marks, P. J., Stephens, D. P., Lum, G. D., Jacups, S. P., and Krause, V. L. (2000) Endemic melioidosis in tropical northern Australia: a 10-year prospective study and review of the literature, *Clin. Infect. Dis.*, **31**, 981–986.

200. Woods, M. L. 2nd, Currie, B. J., Howard, D. M., Tierney, A., Watson, A., Anstey, N. M., Philpott, J., Asche, V., and Withnall, K. (1992) Neurological melioidosis: seven cases from the Northern territory of Australia, *Clin. Infect. Dis.*, **15**(1), 163–169.

201. Currie, B., Fisher, D. A., Howard, D. M., and Burrow, J. N. (2000) Neurological melioidosis, *Acta Trop.*, **74**(2–3), 145–151.

202. World Health Organization (1976) Ebola haemorrhagic fever in Zaire, *Bull. World Health Organization*, **56**, 271–293.

203. Bowen, E. T. W., Platt, G. S., Lloyd, G., Baskerville, A., Harris, W. J., and Vella, E. C. (1977) Viral haemorrhagic fever in southern Sudan and northern Zaire: preliminary studies on the aetiologic agent, *Lancet*, **1**, 571–573.

204. Baron, R. C., McCormick, J. B., and Zubeir, O. A. (1983) Ebola virus disease in southern Sudan: hospital dissemination and intrafamilial spread, *Bull. World Health Organization*, **62**, 997–1003.

205. Sanchez, A., Ksiazek, T. G., Rollin, P. E., Peters, C. J., Nichol, S. T., Khan, A. S., and Mahy, B. W. J. (1995) Reemergence of Ebola virus in Africa, *Emerg. Infect. Dis.*, **1**(3), 96–97.

206. Centers for Disease Control and Prevention (1995) Outbreak of Ebola viral hemorrhagic fever – Zaire, *Morb. Mortal. Wkly Rep.*, **44**, 381–382.

207. Centers for Disease Control and Prevention (1995) Update: outbreak of ebola viral hemorrhagic fever – Zaire, *Morb. Mortal. Wkly Rep.*, **44**, 399.

208. Formenty, P., Boesch, C., Wyers, M., Steiner, C., Donati, F., Dind, F., Walker, F., and Le Guenno, B. (1999) Ebola virus outbreak among wild chimpanzees living in a rain forest of Côte d'Ivoire, *J. Infect. Dis.*, **179**(Suppl. 1), S120–S126.

209. Le Guenno, B., Formenty, P., Wyers, M., Gounon, P., Walker, F., and Boesch, C. (1995) Isolation and partial characterization of a new strain of Ebola virus, *Lancet*, **345**(8960), 1271–1274.

210. Jahrling, R. B., Geisbert, T. W., Jaax, N. K., Hanes, M. A., Ksiazek, T. G., and Peters, C. J. (1996) Experimental infection of cynomolgus macaques with Ebola-Reston filoviruses from the 1989–1990 U.S. epizootic, *Arch. Virol. Suppl.*, **11**, 115–134.

211. World Health Organization (1992) Viral haemorrhagic fever in imported monkeys, *Wkly Epidemiol. Rec.*, **67**, 142–143.

212. Francesconi, P., Yoti, Z., Declich, S., Onek, P. A., Fabiani, M., Olango, J., Andreghetti, R., Rollin, P. E., Opira, C., Greco, D., and Salmaso, S. (2003) Ebola hemorrhagic fever transmission and risk factors of contact, Uganda, *Emerg. Infect. Dis.*, **9**(11), 1430–1437.

213. Sanchez, A., Kiley, M. P., Holloway, B. P., and Auperin, D. D. (1993) Sequence analysis of the Ebola genome: organization, genetic elements, and comparison with the genome of Marburg virus, *Virus Res.*, **29**, 215–240.

214. Yaddanapudi, K., Palacios, G., Towner, J. S., Chen, I., Sariol, C. A., Nichol, S. T., and Lipkin, W. I. (2006) Implication of a retrovirus-like glycoprotein peptide in the immunopathogenesis of Ebola and Marburg viruses, *FASEB J.*, **20**, 2519–2530.

215. Baize, S., Leroy, E. M., Georges-Courbot, M. C., Capron, M., Lansoud-Soukate, J., Debre, P., Fisher-Hoch, S. P., McCormick, J. B., and Georges, A. J. (1999) Defective humoral responses and extensive intravascular apoptosis are associated with fatal outcome in Ebola virus-infected patients, *Nat. Med.*, **5**, 423–426.

216. Leroy, E. M., Baize, S., Volchkov, V. E., Fisher-Hoch, S. P., Georges-Courbot, M. C., Lansoud-Soukate, J., Capron, M., Debre, P., McCormick, J. B., and Georges, A. J. (2000) Human asymptomatic Ebola infection and strong inflammatory response, *Lancet*, **355**, 2210–2215.

217. Villinger, F., Rollin, P. E., Brar, S. S., Chikkala, N. F., Winter, J., Sundstrom, J. B., Zaki, S. R., Swanepoel, R., Ansari, A. A., and Peters, C. J. (1999) Markedly elevated levels of interferon (IFN)-gamma, INF-alpha, interleukin (IL)-2, IL-10, and tumor necrosis factor-alpha associated with fatal Ebola virus infection, *J. Infect. Dis.*, **179**(Suppl.), S188–S191.

218. Yang, Z. Y., Duckers, H. J., Sullivan, N. J., Sanchez, A., Nabel, E. G., and Nabel, G. J. (2000) Identification of the Ebola virus glycoprotein as the main determinant of vascular cell cytotoxicity and injury, *Nat. Med.*, **6**, 886–889.

219. Volchkov, V. E., Volchkova, V. A., Muhlberger, E., Kolesnikova, L. V., Weik, M., Dolnik, O., and Klenk, H. D. (2001) Recovery of infectious Ebola virus from complementary DNA: RNA editing of the GP gene and viral cytotoxicity, *Science*, **291**, 1965–1969.

220. Feldman, H., Volchkov, V. E., Volchkova, V. A., Stroher, U., and Klenk, H. D. (2001) Biosynthesis and role of filoviral glucoproteins, *J. Gen. Virol.* **82**, 2839–2848.

221. Yaddanapudi, K., Palacios, G., Towner, J. S., Chen, I., Sariol, C. A., Nichol, S. T., and Lipkin, W. I. (2006) Implication of a retrovirus-like glycoprotein peptide in the immunopathogenesis of Ebola and Marburg viruses, *FASEB J.*, **20**, 2519–2530.

222. Denner, J., Norley, S., and Kurth, R. (1994) The immunosuppressive peptide of HIV-1: functional domains and immune response in AIDS patients, *AIDS*, **8**, 1063–1072.

223. Haraguchi, S., Good, R. A., and Day, N. K. (1995) Immunosuppressive retroviral peptides: cAMP and cytokine patterns, *Immunol. Today*, **16**, 595–603.

224. Cianciolo, G. J., Copeland, T. D., Oroszlan, S., and Snyderman, R. (1985) Inhibition of lymphocyte proliferation by a synthetic peptide homologous to retroviral envelope proteins, *Science*, **230**, 453–455.

225. Haraguchi, S., Good, R. A., James-Yarish, M., Cianciolo, G. J., and Day, N. K. (1995) Induction of intracellular cAMP by a synthetic retroviral envelope peptide: a possible mechanism of immunopathogenesis in retroviral infections, *Proc. Natl. Acad. Sci. U.S.A.*, **92**, 5568–5571.

226. Haraguchi, S., Good, R. A., James-Yarish, M., Cianciolo, G. J., and Day, N. K. (1995) Differential modulation of Th1- and Th2-related cytokine mRNA expression by a synthetic peptide homologous to a conserved domain within retroviral envelope protein, *Proc. Natl. Acad. Sci. U.S.A.*, **92**, 3611–3615.

227. Gottlieb, R. A., Kleinerman, A. S., O'Brien, C. A., Tsujimoto, S., Cianciolo, G. J., and Lennarz, W. J. (1990) Inhibition of protein kinase G by a peptide conjugate homologous to a domain of the retroviral protein p15E, *J. Immunol.*, **145**, 2566–2570.

228. Kadota, J., Cianciolo, G. J., and Snyderman, R. (1991) A synthetic peptide homologous to retroviral transmembrane envelope proteins depresses protein kinase C mediated lymphocytic proliferation and directly inactivated protein kinase C: a potential mechanism for immunosuppression, *Microbiol. Immunol.*, **35**, 443–459.

229. Feldman, H. and Klenk, H.-D. Filoviruses. In: *Medmicro Chapter 72* (http://www.gsbs.utmb.edu/microbook/ch072.htm).

230. Sullivan, N. J., Sanchez, A., Rollin, P. E., Yang, Z. Y, and Nabel, G. J. (2000) Development of preventive vaccine for Ebola virus infection in primates, *Nature*, **408**(6812), 605–609.

231. Kudoyarova-Zubavichene, N. M., Sergeyev, N. N., Chepurnov, A. A., and Netesov, S. V. (1999) Preparation and use of hyperimmune serum for prophylaxis and therapy of Ebola virus infection, *J. Infect. Dis.*, **179**(Suppl.), S218–S223.

232. Jahrling, P. B., Geisbert, T. W., Geisbert, J. B., Swearengen, J. R., Bray, M., Jaax, N. K., Huggins, J. W., LeDuc, J. W., and Peters, C. J. (1999) Evaluation of immune globulin and recombinant interferon-α2b for treatment of experimental Ebola virus infections, *J. Infect. Dis.*, **179**(Suppl.), S224–S234.

233. Burton, D. R. and Parren, P. W. H. I. (2000) Fighting the Ebola virus, *Nature*, **408**. 527–528.

234. Hevey, M., Negley, D., Pushko, P., Smith, J., and Schmaljohn, A. (1998) Marburg virus vaccines based upon alphavirus replicons protect guinea pigs and nonhuman primates, *Virology*, **251**(1), 28–37.

235. Elliott, R. M., Bouloy, M., Calisher, C. H., Goldbach, R., Moyer, J. T., Nichol, S. T., Pettersson, R., Plyusnin, A., and Schmaljohn, C. S. (2000) Family *Bunyaviridae*. In: *Virus Taxonomy. Seventh Report of the International Committee on Taxonomy of Viruses* (van Regenmortel, M. H. V., Fauquet, C. M., Bishop, D. H. L.,

Carstens, E. B., Estes, M. K., Lemon, S. M., Maniloff, J., Mayo, M. A., McGeoch, D. J., Pringle, C. R., and Wickner, R. B., eds.), Academic Press, San Diego, pp. 599–621.

236. Elliott, R. M. (1990) Molecular biology of *Bunyaviridae, J. Gen. Virol.*, **71**, 501–522.

237. Bowen, M. D., Trappier, S. G., Sanchez, A. J., Meyer, R. F., Goldsmith, C. S., Zaki, S. R., Dunster, L. M., Peters, C. J., Ksiazek, T. G., and Nichol, S. T. (2001) A reassortant Bunyavirus isolated from hemorrhagic fever cases in Kenya and Somalia, *Virology*, **291**, 185–190.

238. Gerrard, S. R., Li, L., Barrett, A. D., and Nichol, S. T. (2004) Ngari virus is a Bunyamwera virus reassortant that can be associated with large outbreaks of hemorrhagic fever in Africa, *Virology*, **78**, 8922–8926.

239. Flick, R. and Whitehouse, C. A. (2005) Crimean-Congo hemorrhagic fever, *Curr. Mol. Med.*, **5**, 753–760.

240. Clerx-van Haaster, C. M., Clerx, J. P. M., Ushijima, H., Akashi, H., Fuller, F., and Bishop, D. H. L. (1982) The 3′ terminal RNA sequences of Bunyaviruses and Nairoviruses (*Bunyaviridae*): evidence of end sequence generic differences within the virus family, *J. Gen. Virol.*, **61**, 289–292.

241. Flick, R., Elgh, F., and Pettersson, R. F. (2002) Mutational analysis of the Uukuniemi virus (*Bunyaviridae* family) promoter reveals two elements of functional importance, *J. Virol.*, **76**(21), 10849–10860.

242. Bishop, D. H. L., Calisher, C., Casals, J., Chumakov, M. P., Gaidamovich, S. Y., Hannoun, C., Lvov, D. K., Marshall, I. D., Oker-Blom, N. M., Peterrsson, R. F., Porterfield, J. S., Russell, P. K., Shope, R. E., and Westaway, E. G. (1980), *Bunyaviridae, Intervirology*, **14**, 125–143.

243. Kinsella, E., Martin, S. G., Grolla, A., Czub, M., Feldmann, H., and Flick, R. (2002) Sequence determination of the Crimean-Congo hemorrhagic fever virus L segment, *Virology*, **321**(1), 23–28.

244. Honig, J. E., Osborne, J. C., and Nichol, S. T. (2004) Crimean-Congo hemorrhagic fever virus genome L RNA segment and encoded protein, *Virology*, **321**, 29–35.

245. Sanchez, A. J., Vincent, M. J., and Nichol, S. T. (2002) Characterization of the glycoproteins of Crimean-Congo hemorrhagic fever virus, *J. Virol.*, **76**, 7263–7275.

246. Baskerville, A., Fisher-Hoch, S. P., Neild, G. H., and Dowsett, A. B. (1985) Ultrastructural pathology of experimental Ebola haemorrhagic fever virus infection, *J. Pathol.*, **147**(3), 199–209.

247. Vincent, M. J., Sanchez, A. J., Erickson, B. R., Basak, A., Chretien, M., Seidah, N. G., and Nichol, S. T. (2003) Crimean-Congo hemorrhagic fever virus glycoprotein proteolytic processing by subtilase SKI-1, *J. Virol.*, **77**(16), 8640–8649.

248. Haferkamp, S., Fernando, L., Schwartz, T. F., Feldmann, H., and Flick, R. (2005) Intracellular localization of Crimean-Congo hemorrhagic fever (CCHF) virus glycoproteins, *Virol. J.*, **2**, 42.

249. Walpita, P. and Flick, R. (2005) Reverse genetics of negative-stranded RNA viruses: a global perspective, *FEMS Microbiol. Lett.*, **266**(1), 9–18.

250. Lawson, N. D., Stillman, E. A., Whitt, M. A., and Rose, J. K. (1995) Recombinant vesicular stomatitis viruses from DNA, *Proc. Natl. Acad. Sci. U.S.A.*, **92**, 4477–4481.

251. Whelan, S. P. J., Ball, L. A., Barr, J. N., and Wertz, G. T. W. (1995) Efficient recovery of infectious vesicular stomatitis virus entirely from cDNA clones, *Proc. Natl. Acad. Sci. U.S.A.*, **92**, 8388–8392.

252. He, B., Paterson, R. G., Ward, C. D., and Lamb, R. A. (1997) Recovery of infectious SV5 from cloned DNA and expression of a foreign gene, *Virology*, **237**(2), 249–260.

253. Barron, M. D. and Barrett, T. (1997) Rescue of rinderpest virus from cloned cDNA, *J. Virol.*, **71**(2), 1265–1271.

254. Neumann, G., Feldmann, H., Watanabe, S., Lukashevich, I., and Kawaoka, Y. (2002) Reverse genetics demonstrates that proteolytic processing of the Ebola virus glycoprotein is not essential for replication in cell culture, *J. Virol.*, **76**(1), 406–410.

255. Neumann, G., Watanabe, T., Ito, H., Watanabe, S., Goto, H., Gao, P., Hughes, M., Perez, D. R., Donis, R., Hoffmann, E., Hobom, G., and Kawaoka, Y. (1999) Generation of influenza A viruses entirely from cloned cDNAs, *Proc. Natl. Acad. Sci. U.S.A.*, **96**(16), 9345–9350.

256. Flick, R., Flick, K., Feldmann, H., and Elgh, F. (2003) Reverse genetics for Crimean-Congo hemorrhagic fever virus, *J. Virol.*, **77**(10), 5997–6006.

257. Zobel, A., Neumann, G., and Hobom, G. (1993) RNA polymerase I catalyzed transcription of insert viral cDNA, *Nucleic Acids Res.*, **21**(16), 3607–3614.

258. Neumann, G., Zobel, A., and Hobom, G. (1994) RNA polymerase I-mediated expression of influenza viral RNA molecules, *Virology*, **202**(1), 477–479.

259. Talmon, Y., Prasad, B. V. V., Clerx, J. P. M., Wang, G.-J., Chiu, W., and Hewlett, M. J. (1987) Electron microscopy of vitrified-hydrated La Cross virus, *J. Virol.*, **61**, 2319–2321.

260. Eliott, L. H., Kiley, M. P., and McCormick, J. B. (1984) Hantaan virus: identification of virion proteins, *J. Gen. Virol.*, **65**, 1285–1293.

261. Beaty, B. J., Rozhon, E. J., Gensemer, P., and Bishop, D. H. L. (1981) Formation of reassortant bunyaviruses in dually infected mosquitoes, *Virology*, **111**, 662–665.

262. Beaty, B. J., Miller, B. R., Shope, R. E., Rozhon, E. J., and Bishop, D. H. L. (1982) Molecular basis of bunyavirus *per os* infection of mosquitoes: role of middle-sized RNA segment, *Proc. Natl. Acad. Sci. U.S.A.*, **79**, 1295–1297.

263. Beaty, B. J., Sundin, D. R., Chandler, L. J., and Bishop, D. H. L. (1985) Evolution of bunyaviruses by genome reassortment in dually infected mosquitoes (*Aedes triseriatus*), *Science*, **230**, 548–550.

264. Klimas, R. A., Thompson, W. A., Calisher, C. H., Clark, G. G., Grimstad, P. R., and Bishop, D. H. L. (1981) Genotypic varieties of La Cross virus isolated from different geographic regions of the continental United States and evidence of naturally occurring intertypic recombinant La Cross virus, *Am. J. Epidemiol.*, **114**, 112–131.

264a. Ushijima, H., Clerx-van Haaster, C. M., and Bishop, D. H. L. (1981) Analyses of Patois group bunyaviruses: evidence for naturally occurring recombinant bunyaviruses and existence of immune precipitable and nonprecipitable nonvirion proteins induced in bunyavirus-infected cells, *Virology*, **110**, 318–332.

264b. Sall, A. A., de Zanotto, P. M., Sene, O. K., Zeller, H. G., Digoutte, J. P., Thiongane, Y., and Bouloy, M. (1999) Genetic reassortment of Rift Valley fever virus in nature, *J. Virol.*, **73**(10), 8196–8200.

264c. Hoogstraal, H. (1979) The epidemiology of tick-borne Crimean-Congo hemorrhagic fever in Asia, Europe, and Africa, *J. Med. Entomol.*, **15**(4), 307–417.

264d. Leshchinskaya, E. V. (1965) Clinical picture of Crimean haemorrhagic fever in Russia, *Trudy Inst. Polio Virusn. Entsefalitov Akad. Med. Nauk SSSR*, **7**, 226–236. (in English: NAMRU3-1856).

265. Woodall, J. P., Williams, M. C., and Simpson, D. I. (1967) Congo virus: a hitherto underdescribed virus occurring in Africa. II. Identification studies, *East Afr. Med. J.*, **44**(2), 93–98.

266. Casals, J. (1969) Antigenic similarity between the virus causing Crimean hemorrhagic fever and Congo virus, *Proc. Soc. Exp. Biol. Med.*, **131**(1), 233–236.

267. Begum, F., Wisseman, C. L., Jr., and Casals, J. (1970) Tick-borne viruses of West Pakistan. IV. Viruses similar to, or identical with, Crimean Hemorrhagic fever (Congo-Semunya), Wad

medani, and Pak Argas 461 isolated from ticks of the Changa Manga Forest, Lahore District, and Hunza, Gilgit Agency, W. Pakistan, *Am. J. Epidemiol.*, **92**(3), 197–202.

268. Schwartz, T. F., Nitschko, H., Jager, G., Nsanze, H., Longson, M., Pugh, R. N., and Abraham, A. K. (1995) Crimean-Congo haemorrhagic fever in Oman, *Lancet*, **4**(8984), 1230.

269. Whitehouse, C. A. (2004) Crimean-Congo hemorrhagic fever, *Antiviral Res.*, **64**, 145–160.

270. Swanepoel, R., Gill, D. E., Shepherd, A. J., Leman, P. A., Mynhardt, J. H., and Harvey, S. (1989) The clinical pathology of Crimean-Congo hemorrhagic fever, *Rev. Infect. Dis.*, **11**(Suppl. 4), S794–S800.

271. Saijo, M., Tang, Q., Shimayi, B., Han, L., Zhang, Y., Asiguma, M., Tianshu, D., Maeda, A., Kurane, I., and Morikawa, S. (2005) Recombinant nucleoprotein-based serological diagnosis of Crimean-Congo hemorrhagic fever virus infections, *J. Med. Virol.*, **75**(2), 295–299.

272. Saijo, M., Tang, Q., Shimayi, B., Han, L., Zhang, Y., Asiguma, M., Tianshu, D., Maeda, A., Kurane, I., and Morikawa, S. (2005) Antigen-capture enzyme-linked immunosorbent assay for the diagnosis of Crimean-Cong hemorrhagic fever using a novel monoclonal antibody, *J. Med. Virol.*, **77**(1), 83–88.

273. Paragas, J., Whitehouse, C. A., Endy, T. P., and Bray, M. (2004) A simple assay for determining antiviral activity against Crimean-Congo hemorrhagic fever virus, *Antiviral Res.*, **62**(1), 21–25.

274. Tignor, G. H. and Hanham, C. A. (1993) Ribavirin efficacy in an in vivo model of Crimean-Congo hemorrhagic fever virus (CCHF) infection, *Antiviral Res.*, **22**(4), 309–325.

275. Mardani, M., Keshtkar, M., Holakouie Naieni, K., and Zeinali, M. (2003) The efficacy of oral ribavirin in the treatment of Crimean-Congo hemorrhagic fever in Iran, *Clin. Infect. Dis.*, **36**, 1613–1618.

276. Papa, A., Bozovi, B., Pavlidou, V., Papadimitriou, E., Pelemis, M., and Antoniadis, A. (2002) Genetic detection and isolation of Crimean-Congo hemorrhagic fever virus, Kosovo, Yugoslavia, *Emerg. Infect. Dis.*, **8**(8), 852–854.

277. Tang, Q., Saijo, M., Zhang, Y., Asiguma, M., Tianshu, D., Han, L., Shimayi, B., Maeda, A., Kurane, I., and Morikawa, S. (2003) A patient with Crimean-Congo hemorrhagic fever serologically diagnosed by recombinant nucleoprotein-based antibody detection systems, *Clin. Diagn. Lab. Immunol.*, **10**(3), 489–491.

278. Fisher-Hoch, S. P., Khan, J. A., Rehman, S., Mirza, S., Khurshid, M., and McCormick, J. B. (1995) Crimean-Congo-haemorrhagic fever treated with oral ribavirin, *Lancet*, **346**(8973), 472–475.

279. Centers for Disease Control (1988) Management of patients with suspected viral hemorrhagic fever, *Morb. Mortal. Wkly Rep.*, **37**(Suppl. 3) 1–16.

280. Vassilenko, S. M., Vassilev, T. L., Bozadjiev, L. G., Bineva, I. L., and Kazarov, G. Z. (1990) Specific intravenous immunoglobulin for Crimean-Congo haemorrhagic fever, *Lancet*, **335**(8692), 791–792.

281. Vassilev, T., Valchev, V., Kazarov, G., Razsukanova, L., and Vitanov, T. (1991) A reference preparation for human immunoglobulin against Crimean/Congo hemorrhagic fever, *Biologicals*, **19**(1), 57.

282. Papa, A., Christova, I., Papadimitriou, E., and Antoniadis, A. (2004) Crimean-Congo hemorrhagic fever in Bulgaria, *Emerg. Infect. Dis.*, **10**(8), 1465–1467.

283. Kovacheva, T., Velcheva, D., and Katzarov, G. (1997) Studies on the morbidity of Congo-Crimean hemorrhagic fever before and after specific immunoprophylaxis [in Bulgarian], *Infectology*, **34**, 34–35.

284. Flick, R. and Bouloy, M. (2005) Rift Valley virus, *Curr. Mol. Med.*, **5**, 827–834.

285. Gerdes, G. H. (2004) Rift Valley fever, *Rev. Sci. Tech. Off. Int. Epiz.*, **23**, 613–623.

286. Bird, B. H., Albariño, C. G., and Nichol, S. T. (2007) Rift Valley fever virus lacking NSm proteins retains high virulence in vivo and may provide a model of human delayed onset neurologic disease, *Virology*, **362**(1), 10–15.

287. Ikegami, T., Peters, C. J., and Makino, S. (2005) Rift Valley fever virus nonstructural protein NSs promotes viral RNA replication and transcription in a minigenome system, *J. Virol.*, **79**(9), 5606–5615.

288. Neumann, G., Zobel, A., and Hobom, G. (1994) RNA polymerase I-mediated expression of influenza viral RNA molecules, *Virology*, **202**, 477–479.

289. Zobel, A., Neumann, G., and Hobom, G. (1993) RNA polymerase I catalyzed transcription of insert viral cDNA, *Nucleic Acids Res.*, **21**(16), 3607–3614.

290. Gauliard, N., Billecocq, A., Flick, R., and Bouloy, M. (2006) Rift Valley fever virus noncoding regions of L, M and S segments regulate RNA synthesis, *Virology*, **351**(1), 170–179.

291. Billecock, A., Spiegel, M., Vialat, P., Kohl, A., Weber, F., Bouloy, M., and Haller, O. (2004) NSs protein of Rift Valley fever virus blocks interferon production by inhibiting host gene transcription, *J. Virol.*, **78**(18), 9798–9806.

292. Haller, O., Kochs, G., and Weber, F. (2006) The interferon response circuit: induction and suppression by pathogenic viruses, *Virology*, **344**, 119–130.

293. Marie, I., Durbin, J. E., and Levy, D. E. (1998) Differential viral induction of distinct interferon-alpha genes by positive feedback through interferon regulatory factor-7, *EMBO J.*, **17**(22), 6660–6669.

294. Samuel, C. E. (2001) Antiviral actions of interferons, *Clin. Microbiol. Rev.*, **14**(4), 778–809.

295. de Veer, M. J., Holko, M., Frevel, M., Walker, E., Der, S., Paranjape, J. M., Silverman, R. H., and Williams, B. R. (2001) Functional classification of interferon-stimulated genes identified using microarray, *J. Leukocyte Biol.*, **69**(6), 912–920.

296. Geisbert, T. W. and Jahrling, P. B. (2004) Exotic emerging viral disease: progress and challenges, *Nat. Med.*, **10**(12 Suppl.), S110–S121.

297. Collett, M. S. (1986) Messenger RNA of the M segment of RNA of Rift Valley fever virus, *Virology*, **151**(1), 151–156.

298. Bridgen, A. and Elliott, R. M. (1996) Rescue by a segmented negative-strand virus entirely from cloned complentary DNAs, *Proc. Natl. Acad. Sci. U.S.A.*, **93**, 15400–15404.

299. Le May, N., Dubaele, S., Proietti De Santis, L., Billecock, A., Bouloy, M., and Egly, J.-M. (2004) TFIIF transcription factor, a target for the Rift Valley hemorrhagic fever virus, *Cell*, **116**, 541–550.

300. Peters, C. J., Reynolds, J. A., Slone, T. W., Jones, D. E., and Stephen, E. L. (2001) Prophylaxis of Rift Valley fever with antiviral drugs, immune serum, an interferon inducer, and a macrophage activator, *Antiviral Res.*, **6**(5), 285–297.

301. Khaiboullina, S. F., Morzunov, S. P., and St. Jeor, S. C. (2005) Hantaviruses: molecular biology, evolution and pathogenesis, *Curr. Mol. Med.*, **5**, 773–790.

302. Schmaljohn, C. S. (1996) *Bunyaviridae:* the viruses and their replication. In: *Fields Virology* (Fields, B. N., Knipe, D. M., and Howley, P. M., eds.), Lippincott-Raven, Philadelphia, pp. 1447–1471.

303. LeDuc, J. W., Childs, J. E., and Glass, G. E. (1992) The hantaviruses, etiologic agents of hemorrhagic fever with renal syndrome: a possible cause of hypertension and chronic renal disease in the United States, *Annu. Rev. Publ. Health*, **13**, 79–98.

304. Peters, C. J., Simpson, G. L., and Levy, H. (1999) Spectrum of hantavirus infection: hemorrhagic fever with renal syndrome and hantavirus pulmonaty syndrome, *Annu. Rev. Med.*, **50**, 531–545.

305. Plyusnin, A., Vapalahti, O., and Vaheri, A. (1996) Hantaviruses: genome structure, expression and evolution, *J. Gen. Virol.*, **77**, 2677–2687.

306. Alfadhli, A., Steel, E., Finlay, L., Bächinger, H. P., and Barklis, E. (2002) Hantavirus nucleocapsid protein coiled-coil domains, *J. Biol. Chem.*, **277**(30), 27103–27108.

307. Pensiero, M. N. and Hay, J. (1992) The Hantaan virus M-segment glycoproteins G1 and G2 can be expressed independently, *J. Virol.*, **66**, 1907–1914.

308. Deyde, V. M., Rizvanov, A. A., Chase, J., Otteson, E. W., and St. Jeor, S. C. (2005) Hantaan virus replication: effects of monensin, tunicamycin and endoglycosidases on the structural glycoproteins, *Virology*, **331**, 307–315.

309. Schmaljohn, C. S., Hasty, S. E., Rasmussen, L., and Dalrymple, J. M. (1986) Interaction and trafficking of Andes and Sin Nombre hantavirus glycoproteins G1 and G2, *J. Gen. Virol.*, **67**(Pt. 4), 707–717.

310. Tsai, T. F., Tang, Y. W., Hu, S. L., Ye, K. L., Chen, G. L., and Xu, Z. Y. (1984) Hemagglutination-inhibiting antibody in hemorrhagic fever with renal syndrome, *J. Infect. Dis.*, **150**, 895–898.

311. Arikawa, J., Takashima, I., and Hashimoto, N. (1985) Cell fusion by hemorrhagic fever with renal syndrome (HFRS) viruses and its application for titration of virus infectivity and neutralizing antibody, *Arch. Virol.*, **86**, 303–313.

312. Okuno, Y., Yamanishi, K., Takahashi, Y., Tanishita, O., Nagai, T., Dantas, J. R., Jr., Okamoto, Y., Tadano, M., and Takahashi, M. (1986) Haemagglutination-inhibition test for hemorrhagic fever with renal syndrome using virus antibody prepared from infected tissue culture fluid, *J. Gen. Virol.*, **67**(Pt. 1), 149–156.

313. Gavrilovskaya, I. N., Brown, E. J., Ginsberg, M. H., and Mackow, E. R. (1999) Cellular entry of hantaviruses which cause hemorrhagic fever with renal syndrome is mediated by β_3 integrins, *J. Virol.*, **73**(5), 3951–3959.

314. Kolakofsky, D. and Hacker, D. (1991) Bunyavirus RNA synthesis: transcription and replication, *Curr. Top. Microbiol. Immunol.*, **169**, 143–159.

315. Peng, G., Hongo, S., Kimura, H., Muraki, Y., Sugawara, K., Kitame, F., Numazaki, Y., Suzuki, H., and Nakamura, K. (1996) Frequent occurence of genetic reassortment between influenza C virus strains in nature, *J. Gen. Virol.*, **77**(Pt. 7), 1489–1492.

316. Li, D., Schmaljohn, A. L., Anderson, K., and Schmaljohn, C. S. (1995) Complete nucleotide sequence of the M and S segments of two hantavirus isolates from California: evidence for reassortment in nature among viruses related to hantavirus pulmonary syndrome, *Virology*, **206**, 973–983.

317. Webster, R. G. and Laver, W. G. (1971) Antigenic variation in influenza virus. Biology and chemistry, *Prog. Med. Virol.*, **13**, 271–338.

318. Beaty, B. J., Sundin, D. R., Chandler, L. J., and Bishop, D. H. (1985) Evolution of bunyaviruses by genome reassortment in dually infected mosquitoes (*Aedes triseriatus*), *Science*, **230**, 548–550.

319. Urquidi, V. and Bishop, D. H. (1992) Non-random reassortment between the tripartite RNA genomes of La Crosse and snowshoe hare viruses, *J. Gen. Virol.*, **73**(Pt. 9), 2255–2265.

320. Sall, A. A., Zanotto, P. M., Sene, O. K., Zeller, H. G., Digoutte, J. P., Thiongane, Y., and Bouloy, M. (1999) Genetic reassortment of Rift Valley fever virus in nature, *J. Virol.*, **73**, 8196–8200.

321. Khaiboullina, S. F., Rizvanov, A. A., Otteson, E., Miyazato, A., Maciejewski, J., and St. Jeor, J. S. (2004) Regulation of cellular gene expression in endothelial cells by Sin Nombre and prospect hill viruses, *Viral Immunol.*, **17**, 234–251.

322. Geimonen, E., Neff, S., Raymond, T., Kocer, S. S., Gavrilovskaya, I. N., and Mackow, E. R. (2002) Pathogenic and nonpathogenic hantaviruses differentially regulate endothelial cell responses, *Proc. Natl. Acad. Sci. U.S.A.*, **99**, 13837–13842.

323. Gavrilovskaia, I. N., Podgorodnichenko, V. K., Apekina, N. S., Gorbachkova, E. A., and Bogdanova, S. B. (1987) Determination of specific immune complexes and dynamics of their circulation in patients with hemorrhagic fever with renal syndrome, *Mikrobiol. Zh.*, **49**, 71–76.

324. Penttinen, K., Lahdevirta, J., Kekomaki, R., Ziola, B., Salmi, A., Hautanen, A., Lindstrom, P., Vaheri, A., Brummer-Korvenkontio, M., and Wager, O. (1981) Circulating immune complexes, immunoconglutinins, and rheumatoid factors in nephropathia epidemica, *J. Infect. Dis.*, **143**(1), 15–21.

325. Jokinen, E. J., Lahdevirta, J., and Collan, Y. (1978) Nephropathia epidemica: immunohistochemical study of pathogenesis, *Clin. Nephrol.*, **9**, 1–5.

326. Lahdevirta, J. (1971) Nephropathia epidemica in Finland. A clinical histological and epidemiological study, *Ann. Clin. Res.*, **3**, 1–54.

327. Ferrer, J. F., Jonsson, C. B., Esteban, E., Galligan, D., Basombrio, M. A., Peralta-Ramos, M., Bharadwaj, M., Torrez-Martinez, N., Callahan, J., Segovia, A., and Hjelle, B. (1998) High prevalence of hantavirus infection in Indian communities of Paraguyan and Argentinean Gran Chaco, *Am. J. Trop. Med. Hyg.*, **59**, 438–444.

328. Lundkvist, A., Horling, J., and Niklasson, B. (1993) The humoral response to Puumala virus infection (nephropathia epidemica) investigated by viral protein specific immunoassays, *Arch. Virol.*, **130**, 121–130.

329. Ulrich, R., Lundkvist, A., Meisel, H., Koletzki, D., Sjolander, K. B., Gelderblom, H. R., Borisova, G., Schnitzler, P., Darai, G., and Kruger, D. H. (1998) Chimaeric HBV core particles carrying a defined segment of Puumala hantavirus nucleocapsid protein evoke protective immunity in an animal model, *Vaccine*, **16**, 272–280.

330. Alexeyev, O. A., Ahlm, C., Billheden, J., Settergren, B., Wadell, G., and Juto, P. (1994) Elevated levels of total and Puumala virus-specific immunoglobulin E in the Scandinavian type of hemorrhagic fever with renal syndrome, *Clin. Diagn. Lab. Immunol.*, **1**, 269–272.

331. Araki, K., Yoshimatsu, K., Lee, B. H., Kariwa, H., Takashima, I., and Arikawa, J. (2003) Hantavirus-specific CD8(+)-T-cell responses in newborn mice persistently infected with Hantaan virus, *J. Virol.*, **77**, 8408–8417.

332. Ennis, F. A., Cruz, J., Spiropoulou, C. F., Waite, D., Peters, C. J., Nichol, S. T., Kariwa, H., and Koster, F. T. (1997) Hantavirus pulmonary syndrome: CD8$^+$ and CD4$^+$ cytotoxic T lymphocytes to epitopes on Sin Nombre virus nucleocapsid protein isolated during acute illness, *Virology*, **238**, 380–390.

333. Kagi, D., Vignaux, F., Ledermann, B., Burki, K., Depraetere, V., Nagata, S., Hengartner, H., and Golstein, P. (1994) Fas and perforin pathways as major mechanisms of T cell-mediated cytotoxicity, *Science*, **265**, 528–530.

334. Ishak, K. G. (1976) Light microscopic morphology of viral hepatitis, *Am. J. Clin. Pathol.*, **65**, 787–827.

335. Lowin, B., Hahne, M., Mattmann, C., and Tschopp, J. (1994) Cytolytic T-cell cytotoxicity is mediated through perforin and Fas lytic pathways, *Nature*, **370**, 650–652.

336. Belz, G. T., Xie, W., and Doherty, P. C. (2001) Diversity of epitope and cytokine profiles for primary and secondary influenza a virus-specific CD8$^+$ T cell responses, *J. Immunol.*, **166**, 4627–4633.

337. Kakimi, K., Lane, T. E., Wieland, S., Asensio, V. C., Campbell, I. L., Chisari, F. V., and Guidotti, L. G. (2001) Blocking CRG2/IP10 and Mig activity in vivo reduces the pathogenetic but not the antiviral potential of hepatitis B virus (HBV)-specific CTLs, *J. Exp. Med.*, **194**, 1755–1766.

338. Zaki, S. R., Greer, P. W., Coffield, L. M., Goldsmith, C. S., Nolte, K. B., Foucar, K., Feddersen, R. M., Zumwalt, R. E., Miller,

G. L., Khan, A. S., et al. (1995) Hantavirus pulmonary syndrome. Pathogenesis of an emerging infectious disease, *Am. J. Pathol.*, **146**, 552–579.

339. Lee, H. W. and Lee, P. W. (1976) Korean hemorrhagic fever. Demonstration of causative antigen and antibodies, *Kor. J. Med.*, **19**, 371–383.

340. Lee, H. W. and Lee, P. W. (1977) Korean hemorrhagic fever. Isolation of the etiologic agent, *J. Kor. Soc. Virol.*, **7**, 1–9.

341. Glass, G. E., Watson, A. J., LeDuc, J. W., and Childs, J. E. (1994) Domestic cases of hemorrhagic fever with renal syndrome in the United States, *Nephron*, **68**, 48–51.

341a. Bugert, J. J., Welzel, T. M., Zeiler, M., and Darai, G. (1999) Hantavirus infection-haemorrhagic fever in the Baikans-potential nephrological hazards in the Kosovo war, *Nephrol. Dial. Transplant.*, **14**, 1843–1844.

341b. Sibold, C., Ulrich, R., Labuda, M., et al. (2001) Dobrava hantavirus causes hemorrhagic fever with renal syndrome in central Europe and carried by two different *Apodemus* mice species, *J. Med. Virol.*, **63** (2), 158–167.

342. Huggins, J. W., Hsiang, C. M., Cosgriff, T. M., et al. (1991) Prospective, double-blind, concurrent, placebo-controlled clinical trial of intravenous ribavirin therapy of hemorrhagic fever with renal syndrome, *J. Infect. Dis.*, **164**, 1119–1127.

343. Lee, H. W. and van der Groen, G. (1989) Hemorrhagic fever with renal syndrome, *Prog. Med. Virol.*, **36**, 62–102.

344. Vaheri, A. (2002) The Fifth International Conference on hemorrhagic fever with renal syndrome, hantavirus pulmonary syndrome, and hantaviruses, *Emerg. Infect. Dis.*, **8**(1), 109.

344a. Hooper, J. W., Custer, D. M., Thompson, E., and Schmaljohn, C. S (2001) DNA vaccination with the Hantaan virus M gene protects hamsters against three of four HFRS hantaviruses and elicits a high-titer neutralizing antibody response in rhesus monkeys, *J. Virol.*, **75** (18), 8469–8477.

345. Lee, H. W., Ahn, C. N., Song, J. W., Baek, L. J., Seo, T. J., and Park, S. C. (1990) Field trial of an inactivated vaccine against hemorrhagic fever with renal syndrome, *Arch. Virol.*, **1** (Suppl 1), 35–47.

346. Yamanishi, K., Tanishita, O., Tamura, M., Asada, H., Kondo, K., et al. (1988) Development of inactivated vaccine against virus causing haemorrhagic fever with renal syndrome, *Vaccine*, **6**, 278–282.

347. Khan, A. S., Spiropoulou, C. S., Morzunov, S., et al. (1995) A fatal illness associated with a new hantavirus in Louisiana, *J. Med. Virol.*, **46**, 281–286.

348. Khan, A. S., Gaviria, M., Rollin, P. E., et al. (1966) Hantavirus pulmonary syndrome in Florida: association with the newly identified Black Creek Canal virus, *Am. J. Med.*, **100**, 46–48.

349. Hjelle, B., Goade, D., Torrez-Martinez, N., et al. (1996) Hantavirus pulmonary syndrome, renal insufficiency, and myositis associated with infection by bayou hantavirus, *Clin. Infect. Dis.*, **23**(3), 495–500.

350. Torrez-Martinez, N., Bharadwaj, M., Goade, D., et al. (1998) Virus-associated hantavirus pulmonary syndrome in eastern Texas: identification of the rice rat, *Orysomys palustris*, as reservoir host, *Emerg. Infect. Dis.*, **4**(1) 105–111.

351. Peters, C. J. and Khan, A. S. (2002) Hantavirus pulmonary syndrome: the new American hemorrhagic fever, *Clin. Infect. Dis.*, **34**, 1224–1231.

352. Wells, R. M., Sosa, E. S., Yadon, Z. E., et al. (1997) An unusual hantavirus outbreak in southern Argentina: person-to-person transmission? *Emerg. Infect. Dis.*, **3**, 171–174.

353. Padula, P. J., Edelstein, A., Miguel, S. D., et al. (1998) Hantavirus pulmonary syndrome outbreak in Argentina: molecular evidence for person-to-person transmission of Andes virus, *Virology*, **241**(2), 323–330.

354. Charrel, R. N. and de Lamballerie, X. (2003) Arenaviruses other than Lassa virus, *Antiviral Res.*, **57**, 89–100.

355. Peters, C. J., Kuehne, R. W., Mercado, R. R., Le Bow, R. H., Spertzel, R. O., and Webb, P. A. (1974) Hemorrhagic fever in Cochabamba, Bolivia, 1971, *Am. J. Epidemiol.*, **99**, 425–433.

356. de Manzione, N., Salas, R. A., Paredes, H., Godoy, O., Rojas, L., Araoz, F., Fulhorst, C. F., Ksiazek, T. G., Mills, J. N., Ellis, B. A., Peters, C. J., and Tesh, R. B. (1998) Venezuelan hemorrhagic fever: clinical and epidemiological studies of 165 cases, *Clin. Infect. Dis.*, **26**, 308–313.

357. Buchmeier, M., Adam, E., and Rawls, W. E. (1974) Serological evidence of infection by Pichinde virus among laboratory workers, *Infect. Immun.*, **9**, 821–823.

358. Peters, C. J., Buchmeier, M., Rollin, P. E., and Ksiazek, T. G. (1996) Arenaviruses. In: *Fields Virology*, 3rd ed. (Fields, B. N., Knipe, D. M., Howley, P. M., Chanock, R. M., Melnick, J. L., Monath, T. P., Roizman, R., and Straus, S. E., eds.), Lippincott-Raven Publishers, Philadelphia, pp. 1521–1551.

359. Peters, C. J., Jahrling, P. B., and Khan, A. S. (1996) Patients infected with high-hazard viruses: scientific basis for infection control, *Arch. Virol.*, **11**, 141–168.

360. Centers for Disease Control (1990) Fatal illnesses associated with a New World arenavirus – California, 1999–2000, *Morb. Mortal. Wkly Rep.*, **49**, 709–711.

361. Cao, W., Henry, M. D., Borrow, P., Yamada, H., Elder, J. H., Ravkov, E. V., Nichol, S. T., Compans, R. W., Campbell, K. P., and Oldstone, M. B. A. (1998) Identification of α-dystroglycan as a receptor for lymphocytic choriomeningitis virus and Lassa virus, *Science*, **282**, 2079–2081.

362. Radoshitzky, S. R., Abraham, J., Spiropoulou, C. F., Kuhn, J. H., Nguyen, D., Li, W., Nagel, J., Schmidt, P. J., Nunberg, J. H., Andrews, N. C., Farzan, M., and Choe, H. (2007) Transferrin receptor 1 is the cellular receptor for New World haemorrhagic fever arenaviruses, *Nature*, **446**, 92–96.

363. Castilla, V. and Mersich, S. E. (1996) Low-pH-induced fusion of Vero cells infected with Junin virus, *Arch. Virol.*, **141**, 1307–1317.

364. Oldstone, M. B. (2002) Arenaviruses. II. The molecular pathogenesis of arenavirus infections. Introduction, *Curr. Top. Microbiol. Immunol.*, **263**, V–XII.

365. Daniels, T. T., Delgado, T., Rodriguez, J. A., Helguera, G., and Penichet, M. L., (2006) The transferring receptor, part I: biology and targeting with cytotoxic antibodies for the treatment of cancer, *Clin. Immunol.*, **121**, 144–158.

366. Soda, R. and Tavassoli, M. (1984) Liver endothelium and not hepatocytes or Kupfer cells have transferring receptors, *Blood*, **63**, 270–276.

367. Jefferies, W. A., Brandon, M. R., Hunt, S. V., Williams, A. F., Gatter, K. G., and Mason, D. Y. (1984) Transferrin receptor on endothelium of brain capillaries, *Nature*, **312**, 162–163.

368. Peters, C. J. and Zaki, S. R. (2002) Role of the endothelium in viral hemorrhagic fever, *Crit. Care Med.*, **30**, 5268–5273.

369. Lawrence, C. M., Ray, S., Babyonyshev, M., Galluser, R., Borhani, D. W., and Harrison, S. C. (1999) Crystal structure of the ectodomain of human transferring factor, *Science*, **286**, 779–782.

370. Cheng, Y., Zak, O., Aisen, P., Harrison, S. C., and Walz, T. (2004) Structure of the human transferring receptor-transferrin complex, *Cell*, **116**, 565–576.

371. Harrison, L. H., Halsey, N. A., McKee, K. T., Jr., Peters, C. J., Barrera Oro, J. G., Briggiler, A. M., Feuillade, M. R., and Maiztegui, J. I. (1999) Clinical case definition for Argentine hemorrhagic fever, *Clin. Infect. Dis.*, **28**, 1091–1094.

372. Vainrub, B. and Salas, R. (1994) Latin American hemorrhagic fever, *Infect. Dis. Clin. North Am.*, **8**, 47–59.

373. Johnson, K. M., Halstead, S. B., and Cohen, S. N. (1967) Hemorrhagic fevers of Southeast Asia and South America: a comparative appraisal, *Prog. Med. Virol.*, **9**, 105–158.

374. Enria, D. A., Brigiller, A. M., Fernandez, N. J., Levis, S. C., and Maiztegui, J. I. (1984) Importance of dose of neutralizing antibodies in treatment of Argentine hemorrhagic fever with immune plasma, *Lancet*, **2**, 255–256.

375. Maizfegui, J. I., Fernandez, N. J., and de Damilano, A. J. (1979) Efficacy of immune plasma in treatment of Argentine haemorrhagic fever and association between treatment and a late neurological syndrome, *Lancet*, **2**, 1216–1217.

376. Streeter, D. G., Witkowski, J. T., Khare, G. P., Sidwell, R. W., Bauer, R. J., Robins, R. K., and Simon, L. N. (1973) Mechanism of action of 1-β-*D*-ribofuranosyl-1,2,4-triazole-3-carboxamide (Virazole), a new broad spectrum antiviral agent, *Proc. Natl. Acad. Sci. U.S.A.*, **70**, 1174–1178.

377. Ericksson, B., Helgestrand, E., Johansson, N. G., Larsson, A., Misiorny, A., Noren, J. O., Philipson, L., Stenberg, G., Stridt, S., and Oberg, B. (1977) Inhibition of influenza virus ribonucleic acid polymerase by ribavirin triphosphate, *Antimicrob. Agents Chemother.*, **11**, 946–951.

378. Johnson, K. M., Ksiazek, T. G., Rollin, P. E., Mills, J. N., Villagra, M. R., Montenegro, M. J., Costales, M. A., Peredes, L. C., and Peters, C. J. (1997) Treatment of Bolivian hemorrhagic fever with intravenous ribavirin, *Clin. Infect. Dis.*, **24**, 718–722.

379. Barry, M., Russi, M., Armstrong, L., Geller, D., Tesh, R., Dembry, L., Gonzalez, J. P., Khan, A. S., and Peters, C. J. (1995) Brief report: treatment of a laboratory-acquired Sabia virus infection, *N. Engl. J. Med.*, **333**, 294–296.

380. Carballal, G., Calello, M. A., Laguens, R. P., and Weissenbacher, M. C. (1987) Tacaribe virus: a new alternative for Argentine hemorrhagic fever vaccine, *J. Med. Virol.*, **23**, 257–263.

381. Carballal, G., Oubina, J. R., Molinas, F. C., Nagle, C., de la Vega, M. T., Videla, C., and Elsner, B. (1987) Intracerebral infection of *Cebus paella* with the XJ-Clone 3 strain of Junin virus, *J. Med. Virol.*, **21**, 257–268.

382. Barrera Oro, J. G. and McKee, K. T., Jr. (1991) Toward a vaccine against Argentine hemorrhagic fever, *Bull. Pan Am. Health Organ.*, **25**, 118–126.

383. McKee, K. T., Jr., Huggins, J. W., Trahan, C. J., and Mahlandt, B. G. (1988) Ribavirin prophylaxis and therapy for experimental Argentine hemorrhagic fever, *Antimicrob. Agents Chemother.*, **32**, 1304–1309.

384. Peters, C. J., Jahrling, P. B., Liu, C. T., Kenyon, R. H., McKee, K. T., Jr., and Barrera Oro, J. G. (1987) Experimental studies of arenaviral hemorrhagic fevers, *Curr. Top. Microbiol Immunol.*, **134**, 5–68.

385. Maiztegui, J. I., McKee, K. T., Jr., Barrera Oro, J. G., Harrison, L. H., Gibbs, P. H., Feuillade, M. R., Enria, D. A., Briggiler, A. M., Levis, S. C., Ambrosio, A. M., Halsey, N. A., and Peters, C. J. (1998) Protective efficacy of a live attenuated vaccine against Argentine hemorrhagic fever. AHF Study Group, *J. Infect. Dis.*, **177**, 277–283.

386. Ambrosio, A. M., Riere, L. M., del Carmen Saavedras, M., and Sabattini, M. S. (2006) Immune response to vaccination against Argentine hemorrhagic fever an area where different arenaviruses coexist, *Viral Immunol.*, **19**(2), 196–201.

387. Sanchez, A., Pifat, D. Y., Kenyon, R. H., Peters, C. J., McCormick, J. B., and Kiley, M. P. (1989) Junin virus monoclonal antibodies: characterization and cross-reactivity with other arenaviruses, *J. Gen. Virol.*, 70, 1125–1132.

388. Kunz, S., Rojek, J. M., Perez, M., Spiropoulou, C. F., and Oldstone, M. B. (2005) Characterization of the interaction of Lassa fever virus with its cellular receptor alpha-dystroglycan, *J. Virol.*, **79**(10), 5979–5987.

389. Fisher, S. A., Graham, M. B., Kuehnert, M. J., Kotton, C. N., Srinivasan, A., Marty, F. M., Comer, J. A., Guarner, J., Paddock, C. D., Demeo, D. L., Shieh, W.-J., Erickson, B. R., Bandy, U., Demaria, A., Davis, J. P., Delmonico, F. L., Pavlin, B., Likos, A., Vincent, M. J., Sealy, T. K., Goldsmith, C. S., Jernigan, D. B., Rollin, P. E., Packard, M. M., Patel, M., Rowland, C., Helfand, R. F., Nichol, S. T., Fishman, J. A., Ksizek, T., Zaki, S. R., and the LCMV in Transplant Recipients Investigation Team (2006) Transmission of lymphocytic choriomeningitis virus by organ transplantation, *N. Engl. J. Med.*, **354**(21), 2235–2249.

390. Barton, L. L. and Hyndman, N. J. (2000) Lymphocytic choriomeningitis virus: reemerging central nervous system pathogen, *Pediatrics*, **105**(3), E35.

391. Childs, J. E., Glass, G. E., Ksiazek, T. G., Rossi, C. A., Barrera Oro, J. G., and LeDuc, J. W. (1991) Human-rodent contact and infection with lymphocytic choriomeningitis and Seoul viruses in an inner-city population, *Am. J. Trop. Med. Hyg.*, **44**, 117–121.

392. Stephensen, C. B., Blount, S. R., Lanford, R. E., Holmes, K. V., Montali, R. J., Fleenor, M. E., and Shaw, J. F. (1992) Prevalence of serum antibodies against lymphocytic choriomeningitis virus in selected populations from two US cities, *J. Med. Virol.*, **38**, 27–31.

392a. Casals, J. (1977) Serologic reactions with arenaviruses, *Medicina (Buenos Aires)*, **37** (suppl. 3), 59–68.

393. Filomatori, C. V., Lodeiro, M. F., Alvarez, D. E., Samsa, M. M., Pietrasanta, L., and Gamarnik, A. V. (2006) A 5′ RNA element promotes dengue virus RNA synthesis on a circular genome, *Genes Dev.*, **20**, 2238–2249.

394. Theiler, M. and Smith, H. H. (1937) Use of yellow fever virus modified by in vitro cultivation for human immunization, *J. Exp. Med.*, **65**, 787–800.

395. World Health Organization (1945) Standards for the manufacture and control of yellow fever vaccine. United Nations Relief and Rehabilitation Administration, *WHO Epidemiological Information Bulletin*, **1**, 365.

396. Monath, T. P., Kinney, R. M., Schlesinger, J. J., Brandriss, M. W., and Brès, P. (1983) Ontogeny of yellow fever 17D vaccine: RNA oligonucleotide fingerprint and monoclonal antibody analyses of vaccines produced worldwide, *J. Gen. Virol.*, **64**, 627–637.

397. Martin, M., Tsai, T. F., Cropp, B., Chang, G. J., Holmes, D. A., Tseng, J., Shieh, W., Zaki, S. R., Al-Sanouri, I., Cutrona, A. F., Ray, G., Weld, L. H., and Cetron, M. S. (2001) Fever and multisystem organ failure associated with 17D-204 yellow fever: a report of four cases, *Lancet*, **358**, 98–104.

398. Chan, R. C., Penney, D. J., Little, D., Carter, I. W., Roberts, J. A., and Rowlinson, W. D. (2001) Hepatitis and death following vaccination with 17D-204 yellow fever vaccine, *Lancet*, **358**, 121–123.

399. Vasconcelos, P. F., Luna, E. J., Galler, R., Silva, L., Coimbra, T., Barros, V., Monath, T., Rodrigues, S., Laval, C., and Costa, Z. (2001) Serious adverse events associated with yellow fever 17D vaccine in Brazil: a report of two cases, *Lancet*, **358**, 91–97.

400. Centers for Disease Control (2002) Adverse events associated with 17-derived yellow fever vaccination – United States, 2001–2002, *Morb. Mortal. Wkly Rep.*, **51**(44), 989–993.

401. Centers for Disease Control (2002) Yellow fever vaccine: recommendation of the Advisory Committee on Immunization Practices (ACIP), *Morb. Mortal. Wkly Rep.*, **51**(RR-17), 51.

402. Sabin, A. B. and Schlesinger, R. W. (1945) Production of immunity to dengue with virus modified by propagation in mice, *Science*, **101**, 640–642.

403. Gubler, D. J. (1998) Dengue and dengue hemorrhagic fever, *Clin. Microbiol. Rev.*, **11**(3), 480–496.

404. Halstead, S. B. (1980) Dengue hemorrhagic fever – public health problem and a field of research, *Bull. World Health Organization.*, **58**, 1–21.

405. Gubler, D. J. (1988) Dengue. In: *Epidemiology of Arthropod-Borne Viral Disease* (Monath, T. P., ed.), CRC Press, Boca Raton, FL, pp. 223–260.

406. Gubler, D. J. (1998) The global pandemic of dengue/dengue hemorrhagic fever: current status and prospect for the future, *Ann. Acad. Med. Singapore*, **27**(2), 227–234.

407. Gubler, D. J. (1997) Dengue and dengue hemorrhagic fever: its history and resurgence as a global public health problem. In: *Dengue and Dengue Hemorrhagic Fever* (Gubler, D. J. and Kuno, G., eds.), CAB International, London, pp. 1–22.

408. Pinheiro, F. P. and Corber, S. J. (1997) Global situation of dengue and dengue hemorrhagic fever, and its emergence in the Americas, *World Health Stat. Q.*, **50**, 161–169.

409. Centers for Disease Control and Prevention (1995) Imported dengue – United States, 1993 and 1994, *Morb. Mortal. Wkly Rep.*, **44**, 353–356.

410. Gubler, D. J. (1996) Arboviruses as imported disease agents: the need for increased awareness, *Arch. Virol.*, **11**, 21–32.

411. Westaway, E. G. and Blok, J. (1997) Taxonomy and evolutionary relationships of flaviviruses. In: *Dengue and Dengue Hemorrhagic Fever* (Gubler, D. J. and Kuno, G., eds.), CAB International, London, pp. 147–173.

412. Rico-Hesse, R. (1990) Molecular evolution and distribution of dengue viruses type 1 and 2 in nature, *Virology*, **174**, 479–493.

413. Gubler, D. J. and Rosen, L. (1976) A simple technique for demonstrating transmission of dengue viruses by mosquitoes without the use of vertebrate hosts, *Am. J. Trop. Med. Hyg.*, **25**, 146–150.

414. Barnes, W. J. S. and Rosen, L. (1974) Fatal hemorrhagic disease and shock associated with primary dengue infection on a Pacific island, *Am. J. Trop. Med. Hyg.*, **23**, 495–506.

415. Halstead, S. B. (1970) Observations related to pathogenesis of dengue hemorrhagic fever. VI. Hypotheses and discussion, *Yale J. Biol. Med.*, **42**, 350–362.

416. Halstead, S. B. (1988) Pathogenesis of dengue: challenged to molecular biology, *Science*, **239**, 476–481.

417. Mongkolsapaya, J., Dejnirattsai, W., Xu, X., Vasanawathana, S., Tangthawornchaikul, N., Chairunsri, A., Sawasdivorn, S., Duangchinda, T., Dong, T., Rowland-Jones, S., Yenchitsomanus, P., McMichael, A., Malasit, P., and Screaton, G. (2003) Original antigenic sin and apoptosis in the pathogenesis of dengue hemorrhagic fever, *Nat. Med.*, **9**, 921–927.

418. Waterman, S. H. and Gubler, D. J. (1989) Dengue fever, *Clin. Dermatol.*, **7**, 117–122.

419. Dietz, V., Gubler, D. J., Ortiz, S., Kuno, G., Casta-Velez, A., Sather, G. E., Gomez, I., and Vergne, E. (1996) The 1986 dengue and dengue hemorrhagic fever epidemic in Puerto Rico: epidemiologic and clinical observation, *P. R. Health Sci. J.*, **15**, 201–210.

420. Innis, B. L. (1995) Dengue and dengue hemorrhagic fever. In: *Exotic Viral Infections – 1995* (Porterfield, J. S., ed.), Chapman & Hall, London, pp. 103–146.

421. Halstead, S. B. and O'Rourke, E. J. (1977) Antibody-enhanced dengue virus infection in primate leukocytes, *Nature*, **265**, 739–741.

422. Halstead, S. B. and O'Rourke, E. J. (1977) Dengue viruses and mononuclear phagocytes. I. Infection enhancement by non-neutralizing antibody, *J. Exp. Med.*, **146**, 210–217.

423. Morens, D. M., Venkateshan, C. N., and Halstead, S. B. (1987) Dengue 4 virus monoclonal antibodies identify epitopes that mediate immune enhancement of dengue 2 viruses, *J. Gen. Virol.*, **68**, 91–98.

424. Gubler, D. J., Reed, D., Rosen, L., and Hitchcock, J. C. J. (1978) Epidemiologic, clinical and virologic observations on dengue in the Kingdom of Tonga, *Am. J. Trop. Med. Hyg.*, **27**, 581–589.

425. Rosen, L. (1977) The Emperor's new clothes revisited, or reflections on the pathogenesis of dengue hemorrhagic fever, *Am. J. Trop. Med. Hyg.*, **26**, 337–343.

426. Pang, T., Cardosa, M. J., and Guzman, M. G. (2007) Of cascade and perfect storms: the immunopathogenesis of dengue haemorrhagic fever-dengue shock syndrome (DHF/DSS), *Immunol. Cell Biol.*, **85**, 43–45.

427. Busygin, F. F. (2000) Omsk hemorrhagic fever – current status of the problem, (in Russian), *Vopr. Virusol.*, **45**(3), 4–9.

428. Gritsun, T. S., Lashkevich, V. A., and Gould, E. A. (1993) Nucleotide and amino acid sequence of the envelope glycoprotein of Omsk haemorrhagic fever virus: comparison with other flaviviruses, *J. Gen. Virol.*, **74**, 287–291.

429. Holzmann, H., Heinz, F. X., Mandl, C. W., Guirakhoo, F., and Kunz, C. (1990) A single amino acid substitution in envelope protein E of tick-borne encephalitis virus leads to attenuation in the mouse model, *J. Virol.*, **64**, 5156–5159.

430. Cecilia, D. and Gould, E. A. (1991) Nucleotide changes responsible for loss of neuroinvasiveness in Japanese encephalitis virus neutralization-resistant mutants, *Virology*, **181**, 70–77.

431. Rice, C. M., Lenches, E. M., Eddy, S. R., Shin, S. J., Sheets, R. L., and Strauss, J. H. (1985) Nucleotide sequence of yellow fever virus: implications for flavivirus gene expression and evolution, *Science*, **229**, 726–733.

432. Work, T. H. and Trapido, H. (1957) Kyasanur Forest disease, a new virus disease in India, *Ind. J. Med. Sci.*, **11**, 341–345.

433. Work, T. H. and Trepido, H. (1957) Kyasanur Forest disease: a new infection of man and monkeys in tropical India by a virus of the Russian spring-summer complex, *Proceedings IXth Pacific Science Congress, Bangkok*, vol. 17, 80–84 (Public Health and Medical Sciences).

434. D'Lima, L. V. and Pavri, K. M. (1969) Studies on antigenicity of six Kyasanur Forest disease virus strains isolated from various sources, *Ind. J. Med. Res.*, **57**, 1832–1839.

435. Danes, L. (1962) Contribution to the antigenic relationship between tick-borne encephalitis and Kyasanur Forest disease viruses. In: *CSAV Symposium on the Biology of Viruses of the Tick-borne Encephalitis Complex* (Libikova, H., ed.), Czechoslovak Academy of Sciences, Prague, p. 81.

436. Shah, K. V. and Buescher, E. (1962) Discussion. In: *CSAV Symposium on the Biology of Viruses of the Tick-Borne Encephalitis Complex* (Libikova, H., ed.), Czechoslovak Academy of Sciences, Prague, p. 85.

437. Venugopal, K., Gritsun, T., Lashkevich, V. A., and Gould, E. A. (1994) Analysis of the structural protein gene sequence shows Kyasanur Forest disease virus as a distinct member in the tick-borne encephalitis virus serocomplex, *J. Gen. Virol.*, **75**, 227–232.

438. Adhikari Prabha, M. R., Prabhu, M. G., Raghuveer, C. V., Bai, M., and Mala, M. A. (1993) Clinical study of 100 cases of Kyasanur Forest disease with clinico-pathological correlation, *Ind. J. Med. Sci.*, **47**(5), 124–130.

439. Millard, C. B. (2004) Medical defense against protein toxin weapons. In: *Biological Weapons Defense: Infectious Diseases and Counterterrorism* (Lindler, L. E., Lebeda, F. J., and Korch, G. W., eds.), Humana Press, Totowa, NJ, pp. 255–283.

440. Franz, D. R. (1997) Defense against toxin weapons. In: *Medical Aspects of Chemical and Biological Warfare* (Sidell, F. R., Takafuji, E. T., and Franz, D. R., eds.), Office of the Surgeon General, Department of the Army, Washington, DC, pp. 603–620.

441. Simpson, L. L. (1981) The origin, structure, and pharmacological activity of botulinum toxin, *Pharmacol. Rev.*, **33**(3), 155–188.

442. Hathaway, C. L. (1990) Toxigenic clostridia, *Clin. Microbiol. Rev.*, **3**(1), 66–98.

443. Umland, T. C., Wingert, L. M., Swaminathan, S., Furey, W. F., Schmidt, J. J., and Sax, M. (1997) Structure of receptor binding fragment HC of tetanus neurotoxin, *Nat. Struct. Biol.*, **4**(10), 788–792.

444. Lacy, D. B., Tepp, W., Cohen, A. C., DasGupta, B. R., and Stevens, R. C. (1988) Crystal structure of botulinum neurotoxin type A and implications for toxicity, *Nat. Struct. Biol.*, **5**(10), 898–902.

445. Lacy, D. B. and Stevens, R. C. (1999) Sequence homology and structural analysis of the clostridial neurotoxins, *J. Mol. Biol.*, **291**(5), 1091–1104.

446. Eswaramoorthy, S., Kumaran, D., and Swaminathan, S. (2001) Crystallographic evidence for doxorubicin binding to the receptor-binding site of *Clostridium botulinum* neurotoxin B, *Acta Crystallogr. D Biol. Crystallogr.*, **57**(Part 11), 1743–1746.

447. Hanson, P. I., Heuser, J. E., and Jahn, R. (1997) Neurotransmitter release – four years of SNARE complexes, *Curr. Opin. Neurobiol.*, **7**(3), 310–315.

448. Rizo, J. (2003) SNARE function revisited, *Nat. Struct. Biol.*, **10**(6), 417–419.

449. Shapiro, R. L., Hathway, C., and Swerdlow, D. L. (1998) Botulism in the United States: a clinical and epidemiological review, *Ann. Intern. Med.*, **129**(3), 221–228.

450. Arnon, S. S., Schechter, R., Inglesby, T. V., Henderson, D. A., Bartlett, J. G., Ascher, M. S., Aitzen, E., Fine, A. D., Hauer, J., Layton, M., Lillybridge, S., Osterholm, M., T., O'Toole, T., Parker, G., Perl, T. M., Russell, P. K., Swerdlow, D. L., Tonat, K., for the Working Group on Civilian Biodefense (2001) Botulinum toxin as a biological weapon. Medical and public health management, *J. Am. Med. Assoc.*, **8**(8), 1059–1070.

451. Simpson, L. L. (1984) Fragment C of tetanus toxin antagonizes the neuromuscular blocking properties of native tetanus toxin, *J. Pharmacol. Exp. Ther.*, **228**(3), 600–604.

452. Simpson, L. L. (1984) Botulinum toxin and tetanus toxin recognize similar membrane determinants, *Brain Res.*, **305**(1), 177–180.

453. Dertzbaugh, M. T. and West, M. W. (1996) Mapping of protective and cross-reactive domains of the type A neurotoxin of *Clostridium botulinum, Vaccine*, **14**(16), 1538–1544.

454. Middlebrook, J. L. (1995) Protection strategies against botulinum toxin, *Adv. Exp. Med. Biol.*, **383**, 93–98.

455. Potter, K. L., Bevins, M. A., Vassilieva, E. V., Chiruvolu, V. R., Smith, T., Smith, L. A., and Meagher, M. M. (1998) Production and purification of the heavy-chain fragment C of the botulinum neurotoxin, serotype B, expressed in the methylotrophic yeast *Pichia pastoris, Protein Expr. Purif.*, **13**(3), 357–365.

456. Byrne, M. P., Smith, T. J., Montgomery, V. A., and Smith, L. A. (1998) Purification, potency, and efficacy of the botulinum neurotoxin type A binding domain from *Pichia pastoris* as a recombinant vaccine candidate, *Infect. Immun.*, **66**(10), 4817–4822.

457. Byrne, M. P., Titball, R. W., Holey, J., and Smith, L. A. (2000) Fermentation, purification, and efficacy of a recombinant vaccine candidate against botulinum neurotoxin type B from *Pichia pastoris, Protein Expr. Purif.*, **18**(3), 327–337.

458. Potter, K. J., Zhang, W., Smith, L. A., and Meagher, M. M. (2000) Production and purification of the heavy chain fragment C of botulinum neurotoxin, serotype A, expressed in the methylotrophic yeast *Pichia pastoris, Protein Expr. Purif.*, **19**(3), 393–402.

459. Woodward, L. A., Arimitsu, H., Hirst, R., and Oguma, K. (2003) Expression of H_C subunits from *Clostridium botulinum* types C and D and their evaluation as candidate vaccine antigens in mice, *Infect. Immun.*, **71**(5), 2941–2944.

460. Lee, J. S., Pushko, P., Parker, M. D., Dertzbaugh, M. T., Smith, L. A., and Smith, J. F. (2001) Candidate vaccine against botulinum neurotoxin serotype A derived from a Venezuelan equine encephalitis virus vector system, *Infect. Immun.*, **69**(9), 5709–5715.

461. Park, J. B. and Simpson, L. L. (2003) Inhalational poisoning by botulinum toxin and inhalation vaccination with its heavy-chain component, *Infect. Immun.*, **71**(3), 1147–1154.

462. Bennett, A. M., Perkins, S. D., and Holley, J. L. (2003) DNA vaccination protects against botulinum neurotoxin type F, *Vaccine*, **21**(23), 3110–3117.

463. Foynes, S., Holley, J. L., Garmory, H. S., Titball, R. W., and Fairweather, N. F. (2003) Vaccination against type F botulinum toxin using attenuated *Salmonella enterica* var Typhimurium strains expressing the BoTN/F H(c) fragment, *Vaccine*, **21**(11–12), 1052–1059.

464. Kiyatkin, N., Maksymowych, A. B., and Simpson, L. L. (1997) Induction of an immune response by oral administration of recombinant botulinum toxin, *Infect. Immun.*, **65**(11), 4586–4591.

465. Simpson, L. L., Maksymowych, A. B., and Kiyatkin, N. (1999) Botulinum toxin as a carrier for oral vaccine, *Cell Mol. Life Sci.*, **56**(1–2), 47–61.

466. Arnon, S. S., Schechter, R., Inglesby, T. V., Henderson, D. A., Bartlett, J. G., Ascher, M. S., Aitzen, E., Fine, A. D., Hauer, J., Layton, M., Lillybridge, S., Osterholm, M. T., O'Toole, T., Parker, G., Perl, T. M., Russell, P. K., Swerdlow, D. L., Tonat, K., for the Working Group on Civilian Biodefense (2001) Botulinum toxin as a biological weapon. Medical and public health management, *J. Am. Med. Assoc.*, **8**(8), 1059–1070.

467. Ulrich, R. G., Bavari, S., and Olson, M. A. (1995) Bacterial superantigens in human disease: structure, function and diversity, *Trends Microbiol.*, **3**(12), 463–468.

468. Swaminathan, S., Yang, D. S., Furey, W., Abrams, L., Pletcher, J., and Sax, M. (1988) Crystallization and preliminary X-ray study of staphylococcal enterotoxin B, *J. Mol. Biol.*, **199**(2), 397.

469. Swaminathan, S., Furey, W., Pletcher, J., and Sax, M. (1992) Crystal structure of staphylococcal enterotoxin B, a superantigen, *Nature*, **359**(6398), 801–806.

470. Swaminathan, S., Furey, W., Pletcher, J., and Sax, M. (1995) Residues defining the V beta specificity in staphylococcal enterotoxins, *Nat. Struct. Biol.*, **2**(8), 680–686.

471. Schantz, E. J., Roessler, W. G., Wagman, J., Spero, L., Dunnery, D. A., and Bergdoll, M. S. (1965) Purification of staphylococcal enterotoxin B, *Biochemistry*, **4**, 1011–1016.

472. Ulrich, R. G., Olson, M. A., and Bavari, S. (1998) Development of engineered vaccines effective against structurally related bacterial superantigens, *Vaccine*, **16**(19), 1857–1864.

473. Ulrich, R. G., Bavari, S., and Olson, M. A. (1995) Staphylococcal enterotoxins A and B share a common structural motif for binding class II major histocompatibility complex molecules, *Nat. Struct. Biol.*, **2**(7), 554–560.

474. Leder, L., Llera, A., Lavoie, P. M., Lebedeva, M. I., Li, H., Sékaly, R.-P., Bohach, G. A., Gahr, P. J., Schlievert, P. M., Kajalainen, K., and Mariuzza, R. A. (1998) A mutational analysis of the binding of staphylococcal enterotoxins B and C3 to the T cell receptor beta chain and major histocompatibility complex class II, *J. Exp. Med.*, **187**(6) 823–833.

475. LeClaire, R. D. and Pitt, M. L. M. (2004) Biological weapons defense. In: *Biological Weapons Defense: Infectious Diseases and Counterterrorism* (Lindler, L. E., Lebeda, F. J., and Korch, G. W., eds.), Humana Press, Totowa, NJ, pp. 41–61.

476. Rood, J. I., McClane, B. A., Songer, J. G., and Titball, R. W. (1997) *The Clostridia Molecular Biology and Pathogenesis of the Clostridia*, Academic Press, London.

477. Baldwin, L., Henderson, A., Wright, M., and Whitby, M. (1993) Spontaneous *Clostridium perfringens* lung abscess unresponsive to penicillin, *Anaesth. Intensive Care*, **21**, 117–119.

478. Kwan, W. C., Lam, S. C., Chow, A. W., Lepawski, M., and Glanzberg, M. M. (1983) Empiema caused by *Clostridium perfringens, Can. Med. Assoc. J.*, **128**, 1420–1422.

479. Crompton, R. and Gall, D. (1980) Georgi Markov – death in a pellet, *Med. Leg.*, **48**(2), 51–62.

480. Franz, D. R. and Jaax, N. K. (1997) Ricin toxin. In: *Medical Aspects of Chemical and Biological Warfare* (Sidell, F. R., Takafuji, E. T., and Franz, D. R., eds.), Office of the Surgeon General, Department of the Army, Washington, DC, pp. 631–642.

481. Stillmark, R.: Ueber Ricen. Arbeiten des Pharmakologischen Institutes zu Dorpat, iii, 1889. Cited in: Flexner, J. (1897) The histological changes produced by ricin and abrin intoxications, *J. Exp. Med.*, **2**, 197–316.

482. Ucken, F. and Frankel, A. (1993) The current status of immunotoxins: an overview of experimental and clinical studies as presented at the 3rd International Symposium on Immunotoxins, *Leukemia*, **7**, 341–348.

483. Vitetta, E., Thorpe, P., and Uhr, J. (1993) Immunotoxins: magic bullets or misguided missiles? *Trends Pharmacol Sci.*, **14**(5), 148–154.

484. Vitetta, E., Krolick, K., Muneo, M., Cushley, W., and Uhr, J. (1983) Immunotoxins: a new approach to cancer therapy, *Science*, **219**, 644–649.

485. Thorpe, P. E., Mason, D. W., and Brown, A. N. (1982) Selective killing of malignant cells in leukemic rat bone marrow using an antibody-ricin conjugate, *Nature*, **297**, 594–596.

486. Knight, B. (1979) Ricin – a potent homicidal poison, *Br. Med. J.*, **278**, 350–351.

487. Rutenber, E., Katzin, B. J., Ernest, S., Collins, E. J., Mlsna, D., Ready, M. P., and Robertus, J. D. (1991) The crystallographic refinement of ricin at 2.5Å resolution, *Proteins*, **10**, 240–250.

488. Audi, J., Belson, M., Patel, M., Schier, J., and Osterloh, J. (2005) Ricin poisoning. A comprehensive review, *J. Am. Med. Assoc.*, **294**, 2342–2351.

489. Cope, A. C. (1946) Chapter 12: Ricin in Summary Technical Report of Division 9 on chemical warfare and related problems. Parts I–II. National Defense Research Committee, Office of Scientific Research and Development, Washington, DC, pp. 179–203.

490. Griffiths, G. D., Rice, P., Allenby, A. C., and Upshall, D. G. (1996) The inhalation toxicology of the castor bean toxin, ricin, and protection by vaccination, *J. Defense Sci.*, **1**(2), 227–235.

491. Griffiths, G. D., Phillips, G. J., and Bailey, S. C. (1999) Comparison of the quality of protection elicited by toxoid and peptide liposomal vaccine formulations against ricin as assessed by markers of inflammation, *Vaccine*, **17**(20–21), 2562–2568.

492. Smallshaw, J. E., Firan, A., Fulmer, J. R., Ruback, S. L., Ghettie, V., and Vitetta, E. S. (2002) A novel recombinant vaccine which protects mice against ricin intoxication, *Vaccine*, **20**, 3422–3427.

493. Soler-Rodriguez, A. M., Uhr, J. W., Richardson, J., and Vitetta, E. S. (1992) The toxicity of chemically deglycosylated ricin A-chain in mice, *Int. J. Immunopharmacol.*, **14**(2), 281–291.

494. Lord, J. M., Gould, J., Griffiths, D., O'Hare, M., Prior, B., Richardson, P. T., and Robertson, L. M. (1987) Ricin: cytotoxicity, biosynthesis and use in immunoconjugates, *Prog. Med. Chem.*, **24**, 1–28.

495. Lemley, P. V. and Creasia, D. A. (1995) Vaccine against ricin toxin, *U.S. Patent 5453271*.

496. Aboud-Pirak, E., et al. (1993) Identification of a neutralizing epitope on ricin A chain and application of its 3D structure to design peptide vaccines that protect against ricin intoxication. In: *1993 Medical Defense Bioscience Review*, U.S. Army Medical Research & Materiel Command, Baltimore, Maryland. Cited in: Olson, M. A., Carra, J. H., Roxas-Duncan, V., Wannemacher, R. W., Smith, L. A., and Millard, C. B. (2004) Finding a new vaccine in the ricin protein fold, *Protein Eng. Des. Sel.*, **17**(4), 391–397.

497. Griffiths, G. D., Bailey, S. C., Hambrook, J. L., and Keyte, M. P. (1998) Local and systemic responses against ricin toxin promoted by toxoid or peptide vaccines alone or in liposomal formulations, *Vaccine*, **16**(5), 530–535.

498. Olson, M. A. (1997) Ricin A-chain structural determinant for binding substrate analogues: a molecular dynamics simulation analysis, *Proteins*, **27**(1), 80–95.

499. Olson, M. A. and Cuff, L. (1999) Free energy determinants of binding the rRNA substrate and small ligands to ricin A-chain, *Byophys. J.*, **76**(1 Part 1), 28–39.

500. Olson, M. A. (2001) Electrostatic effects on the free-energy balance in folding a ribosome-inactivating protein, *Biophys. Chem.*, **91**(3), 219–229.

501. Sharon, N. and Lis, H. Z (1972) Cell-agglutinating and sugar-specific proteins, *Science*, **177**, 949–959.

502. Olsnes, S. and Pihl, A. (1976) Kinetics of binding of the toxic lectins abrin and ricin to surface receptors of human cells, *J. Biol. Chem.*, **251**, 3977–3984.

503. Chen, Y. L., Chow, L. P., Tsugita, A., and Lin, J. Y. (1992) The complete primary structure of abrin-a B chain, *FEBS J.*, **309**, 115–118.

504. Kimura, M., Sumizawa, T., and Funatsu, G. (1993) The complete amino acid sequences of the B-chains of abrin-a and abrin-b, toxic proteins from the seeds of *Abrus precatorius, Biosci. Biotechnol. Biochem.*, **57**, 166–169.

505. LeClaire, R. D. and Pitt, M. L. M. (2004) Biological weapons defense. In: *Biological Weapons Defense: Infectious Diseases and Counterterrorism* (Lindler, L. E., Lebeda, F. J., and Korch, G. W., eds.), Humana Press, Totowa, NJ, pp. 41–61.

506. Wannamacher, R. W. and Wiener, S. L. (1997) Trichothecene mycotoxins. In: *Textbook of Military Medicine: Medical Aspects of Chemical and Biological Warfare* (Zatjchuk, R., ed.), Borden Institute, Washington, DC, p. 658.

507. Rood, J. I., McClane, B. A., Songer, J. G., and Titball, R. W. (1997) *The Clostridia. Molecular Biology and Pathogenesis of the Clostridia*, Academic Press, London.

508. Peters, C. J. and Dalrymple, J. M. (1990) Alphaviruses. In: *Fields Virology*, 2nd ed. (Fields, B. N., Knipe, D. M., Chanock, R. M., Hirsch, M. S., Melnick, J. L., Monath, T. P., and Roizman, B., eds.), Raven Press, New York, pp. 713–761.

509. Pialoux, G., Gaüzère, B. A., Jauréguiberry, S., and Strobel, M. (2007) Chikungunya, an epidemic arvovirosis, *Lancet Infect. Dis.*, **7**(5), 319–327.

510. Khan, A. H., Morita, K., del Carmen Parquet, M., Hasabe, F., Mathenge, E. G. M., and Igarashi, A. (2002) Complete nucleotide sequence of chikungunya virus and evidence for an internal polyadenylation site, *J. Gen. Virol.*, **83**, 3075–3084.

511. Schuffenecker, I., Iteman, I., Michault, A., Murri, S., Vaney, M.-C., Lavenir, R., Pardigon, N., Reynes, J.-M., Pettinelli, F., Biscornet, L., Diancourt, L., Michel, S., Duquerroy, S., Guidon, G., Frenkiel, M.-P., Bréhin, A.-C., Cubito, N., Desprès, Kunst, F., Rey, F. A., Zeller, H., and Brisse, S. (2006) Genome microevolution of chikungunya viruses causing the Indian Ocean outbreak, *PLoS Med.*, **3**(7), e263.

512. Charrel, R. N., de Lamballerie, X., and Raoult, D. (2007) Chikungunya outbreaks – the globalization of vector-borne diseases, *N. Engl. J. Med.*, **356**, 769–771.

513. Brisse, S., Iteman, I., and Schuffenecker, I. (2007) Chikungunya outbreaks, *N. Engl. J. Med.*, **356**(25), 2650–2652.

514. Simon, F., Parola, P., Grandadam, M., Fourcade, S., Oliver, M., Brouqui, P., Hance, P., Kraemer, P., Mohamed, A. A., de Lamballerie, X., Charrel, R., and Tolou, H. (2007) Chikungunya infection: an emerging rheumatism among travelers returned from Indian Ocean islands. Report of 47 cases, *Medicine (Baltimore)*, **86**(3), 123–137.

515. Mavalankar, D., Shastri, P., and Raman, P. (2007) Chikungunya epidemic in India: a major public-health disaster, *Lancet Infect. Dis.*, **7**(5), 306–307.

516. Saxena, S. K., Singh, M., Mishra, N., and Lakshmi, V. (2006) Resurgence of chikungunya virus in India: an emerging threat, *Euro Surveill.*, **11**(8), E060810.2.

517. Higgs, S. (2006) The 2005–2006 chikungunya epidemic in the Indian ocean, *Vector Borne Zoonotic Dis.*, **6**, 115–116.

518. Josseran, L., Paquet, C., Zehgnoun, A., Caillere, N., Le Tertre, A., Solet, J.-L., and Ledrance, M. (2006) Chikungunya disease outbreak, Reunion Island, *Emerg. Infect. Dis.*, **12**, 1994–1995.

519. Yergolkar, P. N., Tandale, B. V., Arankalle, V. A., Sathe, P. S., Sudeep, A. B., Gandhe, S. S., Gokhle, M. D., Jacob, G. P., Hundekar, S. L., and Mishra, A. C. (2006) Chikungunya outbreaks caused by African genotype, India, *Emerg. Infect. Dis.*, **12**, 1580–1583.

520. Powers, A. M., Brault, A. C., Tesh, R. B., and Weaver, S. C. (2000) Re-emergence of chikungunya and o'nyong-nyong viruses: evidence for distinct geographical lineages and distinct evolutionary relationships, *J. Gen. Virol.*, **81**, 177–191.

521. Haddow, A. J., Davies, C. W., and Walker, A. J. (1960) O'nyong-nyong fever: an epidemic virus disease in East Africa, *Trans. R. Soc. Trop. Med. Hyg.*, **54**, 517–522.

522. Shore, H. (1961) O'nyong-nyong fever: an epidemic virus disease in East Africa. III. Some clinical and epidemiological observations in the northern province of Uganda, *Trans. R. Soc. Trop. Med. Hyg.*, **55**, 361–373.

523. Johnson, B. K., Gichogo, A., Gitau, G., Patel, N., Ademba, G., and Kurui, R. (1981) Recovery of O'nyong-nyong virus from *Anopheles funestis* in western Kenya, *Trans. R. Soc. Trop. Med.*, **75**, 239–241.

524. Yang, G., Pevear, D. C., Davies, M. H., Collett, M. S., Bailey, T., Rippen, S., Barone, L., Burns, C., Rhodes, G., Tohan, S., Huggins, J. W., Baker, R. O., Buller, R. L., Touchette, E., Waller, K., Schriewer, J., Neyts, J., DeClercq, E., Jones, K., Hruby, D., and Jordan, R. (2005) An orally bioavailable antipoxvirus compound (ST-246) inhibits extracellular virus formation and protects mice from lethal orthopoxvirus challenge, *J. Virol.*, **79**(20), 13139–13149.

525. Prichard, M. N., Keith, K. A., Quenelle, D. C., and Kern, E. R. (2006) Activity and mechanism of action of *N*-methanocarbathymidine agains herpesvirus and orthopoxvirus infection, *Antimicrob Agents Chemother.*, **50**(4), 1336–1341.

526. Kuhn, J. H., Radoshitzky, S. R., Guth, A. C., Warfield, K. L., Li, W., Vincent, M. J., Towner, J. S., Nichol, S. T., Bavari, S., Choe, H., Aman, M. J., and Farzan, M. (2006) Conserved receptor-binding domains of Lake Victoria Margburg virus and Zaire Ebola virus bind a common receptor, *J. Biol. Chem.*, **281**(23), 15951–15958.

527. Dong, M., Yeh, F., Tepp, W. T., Dean, C., Johnson, E. A., Janz, R., and Chapman E. R. (2006) SV2 is the protein receptor for botulinum neurotoxin A, *Science*, **312**(5773), 595–596.

528. Bolken, T. C., Laquerre, S., Zhang, Y., Bailey, T. R., Pevear, D. C., Kickner, S. S., Sperzel, L. E., Jones, K. F., Warren, T. K., Lund, S. A., Kirkwood-Watts, D. L., King, D. S., Shurtleff, A. C., Guttiere, M. C., Deng, Y., Bleam, M., and Hruby, D. E. (2006) Identification and characterization of potent small molecule inhibitor of hemorrhagic fever, New World arenaviruses, *Antiviral Res.*, **69**(2), 86–97.

529. Puig-Basagoiti, F., Deas, T. S., Ren, P., Tilgner, M., Ferguson, D. M., and Shi, P.-Y. (2005) High-throughput assays using a luciferase-expressing replicon, virus-like particles, and full-length virus for West Nile discovery, *Antimicrob. Agents Chemother.*, **49**, 4980–4988.

530. Puig-Basagoiti, F., Tilgner, M., Forshey, B. M., Philpott, S. M., Espina, N. G., Wentworth, D. E., Goebel, S. J., Masters, P. S., Falgout, B., Ren, P., Ferguson, D. M., and Shi, P.-Y. (2006) Triaryl pyrazoline compound inhibits flavivirus RNA replication, *Antimicrob. Agents Chemother.*, **50**, 1320–1329.

531. Goodell, J. R., Puig-Basagoiti, F., Forshey, B. M., Shi, P.-Y., and Ferguson, D. M. (2006) Identification of compounds with anti-West Nile virus activity, *J. Med. Chem.*, **49**, 2127–2137.

532. Gu, B., Ouzunov, S., Wang, L., Mason, P., Bourne, N., Cuconati, A., and Block, T. M. (2006) Discovery of small molecule inhibitors of West Nile virus using a high-throughput sub-genomic replicon screen, *Antiviral Res.*, **70**(2), 39–50.

533. Li, G., Chen, N., Feng, Z., Buller, R. M. L., Osborn, J., Harms, T., Damon, I., Upton, C., and Esteban, D. J. (2006) Genomic sequence and analysis of a vaccinia virus isolate from a patient with a smallpox vaccine-related complication, *Virol. J.*, **3**, 88–97.

534. Artenstein, A. W., Johnson, C., Marbury, T. C., Morrison, D., Blum, P. S., Kemp, T., Nichols, R., Balser, J. P., Currie, M., and Monath, T. P. (2005) A novel, cell culture-derived smallpox vaccine in vaccinia-naïve adults, *Vaccine*, **23**(25), 3301–3309.

535. Vollmar, J., Arndtz, N., Eckl, K. M., Thomsen, T., Petzold, B., Mateo, L., Schlereth, B., Handley, A., King, L., Hulsemann, V., Tzatzaris, M., Merkl, K., Wulff, N., and Chaplin, P. (2006) Safety and immugenicity of IMVAMUNE, a promising candidate as a third generation smallpox vaccine, *Vaccine*, **24**(12), 2065–2070.

536. Stittelaar, K. J., van Amerongen, G., Kondova, I., Kuiken, T., van Lavieren, R. F., Pistoor, F. H. M., Niesters, H. G. M., van Doornum, G., van der Zeijst, B. A. M., Mateo, L., Chaplin, P. J., and Osterhaus, A. D. M. E. (2005) Modified vaccinia virus Ankara protects macaques against respiratory challenge with monkeypox virus, *J. Virol.*, **79**(12), 7845–7851.

537. Deziel, M. R., Heine, H., Louie, A., Kao, M., Byrne, W. R., Basset, J., Miller, L., Bush, K., Kelly, M., and Drusano, G. L., (2005) Effective antimicrobial regimens for use in humans for therapy of *Bacillus anthracis* infections and postexposure prophylaxis, *Antimicrob. Agents Chemother.*, **49**(12), 5099–5106.

538. Crane, J. K., Choudhari, S. S., Naeher, T. M., and Duffey, M. E. (2006) Mutual enhancement of virulence by enterotoxigenic and enteropathogenic *Escherichia coli, Infect. Immun.*, **74**(3), 1505–1515.

539. Lu, X., Wang, M., Qi, J., Wang, H., Li, X., Gupta, D., and Dziarski, D. (2006) Peptidoglycan recognition proteins are a new class of human bactericidal proteins, *J. Biol. Chem.*, **281**(9), 5895–5907.

540. Tabeta, K., Hoebe, K., Janssen, E. M., Du, X., Georgel, P., Crozat, K., Mudd, S., Mann, N., Sovath, S., Goode, J., Shamel, L., Herskovits, A. A., Portnoy, D. A., Cooke, M., Tarantino, L. M., Wiltshire, T., Steinberg, B. E., Grinstein, S., and Beutler, B. (2006) The Unc93b1 mutation 3d disrupts exogenous antigen presentation and signaling via Toll-like receptors 3, 7, and 9, *Nat. Immunol.*, **7**, 156–164.

541. Gilchrist, M., Thorsson, V., Li, B., Rust, A. G., Korb, M., Kennedy, K., Hai, T., Bolouri, H., and Aderem, A. (2006) Systems biology approaches identify ATF3 as a negative regulator of Toll-like receptor 4, *Nature*, **441**,173–178.

542. Howell, M. D., Gallo, R. L., Boguniewicz, M., Jones, J. F., Wong, C., Streib, J. E., and Leung, D. Y. (2006) Cytokine milieu of atopic dermatitis skin subverts the innate immune response to vaccinia virus, *Immunity*, **24**, 341–348.

543. Sullivan, N. J., Geisbert, T. W., Geisbert, J. B., Shedlock, D. J., Xu, L., Lamoreaux, L., Custers, J. H., Popernack, P. M., Yang, Z. Y., Pau, M. G., Roederer, M., Koup, R. A., Goudsmit, J., Jahrling, P. B., and Nabel, G. J. (2006) Immune protection of nonhuman primates against Ebola virus with single low-dose adenovirus vectors encoding modified GPs, *PLoS Med.*, **3**(6), e177.

544. Epstein, S. L., Kong, W. P., Misplon, J. A., Lo, C. Y., Tumpey, T. M., Xu, L., and Nabel, G. J. (2005) Protection against multiple influenza a subtypes by vaccination with highly conserved nucleoprotein, *Vaccine*, **23**(46–47), 5404–5410.

Chapter 24

Antimicrobial Resistance and Health Care–Acquired Infections

Since the time antibiotics and other antimicrobial drugs first became widely used in the World War II era, they have saved countless lives and blunted serious complications of many feared diseases and infections. The success of antimicrobials against disease-causing microbes is among modern medicine's great achievements. After more than 50 years of widespread use, however, many antimicrobials are not as effective as they used to be (http://www.niaid.nih.gov/factsheets/antimicro.htm).

Over time, some bacteria have developed ways to circumvent the effects of antibiotics. Widespread use of antibiotics is thought to have spurred evolutionary adaptations that enable bacteria to survive these powerful drugs. Other pathogens, such as viruses, fungi, and parasites, have developed resistance as well. Antimicrobial resistance provides a survival benefit to pathogens and makes it harder to eliminate infections from the body. Ultimately, the increasing difficulty in fighting off pathogens leads to an increased risk of acquiring infections in a hospital or other setting (http://www3.niaid.nih.gov/topics/AntimicrobialResistance/basics/antibiotic.htm).

Diseases such as tuberculosis, gonorrhea, malaria, and childhood ear infections are now more difficult to treat than they were just a few decades ago. Drug resistance is an especially difficult problem for hospitals harboring critically ill patients, who are less able to fight off infections without the help of antibiotics. And heavy use of antibiotics in these patients selects for changes in bacteria that bring about drug resistance. Unfortunately, this worsens the problem by producing bacteria with greater ability to survive even in the presence of our strongest antibiotics. These even stronger drug-resistant bacteria continue to prey on vulnerable hospital patients.

To help curb this problem, the Centers for Disease Control and Prevention (CDC) has provided U.S. hospitals with prevention strategies and educational materials to reduce antibiotic resistance in health care settings (http://www.niaid.nih.gov/factsheets/antimicro.htm). According to CDC statistics:

- Nearly 2 million patients in the United States get an infection in the hospital each year.
- About 90,000 of those patients die each year as a result of their infections, up from 13,300 patient deaths in 1992.
- More than 70% of the bacteria that cause hospital-acquired infections are resistant to at least one of the antibiotics most commonly used to treat them.
- People infected with antibiotic-resistant organisms are more likely to have longer hospital stays and require treatment with second- or third-choice medicines that may be less effective, more toxic, and more expensive.

The burden of health care–associated infections has increased during the past decade due to the increase in immunocompromised patients in hospitals, the development of more delicate life-support treatments, advanced surgical operations, increasing numbers of elderly patients, more complex hospital environments, and failures in infection control measures. In addition, antibiotic resistance has emerged in virtually all health care–associated (*nosocomial*) pathogens. The most common nosocomial infections currently occurring in the United States are those caused by coagulase-negative staphylococci (CNS), *Staphylococcus aureus*, *Enterococcus*, and *Candida*. Gram-positive bacteria account for more than 60% of the total.

Because of the emergence and spread of antimicrobial resistance, several bacterial infections, such as methicillin-resistant *Staphylococcus aureus* (MRSA), vancomycin-resistant *Staphylococcus aureus* (VRSA), vancomycin-resistant *Enterococcus* (VRE), multidrug-resistant *Mycobacterium tuberculosis*, and penicillin-resistant *Streptococcus pneumoniae* (PRSP), are difficult to treat and have negative clinical outcomes and increased treatment costs.

After the introduction of penicillin in 1944 to treat *S. aureus* infections, resistance to the drug evolved rapidly in the 1950s. The next drug developed to treat these infections was methicillin, with MRSA emerging and becoming endemic in hospitals in the 1980s. This trend led to the

V. St. Georgiev, *National Institute of Allergy and Infectious Diseases, NIH: Impact on Global Health*, vol. 2, DOI 10.1007/978-1-60327-297-1_24, © Humana Press, a part of Springer Science+Business Media, LLC 2009

increasing use of vancomycin. In 1996, the first reported case of a S. aureus infection partially resistant to vancomycin was reported in Japan, with subsequent occurrences reported around the world (1). The first clinical infection with a VRSA in the United States was reported in Michigan in July 2002, when, in a clinical setting, a genetic element carrying vancomycin resistance appears to have transferred from VRE to MRSA in a patient with co-infections with each organism at a single site (2). Later that year, the second documented clinical VRSA case occurred in a patient in Pennsylvania (3). A third case of VRSA was reported in New York in 2004 (4), and three additional cases have been reported in Michigan. Each of these events is believed to be the result of natural exchange of genetic material among bacteria; hence, additional VRSA infections are anticipated, necessitating improved infection control practices and alternative therapeutic approaches. In this context, these cases also highlighted the failure of several standard automated susceptibility tests to identify vancomycin resistance in VRSA isolates and suggested that additional VRSA cases may have occurred in the United States but escaped detection. The failure of standard procedures clearly indicates the need to conduct specific vancomycin-resistance testing using nonautomated culture methods (4).

Several reported clusters of MRSA skin infections have been reported among participants in competitive sports. In February 2003, five cases of MRSA occurred in a Colorado fencing club. Since September 2000, other similar outbreaks have been reported in California, Indiana, and Pennsylvania in high school–aged football players and wrestlers. Poor hygiene and sharing of sports equipment and towels were risk factors for these infections. Other factors contributing to transmission of MRSA include abrasions to the skin and direct person-to-person contact (5).

Community-acquired MRSA is now being associated with necrotizing fasciitis, which is a life-threatening infection requiring urgent surgical and medical therapy (6). Data collected from January 2003 to April 2004 in Los Angeles have shown that all recovered MRSA isolates were type USA300 carrying the mec IV cassette along with the Panton-Valentine leukocidin and other toxin genes (6).

Statistics reported by hospitals participating in the National Nosocomial Infections Surveillance (NNIS) System show high rates of resistant bacterial infections in intensive care units (ICUs) nationwide. The most recent prevalence data (2003) for selected antimicrobial-resistant pathogens associated with nosocomial infections reported were

- MRSA: 59.5% (11% increase over 1998–2002 mean)
- MCNS [methicillin-resistant coagulase negative staphylococci (7)]: 89.1% (1% increase over 1998–2002 mean)
- VRE: 28.5% (12% increase over 1998–2002 mean)

Several studies using different methodologies have concluded that MSRA infections are more frequently fatal than are methicillin-sensitive infections. One retrospective cohort analysis revealed a 22% difference between mortality in MRSA bacteremia (35.3%) compared with that in methicillin-sensitive bacteria (8.8%). Another study, looking at the health and economic impact of VRE infections, showed increases in case fatality rates and hospital costs in the VRE group compared with those of matched controls, respectively (8–10).

24.1 Environmental Factors of Drug Resistance

A key factor in the development of antibiotic resistance is the ability of infectious organisms to adapt quickly to new environmental conditions. Bacteria are single-celled organisms that, compared with higher life forms, have small numbers of genes. Therefore, even a single random genetic mutation can greatly affect their ability to cause disease. And because most microbes reproduce by dividing every few hours, bacteria can evolve rapidly. A mutation that helps a microorganism survive exposure to an antibiotic will quickly become dominant throughout the microbial population. Microorganisms also often acquire genes from each other, including genes that confer resistance.

The advantage that microorganisms gain from their innate adaptability is augmented by the widespread and sometimes inappropriate use of antibiotics. A physician, wishing to placate an insistent patient who has a virus or an as-yet undiagnosed condition, sometimes inappropriately prescribes antibiotics. Also, when a patient does not finish taking a prescription for antibiotics, some bacteria may remain. These bacterial survivors are more likely to develop resistance and spread. Hospitals also provide a fertile environment for antibiotic-resistant germs, as close contact among sick patients and extensive use of antibiotics select for resistant bacteria. Scientists also believe that the practice of adding antibiotics to agricultural feed promotes drug resistance (http://www.niaid.nih.gov/factsheets/antimicro.htm).

24.2 Methicillin-Resistant Staphylococcus aureus

During the past four decades, a type of bacterium has evolved from a controllable nuisance into a serious public health concern. This bacterium is known as methicillin-resistant Staphylococcus aureus (MRSA). About one third of people in the world have S. aureus bacteria on their bodies at any given time, primarily in the nose and on the skin. The bacteria can be present but not causing active infection. According to the CDC, of the people with *S. aureus* present, about 1% have MRSA. Life-threatening MRSA infections can involve anyone, including people living in confined areas or those who have close skin-to-skin contact with others, such as athletes involved in football and wrestling, soldiers kept in close quarters, inmates, childcare workers, and residents of long-term care facilities.

MRSA has attracted the attention of the medical research community, underscoring the urgent need to develop better ways to diagnose and treat bacterial infections (http://www3.niaid.nih.gov/topics/AntimicrobialResistance/basics/methicillin.htm).

Cause of MRSA Drug Resistance. The *S. aureus* bacterium, commonly known as "staph," was discovered in the 1880s. During this era, *S. aureus* infection was known to cause painful skin and soft tissue conditions, such as boils, scalded-skin syndrome, and impetigo. *S. aureus* acquired from improperly prepared or stored food can also cause a form of food poisoning. More serious forms of *S. aureus* infection can progress to bacterial pneumonia or to bacteria in the bloodstream, for example, both of which can be fatal.

In the 1940s, medical treatment for *S. aureus* infections became routine and successful with the discovery and introduction of antibiotics such as penicillin.

From that point on, however, use of antibiotics—including misuse and overuse—has aided natural bacterial evolution by helping microoorganisms become resistant to drugs designed to help fight these infections.

In the late 1940s and throughout the 1950s, *S. aureus* developed resistance to penicillin. Methicillin, a congener of penicillin, was introduced to counter the increasing problem of penicillin-resistant *S. aureus*. Methicillin was one of the most common classes of antibiotics used to treat *S. aureus* infections until 1961 when British scientists identified the first strains of *S. aureus* bacteria that resisted methicillin. This was the so-called birth of MRSA.

The first reported human case of MRSA in the United States came in 1968. Subsequently, new strains of bacteria have developed that can now resist previously effective drugs, such as methicillin and most other related antibiotics.

MRSA is actually resistant to an entire class of penicillin-like antibiotics, the β-lactams, including such drugs as penicillin, amoxicillin, oxacillin, and methicillin.

Two Types of MRSA: Hospital-Associated and Community-Associated. Today, *S. aureus* has evolved to the point where experts refer to MRSA in terms ranging from a considerable burden to a crisis. The bacteria have been classified into two categories based on where it is believed infection first occurred.

One classification has been recognized for decades and primarily affects people in health care settings, such as those who have had surgery or medical devices surgically implanted. Referred to as hospital-associated (HA-MRSA), this source of MRSA is typically problematic for people with weak immune systems and those undergoing kidney dialysis or using venous catheters or prosthetics.

Another source of MRSA is the community-associated MRSA (CA-MRSA). Its existence has only been known since the 1990s. CA-MRSA is of great concern to public health professionals because of whom it can affect. Unlike the hospital sources, which usually can be traced to a specific exposure, the origin of CA-MRSA infection is elusive. In addition, the disease is more difficult to treat and has greater potential for serious outcomes.

A study published in 2005 found that nearly 1% of all hospital inpatient stays, or 292,045 per year, were associated with *S. aureus* infection. The study reviewed nearly 14 million patient discharge diagnoses from 2000 and 2001. Patients with diagnoses of *S. aureus* infection, when compared with those without the infection, had about three times the length of stay, three times the total cost, and five times the risk of in-hospital death. Notably, the *S. aureus* infections in this hospital study resulted in 14,000 deaths (http://www3.niaid.nih.gov/topics/AntimicrobialResistance/basics/methicillin.htm).

S. aureus is evolving even more and has begun to show resistance to additional antibiotics. In 2002, physicians in the United States documented the first *S. aureus* strains resistant to the antibiotic vancomycin, which had been one of a handful of antibiotics of last resort for use against *S. aureus*. Originally feared to quickly become a major issue in antibiotic resistance, vancomycin-resistant strains are rare at this time.

CA-MRSA. Outbreaks of CA-MRSA have involved strains with specific microbiologic and genetic differences from traditional HA-MRSA strains. These differences suggest that community strains might spread more easily and cause more skin disease than does HA-MRSA, although comparative studies remain under way.

CA-MRSA most often appears in the form of a skin or soft tissue infection, such as a boil or abscess. People with CA-MRSA often presume they were bitten by a spider. The involved site is red, swollen, and painful and may have pus or other drainage. CA-MRSA also can cause more serious infections, such as bloodstream infections or pneumonia, leading to a variety of other symptoms including shortness of breath, fever, chills, and death.

Transmission. CA-MRSA often enters the body through a cut or scrape and can quickly cause a widespread infection. CA-MRSA can be particularly dangerous in children. Children may be susceptible because their immune systems are not fully developed or they have not developed the specific infection-fighting antibodies to fight off these germs. Living in close quarters with others and poor hygiene may also contribute to a child's susceptibility. Children and young adults are also much more likely to develop dangerous forms of pneumonia than are older people.

Contact-sport participants are also at risk since the bacteria spread easily through cuts and abrasions, skin-to-skin contact, and even through sharing of sweaty towels.

Outbreaks of CA-MRSA also have occurred in military training camps, prisons, childcare and long-term care facilities, and generally in places where crowding and unsanitary conditions are present.

Health care workers, and people in close contact with health care workers, are also at increased risk of serious staph infections.

24.3 Drug Resistance and Nosocomial Infections

Many factors are believed to contribute to the emergence of resistance among nosocomial pathogens, including the indiscriminate use of broad-spectrum antibiotics (both inside and outside the intensive care unit); increasing numbers of susceptible, immunocompromised patients; technologic changes (implants, catheters, intravenous lines); and the breakdown in hygiene, infection control, and disease control programs that leads to increased transmission of resistant bacteria. A disturbing trend is increasing reports of MRSA, historically considered a hospital pathogen, causing serious skin and soft tissue infections in community settings. Over the past several years, there have been reports of MRSA infection affecting prison inmates and military units (11), children attending daycare, sports teams (12), and men who have sex with men. Studies of the genetic and epidemiologic association between hospital-associated MRSA strains and community-associated MRSA strains are under way.

24.3.1 Incidence and Prevalence of Morbidity and Mortality in Nosocomial Infections

Currently, 5% to 10% of patients admitted to acute-care hospitals acquire health care–associated infections, and the risks have increased steadily during the recent decades (13).

A study on the epidemiology of blood and tissue infections (sepsis) in the United States from 1979 through 2000 has shown that the incidence of sepsis and the number of sepsis-related deaths are increasing, although the overall mortality rate among patients with sepsis is declining (14). The incidence of sepsis nearly tripled, increasing from 82.7 cases per 100,000 to 240.4 cases per 100,000 for an annualized increase of 8.7% over the study period. Sepsis is often lethal, killing 20% to 50% of severely affected

patients. The overall sepsis mortality rate at the end of this study period was 17.9%. Because the incidence of sepsis is increasing, the number of deaths due to sepsis tripled over the 22-year study period. Furthermore, sepsis is the second leading cause of death among patients in noncoronary ICUs and the 10th leading cause of death overall in the United States. Care of patients with sepsis costs as much as US$50,000 per patient, adding up to US$17 billion annually in the United States (14).

The National Nosocomial Infections Surveillance (NNIS) System (http://www.cdc.gov/ncidod/hip/SURVEILL/NNIS. HTM) reports health care–associated infections data collected from more than 300 hospitals that enter standardized surveillance components to the system. The NNIS data are collected from adult and pediatric ICUs, high-risk nurseries (HRN), and surgical patients, and its most recent report is available at http://www.cdc.gov/ncidod/hip/NNIS/ 2004NNISreport.pdf) (15). In adults, urinary tract infections are the most common nosocomial infections, whereas bloodstream infections predominate in neonates and children. Blood catheter–acquired infections vary depending on the clinical setting and the type of intensive care, and risk of surgical infection varies with the type of surgery.

24.4 Cellular Physiology and Genetics of Antimicrobial Resistance

On the cellular level, antimicrobial drug resistance derives from changes in two interrelated processes: cellular physiology and genetic coding (16). Microorganisms use a number of physiologic mechanisms based on modifications of their normal molecular pathways to resist being killed by antimicrobial agents. Each alteration in cellular physiology derives from a change in the genetic encoding (16).

24.4.1 Mechanisms of Cellular Physiology

Three basic physiologic mechanisms cause most antimicrobial resistance: (i) enzymatic modification of the antibiotic; (ii) alteration of antibiotic target sites; and (iii) changes in antibiotic uptake or efflux. Each microorganism may use one or more of these strategies to evade antimicrobial agents (16–20).

Enzymatic Modifications. A classic example of a microorganism that depends on antibiotic modification is *Staphylococcus aureus*, which has been known to produce the enzyme β-lactamase. This enzyme will cleave the β-lactam ring of antibiotics to inactivate them (18, 20).

Target Site Alteration. Resistance by target site alteration will occur when the antibiotic can reach its usual target but is unable to act because of a change in the target. For example, for penicillin to act against streptococci, the drug depends on binding to the target penicillin-binding proteins (PBPs). However, the penicillin-resistant *Streptococcus pneumoniae* produces a different PBP with low affinity for penicillin, which would enable the bacterium to evade the drug effect *(18, 20)*.

Changes in Antibiotic Uptake or Efflux. Bacteria can have decreased antibiotic uptake as a result of reduced permeability of their outer layer. Thus, *Pseudomonas aeruginosa* and *Escherichia coli* have an outer membrane with low permeability to antibiotics *(21)*. Because antibiotics must use bacterial porins to penetrate the bacterial cell, the diffusion rate of the drug will be altered by changes in these porin channels. It is the loss of the porin required for imipenem to enter the cell that causes *P. aeruginosa* to develop imipenem resistance *(21)*. Alternatively, the drug's exit from the cell may be enhanced. Thus, the tetracycline resistance for a number of bacteria, including many Enterobacteriaceae, some staphylococci, and some streptococci is the result of active export of the antibiotic out of the bacterial cell (*drug efflux*) *(18, 22)*. In another example, increased drug efflux is also a mechanism of chloroquine resistance in *Plasmodium falciparum* *(23–25)*.

24.4.2 Genetic Basis for Antimicrobial Drug Resistance

The genetic changes leading to the cellular physiology of resistance are complex and varied, but there are three main types: (i) chromosomal mutations of common resistance genes; (ii) acquisition of resistance genes carried on plasmids and other exchangeable genetic segments; and (iii) inducible expression of existing genes *(16, 20, 21, 26, 27)*.

Chromosomal Mutations. Chromosomal mutations in common resistance genes can be spontaneous or complex accumulated mutations *(16)*. Multidrug-resistant tuberculosis (MDR TB) will develop when mutations in individual chromosomal genes accumulate—the likelihood of a *M. tuberculosis* mutant to be simultaneously resistant to two or more drugs is the product of individual probabilities of a single mutation *(28)*.

Plasmids and Exchangeable Gene Segments. Plasmids and other exchangeable segments of genes such as transposons, gene cassettes, integrons, and phage genes are more rapidly disseminated than are the chromosomal mutations *(16)*. *Transposons* are segments of DNA that have a repeat of an insertion sequence element at each end and can migrate from one plasmid to another within the same bacterium, to a bacterial chromosome, or to a bacteriophage. *Gene cassettes* represent a family of discrete mobile genetic elements that each contain an antibiotic resistance gene and are dependent on integrons for integration in chromosomes *(29)*. *Integrons* are receptor elements on the chromosome that provide the site into which the gene cassette is integrated and provide the enzyme for integration *(29)*.

One example of the role of these exchangeable gene segments is the plasmid-encoded, extended-spectrum β-lactamases (ESBLs) in Gram-negative microorganisms. The ESBLs confer resistance to ampicillin, carbenicillin, ticarcillin, and the extended-spectrum cephalosporins *(16)*. Their broad activity arises from amino acid substitutions that alter the configuration around the active site of the β-lactamase enzyme and thus increase the enzyme affinity for broad-spectrum β-lactam antibiotics *(18)*.

The rapid exchangeability of plasmids or other exchangeable gene segments has several implications: (i) surveillance systems need to detect sudden changes in resistance patterns in a community; (ii) drug resistance may be easily transferred between bacterial species; and (iii) resistance to several different drugs may travel together *(16)*.

The coexistence of resistance to several drugs should always be expected, especially when it is known that the resistance is carried on an exchangeable element. Thus, in 1998, 32% of *Salmonella* isolates in the United States demonstrated a linked five-drug resistance pattern, in contrast with fewer than 1% in 1979–1980 *(30–32)*. Of *Streptococcus pneumoniae* isolates that were resistant to penicillin, two thirds were also resistant to crythromyom, and 93% were nonsusceptible to trimethoprim-sulfamethoxazole *(32)*. Although *S. pneumoniae* co-resistances are not plasmid-borne, they are complex gene mosaics that appear to be tightly linked like those on plasmids *(16)*.

Inducible Mechanisms. Inducible mechanisms cause resistance that arises during treatment with a given antimicrobial agent *(16)*. For example, treatment of influenza A virus with rimantadine regularly results in the rapid emergence of resistant virus in the affected patient *(33, 34)*. Also, several Enterobacteriaceae possess a cephalosporinase that is not normally expressed, but certain cephalosporins will trigger expression of high concentrations of the enzyme *(35)*. However, effective surveillance for these inducible mechanisms is not possible because they are not expressed phenotypically at baseline *(16)*.

24.5 NIAID Involvement in Research on Antimicrobial Drug Resistance

The increasing use of antimicrobial drugs in humans, animals, and agriculture has resulted in many pathogens developing resistance to these powerful drugs. All major groups of pathogens—viruses, fungi, parasites, and bacteria—can become resistant to antimicrobials. Many diseases are increasingly difficult to treat because of the emergence of drug-resistant organisms, including HIV and other viruses; bacteria such as staphylococci, enterococci, and *Escherichia coli*; respiratory infections such as tuberculosis and influenza; food-borne pathogens such as *Salmonella* and *Campylobacter*; sexually transmitted organisms such as *Neisseria gonorrhoeae*; fungal infections such as *Candida*; and parasites such as *Plasmodium falciparum*, the cause of malaria (http://www3.niaid.nih.gov/research/topics/antimicrobial/introduction.htm).

24.5.1 Plans, Priorities, and Goals

NIAID manages research funding specifically aimed at the problem of antibiotic resistance and hospital-acquired infections (http://www3.niaid.nih.gov/research/topics/ antimicrobial/introduction.htm).

Antimicrobial Resistance Program. This program is designed to support research in several areas, including:

- Studies on antimicrobial resistance in major viral, bacterial, fungal, and parasitic pathogens, including the major health care–associated bacterial pathogens.
- Identification of new diagnostic techniques, novel therapeutics, and preventive measures to minimize infection with resistant pathogens; prevent the acquisition of resistant traits; and control the spread of resistance factors and resistant pathogens, with a focus on health care settings.
- Basic research into the molecular biology and genetics of the acquisition, maintenance, and transmission of resistance genes.
- Collaborations with academic researchers and biotechnology companies to explore novel therapeutic approaches such as bacteriophage therapy and natural antimicrobial peptides.

Medical Bacteriology Program. The major objectives of this program are to support research to:

- Control and prevent the spread of bacterial infections in patient care facilities.
- Facilitate development of interventions for health care–associated bacterial infections.
- Understand the biology of bacterial species most often involved in hospital-acquired infections.
- Control and prevent bacterial sepsis.
- Control and prevent bacterial urinary tract infections.

- Develop diagnostics platforms for novel detection of key pathogens responsible for sepsis and community acquired pneumonia.

24.6 Recent Programmatic Accomplishments/Developments

- In 2005, the *Interagency Task Force on Antimicrobial Resistance* has reviewed the progress in implementing "A Public Health Action Plan to Combat Antimicrobial Resistance Part 1: Domestic Issues." The action plan, which reflects a broad-based consensus of federal agencies on actions needed to address antimicrobial resistance, is based on input from a wide variety of constituents and collaborators. The Task Force, which is chaired by NIH (NIAID), the CDC, and the Food and Drug Administration (FDA), also includes representatives from the Agency for Healthcare Research and Quality, the Department of Agriculture, the Department of Defense, the Department of Veterans Affairs, the Environmental Protection Agency, the Center for Medicare and Medicaid Services, and the Health Resources and Services Administration.
- NIAID jointly supports a contract "Network on Antimicrobial Resistance in *Staphylococcus aureus* (NARSA)," with FOCUS Bio-Inova, Inc., in Herndon, Virginia. The network includes more than 200 domestic and international investigators including basic researchers, clinical laboratory scientists, epidemiologists, and infectious disease clinicians involved in staphylococcal and antimicrobial resistance research. Major functions of NARSA include support of electronic sharing of information and meetings, integration with the CDC's surveillance system on antibiotic resistance, and support of a case registry and extensive repository of staphylococcal clinical, research, resistant, and historical isolates. The repository has available more than 200 strains of *S. aureus* including the first three VRSA isolates identified in the United States *(2–4)*. A special application and approval is required to procure these isolates. Additional information is available through www.narsa.net and http://www.niaid.nih.gov/dmid/antimicrob/.
- A new research initiative, "Sepsis and community-acquired pneumonia (CAP): Partnerships for Diagnostics Development" (http://grants1.nih.gov/grants/guide/rfa-files/RFA-AI-04-043.html), was recently funded by NIAID. The purpose of the initiative is to support development by industry of broad diagnostic technologies that provide early detection of select major causes of septicemia, bacteremia, candidemia, and community-acquired pneumonia (CAP) (http://www.niaid.nih.gov/factsheets/antimicro.htm).

- ICUs are the most frequently identified sources of nosocomial infections within the hospital, with infection and antimicrobial resistance rates significantly higher than in the general wards. In current clinical practice, these patients often receive antibiotics for an extended time, even though the likelihood of infection is low. In a trial entitled "Randomized, Multicenter Comparative Trial of Short-Course Empiric Antibiotic Therapy versus Standard Antibiotic Therapy for Subjects with Pulmonary Infiltrates in the Intensive Care Unit," NIAID investigators compared a "short course" antibiotic regimen (3 days) to the common-practice treatment of 8 days or more. The results of the study may lead to reduced use of antimicrobials in ICUs and a subsequent drop in antimicrobial resistance.

The "Partnerships to Improve Diagnosis and Treatment of Selected Drug-Resistant Healthcare-Associated Infections (U01)" initiative (http://grants.nih.gov/grants/guide/rfa-files/RFA-AI-06-036.html) is designed to support the development of therapeutics to treat, or rapid diagnostics to identify, specific bacterial strains and drug-resistant phenotypes for the following health care–associated pathogens: *Clostridium difficile, Pseudomonas, Acinetobacter, Enterobacter, Klebsiella, Serratia, Proteus,* and *Stenotrophomonas (Pseudomonas) maltophilia.*

The "Clinical Trial for Community-Acquired Methicillin-Resistant *Staphylococcus aureus* (CA-MRSA) Infections" initiative was released in response to the increasing prevalence of CA-MRSA in various areas of the United States. This initiative is aimed to define the optimal outpatient treatment with skin and soft tissue infection in areas where prevalence of CA-MRSA was high. The efficacy of off-patent antimicrobials such as clindamycin and trimethoprim-sulfamethoxazole is being evaluated.

24.7 Resources for Researchers

NIAID has made the following resources available to researchers http:// www3. niaid. nih. gov/ research/ topicsantimicrobial/ resources.htm):

- The Alliance for the Prudent Use of Antibiotics, Reservoirs of Antibiotic Resistance (ROAR) Network
- Bacteriology and Mycology Study Group
- Bioinformatics Resource Centers
- Microbial Sequencing Centers
- Mycoses Study Group
- Network on Antimicrobial Resistance in *Staphylococcus aureus* (NARSA)

NARSA is a multidisciplinary international cadre of scientists conducting basic and clinical research focused on combating antimicrobial-resistant *S. aureus* and related staphylococcal bacterial infections.

- Proteomics Research Centers
- Pathogen Functional Genomics Resource Center

24.8 Recent Scientific Advances

- *Immunization with Staphylococcus aureus Clumping Factor B, a Major Determinant in Nasal Carriage, Reduces Nasal Colonization in a Murine Model.* Staphylococcus aureus is a human pathogen that can cause life-threatening infections of the skin, bone, heart, and other vital organs. Staphylococcal pathogenicity is the result of a coordinated expression of a few dozen different genes, including those for toxins, enzymes, structural molecules, and other proteins. Nasal carriage of *S. aureus*, which is a major risk factor for infection and a major determinant for nasal colonization by *S. aureus*, is linked with the expression of a bacterial surface protein called *clumping factor B*. In a recent study, mice immunized systemically or intranasally with a clumping factor B recombinant vaccine showed a lower level of *S. aureus* colonization than did control animals *(36)*. It is believed that with reduced nasal colonization, the risk of infection will be reduced. The use of vaccines is also important because of the high incidence of multiple antibiotic resistances in *S. aureus*, complicating treatment with traditional antibiotics.

References

1. Hiramatsu, K. (2001) Vancomycin-resistant Staphylococcus aures: a new model of antibiotic resistance, *Lancet Infect. Dis.*, **1**(3), 147–155.
2. Sievert, D. M., Boulton, M. L., Stoltman, G., et al. (2002) *Staphylococcus aureus* resistant to vancomycin – United States, 2002, *Morb. Mortal. Wkly Rep.*, **51**(26), 565–567.
3. Miller, D., Urdaneta, V., Weltman, A., and Park, S. (2002) Vancomycin-resistant *Staphylococcus aureus* – Pennsylvania, 2002, *Morb. Mortal. Wkly Rep.*, **51**(40), 902.
4. Kacica, M. and McDonald, L. C. (2004) Vancomycin-resistant *Staphylococcus aureus* – New York, 2004, *Morb. Mortal. Wkly Rep.*, **53**(15), 322–323.
5. Centers for Disease Control and Prevention. Immunity-associated methicillin-resistant *Staphylococcus aureus* skin infections – Los Angeles County, California, 2002–2003, *Morb. Mortal. Wkly Rep.*, **52**, 88.
6. Miller, L. G., Perdreau-Remington, F., Rieg, G., Mehdi, S., Perlroth, J., Bayer, A. S., Tang, A. W., Fung, T. O., and Spielberg, B. (2005) Necrotizing fasciitis caused by community-associated methicillin-resistant Staphylococcus aureus, in Los Angeles, *N. Engl. J. Med.*, **352**, 1445–1453.

7. Cardo, D., Horan, T., Andrus, M., Dembinski, M., Edwards, J., Peavy, G., Tolston, J., and Wagner, D. (2004) National Nosocomial Infections Surveillance (NNIS) System report, data summary from January 1992 through June 2004, issued October 2004, *Am. J. Infect. Control*, **32**(8), 470–485.

8. Blot, S. I., Vandewoude, K. H., Hoste, E. A., and Colardyn, F. A. (2002) Outcome and attributable mortality of ill patients with bacteremia involving methicillin-susceptible and methicillin-resistant *Staphylococcus aureus*, *Arch. Intern. Med.*, **62**(19), 2229–2235.

9. Cosgrove, S. E., Sakoulas, G., Perencevich, E. N., Schwaber, M. J., Karchmer, A. W., and Carmeli, Y. (2003) Comparison of mortality associated with methicillin-susceptible and methicillin-resistant *Staphylococcus aureus* bacteremia: a meta-analysis, *Clin. Infect. Dis.*, **36**, 53–59.

10. Carmeli, Y., Eliopoulos, G., Mozaffari, E., and Samore, M. (2002) Health and economic outcomes of vancomycin-resistant enterococci, *Arch. Intern. Med.*, **162**, 2223–2228.

11. Aiello, A. E., Lowy, F. D., Wright, L. N., and Larson, E. L. (2006) Methicillin-resistant *Staphylococcus aureus* among US prisoners and military personnel: review and recommendation for future studies, *Lancet Infect. Dis.*, **6**(6), 335–341.

12. Kazakova, S. V., Hageman, J. C., Matava, M., et. al. (2005) A clone of *Staphylococcus aureus* among professional football players, *N. Engl. J. Med.*, **352**(5), 468–475.

13. Burke, J. P. (2003) Infection control – a problem of patient safety, *N. Engl. J. Med.*, **347**(7), 651–656.

14. Martin, G. S., Mannino, D. M., Eaton, S., and Moss, M. (2003) The epidemiology of sepsis in the United States from 1979 through 2000, *N. Engl. J. Med.*, **348**(16), 1546–1554.

15. Solomon, S., Horan, T., Andrus, M., Edwards, J., Fridkin, S., Koganti, J., Peavy, G., and Tolston, J. (2003) National Nosocomial Infections Surveillance (NNIS) System report, data summary from January 1992 through June 2003, issued August 2003, *Am. J. Infect. Control*, **31**(8), 481–498.

16. Benin, A. L. and Dowell, S. F. (2001) Antibiotic resistance and implications for the appropriate use of antimicrobial agents. In: *Management of Antimicrobials in Infectious Diseases* (Mainous, A. G. III and Pomeroy, C., eds.), Humana Press, Totowa, NJ, pp. 3–25.

17. Tenover, F. C. and Hughes, J. M. (1996) The challenges of emerging infectious diseases: development and spread of multiply-resistant bacterial pathogens, *J. Am. Med. Assoc.*, **275**, 300–304.

18. Jacoby, G. A. and Archer, G. L. (1991) New mechanisms of bacterial resistance to antimicrobial agents, *N. Engl. J. Med.*, **324**, 601–612.

19. Shlaes, D. M., Gerding, D. N., John, J. F., Craig, W. A., Bornstein, D. L., Duncan, R. A., et al. (1997) Society for healthcare epidemiology of America and Infectious Diseases Society of America Joint Committee on the Prevention of Antimicrobial Resistance: guidelines for the prevention of antimicrobial resistance in hospitals, *Clin. Infect. Dis.*, **25**, 584–599.

20. Hawkey, P. M. (1998) The origins and molecular basis of antibiotic resistance, *Br. Med. J.*, **317**, 657–660.

21. Nikaido, H. (1994) Prevention of drug access to bacterial targets: permeability barriers and active efflux, *Science*, **264**, 382–388.

22. Levy, S. B. (1992) Active efflux mechanisms for antimicrobial resistance, *Antimicrob. Agents Chemother.*, **36**, 695–703.

23. Barat, L. M. and Bloland, P. B. (1997) Drug resistance among malaria and other parasites, *Infect. Dis. Clin. North Am.*, **11**, 969–987.

24. Krogstad, D. J. (1996) Malaria as a reemerging disease, *Epidemiol. Rev.*, **18**, 77–89.

25. White, N. J. (1992) Antimalarial drug resistance: the pace quickens, *J. Antimicrob. Chemother.*, **30**, 571–585.

26. Davies, J. (1994) Inactivation of antibiotics and the dissemination of resistance genes, *Science*, **264**, 375–382.

27. Gold, H. S. and Moellering, R. C. (1996) Antimalarial-drug resistance, *N. Engl. J. Med.*, **335**, 1445–1453.

28. Rattan, A., Kalia, A., and Ahmad, N. (1998) Multidrug-resistant *Mycobacterium tuberculosis*: molecular perspectives, *Emerg. Infect. Dis.*, **4**, 195–209.

29. Hall, R. M. (1997) Mobile gene cassettes and integrons: moving antibiotic resistance genes in gram-negative bacteria, *Ciba Foundation Symposium 1997*, **207**, 192–202; discussion: 202–205.

30. Centers for Disease Control and Prevention (1999) National antimicrobial resistance monitoring system: enteric bacteria, 1998 Annual report (http://www.cdc.gov/ncidod/dbmd/narms.htl).

31. Glynn, M. K., Bopp, C., Dewitt, W., Dabney, P., Mokhtar, M., and Angulo, F. J. (1998) Emergence of multidrug-resistant *Salmonella enterica* serotype typhimurium DT104 infections in the United States, *N. Engl. J. Med.*, **338**, 1333–1338.

32. Doern, G. V., Brueggemann, A., Huynh, H., Wingert, E., and Rhomberg, P. (1999) Antimicrobial resistance with *Streptococcus pneumoniae* in the United States, 1997–1998, *Emerg. Infect. Dis.*, **5**, 757–765.

33. Hayden, F. G., Belshe, R. B., Clover, R. D., Hay, A. J., Oakes, M. G., and Soo, W. (1989) Emergence and apparent transmission of rimantadine-resistant influenza A virus in families, *N. Engl. J. Med.*, **321**, 1696–1702.

34. Hall, C. B., Dolin, R., Gala, C. L., Markovitz, D. M., Zhang, Y. Q., Madore, P. H., et al. (1987) Children with influenza A infection: treatment with ramantidine, *Pediatrics*, **80**, 275–282.

35. Neu, H. C. (1992) The crisis in antibiotic resistance, *Science*, **257**, 1064–1073.

36. Schaffer, A. C., Solinga, R. M., Cocchiaro, J., Portoles, M., Kiser, K. B., Risley, A., Randall, S. M., Valtulina, V., Speziale, P., Walsh, E., Foster, T., and Lee, J. C. (2006) Immunization with *Staphylococcus aureus* clumping factor B, a major determinant in nasal carriage, reduces nasal colonization in a murine model, *Infect. Immun.*, **74**, 2145–2153.

Chapter 25

Genomic and Postgenomic Research

The word *genomics* was first coined by T. Roderick from the Jackson Laboratories in 1986 as the name for the new field of science focused on the analysis and comparison of complete genome sequences of organisms and related high-throughput technologies.

A sequence provides the most fundamental information about an organism, and the genes and the regulatory sites encoded in the sequence will reveal the complete profile of the organism and information about its evolution *(1)*.

The development of genomics should be considered one of the most dramatic results of the advances in biomedical sciences in the 20th century.

25.1 Computational Methods for Genome Analysis

Two basic computational methods are used for genome analysis: gene finding and whole genome comparison *(2)*.

Gene Finding. Using a computational method that can scan the genome and analyze the statistical features of the sequence is a fast and remarkably accurate way to find the genes in the genome of prokaryotic organisms (bacteria, archaea, viruses) compared with the still difficult problem of finding genes in higher eukaryotes. By using modern bioinformatics software, finding the genes in a bacterial genome will result in a highly accurate, rich set of annotations that provide the basis for further research into the functions of those genes.

The absence of introns—those portions of the DNA that lie between two exons and are transcribed into a RNA but will not appear in that RNA after maturation and therefore are not expressed (as proteins) in the protein synthesis—will remove one of the major barriers to computational analysis of the genome sequence, allowing gene finding to identify more than 99% of the genes of most genomes without any human intervention. Next, these gene predictions can be further refined by searching for nearby regulatory sites such as the ribosome-binding sites, as well as by aligning protein sequences to other species. These steps can be automated using freely available software and databases *(2)*.

Gene finding in single-cell eukaryotes is of intermediate difficulty, with some organisms, such as *Trypanosoma brucei*, having so few introns that a bacterial gene finder is sufficient to find their genes. Other eukaryote organisms (e.g., *Plasmodium falciparum*) have numerous introns and would require the use of special-purpose gene finder, such as GlimmerM *(3, 4)*.

Whole Genome Comparison. This computational method refers to the problem of aligning the entire deoxyribonucleic acid (DNA) sequence of one organism to that of another, with the goal of detecting all similarities as well as rearrangements, insertions, deletions, and polymorphisms *(2)*. With the increasing availability of complete genome sequences from multiple, closely related species, such comparisons are providing a powerful tool for genomic analysis. Using *suffix trees*—data structures that contains all of the subsequences from a particular sequence and can be built and searched in linear time—this computational task can be accomplished in minimal time and space. Because the suffix tree algorithm is both time and space efficient, it is able to align large eukaryotic chromosomes with only slightly greater requirements than those for bacterial genomes *(2)*.

Bacterial Genome Annotation. The major goal of the bacterial genome annotation is to identify the functions of all genes in a genome as accurately and consistently as possible by using initially automated annotation methods for preliminary assignment of functions to genes, followed by a second stage of manual curation by teams of scientists.

25.2 Genomes of Pathogenic Enterobacteria

The family Enterobacteriaceae encompasses a diverse group of bacteria including many of the most important human pathogens (*Salmonella, Yersinia, Klebsiella, Shigella*), as well as one of the most enduring laboratory research organisms, the nonpathogenic *Escherichia coli* K12. Many of

V. St. Georgiev, *National Institute of Allergy and Infectious Diseases, NIH: Impact on Global Health*, vol. 2, DOI 10.1007/978-1-60327-297-1_25, © Humana Press, a part of Springer Science+Business Media, LLC 2009

these pathogens have been subject to genome sequencing or are under study. Genome comparisons among these organisms have revealed the presence of a core set of genes and functions along a generally collinear genomic backbone. However, there are also many regions and points of difference, such as large insertions and deletions (including pathogenicity islands), integrated bacteriophages, small insertions and deletions, point mutations, and chromosomal rearrangements *(5)*.

25.2.1 *Escherichia coli K12*

The first genome sequence of *Escherichia coli* K12 (reference strain MG1655) was completed and published in 1997 *(6)*. Later, the genome sequence of two other genotypes of *E. coli*, the enterohemorrhagic *E. coli* O157:H7 (EHEC; strains EDL933 and RIMD 0509952-Sakai) *(7, 8)* and the uropathogenic *E. coli* (UPEC; strain CFT073) *(9)*, were sequenced and the information published. Currently, it is accepted that shigellae are part of the *E. coli* species complex, and information on the genome of *Shigella flexneri* strain 2a has been published *(10)*.

A comparison of all three pathogenic *E. coli* with the archetypal nonpathogenic *E. coli* K12 revealed that the genomes were essentially collinear, displaying both conservation in sequence and gene order *(5)*. The genes that were predicted to be encoded within the conserved sequence displayed more than 95% sequence identity and have been termed the *core genes*. Similar observations were made for the *Shigella flexneri* genome, which also shares 3.9 Mb of common sequence with *E. coli (10)*.

A comparison of the three *E. coli* genomes revealed that genes shared by all genomes amounted to 2,996 *(9)* from a total of 4,288, and about 5,400 and 5,500 predicted protein-coding sequences for *E. coli* K12, EHEC, and UPEC, respectively *(5)*. The region encoding these core genes is known as the *backbone sequence.*

It was also apparent from these comparisons that interdispersed throughout this backbone sequence were large regions unique to the different genotypes. Moreover, several studies had shown that some of these unique loci were present in clinical disease–causing isolates but were apparently absent from their comparatively benign relatives *(11)*. One such well-characterized region is the *locus of enterocyte effacement (LEE)* in the enteropathogenic *E. coli* (EPEC). Thus, an EPEC infection results in effacement of the intestinal microvilli and the intimate adherence of bacterial cells to enterocytes. Furthermore, EPEC also subverts the structural integrity of the cell and forces the polymerization of actin, which accumulates below the adhered EPEC cells, forming cup-like pedestals *(12)*. This is called an *attachment and effacing (AE)* lesion. Subsequently, LEE was found in all bacteria known to be able to elicit an AE lesion *(5)*.

25.2.1.1 Pathogenicity Islands

The presence of many regions in the backbone sequence similar to LEE have been characterized in both Gram-negative and Gram-positive bacteria *(13)*. This led to the concept of *pathogenicity islands (PAIs)* and the formulation of a definition to describe their features *(5)*.

Typically, PAIs are inserted adjacent to stable RNA genes and have an atypical G+C content. In addition to virulence-related functions, the pathogenicity islands often carry genes encoding transposase or integrase-like proteins and are unstable and self-mobilizable *(13, 14)*. It was also noted that PAIs possess a high proportion of gene fragments or disrupted genes when compared with the backbone regions *(15)*.

It is generally accepted that the pathogenic *E. coli* genotypes have evolved from a much smaller nonpathogenic relative by the acquisition of foreign DNA. This laterally acquired DNA has been attributed with conferring on the different genotypes the ability to colonize alternative niches in the host and the ability to cause a range of different disease outcomes *(5)*.

Although sharing some of the features of PAIs and considered to be parts of the PAIs, some genomic loci are unlikely to impinge on pathogenicity. To take account of this, the concept of PAIs has been extended to include islands or strain-specific loops, which represent discrete genetic loci that are lineage-specific but are as yet not known to be involved in virulence *(7, 8)*.

25.2.2 *Salmonella Pathogenicity Islands*

Currently, there are more than 2,300 *Salmonella* serovars in two species, *S. enterica* and *S. bongori*. All salmonellae are closely related, sharing a median DNA identity for the reciprocal best match of between 85% and 95% *(16, 17)*. Despite their homogeneity, there are still significant differences in the pathogenesis and host range of the different *Salmonella* serovars. Thus, whereas *S. enterica* subspecies *enterica* serovar Typhi (*S. typhi*) is only pathogenic to humans causing severe typhoid fever, *S. typhimurium* causes gastroenteritis in humans but also a systemic infection in mice and has a broad host range *(16)*.

Like *E. coli*, the salmonellae are also known to possess PAIs, known as *Salmonella* pathogenicity islands (SPIs). It is thought that SPIs have been acquired laterally. For example, the gene products encoded by SPI-1 *(18, 19)* and SPI-2

(20, 21) have been shown to play important roles in the different stages of the infection process. Both of these islands possess type III secretion systems and their associated secreted protein effectors. SPI-1 is known to confer on all salmonellae the ability to invade epithelial cells. SPI-2 is important in various aspects of the systemic infection, allowing *Salmonella* to spread from the intestinal tissue into the blood and eventually to infect, and survive within, the macrophages of the liver and spleen *(22)*.

SPI-3, like LEE and PAI-1 of UPEC, is inserted alongside the *selC* tRNA gene and carries the gene *mgtC*, which is required for the intramacrophage survival and growth in the low-magnesium environment thought to be encountered in the phagosome *(23)*.

Other *Salmonella* SPIs encode type III–secreted effector proteins, chaperone-usher fimbrial operons, Vi antigen biosynthetic gene, a type IVB pilus operon, and many other determinants associated with the salmonellae enteropathogenicity *(15)*.

25.2.3 Yersinia High-Pathogenicity Island

Although the mobile nature of PAIs is frequently discussed in the literature, there is little direct experimental evidence to support these observations. One possible explanation for this may be that on integration, the mobility genes of the PAIs subsequently become degraded, thereby fixing their position *(5)*. Certainly, there is evidence to support this hypothesis, as many proposed PAIs carry integrase or transposase pseudogenes or remnants. One excellent example of this is the high-pathogenicity island (HPI) first characterized in *Yersinia (24)*.

The *Yersinia* HPIs can be split into two lineages based on the integrity of the phage integrase gene (*int*) carried in the island: (i) *Y. enterocolitica* biotype 1B and (ii) *Y. pestis* and *Y. pseudotuberculosis*. The *Y. enterocolitica* HPI *int* gene carries a point mutation, whereas the analogous gene is intact in the *Y. pestis* and *Y. pseudotuberculosis* HPIs.

The *Yersinia* HPI is a 35- to 43-kb island that possesses genes for the production and uptake of the siderophore yersiniabactin, as well as genes, such as *int*, thought to be involved in the mobility of the island. HPI-like elements are widely distributed in enterobacteria, including *E. coli, Klebsiella, Enterobacter,* and *Citrobacter* spp., and like many prophages, these HPIs are found adjacent to *asn*-tRNA genes *(8)*. tRNA genes are common sites for bacteriophage integration into the genome *(25)*.

Integration at these sites typically involves site-specific recombination between short stretches of identical DNA located on the phage (*attP*) and at the integration site on the bacterial genomes (*attB*). The tRNA genes represent common sites for the integration of many other PAIs and bacteriophages, with the *secC* tRNA locus being the most heavily used integration site in the enterics *(9)*.

25.2.4 Bacteriophages (Prophages)

Integrated bacteriophages, also known as prophages, are also commonly found in bacterial genomes *(5)*. For example, in the S loops of the *E. coli* O157:H7 strain EDL933 (EHEC) unique regions, nearly 50% were phage related. In addition to the 18 prophage sequences detected in the genome of EHEC strain Sakai *(8)*, the genomes of *E. coli* K12, UPEC, and *S. flexneri* have all been shown to carry multiple prophage or prophage-like elements *(6, 7, 9, 10)*. Moreover, comparison of the genome sequences of EHEC O157:H7 strain EDL933 and strain Sakai revealed marked variations in the complement and integration sites of the prophages, as did internal regions within highly related phages *(8, 26)*.

In addition to genes essential for their own replication, phages often carry genes that, for example, prevent superinfection by other bacteriophages, such as *old* and *tin (27, 28)*. However, other genes carried in prophages appear to be of nonphage origin and can encode determinants that enhance the virulence of the bacterial host by a process known as *lysogenic conversion (29)*.

In addition to the presence of the LEE PAI and the ability to elicit AE lesion, another defining characteristics of the enterohemorrhagic *E. coli* (EHEC) is the production of Shiga toxins (Stx). The Shiga toxins represent a family of potent cytotoxins that, on entry into the eukaryotic cell, will act as glycosylases by cleaving the 28S ribosomal RNA (rRNA) thereby inactivating the ribosome and consequently preventing the protein synthesis *(30)*.

Other enteric pathogens such as *S. typhi, S. typhimurium,* and *Y. pestis* are also known to possess significant numbers of prophages *(15, 16, 31)*. Thus, the principal virulence determinants of the salmonellae are the type III secretion systems, carried by SPI-1 and SPI-2, and their associated protein effectors *(32, 33)*. A significant number of these type III secreted effector proteins are present in the genomes of prophages and have a dramatic influence on the ability of their bacterial hosts to cause disease *(5)*.

25.2.5 Other Characteristic Features of the Enterobacterial Genomes

Small Insertions and Deletions. Even though the large PAIs play a major role in defining the phenotypes of different strains of the enteric bacteria, there are many other differences resulting from small insertions and deletions, which must be taken into account when considering the overall genomic picture of Enterobacteriaceae *(5)*.

Thus, the comparisons between *E. coli* K12 and *E. coli* O157:H7 and between *S. typhi* and *S. typhimurium* have indicated the existence of many small differences that exist aside from the large pathogenicity islands. For example, the number of separate insertion and deletion events has shown that there are 145 events of 10 genes or fewer compared with 12 events of 20 genes or more for the *S. typhi* and *S. typhimurium* comparison. Furthermore, comparison between *S. typhi* and *E. coli* revealed 504 events of 10 genes or fewer compared with just 25 events of 20 genes or more. Even taking into account that the larger islands contain many more genes per insertion or deletion event, it becomes clear that nearly equivalent numbers of species-specific genes are attributable to insertion or deletion events involving 10 genes or fewer as are due to events involving 20 genes or more. These data should lend credence to the assertion that the acquisition and exchange of *small islands* is important in defining the overall phenotype of the organism *(5)*. In the majority of cases studied to date, there is no evidence to suggest the presence of genes that may allow these small islands to be self-mobile. It is far more likely that small islands of this type are exchanged between members of a species and constitute part of the species gene pool. Once acquired by one member of the species, they can be easily exchanged by generalized transduction mechanisms, followed by homologous recombination between the near identical flanking genes to allow integration into the chromosome *(5)*.

This sort of mechanism of genetic exchange would also make possible nonorthologous gene replacement, involving the exchange of related genes at identical regions in the backbone. A specific example to illustrate such a possibility is the observed *capsular switching* of *Neisseria meningitides (34)* and *Streptococcus pneumoniae (35, 36)* for which different sets of genes responsible for the biosynthesis of different capsular polysaccharides are found at identical regions in the chromosome and flanked by conserved genes. The implied mechanism for capsular switching involves replacement of the polysaccharide-specific gene sites by homologous recombination between the chromosome and exogenous DNA in the flanking genes *(5)*.

Point Mutations and Pseudogenes. One of the most surprising observations to come from enterobacterial genome research has been the discovery of a large number of *pseudogenes*. The pseudogenes appeared to be untranslatable due to the presence of stop codons, frameshifts, internal deletions, or insertion sequence (IS) element insertions. The presence of pseudogenes seems to run contrary to the general assumption that the bacterial genome is a highly "streamlined" system that does not carry "junk DNA" *(5)*.

For example, *Salmonella typhi*, the etiologic agent of typhoid fever, is host restricted and appears only capable of infecting a human host, whereas *S. typhimurium*, which causes a milder disease in humans, has a much broader host range. Upon analysis, the genome of *S. typhi* contained more than 200 pseudogenes *(15)*, whereas it was predicted that the number of pseudogenes in the genome of *S. typhimurium* would be around 39 *(16)*. From this observation, it becomes clear that the pseudogenes in *S. typhi* were not randomly spread throughout its genome—in fact, they were overrepresented in genes that were unique to *S. typhi* when compared with *E. coli*, and many of the pseudogenes in *S. typhi* have intact counterparts in *S. typhimurium* that have been shown to be involved in aspects of virulence and host interaction. Given this distribution of pseudogenes, it has been suggested that the host specificity of *S. typhi* may be the result of the loss of its ability to interact with a broader range of hosts caused by functional inactivation of the necessary genes *(15)*. In contrast with other microorganisms containing multiple pseudogenes, such as *Mycobacterium leprae (37)*, most of the pseudogenes in *S. typhi* were caused by a single mutation, suggesting that they have been inactivated relatively recently.

Taken together, these observations suggest an evolutionary scenario in which the recent ancestor of *S. typhi* had changed its niche in a human host, evolving from an ancestor (similar to *S. typhimurium*) limited to localized infection and invasion around the gut epithelium into one capable of invading the deeper tissues of the human hosts *(5)*.

A similar evolutionary scenario has been suggested for another recently evolved enteric pathogen, *Yersinia pestis*. This bacterium has also recently changed from a gut bacterium (*Y. pseudotuberculosis*), transmitted via the fecal-oral route, to an organism capable of using a flea vector for systemic infection *(38, 39)*. Again, this change in niche was accompanied by pseudogene formation, and genes involved in virulence and host interaction are overrepresented in the set of genes inactivated *(31)*.

Yet another example of such an evolutional scenario is *Shigella flexneri* 2a, a member of the species *E. coli* (which is predicted to have more than 250 pseudogenes), and is again restricted to the human body *(10)*.

All of these organisms demonstrate that the enterobacterial evolution has been a process that has involved both gene loss and gene gain, and that the remnants of the genes lost in the evolutionary process can be readily detected *(5)*.

25.3 Bacterial Proteomes as Complements of Genomes

The focus in the postgenomic era is on functional genomics, in which proteomics plays an essential role. The living cell is a dynamic and complex system that cannot be predicted from the genome sequence. Whereas genomes will disclose important information on the biological importance of the organism, it is still static and will not reveal information on the expression of a particular gene or of posttranslational modifications or on how a protein is regulated in a specific biological situation *(40)*.

Thus, whereas the complete genome sequence provides the basis for experimental identification of expressed proteins at the cellular level, very little has been accomplished to identify all expressed and potentially modified proteins.

Direct investigation of the total content of proteins in a cell is the task of proteomics. Proteomics is defined as the complete set of posttranslationally modified and processed proteins in a well-defined biological environment under specific circumstances, such as growth conditions and time of investigation *(40, 41)*.

Proteomics can be studied by following two separate steps: separation of the proteins in a sample, followed by identification of the proteins. The common methodology used for separating proteins is two-dimensional polyacrylamide gel electrophoresis (2D PAGE). The principal method for large-scale identification is mass spectroscopy (MS), but other identification methods, such as *N*-terminal sequencing, immunoblotting, overexpression, spot colocalization, and gene knockouts, can also be used.

25.3.1 Two-Dimensional Polyacrylamide Gel Electrophoresis

Because of its high-resolution power, 2D PAGE is currently the best methodology to achieve global visualization of the proteins of a microorganism. In the first dimension, isoelectric focusing is carried out to separate the proteins in a pH gradient according to their isoelectric point (p*I*). In the second dimension, the proteins are separated according to their molecular weight by SDS-PAGE (sodium dodecyl sulfate–PAGE). The resulting gel image presents itself as a pattern of spots in which p*I* and the relative molecular weight (M_r) can be recognized as in a coordinate system *(40)*. A critical step during the 2D PAGE procedure is the sample preparation, as there is no single method that can be universally applied because different reagents are superior with respect to different samples. To this end, chaotropes such as urea, which act by changing the parameters of the solvent, are used in most 2D PAGE procedures.

Major problems to overcome in 2D PAGE sample preparation arise because of limited entry into the gel of high-molecular-weight proteins and the presence of highly hydrophobic and/or basic proteins *(42, 43)*.

For protein separation, the protein mixture is loaded onto an acrylamide gel strip in which a pH gradient is established. When a high voltage is applied over the strip, the proteins will focus at the pH at which they carry zero net charge. The pH gradient is established during the focusing using either carrier ampholytes in a slab gel *(44)* or a precast polyacrylamide gel with an immobilized pH gradient (IPG) *(45)*. The latter method is advantageous because of improved reproducibility. Samples can be applied to IPG dry strips preferably by rehydration. Rehydration of dried IPGs under application of a low voltage (10 to 50 V) has significantly improved the recovery especially of high-molecular-weight proteins.

25.3.2 Mass Spectrometry

Mass spectrometry is the method of choice for identifying proteins in proteomics. The proteins are converted into gas phase ions that can be measured with an accuracy better than 50 ppm *(40)*. Two widely used techniques for ionization are matrix-assisted laser desorption ionization (MALDI) *(46)* and electrospray ionization *(47)*. MALDI is usually coupled with a TOF (time of flight) device for measuring the masses. The ionized peptides are then accelerated by the application of accelerated field and the TOF until they reach a detector to calculate their mass/charge ratio *(40)*.

In electrospray ionization, the peptides are sprayed into the spectrometer *(47)*. Ionization is achieved when the charged droplets evaporate. An alternative procedure for measuring masses is the ion trap *(48)*, which selects ions with certain mass/charge ratios by keeping them in sinusoidal motion between two electrodes.

25.4 NIAID Research Programs in Genomic Research

In 1995, the first microbe sequencing project, *Haemophilus influenzae* (a bacterium causing upper respiratory infection), was completed with a speed that stunned scientists (http://www3.niaid.nih.gov/research/topics/pathogen/Introduction.htm). Encouraged by the success of that initial effort, researchers have continued to sequence an astonishing array of other medically important microorganisms. To this end, NIAID has made significant investments in large-scale sequencing projects, including projects to sequence the complete genomes of many pathogens, such as the bacteria that cause tuberculosis, gonorrhea, chlamydia, and cholera, as well as organisms that are considered agents of bioterrorism. In addition, NIAID is collaborating with other funding agencies to sequence larger genomes of protozoan pathogens such as the organism causing malaria.

The availability of microbial and human DNA sequences opens up new opportunities and allows scientists to perform functional analyses of genes and proteins in whole genomes and cells, as well as the host's immune response and an individual's genetic susceptibility to pathogens. When scientists identify microbial genes that play a role in disease, drugs can be designed to block the activities controlled by those genes. Because most genes contain the instructions for making proteins, drugs can be designed to inhibit specific proteins or to use those proteins as candidates for vaccine testing. Genetic variations can also be used to study the spread of a virulent or drug-resistant form of a pathogen.

25.4.1 Genomic Initiatives

NIAID has launched initiatives to provide comprehensive genomic, proteomic, and bioinformatic resources. These resources, listed below, are available to scientists conducting basic and applied research on a broad array of pathogenic microorganisms (http://www3.niaid.nih.gov/research/topics/pathogen/initiatives.htm):

- *NIAID's Microbial Sequencing Centers (NSCs)*. The NIAID's Microbial Sequencing Centers are state-of-the-art high-throughput DNA sequencing centers that can sequence genomes of microbes and invertebrate vectors of infectious diseases. Genomes that can be sequenced include microorganisms considered agents of bioterrorism and those responsible for emerging and re-emerging infectious diseases.
- *NIAID's Pathogen Functional Genomics Resource Center (PFGRC)*. NIAID's Pathogen Functional Genomics Resource Center is a centralized facility that provides scientists with the resources and reagents necessary to conduct functional genomics research on human pathogens and invertebrate vectors at no cost. The PFGRC provides scientists with genomic resources and reagents such as microarrays, protein expression clones, genotyping, and bioinformatics services. The PFGRC supports the training of scientists in the latest techniques in functional genomics and emerging genomic technologies.
- *NIAID's Proteomics Centers*. The primary goal of these centers is to characterize the pathogen and/or host cell proteome by identifying proteins associated with the biology of the microorganisms, mechanisms of microbial pathogenesis, innate and adaptive immune responses to infectious agents, and/or non–immune-mediated host

responses that contribute to microbial pathogenesis. It is anticipated that the research programs will discover targets for potential candidates for the next generation of vaccines, therapeutics, and diagnostics. This will be accomplished by using existing proteomics technologies, augmenting existing technologies, and creating novel proteomics approaches as well as performing early-stage validation of these targets.

- *Administrative Resource for Biodefense Proteomic Centers (ARBPCs)*. The ARBPCs consolidate data generated by each proteomics research center and make it available to the scientific community through a publicly accessible Web site. This database (www.proteomicsresource.org) serves as a central information source for reagents and validated protein targets and has recently been populated with the first data released.
- *NIAID's Bioinformatics Resource Centers*. The NIAID's Bioinformatics Resource Centers will design, develop, maintain, and continuously update multiorganism databases, especially those related to biodefense. Organisms of particular interest are the NIAID Category A to C priority pathogens and those causing emerging and re-emerging diseases. The ultimate goal is to establish databases that will allow scientists to access a large amount of genomic and related data. This will facilitate the identification of potential targets for the development of vaccines, therapeutics, and diagnostics. Each contract will include establishing and maintaining an analysis resource that will serve as a companion to the databases to provide, develop, and enhance standard and advanced analytical tools to help researchers access and analyze data.
- A joint collaboration between NIAID and the National Institute of General Medical Sciences (NIGMS) is providing research funding for the *Protein Structure Initiative (PSI) Centers*:

  ○ *TB Structural Genomics Consortium*. A collaboration of scientists in six countries formed to determine and analyze the structures of about 400 proteins from *Mycobacterium tuberculosis*. The group seeks to optimize the technical and management aspects of high-throughput structure determination and will develop a database of structures and functions. NIAID, which is co-funding this project with NIGMS, anticipates that this information will also lead to the design of new and improved drugs and vaccines for tuberculosis.
  ○ *Structural Genomics of Pathogenic Protozoa Consortium*. This consortium is aiming to develop new ways to solve protein structures from organisms known as protozoans, many species of which cause

deadly diseases such as sleeping sickness, malaria, and Chagas' disease.

25.4.2 Recent Programmatic Accomplishments

25.4.2.1 Genome Sequencing

The National Institute of Allergy and Infectious Diseases is providing support to the *Microbial Genome Sequencing Centers* (MSCs) at the J. Craig Venter Institute [formerly, the Institute for Genomic Research (TIGR)], the Broad Institute at the Massachusetts Institute of Technology (MIT), and Harvard University for a rapid and cost-efficient production of high-quality, microbial genome sequences and primary annotations. NIAID's MSCs (http://www.niaid.nih.gov/dmid/genomes/mscs/) are responding to the scientific community and national and federal agencies' priorities for genome sequencing, filling in sequence gaps, and therefore providing genome sequencing data for multiple uses including understanding the biology of microorganisms, forensic strain identification, and identifying targets for drugs, vaccines, and diagnostics. In addition, the NIAID's MSCs have developed Web sites that provide descriptive information about the sequencing projects and their progress (http://www.broad.mit.edu/seq/msc/ and http://msc.tigr.org/status.shtml).

Genomes to be sequenced include microorganisms considered to be potential agents of bioterrorism (NIAID Category A, B, and C), related organisms, clinical isolates, closely related species, and invertebrate vectors of infectious diseases and microorganisms responsible for emerging and re-emerging infectious diseases.

In addition, in response to a recommendation from a 2002 NIAID-sponsored Blue Ribbon Panel on Bioterrorism and its Implication for Biomedical Research to support genomic sequencing of microorganisms considered agents of bioterrorism and related organisms, the MSCs will address the institute's need for additional sequencing of such microorganisms and invertebrate vectors of disease and/or those that are responsible for emerging and re-emerging diseases (http://www.niaid.nih.gov/dmid/genomes/mscs/overview.htm). The panel's recommendation included careful selection of species, strains, and clinical isolates to generate genomic data for different uses such as identification of strains and targets for diagnostics, vaccines, antimicrobials, and other drug developments.

The MSCs have the capacity to rapidly and cost-effectively sequence genomic DNA and provide preliminary identification of open reading frames and annotation of gene function for a wide variety of microorganisms, including viruses, bacteria, protozoa, parasites, and fungi. Sequencing projects will be considered for both complete, finished genome sequencing and other levels of sequence coverage. The choice and justification of complete versus draft sequence is likely to depend on the nature and scope of the proposed project.

Large-scale prepublication information on genome sequences is a unique research resource for the scientific community, and rapid and unrestricted sharing of microbial genome sequence data is essential for advancing research on infectious agents responsible for human disease. Therefore, it is anticipated that prepublication data on genome sequences produced at the NIAID Microbial Sequencing Centers will be made freely and publicly available via an appropriate publicly searchable database as rapidly as possible.

Completed Genome Sequencing Projects in 2006

NIAID-supported investigators have completed 131 genome sequencing projects for 105 bacteria, 8 fungi, 15 parasitic protozoa, 2 invertebrate vectors of infectious diseases, and one plant (http://www.niaid.nih.gov/dmid/genomes/mscs/req_process.htm). In addition, NIAID completed the sequence for 1,467 influenza genomes. In 2006, genome sequencing projects were completed for 22 pathogens as described in Section 23.16.2. Genome sequencing data is publicly available through Web sites such as GenBank, and data for the influenza genome sequences have been published in 2006.

Furthermore, through the NIAID's Microbial Sequencing Centers, the NIAID has funded the sequence, assembly, and annotation of three invertebrate vectors of infectious diseases. In 2006, the final sequence, assembly, and the annotation of *Aedes aegyptii* were released, as well as the preliminary sequence and assembly of the genomes for *Ixodes scapularis* and *Culex pipiens*; the final results for *I. scapularis* and *C. pipiens* will be released in 2007.

Genome Sequencing Projects in Progress

In 2006, NIAID supported nearly 40 large-scale genome sequencing projects for additional strains of viruses, bacteria, fungi, parasites, viruses, and invertebrate vectors. New projects included additional strains of *Borrelia, Clostridium, Escherichia coli, Salmonella, Streptococcus pneumonia, Ureaplasma, Coccidioides, Penicillium marneffei, Talaromyces stipitatus, Lacazia loboi, Histoplasma capsulatum, Blastomyces dermatitidis, Cryptosporidium muris,* and dengue viruses, as well as additional sequencing and annotation of *Aedes aegyptii*.

25.4.2.2 Influenza Genome Sequencing Project

In 2004, NIAID launched the *Influenza Genome Sequencing Project (IGSP)* (http://www.niaid.nih.gov/dmid/genomes/mscs/influenza.htm), which has provided the scientific community with complete genome sequence data for thousands of human and animal influenza viruses. The influenza sequence data has been rapidly placed in the public domain, through GenBank, an international searchable database, and the NIAID-funded Bioinformatics Resource Center with accompanying data analysis tools. All of the information will enable scientists to further study how influenza viruses evolve, spread, and cause disease and may ultimately lead to improved methods of treatment and prevention. This sequence information is now providing a larger and more representative sample of influenza than was previously publicly available. The Influenza Genome Sequencing Project has the capacity to sequence more than 200 genomes per month and is a collaborative effort among NIAID (including the NIAID's Division of Intramural Research), the National Center for Biotechnology Information at the National Library of Medicine, NIH (NCBI/NLM/NIH), the J. Craig Venter Institute, the Wadsworth Center at the New York State Department of Health, St. Jude Children's Research Hospital in Memphis, Ohio State University, the Canterbury Health Laboratories (New Zealand), Los Alamos National Laboratories, OIE/FAO International Reference Laboratory, Baylor College of Medicine, and others. As of September 2006, 1,467 complete genome sequences for influenza viruses were released to GenBank, including the H1N1, H1N2, and H3N2 viruses from human clinical isolates collected globally from 1931 to 2006, as well as other isolates from different hosts including birds, horses, swine, and ducks. Additional information can be found at http://www.ncbi.nlm.nih.gov/genomes/FLU/Database/shipment.cgi

25.4.2.3 Functional Genomics

NIAID is continuing its support for the *Pathogen Functional Genomics Resource Center (PFGRC)* (http://www.niaid.nih.gov/dmid/genomes/pfgrc/default.htm) at The Institute for Genomic Research (TIGR) (currently part of the J. Craig Venter Institute). The PFGRC was established in 2001 to provide and distribute to the broader research community a wide range of genomic resources, reagents, data, and technologies for the functional analysis of microbial pathogens and invertebrate vectors of infectious diseases. In addition, the PFGRC was expanded to provide the research community with the resources and reagents needed to conduct both basic and applied research on microorganisms responsible for emerging and re-emerging infectious diseases and those considered agents of bioterrorism.

Bioinformatic Software Tools and Web Site Enhancements

One of the priorities for the PFGRC has been to provide the scientific community with access to the reagents and genomic and proteomic data that the PFGRC generated. A new software tool, called *SNP filtering tool*, was developed for Affymetrix resequencing arrays to analyze the single nucleotide polymorphism (SNP) data. Enhancements have been made to other tools for microarray data analysis, including a tool for analyzing slide images. A new layout for the TIGR-PFGRC Web site (http://pfgrc.tigr.org/) has been developed and launched and has the potential to be more user-friendly for the scientific community to access the PFGRC research and development projects, poster presentations, publications, reagents, and their descriptions and data.

DNA Microarrays

The number of organism-specific microarrays produced and distributed to the scientific community increased to 28 in 2006 and now includes arrays for viruses, bacteria, fungi, and parasites. The available organism-specific arrays include *Aspergillus fumigatus, Aspergillus nidulans, Candida albicans, Chlamydia,* coronaviruses (animal and human), human SARS chip, *Helicobacter pylori, Mycobacterium smegmatis, Neisseria gonorrhoeae, Plasmodium falciparum, Plasmodium vivax, Pseudomonas aeruginosa, Staphylococcus aureus, Streptococcus agalactiae, Streptococcus pneumoniae, Trypanosoma brucei,* and *Trypanosoma cruzi.* In addition, organism-specific microarrays were produced and distributed for organisms considered agents of bioterrorism, including *Bacillus anthracis, Burkholderia, Clostridium botulinum, Francisella tularensis, Giardia lamblia, Listeria monocytogenes, Mycobacterium tuberculosis, Rickettsia prowazekii, Salmonella typhimurium, Vibrio cholerae,* and *Yersinia pestis.*

PFGRC has continued to collaborate with the National Institute of Dental and Craniofacial Research (NIDCR/NIH) in producing and distributing five organism-specific microarrays, including arrays for *Actinobacillus actinomycetemcomitans, Fusobacterium nucleatum, Porphyromonas gingivalis, Streptococcus mutans,* and *Treponema denticola.*

Protein Expression Clones

PFGRC has also developed the methods and pipeline for generating organism-specific clones for protein expression.

Seven complete clone sets are now available for human severe acute respiratory syndrome coronavirus (SARS-CoV), *Bacillus anthracis, Yersinia pestis, Francisella tularensis, Streptococcus pneumoniae, Staphylococcus aureus*, and *Mycobacterium tuberculosis.* In addition, individual custom clone sets are available for more than 20 organisms upon request.

Comparative Genomics

Comparative genomics analysis using the available *Bacillus anthracis* sequence data and the discovery of the SNPs were used to develop a new bacterial typing system for screening anthrax strains. This system allowed NIAID-funded scientists to define detailed phylogenetic lineages of *Bacillus anthracis* and to identify three major lineages (A, B, C) with the ancestral root located between the A+B and C branches. In addition, a genotyping Genechip, which has been developed and validated for *Bacillus anthracis*, will be used to genotype about 300 different strains of *Bacillus anthracis.*

PFGRC has developed additional comparative genomic platforms for both facilitating the resequencing a bacterial genome on a chip to identify sequence variation among strains and to discover novel genes. A pilot project has been completed with *Streptococcus pneumoniae* for sequencing different strains using resequencing chip technology. In collaboration with the Department of Homeland Security (DHS), a resequencing chip has been developed and is now being used to screen a number of *Francisella tularensis* strains to identify SNPs and genetic polymorphisms. Sixteen *Francisella tularensis* strains are being genotyped by using the newly developed resequencing chip. Additional collaboration with DHS led to the development of a gene discovery platform aimed at discovering novel genes among different strains of *Yersinia pestis*. To this end, nine strains are being analyzed using this platform to discover novel gene sets.

Proteomics

PFGRC is developing proteomics technologies for protein arrays and comparative profiling of microbial proteins. A protein expression platform is under development, and a pilot comparative protein profiling project using *Staphylococcus aureus* has already been completed and published. A protein profiling project using *Yersinia pestis* to compare proteomes in different strains is now under way, complementing ongoing proteomics projects supported by NIAID; numerous proteins are currently being identified that are differently abundant during different growth conditions.

A new project was added in 2006 for comparative profiling of proteins on the proteomes of *E. coli* and *Shigella dysenteriae* to provide the scientific community with reference data on differential protein expression in animal models versus cultured systems infected with the pathogen.

25.4.2.4 Population Genetics Analysis Program: Immunity to Vaccines/Infections

In 2006, NIAID continued to support the *Population Genetics Analysis Program: Immunity to Vaccines/Infections.* A joint project between NIAID's Division of Allergy, Immunity, and Transplantation (DAIT) and the Division of Microbiology and Infectious Diseases (DMID), this program is aimed to identify associations between specific genetic variations or polymorphisms in immune response genes and the susceptibility to infection or response to vaccination, with a focus on one or more NIAID Category A to C pathogens and influenza.

NIAID awarded six centers to study the genetic basis for the variable human response to immunization (smallpox, typhoid fever, cholera, and anthrax) and susceptibility to disease (tuberculosis, influenza, encapsulated bacterial diseases, and West Nile virus infection). The centers are comparing genetic variance in specific immune response genes as well as more generally associated genetic variance across the whole genome in affected and nonaffected individuals. The physiologic differences associated with these genome variations will also be studied. In 2006, these centers focused on recruiting the samples needed for genotyping. For example, more than 1,100 smallpox-vaccinated individuals and controls were recruited and blood and peripheral blood mononuclear cell (PBMC) samples were obtained for whole genome association studies, which were conducted in 2007.

In another example, one of the centers used genome-wide linkage approaches to map, isolate, and validate human host genes that confer susceptibility to influenza infection. Nearly 1,000 individuals with susceptibility to influenza and 2,000 control individuals were recruited using an Iceland genealogy database. By late 2006, the center had recruited more than 600 individuals and had genotyped more than 500 in this subproject of the study.

25.4.2.5 Microbial Bioinformatics

During 2006, NIAID continued its support of the eight *Bioinformatics Resource Centers (BRCs)* (http://www. niaid.nih.gov/dmid/genomes/brc/default.htm) with the goal of providing the scientific community with a publicly accessible resource that allows easy access to genomic and related data for the NIAID Category A to C priority pathogens, invertebrate vectors of infectious diseases, and pathogens causing emerging and re-emerging infectious diseases. The

BRCs are supported by multidisciplinary teams of scientists to develop new and improved computational tools and interfaces that can facilitate the analysis and interpretation of the genomic-related data by the scientific community. In 2006, each publicly accessible BRC Web site continued to be developed, the user interfaces were improved, and a variety of genomics data types were integrated, including gene expression and proteomics information, host/pathogen interactions, and signaling/metabolic pathways data. A public portal of information, data, and open-source software tools generated by all the BRCs is available at http://www.brc-central.org/. In 2006, many genomes of microbial species were sequenced by the NIAID's Microbial Sequencing Centers as well as by other national and international sequencing efforts, and the BRCs provided either long-term maintenance of the genome sequence data and annotation or the initial annotation for a number of particular microbial genomes. For example, NIAID's BRC VectorBase collaborated with NIAID's MSCs to annotate the genome of *Aedes aegyptii* with the scientific community and will continue the curation of this genome.

25.4.2.6 Microbial Proteomics

In 2006, NIAID continued to support contracts for seven *Biodefense Proteomics Research Centers (BPRCs)* to characterize the proteome of NIAID Category A to C bioweapon agents and to develop and enhance innovative proteomic technologies and apply them to the understanding of the pathogen and/or host cell proteome (http://www.niaid.nih.gov/dmid/genomes/prc/default.htm). These centers conducted a range of proteomics studies, including six Category A pathogens, six Category B pathogens, and one Category C emerging disease organism. Data, reagents, and protocols developed in the research centers are released to the NIAID-funded Administrative Resource for Biodefense Proteomics Research Centers (www.proteomicsresource.org) Web site within 2 months of validation. The Administrative Resource Web site was created to integrate the diverse data generated by the BPRCs. In 2005, more than 700 potential targets for vaccines, therapeutics, and diagnostics were generated. Examples of progress include:

(i) The elucidation of five SARS-CoV open reading frame (ORF) structures.
(ii) Cloning for expression studies of 99% of the ORFs for *V. cholerae*.
(iii) Development of multiple protocols for extracellular components and membrane subfractionation prior to mass spectroscopy.
(iv) Accurate time and mass tag databases have been populated for *Salmonella typhimurium*.

In 2006, more than 2,400 potential new pathogen targets for vaccines, therapeutics, and diagnostics were identified, and more than 5,700 new corresponding host targets were generated. In addition:

(i) Two more SARS-CoV structures were solved.
(ii) Ninety-six percent of the ORFs for *B. anthracis* were cloned with 47% sequence validated.
(iii) A custom *B. anthracis* Affymetrix GeneChip was developed.
(iv) Fifty-three polyclonal sera generated against novel *Toxoplasma gondii* and *Cryptosporidium parvum* proteins were characterized, and accurate time and mass tag databases were populated for *Salmonella typhi*, monkeypox, and vaccinia virus.

25.4.2.7 Transgenomic Activities

● NIAID staff are participating in two related NIH-wide genomic initiatives that focus on examining and identifying genetic variations across the human genome (genes) that may be linked or influence susceptibility or risk to a common human disease, such as asthma, autoimmunity, cancer, eye diseases, mental illness, and infectious diseases, or response to treatment as a vaccine. The approach is to conduct genome-wide association studies in which a dense set of SNPs across the human genome is genotyped in a large defined group of controls and diseases samples to identify genetic variations that may contribute to or have a role in the disease, with the hope of identifying an association between a genetic variant in a gene or group of genes and the disease.

○ *GAIN (Genome Association Identification Network).* GAIN is a public-private partnership alliance with Pfizer Corp., Affymetrix, and NIH and managed by the NIH Foundation to bring new scientific and financial resources to NIH for genome-wide association studies (www.fnih.org/GAIN/GAIN_home.shtml). Initially, Pfizer Corp. has committed US$20 million for management and genotyping capacity for five common diseases in partnership with Perlegen Sciences. Investigators were invited initially to submit applications to have genotyping performed on existing DNA samples from patients with specific diseases and control individuals in case control studies. The GAIN initiative proposes to raise additional private funds for genotyping of more common diseases.

○ *GWAS (Genome-Wide Association Studies).* GWAS is a trans-NIH committee that is focused on developing an NIH-wide policy for sharing data obtained in NIH-supported or conducted Genome-Wide Association Studies. The policy is to focus on data sharing procedures, data access principles, intellectual policy, and issues related to protection of research participants. In 2006, the proposed policy has been shared with the scientific community for public comment as a NIH Guide Request for Information (RFI).

- NIAID has continued to participate in a coordinated federal effort in biodefense genomics and is a major participant in the *National Inter-Agency Genomics Sciences Coordinating Committee (NIGSCC)*, which includes many federal agencies. This committee was formed in 2002 to address the most serious gaps in the comprehensive genomic analysis of microorganisms considered agents of bioterrorism. A comprehensive list of microorganisms considered agents of bioterrorism was developed that identifies species, strains, and clinical and environmental isolates that have been sequenced, that are currently being sequenced, and that should be sequenced.

In 2003, the committee focused on Category A agents and provided the CDC with new technological approaches for sequencing additional smallpox viral strains. Affymetrix-based microarray technology for genome sequencing was established, as well as additional bioinformatics expertise for analyzing the genomic sequencing data. In 2004, as a result of this continuing coordination of federal agencies in genome sequencing efforts for biodefense, NIAID developed a formal interagency agreement with the Department of Homeland Security (DHS) to perform comparative genomics analysis to characterize biothreat agents at the genetic level and to examine polymorphisms for identifying genetic variations and relatedness within and between species.

- NIAID continues to participate in the *Microbe Project Interagency Working Group (IWG)*, which has developed a coordinated, interagency, 5-year action plan on microbial genomics, including functional genomics and bioinformatics in 2001 (http://www.ostp.gov/html/microbial/start.htm). In 2003, the Microbe Project Interagency Working Group developed guidelines for sharing prepublication genomic sequencing data that serve as guiding principles, so that federal agencies have consistent policies for sharing sequencing data with the scientific community and can then implement their own detailed version of the data release plan. In 2004, the Microbe Project IWG supported a workshop on "An Experimental Approach to Genome Annotation," which was coordinated by the American Society for Microbiology, and discussed issues faced in annotating microbial genome sequences that have been completed or will be completed in the next few years. In 2005, the Microbe Project IWG developed a Strategic Plan and Implementation Steps as an updated action plan

for coordinating microbial genomics among federal agencies, and the plan was finalized in 2006.

- NIAID continues to participate with other federal agencies in coordinating medical diagnostics for biodefense and influenza across the federal government and in facilitating the development of a set of contracts to support advanced development toward the approval of new or improved point-of-care diagnostic tests for the influenza virus and early manufacturing and commercialization.

- NIAID continues to participate in the NIH Roadmap Initiatives, including Lead Science Officers for one of the National Centers for Biomedical Computation and one of the National Technology Centers for Networks and Pathways. Seven biomedical computing centers are developing a universal computing infrastructure and creating innovative software programs and other tools that would enable the biomedical community to integrate, analyze, model, simulate, and share data on human health and disease. Five technology centers were created in 2004 and 2005 to cooperate in a U.S. national effort to develop new technologies for proteomics and the study of dynamic biological systems.

25.4.3 Resources for Researchers

25.4.3.1 NIAID-Supported Sequencing Centers

- Bioinformatics Resource Centers
- Microbial Sequencing Centers
- Pathogen Functional Genomics Resource Center
- Proteomics Research Centers

25.4.3.2 Genome Sequence Databases

- Administrative Resource for Biodefense Proteomic Centers
- ATCC Animal Virology Collection
- BRC (Bioinformatics Research Centers) Central
- Malaria Research and Reference Reagent Resource (MR4) Center

25.4.3.3 Sequencing Projects

- NIAID Influenza Genome Sequencing Project
- The Microbe Project: U.S. Federal Efforts in Microbial Research
- Network on Antimicrobial Resistance in *Staphylococcus aureus* (NARSA)

25.5 Recent Scientific Advances

- *Supramolecular Architecture of Severe Acute Respiratory Syndrome Coronavirus (SARS-CoV)*. Coronaviruses derive their name from their protruding oligomers of the spike glycoprotein (S), which forms a coronal ridge around the virion. The understanding of the virion and its organization has previously been limited to x-ray crystallography of homogenous symmetric virions, whereas coronaviruses are neither homogenous nor symmetric. In this study, a novel methodology of single-particle image analysis was applied to selected coronavirus features to obtain a detailed model of the oligomeric state and spatial relationships among viral structural proteins. The two-dimensional structures of S, M, and N structural proteins of SARS-CoV and two other coronaviruses were determined and refined to a resolution of approximately 4 nm. These results demonstrated a higher level of supramolecular organization than was previously known for coronaviruses and provided the first detailed view of the coronavirus ultrastructure. Understanding the architecture of the virion is a necessary first step to defining the assembly pathway of SARS-CoV and may aid in developing new or improved therapeutics *(49)*.

- *Large-Scale Sequence Analysis of Avian Influenza Isolates*. Avian influenza is a significant global human health threat because of its potential to infect humans and result in a global influenza pandemic. However, very little sequence information for avian influenza virus (AIV) has been in the public domain. A more comprehensive collection of publicly available sequence data for AIV is necessary for research on influenza to understand how flu evolves, spreads, and causes disease, to shed light on the emergence of influenza epidemics and pandemics, and to uncover new targets for drugs, vaccines, and diagnostics. In this study, the investigators released genomic data from the first large-scale sequencing of AIV isolates, doubling the amount of AIV sequence data in the public domain. These sequence data include 2,196 AIV genes and 169 complete genomes from a diverse sample of birds. The preliminary analysis of these sequences, along with other AIV data from the public domain, revealed new information about AIV, including the identification of a genome sequence that may be a determinant of virulence. This study provides valuable sequencing data to the scientific community and demonstrates how informative large-scale sequence analysis can be in identifying potential markers of disease *(50)*.

First Large-Scale Sequencing and Analysis of Human Influenza Viruses Supported by the NIAID-Funded Influenza Genome Sequencing Project. The analysis of the first 209 full genome sequences from human influenza strains, deposited in GenBank through the NIAID Influenza Genome Sequencing Project, was published in 2006 *(51)*. Influenza isolates were chosen in a relatively unbiased manner, allowing a comprehensive look at the influenza virus population circulating within the same geographic region over several seasons, which provided a real picture of the dynamics of influenza virus mutation and evolution. Analysis demonstrated that the circulating strains of influenza included alternative minor lineages that could provide genetic variation for the dominant strain. This may allow a novel strain to emerge within a human host and would explain the unexpected emergence of the Fujian influenza strain in 2003–2004 that resulted in a vaccine mismatch. These findings demonstrate the usefulness of full genomic sequences for providing new information on influenza viruses and lend further support for the need for large-scale influenza sequencing and the availability of sequence data in the public domain. Within the influenza community, public availability of influenza sequence data and sharing of strains has been an important issue. The NIAID has been instrumental in promoting the sharing of influenza sequence information, notably by sequencing more than 1,400 complete influenza genome sequences and depositing the sequences in the public domain through GenBank as soon as sequencing has been completed.

References

1. Smith, H. O. (2004) History of microbial genomics. In: *Microbial Genomes* (Fraser, C. M., Read, T. D., and Nelson, K. E., eds.), Humana Press, Totowa, NJ, pp. 3–16.
2. Salzberg, S. L. and Delcher, A. L. (2004) Tools for gene finding and whole genome comparison. In: *Microbial Genomes* (Fraser, C. M., Read, T. D., and Nelson, K. E., eds.), Humana Press, Totowa, NJ, pp. 19–31.
3. Salzberg, S. L., Pertea, M., Delcher, A. L., Gardner, M. J., and Tettelin, H. (1999). Interpolated Markov models for eukaryotic gene finding, *Genomics*, **59**, 24–31.
4. Pertea, M. and Salzberg, S. L. (2002) Computational gene finding in plants, *Plant Mol. Biol.*, **48**, 39–48.
5. Parkhill, J. and Thomson, N. R. (2004) The genomes of pathogenic Enterobacteria. In: *Microbial Genomes* (Fraser, C. M., Read, T. D., and Nelson, K. E., eds.), Humana Press, Totowa, NJ, pp. 269–289.
6. Blattner, F. R., Plunkett, G., Bloch, C. A., et al. (1997) The complete genome sequence of *Escherichia coli* K-12, *Science*, **277**, 1453–1474.
7. Perna, N. T., Plunkett, G., 3rd, Burland, V., et al. (2001) Genome sequence of enterohemorrhagic *Escherichia coli* O157:H7, *Nature*, **409**, 529–533.
8. Hayashi, T., Makino, K., Ohnishi, M., et al. (2001) Complete genome sequence of enterohemorrhagic *Escherichia coli* O157:H7 and genomic comparison with a laboratory strain K-12, *DNA Res.*, **8**, 11–22.
9. Welch, R. A., Burland, V., Plunkett, G. 3rd, et al. (2002) Extensive mosaic structure revealed by the complete genome sequence of uropathogenic *Escherichia coli*, *Proc. Natl. Acad. Sci. U.S.A.*, **99**, 17020–17024.

10. Jin, Q., Yuan, Z., Xu, J., et al. (2002) Genome sequence of *Shigella flexneri* 2a: insights into pathogenicity through comparison with genomes of *Escherichia coli* K12 and O157, *Nucleic Acids Res.*, **30**, 4432–4441.

11. Knapp, S., Hacker, J., Jarchau, T., and Goebel, W. (1986) Large, unstable inserts in the chromosome affect virulence properties of uropathogenic *Escherichia coli* O6 strain 536, *J. Bacteriol.*, **168**, 22–30.

12. Levine, M. M. (1987) *Escherichia coli* that cause diarrhea: enterotoxigenic, enteropathogenic, enteroinvasive, enterohemorrhagic, and enteroadherent, *J. Infect. Dis.*, **155**, 377–389.

13. Hacker, J., Blum-Oehler, G., Muhldorfer, I., and Tschape, H. (1997) Pathogenicity islands of virulent bacteria: structure, function and impact on microbial evolution, *Mol. Microbiol.*, **23**, 1089–1097.

14. Blum, G., Ott, M., Lischewski, A., et al. (1994) Excision of large DNA regions termed pathogenicity islands from tRNA-specific loci in the chromosome of an *Escherichia coli* wild-type pathogen, *Infect. Immunol.*, **62**, 606–614.

15. Parkhill, J., Dougan, G., James, K. D., et al. (2001) Complete genome sequence of multiple drug resistant *Salmonella enterica* serovar Typhi CT18, *Nature*, **413**, 848–852.

16. McClelland, M., Sanderson, K. E., Spieth, J., et al. (2001) Complete genome sequence of *Salmonella enterica* serovar Typhimurium LT2, *Nature*, **413**, 852–856.

17. Reeves, P. and Stevenson, G. (1989) Cloning and nucleotide sequence of the *Salmonella typhimurium* LT2 gnd gene and its homology with the corresponding sequence of *Escherichia coli* K12, *Mol. Gen. Genet.*, **217**, 182–184.

18. Mills, D. M., Bajaj, V., and Lee, C. A. (1995) A 40 kb chromosomal fragment encoding *Salmonella typhimurium* invasion genes is absent from the corresponding region of the *Escherichia coli* K-12 chromosome, *Mol. Microbiol.* **15**, 749–759.

19. Galan, J. E. (1996) Molecular genetic bases of *Salmonella* entry into host cells, *Mol. Microbiol.*, **20**, 263–271.

20. Shea, J. E., Hensel, M., Gleeson, C., and Holden, D. W. (1996) Identification of a virulence locus encoding a second type III secretion system in *Salmonella typhimurium*, *Proc. Natl. Acad. Sci. U.S.A.*, **93**, 2593–2597.

21. Ochman, H., Soncini, F. C., Solomon, F., and Groisman, E. A. (1996) Identification of a pathogenicity island required for *Salmonella* survival in host cells, *Proc. Natl. Acad. Sci. U.S.A.*, **93**, 7800–7804.

22. Kingsley, R. A. and Baumler, A. J. (2002) Pathogenicity islands and host adaptation of *Salmonella* serovars, *Curr. Top. Microbiol. Immunol.*, **264**, 67–87.

23. Blanc-Potard, A. B. and Groisman, E. A. (1997) The *Salmonella selC* locus contains a pathogenicity island mediating intramacrophage survival, *EMBO J.*, **16**, 5376–5385.

24. Buchrieser, C., Prentice, M., and Carniel, E. (1998) The 102-kb unstable region of *Yersinia pestis* comprises a high-pathogenicity island linked to a pigmentation segment which undergoes internal rearrangement, *J. Bacteriol.*, **180**, 2321–2329.

25. Reiter, W. D., Palm, P., and Yeats, S. (1989) Transfer RNA genes frequently serve as integration sites for prokaryotic genetic elements, *Nucleic Acid Res.*, **17**, 1907–1914.

26. Makino, K., Yokoyama, K., Kubota, Y., et al. (1999) Complete nucleotide sequence of the prophage VT2-Sakai carrying the verotoxin 2 genes of the enterohemorrhagic *Escherichia coli* O157:H7 derived from the Sakai outbreak, *Genes Genet. Syst.*, **74**, 227–239.

27. Mosig, G., Yu, S., Myung, H., et al. (1997) A novel mechanism of virus-virus interactions: bacteriophage P2 Tin protein inhibits phage T4 DNA synthesis by poisoning the T4 single-stranded DNA binding protein, go32, *Virology*, **230**, 72–81.

28. Myung, H. and Calendar, R. (1995) The *old* exonuclease of bacteriophage P2, *J. Bacteriol.*, **177**, 497–501.

29. Davis, B. M. and Waldor, M. K. (2003) Filamentous phages linked to virulence of *Vibrio cholerae*, *Curr. Opin. Microbiol.*, **6**, 35–42.

30. Donohue-Rolfe, A., Acheson, D. W., and Keusch, G. T. (1999) Shiga toxin: purification, structure, and function, *Rev. Infect. Dis.*, **13**(Suppl. 4), S293–S297.

31. Parkhill, J., Wren, B. W., Thomson, N. R., et al. (2001) Genome sequence of Y*ersinia pestis*, the causative agent of plague, *Nature*, **413**, 523–527.

32. Hansen-Wester, I. and Hensel, M. (2001) *Salmonella* pathogenicity islands encoding type III secretion systems, *Microbes Infect.*, **3**, 549–559.

33. Lostroh, C. P. and Lee, C. A. (2001) The *Salmonella* pathogenicity island-1 type III secretion system, *Microbes Infect.*, **3**, 1281–1291.

34. Swartley, J. S., Marfin, A. A., Edupuganti, S., et al. (1997) Capsule switching of *Neisseria meningitides*, *Proc. Natl. Acad. Sci. U.S.A.*, **94**, 271–276.

35. Dillard, J. P., Caimano, M., Kelly, T., and Yother, J. (1995) Capsules and cassettes: genetic organization of the capsule locus of *Streptococcus pneumoniae*, *Dev. Biol. Stand.*, **85**, 261–265.

36. Dillard, J. P. and Yother, J. (1994) Genetic and molecular characterization of capsular polysaccharide biosynthesis in *Streptococcus pneumoniae* type 3, *Mol. Microbiol.*, **12**, 959–972.

37. Cole, S. T., Eiglmeier, K., Parkhill, J., et al. (2001) Massive gene decay in the leprosy bacillus, *Nature*, **409**, 1007–1011.

38. Perry, R. D. and Fetherston, J. D. (1997) *Yersinia pestis* – etiologic agent of plague, *Clin. Microbiol. Rev.*, **10**, 35–66.

39. Achtman, M., Zurth, K., Morelli, G., Torrea, G., Guiyoule, A., and Carniel, E. (1999) *Yersinia pestis*, the cause of plague, is a recently emerged clone of *Yersinia pseudotuberculosis*, *Proc. Natl. Acad. Sci. U.S.A.*, **96**, 14043–14048.

40. Birkelund, S., Vandahl, B. B., Shaw, A. C., and Christiansen, G. (2004) Microbial proteomics. In: *Microbial Genomes* (Fraser, C. M., Read, T. D., and Nelson, K. E., eds.), Humana Press, Totowa, NJ, pp. 517–530.

41. Wilkins, M. P., Pasquali, C., Appel, R. D., et al. (1996) From proteins to proteomes: large scale protein identification by two-dimensional electrophoresis and amino acid analysis, *Biotechnology (NY)*, **14**, 61–65.

42. Santoni, V., Molloy, M., and Rabilloud, T. (2000) Membrane proteins and proteomics: un amour impossible? *Electrophoresis*, **21**, 1054–1070.

43. Adessi, C., Miege, C., Albrieux, C., and Rabilloud, T. (1997) Two-dimensional electrophoresis of membrane proteins: a current challenge for immobilized pH gradients, *Electrophoresis*, **18**, 127–135.

44. Righetti, P. G. and Gianazza, E. (1980) New developments in isoelectric focusing, *J. Chromatogr.*, **184**, 415–456.

45. Bjellqvist, B., Ek, K., Righetti, P. G., et al. (1982) Isoelectric focusing in immobilized pH gradients: principle, methodology and some applications, *J. Biochem. Biophys. Methods*, **6**, 317–339.

46. Karas, M. and Hillenkamp, F. (1988) Laser desorption ionization of proteins with molecular masses exceeding 10,000 daltons, *Analyt. Chem.*, **60**, 2299–2301.

47. Fenn, J. B., Mann, M., Meng, C. K., Wong, S. F., and Whitehouse, C. M. (1989) Electrospray ionization for mass spectrometry of large biomolecules, *Science*, **246**, 64–71.

48. Cooks, R. G., Glish, G. L., Kaiser, R. E., and McLuckey, S. A. (1991) Ion trap mass spectrometry, *Chem. Eng. News*, **69**, 26–41.

49. Neuman, B. W., Adair, B. D., Yoshioka, C., Quispe, J. D., Orca, G., Kuhn, P., Milligan, R. A., Yeager, M., and Buchmeier, M. J. (2006) Supramolecular architecture of severe acute respiratory syndrome coronavirus revealed by electron cryomicroscopy, *J. Virol.*, **80**(16), 7918–7928.

50. Obenauer, J. C., Denson, J., Mehta, P. K., Su, X., Mukatira, S., Finkelstein, D. B., Xu, X., Wang, J., Ma, J., Fan, Y., Rakestraw, K. M., Webster, R. G., Hoffmann, E., Krauss, S., Zheng, J., Zhang, Z., and Naeve, C. W. (2006) Large-scale sequence analysis of avian influenza isolates, *Science*, **311,**1576–1580.

51. Ghedin, E., Sengamalay, N. A., Shumway, M., Zaborsky, J., Feldblyum, T., Subbu, V., Spiro, D. J., Sitz, J., Koo, H., Bolotov, P., Dernovoy, D., Tatusova, T., Bao, Y., St. George, K., Taylor, J., Lipman, D. J., Fraser, C.M., Taubenberger, J. K., and Salzberg, S. L. (2005) Large-scale sequencing of human influenza reveals the dynamic nature of viral genome evolution, *Nature*, **437**, 1162–1166.

Chapter 26

Drug Development Research

Infectious diseases are significant causes of human mortality, morbidity, and economic loss. Although effective antimicrobial agents are available for treating bacterial infections, as are limited agents for viral, fungal, and parasitic infections, many diseases are still very difficult to treat effectively and may present serious health concerns. The emergence of drug resistance among common pathogens continues to render ineffective many previously frontline therapies, and the use of many drugs is often limited by toxicity concerns. Emergence of diseases caused by new or drug-resistant pathogens demands more effective drugs. However, current advances in chemistry, bioinformatics, and structural biology should make it possible to discover or design novel anti-infective agents that target specific functions required for pathogen growth and pathogenesis (http://www3.niaid.nih.gov/about/organization/dmid/overview.htm).

One major research goal of NIAID is to facilitate the discovery and evaluation of clinically effective drugs for a host of infectious diseases by supporting research at three levels: basic research and drug discovery; preclinical evaluation; and clinical evaluation (http://www.niaid.nih.gov/dmid/meetings/anti_infective_mttg_2004.pdf), as follows:

Basic Research

- Continue strong support of basic research, including focused emphasis on mechanisms of antimicrobial resistance and microbial membrane biophysics.
- Continue support for basic discovery research, including identification of targets and development of assays and diagnostic tools for more rapid, earlier detection of antimicrobial resistance.
- Expand support for preclinical toxicology (e.g., *in vitro* toxicology, animal toxicology) and drug metabolism studies.
- Continue strong support of genomic research, including analysis, proteomics capabilities, and protein structure.
- Support the involvement of medicinal chemists and molecular biophysicists in research on anti-infective drugs.

Translational Research

- Establish a prioritization process for allocating resources. Criteria could include public health priorities; feasibility of scientific and clinical research paths to product licensure; feasibility of product production; and feasibility of product distribution.
- Support resources for developing models for pharmacokinetic and/or pharmacodynamic analysis and development of nonmurine animal models.
- Provide resources for medicinal chemistry and formulation methodologies. Provide support for developing new statistical tools for analyzing clinical trial data.
- Support the conduct of early-phase clinical trials, including pharmacokinetic studies in special populations, in low incidence diseases, or difficult indications.
- Provide support for assessing the impact of the use of diagnostics on drug resistance.
- Support development of improved methodologies, including statistical tools to allow more efficient use of clinical trial resources.
- Establish collaborations with FDA and the pharmaceutical industry to evaluate possible alternative end points for prospective clinical trials.
- Promote the evaluation of drugs not developed as anti-infectives for use as anti-infectives and discontinued candidates for potential niche indications.

26.1 Recent Programmatic Accomplishments/Developments

26.1.1 Antiviral Drug Development

NIAID is continuing to support both *in vitro* and *in vivo* antiviral screening programs, preclinical evaluation of antiviral lead compounds, and clinical evaluation of antiviral drugs for medically important, emerging/re-emerging, and rare viral diseases.

V. St. Georgiev, *National Institute of Allergy and Infectious Diseases, NIH: Impact on Global Health*, vol. 2, DOI 10.1007/978-1-60327-297-1_26, © Humana Press, a part of Springer Science+Business Media, LLC 2009

26.1.1.1 The Collaborative Antiviral Testing Group

The Collaborative Antiviral Testing Group (CATG) (http://www.niaid.nih.gov/dmid/viral) continues to support a number of contracts that perform *in vitro* screening and *in vivo* testing in animal models and that conduct preliminary studies of efficacy, pharmacology, toxicology, and drug delivery:

In Vitro Screening Systems. Currently, CATG supports the following antiviral *in vitro* screening systems:

- Orthopoxviruses: vaccinia, cowpox
- Herpesviruses: HSV-1, HSV-2, VZV, EBV, CMV, HHV-6, HHV-8
- BK virus
- Papillomaviruses
- Hepatitis B virus
- Hepatitis C virus
- Respiratory viruses: influenza A, influenza B, respiratory syncytial virus (RSV), parainfluenza, rhinoviruses, measles, human coronaviruses, SARS coronavirus (SARS-CoV)
- Biodefense viral hemorrhagic fevers and encephalitides: dengue virus, yellow fever virus, West Nile virus, Venezuelan equine encephalitis virus (a Togavirus), Pichinde virus (an Arenavirus), Punta Toro virus (a Bunyavirus)

In Vivo Animal Models. Currently, CATG also supports the following *in vivo* animal disease models:

- Orthopoxviruses: murine models of vaccinia, cowpox, and ectromelia
- Herpesviruses: murine models of herpes simplex virus (HSV)-1, HSV-2; guinea pig HSV-1, HSV-2; murine cytomegalovirus (CMV); guinea pig CMV; human CMV in SCID-hu mice
- Hepatitis viruses: woodchuck hepatitis in woodchucks; hepatitis B virus (HBV) transgenic mice
- Respiratory viruses: murine model of SARS-CoV; murine models of influenza A and influenza B; cotton rat models of RSV, measles, bovine parainfluenza type3 (PIV3), and human metapmeumovirus (hMPV)
- Papillomaviruses: Shope papilloma in rabbits; human papillomavirus 6 (HPV6) or HPV11 in SCID-hu mice
- Hamster scrapie: in hamster-prion transgenic mice
- Biodefense: Pichinde virus in hamsters; Banzi virus in mice; Punta Toro virus in mice and hamsters; Semliki Forest virus in mice; West Nile virus in mice and hamsters; Venezuelan equine encephalitis in mice; Western equine encephalitis in hamsters; yellow fever virus in hamsters

26.1.1.2 The Collaborative Antiviral Study Group

The Collaborative Antiviral Study Group (CASG) (http://www.niaid.nih.gov/daids/PDATguide/casg.htm) — which consists of a multi-institute infrastructure comprising more than 90 sites in the United States and internationally—is continuing its support for clinical studies on antiviral compounds. Clinical studies on therapies for the following viral infections are under way: cytomegalovirus; herpes simplex virus; BK virus; West Nile virus; and influenza. Specific activities include:

- A protocol has been developed to use cidofovir as a contingency to treat smallpox in the event of an outbreak. More information can be found at the CASG Web site: http://www.peds.uab.edu/casg/.
- In 2005, CASG initiated a chart review in selected pediatric practices that used oseltamivir in infants with influenza to gather safety data to help inform prospective users. Data have been collected and partially analyzed on 120 subjects up to October 2006. By November 2006, data were collected and analyzed on 150 to 200 subjects.
- In July 2006, CASG, in collaboration with Hoffmann-LaRoche, Inc., developed a protocol for a safety and pharmacokinetic/pharmacodynamic (PK/PD) prospective study of oseltamivir for the treatment of children under the age of 2 with documented influenza. CASG opened a study in October 2006 in as many as 25 centers across the United States.
- Recently, CASG initiated a study to evaluate the safety and tolerability of cidofovir as a treatment for BK virus renal nephropathy in renal transplant patients.

26.1.1.3 Development of Therapeutic Agents for Selected Viral Diseases

In 2006, NIAID awarded four new contracts to biotechnology companies to develop antiviral therapeutics against biodefense viral pathogens:

- To Alnylam Pharmaceuticals, Inc. (Cambridge, MA) to perform preclinical development and Investigational New Drug (IND)-enabling studies on RNA interference (RNAi)-based therapeutic agents designed to treat hemorrhagic fever caused by Ebola virus.
- To Macrogenics, Inc. (Rockville, MD) to perform pivotal nonclinical animal efficacy and IND-enabling studies, Phase I human safety trials, and biologic license application (BLA)-enabling studies on a therapeutic monoclonal antibody to treat West Nile virus infection.
- To SIGA Technologies, Inc. (Corvallis, OR) to perform Phase I human safety trials and NDA-enabling studies

on a small-molecule compound, ST-246, as a preexposure and postexposure therapeutic against smallpox virus.

- To NexBio, Inc. (San Diego, CA) to perform Phase I human safety and Phase II clinical trials and other NDA-enabling studies on a recombinant therapeutic enzyme, Fludase, as a preexposure/treatment therapeutic against influenza virus.

26.1.2 Antibacterial and Antitoxin Drug Development

NIAID is continuing its support of *in vitro* and *in vivo* antibacterial screening programs, preclinical evaluation of antibacterial lead compounds, and clinical evaluation of antibacterial drugs for medically important, emerging/re-emerging, and rare bacterial and toxin-caused diseases.

- *Monoclonal Antibody Therapeutic for Botulinum Neurotoxin Serotype A*. In 2006, NIAID awarded a 3-year contract to XOMA LLC to formulate, finish, and release a mixture of the botulinum neurotoxin A monoclonal antibodies, to perform long-term stability studies and investigational new drug-enabling nonclinical safety studies, and to develop analytical assays that support future Phase I clinical trials.
- *The Bacteriology and Mycology Study Group (BAMSG)* and *Bacteriology and Mycology Biostatistical and Operations Unit (BAMBU)*. The BAMSG is managed under a contract awarded to the University of Alabama at Birmingham and supports clinical studies to evaluate interventions for serious fungal diseases, as well as health care–associated resistant bacterial infections. The BAMBUs are providing biostatistical and administrative support for the clinical studies. The BAMBU contract is managed by Rho Federal Systems Division, Inc. Under the BAMSG resource, a reserve fund has been established to support orphan studies that cannot be funded through industrial sponsors.

26.1.3 Antiparasitic Drug Development

Identification, validation, and evaluation of new antimalarial therapies remain NIAID priority activities. Highlights of specific activities are summarized below.

- The objective of the *Tropical Diseases Research Units (TDRU)* program is to support translational research leading to the discovery and preclinical development of new drugs or vector control methods to reduce or eliminate morbidity and mortality resulting from parasitic infection.

One of the three awards made under this program focuses on development of novel antimalarial drugs.

- NIAID is continuing its support for investigator-initiated research on preclinical development and evaluation of novel compounds and has released a new initiative (RFA) seeking applications from public-private partnerships that are engaged in developing therapeutic or diagnostic products directed against neglected diseases, including malaria. NIAID is also supporting preclinical and clinical studies of combination therapies for malaria, especially those including artesunate. In December 2005, NIAID and the *Medicines for Malaria Venture (MMV)* jointly convened a meeting, including participants from FDA, CDC, and international drug regulatory agencies, to establish consensus regarding the appropriate design of Phase III clinical trials for new antimalarial drug combinations.
- Identifying, validating, and evaluating new vector control compounds and strategies remain NIAID priority activities. Under the partnership initiatives (RFAs), these projects will explore the role of strategies to control larva and mosquitoes in reducing the transmission of malaria and will develop new and safe insecticides targeting mosquito activities, including those aimed at mitigating resistance to insecticides.

26.1.4 Research Resources

NIAID is also maintaining several contracts that provide a broad range of services to support the nonclinical and clinical development of new drugs.

- *Services for the Preclinical Development of Therapeutic Agents*. In 2006, SRI International was awarded a contract from NIAID to provide a suite of services for preclinical development of therapeutic agents. This resource is intended to rapidly and efficiently close gaps in the preclinical development of promising new therapeutic agents that emerge from academia, the private sector, and other areas. This will allow for the commercial development of new therapeutics against potential agents of bioterrorism, drug-resistant pathogens, emerging and re-emerging infectious diseases, and diseases prevalent in resource-limited countries.
- *The In Vitro and Animal Models for Emerging Infectious Diseases and Biodefense Program*. This program continues to provide a wide range of resources for *in vitro* and *in vivo* nonclinical testing of new therapies and vaccines. These contracts provide resources for developing and validating small laboratory animal and non-human primate infection models for licensure of therapeutics.

Specific projects include the following:

- *Anthrax*: (i) Screening of existing FDA-approved antimicrobials and immunomodulators for efficacy against inhalational anthrax; (ii) evaluating whether immunization with recombinant Protective Antigen (rPA) vaccines can reduce the course of antibiotic therapy; and (iii) developing therapeutic animal models in rabbits and non-human primates.
- *Plague*: (i) Screening of existing FDA-approved antimicrobials for efficacy; and (ii) developing alternative non-human primate and mouse models.
- *Smallpox*: (i) Performing therapeutic efficacy studies in non-human primates; and (ii) evaluating toxicology of specific antiviral agents.
- *Tularemia*: Developing alternative non-human primate and mouse models.
- *Botulinum neurotoxin*: Developing small laboratory animal assay and therapeutic efficacy model.
- *Ricin*: Determining toxicokinetics in small animals.
- *SARS*: Developing small laboratory animal and non-human primate models.
- *Avian influenza*: Developing ferret model and testing its efficacy; evaluating toxicology.
- *Antimicrobials*: Performing *in vitro* screening.

26.2 Recent Research Programs in Drug Development

Several awards were made in 2006 to drug development–related programs:

- *NIAID's Cooperative Research for the Development of Vaccines, Adjuvants, Therapeutic Immunotherapeutics, and Diagnostics for Biodefense and SARS Program.* This program supports discovery/design and development of vaccines, therapeutics, adjuvants, and diagnostics for biodefense. The program will help translate research from the target identification stage through target validation to early product development. In 2006, 27 awards were made, several of which focused on therapeutic development.
- *NIAID's Small Business Advanced Technology Program.* This program is designed to encourage SBIR/STTR applications to develop therapeutics, vaccines, adjuvants/immunostimulants, diagnostics, and selected resources for biodefense. Several grants related to therapeutic development were made in 2006. A small-molecule inhibitor, ST-294, against viral hemorrhagic fever caused by New World arenaviruses was advanced through preclinical development through this program.

26.3 Recent NIAID-Supported Scientific Advances

- *New Developments in Yellow Fever Virus Research.* A hamster model for evaluating compounds against yellow fever virus (YFV) was developed and characterized *(1)*. Challenge with yellow fever virus resulted in 50% to 80% mortality in female hamsters with virus detected in many organs, including the liver, kidney, and spleen. Treatment of hamsters with interferon, viramidine or ribavirin, initiated 4 hours prior to YFV infection, resulted in significant improvement in survival and liver enzyme levels.
- *Derivatives of Cidofovir Inhibit Polyomavirus BK Replication In Vitro.* Polyomavirus BK is a significant pathogen in transplant recipients, but no effective antiviral therapy is available. Esterification of cidofovir with hexadecyloxypropyl, octadecyloxyethyl, and oleyloxyethyl groups resulted in significantly enhanced activity against BK virus replication *in vitro (2)*. These lipid esters of cidofovir are orally bioavailable and are not nephrotoxic; thus, they are promising new antivirals for BK virus infection in transplant recipients.
- *Development of New Cell-Based Screen May Help Identify New Antivirals.* Identification of new antiviral lead compounds depends on robust primary assays for high-throughput screening (HTS) of large compound libraries. In a recent study, researchers developed a cell-based screen in 384-well plates to identify potential antiviral agents against influenza by measuring the cytopathic effect (CPE) induced by influenza virus (A/Udorn/72, H3N2) infection in Madin Darby canine kidney (MDCK) cells using the luminescent-based CellTiter Glo system *(3)*. This assay is translatable for screening against other influenza strains, such as avian flu, and may facilitate identification of antivirals for other viruses that induce CPE, such as West Nile or dengue.
- *Development of Alternative Approaches to Treating Influenza.* To provide an urgently needed alternative treatment modality for influenza, NIAID-supported investigators have generated a recombinant fusion protein composed of a sialidase catalytic domain derived from *Actinomyces viscosus* fused with a cell surface–anchoring sequence *(4)*. The sialidase fusion protein is to be applied as an inhalant to remove the influenza viral receptors, sialic acids, from the airway epithelium. Thus, a specific sialidase fusion construct, DAS181, effectively cleaved sialic acid receptors used by both human and avian influenza viruses. The treatment provided a long-lasting effect and is nontoxic to the cells. DAS181 demonstrated potent antiviral and cell protective efficacies against a panel of laboratory strains and clinical isolates of influenza A and B. Mouse and ferret studies confirmed

significant *in vivo* efficacy of the sialidase fusion in both prophylactic and treatment modes.

- *Potential Therapeutic for Orthopoxvirus and Herpesvirus Infections.* *N*-Methanocarbathymidine [(N)-MCT] is a novel nucleoside analogue that was found active against some herpesviruses and orthopoxviruses *in vitro (5)*. The antiviral activity of this molecule was dependent on the type I thymidine kinase (TK) in herpes simplex virus and also appeared to be dependent on the type II TK expressed by cowpox and vaccinia viruses. (N)-MCT was also a good inhibitor of viral DNA synthesis in both viruses and was consistent with inhibition of the viral DNA polymerase once it had been activated by the viral TK homologues. The compound was nontoxic *in vivo* and effectively reduced the mortality of mice infected with orthopoxviruses, as well as those infected with herpes simplex virus type 1 when treatment was initiated 24 hours after infection. These results indicated that (N)-MCT is active *in vitro* and *in vivo*, and its mechanism of action suggested that the molecule may be an effective therapeutic agent for orthopoxvirus and herpesvirus infections, thus warranting further development.

- *Elusive Drug Target in Mycobacterium tuberculosis Is Identified.* Isoniazid (INH) is one of the most effective drugs against tuberculosis (TB), but *Mycobacterium tuberculosis* (Mtb), the bacterium that causes TB, has found ways to resist this drug. Over the past decade, several proteins have been suggested to be the target for INH, but researchers have not been able to define exactly which one is attacked by INH and is responsible for the drug's action on the bacteria. To define whether one or more proteins are directly affected by the drug, it was important to change these targets one at a time to demonstrate which one is primarily attacked by INH. Using new molecular tools that were developed, a team of researchers introduced, for the first time, a small but defined change (mutation) in the protein InhA alone, which was thought to be the primary target for INH *(6)*. This small change is the same that is seen in this protein when the bacteria become resistant to INH. The bacteria with the changed protein InhA could no longer be killed with therapeutic amounts of INH. Furthermore, the altered InhA protein from Mtb was also isolated, and it was determined that it lost the ability to effectively bind to isoniazid. To make sure that this changed protein was indeed the primary target of INH, the same techniques were applied to create Mtb bacteria with defined changes in one other protein that had been hypothesized to be a target of INH. This change, however, could not alter the way the bacteria responded to the drug. With this information, scientists can now study the exact interaction between INH and its target in the bacterial cell and can start designing new versions of the drug that are still effective even if the

bacterium changes the makeup of the InhA protein—as it has done to become resistant to this drug *(6)*. INH remains the most effective drug against TB. However, resistance against INH is increasing despite the use of multidrug regimens against this disease. Because it cannot be presumed that a drug has only one target, it is important to characterize what bacterial components are primarily responsible for its action. With this information, it is now possible to characterize the exact effect of the drug on the bacterial metabolism, to better understand how bacteria create resistance against INH, to construct new versions of the drug that are effective even against mutated target drugs, and also to generate appropriate companion drugs to INH that make it more difficult for Mtb to become resistant. The proof that InhA is the primary target for INH is a new milestone in TB research that has been the focus of intense investigation since the early 1990s.

- *Effective Antimicrobial Regimens for Use in Humans for Therapy for Bacillus anthracis Infections and Postexposure Prophylaxis.* Expanded options for treatments directed against pathogens that can be used for bioterrorism are urgently needed. Treatment regimens directed against such pathogens can be identified only by using data derived from *in vitro* and animal studies. It is crucial that these studies reliably predict the efficacy of proposed treatments in humans. The objective of this study was to identify a levofloxacin treatment regimen that will serve as an effective therapy for *Bacillus anthracis* infections and postexposure prophylaxis. An *in vitro* hollow-fiber infection model that replicates the pharmacokinetic profile of levofloxacin observed in humans (half-life [$t_{1/2}$], 7.5 hours) or in animals such as the mouse or the rhesus monkey ($t_{1/2}$, ~2 hours) was used to evaluate a proposed indication for levofloxacin (500 mg once daily) for treating *Bacillus anthracis* infections *(7)*. The results obtained with the *in vitro* model served as the basis for the doses and the dose schedules that were evaluated in the mouse inhalational anthrax model. The effects of levofloxacin and ciprofloxacin treatment were compared with those of no treatment (untreated controls). The main outcome measure in the *in vitro* hollow-fiber infection model was a persistent reduction of culture density (≥ 4 $\log_{10}$ reduction) and prevention of the emergence of levofloxacin-resistant organisms. In the mouse inhalational anthrax model, the main outcome measure was survival. The results indicated that levofloxacin given once daily with simulated human pharmacokinetics effectively sterilized *Bacillus anthracis* cultures. By using a simulated animal pharmacokinetic profile, a once-daily dosing regimen that provided a human-equivalent exposure failed to sterilize the cultures. Dosing regimens that "partially humanized" levofloxacin exposures within the constraints of animal pharmacokinetics reproduced the antimicrobial efficacy seen with human pharmacokinetics. In a mouse inhalational anthrax model, once-daily dosing was significantly inferior (survival end point) to regimens of dosing every 12 hours or every 6 hours with identical total daily levofloxacin doses. These results demonstrated the predictive value of the *in vitro* hollow-fiber infection model with respect to the success or the failure of treatment regimens in animals. Furthermore, the model permits the evaluation of treatment regimens that "humanize" antibiotic exposures in animal models, enhancing the confidence with which animal models may be used to reliably predict the efficacies of proposed antibiotic treatments in humans in situations where human trials cannot be performed (e.g., the release of pathogens as agents of bioterrorism or emerging infectious diseases). A treatment regimen effective in rhesus monkeys was identified *(7)*.

This study demonstrated the combinational use of *in vitro* hollow-fiber and animal models to evaluate the effectiveness of certain antibiotics for treating human infection for diseases where human trials cannot be performed, such as anthrax and plague. Such systemic pharmacokinetic and pharmacodynamic characterization of existing antibiotics will make it possible to identify active anti-infective agents and to design effective treatment regimens. The findings gained from this study will provide the public with options of more than one antibiotic if there is an urgent need to counteract a bioterror attack or other unexpected outbreak of an emerging infectious disease.

- *RNA Interference as a Potential Antiviral Therapy Against West Nile Virus.* RNA interference (RNAi) is a recently discovered cellular mechanism in which small pieces of double-stranded RNA (small interfering RNAs, or siRNAs) suppress the expression of genes with sequence homology. A team of investigators has been able to harness RNA interference to protect laboratory animals against lethal infection with important human pathogens like the herpes simplex virus 2 (HSV-2), West Nile virus (WNV), and the Japanese encephalitis virus (JEV) *(8)*. It was demonstrated that a single siRNA, targeting a conserved sequence present in both WNV and JEV, protected mice infected with WNV or JEV from lethal encephalitis

when administered before or after infection. WNV and JEV, both mosquito-borne flaviviruses that cause acute encephalitis, are important re-emerging viruses that cause tens of thousands of infections in the world and significant morbidity and mortality. Currently, no drugs exist to treat WNV or JEV. This study supports the further development of siRNAs as a novel, broad-spectrum antiviral therapy against emerging flaviviruses.

References

1. Julander, J. G., Siddharthan, V., Blatt, L. M., Schafer, K., Sidwell, R. W., and Morrey, J. D. (2007) Comparison of the inhibitory effects of interferon alfacon-1 and ribavirin on yellow fever virus infection in a hamster model, *Antiviral Res.*, **73**(2), 140–146.
2. Randhawa, P., Farasati, N.A., Shapiro, R., and Hostetler, K. Y. (2006) Ether lipid ester derivatives of cidofovir inhibit polyomavirus BK replication *in vitro*, *Antimicrob. Agents Chemother.*, **50**, 1564–1566.
3. Noah, J. W., Severson, W., Noah, D. L., Rasmussen, L., White, E. L., and Jonsson, C.B. (2006) A cell-based luminescence assay is effective for high-throughput screening of potential influenza antivirals, *Antiviral Res.*, **73**(1), 50–59.
4. Malakhov, M. P., Aschenbrenner, L. M., Smee, D. F., Wandersee, M. K., Sidwell, R. W., Gubareva, L. V., Mishin, V. P., Hayden, F. G., Kim, D. H., Ing, A., Campbell, E. R., Yu, M., and Fang, F. (2006) Sialidase fusion protein as a novel broad-spectrum inhibitor of influenza virus infection, *Antimicrob. Agents Chemother.*, **50**, 1470–1479.
5. Prichard, M. N., Keith, K. A., Quenelle, D. C., and Kern, E. R. (2006) Activity and mechanism of action of *N*-methanocarbathymidine against herpesvirus and orthopoxvirus infections, *Antimicrob Agents Chemother.*, **50**, 1336–1341.
6. Vilcheze, C., Wang, F., Arai, M., Hazbon, M. H., Colangeli, R., Kremer, L., Weisbrod, T. R., Alland, D., Sacchettini, J. C., and Jacobs, W. R. Jr. (2006) Transfer of a point mutation in *Mycobacterium tuberculosis* inhA resolves the target of isoniazid, *Nat. Med.*, **12**(9), 1027–1029.
7. Deziel, M. R., Heine, H., Louie, A., Kao, M., Byrne, W. R., Basset, J., Miller, L., Bush, K., Kelly, M., and Drusano, G. L. (2005) Effective antimicrobial regimens for use in humans of *Bacillus anthracis* infections and postexposure prophylaxis, *Antimicrob. Agents Chemother.* **49**, 5099–5106.
8. Kumar, P., Lee, S. K., Shankar, P., and Swamy, M. (2006) A single siRNA suppresses fatal encephalitis induced by two different flaviviruses, *PLoS Med.*, **3**(4), e96.

Part II
Human Immunodeficiency Virus and Acquired
Immunodeficiency Syndrome

Chapter 27

Introduction

For nearly three decades, the human immunodeficiency virus (HIV) and the acquired immunodeficiency syndrome (AIDS) pandemic has claimed the lives of many millions of people to have a devastating impact on global health by changing its disease progression patterns *(1)*.

During the period 1982–2006, the National Institutes of Health (NIH) cumulative funding for HIV/AIDS research reached nearly US$30 billion *(2)*. The National Institutes of Allergy and Infectious Diseases (NIAID), through its Division of AIDS (DAIDS), remains the world's leading institution in supporting HIV/AIDS research, including (i) basic science, biology, and pathogenesis; (ii) therapeutics; (iii) vaccines; (iv) prevention (other than vaccines and microbicides); (v) natural history; (vi) training and infrastructure; and (vii) HIV topical microbicides (http://www3.niaid.nih.gov/research/topics/HIV/).

Since the early 1990s, the tuberculosis epidemic has largely been driven by the HIV/AIDS pandemic. However, fueled by growing antibiotic resistance, inappropriate prescription of ineffective drugs, and poor adherence to medication regimens, tuberculosis—which once was believed to be under control—has re-emerged as a major global threat.

The primary research priorities of NIAID can be summarized as follows:

- Discovering and developing safe, efficacious, and cost-effective vaccines to prevent HIV infection and/or disease
- Translating research and developing drugs
- Preventing mother-to-child transmission
- Preventing HIV infection (other than vaccines and microbicides)
- Developing topical microbicides
- Optimizing clinical management

In supporting HIV/AIDS research, DAIDS has identified a number of important *cross-cutting issues* that need to be studied. They can be summarized as follows:

- Identifying the highest risk populations for studies and trials
- Identifying and studying intervention on co-morbidities

- Conducting behavioral interventions and research in all areas of HIV/AIDS studies
- Clarifying the role(s) that host differences play in the outcome of HIV disease (e.g., HLA/other genetics, age, gender, etc.)
- Exchanging information on seroconverters in the context of vaccine, prevention, and treatment
- Referring HIV-positive individuals during screening and trials to care and treatment programs or research studies
- Identifying underserved, disenfranchised, and/or vulnerable populations (e.g., women, minorities, adolescents, young children) and specifying barriers to participation in clinical research for these and other special populations; developing strategies to address these populations

Finally, whereas advances in the therapy of HIV/AIDS continue to be made, there remains an urgent need for identifying new host and viral targets based on new insights into HIV pathogenesis, novel drugs and delivery systems, and immunologic approaches to address the dual problems of drug resistance and toxicity.

27.1 Human Immunodeficiency Virus

The genome and proteins of HIV have been the subject of extensive research since the discovery of the virus in 1983. It is a well-known fact that no two HIV genomes are the same, not even from the same person, causing some to speculate that HIV is a "quasispecies" of a virus *(3, 4)*.

27.1.1 Structure and Expression of HIV Genome

Structure. The HIV structure is different from that of other retroviruses. It is around 120 nm in diameter (120 billionths of a meter; around 60 times smaller than a red blood cell) and roughly spherical. HIV-1 is composed of two copies of single-stranded RNA enclosed by a conical capsid comprising the viral protein p24, typical of lentiviruses. The RNA component is 9,749 nucleotides long. This, in turn, is surrounded by a plasma membrane of host-cell origin. The single-strand RNA is tightly bound to the nucleocapsid protein, p7, and enzymes that are indispensable for the virus' replication, such as reverse transcriptase and integrase. The nucleocapsid protein p7 associates with the genomic RNA (one molecule per hexamer) and protects the RNA from being digested by nucleases. A matrix composed of an association of the viral protein p17 surrounds the capsid, ensuring the integrity of the virion particle. Also enclosed within the virion particle are Vif, Vpr, Nef, p7, and the viral protease. The envelope (composed of glycoproteins p120 and p41) is incorporated when the capsid buds from the host cell, taking some of the host cell's membrane with it *(5, 6)*.

Genome Organization. HIV has several major genes coding for structural proteins that are found in all retroviruses and several nonstructural ("accessory") genes that are unique to HIV *(7)*. The *gag* gene provides the basic physical infrastructure of the virus, and the *pol* gene provides the basic mechanism by which retroviruses reproduce, whereas the others help HIV to enter the host cell and enhance its reproduction. Although they may be altered by mutation, all of these genes except *tev* exist in all known variants of HIV:

- *gag* (group-specific antigen): codes for p24, the viral capsid p6; p7, the nucleocapsid protein; and p17, the matrix protein
- *pol*: codes for viral enzymes, the most important of which are reverse transcriptase, integrase, and the protease that cleaves the proteins derived from *gag* and *pol* into functional proteins
- *env*: codes for the precursor to gp120 and gp41, proteins embedded in the viral envelope that enable the virus to attach to and fuse with target cells
- *tat, rev, nef, vif, vpr, vpu*: each of these genes codes for a single protein with the same name; see Tat, Rev, Nef, Vif, Vpr, Vpu
- *tev*: this gene is present in only a few HIV-1 isolates. It is a fusion of parts of the *tat, env*, and *rev* genes and codes for a protein with some of the properties of Tat, but few or none of the properties of Rev. [*Note*: After being first published in the late 1980s *(8, 9)*, the role of the Tev protein in HIV replication and pathogenesis has not been firmly established in subsequent studies.]

Recently, an Anglo-German team compiled a three-dimensional structure of HIV by combining multiple images *(10)*. HIV buds from the membrane of an infected cell in an immature, noninfectious form *(11)*. The viral particles are mostly spherical and have a variable diameter *(12–14)*. This heterogeneity is a general feature of retroviruses *(15–17)*.

In immature HIV particles, the major structural protein, Gag, is arranged in a radial fashion, with the *N*-terminal matrix (MA) domain associated with the viral membrane, followed by the internal capsid (CA) domain and the *C*-terminal nucleocapsid (NC) domain pointed toward the center *(13, 14)*. During or shortly after budding, Gag is cleaved by the viral protease, leading to maturation of the virus, which is reflected in a dramatic morphologic change required for infectivity *(11, 18)*. Maturation requires disassembly of the immature Gag shell, followed by a second assembly step leading to the mature core *(19)*. The MA domains remain associated with the viral membrane, and the ribonucleoprotein (RNP) complex of NC and genomic RNA condense in the center. The CA domains form the typical cone-shaped core of mature HIV encasing the RNP. Formation of the mature core requires only a fraction of the available CA molecules *(19)*, and it may depend on nucleation by the viral genome *(11)*.

Infectious HIV particles contain a characteristic cone-shaped core encasing the viral RNA and replication proteins *(10)*. The core exhibits significant heterogeneity in size and shape, yet consistently forms a well-defined structure. In general, the mechanism by which the core is assembled in the maturing virion remains poorly understood. However, recent studies have shown that using cryoelectron tomography makes it possible to produce three-dimensional reconstructions of authentic, unstained HIV-1 by revealing viral morphology with unprecedented clarity. It also suggests a mechanism for core formation inside the extracellular virion, in which core growth initiates at the narrow end of the cone and proceeds toward the distal side of the virion until limited by the viral membrane. Curvature and closure of the broad end of the core are then directed by the inner surface of the viral membrane. This mechanism accommodates significant flexibility in lattice growth while ensuring that cores of variable size and shape are closed *(10)*. It is hoped that this new information will contribute to scientific understanding of the virus and help in identifying new targets for therapeutic and preventive intervention. However, the validity of this work *(10)* still remains a matter of debate *(20)*, as a conflicting model has been produced by another team of researchers from the United States *(21)*.

HIV Proteins and Their Functions. The integrated form, also known as the provirus, is approximately 9.8 kilobases in length *(22)*. The viral genes are located in the central region of the proviral DNA and encode at least nine proteins *(23)*. Flanking the nine HIV genes on both sides are the *long terminal repeats (LTRs)* (see Section 27.1.2). The LTRs are divided into three regions (U5, R, and U3) and serve to initiate the expression of the viral genes with the help of the cellular RNA polymerase II and the auxiliary transcription factors (Sp1, NF-κB) *(7)*.

The viral proteins are divided into three classes: (i) major structural proteins (Gag, Pol, and Env); (ii) regulatory proteins (Tat and Rev); and (iii) accessory proteins (Vpu, Vpr, Vif, and Nef).

- *Structural Proteins*

  o *Gag Protein.* The *gag* gene gives rise to the 55-kDa Gag precursor protein (Pr55^{gag}), which is expressed from the unspliced viral mRNA. During the translation, the *N*-terminus of p55 is myristoylated *(24)*, triggering its association with the cytoplasmic aspect of the cell membranes. Next, the membrane-associated Gag polyprotein recruits two copies of the viral genomic RNA along with other viral and cellular proteins that initiate the budding of the viral particle from the surface of an infected cell. After budding, the p55 protein is cleaved by the virally encoded protease *(25)* (generated by the *pol* gene) during the process of viral maturation into four smaller proteins designated as MA (matrix [p17]), CA (capsid [p24]), NC (nucleocapsid [p7]), and p6 *(7, 25)*.

    ▪ *p17 (MA)*—the MA polypeptide is derived from the *N*-terminal myristoylated end of p55 *(7)*. Most MA molecules remain attached to the inner surface of the virion lipid bilayer, stabilizing the particle. A subset of MA is recruited inside the deeper layers of the virion where it becomes part of the complex that escorts the viral DNA to the nucleus *(26)*. These MA molecules facilitate the nuclear transport of the viral genome because a karyophilic signal on MA is recognized by the cellular nuclear import machinery. This phenomenon allows HIV to infect nondividing cells, an unusual property for a retrovirus *(27)*.

    ▪ *p24 (CA)*—p24 makes up the conical core of the viral capsid. When a Western blot test is used to detect HIV infection, p24 is one of the three major proteins tested for, along with gp120/gp160 and gp41.

    ▪ *p7 (NC)*—the NC region of Gag is responsible for specifically recognizing the so-called packaging signal of HIV *(28)*. The packaging signal consists of four stem-loop structures located near the 5′ end of the viral RNA and is sufficient to mediate the incorporation of a heterologous RNA into HIV-1 virions *(29)*. NC binds to the packaging signal through interactions mediated by two zinc-finger motifs. NC also facilitates reverse transcription *(30)*.

    ▪ *p6*—p6 mediates interactions between p55 Gag and the accessory protein Vpr, leading to the incorporation of Vpr into assembling virions *(31)*. The p6 region also contains the so-called late domain, which

is required for the efficient release of budding virions from an infected cell *(7)*.

  o *Gag-Pol Precursor.* The viral protease (Pro), integrase (IN), RNase H, and reverse transcriptase (RT) are always expressed within the context of a Gag-Pol fusion protein *(32)*. The Gag-Pol precursor (Pr160$^{gag-pol}$) is generated by a ribosomal frameshifting event, which is triggered by a specific *cis*-acting RNA motif *(33)* (a heptanucleotide sequence followed by a short stem-loop in the distal region of the Gag RNA). When ribosomes encounter this motif, they shift approximately 5% of the time to the *pol* reading frame without interrupting translation. The frequency of ribosomal frameshifting explains why the Gag and the Gag-Pol precursor are produced at a ratio of approximately 20:1. During viral maturation, the virally encoded protease cleaves the Pol polypeptide away from Gag and further digests it to separate the protease (p10), RT (p55/66), RNase H (p15), and integrase (p31) activities. However, these cleavages do not all occur efficiently; for example, roughly 50% of the RT protein remains linked to RNase H as a single polypeptide (p65) *(7)*.

  o *Protease.* The HIV-1 protease is an aspartyl protease *(34)* that acts as a dimer. Protease activity is required for cleavage of the Gag and Gag-Pol polyprotein precursors during virion maturation. The three-dimensional structure of the protease dimer has been determined *(35, 36)*. Knowledge of this structure has led to a class of drugs directed toward inhibiting the HIV protease function. These antiviral compounds have greatly improved treatment for HIV-infected individuals (see Section 34.6 in Chapter 34).

  o *Reverse Transcriptase.* The *pol* gene encodes reverse transcriptase. Pol has RNA-dependent and DNA-dependent polymerase activities. During the process of reverse transcription, the polymerase makes a double-stranded DNA copy of the dimer of single-stranded genomic RNA present in the virion. RNase H removes the original RNA template from the first DNA strand, allowing synthesis of the complementary strand of DNA. Viral DNA can be completely synthesized within 6 hours after viral entry, although the DNA may remain unintegrated for prolonged periods *(37)*. Many *cis*-acting elements in the viral RNA are required for generating viral DNA. For example, the TAR element, a small RNA stem-loop structure located at the 5′ end of viral RNAs and containing the binding site for Tat, is required for initiating reverse transcription *(38)*. The predominant functional species of the polymerase is a heterodimer of p65 and p50/66. All of the pol gene products can be found within the capsid of free

HIV-1 virions. Because the polymerase does not contain a proofreading activity, replication is error-prone and introduces several point mutations into each new copy of the viral genome. The crystal structure of HIV-1 RT has been determined *(39)*.

○ *Integrase.* This enzyme integrates the insertion of the proviral DNA produced by reverse transcriptase into the genome of the host's infected cell *(7)*. This process is mediated by three distinct functions of integrase *(40)*. First, an exonuclease activity trims two nucleotides from each 3′ end of the linear viral DNA duplex. Then, a double-stranded endonuclease activity cleaves the host DNA at the integration site. Finally, a ligase activity generates a single covalent linkage at each end of the proviral DNA. It is believed that cellular enzymes then repair the integration site. No exogenous energy source, such as ATP, is required for this reaction. The accessibility of the chromosomal DNA within chromatin, rather than specific DNA sequences, seems to influence the choice of integration sites *(41)*. Sites of DNA kinking within chromatin are thus "hotspots" for integration, at least *in vitro (42)*. It is possible to promote integration within specific DNA regions by fusing integrase to sequence-specific DNA binding proteins *(43)*. Preferential integration into regions of open, transcriptionally active, chromatin may facilitate the expression of the provirus. The viral genes are not efficiently expressed from nonintegrated proviral DNA *(44)*.

○ *Envelope Protein (Env).* The 160-kDa Env protein (gp160) is expressed from singly spliced mRNA *(7)*. First synthesized in the endoplasmic reticulum, the Env migrates through the Golgi complex where it undergoes glycosylation with the addition of 25 to 30 complex *N*-linked carbohydrate side chains that are added at asparagine residues. The Env glycosylation is required for infectivity *(45)*. A cellular protease cleaves gp160 to generate the gp41 and gp120 proteins. The gp41 moiety contains the transmembrane domain of Env, and gp120 is located on the surface of the infected cell and of the virion through noncovalent interactions with gp41. The Env protein exists as a trimer on the surface of infected cells and virions *(46)*

■ *gp120*—exposed on the surface of the viral envelope, the glycoprotein gp120 binds to the CD4 receptor on any target cell that has such a receptor, particularly the helper T-cell. Because CD4 receptor binding is the most obvious step in HIV infection, gp120 was among the first targets of HIV vaccine research. These efforts have been hampered by its chemical properties, which make it difficult for antibodies to

bind to gp120; also, it can easily be shed from the virus due to its loose binding with gp41.

Interactions between HIV and the virion receptor CD4 are mediated through specific domains of gp120 *(47)*. The structure of gp120 has recently been determined *(48)*. The gp120 moiety has nine highly conserved intrachain disulfide bonds. Also present in gp120 are five hypervariable regions, designated V1 through V5, whose amino acid sequences can vary greatly among HIV-1 isolates. One such region, called the V3 loop, is not involved in CD4 binding, but is rather an important determinant of the preferential tropism of HIV-1 for either T-lymphoid cell lines or primary macrophages *(49)*. Sequences within the V3 loop interact with the HIV coreceptors CXCR4 and CCR5, which belong to the family of chemokine receptors and partially determine the susceptibility of cell types to given viral strains *(50, 51)*. The V3 loop is also the principal target for neutralizing antibodies that block HIV-1 infectivity *(52)*. The gp120 moiety also interacts with the protein DC-SIGN, which is expressed on the cell surface of dendritic cells. Interaction with DC-SIGN increases the efficiency of infection of CD4-positive T cells *(53)*. Further, it is believed that DC-SIGN can facilitate mucosal transmission by transporting HIV to lymphoid tissues.

● *gp41*—the glycoprotein gp41 is noncovalently bound to gp120 and provides the second step by which HIV enters the cell. It is originally buried within the viral envelope, but when gp120 binds to a CD4 receptor, gp120 changes its conformation, causing gp41 to become exposed, where it can assist in fusion with the host cell. Fusion inhibitor drugs such as enfuvirtide block the fusion process by binding to gp41.

The gp41 moiety contains an *N*-terminal fusogenic domain that mediates the fusion of the viral and cellular membranes, thereby allowing the delivery of the virion's inner components into the cytoplasm of the newly infected cell *(54)*. A new class of antiviral therapeutics that prevent membrane fusion has shown promise in clinical trials. The *env* gene does not actually code for gp120 and gp41 but for a precursor to both, gp160. During HIV replication, the host cell's own enzymes cleave gp160 into gp120 and gp41 *(7)*.

● *Regulatory (Transactivator) Proteins*

○ *Tat (Transactivator of Transcription).* Tat is a transcriptional transactivator that is essential for the replication of HIV-1 *(55)*. The 72- and 101-amino-acid-long forms of Tat are expressed by early fully spliced mRNAs or late incompletely spliced HIV mRNAs, respectively. Both forms function as transcriptional activators and are found within the nuclei and nucleoli of infected cells *(7)*. Tat is an RNA binding protein, unlike conventional transcription factors that interact with DNA *(56, 57)*. Tat binds to a short-stem loop structure, known as the *transactivation response element (TAR)*, which is located at the 5′ terminus of HIV RNAs. Tat binding occurs in conjunction with cellular proteins that contribute to the effects of Tat. The binding of Tat to TAR activates transcription from the HIV LTR at least 1000-fold *(7)*.

The mechanism of Tat function has recently been elucidated. Tat acts principally to promote the elongation phase of HIV-1 transcription, so that full-length transcripts can be produced *(58, 59)*. In the absence of Tat expression, HIV generates primarily short (<100 nucleotides) transcripts. Polymerase elongation is stimulated by the recruitment of a serine kinase that phosphorylates the carboxyl-terminal domain (CTD) of RNA polymerase II. This kinase, which is known as CDK9, is part of a complex that binds directly to Tat *(60)*. Tat function requires a cellular cofactor, known as *Cyclin T*, which facilitates the recognition of the TAR loop region by the cyclin T-Tat complex *(61)*. The cellular uptake of Tat released by infected cells has been observed *(59)*, although the impact of this phenomenon on pathogenesis is unknown. Tat has been shown to activate the expression of a number of cellular genes including the tumor necrosis factor-β *(62)* and transforming growth factor-β *(63)* and to downregulate the expression of other cellular genes including bcl-2 *(64)* and the chemokine MIP-1α *(65)*.

- *Rev (Regulator of Virion) Protein*. Rev is a 13-kDa sequence-specific RNA binding protein *(7, 66)*. Produced from fully spliced mRNAs, Rev induces the transition from the early to the late phase of HIV gene expression *(67)*. Rev, which is encoded by two exons, accumulates within the nuclei and nucleoli of infected cells and binds to a 240-base region of complex RNA secondary structure, the so-called *Rev Response Element (RRE)*, which lies within the second intron of HIV *(68)*. Furthermore, Rev binds to a "bubble" within a double-stranded RNA helix containing a non–Watson-Crick G-G base pair *(69)*. This structure, known as the *Rev high affinity binding site*, is located in a region of the RRE known as stem loop 2 *(7)*.

The binding of Rev to the RRE facilitates the export of unspliced and incompletely spliced viral RNAs from the nucleus to the cytoplasm. Normally, RNAs that contain introns (i.e., unspliced or incompletely spliced RNA) are retained in the nucleus. High levels of Rev expression can lead to excessive export of intron containing viral RNA so that the amount of RNA available for complete splicing is decreased, which, in turn, reduces the levels of Rev expression. Therefore, this ability of Rev to decrease the rate of splicing of viral RNA generates a *negative feedback loop* whereby Rev expression levels are tightly regulated *(70)*.

Rev, which is believed to exist as a homotetramer in solution *(71)*, has been shown to contain at least three functional domains *(72)*: an arginine-rich RNA binding that mediates interactions with the RRE; a multimerization domain that is required for Rev to function *(73)*; and an effector domain that is a specific *nuclear export signal (NES) (74, 75)*.

Viral RNA is exported by Rev through a pathway typically used by the small nuclear RNAs (snRNAs) and the ribosomal 5s RNA, rather than through the normal pathway for cellular mRNAs *(75)*. The Rev export is mediated through interactions with the NES receptor known as CRM1. NES mutants of Rev are dominant negative *(72)*. Inhibition is caused by the formation of nonfunctional multimers between NES-mutant and wild type Rev monomers *(76)*.

Overall, Rev is absolutely required for HIV-1 replication: proviruses that lack Rev function, though transcriptionally active, do not express viral late genes and thus do not produce virions *(7)*.

- *Accessory Proteins*. In addition to the *gag*, *pol*, and *env* genes contained in all retroviruses, and the *tat* and *rev* regulatory genes, HIV-1 contains four additional genes: *nef*, *vif*, *vpr*, and *vpu*, which encode the so-called accessory proteins *(7)*. HIV-2 does not contain *vpu*, but instead harbors another gene, *vpx*. Although the accessory proteins are not absolutely required for viral replication in all *in vitro* systems, they represent critical infectivity factors *in vivo*. Nef is expressed from a multiply spliced mRNA and is, therefore, Rev-independent. In contrast, Vpr, Vpu, and Vif are the product of incompletely spliced mRNA and thus are expressed only during the late, Rev-dependent phase of infection from singly spliced mRNAs. Most of the small accessory proteins of HIV have multiple functions, as described below *(7)*.

  ○ *Nef (Negative Regulation Factor)*. Nef is a 27-kDa myristoylated protein that is encoded by a single exon and extends into the 3′ LTR. Nef, an early gene of HIV, is the first viral protein to accumulate to detectable levels in a cell after HIV-1 infection *(67)*. Its name is a consequence of early reports claiming that Nef downregulated transcriptional activity of the HIV-1 LTR. However, it is no longer believed that Nef has a direct effect on HIV gene expression. Instead, Nef has been shown to have multiple activities, including the downregulation of the cell surface expression of CD4, the perturbation of T-cell activation, and the stimulation of HIV infectivity *(7)*.

Nef acts posttranslationally to decrease the cell-surface expression of CD4, the primary receptor for HIV *(77)*. Furthermore, it increases the rate of CD4 endocytosis and lysosomal degradation *(78)*. The cytoplasmic tail of CD4, and in particular, a di-leucine repeat sequence contained in its membrane proximal region, plays a pivotal role in the effect of Nef on CD4 *(78)*. CD4 downregulation appears to be advantageous to viral production because an excess of CD4 on the cell surface has been found to inhibit Env incorporation and virion budding *(79, 80)*. Nef also downregulates the cell surface expression of class I major histocompatibility complex (MHC), albeit to a lesser degree *(81)*. The downregulation of class I MHC decreases the efficiency of the killing of HIV-infected cells by cytotoxic T cells *(7)*.

In another function, Nef also perturbs the activation of T cells *(7)*. Studies in the Jurkat T-cell line indicated that Nef expression has a negative effect on the induction of the transcription factor NF-κB and on the IL-2 expression *(82)*. In contrast, results obtained in Nef transgenic mice revealed that Nef led to elevated T-cell signaling *(83)*. The expression of a CD8-Nef chimeric molecule in Jurkat cells had either positive or negative effects depending on the cellular localization of the hybrid Nef molecule *(84)*. The accumulation of the CD8-Nef protein in the cytoplasm results in blocking of the normal signaling through the T-cell receptor. When the CD8-Nef chimera was expressed at high levels on the cell surface, however, spontaneous activation followed by apoptosis was detected. Together, these observations suggest that Nef can exert pleiomorphic effects on T-cell activation, depending on the context of expression *(7)*. Consistent with this model, Nef has been found to associate with several different cellular kinases that are present in helper T lymphocytes.

Nef also stimulates the infectivity of HIV virions *(85)*. HIV-1 particles produced in the presence of Nef can be up to 10 times more infectious than virions produced in the absence of Nef. Nef is packaged into virions, where it is cleaved by the viral protease during virion maturation *(86)*. The importance of this event, however, is not clear. Virions produced in the absence of Nef are less efficient for proviral DNA synthesis, although Nef does not appear to influence directly the process of reverse transcription *(87)*. The downregulation of CD4 and the effect on virion infectivity by Nef are genetically distinct, as demonstrated by certain mutations that affect only one of these two activities *(88)*.

There is compelling genetic evidence that the Nef protein of simian immunodeficiency virus is absolutely required for high-titer growth and the typical development of disease in adult animals *(89)*. It is possible, however, for Nef-defective mutants of simian immunodeficiency virus (SIV) to cause disease in newborn animals *(90)*. Furthermore, Nef-defective virions may also cause an AIDS-like disease in infected animals, although onset is delayed *(91)*.

- *Vpr (Viral Protein R) Protein.* The Vpr protein is incorporated into viral particles. Approximately 100 copies of Vpr are associated with each virion *(92)*. Incorporation of Vpr into virions is mediated through specific interactions with the carboxyl-terminal region of p55 Gag *(37)*,

which corresponds with p6 in the proteolytically processed protein *(7)*.

Functionally, Vpr plays a role in the ability of HIV-1 to infect nondividing cells by facilitating the nuclear localization of the *pre-integration complex (PIC) (93)*. Vpr is present in the PIC. However, rather than tethering additional nuclear localization signals to the PIC, Vpr may act as a nucleocytoplasmic transport factor by directly tethering the viral genome to the nuclear pore. Consistent with this model, Vpr expressed in cells is found associated with the nuclear pore and can be biochemically demonstrated to bind to components of the nuclear pore complex *(94)*. Vpr can also block cell division *(95)*. Cells expressing Vpr accumulate in the G2 phase of the cell cycle *(96)*. The expression of Vpr has been shown to prevent the activation of the p34cdc2/cyclin B complex, which is a regulator of the cell cycle important for entry into mitosis *(97, 98)*. Accordingly, expression of a constitutively active mutant of p34cdc2 prevents the Vpr-induced accumulation of cells in the G2 phase of the cell cycle *(99)*.

Vpr has also been shown to interact with the cellular protein uracil-DNA glycosylase (UNG) *(100)*. The biological consequences of this phenomenon have yet to be determined. Another enzyme involved with the modification of deoxyuracil (dUTP), deoxyuracil phosphatase (dUTPase), is expressed by two lentiviruses that do not contain a *vpr* gene: equine infectious anemia virus and feline immunodeficiency virus. It is believed that the dUTPase depletes the dUTP within the cell, thereby preventing the deleterious consequences of dUTP incorporation into viral DNA *(101)*.

- *Vpu (Viral Protein U).* Vpu is involved in viral budding, enhancing virion release from the cell. The 16-kDa Vpu polypeptide is an integral membrane phosphoprotein that is primarily localized in the internal membranes of the cell *(102)*. Vpu, which is expressed from the mRNA that also encodes *env*, is translated from this mRNA at levels 10 times lower than that of Env because the Vpu translation initiation codon is not efficient *(103)*. The two functions of Vpu, the down-modulation of CD4 and the enhancement of virion release, can be genetically separated *(104)*.

In HIV-1–infected cells, complexes form between the viral receptor, CD4, and the viral envelope protein in the endoplasmic reticulum, causing both proteins to be trapped within this compartment. The formation of intracellular Env-CD4 complexes will therefore interfere with the virion assembly. Vpu liberates the viral envelope by triggering the ubiquitin-mediated degradation of CD4 molecules complexed with Env *(105)*.

Furthermore, Vpu also increases the release of HIV from the surface of an infected cell. In the absence of Vpu, large numbers of virions can be seen attached to the surface of infected cells *(106)*.

- *Vif (Viral Infectivity Factor) Protein.* Vif is a 23-kDa polypeptide that is essential for the replication of HIV in peripheral blood lymphocytes, macrophages, and certain cell lines *(107)* and is incorporated into the HIV virions *(108)*. In most cell lines, Vif is not required, suggesting that these cells may express a protein that can complement Vif function. These cell lines are called permissive for the Vif mutants of HIV. Virions generated in permissive cells can infect nonpermissive cells but the virus subsequently produced is noninfectious *(7)*.

Complementation studies indicate that it is possible to restore the infectivity of HIV Vif mutants by expression of Vif in producer cells but not in target cells *(109)*. These results indicate that Vif must be present during virion assembly. However, this phenomenon may be nonspecific because Vif is also incorporated into heterologous retroviruses such as murine leukemia viruses *(110)*. Studies producing HIV from heterokaryons generated by the fusion of permissive and nonpermissive cells revealed that nonpermissive cells contain a naturally occurring antiviral factor that is overcome by Vif *(111)*. Further support for a model demonstrating that Vif counteracts an antiviral cellular factor comes from the observation that Vif proteins from different lentiviruses are species specific *(112)*. For example, the HIV Vif can modulate the infectivity of HIV-2 and SIV in human cells, whereas the SIV Vif protein does not function in human cells. This observation indicates that cellular factors, rather than viral components, are the target of Vif action. Vif-defective HIV strains can enter cells but cannot efficiently synthesize the proviral DNA *(109)*. It is not clear whether the Vif defect affects reverse transcription *per se*, viral uncoating, or the overall stability of the viral nucleoprotein complex. Vif mutant virions have improperly packed nucleoprotein cores, as revealed by electron microscopic analyses *(113)*.

27.1.2 Regulation of HIV Gene Expression

HIV gene expression is regulated by a combination of both cellular and viral factors, at both the transcriptional and post-transcriptional levels *(7)*. The HIV genes can be divided into the early genes and the late genes *(86, 87)*. The early genes, *tat*, *rev*, and *nef*, are expressed in a Rev-independent manner. The mRNAs encoding the late genes, *gag*, *pol*, *env*, *vpr*, *vpu*, and *vif*, require Rev in order to be cytoplasmically localized and expressed (see Section 27.1.1).

Transcription of the Proviral Genome. The HIV transcription is mediated by a single promoter in the 5′ LTR. Expression from the 5′ LTR generates a 9-kb primary transcript that has the potential to encode all nine HIV genes. The primary transcript is roughly 600 bases shorter than the provirus. The primary transcript can be spliced into one of more than 30 mRNA species *(114)* or packaged without further mod-

ification into virion particles (to serve as the viral RNA genome) *(7)*.

The long terminal repeats (LTRs) are composed of three subregions designated (according to their location within the primary transcript of HIV) as U3, R, and U5 *(115)*. The U3 region (for unique 3′ sequence) is approximately 450 base pairs (bp) in length and is located at the 5′ end of each LTR. The U3 region contains most of the *cis*-acting DNA elements, which are the binding sites for cellular transcription factors. The central region of each LTR contains the 100-bp R (for repeated sequence) region. Transcription begins at the first base of the R region and polyadenylation occurs immediately after the last base of R. The U5 region (for unique 5′ sequence) is 180-bp in length and contains the Tat binding site and the packaging sequences of HIV. The 3′ end of U5 is defined by the location of a lysyl tRNA binding site. The lysyl tRNA acts as a primer for reverse transcription *(7)*.

Regulation of Transcription. The LTR of HIV contains DNA binding sites for several cellular transcription factors. Key among the DNA binding sites required for activating the transcription of the HIV provirus are those for the NF-κB family of transcription factors *(116)*. Two adjacent NF-κB sites are present in the U3 region of the HIV-1 LTR. The NF-κB protein allows the virus to be responsive to the activation state of the infected T cell. Stimulation of the T-cell receptor (TCR) causes the inactive form of NF-κB, localized in the cytoplasm, to be translocated into the nucleus where it induces the expression of a series of T-cell activation–specific genes. NF-κB and subsequent activation of HIV transcription can also be induced by the cytokines tumor necrosis factor-α (TNF-α) *(117)* and interleukin-1 (IL-1) *(118)*. The HIV LTR also contains binding sites for the constitutive transcription factors SP-1, Lef, and Ets, along with binding sites for the inducible transcription factors NF-AT and AP-1 *(119, 120)*. Lef and NF-At are T-cell–specific factors. The SP-1 binding sites are essential to the function of the HIV promoter *(7)*.

The initial activation of the HIV LTR is a consequence of inducible and constitutive cellular transcription factors *(7)*. Activation of the LTR by cellular transcription factors leads primarily to the generation of short transcripts *(58)*. These short transcripts are caused in part by an element located just downstream from the site of the initiation of transcription, known as the *inducer of short transcripts (IST)* *(121)*. Some complete transcripts, however, are generated and allow the production of the Tat protein. The Tat protein then interacts with the TAR element to greatly increase the levels of transcription of viral RNAs. The Tat protein would thereby play a key role in the activation and maintenance of high levels of transcription from the proviral DNA *(7)*.

mRNA Splicing and Cellular Localization. The primary HIV-1 transcript contains multiple splice donors (5′ splice sites) and splice acceptors (3′ splice sites), which can be processed to yield more than 30 alternative mRNAs *(114)*. Many of the mRNAs are polycistronic (i.e., they contain the open reading frame of more than one protein). The polycistronic mRNAs typically express a single gene product, and the open reading frame choice is governed by the efficiency of the initiation codon and the proximity of the initiation codon to the 5′ end of the mRNA *(122)*.

The HIV-1 mRNAs fall into three size classes:

- *Unspliced RNAs.* The unspliced 9-kb primary transcript can be expressed to generate the Gag and Gag-Pol precursor proteins or be packaged into virions to serve as the genomic RNA *(7)*.
- *Incompletely spliced RNAs.* These mRNAs will use the splice donor site located nearest the 5′ end of the HIV RNA genome in combination with any of the splice acceptors located in the central region of the virus. Furthermore, these RNAs can potentially express Env, Vif, Vpu, Vpr, and the single-exon form of Tat. These heterogeneous mRNAs are 4- to 5-kb long and retain the second intron of HIV *(7)*.
- *Fully spliced RNAs.* These mRNAs have spliced out both introns of HIV and have the potential to express Rev, Nef, and the two-exon form of Tat. These heterogeneous mRNAs do not require the expression of the Rev protein *(7)*.

Normally, intron-containing RNAs must be completely spliced before they can exit the nucleus *(7)*. This regulation is essential because it prevents the translation of intronic sequences contained in partially spliced mRNAs. The Rev protein binds to viral RNAs that retain intron sequences and directs their export from the nucleus. This export allows the unconventional viral RNAs to bypass the normal "check point" of RNA splicing. The fully spliced viral mRNAs will exit the nucleus by using the export pathway followed by the majority of cellular mRNAs. Threshold levels of Rev are necessary for exporting intron-containing HIV mRNAs, which explains why those encode the viral late gene products. In contrast, the proteins encoded by the fully spliced mRNAs, Nef, Tat, and Rev, can be produced immediately and are thus considered to be early viral gene products *(7)*.

27.1.3 HIV Viral Entry: Host Cell Receptor and Coreceptors

HIV-1 enters target cells by direct fusion of the viral and target cell membranes. The fusion reaction is mediated by the viral envelope glycoprotein (Env), which binds with high affinity to CD4, the primary receptor on the target cell surface *(123)*. By a similar or identical mechanism, cells expressing Env can fuse with CD4$^+$ target cells, sometimes leading to the formation of giant cells (syncytia) *(124)*.

In addition to CD4, HIV requires a coreceptor for entry into target cells *(124)*. The chemokine receptors CXCR4 and CCR5, members of the G protein–coupled receptor superfamily, have been identified as the principal coreceptors for T-cell line-tropic and macrophage-tropic HIV-1 isolates, respectively. The updated coreceptor repertoire includes numerous members, mostly chemokine receptors and related orphans *(124)*. These discoveries provide a new framework for understanding critical features of the basic biology of HIV-1, including the selective tropism of individual viral variants for different CD4$^+$ target cells and the membrane fusion mechanism governing virus entry. In addition, the coreceptors also provide molecular perspectives on central puzzles of HIV-1 disease, including the selective transmission of macrophage-tropic variants, the appearance of T-cell line-tropic variants in many infected persons during the disease's progression to AIDS, and differing susceptibilities of individuals to infection and disease progression. Genetic findings have yielded major insights into the *in vivo* roles of individual coreceptors and their ligands; of particular importance is the discovery of an inactivating mutation in the CCR5 gene that, in homozygous form, confers strong resistance to HIV-1 infection. Beyond providing new perspectives on fundamental aspects of the transmission and pathogenesis of HIV-1, the coreceptors suggest new avenues for developing novel therapeutic and preventive strategies to combat the AIDS epidemic *(124)*.

HIV-2 and the simian immunodeficiency virus have also been shown to use chemokine receptors and related orphans as coreceptors *(125, 126)*.

Coreceptor for T-Cell Line (TCL)-Tropic HIV-1. The first HIV-1 coreceptor was identified by using an unbiased functional cDNA cloning strategy based on the ability of a cDNA library to render a CD4-expressing murine cell permissive for fusion with cells expressing Env from a TCL-adapted strain *(127)*. A single cDNA was isolated, and sequence analysis indicated that the protein product was a member of the superfamily of the seven transmembrane domain G protein–coupled receptors, the largest receptor superfamily in the human genome. The cDNA previously had been isolated and sequenced by several laboratories investigating G protein–coupled receptors, but no ligands or functional activities had been found; the protein was thus considered an "orphan" receptor. Because of its new-found activity in HIV-1 Env-mediated fusion, the protein was named "fusin" *(127)*. Its role as a coreceptor was based on both gain-of-function experiments demonstrating that coexpression of fusin along with CD4 rendered non-human cells permissive for Env-mediated cell fusion and infection and on loss-of-function experiments showing that antifusin antibodies potently inhibited fusion and infection of primary human CD4$^+$ T lymphocytes. Most importantly, both types of analyses indicated that fusin functioned for TCL-tropic, but not M-tropic, HIV-1 strains. Fusin thus fit the criteria for the TCL-tropic HIV-1 coreceptor *(124)*.

Coreceptor for M-Tropic HIV-1. The discovery of fusin, a putative chemokine receptor, as the coreceptor for TCL-tropic HIV-1 strains provided an impetus and direction for identifying the coreceptor for M-tropic isolates. The focus was narrowed to CC chemokine receptors by a link with an earlier study directed at a seemingly unrelated problem, namely the identity of soluble HIV-1 suppressor factor(s) released by $CD8^+$ T lymphocytes, a phenomenon first described in the late 1980s *(128)*. The first success was achieved in 1995 with the demonstration that the CC chemokines RANTES, MIP-1α, and MIP-1β are major suppressive factors released by $CD8^+$ T-lymphocytes *(129)*. Particularly intriguing was the fact that these CC chemokines potently suppressed infection by M-tropic HIV-1 strains but had little effect on a TCL-tropic strain. Because fusin, the coreceptor for TCL-tropic strains, was a putative chemokine receptor, an obvious mechanism for inhibiting infection by CC chemokines was suggested, namely, that they bind to and block a chemokine receptor that functions as a coreceptor for M-tropic HIV-1. Fortuitously, at approximately the same time, a chemokine receptor was identified with precisely the corresponding specificity for RANTES, MIP-1α, and MIP-1β *(130–132)*; it was designated *CCR5*, in keeping with the standard nomenclature system for chemokine receptors (fifth receptor for CC chemokines). Shortly thereafter, five independent reports demonstrated that CCR5 is a major coreceptor for M-tropic HIV-1 strains *(133–137)*; the evidence was based on both gain-of-function studies with recombinant CCR5 and loss-of-function studies using CCR5 chemokine ligands as blocking agents *(124)*.

Fusin as a Chemokine Receptor (CXCR4). The discoveries of coreceptors were soon followed by the demonstration that fusin is indeed a chemokine receptor, specific for the functionally equivalent CXC chemokines SDF-1α and SDF-1β *(138, 139)*, which are formed by alternative splicing. Fusin was therefore renamed CXCR4 (fourth receptor for CXC chemokines). SDF-1 was shown to be a selective inhibitor of TCL-tropic HIV-1 strains *(124)*.

The Integrin α4β7 Coreceptor. Gut-associated lymphoid tissue (GALT) is the principal site where HIV-1 replicates *(140–145)*. Regardless of the route of transmission, HIV-1 rapidly establishes infection in GALT *(140)*. It has been postulated that the distinct tropism of HIV-1 for GALT results from the high frequency of activated $CD4^+CCR5^+$ T cells, which, it is argued, provide a target-rich environment *(145)*. Yet CCR5 expression, as measured by flow cytometry, did not correlate with the frequency of infected memory $CD4^+$ T cells in the gut *(144)*. Moreover, infection of resting memory $CD4^+$ T cells in the gut is thought to be vital to the establishment of infection *(146)*. Soon after HIV-1 is seeded in the gut, it will undergo substantial depletion of $CD4^+$ T-cells. It has been proposed that this depletion represents an irreversible insult to the immune system, which ultimately would result in AIDS *(147)*. The mechanisms underlying $CD4^+$ T-cell depletion in the gut remain controversial. T-cell depletion may result from either direct infection *(145)* or, alternatively, through bystander effects mediated by the HIV-1 envelope *(143)*. It is apparent that much is not yet understood about HIV-1 replication in the gut and the concomitant depletion of $CD4^+$ T cells from the gut. Yet understanding of these events is fundamental to an accurate description of HIV-1 pathogenesis and possibly to the development of an effective HIV-1 vaccine. Results from recent experiments have shown that the HIV-1 envelope protein gp120 bound to and signaled by means of an activated form of integrin α4β7 on $CD4^+$ T lymphocytes *(148)*. Furthermore, the gp120 rapidly activated LFA-1, an integrin that facilitates HIV-1 infection, on $CD4^+$ T cells in α4β7-dependent way. Functioning principally as a homing receptor, α4β7 would mediate the migration of leukocytes to and retention of leukocytes in the lamina propria of the gut *(149, 150)*. Thus, in the tissue where HIV-1 "preferentially" replicates, its envelope would interact directly with an adhesion receptor that is specifically linked to the function of $CD4^+$ T cells in that tissue *(148)*.

27.1.4 HIV-1 Genetic Diversity

HIV-1 is characterized by a very high degree of genetic diversity *(151–153)*. Even in a single infected individual, the virus can be best described as a population of distinct, but closely related, genetic variants, referred to as a *quasispecies* *(154, 155)*. A deterministic evolutionary model of HIV-1 has been proposed to describe its evolution. This model assumes a large population size of HIV-1 *(156–159)*, in which competition among constantly generated viral variants with slight fitness differences determines the exact frequency of mutants *(160)*. According to this model, evolution will be inevitable and, in principle, predictable. Recently, however, it has been argued that chance may play a significant role in the evolution of HIV-1, because the *effective population size* (N_e) in an infected individual may be small *(161, 162)*. N_e is defined as an ideal population that is drawn randomly from the total population and that has the same statistical characteristics as the total population. In the case of HIV-1, N_e can be described as the average number of virus variants that produce infectious progeny. A stochastic evolutionary model would take into account the impact of chance on the evolution of HIV-1 *(163)*.

27.1.5 APOBEC3 Protein Family

Apolipoprotein B mRNA editing enzyme, catalytic polypeptide-like 3C, also known as APOBEC3C, is a human gene *(164)*.

The genomes of humans and other primates encode at least five, and possibly up to seven, APOBEC3 proteins, all of which are encoded by a single gene cluster on chromosome 22 *(165, 166)*. This gene cluster appears to be unique to primates, as the genomes of several other mammalian species, such as mice, cats, and cows, encode only a single APOBEC3 protein *(167, 168)*.

The APOBEC3 protein family was so named because all APOBEC3 proteins display significant homology to APOBEC1 and to two other human gene products, APOBEC2 and activation-induced deaminase (AID) *(166)*. APOBEC1, the founding member of this extended protein family, edits a single C residue to U on the mRNA encoding apolipoprotein B (ApoB), thereby introducing a premature stop codon and inducing production of a truncated form of ApoB that has a different biological function *(164)*. Though the role of APOBEC2 remains unclear, AID functions in activated B cells, where it randomly edits dC residues to dU in the immunoglobulin gene locus *(169)*.

The initial characterization and sequencing of the human APOBEC3 gene family led to the proposal that these genes encoded a novel set of orphan cytidine deaminases, based on their similarity to APOBEC1 and AID *(166)*. However, the subsequent observation that APOBEC3 proteins can function as innate inhibitors of retroviral replication came from unrelated studies focused on the pathogenic lentivirus, human immunodeficiency virus type 1 (HIV-1), and, more specifically, on the role and mechanism of action of the HIV-1 virion infectivity factor (Vif) gene product, an ∼192-aa cytoplasmic protein.

A key aspect of the mechanism of action of hA3G and the other APOBEC3 proteins is their specific incorporation into retroviral virions, as well as HBV virions and LTR-retrotransposon VLPs (virus-like particles). Only after incorporation can the APOBEC3 proteins interfere with virion or VLP function, by inducing deamination of dC residues present on reverse transcripts and/or by interfering with aspects of virion or VLP morphogenesis. The APOBEC3 proteins, and hA3G in particular, inhibit a wide range of retroviruses and LTR retrotransposons, so it is important to understand how the APOBEC3 proteins are able to target all of these disparate viruses or genomic parasites (i.e., to understand what defines the pathogen-associated molecular patterns (PAMP) shared by these viruses and virus-like elements that is recognized by the APOBEC3 protein family) *(165)*.

This question has been partly addressed by work analyzing the packaging of hA3G into HIV-1 virions. This research demonstrated that hA3G binds to the nucleocapsid (NC) domain of the Gag polyprotein during virion assembly *(170–175)*. As a result, HIV-1 Gag derivatives lacking NC, which can still assemble into VLPs, fail to package hA3G *(168, 169)*. Interestingly, the Gag-hA3G interaction depends on the presence of RNA *(172, 174–176)*. Though

viral RNA may be ideal, nonspecific cellular RNA seems almost as effective at mediating the Gag-hA3G interaction. Of note, a key role of the NC domain of Gag is to recruit the viral RNA genome into virion particles, and NC to display both specific and nonspecific RNA binding properties *(171)*. Similarly, hA3G has also been shown to bind RNA nonspecifically *(177)*.

The APOBEC3 cytidine deaminases, which are unique to mammals, have been identified as potent innate cellular defenses against both endogenous retroelements and diverse retroviruses *(178, 179)*.

A variety of mechanisms of innate immunity that protect organisms from retroviral infections, including HIV, are known. Lentiviruses express viral infectivity factor (Vif) protein, which has the ability to counter antiviral activity exhibited by the recently discovered host cytidine deaminases, APOBEC3G and 3F. Although these host factors are present in diverse mammalian species and have been shown to act against various organisms, their importance in HIV infection has been highlighted because of their suggested activities against HIV *in vivo* and the strong conservation of the HIV *vif* gene encoding the Vif protein capable of countering this innate activity *(180)*.

Wild-type HIV-1 is clearly resistant to inhibition by all human APOBEC3 proteins except hA3B, which did not appear to be expressed in the human tissues normally infected by HIV-1. It is, however, possible that the inhibition of hA3G and/or hA3F function by HIV-1 Vif may not always be complete, especially in cells that express unusually high levels of these proteins. Moreover, HIV-1 would undergo rapid sequence evolution in infected patients, presumably due largely to the error-prone viral reverse transcriptase but also potentially due to editing by hA3G and/or hA3F. If the *vif* gene were to be fully or partially inactivated as a result of mutation, then one might predict that hypermutated HIV-1 proviruses would arise *(165)*.

To evade such host defenses, retroviruses have developed multiple strategies. Recent findings have suggested several mechanisms of these viral counterdefenses. For example: (i) primate lentiviruses did encode a virion-infectivity factor that induced targeted destruction of APOBEC3 proteins by hijacking the cellular ubiquitin-proteasome pathway; (ii) virion-infectivity factor molecules of HIV-1 and SIV such as the newly identified substrate receptor proteins that assemble with Cul5, ElonginB, ElonginC, and Rbx1 did form an E3 ubiquitin ligase that targeted selected APOBEC3 proteins for polyubiquitination; (iii) the foamy viruses did use a different viral protein, Bet, which would bind and sequester APOBEC3 away from the assembling virions; and (iv) simple retroviruses such as murine leukemia virus may avoid virion packaging of cognate APOBEC3 protein through yet another novel mechanism, in the absence of a viral regulatory factor *(165)*.

As a result, these retroviruses and APOBEC3 proteins maintain an equilibrium that allows regulated viral replication. These viral counterdefenses thus represent vulnerable targets for the design of new classes of antiviral inhibitors *(165)*.

27.1.6 TRIM5α Restriction Factor

The tripartite motif (TRIM) family is a well-conserved family of proteins characterized by a structure comprising a RING domain, one or two B-boxes, and a predicted coiled-coil region *(181, 182)*. In addition, most TRIM proteins have additional C-terminal domains.

Members of the TRIM protein family are involved in various cellular processes, including cell proliferation, differentiation, development, oncogenesis, and apoptosis *(183, 184)*. Some TRIM proteins display antiviral properties—targeting retroviruses in particular—targeting the early steps of cellular infection *(185)*.

The control of retroviral infection by antiviral factors referred to as restriction factors has become an exciting area in infectious disease research. TRIM5α has emerged as an important restriction factor affecting retroviral replication, including HIV-1 replication in primates. TRIM5α has a tripartite motif comprising RING, B-box, and coiled coil domains. The antiviral α splice variant additionally encodes a B30.2 domain that is recruited to incoming viral cores and determines antiviral specificity *(186)*.

TRIM5α is ubiquitinylated and rapidly turned over by the proteasome in a RING-dependent way. It protects restricted virus from degradation by inhibiting the proteasome. Furthermore, TRIM5α rescues DNA synthesis, but not infectivity, indicating that restriction of infectivity by TRIM5α did not depend on the proteasome but on the early block to DNA synthesis, which is likely to be mediated by rapid degradation of the restricted cores *(186)*. To this end, the peptidyl prolyl isomerase enzyme cyclophilin A has been found to isomerize a peptide bond on the surface of the HIV-1 capsid and to affect sensitivity to restriction by TRIM5α from Old World monkeys *(186)*. This finding suggests that TRIM5α from Old World monkeys might have a preference for a particular capsid isomer and also suggests a role for cyclophilin A in innate immunity in general. Whether there are more human antiviral TRIMs remains uncertain, although the evidence for TRIM19's (PML) antiviral properties continues to grow. A TRIM5-like molecule with broad antiviral activity in cattle suggests that TRIM-mediated innate immunity may be common in mammals *(186)*.

TRIM5α is characterized by marked amino acid diversity among primates, including specific clusters of residues under positive selection *(181, 187, 188)*. TRIM5α restricts retroviral infection by specifically recognizing the capsid and promotes its premature disassembly *(189)*. Human TRIM5α (huTRIM5α) has limited efficacy against HIV-1, whereas some primate TRIM5α orthologues can potently restrict lentivirus *(183, 184)*.

Analysis of huTRIM5α polymorphism in blood donors identified more than 20 common genetic variants *(181, 182)* and several rare non-synonymous variants *(187, 188)*. The identification of multiple non-synonymous changes in humans suggests that TRIM5α variants might be relevant to retroviral pathogenesis *(181)*.

Antiretroviral Activity of TRIM5α. TRIM5α has recently emerged as an important restriction factor in mammals, blocking infection by retroviruses in a species-specific way *(186)*. Early evidence for TRIM5α's antiviral activity included the species-specific infectivity of retroviral vectors, even when specific envelope/receptor requirements were obviated by the use of the vesicular stomatitis virus (VSV-G) envelope. Notable examples include the poor infectivity of certain murine leukemia viruses (MLVs) on cells from humans and primates and the poor infectivity of HIV-1 on cells from Old World monkeys *(190–192)*. The notion that a dominant antiviral factor was responsible was suggested by the demonstration that the block to infection could be saturated, or abrogated, by high doses of retroviral cores *(193–195)*. The putative human antiviral factor was named Ref1 and the simian factor Lv1 *(190, 195)*. TRIM5α was identified in 2004 by screening rhesus cDNAs for those with antiviral activity against HIV-1 *(185)*. Shortly afterwards, several groups demonstrated that Ref1 and Lv1 were encoded by species-specific variants of TRIM5α *(196–199)*. TRIM5α, therefore, represents a hitherto undescribed *arm of the innate immune system*, blocking infection by an incompletely characterized mechanism. Its expression is induced by interferon via an IRF3 site in the TRIM5 promoter linking it to the classic innate immune system *(200)*.

Recently, two studies have addressed the potential role of huTRIM5α variants in modulating susceptibility to HIV-1 *(187, 188)*. The first study identified several non-synonymous SNPs in huTRIM5α, but only one of these (H43Y) was found to have a functional consequence *(187)*]. H43Y, which was found in the RING domain of TRIM5α, may negatively affect its putative E3 ubiquitin ligase activity. Although huTRIM5α weakly restricts HIV-1, H43Y might further reduce viral restriction to a level similar to that of cells expressing no exogenous huTRIM5α *(187)*. To assess whether the impaired retroviral restriction seen with exogenously expressed huTRIM5α H43Y resulted in altered susceptibility in human cells, researchers tested B-lymphocytes from four individuals: one homozygous for H43, two homozygous for 43Y, and one heterozygous at this site. Challenge with HIV-1 failed to demonstrate a significant effect of the H43Y change, although 43Y homozygous cells could be infected with N-MLV about 100-fold more efficiently than cells with the common H43 allele *(187)*.

A second study assessed the association of various non-synonymous variants with susceptibility to HIV-1 among 110 HIV-1-infected subjects and 96 exposed seronegative persons *(188)*. This study identified possible associations between specific haplotypes and alleles and susceptibility to infection and viral setpoint after acute infection.

In a third study, data were analyzed from a large cohort of subjects infected with HIV-1 to explore whether different huTRIM5α variants are associated with long-term disease evolution. The study was complemented by analysis of CD4 cell susceptibility to HIV-1 and the *in vitro* functionality of selected huTRIM5α variants. The results showed that there was no impact for some and negligible to modest impact for other common human variants of TRIM5α on disease progression *(181)*. Modest differences were observed in disease progression for evolutionary branches carrying R136-derived haplotypes, and with the non-synonymous polymorphisms G249D and H419Y. *In vitro* analysis of susceptibility of donor CD4 T-cells, and of the various transduced HeLa cell lines, supported the absence of significant differential restriction of HIV-1 infection by the various huTRIM5α alleles. Common human variants of TRIM5α have no effect or modest effect on HIV-1 disease progression. These variants occurred at sites conserved throughout evolution and were remote from clusters of positive selection in the primate lineage. The evolutionary value of the substitutions remains unclear *(181)*.

The Tripartite Motif. TRIM5 has a *tri*partite *mo*tif, also known as an RBCC domain, comprising a RING domain, a B-box2 domain, and a coiled-coil *(182, 201)*. The RING is a zinc-binding domain, typically involved in specific protein-protein interactions. Many RING domains have E3 ubiquitin ligase activity, and TRIM5 can mediate RING-dependent auto-ubiquitinylation *in vitro* *(203)*. B-boxes are of two types, either B-box1 or B-box2, and TRIM5 encodes a B-box2. B-boxes have a zinc-binding motif and are putatively involved in protein-protein interactions. The two types of B-box have distinct primary sequences but similar tertiary structures and are structurally similar to the RING domain. The coiled-coil is involved in homo- and hetero-multimerization of TRIM proteins *(202, 203)*. TRIM5 exists as a trimer with the coiled-coil facilitating homo- and hetero-multimerization with related TRIM proteins *(204–206)*.

TRIM5 RNA is multiply spliced, generating a family of isoforms, each shorter from the *C*-terminus. The longest, TRIM5α, encodes a *C*-terminal B30.2 domain that interacts directly with viral capsid and determines antiviral specificity *(204, 207, 208)*. The shorter isoforms, TRIM5γ and TRIM5δ, do not have B30.2 domains and act as dominant negatives to TRIM5α and rescue restricted infectivity when overexpressed *(185, 209)*. It is assumed that the shorter forms form heteromultimers via the coiled-coil and titrate the viral binding B30.2 domains. It is, therefore, possible that the antiviral activity of TRIM5 is regulated by splicing *(199)*.

27.1.7 Retroviral Superinfection Resistance

The retroviral phenomenon of superinfection resistance defines an interference mechanism that is established after primary infection, preventing the infected cell from being superinfected by a similar type of virus *(210)*.

Viral entry and replication is a complex process that involves multiple viral and host proteins. Many host gene products can interfere with virus infection at the cellular level *(211)*. These proteins are encoded by variants of essential genes (which cannot support viral infection), or represent true antiviral factors (gene products whose main role is to protect the cell from a productive virus infection). A special form of virus resistance is the capacity of cells to prevent a second infection by a virus that is closely related to the virus that has already established an infection. In most cases, virus-encoded proteins are responsible for this phenomenon, which is termed *superinfection resistance (SIR)*, or *viral interference (210)*. A simple form of SIR is receptor occupancy by viral Env proteins, preventing the binding of a second virus, but many additional mechanisms have been described. Although SIR is not restricted to retroviruses, it has been studied in depth for this class of viruses.

HIV-1 Superinfection. HIV-1 superinfection in patients is defined as the re-infection of an individual with a second heterologous strain of HIV-1 *(212)*. Since the identification of the AIDS virus, various strategies have been proposed to prevent the spread of HIV infection. The underlying mechanisms of SIR in HIV-infected cells are of particular interest for developing novel antiviral approaches related to SIR. However, as a caveat, it should be noted that several studies have described the occurrence of HIV superinfection in HIV-infected patients *(210)*.

Like all other retroviruses, the HIV virion contains two copies of an RNA genome that is encapsulated by CA(p24) and Env proteins. The Env glycoproteins gp120 and gp41 mediate viral entry by interacting with CD4 molecules on susceptible cells. The CD4 receptor is a type 1 transmembrane glycoprotein and is mainly found on primary T lymphocytes, dendritic cells, and macrophages. Interaction of gp120 with CD4 induces conformational changes in the Env protein structure, which enables Env to interact with a coreceptor, such as the CCR5 or CXCR4 chemokine receptor, which leads to HIV entry into the target cell *(213)*. Several host factors have been identified that interfere with early steps during entry or replication of HIV-1 (e.g., APOBEC3G/CEM15, Lv1, Lv2, and TRIM5α) *(214)*.

CD4-Mediated Resistance to HIV Superinfection. One of the major characteristics of HIV-infected cells is the down-modulation of the CD4 receptor *(215–217)*. To date, three viral HIV proteins, Vpu, Env, and Nef, have been identified that mediate CD4 downregulation by distinct mechanisms *(218, 219)*, indicating the importance of CD4 down-regulation for HIV infection. As receptor down-modulation is a simple way of preventing a second viral infection and a method that is successfully used by other retroviruses, CD4 down-modulation was initially assumed to be the main SIR mechanism in HIV infection *(210)*.

All primate lentiviruses, HIV-1, HIV-2, and simian immunodeficiency virus (SIV), encode the Nef protein *(218)*. Nef binds directly to a di-leucine-like motif in the cytoplasmic domain of CD4. Nef is able to bind different members of the adaptor proteins (AP-1, AP-2, AP-3, and AP-4), which contain distinct transport signals. Simultaneous binding of Nef to CD4 and AP-2 at the cell surface induces endocytosis of CD4. In addition, Nef binding of AP-1 and AP-3 in the trans-Golgi network may mediate trafficking of newly synthesized CD4 directly to lysosomes. Stable transfection of the SIV *nef* gene in a CD4$^+$T-cell line reduced cell surface expression of CD4 and rendered the cells resistant to subsequent HIV-1 infection *(220)*. HIV-2 infected cells do not seem to resist subsequent HIV-1 infection, which may be explained by the inability of HIV-2 to induce CD4 down-modulation *(210)*.

In contrast with Nef, Env and Vpu mediate CD4 down-modulation by preventing the intracellular transport of newly synthesized CD4 molecules *(219)*. Binding of CD4 by the Env precursor protein gp160 in the endoplasmic reticulum (ER) triggers the formation of aggregates, which block further CD4 transport to the cell surface. In addition, Vpu mediates CD4 down-modulation by directing newly synthesized CD4 to proteosomes for degradation. Among the immunodeficiency viruses, Vpu is encoded nearly exclusively by HIV-1. It has been suggested that Vpu redirects CD4 trafficking by acting as an adaptor between CD4 and the h-βTrCP protein that is a key connector in the ubiquitin-mediated proteolysis machinery. Restriction of Vpu-mediated CD4 down-modulation either by inhibition of the proteosome activity or mutation of putative ubiquitination sites in the CD4 cytoplasmic domain supports this hypothesis *(210)*.

The most important physiologic purpose of CD4 down-modulation is likely not to resist superinfection but rather to increase viral replication and to promote the release of progeny virions *(220, 221)*. Reduction of CD4 cell surface expression results in particles with less CD4 and more Env molecules, which probably eases their release from the cell. When using HIV-1 variants with different coreceptor usage obtained from patients, it was found that down-modulation

of CD4 was not associated with CCR5-using viruses that are present early in infection, but were characteristic of CXCR4- or CXCR4/CCR5-using viruses that are mostly seen later in infection during the onset of AIDS *(222)*. In line with this, it was found that a macrophage-tropic, non-cytopathic strain of HIV-1 that did not downregulate CD4 also did not resist subsequent superinfection with a cytopathic HIV-1 strain in a CD4$^+$ T-cell clone (PM1) susceptible to a wide variety of HIV isolates *(223)*. Furthermore, *nef* genes from AIDS patients were far more efficient in downregulating CD4 than were *nef* alleles from asymptomatic patients *(221)*. Together, these results raised the question whether CD4 down-modulation *in vivo* is a significant cause of SIR in HIV-1 infection *(210)*.

Downregulation of coreceptors could be an alternative SIR mechanism *(210)*. However, downregulation of CXCR4 was not observed in culture, and although chronic infection with CCR5-using viruses abrogated CCR5 expression, the effect on superinfection was not tested *(222)*. A single study suggested that CCR5 down-modulation in an HIV-2–infected cohort of Senegalese women protected them from HIV-1 superinfection *(224)*.

CD4-Independent Mechanisms Contributing to HIV SIR. A few studies have shown cellular resistance to HIV superinfection by mechanisms unrelated to CD4 *(225, 226)*. Experimental results have demonstrated SIR in HIV-1–infected T cells that still expressed substantial levels of CD4 *(227)*. Moreover, nonfunctional HIV-1 mutants and HIV-1 mutants that could only bind CD4, but not enter the T cells, did not restrict superinfection of HIV-1 in these cells. The mechanism was HIV-1-specific, as the cells could be infected by other (retro)viruses, indicating that the results could not be explained by a general block of virus replication. HIV-1 mutants that encode inactive *vpu, vpr,* and *nef* genes were fully active in SIR, ruling out these genes as contributing to HIV SIR *(210)*.

Another study demonstrated CD4-independent SIR mechanisms in cells infected with a nonproducer HIV mutant *(228)*. CD4 down-modulation in these F12-HIV–infected cells did not change their susceptibility to a challenge HIV strain. However, SIR was established by inhibiting the replication of the superinfecting HIV strain.

An additional study evaluated SIR in cells transfected with distinct vectors containing a particular HIV protein *(229)*. The F12-HIV genes *gag, vif,* and *nef* were all found to alter replication of the superinfecting HIV-1 strain. Moreover, expression of Nef established complete resistance against the challenge by inhibiting HIV-1 replication at a late stage. Nef-mediated inhibition of viral replication has been associated with interference of Gag processing by preventing the cleavage of the p41 Gag precursor protein into p17 (MA) and p24 (CA) *(230)*. Moreover, the disturbed processing of Gag has been correlated with an altered subcellular distribution of F12-Nef compared with that of the wild-type Nef protein.

CD8 T-Cells and HIV Superinfection Resistance. In animals, antiviral effects, either to the initial or to a second viral infection, are in large part mediated by the immune system, making superinfections of animals greatly different from SIR in cells. A 100% effective SIR mechanism could prevent superinfection of a given cell in an animal, but a second virus could infect another, noninfected cell, leading to superinfection of the animal, but not to superinfection of the already infected cell *(210)*.

Neutralizing antibodies did restrict re-infection of cells from seropositive donors in culture *(231)*, and cytokines induced by the first viral infection can have a negative effect on subsequent infections *(232)*. An important immune-mediated inhibition of viral replication is exerted by noncytotoxic $CD8^+$ T cells. These cells belong to the innate immune system and were found to suppress replication of HIV-1 in $CD4^+$ T cells by a noncytotoxic mechanism mediated by a soluble antiviral factor, provisionally named CAF *(233–236)*. Until now, the identity of *CAF*, short for $CD8^+$-*cell antiviral factor*, has not been resolved, but it suppresses transcription of viral RNA *(237, 238)*, is found in both healthy persons and in asymptomatic HIV-1–infected patients *(239)*, can be inhibited by protease inhibitors *(240)*, and strongly suppresses HIV-1/HIV-2 superinfection in culture *(241)*. The mechanism is not virus- or species-specific and is also operational *in vivo*. It has been found in HIV-2–infected baboons *(242)* and in feline immunodeficiency virus (FIV)-infected cats *(243)*.

HIV-2–infected PBMCs from pig-tailed macaques, however, can be superinfected with another strain of HIV-2 *in vitro* in the presence of $CD8^+$ T cells *(244)*. Furthermore, 80% to 100% of chimpanzees experimentally infected with HIV-1 could be superinfected after 8 to 64 months with the same or a different viral subtype despite a fully functional immune system *(245)*.

Besides CAF as soluble factor, it has been suggested that contact between $CD4^+$ and $CD8^+$ cells is important for inhibiting viral replication, including HIV-1 superinfection *(242, 246)*. During disease progression, the anti-HIV effect of the CD8 T-cells was gradually lost *(239, 247)*, as was their ability to suppress superinfection *(241)*, probably due to a functional impairment of the (HIV-specific) $CD8^+$ cells in the AIDS phase *(248)*.

The studies described have clearly demonstrated HIV-1 superinfection in humans both with different HIV-1 strains and with closely related HIV-1 subtypes *(210)*. In an asymptomatic patient, a large reservoir of uninfected cells is available for infection by a second virus, as only 1:2,500 to 1:100,000 CD4 cells are estimated to be infected by HIV *(249, 250)*. During disease progression, substantially more virus is produced, and more $CD4^+$ cells become infected

(250). Thus, in the later stages of HIV infection, when both viruses produce a significant amount of progeny, uninfected cells can become dually infected with both virus strains, enabling the formation of recombinant forms. In other cells of the same organism, SIR might be operational and prevent a second infection. Indeed, in splenocytes of two HIV patients, an average of three to four HIV-1 proviruses were found *(251)*. Sequence analysis showed that proviruses in a single cell were often genetically distinct and gave rise to recombinants *(251)*.

27.2 HIV/AIDS Global Pandemic

Since the first cases of AIDS were reported in 1981, infection with HIV has grown to pandemic proportions, resulting in an estimated 65 million infections and 25 million deaths *(252–254)*. HIV continues to disproportionately affect certain geographic regions, such as sub-Saharan Africa and the Caribbean, and subpopulations [e.g., women in sub-Saharan Africa, men who have sex with men (MSM), injection-drug users (IDUs), and sex workers]. However, effective treatment of HIV infection with antiretroviral therapy (ART) is now available, even in countries with limited resources *(254)*. Nonetheless, comprehensive programs are needed to reach all persons who require treatment and to prevent transmission of new infections.

A recent report has summarized selected regional trends in the HIV/AIDS pandemic, based on data from the *2007 Report on the Global AIDS Epidemic* by the Joint United Nations Program on HIV/AIDS (UNAIDS) *(254)*.

Sub-Saharan Africa. Approximately 10% of the world population lives in sub-Saharan Africa, but the region is home to approximately 64% of the world population living with HIV *(254)*. Transmission is primarily through heterosexual contact, and more women are HIV-infected than men. Southern Africa is the epicenter of the AIDS epidemic; all countries in the region except Angola have an estimated prevalence of adult (i.e., aged 15 to 49 years) HIV exceeding 10% *(254)*. In Botswana, Lesotho, Swaziland, and Zimbabwe, the estimated adult HIV prevalence exceeds 20% *(254)*. South Africa, with an HIV prevalence of 18.8% and 5.5 million persons living with HIV, has, along with India, the largest number of persons living with HIV in the world *(254)*. Recently, declines in adult HIV prevalence have been observed in Kenya, Uganda, Zimbabwe, and urban areas of Burkina Faso. Although in these countries HIV-related sexual risk behaviors and HIV incidence have decreased, AIDS death rates continue to rise. In sub-Saharan Africa, only 17% of the estimated number of persons in need of ART received it in 2005 *(255)*.

Asia. Adult HIV prevalence is lower in Asian countries than in countries in sub-Saharan Africa, and the epidemic in most Asian countries is attributable primarily to various high-risk behaviors (e.g., unprotected sexual intercourse with sex workers, IDUs, or MSM and injection-drug use) *(252)*. Of the 8.3 million HIV-infected persons in Asia, 5.7 million live in India, where the prevalence varies by state. Approximately 80% of HIV infections in India are acquired heterosexually. Recent data from four Indian states indicated a decline in the prevalence of HIV among pregnant women aged 15 to 24 years, from 1.7% in 2000 to 1.1% in 2004 *(256)*. In China, currently 650,000 IDUs account for approximately half of those living with HIV infection. In contrast, the epidemics in Thailand and Cambodia have been driven largely by commercial sex. In Thailand, HIV prevalence in pregnant women declined from 2.4% in 1995 to 1.2% in 2003. However, HIV prevalence among MSM in Bangkok increased from 17% in 2003 to 28% in 2005 *(257)*. Only 16% of persons in need of ART in Asia received it in 2005 *(255)*.

The Americas. HIV infections are reported mostly among MSM, IDUs, and sex workers in the Americas *(252)*. Brazil, the second most populous country in the Americas (after the United States), has an adult HIV prevalence of 0.5%, and has approximately 30% of the population living with HIV in South and Central America and the Caribbean. High-risk behavior among Brazilians aged 15 to 24 years remains high; one in three persons report initiating sexual activity before age 15 years, and one in five report having had more than 10 sex partners. Brazil provides free ART to all in need of treatment, and approximately 83% of HIV-infected persons receive therapy.

After sub-Saharan Africa, the Caribbean is the second most HIV-affected region of the world. Like sub-Saharan Africa, HIV transmission in the Caribbean is largely heterosexual. HIV prevalence has declined in the urban areas of Haiti but has remained constant in other areas of the Caribbean. Overall in South and Central America and the Caribbean, approximately 68% of persons in need of ART received it in 2005 *(255)*.

In the United States, recent evidence suggests a resurgence of HIV transmission among MSM; during the period 2001–2004, an estimated 44% of new HIV infections were in MSM, and 17% were in IDUs *(258)*. In addition, blacks and Hispanics together account for 69% of all reported HIV/AIDS cases. In the United States, 55% of persons in need of ART received it in 2005 *(252)*.

Early in the epidemic, HIV infection and AIDS were diagnosed in relatively few women and female adolescents—although it is known now that many women were infected with HIV through injection drug use but that their infections were not diagnosed *(259)*. Today, according to 2007 data from the CDC, women account for more than one quarter of all new HIV/AIDS diagnoses (http://www.cdc.gov/hiv/ topics/women/resources/factsheets/women.htm). Women of color are especially affected by HIV infection and AIDS. In 2004 (the most recent year for which data are available), HIV infection was the leading cause of death for black women (including African-American women) aged 25 to 34 years:

- the third leading cause of death for black women aged 35 to 44 years;
- the fourth leading cause of death for black women aged 45 to 54 years;
- the fourth leading cause of death for Hispanic women aged 35 to 44 years.

In the same year, HIV infection was the fifth leading cause of death among all women aged 35 to 44 years and the sixth leading cause of death among all women aged 25 to 34 years. The only diseases causing more deaths of women were cancer and heart disease *(260)*.

References

1. World Health Organization, UNAIDS, UNICEF (2007) Towards universal access scaling up priorities in HIV/AIDS intervention in the health sector: progress report (http://www.who.int/ hiv/mediacentre/universal_access_progress_report_en.pdf).
2. Fauci, A. S. (2007) The expanding global health agenda: a welcome development, *Nat. Med.*, **13**(10), 21–23.
3. Wain-Hobson, S. (1989) HIV genome variability in vivo, *AIDS*, **3**(Suppl. 1), 13–19.
4. Wain-Hobson, S. (1992) Human immunodeficiency virus type 1 quasispecies in vivo and ex vivo, *Curr. Top. Microbiol. Immunol.*, **176**, 181–193.
5. Gelderbloom, H. R., Özel, M., and Pauli, G. (1989) Morphogenesis and morphology of HIV. Structure-function relations, *Arch. Virol.*, **106**, 1–13.
6. Wong-Stall, F. and Klotman, M. E. (1991) Human immunodeficiency virus (HIV) gene structure and genetic diversity. In: *The Human Retroviruses* (Gallo, R. C. and Jay, G., eds.), Academic Press, San Diego, CA, pp. 35–68.
7. Hope, T. J. and Trono, D. (2000) Structure, expression, and regulation of the HIV genome, HIV InSite Knowledge Base Chapter (http://hivinsite.ucsf.edu/InSite?page=kb-02-01-02).
8. Felber, B. K., Hadzopoulou-Cladaras, M., Cladaras, C., Copeland, T., and Pavlakis, G. N. (1989) Rev protein of the human immunodeficiency virus type 1 affect the stability and transport of viral mRNA, *Proc. Natl. Acad. Sci. U.S.A.*, **86**, 1495–1499.
9. Hadzopoulou-Cladaras, M., Felber, B. K., Cladaras, C., Athanassopoulos, A., Tse, A., and Pavlakis, G. N. (1980) The *rev* (*trs/art*) protein of the human immunodeficiency virus type 1 affects viral mRNA via a *cis*-acting sequence in the *env* region, *J. Virol.*, **63**, 1265–1274.
10. Briggs, J. A. G., Grünewald, K., Glass, B., Förster, F., Kräusslich, H.-G., and Fuller, S. D. (2006) The mechanism of HIV-1 core assembly: insights from three-dimensional reconstructions of authentic virions, *Structure*, **14**, 15–20.
11. Swanstrom, R. and Wills, J. W. (1997) Synthesis, assembly, and processing of viral proteins. In: *Retroviruses* (Coffin, J. M., Hughes, S. H., and Varmus, H. E., eds.), Cold Spring Harbor Laboratory Press, Cold Spring Harbor, NY, pp. 263–334.

12. Briggs, J. A. G., Wilk, T., Welker, R., Kräusslich, H. G., and Fuller, S. D. (2003) Structural organization of authentic, mature HIV-1 virions and cores, *EMBO J.*, **22**, 1707–1715.

13. Fuller, S. D., Wilk, T., Gowen, B. E., Kräusslich, H. G., and Vogt V. M. (1997) Cryo-electron microscopy reveals ordered domains in the immature HIV-1 particle, *Curr. Biol.*, **7**, 729–738.

14. Wilk, T., Gross, I., Gowen, B. E., Rutten, T., de Haas, F., Welker, R., Kräusslich, H. G., Boulanger, P., and Fuller, S. D. (2001) Organization of immature human immunodeficiency virus type 1, *J. Virol.*, **75**, 759–771.

15. Briggs, J. A. G., Watson, B. E., Gowen, B. E., and Fuller, S. D. (2004) Cryoelectron microscopy of mouse mammary tumor virus, *J. Virol.*, **78**, 2606–2608.

16. Kingston, R. L., Olson, N. H., and Vogt, V. M. (2001) The organization of mature Rous sarcoma virus as studied by cryoelectron microscopy, *J. Struct. Biol.*, **136**, 67–80.

17. Yeager, M., Wilson-Kubalek, E. M., Weiner, S. G., Brown, P. O., and Rein, A. (1998) Supramolecular organization of immature and mature murine leukemia virus revealed by electron cryomicroscopy: implications for retroviral assembly mechanisms, *Proc. Natl. Acad. Sci. U.S.A.*, **95**, 7299–7304.

18. Vogt, V. M. (1997) Retroviral virions and genomes. In: *Retroviruses* (Coffin, J. M., Hughes, S. H., and Varmus, H. E., eds.), Cold Spring Harbor Laboratory Press, Cold Spring Harbor, NY, pp. 27–69.

19. Briggs, J. A. G., Simon, M. N., Gross, I., Kräusslich, H. G., Fuller, S. D., Vogt, V. M., and Johnson, M. C. (2004) The stoichiometry of Gag protein in HIV-1, *Nat. Struct. Mol. Biol.*, **11**, 672–675.

20. Feinberg, M. B., Baltimore, D., and Frankel, A. D. (1991) The role of Tat in the human immunodeficiency virus life cycle indicates a primary effect on transcriptional elongation, *Proc. Natl. Acad. Sci. U.S.A.*, **88**, 4045–4049.

21. Zhu, Y., Pe'ery, T., Peng, J., Ramanathan, Y., Marshall, N., Marshall, T., Amendt, B., Mathews, M. B., and Price, D. H. (1997) Transcription elongation factor P-TEFb is required for HIV-1 tat transactivation in vitro, *Genes Dev.*, **11**, 2622–2632.

22. Muesing, M. A., Smith, D. H., Cabradilla, C. D., et al. (1985) Nucleic acid structure and expression of the human AIDS/lymphodenopathy virus, *Nature*, **313**, 450–458.

23. Gallo, R., Wong-Staal, F., Montagnier, L., et al (1988) HIV/HTLV gene nomenclature, *Nature*, **333**, 504.

24. Bryant, M. and Ratner, L. (1990) Myristoylation-dependent replication and assembly of human immunodeficiency virus, *Proc. Natl. Acad. Sci. U.S.A.*, **87**, 523–527.

25. Gottlinger, H. G., Sodroski, J. G., and Haseltine, W. A. (1989) Role of capsid precursor processing and myristoylation in morphogenesis and infectivity of human immunodeficiency virus type 1, *Proc. Natl. Acad. Sci. U.S.A.*, **86**, 5781–5785.

26. Gallay, P., Swingler, S., Song, J., et al. (1995) HIV nuclear import is governed by the phosphotyrosine-mediated binding of matrix to the core domain of integrase, *Cell*, **83**, 569–576.

27. Lewis, P., Hensel, M., and Emerman, M. (1992) Human immunodeficiency virus infection of cells arrested in the cell cycle, *EMBO J.*, **11**, 3053–3058.

28. Harrison, G. P., and Lever, A. M. (1992) The human immunodeficiency virus type 1 packaging signal and major splice donor region have a conserved stable secondary structure, *J. Virol.*, **66**, 4144–4153.

29. Poznansky, M., Lever, A., Bergeron, L., et al. (1991) Gene transfer into human lymphocytes by a defective human immunodeficiency virus type1 vector, *J. Virol.*, **65**, 532–536.

30. Lapadat-Tapolsky, M., De Rocquigny, H., Van Gent, D., et al. (1993) Interactions between HIV-1 nucleocapsid protein and viral DNA may have important functions in the viral life cycle, *Nucleic Acids Res.*, **21**, 831–839.

31. Paxton, W., Connor, R. I., and Landau, N. R. (1993) Incorporation of Vpr into human immunodeficiency virus type 1 virions: requirement for the p6 region of gag and mutational analysis, *J. Virol.*, **67**, 7229–7237.

32. Jacks, T., Power, M. D., Masiarz, F. R., et al. (1988) Characterization of ribosomal frameshifting in HIV-1 gag-pol expression, *Nature*, **331**, 280–283.

33. Parkin, N. T., Chamorro, M., and Varmus, H. E. (1992) Human immunodeficiency virus type 1 gag-pol frameshifting is dependent on mRNA secondary structure: demonstration by expression in vivo, *J. Virol.*, **66**, 5147–5151.

34. Ashorn, P., McQuade, T. J., Thaisrivongs, S., et al. (1990) An inhibitor of the protease blocks maturation of human and simian immunodeficiency viruses and spread of infection, *Proc. Natl. Acad. Sci. U.S.A.*, **87**, 7472–7476.

35. Miller, M., Jaskolski, M., Rao, J. K., et al. (1989) Crystal structure of retroviral protease proves relationship to aspartic protease family, *Nature*, **337**, 576–579.

36. Navia, M. A., Fitzgerald, P. M., McKeever, B. M., et al. (1989) Three-dimensional structure of aspartyl protease from human immunodeficiency virus HIV-1, *Nature*, **337**, 615–620.

37. Zack, J. A., Arrigo, S. J., Weitsman, S. R., et al. (1990) HIV-1 entry into quiescent primary lymphocytes: molecular analysis reveals a liable, latent viral structure, *Cell*, **61**, 213–222.

38. Harrich, D., Ulich, C., and Gaynor, R. B. (1996) A critical role for the TAR element in promoting efficient human immunodeficiency virus type 1 reverse transcription, *J. Virol.*, **70**, 4017–4027.

39. Kohlstaedt, L. A., Wang, J., Friedman, J. M., Rice, P. A., and Steitz, T. A. (1992) Crystal structure at 3.5 Å resolution of HIV-1 reverse transcriptase complexed with an inhibitor, *Science*, **256**, 1783–1790.

40. Bushman, F. D., Fujiwara, T., and Craigie, R. (1990) Retroviral DNA integration directed by HIV integration protein in vitro, *Science*, **249**, 1555–1558.

41. Pryciak, P. M. and Varmus, H. E. (1992) Nucleosomes, DNA-binding proteins, and DNA sequence modulate retroviral integration target site selection, *Cell*, **69**, 769–780.

42. Pruss, D., Bushman, F. D., and Wolffe, A. P. (1994) Human immunodeficiency virus integrase directs integration to sites of severe DNA distortion within the nucleosome core, *Proc. Natl. Acad. Sci. U.S.A.*, **91**, 5913–5917.

43. Bushman, F. D. (1994) Tethering human immunodeficiency virus 1 integrase to a DNA site directs integration to nearby sequences, *Proc. Natl. Acad. Sci. U.S.A.*, **91**, 9233–9237.

44. Wiskerchen, M. and Muesing, M. A. (1995) Human immunodeficiency virus type 1 integrase: effects of mutations on viral ability to integrate, direct viral expression from unintegrated viral DNA templates, and sustain viral propagation in primary cells, *J. Virol.*, **69**, 376–386.

45. Capon, D. J. and Ward, R. H. (1991) The CD-4-gp120 interaction and AIDS pathogenesis, *Annu. Rev. Immunol.*, **9**, 649–678.

46. Bernstein, H. B., Tucker, S. P., Kar, S. R., et al. (1995) Oligomerization of the hydrophobic heptad repeat of gp41, *J. Virol.*, **69**, 2745–2750.

47. Landau, N. R., Warton, M., and Littman, D. R. (1988) The envelope glycoprotein of the human immunodeficiency virus binds to the immunoglobulin-like domain of CD4, *Nature*, **334**, 159–162.

48. Kwong, P. D., Wyatt, R., Robinson, J., Sweet, R. W., Sodroski, J, and Hendrickson, W. A. (1998) Structure of an HIV gp120 envelope glycoprotein in complex with the CD4 receptor and a neutralizing human antibody, *Nature*, **393**, 648–659.

49. Hwang, S. S., Boyle, T. J., Lyerly, H. K., and Cullen, B. R. (1991) Identification of the envelope V3 loop as the primary determinant of cell tropism in HIV-1, *Science*, **253**, 71–74.

50. Feng, Y., Broder, C. C., Kennedy, P. E., et al. (1996) HIV-1 entry cofactor: functional cDNA cloning of a

seven-transmembrane, G protein-coupled receptor, *Science*, **272**, 872–877.

51. Deng, H., Liu, R., Ellmeier, W., et al. (1996) Identification of a major co-receptor for primary isolates of HIV-1, *Nature*, **381**, 661–666.

52. Goudsmit, J., Debouck, C., Meloen, R. H., et al. (1988) Human immunodeficiency virus type 1 neutralization epitope with conserved architecture elicit early type-specific antibodies in experimentally infected chimpanzees, *Proc. Natl. Acad. Sci. U.S.A.*, **85**, 4478–4482.

53. Geijtenbeek, T. B., Kwon, D. S., Torensma, R., van Vliet, S. J., van Duijnhoven, G. C., Middel, J., Cornelissen, I. L., Nottet, H. S., KewalRamani, V. N., Littman, D. R., Figdor, C. G., and van Kooyk, Y. (2000) DC-SIGN, a dendritic cell-specific HIV-1-binding protein that enhances trans-infection of T cells, *Cell*, **100**, 587–597.

54. Camerini, D. and Seed, B. (1990) A CD4 domain important for HIV-mediated syncytium formation lies outside the virus binding site, *Cell*, **60**, 747–754.

55. Ruben, S., Perkins, A., Purcell, R., et al. (1989) Structural and functional characterization of human immunodeficiency virus tat protein, *J. Virol.*, **63**, 1–8.

56. Feng, S. and Holland, E. C. (1988) HIV-1 tat trans-activation requires the loop sequence within tar, *Nature*, **334**, 65–167.

57. Roy, S., Delling, U., Chen, C. H., et al. (1990) A bulge structure in HIV-1 TAR RNA is required for Tat binding and Tat-mediated trans-activation, *Genes Dev.*, **4**, 1365.

58. Kao, S. Y., Calman, A. F., Luciw, P. A., et al. (1987) Antitermination of transcription within the long terminal repeat of HIV-1 by tat gene product, *Nature*, **330**, 489–493.

59. Zhou, Q. and Sharp, P. A. (1996) Tat-SF1: cofactor for stimulation of transcriptional elongation by HIV-1 Tat, *Science*, **274**(5287), 605–610.

60. Zhu, Y., Pe'ery, T., Peng, J., Ramanathan, Y., Marshall, N., Marshall, T., Amendt, B., Mathews, M. B., and Price, D. H. (1997) Transcription elongation factor P-TEFb is required for HIV-1 tat transactivation in vitro, *Genes Dev.*, **11**, 2622–2632.

61. Wei, P., Garber, M. E., Fang, S. M., Fischer, W. H., and Jones, K. A. (1998) A novel CDK9-associated C-type cyclin interacts directly with HIV-1 Tat and mediates its high-affinity, loop-specific binding to TAR RNA, *Cell*, **92**, 451–462.

62. Brother, M. B., Chang, H. K., Lisziewicz, J., et al. (1996) Block of Tat mediated transactivation of tumor necrosis factor beta gene expression by polymeric-TAR decoys, *Virology*, **222**(1), 252–256.

63. Rasty, S., Thatikunta, P., Gordon, J., et al. (1996) Human immunodeficiency virus tat gene transfer to the murine central nervous system using a replication-defective herpes simplex virus vector stimulates transforming growth factor beta 1 gene expression, *Proc. Natl. Acad. Sci. U.S.A.*, **93**, 6073–6078.

64. Sastry, K. J., Marin, M. C., Nehete, P. N., et al. (1996) Expression of human immunodeficiency virus type I tat results in downregulation of bcl-2 and induction of apoptosis in hematopoietic cells, *Oncogene*, **13**, 487–493.

65. Sharma, V., Xu, M., Ritter, L. M., et al. (1996) HIV-1 tat induces the expression of a new hematopoietic cell-specific transcription factor and downregulates MIP-1 alpha gene expression in activated T cells, *Biochem. Biophys. Res. Commun.*, **223**, 526–533.

66. Zapp, M. L. and Green, M. R. (1989) Sequence-specific RNA binding by the HIV-1 Rev protein, *Nature*, **342**, 714–716.

67. Kim, S. Y., Byrn, R., Groopman, J., et al. (1989) Temporal aspects of DNA and RNA synthesis during human immunodeficiency virus infection: evidence for differential gene expression, *J. Virol.*, **9**(63), 3708–3713.

68. Malim, M. H., Hauber, J., Le, S. Y., et al. (1989) The HIV-1 rev trans-activator acts through a structured target sequence to activate nuclear export of unspliced viral mRNA, *Nature*, **338**(6212), 254–257.

69. Bartel, D. P., Zapp, M. L., Green, M. R., et al. (1991) HIV-1 Rev regulation involves recognition of non-Watson-Crick base pairs in viral RNA, *Cell*, **67**, 529–536.

70. Felber, B. K., Drysdale, C. M., and Pavlakis, G. N. (1990) Feedback regulation of human immunodeficiency virus type 1 expression by the Rev protein, *J. Virol.*, **64**, 3734–3741.

71. Zapp, M. L., Hope, T. J., Parslow, T. G., et al. (1991) Oligomerization and RNA binding domains of the type 1 human immunodeficiency virus Rev protein: a dual function for an arginine-rich binding motif, *Proc. Natl. Acad. Sci. U.S.A.*, **88**, 7734–7738.

72. Malim, M. H., Bohnlein, S., Hauber, J., et al. (1989) Functional dissection of the HIV-1 Rev trans-activator-derivation of a transdominant repressor of Rev function, *Cell*, **58**, 205–214.

73. Hope, T. J., McDonald, D., Huang, X. J., et al. (1990) Mutational analysis of the human immunodeficiency virus type 1 Rev transactivator: essential residues near the amino terminus, *J. Virol.*, **64**, 5360–5366.

74. Wen, W., Meinkoth, J. L., Tsien, R. Y., et al. (1995) Identification of a signal for rapid export of proteins from the nucleus, *Cell*, **82**, 463–473.

75. Fischer, U., Huber, J., Boelens, W. C., et al. (1995) The HIV-1 Rev activation domain is a nuclear export signal that accesses an export pathway used by specific cellular RNAs, *Cell*, **82**, 475–483.

76. Hope, T. J., Klein, N. P., Elder, M. E., and Parslow, T. G. (1992) Trans-dominant inhibition of human immunodeficiency virus type 1 Rev occurs through formation of inactive protein complexes, *J. Virol.*, **66**, 1849–1855.

77. Garcia, J. V. and Miller, A. D. (1992) Downregulation of cell surface CD4 by nef, *Res. Virol.*, **143**, 52–55.

78. Aiken, C., Konner, J., Landau, N. R., et al. (1994) Nef induces CD4 endocytosis: requirement for a critical dileucine motif in the membrane-proximal CD4 cytoplasmic domain, *Cell*, **76**, 853–864.

79. Lama, J., Mangasarian, A., and Trono, D. (1999) Cell-surface expression of CD4 reduces HIV-1 infectivity by blocking Env incorporation in a Nef-and Vpu-inhibitable manner, *Curr. Biol.*, **9**, 622–631.

80. Ross, T. M., Oran, A. E., and Cullen, B. R. (1999) Inhibition of HIV1 progeny virion release by cell-surface CD4 is relieved by expression of the viral Nef protein, *Curr. Biol.*, **9**, 613–621.

81. Schwartz, O., Marechal, V., Le Gall, S., et al. (1996) Endocytosis of major histocompatibility complex class I molecules is induced by the HIV-1 Nef protein, *Nat. Med.*, **2**, 338–342.

82. Luria, S., Chambers, I., and Berg, P. (1991) Expression of the type 1 human immunodeficiency virus Nef protein in T cells prevents antigen receptor-mediated induction of interleukin 2 mRNA, *Proc. Natl. Acad. Sci. U.S.A.*, **88**, 5326–5330.

83. Skowronski, J., Parks, D., and Mariani, R. (1993) Altered T cell activation and development in transgenic mice expressing the HIV-1 nef gene, *EMBO J.*, **12**, 703–713.

84. Baur, A. S., Sawai, E. T., Dazin, P., et al. (1994) HIV-1 Nef leads to inhibition or activation of T cells depending on its intracellular localization, *Immunity*, **1**, 373–384.

85. Miller, M. D., Warmerdam, M. T., Gaston, I., et al. (1994) The human immunodeficiency virus-1 nef gene product: a positive factor for viral infection and replication in primary lymphocytes and macrophages, *J. Exp. Med.*, **179**, 101–113.

86. Pandori, M. W., Fitch, N. J., Craig, H. M., et al. (1996) Producer-cell modification of human immunodeficiency virus type 1: nef is a virion protein, *J. Virol.*, **70**, 4283–4290.

87. Schwartz, O., Marechal, V., Danos, O., et al. (1995) Human immunodeficiency virus type 1 Nef increases the efficiency of reverse transcription in the infected cell, *J. Virol.*, **69**, 4053–4059.

88. Goldsmith, M. A., Warmerdam, M. T., Atchison, R. E., et al. (1995) Dissociation of the CD4 downregulation and viral infectivity enhancement functions of human immunodeficiency virus type 1 Nef, *J. Virol.*, **69**, 4112–4121.

89. Kestler, H. W., III, Ringler, D. J., Mori, K., et al. (1991) Importance of the nef gene for maintenance of high virus loads and for development of AIDS, *Cell*, **65**, 651–662.

90. Baba, T. W., Jeong, Y. S., Pennick, D., et al. (1995) Pathogenicity of live, attenuated SIV after mucosal infection of neonatal macaques, *Science*, **267**, 1820–1825.

91. Collins, K. L. and Nabel, G. J. (1999) Naturally attenuated HIV – lessons for AIDS vaccines and treatment, *N. Engl. J. Med.*, **340**, 1756–1757.

92. Cohen, E. A., Dehni, G., Sodroski, J. G., et al. (1990) Human immunodeficiency virus vpr product is a virion-associated regulatory protein, *J. Virol.*, **64**, 3097–3099.

93. Heinzinger, N. K., Bukinsky, M. I., Haggerty, S. A., et al. (1994) The Vpr protein of human immunodeficiency virus type 1 influences nuclear localization of viral nucleic acids in nondividing host cells, *Proc. Natl. Acad. Sci. U.S.A.*, **91**, 7311–7315.

94. Vodicka, M. A., Koepp, D. M., Silver, P. A., and Emerman, M. (1998) HIV-1 Vpr interacts with the nuclear transport pathway to promote macrophage infection, *Genes Dev.*, **12**(2), 175–185.

95. Rogel, M. E., Wu, L. I., and Emerman, M. (1995) The human immunodeficiency virus type 1 vpr gene prevents cell proliferation during chronic infection, *J. Virol.*, **69**, 882–888.

96. Jowett, J. B., Planelles, V., Poon, B., et al. (1995) The human immunodeficiency virus type 1 vpr gene arrests infected T cells in the G2 + M phase of the cell cycle, *J. Virol.*, **69**, 6304–6313.

97. Braaten, D., Franke, E. K., and Luban, J. (1995) Human immunodeficiency virus type 1 Vpr arrests the cell cycle in G2 by inhibiting the activation of p34cdc2-cyclin B, *J. Virol.*, **69**, 6859–6864.

98. He, J., Choe, S., Walker, R., et al. (1995) Human immunodeficiency virus type 1 viral protein R (Vpr) arrests cells in the G2 phase of the cell cycle by inhibiting p34cdc2 activity, *J. Virol.*, **69**, 6705–6711.

99. Starcich, B., Ratner, L., Josephs, S. F., et al. (1985) Characterization of long terminal repeat sequences of HTLV-III, *Science*, **227**, 538–540.

100. Bouhamdan, M., Benichou, S., Rey, F., et al. (1996) Human immunodeficiency virus type 1 Vpr protein binds to the uracil DNA glycosylase DNA repair enzyme, *J. Virol.*, **70**, 697–704.

101. Steagall, W. K., Robek, M. D., Perry, S. T., et al. (1995) Incorporation of uracil into viral DNA correlates with reduced replication of EIAV in macrophages, *Virology*, **10**, 302–313.

102. Sato, A., Igarashi, H., Adachi, A., et al. (1990) Identification and localization of vpr gene product of human immunodeficiency virus type 1, *Virus Genes*, **4**, 303–312.

103. Schwartz, S., Felber, B. K., Fenyo, E. M., et al. (1990) Env and Vpu proteins of human immunodeficiency virus type 1 are produced from multiple bicistronic mRNAs, *J. Virol.*, **64**, 5448–5456.

104. Schubert, U., Bour, S., Ferrer-Montiel, A. V., et al. (1996) The two biological activities of human immunodeficiency virus type 1 Vpu protein involve two separable structural domains, *J. Virol.*, **70**, 809–819.

105. Willey, R. L., Maldarelli, F., Martin, M. A., et al. (1992) Human immunodeficiency virus type 1 Vpu protein induces rapid degradation of CD4, *J. Virol.*, **66**(12), 7193–7200.

106. Klimkait, T., Strebel, K., Hoggan, M. A., et al. (1990) The human immunodeficiency virus type 1-specific protein vpu is required for efficient virus maturation and release, *J. Virol.*, **64**, 621–629.

107. Strebel, K., Daugherty, D., Clouse, K., et al. (1987) The HIV A(sor) gene product is essential for virus infectivity, *Nature*, **328**, 728–730.

108. Liu, H., Wu, X., Newman, M., et al. (1995) The Vif protein of human and simian immunodeficiency viruses is packaged into virions and associates with viral core structures, *J. Virol.*, **69**, 7630–7638.

109. von Schwedler, U., Song, J., Aiken, C., et al. (1993) Vif is crucial for human immunodeficiency virus type 1 proviral DNA synthesis in infected cells, *J. Virol.*, **67**, 4945–4955.

110. Camaur, D. and Trono, D. (1996) Characterization of human immunodeficiency virus type 1 Vif particle incorporation, *J. Virol.*, **70**, 6106–6111.

111. Simon, J. H., Gaddis, N. C., Fouchier, R. A., and Malim, M. H. (1998) Evidence for a newly discovered cellular anti-HIV-1 phenotype, *Nat. Med.*, **4**, 1397–1400.

112. Simon, J. H., Miller, D. L., Fouchier, R. A., Soares, M. A., Peden, K. W., and Malim, M. H. (1998) The regulation of primate immunodeficiency virus infectivity by Vif is cell species restricted: a role for Vif in determining virus host range and cross-species transmission, *EMBO J.*, **17**, 1259–1267.

113. Hoglund, S., Ohagen, A., Lawrence, K., et al. (1994) Role of vif during packing of the core of HIV-1, *Virology*, **201**(2), 349–355.

114. Schwartz, S., Felber, B. K., Benko, D. M., et al. (1990) Cloning and functional analysis of multiply spliced mRNA species of human immunodeficiency virus type 1, *J. Virol.*, **4**, 2519–2529.

115. Starcich, B., Ratner, L., Josephs, S. F., et al. (1985) Characterization of long terminal repeat sequences of HTLV-III, *Science*, **227**, 538–540.

116. Nabel, G. and Baltimore, D. (1987) An inducible transcription factor activates expression of human immunodeficiency virus in T cells, *Nature*, **326**, 711–713.

117. Okamoto, T., Matsuyama, T., Mori, S., et al. (1989) Augmentation of human immunodeficiency virus type 1 gene expression by tumor necrosis factor alpha, *AIDS Res. Hum. Retroviruses*, **5**, 131–138.

118. Kobayashi, N., Hamamoto, Y., Koyanagi, Y., et al. (1989) Effect of interleukin-1 on the augmentation of human immunodeficiency virus gene expression, *Bioch. Biophys. Res. Commun.*, **165**, 715–721.

119. Garcia, J. A., Harrich, D., Soultanakis, E., et al. (1989) Human immunodeficiency virus type 1 LTR TATA and TAR region sequences required for transcriptional regulation, *EMBO J.*, **8**, 765–778.

120. Sheridan, P. L., Sheline, C. T., Cannon, K., et al. (1995) Activation of the HIV-1 enhancer by the LEF-1 HMG protein on nucleosome-assembled DNA in vitro, *Genes Dev.*, **9**, 2090–2104.

121. Sheldon, M., Ratnasabapathy, R., and Hernandez, N. (1993) Characterization of the inducer of short transcripts, a human immunodeficiency virus type 1 transcriptional element that activates the synthesis of short RNAs, *Mol. Cell Biol.*, **13**, 1251–1263.

122. Schwartz, S., Felber, B. K., and Pavlakis, G. N. (1992) Mechanism of translation of monocistronic and multicistronic human immunodeficiency virus type 1 mRNAs, *Mol. Cell Biol.*, **12**, 207–212.

123. Wyatt, R. and Sodroski, J. (1998) The HIV-1 envelope glycoproteins: fusogens, antigens, and immunogens, *Science*, **280**, 1884–1888.

124. Berger, E. A., Murphy, P. M., and Farber, J. M. (1999) Chemokine receptors as HIV-1 coreceptors: roles in viral entry, tropism, and disease, *Annu. Rev. Immunol.*, **17**, 657–700.

125. Unutmaz, D., Kewalramani, V. N., and Littman, D. R. (1998) G protein-coupled receptors in HIV and SIV entry: new perspectives on lentivirus-host interactions and on the utility of animal models, *Semin. Immunol.*, **10**, 225–236.

126. Marx, P. A. and Chen, Z. W. (1998) The function of simian chemokine receptors in the replication of SIV, *Semin. Immunol.*, **10**, 215–223.

127. Feng, Y., Broder, C. C., Kennedy, P. E., and Berger, E. A. (1996) HIV-1 entry cofactor: functional cDNA cloning of a seven-transmembrane, G protein-coupled receptor, *Science*, **272**, 872–877.

128. Levy, J. A., Mackewicz, C. E., and Barker, E. (1996) Controlling HIV pathogenesis: the role of the noncytotoxic anti-HIV response of CD8(+) T cells, *Immunol. Today*, **17**, 217–224.

129. Cocchi, F., DeVico, A. L., Garzino-Demo, A., Arya, S. K., Gallo, R. C., and Lusso, P. (1995) Identification of RANTES, MIP-1α, and MIP-1β as the major HIV-suppressive factors produced by CD8$^+$ T cells, *Science*, **270**, 1811–1815.

130. Samson, M., Labbe, O., Mollereau, C., Vassart, G., and Parmentier M. (1996) Molecular cloning and functional expression of a new human CC-chemokine receptor gene, *Biochemistry*, **35**, 3362–3367.

131. Combadiere, C., Ahuja, S. K., Tiffany, H. L., and Murphy, P. M. (1996) Cloning and functional expression of CC CKR5, a human monocyte CC chemokine receptor selective for MIP-1α, MIP-1β, and RANTES, *J. Leukocyte Biol.* **60**, 147–152.

132. Raport, C. J., Gosling, J., Schweickart, V. L., Gray, P. W., and Charo, I. F. (1996) Molecular cloning and functional characterization of a novel human CC chemokine receptor (CCR5) for RANTES, MIP-1β, and MIP-1α, *J. Biol. Chem.*, **271**, 17161–17166.

133. Deng, H. K., Liu, R., Ellmeier, W., Choe, S., Unutmaz, D., Burkhart, M., Di Marzio, P., Marmon, S., Sutton, R. E., Hill, C. M., Davis, C. B., Peiper, S. C., Schall, T. J., Littman, D. R., and Landau, N. R. (1996) Identification of a major co-receptor for primary isolates of HIV-1, *Nature*, **381**, 661–666.

134. Dragic, T., Litwin, V., Allaway, G. P., Martin, S. R., Huang, Y. X., Nagashima, K. A., Cayanan, C., Maddon, P. J., Koup, R. A., Moore, J. P., and Paxton, W. A. (1996) HIV-1 entry into CD4$^+$ cells is mediated by the chemokine receptor CC-CKR-5, *Nature*, **381**, 667–673.

135. Alkhatib, G., Combadiere, C., Broder, C. C., Feng, Y., Kennedy, P. E., Murphy, P. M., and Berger, E. A. (1996) CC CKR5: a RANTES, MIP-1α MIP-1β receptor as a fusion cofactor for macrophage-tropic HIV-1, *Science*, **272**, 1955–1958.

136. Choe, H., Farzan, M., Sun, Y., Sullivan, N., Rollins, B., Ponath, P. D., Wu, L., Mackay, C. R., Larosa, G., Newman, W., Gerard, N., Gerard, C., and Sodroski, J. (1996) The beta-chemokine receptors CCR3 and CCR5 facilitate infection by primary HIV-1 isolates, *Cell*, **85**, 1135–1148.

137. Doranz, B. J., Rucker, J., Yi, Y. J., Smyth, R. J., Samson, M., Peiper, S. C., Parmentier, M., Collman, R. G., and Doms, R. W. (1996) A dual-tropic primary HIV-1 isolate that uses fusin and the beta-chemokine receptors CKR-5, CKR-3, and CKR-2b as fusion cofactors, *Cell*, **85**, 1149–1158.

138. Bleul, C. C., Farzan, M., Choe, H., Parolin, C., Clark-Lewis, I., Sodroski, J., and Springer, T. A. (1996) The lymphocyte chemoattractant SDF-1 is a ligand for LESTR/fusin and blocks HIV-1 entry, *Nature*, **382**, 829–833.

139. Oberlin, E., Amara, A., Bachelerie, F., Bessia, C., Virelizier, J. L., Arenzana-Seisdedos, F., Schwartz, O., Heard, J. M., Clark-Lewis, I., Legler, D. F., Loetscher, M., Baggiolini, M., and Moser, B. (1996) The CXC chemokine SDF-1 is the ligand for LESTR/fusin and prevents infection by T-cell-line-adapted HIV-1, *Nature*, **382**, 833–835.

140. Brenchley, J. M., Price, D. A., and Douek, D. C. (2006) HIV disease: fallout from a mucosal catastrophe? *Nat. Immunol.*, **7**, 235–239.

141. Brenchley, J. M., Schacker, T. W., Ruff, L. E., et al. (2004) CD4$^+$ T cell depletion during all stages of HIV disease occurs predominantly in the gastrointestinal tract, *J. Exp. Med.*, **200**, 749–759.

142. Guadalupe, M., Reay, E., Sankaran, S., et al. (2003) Severe CD4$^+$ T-cell depletion in gut lymphoid tissue during primary human immunodeficiency virus type 1 infection and substantial delay in restoration following highly active antiretroviral therapy, *J. Virol.*, **77**, 11708–11717.

143. Li, Q., Duan, L., Estes, J. D., et al. (2005) Peak SIV replication in resting memory CD4$^+$ T cells depletes gut lamina propria CD4$^+$ T cells, *Nature*, **434**, 1148–1152.

144. Mattapallil, J. J., Douek, D. C., Hill, B., et al. (2005) Massive infection and loss of memory CD4$^+$ T cells in multiple tissues during acute SIV infection, *Nature*, **434**, 1093–1097.

145. Veazey, R. S., Demaria, M., Chalifoux, L. V., et al. (1998) Gastrointestinal tract as a major site of CD4$^+$ T cell depletion and viral replication in SIV infection, *Science*, **280**, 427–431.

146. Haase, A. T. (2005) Perils at mucosal front lines for HIV and SIV and their hosts, *Nat. Rev. Immunol.*, **5**, 783–792.

147. Picker, L. J. (2006) Immunopathogenesis of acute AIDS virus infection, *Curr. Opin. Immunol.*, **18**, 399–405.

148. Arthos, J., Cicala, C., Martinelli, C., et al. (2008) HIV-1 envelope protein binds to and signals through integrin α$_4$β$_7$, the gut mucosal homing receptor for peripheral T cells, *Nat. Immunol.*, **9**, 301–309.

149. von Andrian, U. H. and Mackay, C. R. (2000) T-cell function and migration. Two sides of the same coin, *N. Engl. J. Med.*, **343**, 1020–1034.

150. Wagner, N., Löhler, J., Kunkel, E. J., et al. (1996) Critical role for β$_7$ integrins in formation of the gut-associated lymphoid tissue, *Nature*, **382**, 366–370.

151. Domingo, E., Escarmis, C., Sevilla, N., et al. (1996) Basic concepts in RNA virus evolution, *FASEB J.*, **10**, 859–864.

152. Coffin, J. M. (1992) Genetic diversity and evolution of retroviruses, *Curr. Top. Microbiol. Immunol.*, **176**, 143–164.

153. Domingo, E. and Holland, J. J. (1997) RNA virus mutations and fitness for survival, *Annu. Rev. Microbiol.*, **51**, 151–178.

154. Eigen, M. (1992) *Steps Toward Life*, Oxford University Press, Oxford, UK.

155. Eigen, M. (1993) The origins of genetic information: viruses as models, *Gene* **135**, 37–47.

156. Piatak, M., Jr., Saag, M. S., Yang, L. C., Clark, S. J., Kappes, J. C., Luk, K. C., Hahn, B. H., Shaw, G. M., and Lifson, J. D. (1993) High levels of HIV-1 in plasma during all stages of infection determined by competitive PCR, *Science*, **259**, 1749–1754.

157. Wei, X., Ghosh, S. K., Taylor, M. E., Johnson, V. A., Emini, E. A., Deutsch, P., Lifson, J. D., Bonhoeffer, S., Nowak, M. A., Hahn, B. H., et al. (1995) Viral dynamics in human immunodeficiency virus type 1 infection, *Nature*, **373**, 117–122.

158. Ho, D. D., Neumann, A. U., Perelson, A. S., Chen, W., Leonard, J. M., and Markowitz, M. (1995) Rapid turnover of plasma virions and CD4 lymphocytes in HIV-1 infection, *Nature*, **373**, 123–126.

159. Perelson, A. S., Neumann, A. U., Markowitz, M., Leonard, J. M., and Ho, D. D. (1996) HIV-1 dynamics in vivo: virion clearance rate, infected cell life-span, and viral generation time, *Science*, **271**, 1582–1586.

160. Coffin, J. M. (1995) HIV population dynamics in vivo: implications for genetic variation, pathogenesis, and therapy, *Science*, **267**, 483–489.

161. Leigh Brown, A. J. and Richman, D. D. (1997) HIV-1: gambling on the evolution of drug resistance? *Nat. Med.*, **3**, 268–271.

162. Leigh Brown, A. J. (1997) Analysis of the HIV-1 env gene sequences reveals evidence for a low effective number in the viral population, *Proc. Natl. Acad. Sci. U.S.A.*, **94**, 1862–1865.

163. Nijhuis, M., Boucher, C. A. B., Schipper, P., Leitner, T., Schuurman, R., and Albert, J. (1998) Stochastic processes strongly influence HIV-1 evolution during suboptimal protease-inhibitor therapy, *Proc. Natl. Acad. Sci. U.S.A.*, **95**(24), 14441–14446.

164. Wedekind, J. E., Dance, G. S., Sowden, M. P., and Smith, H. C. (2003) Messenger RNA editing in mammals: new members of the APOBEC family seeking roles in the family business, *Trends Genet.*, **19**(4), 207–216.

165. Cullen, B. R. (2006) Role and mechanism of action of the APOBEC3 protein family of antiretroviral resistance factors, *J. Virol.*, **80**(3), 1067–1076.

166. Jarmuz, A., Chester, A., Bayliss, J., Gisbourne, J., Dunham, I., Scott, J., and Navaratnam, N. (2002) An anthropoid-specific locus of orphan C to U RNA-editing enzymes on chromosome 22, *Genomics*, **79**, 285–296.

167. Löchelt, M., Romen, F., Bastone, P., et al. (2005) The antiretroviral activity of APOBEC3 is inhibited by the foamy virus accessory Bet protein, *Proc. Natl. Acad. Sci. U.S.A.*, **102**, 7982–7987.

168. Mariani, R., Chen, D., Schröfelbauer, B., et al. (2003) Species-specific exclusion of APOBEC3G from HIV-1 virions by Vif, *Cell*, **114**, 21–31.

169. Bransteitter, R., Pham, P., Scharff, M. D., and Goodman, M. F. (2003) Activation-induced cytidine deaminase deaminates deoxycytidine on single-stranded DNA but requires the action of RNase, *Proc. Natl. Acad. Sci. U.S.A.*, **100**, 4102–4107.

170. Alce, T. M. and Popik, W. (2004) APOBEC3G is incorporated into virus-like particles by a direct interaction with HIV-1 Gag nucleocapsid protein, *J. Biol. Chem.*, **279**, 34083–34086.

171. Cen, S., Guo, F., Niu, M., et al. (2004) The interaction between HIV-1 Gag and APOBEC3G, *J. Biol. Chem.*, **279**, 33177–33184.

172. Khan, M. A., Kao, S., Miyagi, E., et al. (2005) Viral RNA is required for the association of APOBEC3G with human immunodeficiency virus type 1 nucleoprotein complexes, *J. Virol.*, **79**, 5870–5874.

173. Luo, K., Liu, B., Xiao, Z., et al. (2004) Amino-terminal region of the human immunodeficiency virus type 1 nucleocapsid is required for human APOBEC3G packaging, *J. Virol.*, **78**, 11841–11852.

174. Schäfer, A., Bogerd, H. P., and Cullen, B. R. (2004) Specific packaging of APOBEC3G into HIV-1 virions is mediated by the nucleocapsid domain of the gag polyprotein precursor, *Virology*, **328**, 163–168.

175. Zennou, V., Perez-Caballero, D., Göttlinger, H., and Bieniasz, P. D. (2004) APOBEC3G incorporation into human immunodeficiency virus type 1 particles, *J. Virol.*, **78**, 12058–12061.

176. Svarovskaia, E. S., Xu, H., Mbisa, J. L., et al. (2004) Human apolipoprotein B mRNA-editing enzyme-catalytic polypeptide-like 3G (APOBEC3G) is incorporated into HIV-1 virions through interactions with viral and nonviral RNAs, *J. Biol. Chem.*, **279**, 35822–35828.

177. Berkowitz, R. D., Ohagen, A., Hoglund, S., and Goff, S. P. (1995) Retroviral nucleocapsid domains mediate the specific recognition of genomic viral RNAs by chimeric Gag polyproteins during RNA packaging in vivo, *J. Virol.*, **69**, 6445–6456.

178. Yu, X.-F. (2006) Innate cellular defenses of APOBEC3 cytidine deaminases and viral counter-defenses. Host factors, *Curr. Opin. HIV AIDS*, **1**(3), 187–193.

179. Chiu, Y.-L. (2007) The APOBEC3 cytidine deaminases: an innate defensive network opposing exogenous retroviruses and endogenous retroelements, *Ann. Rev. Immunol.*, **26**, 317–353.

180. Arriaga, M. E., Carr, J., Li, P., Wang, B., and Saksena, N. K. (2006) Interaction between HIV-1 and APOBEC3 sub-family of proteins, *Curr. HIV Res.*, **4**(4), 401–409.

181. Goldschmidt, V., Bleiber, G., May, M., et al., and The Swiss HIV Cohort Study (2006) Role of common human TRIM5α variants in HIV-1 disease progression, *Retrovirology*, **3**, 54.; doi: 10.1186/1742-4690-3-54.

182. Surridge, C. (2008) Innate immunity: getting in TRIM to fight retroviruses, *Nat. Rev. Miciobiol.*, **6**, 797

183. Nisole, S., Stoye, J. P., and Saib, A. (2005) TRIM family proteins: retroviral restriction and antiviral defence, *Nat. Rev. Microbiol.*, **3**, 799–808.

184. Towers, G. J. (2006) Restriction of retroviruses by TRIM5 alpha, *Future Virol.*, **1**, 71–78.

185. Stremlau, M., Owens, C. M., Perron, M. J., Kiessling, M., Autissier, P., and Sodroski, J. (2004) The cytoplasmic body component TRIM5alpha restricts HIV-1 infection in Old World monkeys, *Nature*, **427**, 848–853.

186. Towers, G. J. (2007) The control of viral infection by tripartite motif proteins and cyclophilin A, *Retrovirology*, **4**, 40; doi:10.1186/1742-4690-4-40.

187. Sawyer, S. L., Wu, L. I., Akey, J. M., Emerman, M., and Malik, H. S. (2006) High-frequency persistence of an impaired allele of the retroviral defense gene TRIM5alpha in humans, *Curr. Biol.*, **16**, 95–100.

188. Speelmon, E. C., Livingston-Rosanoff, D., Li, S. S., et al. (2006) Genetic association of the antiviral restriction factor TRIM5alpha with human immunodeficiency virus type 1 infection, *J. Virol.*, **80**, 2463–2471.

189. Stremlau, M., Perron, M., Lee, M., et al. (2006) Specific recognition and accelerated uncoating of retroviral capsids by the TRIM5alpha restriction factor, *Proc. Natl. Acad. Sci. U.S.A.*, **103**, 5514–5519.

190. Towers, G., Bock, M., Martin, S., Takeuchi, Y., Stoye, J. P., and Danos, O. (2000) A conserved mechanism of retrovirus restriction in mammals, *Proc. Natl. Acad. Sci. U.S.A.*, **97**, 12295–12299.

191. Shibata, R., Sakai, H., Kawamura, M., Tokunaga, K., and Adachi, A. (1995) Early replication block of human immunodeficiency virus type 1 in monkey cells, *J. Gen. Virol.*, **76**, 2723–2730.

192. Hofmann, W., Schubert, D., LaBonte, J., et al. (1999) Species-specific, postentry barriers to primate immunodeficiency virus infection, *J. Virol.*, **73**, 10020–10028.

193. Towers, G., Collins, M., and Takeuchi, Y. (2002) Abrogation of Ref1 restriction in human cells, *J. Virol.*, **76**, 2548–2550.

194. Besnier, C., Takeuchi, Y., and Towers, G. (2002) Restriction of lentivirus in monkeys, *Proc. Natl. Acad. Sci. U.S.A.*, **99**, 1920–11925.

195. Cowan, S., Hatziioannou, T., Cunningham, T., Muesing, M. A., Gottlinger, H. G., and Bieniasz, P. D. (2002) Cellular inhibitors with Fv1-like activity restrict human and simian immunodeficiency virus tropism, *Proc. Natl. Acad. Sci. U.S.A.*, **99**, 11914–11919.

196. Keckesova, Z., Ylinen, L. M., and Towers, G. J. (2004) The human and African green monkey TRIM5alpha genes encode Ref1 and Lv1 retroviral restriction factor activities, *Proc. Natl. Acad. Sci. U.S.A.*, **101**, 10780–10785.

197. Yap, M. W., Nisole, S., Lynch, C., and Stoye, J. P. (2004) Trim5alpha protein restricts both HIV-1 and murine leukemia virus, *Proc. Natl. Acad. Sci. U.S.A.*, **101**, 10786–10791.

198. Hatziioannou, T., Perez-Caballero, D., Yang, A., Cowan, S., and Bieniasz, P. D. (2004) Retrovirus resistance factors Ref1 and Lv1 are species-specific variants of TRIM5alpha, *Proc. Natl. Acad. Sci. U.S.A.*, **101**, 10774–10779.

199. Perron, M. J., Stremlau, M., Song, B., Ulm, W., Mulligan, R. C., and Sodroski, J. (2004) TRIM5alpha mediates the postentry block to N-tropic murine leukemia viruses in human cells, *Proc. Natl. Acad. Sci. U.S.A.*, **101**, 11827–11832.

200. Asaoka, K., Ikeda, K., Hishinuma, T., Horie-Inoue, K., Takeda, S., and Inoue, S. (2005) A retrovirus restriction factor TRIM5alpha is transcriptionally regulated by interferons, *Biochem. Biophys. Res. Commun.*, **338**, 1950–1956.

201. Borden, K. L., Lally, J. M., Martin, S. R., O'Reilly, N. J., Etkin, L. D., and Freemont, P. S. (1995) Novel topology of a zinc-binding domain from a protein involved in regulating early Xenopus development, *EMBO J.*, **14**, 5947–5956.

202. Surridge, C. (2008) Innate immunity: getting in TRIM to fight retroviruses, *Nat. Rev. Microbiol.*, **6**, 797.

203. Xu, L., Yang, L., Moitra, P. K., et al. (2003) BTBD1 and BTBD2 colocalize to cytoplasmic bodies with the RBCC/tripartite motif protein, TRIM5delta, *Exp. Cell Res.*, **288**, 84–93.

204. Perez-Caballero, D., Hatziioannou, T., Yang, A., Cowan, S., and Bieniasz, P. D. (2005) Human tripartite motif 5{alpha} domains responsible for retrovirus restriction activity and specificity, *J. Virol.*, **79**, 8969–8978.

205. Mische, C. C., Javanbakht, H., Song, B., et al. (2005) Retroviral restriction factor TRIM5alpha is a trimer, *J. Virol.*, **79**, 14446–14450.

206. Zhang, F., Hatziioannou, T., Perez-Caballero, D., Derse, D., and Bieniasz, P. D. (2006) Antiretroviral potential of human tripartite motif-5 and related proteins, *Virology*, **353**(2), 369–409.

207. Yap, M. W., Nisole, S., and Stoye, J. P. (2005) A single amino acid change in the SPRY domain of human Trim5alpha leads to HIV-1 restriction, *Curr. Biol.*, **15**, 73–78.

208. Stremlau, M., Perron, M. J., Welikala, S., and Sodroski, J. (2005) Species-specific variation in the B30.2(SPRY) domain of TRIM5alpha determines the potency of human immunodeficiency virus restriction, *J. Virol.*, **79**, 3139–3145.

209. Passerini, L. D., Keckesova, Z., and Towers, G. J. (2006) Retroviral restriction factors Fv1 and TRM5{alpha} act independently and can compete for incoming virus before reverse transcription, *J. Virol.*, **80**, 2100–2105.

210. Nethe, M., Berkhout, B., and van der Kuyl, A. C. (2005) Retroviral superinfection resistance, *Retrovirology*, **2**, 52; doi: 10.1186/1742-4690-2-52.

211. Goff, S. P. (2004) Genetic control of retrovirus susceptibility in mammalian cells, *Annu. Rev. Genet.*, **38**, 61–85.

212. Allen, T. M. and Altfeld, M. (2003) HIV-1 superinfection, *J. Allergy Clin. Immunol.*, **112**, 829–835.

213. Doms, R. W. and Trono, D. (2000) The plasma membrane as a combat zone in the HIV battlefield, *Genes Dev.*, **14**, 2677–2688.

214. Nisole, S. and Saib, A. (2004) Early steps of retrovirus replicative cycle, *Retrovirology*, **1**, 9; doi: 10.1186/1742-4690-1-9.

215. Hoxie, J. A., Alpers, J. D., Rackowski, J. L., et al. (1986) Alterations in T4 (CD4) protein and mRNA synthesis in cells infected with HIV, *Science*, **234**, 1123–1127.

216. Salmon, P., Olivier, R., Riviere, Y., et al. (1988) Loss of CD4 membrane expression and CD4 mRNA during acute human immunodeficiency virus replication, *J. Exp. Med.*, **168**, 1953–1969.

217. Le Guern, M. and Levy, J. A. (1992) Human immunodeficiency virus (HIV) type 1 can superinfect HIV-2-infected cells: pseudotype virions produced with expanded cellular host range, *Proc. Natl. Acad. Sci. U.S.A.*, **89**, 363–367.

218. Oldridge, J. and Marsh, M. (1998) Nef – an adaptor adaptor? *Trends Cell Biol.*, **8**, 302–305.

219. Lama, J. (2003) The physiological relevance of CD4 receptor down-modulation during HIV infection, *Curr. HIV Res.*, **1**, 167–184.

220. Benson, R. E., Sanfridson, A., Ottinger, J. S., Doyle, C., and Cullen, B. R. (1993) Downregulation of cell-surface CD4 expression by simian immunodeficiency virus Nef prevents viral super infection, *J. Exp. Med.*, **177**, 1561–1566.

221. Arganaraz, E. R., Schindler, M., Kirchhoff, F., Cortes, M. J., and Lama J. (2003) Enhanced CD4 down-modulation by late stage HIV-1 nef alleles is associated with increased Env incorporation and viral replication, *J. Biol. Chem.*, **278**, 33912–33919.

222. Chenine, A. L., Sattentau, Q., and Moulard, M. (2000) Selective HIV-1-induced downmodulation of CD4 and coreceptors, *Arch. Virol.*, **145**, 455–471.

223. Lusso, P., Cocchi, F., Balotta, C., et al. (1995) Growth of macrophage-tropic and primary human immunodeficiency virus type 1 (HIV-1) isolates in a unique CD4+ T-cell clone (PM1): failure to downregulate CD4 and to interfere with cell-line-tropic HIV-1, *J. Virol.*, **69**, 3712–3720.

224. Shea, A., Sarr, D. A., Jones, N., et al. (2004) CCR5 receptor expression is down-regulated in HIV type 2 infection: implication for viral control and protection, *AIDS Res. Hum. Retroviruses*, **20**, 630–635.

225. Potash, M. J. and Volsky, D. J. (1998) Viral interference in HIV-1 infected cells, *Rev. Med. Virol.*, **8**, 203–211.

226. Saha, K., Volsky, D. J., and Matczak, E. (1999) Resistance against syncytium-inducing human immunodeficiency virus type 1 (HIV-1) in selected CD4(+) T cells from an HIV-1-infected nonprogressor: evidence of a novel pathway of resistance mediated by a soluble factor(s) that acts after virus entry, *J. Virol.*, **73**, 7891–7898.

227. Volsky, D. J., Simm, M., Shahabuddin, M., Li, G., Chao, W., and Potash, M. J. (1996) Interference to human immunodeficiency virus type 1 infection in the absence of downmodulation of the principal virus receptor, CD4, *J. Virol.*, **70**, 3823–3833.

228. Federico, M., Nappi, F., Bona, R., D'Aloja, P., Verani, P., and Rossi, G. B. (1995) Full expression of transfected nonproducer interfering HIV-1 proviral DNA abrogates susceptibility of human He-La CD4+ cells to HIV, *Virology*, **206**, 76–84.

229. D'Aloja, P., Olivetta, E., Bona, R., et al. (1998) Gag, vif, and nef genes contribute to the homologous viral interference induced by a nonproducer human immunodeficiency virus type 1 (HIV-1) variant: identification of novel HIV-1-inhibiting viral protein mutants, *J. Virol.*, **72**, 4308–4319.

230. Fackler, O. T., D'Aloja, P., Baur, A. S., Federico, M., and Peterlin, B. M. (2001) Nef from human immunodeficiency virus type 1(F12) inhibits viral production and infectivity, *J. Virol.*, **75**, 6601–6608.

231. Tremblay, M., Numazaki, K., Li, X. G., Gornitsky, M., Hiscott, J., and Wainberg, A. (1990) Resistance to infection by HIV-1 of peripheral blood mononuclear cells from HIV-1-infected patients is probably mediated by neutralizing antibodies, *J. Immunol.*, **145**, 2896–2901.

232. Shirazi, Y. and Pitha, P. M. (1992) Alpha interferon inhibits early stages of the human immunodeficiency virus type 1 replication cycle, *J. Virol.*, **66**, 1321–1328.

233. Walker, C. M., Erickson, A. L., Hsueh, F. C., and Levy, J. A. (1991) Inhibition of human immunodeficiency virus replication in acutely infected CD4+ cells by CD8+ cells involves a noncytotoxic mechanism, *J. Virol.*, **65**, 5921–5927.

234. Mackewicz, C. and Levy, J. A. (1992) CD8+ cell anti-HIV activity: nonlytic suppression of virus replication, *AIDS Res. Hum. Retroviruses*, **8**, 1039–1050.

235. Vella, C. and Daniels, R. S. (2003) CD8+ T-cell-mediated noncytolytic suppression of human immuno-deficiency viruses, *Curr. Drug Targets Infect. Disord.*, **3**, 97–113.

236. Ahmed, R. K., Biberfeld, G., and Thorstensson, R. (2005) Innate immunity in experimental SIV infection and vaccination, *Mol. Immunol.*, **42**, 251–258.

237. Mackewicz, C. E., Blackbourn, D. J., and Levy, J. A. (1995) CD8+ T cells suppress human immunodeficiency virus replication by inhibiting viral transcription, *Proc. Natl. Acad. Sci. U.S.A.*, **92**, 2308–2312.

238. Mackewicz, C. E., Patterson, B. K., Lee, S. A., and Levy, J. A. (2000) CD8(+) cell noncytotoxic anti-human immunodeficiency virus response inhibits expression of viral RNA but not reverse transcription or provirus integration, *J. Gen. Virol.*, **81**, 1261–1264.

239. Mackewicz, C. E., Ortega, H. W., and Levy, J. A. (1991) CD8+ cell anti-HIV activity correlates with the clinical state of the infected individual, *J. Clin. Invest.*, **87**, 1462–1466.

240. Mackewicz, C. E., Craik, C. S., and Levy, J. A. (2003) The CD8$^+$ cell noncytotoxic anti-HIV response can be blocked by protease inhibitors, *Proc. Natl. Acad. Sci. U.S.A.*, **100**, 3433–3438.

241. Barker, E., Bossart, K. N., Locher, C. P., Patterson, B. K., and Levy, J. A. (1996) CD8+ cells from asymptomatic human immunodeficiency virus-infected individuals suppress superinfection of their peripheral blood mononuclear cells, *J. Gen. Virol.*, **77**(Part 12), 2953–2962.

242. Locher, C. P., Blackbourn, D. J., Barnett, S. W., et al. (1997) Superinfection with human immunodeficiency virus type 2 can reactivate virus production in baboons but is contained by a CD8 T cell antiviral response, *J. Infect. Dis.*, **176**, 948–959.

243. Hohdatsu, T., Sasagawa, T., Yamazaki, A., et al. (2002) CD8+ T cells from feline immunodeficiency virus (FIV) infected cats suppress exogenous FIV replication of their peripheral blood mononuclear cells in vitro, *Arch. Virol.*, **147**, 1517–1529.

244. Otten, R. A., Ellenberger, D. L., Adams, D. R., et al. (1999) Identification of a window period for susceptibility to dual infection with two distinct human immunodeficiency virus type 2 isolates in a Macaca nemestrina (pig-tailed macaque) model, *J. Infect. Dis.*, **180**, 673–684.

245. Fultz, P. N. (2004) HIV-1 superinfections: omens for vaccine efficacy? *AIDS*, **18**, 115–119.

246. Chun, T. W., Justement, J. S., Moir, S., et al. (2001) Suppression of HIV replication in the resting CD4+ T cell reservoir by autologous CD8+ T cells: implications for the development of therapeutic strategies, *Proc. Natl. Acad. Sci. U.S.A.*, **98**, 253–258.

247. Blackbourn, D. J., Mackewicz, C. E., Barker, E., et al. (1996) Suppression of HIV replication by lymphoid tissue CD8+ cells correlates with the clinical state of HIV-infected individuals, *Proc. Natl. Acad. Sci. U.S.A.*, **93**(23), 13125–13130.

248. Kostense, S., Vandenberghe, K., Joling, J., et al. (2002) Persistent numbers of tetramer+ CD8(+) T cells, but loss of interferon-gamma+ HIV-specific T cells during progression to AIDS, *Blood*, **99**, 2505–2511.

249. Brinchmann, J. E., Albert, J., and Vartdal, F. (1999) Few infected CD4+ T cells but a high proportion of replication-competent provirus copies in asymptomatic human immunodeficiency virus type 1 infection, *J. Virol.*, **65**, 2019–2023.

250. Yerly, S., Chamot, E., Hirschel, B., and Perrin, L. H. (1992) Quantitation of human immunodeficiency virus provirus and circulating virus: relationship with immunologic parameters, *J. Infect. Dis.*, **166**, 269–276.

251. Jung, A., Maier, R., Vartanian, J. P. O., et al. (2002) Recombination multiply infected spleen cells in HIV patients, *Nature*, **418**, 144.

252. World Health Organization, Interagency Surveillance and Survey Working Group, Office of the U.S. Global AIDS Coordinator, U.S. Department of State; Division of Global AIDS, National Center for HIV, Viral Hepatitis, STDs, and Tuberculosis Prevention (CDC) (2006) The global HIV/AIDS pandemic, 2006, *Morb. Mortal. Wkly Rep.*, **55**(31), 841–844.

253. Centers for Disease Control and Prevention (1981) *Pneumocystis Pneumonia* – Los Angeles, *Morb. Mortal. Wkly Rep.*, **30**(21), 250–252.

254. Joint United Nations Programme on HIV/AIDS (UNAIDS) (2007) 2007 AIDS epidemic update. Geneva, Switzerland: UNAIDS (http://www.unaids.org/en/KnowledgeCentre/ HIV-Data/EpiUpdate/EpiUpdArchive/2007/2007default.asp).

255. World Health Organization (2006) Joint United Nations Programme on antiretroviral therapy: a report on "3 by 5" and beyond (http://www.who.int/hiv/fullreport_en_highres.pdf).

256. Kumar, R., Jha, P., Arora, P., et al. (2006) Trends in HIV-1 in young adults in south India from 2000 to 2004: a prevalence study, *Lancet*, **367**, 1164–1172.

257. Centers for Disease Control and Prevention (2006) HIV prevalence among men who have sex with men – Thailand, 2003 and 2005, *Morb. Mortal. Wkly Rep.*, **55**(31), 844–848.

258. Centers for Disease Control and Prevention (2005) Trends in HIV/AIDS diagnosis – 33 states, 2001–2004, *Morb. Mortal. Wkly Rep.*, **54**(45), 1149–1153.

259. Corea, G. (1992) *The Invisible Epidemic: The Story of Women and AIDS*, HarperCollins, New York.

260. WISQARS (2005) Leading causes of death reports, 1999–2004 (http:// webappa.cdc.gov/sasweb/ncipc/leadcaus10.html).

Chapter 28

NIAID: Extramural Basic Research Programs

NIAID supports a human immunodeficiency virus (HIV) basic science research program that provides valuable scientific information about the basic biology of HIV, the immune response to HIV infection, and potential targets for prevention and therapeutic strategies (http://www3.niaid.nih.gov/research/topics/HIV/BasicScience/).

Much has been learned over the past 25 years since the beginning of the AIDS epidemic about how HIV is transmitted, how the virus invades and is reproduced in the cell, and how HIV causes the progressive disease that leads to acquired immunodeficiency syndrome (AIDS). However, questions still remain about the molecular interactions involved in the regulation of HIV expression and replication in human immune cells, why the host immune response is not fully effective in controlling the infection, and how reservoirs of infection persist in the body despite highly active antiretroviral treatment (HAART; commonly known as ART and/or combination ART). Basic scientific information about how the virus attacks the body and how the body defends itself is critical to feeding the pipeline that generates new agents for therapeutic and preventive interventions.

NIAID's research agenda for HIV basic science research is guided by the *NIH Office of AIDS Research (OAR)*, the entity responsible for the overall scientific, budgetary, legislative, and policy elements of all AIDS research sponsored by NIH. The various institutes and centers at NIH are responsible for implementing OAR's etiology and pathogenesis research agenda, and NIAID has long played a central role in the two major research areas of HIV pathogenesis and HIV targeted interventions (http://www3.niaid.nih.gov/research/topics/HIV/BasicScience/introduction.htm).

28.1 Research Activities

Currently, NIAD is providing support in basic HIV/AIDS research in its intramural research laboratories and through funding of extramural research programs in HIV pathogenesis and HIV targeted interventions.

28.1.1 HIV Pathogenesis

The NIAD portfolio on HIV pathogenesis encompasses a variety of areas, including (i) mechanisms of viral entry, evasion, and replication; (ii) structure, function, and mechanism of action of viral genes and proteins; (iii) roles of cellular accessory molecules in replication; (iv) immunologic and virologic events controlling primary infection and formation of latent reservoirs; (v) development of *in vitro* and *ex vivo* assays to monitor virus growth, immune responses, and reservoir status during HIV disease; (vi) animal models; and (vii) genetic analysis of host factors that modulate viral infection or disease progression (http://www3.niaid.nih.gov/research/topics/HIV/BasicScience/pathogenesis.htm).

To date, NIAID's HIV pathogenesis research efforts have yielded significant scientific information about the basic biology of HIV and the immune response to HIV infection. For example, NIAID-funded investigators have identified the critical steps of how HIV uses the host machinery to enter and exit the cell, as well as the existence of multiple, persistent HIV reservoirs despite HAART. In response to these findings, researchers are focusing their efforts on identifying new strategies to understand and eliminate these reservoirs of latent HIV. Relevant research has also helped identify genetic markers that influence progression to AIDS. Although much has been learned in recent years, questions still remain. Information about how the virus attacks the immune system and which aspects of the immune response are the most helpful in controlling the infection is critical in providing additional targets against which therapeutic interventions and vaccines can be directed.

To this end, the goals of NIAID's HIV pathogenesis research program include:

- Determining the structure, function, and mechanism of action of viral genes and proteins and how they interact with host cell genes and proteins to allow viruses to enter and replicate in cells

- Determining genetic and other factors of the host that modulate the transmission, replication, and establishment of HIV infection and the progression of the disease
- Characterizing all of the elements of the innate and adaptive immune responses to HIV in key anatomic sites (e.g., gut, genital tract, lymph nodes) during primary and chronic infection and their roles in controlling the establishment and progression of disease
- Determining mechanisms of HIV transmission and establishment of infection, especially those involved in mucosal transmission
- Determining host and viral factors modulating persistent cellular and tissue reservoirs of HIV, including compartmentalization of virus in different anatomic sites

28.1.2 Drug Discovery

For nearly two decades, drug discovery efforts have been focused predominately on two viral targets: (i) reverse transcriptase (RT), the enzyme that catalyzes the synthesis of viral DNA from the RNA template present in the incoming, or infecting, virion, and (ii) protease (PR), the enzyme that affects HIV maturation by cleaving and processing viral precursor proteins to their mature form. Whereas viral load can be reduced to undetectable levels by combining RT and PR inhibitors (i.e., HAART), failures of treatment occur due to the development of drug resistance and/or patients' nonadherence to complicated and often toxic regimens. In addition, the current regimens involving RT and PR drugs are costly, complex, and difficult to use worldwide, especially in developing countries. Recently, new drugs such as agents directed at the virus binding and entry process, as well as therapies targeting HIV integrase, various steps of the virus entry process, and virion maturation, have been examined in clinical trials (e.g., Phase II/III). However, new data have emerged suggesting that the development of resistance will continue to be a problem as new agents are introduced into HAART regimens. In addition, extensive research has demonstrated that though effective, HAART cannot totally eliminate HIV-1 and only partially reverses virus-related damage to the immune system.

28.1.3 NIAID Basic Research Initiatives

Targeted areas of NIAID-funded basic research programs include (http://www3.niaid.nih.gov/research/topics/HIV/BasicScience/funding.htm):

- *HIV Proteins and Their Cellular Binding Partners.* This program is designed to support studies that are particularly innovative, novel, possibly high risk/high impact, and that have potential to advance understanding of the interactions of HIV proteins with cognate cellular binding partners. Awarded projects will have milestone "proof-of-concept" studies and then will be evaluated for the expanded development award without the need to submit an additional grant application (http://grants.nih.gov/grants/guide/pa-files/PA-06-388.html).
- *Centers for AIDS Research (CFAR).* Cofunded by six NIH institutes including NIAID, the National Cancer Institute (NCI), the National Institute of Child Health and Human Development (NICHD), the National Heart, Lung, and Blood Institute (NHLBI), the National Institute on Drug Abuse, (NIDA) and the National Institute of Mental Health (NIMH), the CFAR program provides administrative and shared research support to synergistically enhance and coordinate high-quality AIDS research projects. In addition to these six NIH institutes, the CFAR program is also scientifically managed by the National Center for Complementary and Alternative Medicine (NCCAM), the Office of AIDS Research (OAR), and the Fogarty International Center (FIC) of the National Institutes of Health. The various centers will have additional support through core facilities that provide expertise, resources, and services not otherwise readily obtained through more traditional funding mechanisms. The CFAR program emphasizes the importance of interdisciplinary collaboration, especially between basic and clinical investigators, translational research in which findings from the laboratory are brought to the clinic and vice versa, and an emphasis on including minorities and including research on prevention and behavioral change. There are currently 18 CFARs located at academic and research institutions throughout the United States (http://www3.niaid.nih.gov/research/cfar/).
- *HIV Interdisciplinary Network for Pathogenesis Research in Women.* This program is designed to involve either single institutions or consortia to participate in a cooperative, high quality, focused, multidisciplinary pathogenesis research programs in HIV-infected women. The results of this research is expected to enhance knowledge of the pathogenesis of HIV infection in women through investigations of biologic mechanisms that affect HIV transmission, disease acquisition, and the progression and manifestations of HIV in women (http://grants1.nih.gov/grants/guide/rfa-files/RFA-AI-07-009.html).
- *Novel HIV Therapies: Integrated Preclinical/Clinical Program (IPCP).* The IPCP is a program that provides a continuous spectrum of research opportunities. IPCP supports research by collaborative groups seeking to transition from preclinical to clinical studies during the award period, as well as pilot clinical studies of novel treatments. This program is designed to promote creative and original

therapeutic research on diverse facets of HIV infection between multidisciplinary preclinical and clinical research groups from academic or nonprofit institutions and research firms (http://grants.nih.gov/grants/guide/rfa-files/RFA-AI-06-009.html).

- *HIV Vaccine Design and Development Teams (HVDDT).* The HVDDT funds a focused team of scientists with development experience from industry and/or academia who have a mature, promising therapeutic vaccine concept and a plan for targeted development and clinical evaluation. The teams will advance the therapeutic vaccine concept along a well-defined development path in a timely manner toward producing a product and completing a Phase I trial within the 5-year period of the contract. Researchers supported by HVDDT are encouraged but not required to conduct Phase I/II trials in collaboration with NIAID-supported *AIDS Clinical Trials Group (ACTG).* Current HVDDT research projects include:

  o "HIV Expression Plasmids and Molecular Adjuvants" (Wyeth Vaccine Research).
  o "Synthetic CD4 Targeted Therapeutic Vaccine" (United Biomedical, Inc.).
  o "Antigen Message Pulsed Autologous Dendritic Cell Therapies" (Argos Therapeutics, Inc.).

28.1.4 Resources for Researchers

NIAID is currently providing the following resources to researchers (http://www3.niaid.nih.gov/research/topics/HIV/BasicScience/resources.htm):

- AIDS*info* has information on HIV/AIDS-related health topics, treatment and prevention guidelines, information on drugs and vaccines, and a database of all federally funded HIV/AIDS clinical trials.
- *NIH AIDS Research and Reference Reagent Program* provides state-of-the-art biological and chemical materials for the study of HIV and related opportunistic pathogens to registered users worldwide, at no cost.
- *The NIH Tetramer Facility* provides custom synthesis and distribution of soluble MHC-peptide tetramer and CD1d tetramer reagents that can be used to stain antigen-specific T cells.
- *Human HIV Specimens* (e.g., blood, cells, tissues) from U.S.-based and international studies are available for distribution to researchers by (i) providing state-of-the-art storage and computerized inventory management of specimens from domestic and international NIAID-funded HIV/AIDS studies; and (ii) collecting, distribut-

ing, and maintaining a repository of tissues from HIV-positive donors for distribution to qualified biomedical research scientists.

- *HIV Specimen Repository Guidelines* include procedures for investigators seeking to collaborate with NIAID-funded clinical research programs, particularly with regard to gaining access to materials maintained in specimen repositories or databases.
- *AIDS and Cancer Specimen Resource (ACSR)*, funded by the National Cancer Institute, provides HIV-infected human materials from a wide spectrum of HIV-related or associated diseases, including cancer, and from appropriate HIV-negative controls.
- *HIV Molecular Immunology Database* is an annotated, searchable collection of HIV-1 cytotoxic and helper T-cell epitopes and antibody binding sites. These data are also printed in the *HIV Molecular Immunology* compendium, which is updated yearly and provided free of charge to scientific researchers. The goal of this database is to provide a comprehensive listing of defined HIV epitopes.
- *HIV Sequence Database*, based on HIV and SIV sequences from GenBank, allows users to align and analyze sequences by nucleotide, amino acid, or viral subtype using special tools and interfaces.
- *The Center for AIDS Research (CFAR) Network of Integrated Clinical Systems (CNICS)* is a unique resource for HIV clinical, translational, and basic research and will provide the infrastructure and data to address the challenging and rapidly evolving issues in HIV care and research. This project supports a data system that is a central repository of verified and quality-controlled data from the electronic medical records (EMRs) at six CFAR sites. Additional information on how to use this resource is coming soon.
- *Animal models* to evaluate the preclinical efficacy of novel antiviral agents and microbicides are available to investigators through NIAID-supported contracts. The SCID-hu thymus/liver mouse model provides rapid evaluation of *in vivo* antiviral activity and requires relatively small amounts of candidate compounds compared with that for non-human primate models. The simian immunodeficiency virus/simian human immunodeficiency virus (SIV/SHIV) macaque animal models serve as resource to investigators for developing and evaluating therapeutic agents/strategies and topical microbicides for HIV/AIDS using the SIV/SHIV macaque animal models.
- *The HIV/Host Protein Interaction Database* provides scientists with a summary of all known interactions of HIV proteins with host cell proteins, other HIV proteins, or proteins from disease organisms associated with HIV/AIDS. The database is cross-linked to other resources available via the National Center for Biotechnology Information through *Entrez Gene,*

providing a means for searching and understanding the interaction data.

28.2 Recent Scientific Advances

- *Defective Virus Drives HIV Infection, Persistence, and Pathogenesis.* Many aspects of the HIV life cycle are well understood, yet a key paradox remains. The primary targets for HIV are resting $CD4^+$ T lymphocytes that are not permissive to HIV replication unless activated by some external and independent event. Numerous mechanisms for this essential cellular activation step have been proposed, including co-infections, vaccination, cytokines, and endogenous microbial flora. This study proposes scientific evidence revealing a simple and direct source of CD4 cell activation: HIV itself *(1)*. During HIV infection, the great majority of virus produced is noninfectious (i.e., "defective"), primarily as a result of the error-prone process of reverse transcription. Although noninfectious, this defective virus is far from innocuous. It has been proposed that defective HIV particles provide a solution to this paradox, playing a specific, integral role in the HIV life cycle and in driving pathogenesis by (i) preferentially activating $CD4^+$ T-cells, rendering them permissive for productive HIV replication; and (ii) providing a large pool of constantly changing HIV peptides that are presented on major histocompatibility complex (MHC) class II molecules to continuously stimulate resting $CD4^+$ T-cells of different antigen specificities.

References

1. Finzi, D., Plaeger, S. F., and Dieffenbach, C. W. (2006) Defective virus drives HIV infection, persistence and pathogenesis, *Clin. Vaccine Immunol.*, **13**, 715–720.

Chapter 29

NIAID: Programs in HIV Prevention

The development of new and more effective nonvaccine methods and strategies to prevent HIV infection is an important component of NIAID's comprehensive HIV research strategy for disease prevention. To accelerate the identification and evaluation of new concepts, strategies, and products, NIAID has been partnering with community advisory groups, scientific investigators, and other organizations. For example, in an effort to expedite the development of topical microbicides, NIAID recently made a formal agreement with the *International Partnership for Microbicides (IPM)* to increase sharing of information and expertise.

Major research goals that guide NIAID's HIV prevention and microbicide agenda are based on the *Office of AIDS Research (OAR) NIH Plan for HIV-Related Research*, and include (http://www3.niaid.nih.gov/research/topics/HIV/prevention/intro/default.htm):

- Developing and testing promising biomedical and behavioral HIV prevention products and interventions in clinical trials
- Integrating prevention research into the overall HIV/AIDS research agenda
- Identifying opportunities to integrate the planning of HIV prevention research into the existing infrastructures of developing countries
- Developing and implementing effective ways to translate new knowledge into wider practice
- Disseminating information about intervention strategies that can significantly reduce the incidence of new HIV infections

29.1 Research Areas of NIAID Support

The NIAID-funded HIV prevention research is focused on the following areas (http://www3.niaid.nih.gov/research/topics/HIV/prevention/research/):

(i) Prevention of mother-to-child transmission (MTCT).
(ii) Topical microbicides.

(iii) Antiretroviral therapy (ART) to reduce the transmission of HIV.
(iv) Prevention and treatment of sexually transmitted infections (STIs) that play a role in HIV acquisition and transmission.
(v) Integration of biomedical research and behavioral and social sciences research.
(vi) Intervention strategies for injection drug and non-injection drug users to reduce the risk of HIV and other STIs.
(vii) Male circumcision.
(viii) Preexposure prophylaxis and vaginal health intervention.

Several NIAID-supported programs *relevant to HIV prevention* include:

- *HIV Prevention Trials Network (HPTN)* (see Sections 29.1.1 and 29.2.1; and Section 30.3.1 of Chapter 30)
- *Microbicide Trials Network (MTN)* (see Section 29.2.2; and Section 30.3.1 of Chapter 30)
- *Behavioral Science Working Group (BSWG)* (see Section 29.2.3)

29.1.1 Prevention of Mother-to-Child Transmission

Mother-to-child transmission (MTCT) of HIV, which can occur during pregnancy or childbirth or through breast-feeding, accounts for more than 90% of all cases of childhood HIV infection, especially in countries where effective antiretroviral drugs are not available [for information about international MTCT (HIVNET/NPTN) trials, see Chapter 32].

As more women of childbearing age become infected, the number of HIV-infected children is expected to rise (http://www3.niaid.nih.gov/research/topics/HIV/prevention/research/mtct.htm).

V. St. Georgiev, *National Institute of Allergy and Infectious Diseases, NIH: Impact on Global Health*, vol. 2, DOI 10.1007/978-1-60327-297-1_29, © Humana Press, a part of Springer Science+Business Media, LLC 2009

Although opportunities exist to successfully intervene during pregnancy to prevent transmission of HIV from an infected woman to her infant, developing safe, simple, and inexpensive interventions that would be more widely applicable, particularly in the developing world, remains of the highest importance.

NIAID is supporting a number of research studies to optimize and develop strategies to prevent mother-to-child transmission of HIV, including:

- *Perinatal Science Research Strategy* (http://www.hptn. org/prevention_science/perinatal.asp). The current HPTN's perinatal agenda is transitioning to the *International Maternal Pediatric Adolescent AIDS Clinical Trials (IMPAACT)* (http://pactg.s-3.com/). Information on current HPTN perinatal trials will be maintained on the HPTN Web site until this transition process is complete. Successful interventions in the antepartum, intrapartum, and postpartum periods to prevent transmission from an HIV-infected woman to her infant have already been identified and implemented, but there are more opportunities yet to be pursued. Of the highest importance are safe, simple, inexpensive interventions that could be widely applicable, particularly in the developing world

  o *Antepartum.* Now that the efficacy of antiretroviral (ARV) agents to reduce MTCT during the antepartum period has been established, studies of non-antiretroviral or improved antiretroviral regimens must be compared with proven regimens. And discerning an effect from a new intervention requires a significantly increased study size. In the *HIVNET 024* clinical trial, antibiotics given antenatally and at delivery to reduce chorioamnionitis-related HIV infection have shown no added protection against MTCT of HIV beyond that conferred by the *HIVNET 012* regimen. Considerations for antepartum interventions include new ARV agents and regimens, other mechanisms to further reduce maternal viral load, and immunomodulators.

  o *Intrapartum/Neonatal.* As shown in *HIVNET 012*, an intrapartum/neonatal regimen consisting of a single 200 mg dose of nevirapine (NVP) given to the mother at the onset of labor and a single 2 mg/kg dose of NVP given to the infant within 72 hours of life reduced the risk of perinatal transmission among breast-feeding women in Uganda by 47% at 14 to 16 weeks and by 41% at 18 months compared with an intrapartum/neonatal regimen of AZT (600 mg, then 300 mg every 3 hours during labor to mother, and 4 mg/kg twice daily for 1 week to the infant). This regimen has been adopted as the standard of care by the Ministries of Health in many resource-limited

countries. However, inadequate infrastructure has limited widespread implementation. There is concern that use of the single-dose NVP regimen will induce resistance that might diminish the utility of NVP or other non-nucleoside reverse transcriptase inhibitors (NNRTIs) if they become available for use as treatment in a combination antiretroviral regimen. In the *HIVNET 012* trial, resistant virus had faded from detection by 12 months postpartum. It will be important to assess the response to NVP therapy and repeat single-dose NVP prophylaxis in women and children who have been exposed to the single-dose NVP regimen.

  o *Postpartum.* The risk of an infant getting HIV from breast-feeding increases the longer the infant is exposed to HIV in the breast milk. When breast-feeding is stopped at 6 months, the risk of transmission is reduced—some say to as little as 5% (compared with 14% with longer periods of breast-feeding) (http:// www.thebody.com/content/art13590.html). Safe alternatives to breast-feeding are limited or infeasible in resource-poor settings, where the majority of HIV-infected women reside and the benefits of breast-feeding are well known. Therefore, an intervention to reduce the risk of HIV-1 transmission during breast-feeding would be of utmost benefit to women and children in resource-limited settings and is among the highest priorities for the HPTN Behavioral Science Working Group (BSWG). The impact of successful antepartum, intrapartum, and/or neonatal regimens of ARV may be diminished in breast-feeding populations with continual exposure to breast milk. Several important studies by the HPTN and other groups are under way or planned to examine the safety and efficacy of various ARV regimens given for different durations during breast-feeding (e.g., HPTN 046), most in combination with an antepartum and/or intrapartum component. However, the potentially high cost and difficult logistics of continuing ARV therapy in the infant or mother for the duration of breast-feeding may prohibit widespread and routine use in many resource-poor countries. Therefore, active and passive immunization strategies, perhaps combined with antepartum and/or intrapartum ARV regimens, are an attractive and important alternative. Testing appropriate HIV-1– specific antibody products and candidate HIV-1 vaccines as they become available is critical.

Among mothers infected with HIV, infants exclusively breast-fed for 3 months or more have no excess risk of HIV infection over 6 months than that of those who have never been breast-fed, according to latest research. The results could have important implications for public health policy in developing countries, where the total avoidance of breast-feeding is not a realistic option for the vast majority of women. A prospective cohort study was carried out involving 551 pregnant women infected with HIV who chose whether to breast-feed exclusively, use formula feed exclusively, or carry out mixed feeding after being counseled *(1, 2)*. The infants have now been followed for 15 months, and the results confirmed that infants exclusively breast-fed had no excess risk of maternal transmission of HIV over 6 months when compared with infants who were not breast-fed at all. Those at greatest risk were the infants fed on a mixture of breast milk and other foods and liquids. The study is the first to separate women who exclusively breast-feed from those who carry out mixed feeding. The mechanism through which exclusive breast-feeding may be safer than mixed feeding is not known. One possible hypothesis is that contaminated fluids and foods introduced in infants who received mixed feeding may damage the bowel and facilitate entry of HIV in breast milk into the tissues *(1, 2)*

- *HPTN Perinatal Studies*

  (i) *HIVNET 012*: A Phase IIB trial to determine the efficacy of oral zidovudine (AZT) and the efficacy of oral nevirapine for the prevention of vertical transmission of HIV-1 infection in pregnant Ugandan women and their neonates (http://www.hptn.org/research_studies/HIVNET012.asp).

  (ii) *HIVNET 024*: Phase III clinical trial of antibiotics to reduce chorioamnionitis-related perinatal HIV transmission (http://www.hptn.org/research_studies/HIVNET024.asp).

The HIV Network for Prevention Trials (HIVNET) is a multicenter, collaborative research network whose mission is to carry out HIV prevention efficacy trials (http://www.scharp.org/ceg/whatis.html). The HIVNET was established in 1993 by the Division of AIDS (DAIDS) of NIAID. The HIVNET evaluates the safety and effectiveness of promising interventions to prevent the transmission of HIV between sexual and/or needle-sharing partners, as well as from mother to infant during pregnancy and at birth. In most cases, the primary aim of these studies is to measure the effect of prevention interventions on reducing the number of new HIV infections. The methods being evaluated include HIV vaccines, topical gels and lubricants, treatment of other sexually transmitted diseases (such as herpes) that may increase the risk of getting HIV, use of antiviral drugs to prevent mother-to-infant transmission, and ways to help people reduce their risk of getting HIV by changing their behavior.

Field sites are the key organizations that conduct HIVNET studies. To coordinate these field sites in their collaborative

work, five organizations have received contracts funded by DAIDS.

- *The Statistical and Clinical Coordinating Center* is operated by the Fred Hutchinson Cancer Research Center and the University of Washington. This center is responsible for collecting and analyzing the information obtained from HIVNET research. Center staff also are involved in day-to-day coordination of study operations.
- *The Central Laboratory*, operated by the Viral and Rickettsial Disease Laboratory of the California Department of Health Services, provides centralized laboratory testing services for HIVNET studies.
- *The Domestic Master Contractor*, Abt Associates Inc., provides funding for all study sites in the United States. Abt also helps to coordinate study operations and monitors sites to ensure the consistency and quality of the research. In addition, Abt is responsible for coordinating local and national community education efforts.
- *The International Master Contractor* is Family Health International, which subcontracts with study sites outside the United States and oversees their research and related community activities.
- *The Repository Contractor*, Biomedical Research, Inc., provides very low-temperature, long-term storage for biological specimens collected in HIVNET studies.

29.1.2 Topical Microbicides

Topical microbicides are products (e.g., gels, creams, or foams) that are applied either vaginally and/or rectally to prevent HIV and other sexually transmitted infections. Ideally, microbicides would be unnoticeable, fast-acting against HIV and a broad range of other sexually transmitted pathogens, inexpensive, safe for use at least one to two times daily, and easy to store (http://www3.niaid.nih.gov/research/topics/HIV/prevention/research/Microbicides/Introduction+and+Goals/default.htm).

A topical microbicide may prevent HIV transmission by:

- Inactivating cell-free virus
- Strengthening normal defenses at mucosal sites
- Blocking attachment and entry of HIV to susceptible cells
- Preventing dissemination of the virus
- Inhibiting RT or other critical steps in viral replication

The goal of NIAID's HIV Topical Microbicide Program is to support research that leads to identification and development of safe, effective, and acceptable topical microbicides. NIAID's topical microbicide research is outlined in the *NIAID Topical Microbicide Strategic Plan* and includes basic research through preclinical development and clinical trials.

NIAID's microbicide research aims to support:

- Fundamental research to delineate the early steps in HIV infection and transmission at mucosal surfaces in cervico-vaginal and rectal tissues
- Discovery and development of safe and effective formulations and delivery methods
- Development and use of suitable animal models for testing safety and efficacy
- Research into the acceptance and use of microbicides by conducting prevention and behavioral studies
- Exploratory Phase I clinical trials to assess the relevance of and to validate new approaches for determining the safety and efficacy of candidate microbicides
- Iterative preclinical to clinical translational research to evaluate and optimize topical microbicide formulations and strategies
- Clinical trials to determine safety, efficacy, and acceptability of candidate topical microbicides

29.1.2.1 Development and Characteristics of Topical Microbicides

The development process of a microbicide candidate must ensure that it is safe and nonirritating to the genital and anorectal tract while demonstrating that it is effective in preventing HIV infection. After an active agent that can prevent HIV infection has been identified from *in vitro* and *ex vivo* assays designed for specific transmission routes, further studies are conducted to assess potential toxicities. After studies have shown high potency and lack of toxicity, and the candidate displays some of the predetermined criteria for optimal attributes of microbicides, a compatible formulation for its delivery is developed. Additional *in vitro*, *ex vivo*, and *in vivo* studies are undertaken to further characterize the properties of the newly developed topical microbicide before it is tested in clinical trials.

Ultimately, the effectiveness of a microbicide is directly related to its acceptability and any social or cultural factors that might influence its use. Biomedical and behavioral research should be integrated into every stage of microbicidal development.

A summary of the attributes of a candidate microbicide that may predict its transition from preclinical to clinical testing is presented in Table 29.1.

Ideally, topical microbicides should include a combination of agents that should also prevent other STIs, since many have been associated with increased risk of HIV infection or its exacerbation. Some of the STIs or clinical conditions that might increase the risk for HIV infection include (i) herpes simplex virus (HSV-2); (ii) human papillomavirus (HPV);

(iii) hepatitis C virus (HCV); (iv) syphilis; (v) gonorrhea; and (vi) bacterial vaginosis (BV).

After the vaginal microbicide has been tested and shown to prevent transmission in clinical trials and approval has been obtained from appropriate regulatory bodies, the product will be made available to consumers. In light of studies documenting the routine practice of anal intercourse among a considerable number of heterosexuals, and the fact that men who have sex with men (MSM) constitute a significant portion of the HIV-infected population in selected regions of the world, it is anticipated that off-label or unintended use will occur. Thus, products developed as vaginal microbicides also need to be safe for rectal use. Development of safe, effective, and acceptable microbicides specifically for rectal use is proceeding in parallel with vaginal microbicides (http://www3.niaid.nih.gov/research/topics/HIV/prevention/research/Microbicides/Introduction+and+Goals/topical_development.htm).

29.1.2.2 Contraception and Microbicides

In a microbicide strategy, a microbicide's contraceptive capability may be an important factor affecting its acceptance and use in specific populations or ethnic groups. Several microbicides in the pipeline have spermicidal activity (CAP films, Carraguard). Ideally, microbicides would be available in contraceptive and noncontraceptive formulations, in recognition that a woman's reproductive choices may change over her lifetime. This would reduce behavioral and social dilemmas associated with microbicide use and give women the ability to protect themselves and their families from HIV and other STIs in the process of trying to conceive a child (http://www3.niaid.nih.gov/research/topics/HIV/prevention/research/Microbicides/Introduction+and+Goals/topical_contraception.htm).

29.1.2.3 Behavior and Microbicides

The NIAID Topical Microbicide Program has recognized the need to incorporate behavioral and social science research into the microbicide development process. Behavioral and social science research activities can be integrated into all levels of microbicide development, from baseline determinations of acceptability and potential use to collection of specific data on the use of a product in and out of clinical trials. Behavioral and social science research also plays a role in designing clinical trials to test a microbicide's efficacy. By identifying use behaviors or local practices, such as use of vaginal drying agents, which may affect an individual's willingness to use a microbicide or which may influence the level of effectiveness of the microbicide

Table 29.1 Characteristics of topical microbicides

Acceptable	Unacceptable
Safety	
• Administration 6 or more times daily or continuous delivery	• Causes epithelial disruption
• Can be used for extended periods	• Induces inflammation
• Lacks reproductive toxicities	• Is absorbed systemically
Effect	
• Fast	• Unstable
• Long-lasting	• Interval of efficacy between application and coitus is brief (before or after)
• Irreversible	
Acceptability	
• Formulation is stable	• Messy, leaky
• Is acceptable to the user and user's sex partner	• Causes burning, itching
• Is unobtrusive or pleasurable	• Cumbersome
	• Unpleasant odor, taste, color, or texture
	• Delivery vehicle causes trauma or discomfort
Availability	
• Contraceptive/noncontraceptive formulations	• Costly for use and/or manufacturing
• Low cost	• Distribution is regulated (requires M.D. or health care provider)
• Access is unlimited	• Requires special storage/transport
• Ease of scale-up and good manufacturing practice (GMP) production	
Uses	
• Vaginal and/or rectal	• Complicated use
• Unlimited use	
• Compatible with condoms and other STI prevention methods	
Activity	
• Affects STIs in ejaculate and cervicovaginal secretions	• Affects normal vaginal (rectal) microbial ecology
• Broadly active: HIV + other STIs	• Enhances growth of STIs or secondary pathogens

itself, potential confounding factors can be addressed and minimized (http://www3.niaid.nih.gov/research/topics/HIV/prevention/research/Microbicides/Introduction+and+Goals/topical_behavior.htm).

29.1.2.4 The Microbicide Pipeline at NIAID

There are a number of candidate microbicides, including proteins, small-molecule inhibitors, and natural products, which are being supported by the different programs at NIAID. These include:

• Natural Defense Molecules to bolster existing cervicovaginal defenses: *Lactobacillus* delivered CV-N, CD4, RANTES peptides, sIg anti-ICAM, glycerol monolaureate (GML), and PSC-RANTES + immunomodulators
• Acid buffering agents to maintain vaginal pH, such as BufferGel
• Entry inhibitors:

  ○ C-type lectins such as soluble mannans, soluble DC-SIGN, artificial syndecan 1 and 2 agonists

  ○ Agents blocking gp120/CD4 interaction, such as CV-N, 12P1, ISIS 5320, BMS-338806, CD4-IgG(PRO542), monoclonal antibodies b12, 2G12, 2F5, novel dendrimers, CAP, retrocyclins
  ○ Coreceptor inhibitors such as CMPD 167, TAK779, AD-101, PSC-RANTES, and new recombinant analogues, 5P1, 6P4, NB325 (polybiguanide)
  ○ Gp41 inhibitors such as *N*-linked peptides, C52L, T1249, T-20
  ○ Uncharacterized entry target: octylglycerol, ECGC

• Absorption inhibitors that block virus-cell association such as PRO2000
• Reverse transcriptase (RT) inhibitors to block the transcription of HIV RNA to DNA: PMPA (Tenofovir), UC-781, SJ-3366, and SAR series (NNRTI)
• Agents that act on cell-free virus such as NC-p7 inhibitors and anti-HIV catalytic antibodies (gp120 target)
• Combination microbicides that combine multiple mechanisms of action, such as: SJ-3366/SAR+ISIS5320, CV-N+12P1, BufferGel with dendrimers (SPI-7013), NC-p7 inhibitors with CAP, NC-p7 inhibitors +/− ISIS 5320 +/− SJ-3366, ZCM (carrageenan, ZN, MIV150)

29.1.2.5 Programs in Topical Microbicide Research

NIAID is supporting microbicide research through targeted Program Announcements and Request for Applications, which are designed to attract investigators and assemble consortia of scientists and private-sector entities to develop preclinical and early clinical versions of worthy microbicide candidates. Recently, the NIAID Topical Microbicide Program has used or is using the following initiatives to support microbicide research:

- *Microbicide Innovation Program.* This program supports focused innovation and development of microbicides using the R21/R33 phased innovation and development mechanism. This is a milestone-driven program, in which specific milestones are specified for the 2-year R21 portion of the award. If milestones are met and the research still meets program priorities and there are sufficient resources, the award will be quickly transitioned to a 3-year funding through the R33 mechanism.

  - *Integrated Preclinical/Clinical Program for HIV Topical Microbicides.* This program is designed to support preclinical and exploratory Phase I clinical trials aimed at advancing a candidate microbicide or strategy to more advanced clinical trials; it is funded through a collaborative U19 mechanism.

  - *Microbicide Design and Development Teams.* This contract program is supporting microbicide development from initial discovery through exploratory clinical testing (Phase I). It incorporates a commercial partner (private sector) in a multiproject environment under a cooperative agreement (U19) with NIH. It is focused on providing proof-of-concept for new microbicide strategies and approaches and supports critical path development of individual microbicides. Its primary milestone is the initiation of a Phase I clinical trial before the award ends.

29.1.3 Antiretroviral Therapy in HIV Prevention

The advent of antiretroviral therapy (ART) in the early 1980s and highly active antiretroviral therapy (HAART) regimens have dramatically reduced the morbidity and mortality associated with HIV infection through sustained reduction in HIV viral replication. This sustained suppression of viral load has led researchers to consider ARTs as a prevention tool; ARTs would lower the viral load and, thus, the infectiousness of an HIV-infected person to an uninfected partner. This research is particularly relevant for prevention among serodiscordant couples (i.e., one HIV-positive, the other HIV-negative),

many of whom will continue to be sexually active despite their differing infection status.

In addition, researchers are considering the possibility that antiretroviral drugs might be used by uninfected, at-risk persons before exposure to HIV and that these drugs might be able to block or prevent infection from occurring (http://www3.niaid.nih.gov/research/topics/HIV/prevention/research/art.htm).

This potential strategy, called *Preexposure Prophylaxis (PREP)*, does not require participation of a sexual partner (as does condom use) and could also be highly complementary to other prevention strategies, as well as empowering women who wish to protect themselves from HIV. One of NIAID's scientific priorities is to develop PREP approaches as a viable HIV prevention strategy. In this regard, chemoprophylaxis for HIV prevention in men has been a major study focused on reducing the transmission of HIV (e.g., U01-AI064002).

NIAID is supporting research studies that use ART as a strategy to prevent acquisition and transmission of HIV using the *HIV Prevention Trials Network (HPTN)*. For example, HPTN 052 was designed as a randomized trial to evaluate the effectiveness of ART plus HIV primary care versus HIV primary care alone to prevent the sexual transmission of HIV-1 in serodiscordant couples (see Section 29.2.1.1).

29.1.4 Prevention and Treatment of Sexually Transmitted Infections

STIs have been shown to be important cofactors in the transmission and acquisition of HIV infection. An "epidemiologic synergy" exists between STIs and HIV, and thus control of one may have beneficial effects on the control of the other. The primary hypothesis is that interventions designed for more effective control of STIs should reduce the incidence of HIV. However, published results from two community randomized trials that addressed this hypothesis have been *contradictory*—one study showing positive results in decreasing HIV incidence (Mwanza), and the other study showing limited or no effect on HIV incidence (Rakai). Data from a third trial (Musaka) were presented in 2002 at the XIV International AIDS Conference in Barcelona; like the Rakai study, the data showed no impact. Careful analysis of the data from all three trials has shown a unifying theme, namely that these studies need to be done in settings with high incidence of STIs and increasing incidence of HIV (http://www.hptn.org/ prevention_science/std_control.asp).

Effective control of STIs would require both targeted and more generalized strategies. Targeted interventions that reduce transmission in core groups (such as sex workers) with a high rate of partner exchange, and bridging groups (such as migrant workers, truck drivers, etc.), which seed new sexual networks, have led to rapid control of STIs in several areas (e.g., Thailand; South African mining areas; and Nairobi, Kenya). Meanwhile, research has shown that improved access to quality STI services for the general population alone can have a measurable impact on HIV transmission, especially in populations with growing HIV epidemics. These examples provide evidence that control of STIs in the context of HIV transmission may represent an effective HIV prevention strategy. Therefore, as a strategy to reduce the incidence of HIV, one of NIAID's goals is to design interventions that are more effective at controlling STIs that are important cofactors in acquisition and transmission (http://www3.niaid.nih.gov/research/topics/HIV/prevention/research/sti/).

Although the highest research priority identified was a community randomized hybrid study combining these interventions, the HPTN has not had either site capability or funding to approve such a trial. Meanwhile, the emergence of genital herpes, especially in the context of mature HIV epidemics, highlights the evolving nature of the epidemiology of STIs. Recent data from the Rakai trial has shown a nearly fivefold association of HSV-2 with HIV-1 acquisition. Building on the extensive literature that has demonstrated that genital ulcers are a risk factor for acquiring HIV, the HPTN is supporting *HPTN 039*, which examines the effect of acyclovir-mediated suppression of HSV-2 infection on the acquisition of HIV. Because antiretrovirals are still out of reach of the majority of those infected with HIV, and HIV-related immunosuppression facilitates HSV-2 clinical expression, HSV-2 infection is likely to become an important cofactor in mature epidemics and thus increase the risk of HSV transmission (http://www.hptn.org/prevention_science/std_control.asp).

Several key points regarding the interactions of STIs and HIV transmission include:

- Targeted interventions that improve STI treatment and increase condom use in high-risk networks may have the greatest impact on sexual transmission of curable STIs, HSV, and HIV
- Specific, intensive STI interventions, such as treatment of STIs in high-frequency transmitters, can bring about rapid reductions in the prevalence of STIs
- Continuous access to improved STI services may have the greatest impact on HIV transmission
- Treatment of asymptomatic STIs is critical to reducing overall STI prevalence
- STI treatment is critical in populations with early or growing HIV epidemics; the contribution of STIs to the spread of HIV may decline in more mature epidemics
- Genital ulcers, such as those associated with HSV-2, are potent cofactors in both the transmission and acquisition of HIV

- Lack of male circumcision is correlated with higher risks of HIV acquisition

29.1.5 *Integration of Biomedical and Behavioral and Social Science Research*

The behavioral and social sciences play a key role in HIV prevention research because every strategy that can be used for preventing the acquisition or transmission of HIV has associated behavioral components that can influence its effectiveness. These components may affect the adoption and acceptance of a specific prevention approach or may be critical in determining the use, acceptability, and potential efficacy of microbicide strategies in clinical trials (http://www3.niaid.nih.gov/research/topics/HIV/prevention/research/SocialScience.htm).

Research has shown that a wide variety of individual, interpersonal, social, and environmental factors may influence the risk of HIV infection. Individual factors that influence risk may include age, self-esteem, age of sexual debut, willingness to enact prevention behaviors, sexual identity, and substance use or abuse. Interpersonal factors include gender equity and female empowerment, partner status, and ability to negotiate prevention with sexual partners. Social and environmental factors that affect risk may include cultural and religious beliefs about sexuality and sexual behavior, culturally proscribed gender norms, and marginalization of certain populations, such as gay men, drug users, commercial sex workers, and at-risk youth.

Studies have shown that HIV risk behaviors can be reduced in any targeted population through interventions that provide counseling on risk reduction, that stress cognitive approaches to problem solving and behavior change, and that help individuals to build the skills they need to reduce HIV risk. Voluntary counseling and testing (VCT) has also been clearly shown to reduce risky behaviors, especially among HIV-infected persons and in extramarital partnerships.

One of NIAID's major goals is to support research to better understand the effects of social and behavioral factors on the acquisition and transmission of HIV, to develop innovative behavioral prevention strategies that can address the changing contexts of the HIV pandemic, and to use behavioral and social science expertise to improve and effectively implement primarily nonbehavioral clinical prevention and therapeutic trials. Behavioral and social science research needs to address a number of relevant issues in HIV prevention, such as:

- The impact of community-level behavioral interventions on the incidence of HIV at the community level HIV over time

- The HIV prevention needs of adolescents and young adults, particularly young women, girls, and other vulnerable youth in resource-constrained settings
- The prevention needs of HIV-infected persons and the best ways to reach seropositive individuals with prevention messages and interventions
- The early integration of behavioral and social science research into the microbicide development pipeline to facilitate the development and selection of the most acceptable approaches to microbicide use

Through the *HIV Prevention Trial Network (HPTN)*, NIAID, in close collaboration with the National Institute of Mental Health (NIMH), where most of the expertise in this type of research resides, is supporting a number of research studies that aim to better understand the behavioral and social factors that influence HIV risk and to integrate social and behavioral prevention strategies into a more comprehensive portfolio of interventions designed to prevent transmission of HIV.

29.1.6 Intervention Strategies for Injection and Non-injection Drug Users to Reduce the Risk of HIV and Other STIs

Numerous studies have shown that injection drug users who engage in multiperson sharing of needles and syringes have an increased risk for HIV transmission. Drug-related risk behaviors, including exchange of sex for drugs or money, have also been independently associated with HIV infection (http://www3.niaid.nih.gov/research/topics/HIV/prevention/research/intervention.htm).

Injection-related risk behaviors account for the majority of new HIV infections in many parts of the world, including Eastern Europe, Russia, and Southeast Asia. Rapid HIV transmission among populations and social groups associated with injection drug use in low prevalence settings is leading to new epidemics in many countries.

Research has shown that substance-abuse treatment programs, which aim to reduce the frequency of drug use, have made a positive impact on reducing drug-related risk behaviors and subsequent HIV exposure. Risk has been reduced among active drug users in various settings by means of community outreach programs and access to sterile injection equipment.

Nevertheless, preventing HIV transmission among non-injecting and injecting drug users remains an urgent and expanding public health problem in many regions of the world. The NIAID HIV prevention portfolio includes a number of scientific priorities that address risk reduction for HIV

and other STIs among injecting and non-injecting drug users. These priorities include:

- Reducing risk of drug-associated and sexual transmission of HIV among injecting and non-injecting substance users
- Developing and refining primary and secondary prevention interventions for HIV-infected drug users
- Developing interventions designed to overcome structural and community-level barriers to accepting and implementing effective HIV prevention strategies

29.2 Clinical Trials

29.2.1 HIV Prevention Trials Network

The HPTN is a worldwide collaborative clinical trials network that develops and tests the safety and efficacy of primarily nonvaccine interventions designed to prevent the transmission of HIV. Established in 1999 and re-funded in 2006 by the Division of AIDS (DAIDS) of the NIAID, the HPTN carries out its mission through a strong network of expert scientists and investigators from more than two dozen international sites partnered with a leadership group from U.S.-based institutions (http://www.hptn.org/index.htm).

The HPTN comprises a global network of investigators from Clinical Trials Units (CTUs), a Leadership Group consisting of recognized experts in HIV prevention, leadership partners from the network Coordinating and Operations Center (CORE), Network Lab, and Statistical and Data Management Center (SDMC), and various working groups and committees charged with the scientific management and operational support of the network (http://www.hptn.org/hptn_structure.htm).

The HPTN international activities include distributing among sites in developing countries a one-time allocation of funds to support infrastructure, including laboratory, data management, and communications equipment; refurbishing laboratory and clinical space; and providing additional vehicles to support study operations. *International sites:* Brazil, China, India, Malawi, Peru, The Russian Federation, South Africa, Tanzania, Thailand, Uganda, Zambia, and Zimbabwe (http://www.niaid.nih.gov/reposit/hptn.htm).

HPTN-supported areas of research include: antiretroviral therapy, behavioral studies, microbicides, perinatal studies, STIs, and substance abuse (http://www.hptn.org/research_studies/hptn_research_areas.asp).

The strengths of the HPTN include (i) leadership by experts in the prevention sciences; (ii) coordinated domestic-international research agenda; (iii) multidisciplinary study teams of behavioral, clinical, epidemiologic, laboratory, operations, and statistical researchers; (iv) capability to conduct cross-cultural comparisons among different host and viral populations; (v) emphasis on community involvement in all aspects of the research process, from trial development through implementation; and (vi) emphasis on ethical guidelines in research.

Through the HPTN and in close collaboration with the National Institute on Drug Abuse (NIDA) where most of the expertise in this type of research resides, NIAID is supporting a number of research studies to develop strategies to reduce the risk of HIV and other STIs for injecting and non-injecting drug users (see also Section 30.3.1 in Chapter 30).

29.2.1.1 HPTN Trials

- *HPTN 027*: A Phase I study to evaluate the safety and immunogenicity of ALVAC-HIV vCP1521 in infants born to HIV-1–infected women in Uganda (http://www.hptn.org/research_studies/hptn027.asp).
- *HPTN 035*: A Phase II/IIb safety and effectiveness study of the vaginal microbicides BufferGel and 0.5% PRO2000/5 Gel (P) for the prevention of HIV infection in women. *Sites*: Malawi, Zimbabwe, South Africa, Zambia, and the United States. *Note*: The HPTN 035 is no longer a HPTN trial; it is currently included in the Microbicide Trials Network (MTN) (see Section 29.2.2).
- *HPTN 037*: A Phase III randomized controlled study to evaluate the efficacy of an injection drug-user (IDU) network-oriented peer education intervention for the prevention of HIV transmission among IDUs and their network members. *Sites*: Chiang Mai, Thailand, and Philadelphia, U.S.A.
- *HTPN 039*: A Phase III randomized, double-blind, placebo-controlled trial of acyclovir for the reduction of HIV acquisition among high risk HSV-2 seropositive, HIV-seronegative individuals. *Sites*: Peru, South Africa, Zambia, Zimbabwe, and the United States.
- *HTPN 040*: A randomized comparative trial of three antiretroviral regimens for postexposure prophylaxis of HIV-uninfected infants born to HIV-infected women whose HIV status was unknown at the time of delivery and who, therefore, were not exposed to a prenatal or perinatal antiretroviral regimen. *Site*: Brazil.
- *HPTN 043*: A randomized trial of community-based versus clinic-based approaches to voluntary counseling and testing that is being conducted with primary support through an investigator-initiated grant from the NIH's National Institute of Mental Health. *Sites*: 14 communities each in Africa and Thailand.
- *HPTN 046*: Randomized Phase III trial of the efficacy of nevirapine administered to infants during the first 6 months of life to prevent HIV infection through exposure to breast milk of HIV-infected mothers

(http://www.hptn.org/research_studies/HPTN046.asp). *Sites*: South Africa, Tanzania, Uganda, and Zimbabwe.
- *HPTN 052*: A randomized trial to evaluate the effectiveness of antiretroviral therapy plus HIV primary care versus HIV primary care alone to prevent the sexual transmission of HIV-1 in serodiscordant couples. *Sites*: Brazil, India, Malawi, Thailand, Zimbabwe, and the United States.
- *HPTN 057*: A Phase I open-label trial to evaluate the safety and pharmacokinetics of Tenofovir disoproxil fumarate in HIV-1–infected pregnant women and their infants (http://www.hptn.org/research_studies/hptn057.asp).
- *HPTN 058*: A Phase III randomized controlled trial to evaluate the efficacy of buprenorphine/naloxone drug treatment in prevention of HIV infection among opiate-dependent injectors. *Sites*: China and Thailand.
- *HPTN 059*: A Phase II expanded safety and acceptability study of the vaginal microbicide 1% tenofovir gel. *Sites*: India and the United States (http://www3.niaid.nih.gov/research/topics/HIV/prevention/research/Microbicides/).

29.2.2 Microbicide Trials Network

Recognizing the development of microbicides as an important priority in HIV/AIDS research, NIAID established the Microbicide Trials Network (MTN) in 2006 as its newest of six NIAID-funded HIV/AIDS clinical trials networks (http://www.mtnstopshiv.org). The MTN brings together international investigators and community and industry partners who are devoted to reducing the sexual transmission of HIV through the development and evaluation of microbicides, working within a unique infrastructure specifically designed to facilitate research necessary to support licensing topical microbicide products for widespread use.

MTN's research portfolio is designed to face the global urgency of the HIV/AIDS pandemic by including studies considered among the most critically important for advancing the field of HIV prevention. Many of these trials are focused on assessing antiretroviral-based microbicides and include studies designed to evaluate microbicides along with other promising HIV prevention approaches, such as oral antiretroviral prophylaxis. In fact, MTN is the first research group planning an HIV prevention trial that will evaluate both an oral and a topical drug (microbicide) in the same study.

Based at the University of Pittsburgh and Magee-Womens Research Institute in Pittsburgh, MTN's core operations are supported by a network laboratory at the University of Pittsburgh, a statistical and data management center housed within the Statistical Center for HIV/AIDS Research

& Prevention (SCHARP) at the Fred Hutchinson Cancer Research Center, and Family Health International, a global organization with expertise in conducting clinical protocols. In addition, MTN comprises 13 clinical trial units with 18 clinical research sites in seven countries. MTN receives its funding from three NIH institutes: NIAID, the National Institute of Mental Health (NIMH), and the National Institute of Child Health and Human Development (NICHD).

MTN's major focus will be to evaluate nonvaccine strategies for preventing HIV. Major goals of these trials include (i) identifying more practical, safe, and effective approaches to stop the spread of HIV infections, especially in the high risk/incidence populations, and evaluating worldwide the suitability and sustainability of those approaches; (ii) evaluating ART to prevent HIV transmission; (iii) treating or preventing STI; (iv) conducting behavioral interventions to reduce HIV risk behaviors and acquisition or transmission; and (v) conducting interventions to reduce acquisition or transmission of HIV in drug users.

29.2.2.1 MTN Trials

Currently, MTN is implementing a broach spectrum of clinical trials (http://www.mtnstopshiv.org/node/85), including:

- *MTN-004*: A Phase I study evaluating the safety, acceptability, and ease of use of the microbicide candidate VivaGel in sexually active, HIV-negative women ages 18 to 24. It is the first and only trial designed to evaluate a candidate microbicide in young sexually active women, a population in whom HIV rates are steadily increasing. The study, which was launched in July 2007, was paused in October 2007, and researchers are now modifying the protocol to enhance the study's ability to capture relevant safety data. The study will enroll 60 women at two sites and take approximately 1 year to complete. Results of the trial will help researchers determine if the product should be considered for further testing in a larger study, and eventually, in a trial to evaluate whether use of the gel can prevent sexual transmission of HIV in young women (http://www.mtnstopshiv.org/node/64). Also included in MTN's research portfolio are two ongoing trials that prior to 2006 were led by NIAID's HIV Prevention Trials Network:
- *HPTN 035*: A multicenter clinical trial that aims to determine whether the candidate microbicides, BufferGel and PRO 2000, can prevent the sexual transmission of HIV in 3,100 sexually active, HIV-negative women. The trial, which was launched in early 2005, involves six sites in Africa and one U.S. site (http://www.mtnstopshiv.org/node/62).

- *HPTN 059*: A Phase II (expanded safety) trial that aims to assess the safety and acceptability of an antiretroviral-based candidate microbicide called Tenofovir gel. It is the first study evaluating daily use of a gel (non–coitally dependent), an approach to HIV prevention that researchers believe may be more acceptable to women than having to apply a gel at the time of sex (http://www.mtnstopshiv.org/node/63).

29.2.3 Behavioral Science Working Group

Behavioral change remains one of the best available methods of primary prevention of HIV infections in adolescents and adults. High-risk behavior is the main focus of the HPTN Behavioral Science Working Group (BSWG) research agenda because sexual transmission and injection drug use account for the preponderance of cumulative and new HIV infections worldwide (http://www.hptn.org/prevention_science/behavioral.asp). Behavioral science plays a role in HIV prevention research not only through continued development and evaluation of behavioral interventions, but also because almost all other HIV prevention strategies have behavioral components, as do comprehensive methods used to assess and evaluate their efficacy. Whereas individual behavioral scientists participating in HPTN working groups and protocol teams continue to address the behavioral aspects of various biomedical interventions under development, the BSWG's principal focus is on the further identification, development, and evaluation of behavioral interventions associated with reducing risks of acquiring HIV high-risk behavior. To this end, the BSWG is working to identify opportunities for high-priority intervention trials of HIV prevention strategies among at-risk, developing country populations on which HPTN has not previously focused, including high-risk groups, adolescents (especially young women and girls), commercial sex workers, and migrant populations. In addition, BSWG has assumed responsibility for overseeing the *HIVNET 015* protocol conducting a randomized clinical trial of the efficacy of a behavioral intervention to prevent men who have sex with men from acquiring HIV.

A clinical trial "Condom Promotion and Counseling" *(HIVNET/HPTN 016A)* was initiated at three HPTN sites in Zimbabwe and Malawi to evaluate the effectiveness of promoting condom use and providing counseling messages on using condoms as means to prevent HIV transmission.

NIAID/DAIDS-Supported Analyses of Data collected in the community-based trial of the mass treatment of sexually transmitted diseases in the Rakai District in Uganda.

References

1. Coutsoudis, A., Pillay, K., Spooner, E., Kuhn, L., and Coovadia, H. M. (1999) Influence of infant-feeding patterns on early mother-to-child transmission of HIV-1 in Durban, South Africa: a prospective cohort study. South African Vitamin A Study Group, *Lancet*, **354**(9177), 471–476.

2. Coutsoudis, A., Pillay, K., Kuhn, L., Spooner, E., Tsai, W. Y., and Coovadia, H. M., and the South African Vitamin A Study Group (2001) Method of feeding and transmission of HIV-1 from mothers to children by 15 months of age: prospective cohort study from Durban, South Africa, *AIDS*, **15**(3), 379–389 [comments: *AIDS*, **15**(10), 1326–1327 (2001); *AIDS*, **15**(10), 1327–1328 (2001)].

Chapter 30

NIAID: Programs in HIV/AIDS Therapeutics

One of the most important contributions that NIAID has made in the area of HIV/AIDS research has been to give its full support to the discovery and development of new therapeutics that are less toxic and have fewer side effects, promote better adherence, and are readily accessible, particularly in resource-limited settings (http://www3.niaid.nih. gov/research/topics/HIV/therapeutics/intro/default.htm).

Specifically, with the support of NIAID, therapeutic agents have been developed to treat the diseases caused by HIV and its co-infections and to prevent maternal-child transmission of HIV. Therapeutic agents can be small molecules, such as nucleosides, or large biopharmaceutical agents, such as antibodies or therapeutic vaccines. The U.S. Food and Drug Administration (FDA) maintains a current listing of HIV/AIDS therapeutics (http://www.fda. gov/oashi/aids/status.html) that have been approved by that agency.

NIAID's research agenda for developing HIV/AIDS therapeutics is guided by the NIH Office of AIDS Research (OAR), the entity responsible for the overall scientific, budgetary, legislative, and policy elements of all AIDS research sponsored by NIH. NIAID has long played a central role in pursuing the following research goals:

- *Drug Discovery*—to identify and validate new targets critical to the replication of HIV and its co-infections, and to evaluate new therapeutic agents and strategies for potential activity in cell culture and in animal efficacy models.
- *Preclinical Drug Development*—to conduct translational activities (bulk drug synthesis, analytical chemistry, formulation development, animal pharmacology and toxicology) to convert promising lead compounds into pharmaceutical agents suitable for clinical evaluation.
- *Clinical Research*—(i) to conduct clinical research on new therapies and treatment regimens for treating HIV and its co-infections; (ii) to evaluate approaches to prevent the transmission of HIV, improve and sustain an HIV-individual's immune function, overcome drug resistance, and eradicate HIV from latent tissue reservoirs; and

(iii) to investigate the metabolic changes and complications associated with the use of highly active antiretroviral therapy.

30.1 Drug Discovery

30.1.1 HIV Targets

The identification of viral and cellular drug targets relevant to the human immunodeficiency virus is essential for fueling the drug development pipeline (http://www3.niaid.nih.gov/research/topics/HIV/therapeutics/intro/drug_discovery.htm).

Early drug discovery efforts concentrated on a relatively small number of viral targets: HIV reverse transcriptase (an enzyme that catalyzes the synthesis of viral DNA within infected cells from the RNA template carried by infectious virions) and HIV protease (an enzyme that cleaves and processes viral precursor proteins that allow the virion to mature). Treatment regimens containing combinations of reverse transcriptase and protease inhibitors, commonly known as *highly active antiretroviral therapy* (HAART), revolutionized the treatment of people with HIV by markedly lowering viral load and decreasing the incidence of AIDS-associated opportunistic infections. Many patients receiving HAART nevertheless suffer metabolic abnormalities and drug toxicities, have difficulty adhering to the complex drug regimens, and develop strains of HIV resistant to therapy.

Additional viral and cellular targets are now being extensively studied, and therapies targeting HIV integrase, various steps of the virus entry process, and virion maturation have been examined in clinical trials (e.g., Phase II/III) in recent years. Still in the early stages of preclinical investigation are potential inhibitors of Vif/APOBEC; ESCRT I, II, and III (virus assembly); and TRIM5α (virus uncoating) (http://www3.niaid.nih.gov/topics/HIVAIDS/Research/BasicScience/targinter.htm).

30.1.2 Co-infections

HIV-infected individuals without access to effective treatment regimens to combat their HIV infection commonly manifest diseases caused by co-infection with infectious agents, such as *Mycobacterium avium*, *Pneumocystis jirovecii*, *Cryptosporidium parvum*, cryptococci, fungi, and human cytomegalovirus, as well as other HIV/AIDS-associated conditions, such as neuropathy, wasting, and various malignancies.

Diseases caused by opportunistic pathogens are less common nowadays in AIDS patients receiving HAART; however, the incidence of co-infection with hepatitis C virus (HCV) or tuberculosis (TB) has increased, especially in countries where the risk of co-infection is high.

As a result of prolonged survival, greater numbers of HIV-infected individuals are exhibiting the long-term complications of HCV infection, namely end-stage liver disease and hepatocellular carcinoma. Infection by HCV in some instances has been shown to interfere with HAART regimens. TB can accelerate the progress of AIDS and is currently the leading cause of death in persons who are HIV-positive.

30.2 Preclinical Drug Development

Any new therapeutic agent with demonstrated activity in cell culture and in animal efficacy models requires many additional studies to convert it from a promising lead into a pharmaceutical agent suitable for evaluation in clinical trials (http://www3.niaid.nih.gov/research/topics/HIV/therapeutics/intro/preclinical_drug_dev.htm). These product development (or "translational") activities are designed to generate the necessary pharmaceutical-grade materials and preclinical data needed to support the submission of an *Investigational New Drug (IND) application* to the FDA. The types of preclinical studies required include scale-up synthesis of the therapeutic agent, development of analytical assays to detect and quantitate the therapeutic agent and its metabolites, development and manufacture of dosage formulations, and animal pharmacology and toxicology. Many of these studies require compliance with current FDA regulations regarding Good Manufacturing Practices and Good Laboratory Practices.

30.3 Clinical Research

Once a new therapeutic agent or strategy has been thoroughly studied in preclinical studies, the information generated typically is submitted to the FDA as part of an IND application. Evaluation of the therapeutic agent or strategy in human subjects can commence once FDA has approved the IND application.

Clinical trials commonly are designed to investigate the safety and effectiveness of new therapeutic agents for treating HIV and its co-infections. Studies also are conducted to evaluate strategies for the best use of these therapeutic agents in combination with other agents, including ways of minimizing drug-related complications. With the advent of HAART, the complications associated with HIV infection have expanded to include changes in metabolism and morphologic complications caused both by HIV disease and the use of antiretroviral agents. These metabolic changes include altered body fat distribution or lipodystrophy, insulin resistance, elevated triglyceride and cholesterol levels, bone demineralization, and elevated lactate levels. The underlying pathogenic mechanisms of these changes and association with immune activation are unknown or poorly understood, and the long-term consequences, including increased risk of cardiovascular disease, are under investigation (http://www3.niaid.nih.gov/research/topics/HIV/therapeutics/intro/clin_research.htm).

30.3.1 Clinical Trial Units and HIV/AIDS Networks

NIAID is currently supporting the world's largest HIV/AIDS clinical research effort. In a newly restructured system of six HIV/AIDS clinical research networks, NIAID has selected 60 U.S. and international institutions as *HIV/AIDS Clinical Trials Units (CTUs)*—the total number of CTUs is expected to reach 73 (http://www3.niaid.nih.gov/news/newsreleases/2007/ctu07.htm). These Clinical Trials Units are intended to carry out the next generation of HIV/AIDS research on vaccines, prevention, and treatment, and to work with the NIAID clinical research networks in a flexible, collaborative, and coordinated way to tackle the critical research questions that can help accelerate progress against the HIV/AIDS pandemic.

The CTU initiative represents the second step of a two-part restructuring process of NIAID's HIV/AIDS clinical trials networks. NIAID announced the clinical investigators and institutions responsible for leading the new networks in June 2006 (http://www3.niaid.nih.gov/news/newsreleases/2006/leadership.htm). Each CTU is a member of one or more of the six NIAID HIV/AIDS networks: the AIDS Clinical Trials Group, the HIV Prevention Trials Network, the HIV Vaccine Trials Network, the International Maternal Pediatric Adolescent AIDS Clinical Trials

Network, the International Network for Strategic Initiatives in Global HIV Trials, and the Microbicide Trials Network.

- *AIDS Clinical Trials Group (ACTG).* Its major research will focus on optimizing the clinical management of HIV/AIDS, including co-infections and other HIV-related conditions, as well as conducting translational research for new drug development. Major objectives of translational drug research include (i) evaluating antiretroviral therapy (ART) using novel mechanisms of action or aimed at new drug targets; (ii) designing and synthesizing new classes of antiretroviral drugs with unique and/or improved features; (iii) evaluating evolving therapies for HIV/AIDS patients with co-infections; (iv) testing new hypotheses generated by pathogenesis studies; (v) integrating immune-based therapies in treatment regimens, including antiviral effect and immune reconstitution; and (vi) conducting pharmacokinetic studies in children and adolescents to enable licensure of the drugs and to optimize their use. *Site*: University of California at San Diego.
- *HIV Prevention Trials Network (HPTN)* (see Section 29.2.1 in Chapter 29).
- *Microbicide Trials Network (MTN)* (see Section 29.2.2 in Chapter 29).
- *HIV Vaccine Trials Network (HVTN).* The research focus of HVTN will be on evaluating preventive HIV vaccines. The objectives of the HVTN are to (i) identify a safe and effective worldwide vaccine (e.g., all clades, exposures, HLA, etc.); (ii) determine correlate(s) of protection; (iii) develop cohorts to conduct all phases of clinical trials; (iv) develop new assays to measure the full breadth of the induced response; (v) standardize and optimize the trial designs; and (vi) make specimens available to others. *Site*: The Fred Hutchinson Cancer Research Center.
- *International Maternal Pediatric Adolescent AIDS Clinical Trials (IMPAACT).* The trials will focus on children, adolescents, and pregnant women. Major goals include preventing mother-to-child transmission of HIV and optimizing clinical management of HIV/AIDS, co-infections, and other HIV-related conditions. In the context of mother-to-child transmission (MTCT), IMPAACT will aim at (i) identifying safe, practical, and effective approaches to further reduce MTCT; (ii) interrupting transmission through breast-feeding; (iii) achieving safety and efficacy of vaccines to prevent MTCT and transmission through breast-feeding; (iv) evaluating the safety and pharmacokinetics of new drugs or drug combinations in pregnancy and newborn infants; (v) achieving safety and efficacy in passive immunization; and (vi) conducting long-term follow-up of newborn infants. *Site*: Johns Hopkins University School of Medicine.
- *International Network for Strategic Initiatives in Global HIV Trials (INSIGHT).* The trials will be aimed at optimizing the clinical management of HIV/AIDS, including co-infections and other HIV-related conditions. Major goals of INSIGHT include (i) improving the understanding of and optimizing therapies including concurrent evaluation of ART and other therapeutic modalities to manage comorbidities and co-infections, and/or progressive HIV infection; (ii) optimizing therapies for safety, adherence, resistance, durability of response, and prevention of transmission; and (iii) improving ways to use available agents through comparison of dosing regimens, timing of ART—with or without TB therapy, and the impact of traditional medicines on the response to therapy. *Site*: University of Minnesota.

The HIV/AIDS networks and their CTUs will pursue an integrated research approach to conducting clinical trials designed to address the highest priorities in HIV/AIDS research, including:

- Developing a safe and effective HIV vaccine
- Conducting research for new drug development designed to translate laboratory findings into clinical applications
- Optimizing clinical management of HIV/AIDS, including co-infections and other HIV-related conditions
- Developing microbicides to prevent HIV acquisition and transmission
- Creating strategies to prevent mother-to-child HIV transmission
- Developing new methods of preventing HIV

Distinct parts of each unit will be led by a principal investigator and will include an administrative component, community advisory board, and one or more clinical research sites—such as medical schools, academic health centers, hospitals or outpatient clinics—where studies will be conducted (http://www3.niaid.nih.gov/about/organization/daids/Networks/daidsnetworkunits.htm).

The U.S.-based CTUs will be located in the following states and territories: Alabama, California, Colorado, Florida, Georgia, Illinois, Maryland, Massachusetts, Missouri, New Jersey, New York, North Carolina, Ohio, Pennsylvania, Tennessee, Texas, Washington, and Puerto Rico. Additional CTUs are expected in Louisiana and Washington, DC. The CTUs located outside of the United States are in the following countries: the Dominican Republic, Haiti, Jamaica, Peru, South Africa, and Switzerland. Additional CTUs are anticipated in Brazil, China, France, India, and Thailand.

The 145 clinical research sites where clinical trials will be performed may be located in different states or countries from the CTUs to which they are affiliated. In addition to the CTU locations noted above, clinical research sites are also anticipated in Michigan, Oklahoma, Rhode Island, and

Virginia, and internationally in Botswana, Malawi, Panama, Tanzania, Uganda, Vietnam, Zambia, and Zimbabwe.

The selection process for the CTUs has involved a rigorous and extensive scientific review of the proposed clinical programs and capabilities of the CTUs, including access to populations most affected or threatened by the HIV/AIDS epidemic, particularly women, children, adolescents, and people of diverse ethnic or racial backgrounds.

Total funding for the clinical trials networks and the CTUs and their affiliated clinical research sites is expected to reach US$285 million during the first year, which will also include funding for previously existing CTUs and clinical research sites to continue their participation in ongoing studies for a period of time to ensure that there are no gaps in current HIV/AIDS research studies.

The NIAID HIV/AIDS clinical trials networks are also cofunded and supported by a number of other NIH Institutes and Centers that conduct collaborative research studies with the networks. Additional information about the HIV/AIDS clinical trials units can be accessed at http://www3.niaid.nih.gov/news/QA/CTU07QA.htm.

30.4   Resources for Researchers

NIAID has made available the following resources to researchers (http://www3.niaid.nih.gov/research/topics/HIV/therapeutics/resources/):

- AIDS*info* has information on HIV/AIDS-related health topics, treatment and prevention guidelines, information on drugs and vaccines, and a database of all federally funded HIV/AIDS clinical trials (http://www.aidsinfo.nih.gov/).
- *NIH AIDS Research and Reference Reagent Program* provides state-of-the-art biological and chemical materials for the study of HIV and related opportunistic pathogens to registered users worldwide at no cost. Through its Tetramer Facility, the Reagent Program also provides custom synthesis and distribution of soluble MHC I/peptide tetramer reagents that can be used to stain detect antigen specific CD8$^+$ T-cells (http://www.aidsreagent.org/).
- *Human HIV Specimens* (e.g., blood, cells, tissues) from U.S.-based and international studies are available for distribution to researchers through two resources: (i) provides state-of-the-art storage and computerized inventory management of specimens from domestic and international NIAID-funded HIV/AIDS studies; and (ii) collects, distributes, and maintains a repository of tissues from HIV-positive donors for distribution to qualified biomedical research scientists (http://www3.niaid.nih.gov/research/resources/reposit/additionalresources.htm).

- *HIV Specimen Repository Guidelines* include procedures for investigators seeking to collaborate with NIAID-funded clinical research programs, particularly with regard to gaining access to materials maintained in specimen repositories or databases (http://www3.niaid.nih.gov/research/resources/reposit/).
- *Tuberculosis Antimicrobial Acquisition and Coordinating facilities (TAACF)* is a no-cost, multicomponent program that provides *in vitro* and *in vivo* preclinical drug screening and efficacy testing services in order to accelerate new TB drug development (http://www.taacf.org/).
- *HIV/OI/TB Therapeutics Database* includes compounds and testing data for potential inhibitors of HIV, associated opportunistic infections (OIs), and selected viruses of medical importance (http://chemdb2.niaid.nih.gov/struct_search/default.asp).
- *Resource Guide for the Development of AIDS Therapies* contains information about NIAID-funded contracts performing drug development tasks for investigators developing therapies for HIV and its co-infections and microbicide-based prevention strategies (http://www.niaid.nih.gov/daids/PDATguide/overview.htm).
- *BBI Biotech Research, Inc.*, is one of three principal branches of Boston Biomedica, Inc. (BBI), a small business that supports the research needs of the government and industry. Through the NIAID Division of AIDS (DAIDS) specimen repository contract, BBI Biotech provides state-of-the-art storage and computerized inventory management of specimens from domestic and international HIV epidemiology studies, HIV therapeutic and vaccine trials, and other prevention research studies through its central repositories (http://www3.niaid.nih.gov/research/resources/reposit/additionalresources.htm).
- *The National Disease Research Interchange (NDRI)* is a nonprofit organization receiving core support through the *National Center for Research Resources* at the NIH and targeted funding for HIV tissues through DAIDS. The NDRI collects, distributes, and maintains a repository of a wide range of tissues from HIV-positive donors for distribution to qualified biomedical research scientists. Researchers may register for tissues and see the catalog of services at their Web site (http://www3.niaid.nih.gov/research/resources/reposit/additionalresources.htm).

30.5   NIAID Funding Initiatives

Selected targeted programs include:

- *Novel HIV Therapies: Integrated Preclinical/Clinical Program (IPCP).* The IPCP is a program that provides a continuous spectrum of research opportunities (http://

www3.niaid.nih.gov/research/topics/HIV/therapeutics/ funding/). IPCP supports research by collaborative groups seeking to transition from preclinical to clinical studies during the award period, as well as pilot clinical studies of novel treatments. This program is designed to promote creative and original therapeutic research on diverse facets of HIV infection between multidisciplinary preclinical and clinical research groups from academic or nonprofit institutions and research firms. Recent topics of research include:

- ○ "HIV therapy with CCR5 monoclonal antibody PRO 140" (Progenics, Inc.)
- ○ "Lentivirus-based immunogene therapy for HIV infection" (University of Pennsylvania)
- ○ "Lentivirus-based immunotherapy for AIDS" (City of Hope National Medical Center, Duarte, CA)
- ○ "Blocking HIV with aptamers targeted to viral components" (Albert Einstein College of Medicine)

- *Small Business Innovative Research (SBIR).* The SBIR research program provides incentive for biotechnology industry studies of targeted therapies and drug delivery systems (http://www3.niaid.nih.gov/research/topics/ HIV/therapeutics/funding/), such as:

- ○ "HIV-1 envelope phenotype/genotype database resources" (ViroLogic, Inc.)
- ○ "Novel viral load diagnostic for resource-limited settings" (BioScale, Inc.)
- ○ "Mitochondrial dysfunction in HAART: point of care tests" (MitoScience, LLC)
- ○ "High purity Amphotericin B: a safer antimycotic in AIDS" (Cumberland Pharmaceutical, Inc., and the University of Mississippi Mycotic Research Center)
- ○ "Drug susceptibility assay for non-subtype B HIV-1" (ViroLogic, Inc.)
- ○ "Capsid assembly inhibitors for the treatment of AIDS" (Achillion Pharmaceuticals, Inc.)
- ○ "Optimization of HIV-1 entry inhibitors targeting gp41" (Locus Pharmaceuticals, Inc.)

30.6 Clinical Trials

NIAID-funded clinical research pursues clinical research on HIV/AIDS therapeutics through its Division of Intramural Research, individual investigator-initiated grants, and clinical trial networks administered by DAIDS (http://www3. niaid.nih.gov/research/topics/HIV/therapeutics/clinical/).

- *NIAID Division of Intramural Research (DIR).* DIR conducts all of NIAID's in-house research involving basic and clinical research in immunologic, allergic, and

infectious diseases. Patients are frequently admitted into the clinical service to participate in new and promising treatments or diagnostic procedures derived from basic research that was conducted in DIR laboratories.

- *AIDS Clinical Trials Group (ACTG).* The ACTG represents a network of academic research institutions performing all phases of clinical trials to investigate therapeutic interventions to manage HIV infection and its complications, including co-infections and disorders of advancing disease and its therapy (http://www.aactg.org/).
- *International Maternal Pediatric Adolescent AIDS Clinical Trials Group (IMPAACT).* IMPAACT is a network of academic research institutions performing all phases of clinical trials to evaluate clinical interventions for treating HIV infection and HIV-associated illnesses in neonates, infants, children, adolescents, and pregnant women and new approaches to prevent mother-to-infant transmission (http://pactg.s-3.com/).
- *International Network for Strategic Initiatives in Global HIV Trials (INSIGHT).* INSIGHT is an HIV/AIDS clinical trials network composed of international investigators that strive to develop strategies for the optimization of treatment (antiretroviral and immunomodulatory therapies as well as interventions to prevent and treat complications of HIV and antiretroviral therapies) to prolong disease-free survival in a demographically, geographically, and socioeconomically diverse population of individuals infected with HIV (http://insight. ccbr.umn.edu/index.php).

30.6.1 Other NIH-Funded Clinical Trials Networks

Other networks working in collaboration with DAIDS on clinical research pertaining to adolescents and co-infections and complications of HIV, respectively, include:

- *SIDS Malignancy Consortium (AMC)* conducts clinical trials of therapies for AIDS malignancies, including non–Hodgkin's lymphoma, primary central nervous system lymphoma, Kaposi's sarcoma, and cervical cancer (http://www.amc.uab.edu/).
- *Adolescent Trials Network (ATN)* is the only national study of HIV/AIDS in adolescents infected through sex or drug injection. Funded by the National Institute of Child Health and Human Development (NICHD), ATN research will be able to inform the nation's adolescent-specific HIV/AIDS scientific agenda to improve the prevention of HIV infection and the medical treatment of HIV-positive adolescents (https://www.atnonline.org/default.htm).

- *Bacteriology and Mycology Study Group (BAMSG)* directs trials for antimicrobial therapies of systemic fungal infections (http://www.rhofed.com/bambu-bamsg/bambu-bamsg.html).
- *Collaborative Antiviral Study Group (CASG)* conducts studies to evaluate experimental therapies for severe herpes, congenital CMV, human papillomavirus, respiratory viruses, enteroviruses, and hepatitis viruses (http://www.casg.uab.edu/).
- *Neurology AIDS Research Consortium (NARC)* conducts studies on HIV-associated neurologic complications (http://www.neuro.wustl.edu/narc/).
- *Studies of Ocular Complications of AIDS (SOCA)* conducts clinical trials and epidemiologic research on ocular complications of AIDS, primarily CMV retinitis (http://www.jhucct.com/soca/).

30.6.2 *Clinical Trials Guidelines*

The U.S. Department of Health and Human Services (DHHS) provides information on HIV/AIDS treatment, prevention, and research (*AIDSinfo*) at a comprehensive Web site with a database of all federally funded and privately sponsored HIV/AIDS clinical trials. It also provides information on treatment and prevention guidelines for HIV/AIDS and on therapeutic and preventive drugs and vaccines; other HIV/AIDS-related health topics can also be found on the Web site (http://www.aidsinfo.nih.gov). These guidelines are updated periodically by panels of HIV experts and can be accessed at http://www.aidsinfo.nih.gov/Guidelines/Default.aspx?MenuItem=Guidelines.

Chapter 31

NIAID: Programs in HIV Vaccines

According to the latest United Nations estimates, more than 40 million people worldwide are infected with HIV, and the global prevalence of this virus will continue to rise. Historically, vaccines have proved to be the most effective weapon in the fight against infectious diseases, such as smallpox, polio, measles, and yellow fever. Thus, HIV vaccines will provide one of the best hopes to end the HIV pandemic (see also Chapter 32).

To control the alarming spread of HIV, a burning need exists for developing of an effective vaccine that would prevent individuals from becoming infected (http://www3.niaid. nih.gov/research/topics/HIV/vaccines/). Characteristics of a desirable HIV vaccine to control the global spread of AIDS include (i) simple to administer; (ii) inexpensive to produce; (iii) inducing long-lasting immunity; and (iv) effective against all HIV subtypes.

Whereas developing an HIV/AIDS vaccine remains one of NIAID's highest priorities, it still presents a formidable scientific challenge to researchers. NIAID is supporting HIV vaccine development through fundamental basic research (the discovery phase), preclinical screening and animal model development, product development and manufacturing, and clinical research.

HIV vaccine research has progressed from an early focus on HIV surface antigens, particularly the envelope and the role of neutralizing antibodies, to increased attention to cytotoxic T-lymphocytes (CTLs) in HIV immunity. Many novel approaches to elicit anti-HIV neutralizing antibodies and CTLs are now under investigation (http://www3.niaid.nih. gov/research/topics/HIV/vaccines/research/designs/default. htm).

Major goals of the NIAID-funded HIV vaccine research (http://www3.niaid.nih.gov/research/topics/HIV/vaccines/ intro/default.htm#) include:

- *Preclinical Research and Development*

  ○ Identify and develop promising vaccine candidates in animal models that induce (i) broadly neutralizing antibody; (ii) consistent and high level of cytotoxic T lymphocytes; and (iii) strong mucosal immune responses
  ○ Evaluate the candidates for immunogenicity, safety, and efficacy in animal models
  ○ Produce products with the most promise, including those that may not have adequate industry support under good manufacturing conditions, and move these products through the Investigational New Drug (IND) approval process
  ○ Develop and test new adjuvants and cytokines that will increase the magnitude and duration of the immune response when formulated with or given in conjunction with candidate HIV vaccines

- *Vaccine Clinical Research*

  ○ Identify a safe and effective HIV vaccine through clinical trials by (i) harmonizing protocols to allow products, dose, and route of administration to be compared; (ii) ensuring safety of volunteers during trials; and (iii) ensuring compliance with the requirements of regulatory agencies
  ○ Advance knowledge of protective immunity by developing and improving laboratory assays of vaccine-induced human immune responses
  ○ Collaborate with governmental and nongovernmental agencies that conduct HIV vaccine research to expedite the identification of an effective HIV vaccine

31.1 Research Activities

NIAID currently supports preclinical and clinical vaccine research in a variety of areas (http://www3.niaid.nih.gov/ research/topics/HIV/vaccines/research/):

- *NIAID Division of Intramural Research Laboratories.* A number of NIAID intramural laboratories conduct basic biomedical research on HIV/AIDS and the immune system.

- *The Dale and Betty Bumpers Vaccine Research Center (VRC)*. Laboratories at the VRC that conduct biomedical research to facilitate the development of HIV vaccines.
- *Vaccine Designs and Concepts*. Preclinical and clinical vaccine research is supported in a variety of areas. A list and description of vaccine designs currently being investigated by NIAID-supported researchers can be accessed at http://www3.niaid.nih.gov/research/topics/HIV/vaccines/research/designs/default.htm.
- *Vaccine Preclinical Toxicology Testing*. This program provides information to HIV vaccine researchers on preclinical toxicology testing and preclinical product development to aid in translating research concepts into vaccine candidates suitable for human clinical trial testing (http://www3.niaid.nih.gov/daids/vaccine/Science/VRTT/00_Main.htm).
- *Animal Models*. No ideal animal model exists that can imitate the natural history and pathogenesis of HIV infection and AIDS in the human body because the HIV virus exclusively infects and causes disease in humans. Nonetheless, the data from animal models provide better understanding of the immune responses elicited by investigational vaccines, as well as reassurance of safety, guiding preclinical development and decisions to enter into clinical trials with humans.

Non-human primate studies play a leading role in efforts to develop an HIV vaccine. Scientists are using macaque monkeys infected with simian immunodeficiency virus (SIV), a virus closely related to HIV. This model is useful because SIV in macaques follows, albeit slowly, a similar disease course to HIV, and adequate numbers of animals are available. A potential shortcoming is that SIV and HIV, although similar, are different viruses, so that advances made with SIV need to be verified using HIV. Macaques are being used to evaluate a variety of SIV vaccines of the same types as the HIV vaccines being developed for humans. Because the monkeys can be challenged with SIV after immunization, the vaccines can be evaluated for their ability to protect from virus infection or disease in the monkeys.

A hybrid virus created by replacing the SIV envelope with the HIV envelope but retaining the inner core of SIV virus (called SHIVs) replicates acute HIV infection in macaques and causes rapid disease progression leading to death. Monkeys vaccinated with HIV vaccines are challenged with chimeric SHIV to test the ability of the vaccine to protect from infection with the SHIV viruses.

Scientists are also using a number of different animal models to obtain information that can be applied to HIV. Feline immunodeficiency virus (FIV), transgenic mice that contain part of the HIV genome or coreceptors for viral entry, and severe combined immune deficiency (SCID) mice

reconstituted with human immune system cells or tissues are some of the animal models being used to study pathogenesis.

Information about different animal models currently used to study HIV/AIDS can be accessed at http://www3.niaid.nih.gov/research/topics/HIV/vaccines/research/animal/default.htm.

- *Vaccine Assessment*. Developing a safe and effective vaccine requires that laboratories analyzing samples from clinical trials follow good clinical laboratory practices (GCLPs). The laboratories use sensitive, accurate, reproducible, and quantitative assays that provide clear measurements of vaccine-induced immune responses to allow data to be compared across multiple sites and the most promising vaccines to be prioritized. To define the correlates of protection, innovative approaches will be required to correlate immune response with vaccine-induced protection.

The central components of vaccine assessment include:

- *Safety Laboratories*. All phases of clinical trials testing and monitoring the safety of a candidate HIV vaccine help to determine how well the volunteers tolerate the vaccine. Routine safety tests include analyses of blood and urine sample that check blood cell counts, hemoglobin levels, kidney and liver functions, as well as screening for infection with syphilis, HIV, and hepatitis B and C viruses. These tests are performed by laboratories that meet Clinical Laboratory Improvements Amendments (CLIA) standards of certification and accreditation by the College of American Pathologists (CAP), standards that are normative for all clinical laboratories in the United States. Similarly, international laboratories performing assays for HIV vaccine trials that meet local accreditation are enrolled in CAP and in external quality assurance programs to ensure performance standards.
- *PBMC Processing Laboratories*. To ensure the highest possible specimen quality among different clinical settings, optimal methods are required to collect, process, ship, and store blood specimens to ensure appropriate recovery, viability, and function of blood cells. Site-associated laboratories separate and cryopreserve serum and peripheral blood mononuclear cells (PBMCs) from blood within 6 to 8 hours after collection by venipuncture. Appropriate sample volumes are optimally handled to perform immunologic evaluations that indicate immune resistance to HIV infection.
- *End-Point Laboratories*. The immunologic objective of HIV vaccines is to elicit effective humoral, cellular, and mucosal immune responses. To assess the effectiveness of the new generation of vaccines, scientists have expended considerable effort into developing and standardizing reliable assays that analyze and quantify

vaccine-induced immune responses. Specimens from vaccine clinical trials—PBMCs and serum or plasma—are currently evaluated using four optimized and validated assays of immune response to the vaccine. The assays are performed at designated "end-point" laboratories under internationally accepted GCLP guidelines. The end-point laboratories also follow approved quality assurance (QA) and quality control (QC) protocols and have standard operating procedures (SOPs) for the assays. These laboratories participate in external proficiency testing administered by CAP and DAIDS and participate in the transition of assays from R&D into validated assays that are standardized and meant to produce comparable results across different laboratories in different settings. The four validated assays include:

(i) *IFN-γ/ELISPOT Assay.* This assay quantifies the number of fluorescent spots of solid phase–captured interferon gamma (IFN-γ) secreted by individual T cells after stimulation with HIV antigens or peptides.

(ii) *Intracellular Cytokine Staining (ICS) Assay.* This assay uses flow cytometry to separate out T cells from other lymphocytes based on selective expression of surface markers and cytokine secretion upon stimulation with HIV antigens or peptides and after cell activation.

(iii) *Virus Neutralization Assay.* This *in vitro* assay measures the neutralizing immunoglobulin concentration (titer) in serum or plasma that blocks HIV infectivity before entry into target cells.

(iv) *ELISA Binding Antibodies.* This assay detects the presence of binding anti-HIV immunoglobulins in patient's blood, serum, or plasma.

- *New Technology/New Assays.* In addition to the validated assays (see above), there is a need to incorporate new technology platforms into clinical trials of candidate HIV vaccines to comprehensively characterize vaccine-induced responses and to define the correlates of immune protection in large-scale efficacy trials. To accommodate these aims, additional assays currently under development include:

(i) Identification of activated memory CD4 lymphocytes by flow cytometry.

(ii) Measuring of proliferative capacity of lymphocytes by flow cytometry.

Information about safety laboratories, PBMC processing laboratories, end-point laboratories, and new technology or new assays can be accessed at http://www3.niaid.nih.gov/research/topics/HIV/vaccines/research/assessment/.

- *Vaccine Clinical Trials.* NIAID is supporting a number of vaccine trials around the world with a variety of organizations, centers, partnerships, and programs (http://www3.niaid.nih.gov/research/topics/HIV/vaccines/research/clinical/):

o *The Dale and Betty Bumpers Vaccine Research Center (VRC).* The VRC at the National Institutes of Health was established to facilitate research in vaccine development. The VRC is dedicated to improving global human health through the rigorous pursuit of effective vaccines for human diseases (http://www.niaid.nih.gov/vrc/).

o *HIV Vaccine Trials Network (HVTN).* Formed in 1999 by NIAID, the HVTN is an international collaboration of scientists and educators searching for an effective and safe HIV vaccine. The HVTN's mission is to facilitate the process of testing preventive vaccines against HIV/AIDS by conducting all phases of clinical trials, from evaluating experimental vaccines for safety and the ability to stimulate immune responses, to testing vaccine efficacy. Led by investigators and powered by collaborators, the HVTN carries out its research through multicenter clinical trials in a global network of domestic and international sites. Protocols are developed by HVTN investigators and include partnerships between vaccine developers, clinical experts, and biostatisticians. The HVTN works closely with NIH staff in initiating, conducting, funding, and coordinating all vaccine development processes (http://www.hvtn.org/).

o *Partnership for AIDS Vaccine Evaluation (PAVE).* PAVE is a voluntary consortium of U.S. Government agencies and U.S. Government–funded organizations involved in HIV vaccine research. Members of PAVE include NIH, the HIV Vaccine Trials Network, the Dale and Betty Bumpers Vaccine Research Center, the U.S. Military HIV Research Program, and the Centers for Disease Control and Prevention (http://www.hivpave.org/).

o *Center for HIV/AIDS Vaccine Immunology (CHAVI).* CHAVI was established by NIAID as part of the *Global HIV/AIDS Vaccine Enterprise.* Its major goal is to elucidate basic science questions and conduct early-phase clinical trials of HIV vaccine candidates at clinical sites around the world (http://www.chavi.org).

o *U.S. Military HIV Research Program (USMHRP).* Established in 1985 to protect troops entering endemic HIV areas, this program brings together scientists from the Army, Navy, and the Air Force. DAIDS jointly plans and executes HIV/AIDS research projects with the USMHRP through an interagency agreement (http://www.hivresearch.org/).

○ *Global HIV Vaccine Enterprise.* This is a virtual consortium of organizations committed to the development of a preventive HIV/AIDS vaccine. It will implement shared scientific plans, mobilize resources, and improve worldwide collaborations (http://www.hivvaccineenterprise.org/about/index.html).

○ *International AIDS Vaccine Initiative (IAVI).* IAVI was founded in 1996 to speed discovery of an HIV vaccine. It partners with private companies, academic institutions, and government agencies, such as NIH, worldwide (http://www.iavi.org/).

• The list of all federally funded vaccine trials can be accessed at http://www.AIDSinfo.gov. It contains information about collaborators, organizations, centers, partnerships, and programs that are currently conducting HIV vaccine research with NIAID.

• *NIAID HIV Vaccine Research Education Initiative (NHVREI).* NHVREI is designed to increase awareness about the urgent need for an HIV vaccine within communities most affected by HIV/AIDS, creates a supportive environment for current and future HIV vaccine trial volunteers, and improves the public's perceptions and attitudes toward HIV vaccine research (http://www.bethegeneration.org/).

31.2 Resources for Researchers

NIAID has made available to researchers the following resources (http://www3.niaid.nih.gov/research/topics/HIV/vaccines/resources/):

31.2.1 Research

• *Guidelines for Requesting Access to Animal Models and Vaccine Reagents.* This resource describes criteria and procedures for submitting requests for resources to be used for vaccine development.

• *Simian Vaccine Evaluation Unit (SVEU).* SVEU provides resources to evaluate promising SIV and HIV vaccines in non-human primates.

• *Vaccine Reagent Resource.* This resource provides reagents, resources, and quality assurance/quality control analysis.

• *NIH AIDS Research and Reference Reagent Program.* The program provides state-of-the-art biological and chemical materials for studying HIV and related opportunistic infections.

• *Human HIV Specimens.* This resource provides storage and computerized inventory management of HIV/AIDS specimens.

• *HIV Specimen Repository Guidelines* for accessing DAIDS specimen repositories.

• *HIV Databases.* Based at the Los Alamos National Laboratory in New Mexico, the HIV Databases contain a comprehensive list of HIV genetic sequences, immunologic epitopes, drug resistance–associated mutations, and vaccine trials. The Web site (http://www.hiv.lanl.gov/content/index) also gives access to a large number of tools that can be used to analyze these data.

• *NIH Tetramer Facility.* A part of the NIH AIDS Research and Reference Reagent Program, the Tetramer Facility provides custom synthesis and distribution of soluble MHC I/peptide tetramer reagents that can be used to stain antigen-specific CD8 T-cells (http://www.niaid.nih.gov/reposit/tetramer/index.html).

• *National Center for Research Resources (NCRR).* The NCRR supports primary research to create and develop critical resources, models, and technologies (http://www.ncrr.nih.gov/).

• *National Primate Research Centers* represent a network of eight highly specialized facilities for non-human primate research.

31.2.2 Development

Critical Path Resources are available to advance candidates into Phase I trials.

• *Preclinical Master Contract.* NIAID has placed a high priority on the development of safe and effective HIV vaccines for worldwide evaluation and use. A Preclinical Master Contract has been awarded to aid the preclinical development of promising vaccine candidates from the research laboratory to the clinic. This contract offers an array of resources to facilitate development of a promising candidate into a testable product. Resources are available to accomplish three basic functions: (i) manufacture Good Manufacturing Practice (GMP) pilot lots of vaccine for testing in humans, or Good Laboratory Practices (GLP)/reagent-grade vaccine for testing in non-human primates; (ii) perform tests for safety, immunogenicity, and other preclinical testing of GMP-produced candidates; and (iii) prepare FDA submissions leading up to human trials.

Specific vaccines to be produced may include concepts proposed by either industry or academic institutions. Investigators wishing to access these services may submit proposals, following the guidelines found in the *DAIDS Guidelines for Requesting Access to Animal Models,*

Vaccine Reagents and Vaccine Development Resources Web site (http://www3.niaid.nih.gov/research/topics/HIV/vaccines/resources/guidelines/).

31.3   NIAID Research Initiatives

- *Phased Innovation Awards (PIA).* The PIA initiative is aimed at funding exploratory projects to bring new concepts into the research and development "pipeline." Innovation grants involve a high degree of risk, innovation, and novelty with some promise for improving vaccine development. Although there is no requirement for preliminary data, a strong scientific rationale is advisable. Awarded projects will first be tested in milestone-driven exploratory/feasibility "proof-of-concept" studies (R21 phase); and then, if eligible, will be reviewed for the expanded development (R33 phase) award without the need to submit an additional grant application. The phased R21/R33 mechanism offers the potentially successful investigator the opportunity to devote full attention to the research project without the burden of writing additional grant proposals for continued support and will permit promising research to continue with no lapse in funding (http://www3.niaid.nih.gov/research/topics/HIV/vaccines/funding/pia.htm).

- *HIV Research and Design.* The HIVRAD program advances concepts farther toward the development of a prophylactic AIDS vaccine. This grant mechanism accepts projects too advanced for the exploratory Innovation Grant Program, but not yet sufficiently advanced for the production-oriented *Integrated Preclinical/Clinical AIDS Vaccine Development (IPCAVD)* Grant Program. Applicants may target any area of AIDS vaccine research including development of animal models, studies of HIV immunogen structure, studies of mechanisms of vaccine action, development of viral and bacterial vectors, studies of immune responses using existing vaccine cohort samples, or studies that evaluate new assays of immunity.

Neither human clinical studies nor vaccine research focused solely on therapeutic applications are supported by this program. Innovation grantees and investigators with vaccine concepts supported by preliminary data are encouraged to apply. Applications from foreign institutions are also encouraged. HIVRAD grants will be limited to 4 years of funding. Applicants should discuss questions regarding the appropriateness of their research for the HIVRAD grant mechanism and/or funding issues with the NIAID/DAIDS Program contact (http://www3.niaid.nih.gov/research/topics/HIV/vaccines/funding/hivrad.htm).

- *Integrated Preclinical/Clinical AIDS Vaccine Development Program (IPCAVD).* The IPCAVD initiative supports the later stages of concept refinement and testing of preventive HIV/AIDS vaccines, culminating in human studies. Proposed studies can include later-stage preclinical research (vaccine optimization studies, immunogenicity/challenge studies, etc.), GLP/GMP vaccine production, GLP preclinical toxicology and safety studies, pre-IND/IND preparation and submission, and clinical testing. This program will use the NIH Multiproject Cooperative Agreement (U19) mechanism. Under the cooperative agreement, the NIH purpose is to support and/or stimulate the recipient's activity by being involved in and otherwise working jointly with the award recipient in a partner role, but not to assume direction, prime responsibility, or a dominant role in the activity. Applicants are strongly encouraged to discuss questions regarding the appropriateness of their research for the IPCAVD grant mechanism and/or funding issues with the NIAID/DAIDS Program contact (http://www3.niaid.nih.gov/research/topics/HIV/vaccines/funding/ipcavd.htm).

- *HIV Vaccine Design and Development Teams (HVDDT).* The HVDDT is designed to fund consortia of scientists with development experience from industry and/or academia who have identified a promising vaccine concept and envisioned a product worthy of targeted development (http://www3.niaid.nih.gov/research/topics/HIV/vaccines/funding/hvddt.htm).

Chapter 32

NIAID: International Involvement in HIV/AIDS Research

The NIAID commitment to advancing HIV/AIDS research in international settings to prevent, treat, and eventually eradicate this disease has been steadily increasing, reflecting the global impact of the HIV/AIDS pandemic as well as the critical need for cost-effective prevention and treatment strategies. NIAID has supported collaborative international research on HIV/AIDS in more than 40 countries. Many of these projects take place in regions of the world with limited resources and where more than 95% of new HIV infections occur. Important objectives of the NIAID-supported international NIH/AIDS research agenda are to:

- Help identify and characterize the different subtypes of HIV circulating in different regions of the world.
- Support studies on the epidemiology, transmission, and natural history of the HIV disease in different populations in international settings.
- Foster the research, development, and evaluation of novel therapies, combination therapies (including preexposure and postexposure prophylaxis), vaccines, and microbicides.
- Identify cost-effective and culturally appropriate methods of preventing and/or treating HIV/AIDS.
- Evaluate interventions against opportunistic infections in children and adults in international settings.
- Prevent HIV transmission by sexual contact, blood, and blood products, mother-to-child transmission, and injection drug use.
- Translate research findings into practice by providing information based on the latest scientific findings, so that policy and programmatic activities can be informed by the science. This is done through meetings, workshops, and conferences with international visitors as well as grantees, potential grantees, and those requesting information. (Meetings are often with government officials, scientists, educators, students, and nongovernmental organizations. Many of these meetings are done in collaboration with State Department programs.)
- Aid in the development of research infrastructure and capacity at international sites, as well as help to establish collaborations with scientists working in the same interest areas to help foster the development of the research capacity of new international sites and the training and development of young new investigators and clinical site staff.
- Foster collaboration with other partners working in HIV/AIDS internationally.

32.1 The Division of AIDS at NIAID

The Division of AIDS (DAIDS) at NIAID was formed in 1986 to develop and implement the national research agenda to address the HIV/AIDS epidemic. The mission of DAIDS is to help ensure an end to the HIV/AIDS epidemic by increasing basic knowledge of the pathogenesis and transmission of the human immunodeficiency virus (HIV), supporting the development of therapies for HIV infection and its complications and co-infections, and supporting the development of vaccines, topical microbicides, and other prevention strategies. Because the breadth of the division's work is expansive and continually evolving, it is important to keep in mind that what is represented here is a snapshot of the work that is being done, which is supported through DAIDS' extramural program. The mission of DAIDS is accomplished through its HIV/AIDS Clinical Trial Networks, its investigator-initiated grant awards, solicited grant awards, contracts, bilateral and interagency agreements, collaborations through public and private partnerships, as well as serving on working groups and technical expertise panels. More information on DAIDS, as well as NIAID, may be found on the division's Web site at http://www3.niaid.nih.gov/about/organization/daids/default.htm.

32.2 Clinical Trials Network Studies

Throughout the past 20 years, DAIDS programs have evolved to address and respond to the changing HIV/AIDS pandemic. Most recently, during the period 2006–2007, the division restructured its HIV/AIDS Clinical Trial Networks, designing them to address one or more of NIAID's six high-priority areas of research, as follows:

1. Vaccine research and development.
2. Translational research/drug development.
3. Optimization of clinical management, including comorbidities.
4. Microbicides.
5. Prevention of mother-to-child transmission of HIV.
6. Prevention of HIV infection.

The six restructured HIV/AIDS clinical trial networks are outlined below, with some examples of studies that are being conducted under them.

32.2.1 AIDS Clinical Trials Group

The AIDS Clinical Trials Group (ACTG) is a multicenter clinical trials network composed of U.S. and international clinical trials units that conduct translational and therapeutic research. The ACTG was first established in 1987 to pursue therapeutic research. The ACTG now conducts research in the United States and internationally; its highest research priorities are translational research and drug development and optimization of clinical management, including co-infection and comorbidities. In collaboration with other clinical trials networks, the ACTG also pursues therapeutic vaccine research and development, the treatment of pregnant women, and the prevention of HIV infection. The ACTG conducts trials that address specific areas of HIV therapeutic research in collaboration with other NIH institutes, including the National Cancer Institute, the National Institute of Dental and Craniofacial Research, and the National Institute of Neurological Disorders and Stroke.

Translational research and drug development efforts in the ACTG are aimed at the evaluation of:

1. Anti-HIV compounds with novel mechanisms of action or new targets, including small-molecule entry inhibitors, uncoating inhibitors, integrase inhibitors, and maturation inhibitors.
2. New classes of drugs with unique and improved features, such as different resistance profiles or better pharmacologic or toxicologic properties.
3. New therapies for individuals with co-infections, focusing on tuberculosis, hepatitis C, and human papillomavirus (HPV). In addition, the network focuses on the integration of immune-based therapies and treatment regimens, emphasizing mechanisms of antiviral effect and immune reconstitution, and the evaluation of new hypotheses generated by pathogenesis studies.

In the optimization research area, the ACTG evaluates:

1. The effectiveness of new combination regimens or new treatment strategies, particularly those that incorporate agents with novel mechanism of action.
2. Therapies and therapeutic strategies for treating co-infections and complications, including prophylaxis, acute and maintenance treatment, and immune-based therapies. In addition, the ACTG strives to optimize therapies on the basis of safety, adherence, resistance, durability of response, and prevention of transmission.

Some examples of ACTG studies being conducted at international sites include:

- *ACTG A5175*. A Phase IV prospective, randomized, open-label evaluation of the efficacy of once-daily protease inhibitor and once-daily non-nucleoside reverse transcriptase inhibitor–containing therapy combinations for initial treatment of HIV-1–infected individuals from resource-limited settings (PEARLS Trial) (Malawi, South Africa, India, Thailand, Brazil, Haiti, and Peru).
- *ACTG 5208*. Optimal combination therapy after nevirapine exposure (OCTANE) (Botswana, South Africa, Uganda, Zambia, Malawi, Kenya, and Zimbabwe).
- *ACTG 5221*. A strategy study of immediate versus deferred initiation of antiretroviral therapy for HIV-infected persons treated for tuberculosis with CD4 <200 cells/mm^3 (Peru, Thailand, South Africa, Brazil, Zambia, Kenya, India, and Malawi).

More information on the ACTG may be found at the following Web site: http://www.aactg.org.

32.2.2 HIV Prevention Trials Network

The HIV Prevention Trials Network (HPTN) is a worldwide collaborative clinical trials network that develops and tests the safety and efficacy of primarily nonvaccine interventions designed to prevent the transmission of HIV. The HPTN was first established in 2000, building on the work of the HIV Network for Prevention Trials (HIVNET).

The HPTN research agenda is focused primarily on the use of antiretroviral therapy; treatment and prevention of sexually transmitted infections; treatment of substance abuse, particularly injection drug use; and behavioral risk reduction interventions to reduce HIV transmission and acquisition.

HPTN studies evaluate new interventions and strategies for preventing HIV in populations and geographic regions that are bearing a disproportionate burden of infection. These studies are intended to facilitate rapid scale-up and to have the greatest possible impact on the pandemic. In addition, the HPTN has refined and expanded its expertise in the development and validation of tools for the early detection of HIV infection. To maximize their quality and benefits, all HPTN studies are conducted in close partnership with the community.

Some examples of HPTN studies include:

- *HPTN 027.* A Phase I study to evaluate the safety and immunogenicity of ALVAC-HIV vCP1521 in infants born to HIV-1–infected women in Uganda (Uganda).
- *HPTN 046.* A Phase III trial to determine the efficacy and safety of an extended regimen of nevirapine in infants born to HIV-infected women to prevent vertical HIV transmission during breast-feeding (South Africa, Uganda, Tanzania, and Zimbabwe).
- *HPTN 052.* A randomized trial to evaluate the effectiveness of antiretroviral therapy plus HIV primary care versus HIV primary care alone to prevent the sexual transmission of HIV-1 in serodiscordant couples (Thailand, Malawi, Brazil, India, Zimbabwe, and South Africa).
- *HPTN 058.* A Phase III randomized, controlled trial to evaluate the efficacy of drug treatment in prevention of HIV infection among opiate-dependent injectors (Thailand and China).

More information on the HPTN may be found at http://www.hptn.org.

32.2.3   HIV Vaccine Trials Network

The HIV Vaccine Trials Network (HVTN) is an international collaboration of scientists searching for an effective and safe HIV vaccine. The HVTN's mission is to facilitate the process of testing preventive vaccines against HIV/AIDS, conducting all phases of clinical trials, from evaluating experimental vaccines for safety and the ability to stimulate immune responses, to testing vaccine efficacy. The HVTN's priorities include:

1. Performing clinical trials in populations throughout the world to determine if a vaccine candidate or vaccine regimen "qualifies" for further efficacy evaluation.
2. Designing and conducting a program of HIV vaccine efficacy trials that rigorously test critical scientific concepts for the development of HIV vaccines and ultimately characterize the safety and efficacy of a candidate vaccine sufficiently to enable it to be licensed.
3. Developing and maintaining a clinical trials network that will provide an objective and transparent platform to evaluate the safety, immunogenicity, and efficacy of candidate HIV vaccines.
4. Advancing the laboratory and statistical approaches in clinical trial design that will define potential correlates of protection within HIV vaccine efficacy trials.

5. Developing standardized methods of risk reduction counseling that are applicable across all HVTN sites.

The HVTN, like all of the clinical trials networks, includes community members in governing and conducting clinical trials. Involvement is promoted through community representation on HVTN scientific and operational committees and through consultations with trial volunteers and community leaders at conferences and other gatherings of stakeholders in HIV prevention, treatment, and care. In addition, HVTN strives to develop and support collaborations with other relevant NIH networks, federal agencies, and nongovernmental research organizations to advance the highest quality HIV vaccine research, with optimal efficiency and cost-effectiveness.

Some examples of HVTN studies include:

- *HVTN 049.* A Phase I clinical trial to evaluate the safety and immunogenicity of a clade B gag DNA/PLG and env DNA/PLG microparticle prime with a clade B recombinant, oligomeric HIV gp140/MS59 adjuvant boost in healthy, HIV-1–uninfected adult participants (U.S. sites).
- *HVTN 065.* A Phase I clinical trial to evaluate the safety and immunogenicity of pGA2/JS7 DNA vaccine and recombinant modified vaccinia Ankara/HIV62 vaccine in healthy HIV-1–uninfected adult participants (U.S. sites).
- *HVTN 067.* A Phase I clinical trial to evaluate the safety and immunogenicity of DNA vaccine EP-1233 and recombinant MVA-HIV polytope vaccine MVA-mBN32 in a combined prime-boost regimen, and separately, when given to healthy, vaccinia-naïve, HIV-1–uninfected adults (U.S. sites).
- *HVTN 071.* A Phase IB open-label clinical trial to expand the characterization of the immune responses to the Merck adenovirus serotype 5 HIV-1 gag/pol/nef vaccine in healthy, HIV-1–uninfected adult participants (U.S. sites).
- *HVTN 204.* A Phase II clinical trial to evaluate the safety and immunogenicity of a multiclade HIV-1 DNA plasmid vaccine, followed by a multiclade recombinant adenoviral vector HIV-1 vaccine boost, VRC-HIVADV014-00-VP in HIV-1–uninfected adult participants. *Sites*: United States, Jamaica, Haiti, Brazil, and South Africa.
- *HVTN 502.* A multicenter, double-blind, randomized, placebo-controlled Phase II proof-of-concept study to evaluate the safety and efficacy of three-dose regimen of the Merck adenovirus serotype 5 HIV-1 vaccine gag/pol/nef (MRKAd5 HIV-1 gag/pol/nef) in adults at high risk of HIV infection. The NVTN 502 study (also known as the *STEP Study* or *Merck V520-023 Study*), which enrolled 3,000 participants, was conducted by the NIAID-funded HVTN and Merck & Co., Inc. Volunteers were enrolled at sites in Australia, Brazil, Canada, the Dominican Republic, Haiti, Jamaica, Peru, Puerto Rico, and the United States. The Phase IIb "test-of-concept"

study was designed to test Merck's candidate HIV vaccine, the MRKAd5 trivalent vaccine, which aimed to stimulate production of immune system T cells that can kill HIV-infected cells. The goal of the study was to determine if the vaccine could prevent HIV infection, reduce the amount of HIV in those who do become infected, or both. In September 2007, an independent Data and Safety Monitoring Board (DSMB) met to review interim data from a large, international HVTN 502 HIV vaccine clinical trial. The clinical trial, which began enrolling volunteers in December 2004, has been cosponsored by NIAID and Merck & Co. Inc.; the latter also developed and supplied the candidate vaccine.

Based on a review of interim data, the DSMB concluded that the vaccine has not been effective in this trial in preventing HIV infection or affecting the course of the disease in those who become infected with HIV (the vaccine itself cannot cause HIV infection because it contains only synthetically produced snippets of viral material) (http://www.iavireport.org/). *Therefore, Merck & Co., Inc., and NIAID instructed all study sites to cease administering the investigational vaccine but to continue scheduled follow-up visits with all volunteers until the data can be more thoroughly evaluated and a course of action is developed* (http://www3.niaid.nih.gov/news/newsreleases/2007/step_statement.htm).

Based on its first evaluation of interim efficacy data, the DSMB found 24 cases of HIV infection among the 741 volunteers who received at least one dose of the investigational vaccine compared with 21 cases of HIV infection among the 762 volunteers who were vaccinated with a placebo. In volunteers who received at least two vaccinations, the DSMB found 19 cases of HIV infection among the 672 volunteers who received the investigational vaccine and 11 instances of HIV infection among the 691 volunteers who received the placebo. The trial partners will fully evaluate the trial data, provide additional instructions to the STEP trial sites, and provide a detailed scientific analysis of the study results in the near future. The same Merck candidate HIV vaccine is also being tested in South Africa by the HVTN and the South African AIDS Vaccine Initiative in a separate NIAID-sponsored clinical trial known as HVTN 503, or the "Phambili Study." This study was initiated in February 2007 and enrolled 799 individuals. Immunizations and enrollment in the Phambili Study have now been paused. This allows the independent DSMB that oversees the Phambili trial to review all available HVTN 503 and STEP interim findings to determine the next steps. In contrast with the STEP Study where the interim analysis was almost exclusively based on results in volunteers who were men who have sex with men, the Phambili Study primarily enrolled heterosexuals at high risk for HIV. The

study investigators at each site for both the STEP (HVTN 502/Merck V520-023) and Phambili (HVTN 503) vaccine trials have been informed of the decision to cease immunizations and are contacting study volunteers to inform them of the developments. Because HVTN 502 is currently studying the same vaccine as that of HVTN 503, data generated from HVTN 502 may affect the course of the HVTN 503 trial. Data from HVTN 502 will be shared with the NIAID DSMB to help guide and determine the direction of HVTN 503 (http://www3.niaid.nih.gov/news/QA/step_qa.htm).

32.2.3.1 An Update Concerning the HVTN 503/Phambili HIV Vaccine Study

In October 2007, NIAID and the HIV Vaccine Trials Network (HVTN) stopped immunizations and enrollment in the HVTN 503 (Phambili) HIV vaccine study in South Africa. The following are interim data concerning enrollment and the number of HIV infections in the Phambili Study (http://www3.niaid.nih.gov/news/newsreleases/2008/hvtn503_update.htm):

- There were 801 participants in the Phambili Study in October 2007 when immunizations and enrollment were stopped. This included 360 women and 441 men.
- As of January 22, 2008, 11 confirmed HIV infections among the 801 participants had been reported. Seven of these infections were reported among those participants who received the vaccine. Four HIV infections were reported in the placebo group.
- Among the 11 confirmed cases of HIV infection, eight were detected before the study was "unblinded"—that is, when investigators and study participants were told which participants received the vaccine and which received placebo. Two of the cases were detected after unblinding, and the study team is working to clarify whether an additional HIV infection occurred before or after unblinding took place.
- Six cases of HIV infection occurred among vaccine recipients with levels of antibodies against adenovirus type 5 (Ad5 above 18 units) compared with three cases of infection among placebo recipients with similar Ad5 levels. Among vaccine recipients with no detectable antibodies to Ad5 at enrollment, there was one case of HIV infection among vaccine recipients and one case of HIV infection among placebo recipients.
- Ten of the 11 confirmed cases of HIV infection were in women; one male placebo recipient with a high Ad5 level (>18 units) was infected.
- Among the seven vaccine recipients who became HIV infected, two received only one vaccination, four received two vaccinations, and one received all three vaccinations.

These data do not accurately reflect HIV incidence rates within the study because the duration of follow-up of the study volunteers varies considerably by individual and by group. In addition, behavioral risk factors, such as number of sexual partners, have not been accounted for.

To compare HIV incidence in the Phambili Study with HIV incidence in the STEP (HVTN 502) HIV vaccine study will be difficult and may not be possible. The information collected after unblinding may be considered biased by the fact that volunteers may have modified their behaviors based on their knowledge of whether they received the vaccine or the placebo. Furthermore, without substantially more cases of HIV infection, it will not be possible to draw any scientifically valid conclusions about the vaccine's effect on HIV acquisition.

NIAID and the HVTN are committed to conducting further analyses to understand the findings from the HVTN 503 study and use them to inform future research on HIV vaccines. The study investigators will continue to follow all of the Phambili Study volunteers and counsel them on how to reduce HIV exposure to limit the number of any new HIV infections.

Currently, other NIAID-sponsored vaccine studies involving Ad5 are paused or are proceeding only in individuals with Ad5 titers less than 18 units. For a complete listing of these studies, see *Status of NIAID Adenovirus-Based Vaccine Studies*. For more information about the Phambili and STEP HIV vaccine studies, see *Immunizations Are Discontinued in Two HIV Vaccine Trials, An Update Regarding the HVTN 502 and HVTN 503 HIV Vaccine Trials,* and *Questions and Answers: HVTN 502 and HVTN 503 HIV Vaccine Clinical Trials* (see also Section 35.3).

More information on the HVTN may be found at http://www.hvtn.org/.

32.2.4 International Maternal Pediatric Adolescent AIDS Clinical Trials

The International Maternal Pediatric Adolescent AIDS Clinical Trials (IMPAACT) is a merger of the Pediatric AIDS Clinical Trials Group (PACTG) and the Perinatal Scientific Working Group of the HPTN. Together, these two networks have designed and performed clinical trials that have yielded data to set the standards of care for HIV-infected children and for the interruption of vertical transmission throughout the world. The PACTG has been a joint effort between the NIAID and the National Institute of Child Health and Human Development (NICHD) since 1993, and NICHD will continue to work collaboratively with IMPAACT. Specifically, IMPAACT's mission is to significantly decrease the mortality and morbidity associated with HIV disease in children,

adolescents, and pregnant women. To this end, IMPAACT is developing and evaluating safe and cost-effective approaches to interrupt mother-to-infant transmission; evaluating treatments for HIV-infected children, adolescents, and pregnant women, including treatment and prevention of co-infections and comorbidities; and evaluating vaccines for preventing HIV sexual transmission among adolescents. On both a domestic and international scale, IMPAACT's research plan encompasses NIAID's six areas of highest scientific priority including the prevention of mother-to-child transmission (PMTCT), translational research and drug development, optimization of clinical management, including comorbidities, and vaccine development.

32.2.4.1 Mother-to-Child Transmission Agenda

Although perinatal transmission has dropped to less than 2% in the United States, in developing countries approximately 640,000 mother-to-child transmission (MTCT) infections occur each year. Shorter antiretroviral (ARV) regimens have proved to be efficacious, but overall effectiveness is suboptimal due to later transmission via breast-feeding, the limited efficacy of shorter regimens in the antenatal period, and the difficulty of implementing programs for Voluntary Counceling and Testing (VCT) and PMTCT regimens. In addition, even short regimens of nevirapine or 3TC (lamivudine, 3TC is anti-HIV drug) can rapidly select for drug resistance that may potentially limit future treatment options in HIV-positive women and children. The perinatal agenda will evaluate new ARV regimens to prevent MTCT during the perinatal period with special emphasis on low resource areas, evaluate MTCT prevention strategies to minimize development of ARV resistance in mothers and infants, focus on interventions such as use of ARVs and vaccines to prevent transmission via breast-feeding, evaluate strategies to increase population-based coverage of MTCT prevention, and assess ARV pharmacokinetics (PK) and toxicities in pregnant women. Substudies to evaluate the role of HIV subtype, host genetics, drug resistance, pharmacodynamics, HIV-specific immunity, and HIV viral load in compartments in PMTCT are also planned.

32.2.4.2 Translational Agenda

In this priority area, IMPAACT plans to conduct translational research in three areas:

1. Primary antiretroviral therapy for treatment of HIV infection.
2. Prevention and treatment of the complications of HIV infection and ARV drug toxicities.
3. Therapeutic HIV vaccines.

32.2.4.3 Optimization of Clinical Management, Including Comorbidities Agenda

Partners for Appropriate Anti-Infective Community Therapy (PAACT) has identified the following strategic areas of primary therapy, immune-based therapies, and treatment of co-infections/toxicities where carefully constructed clinical studies can yield data that will improve the outcomes for HIV-infected infants, children, and adolescents worldwide:

- *When to Start.* A number of infants and children mount an effective immune response to HIV and do not qualify for treatment under WHO guidelines. Two studies are proposed to evaluate whether early versus deferred treatment makes a significant difference in disease outcome.
- *Treatment Interruption Strategies.* The proportion of HIV-infected children who stop ARV treatment indicates that some children do not progress virologically or immunologically. Studies examining various strategies to maximize immune function, while minimizing ARV toxicities and expense, are needed. Within these studies, parameters that predict success with intermittent antiretroviral therapy (ART) and the need for continuous ART will be identified
- *Strategies to Deal with ARV Resistance.* Three trials will compare specific multidrug regimens or cycling of different highly active antiretroviral therapy (HAART) regimens for suppressing HIV replication. In addition, protocols will examine the efficacy of non-nucleoside reverse transcriptase inhibitors (NNRTI)-ART regimens in nevirapine-exposed versus unexposed infants.
- *Second-Line Therapy for Children Failing NNRTI-Based First-Line Treatment* is a priority within Africa and Asia, including determining which second-line regimen is most efficacious and least toxic.

32.2.5 Vaccines for Preventing Sexual HIV Transmission

Newborn infants of HIV-infected breast-feeding mothers, as well as preadolescents and adolescents, will be the primary target populations of any successful preventive HIV vaccine.

NIAID has conducted more than 60 clinical HIV vaccine trials to date, yet, except for PACTG 218, very few young persons under 18 years of age have been included in trials despite their high risk of infection. In order to license a vaccine for use in this group, safety, immunogenicity, and efficacy data for this population are needed. In parts of sub-Saharan Africa, the annual HIV seroincidence rates in 15- to 19-year-old teenage girls are as high as 18.9%. Many women younger than age 20 access prenatal care at HPTN sites with excellent follow-up rates of retention. We believe that uninfected young women will be ideal for testing the efficacy of an HIV-preventive vaccine, once safety and immunogenicity have been demonstrated in adults. However, the relevant hurdles, such as ethical, legal, regulatory, and feasibility issues, need to be addressed so that this at-risk population can be included in future prevention trials.

Some examples of IMPAACT studies are included in Table 32.1.

More information on IMPAACT may be found at http://pactg.s-3.com/impaact.htm.

32.2.6 International Network for Strategic Initiatives in Global HIV Trials

The International Network for Strategic Initiatives in Global HIV Trials (INSIGHT) is a merger of two existing clinical trials research groups, ESPRIT (Evaluation of Subcutaneous Proleukin® in a Randomized Clinical Trial) and the CPCRA (Terry Beirn Community Programs for Clinical Research on AIDS). This uniquely large network comprises more than 250 clinical sites in 36 countries. INSIGHT will conduct studies in the area of optimizing clinical management of HIV, including HIV-disease and non–HIV-associated comorbidities. The INSIGHT research agenda addresses key issues compromising the health of HIV-infected individuals. The ESPRIT study to determine whether raising CD4 counts by cycles of interleukin-2 in subjects receiving ART confers clinical benefit compared with ART alone and the STALWART study to determine whether cycles of interleukin-2 with or without cycles of ART will permit delay in commencing continuous ART are continuing. A new study is being developed, based on the group's unexpected find-

Table 32.1 Selected landmark international clinical trials conducted by IMPAACT investigators

Sponsor	Number or Name	Type	Location	Brief Description	Outcome
HIVNET	012	Perinatal	INTL	SD NVP vs. ultrashort ZDV to prevent tx	1/2 reduction with NVP
BI	SAINT	Perinatal	INTL	NVP vs. ZDV+3TC to prevent perinatal tx	NVP equivalent to ZDV+3TC
WHO	PETRA	Perinatal	INTL	ZDV+3TC vs. placebo to prevent perinatal tx	1/2 reduction with ZDV+3TC
NICHD	PHPT 2	Perinatal	INTL	Ante/intrapartum ZDV vs. ZDV+NVP	2% tx with ZDV+NVP
NIH DDCF	NVAZ	Perinatal	INTL	Postpartum ZDV+NVP vs. NVP	36% reduction with ZDV/NVP
HPTN	024	Perinatal	INTL	Antibiotics for chorioamnionitis to prevent tx	Not effective

INTL, international; tx, transmission; SD NVP, single-dose nevirapine; ZDV, zidovudine; 3TC, lamivudine.

ings in the Strategies for Management of Anti-Retroviral Therapy (SMART) trial, that individuals interrupting ART experienced a higher rate of both HIV and non-HIV disease progression, especially cardiovascular events. The Strategic Timing of Anti-Retroviral Treatment (START) trial will address when to start therapy for asymptomatic individuals with higher CD4$^+$ T-cell counts. This key pilot study will be conducted over the next 2 years and may then be expanded to a full clinical end-point trial if feasibility and preliminary surrogate marker results are favorable. These trials will help inform clinical practice.

32.2.6.1 Ongoing Studies in INSIGHT

ESPRIT

Evaluation of Subcutaneous Proleukin® in a Randomized International Trial (ESPRIT): ESPRIT is a Phase III, randomized, international, 8- to 9-year, 4,000-person study of interleukin-2 (IL-2) in patients with HIV infection and receiving continuous antiretroviral therapy and a CD4$^+$ cell count of at least 300/mm^3.

- Hypothesis: HAART + intermittent cycles of IL-2 will produce superior immune reconstitution or preservation compared with that of HAART alone, resulting in slower disease progression
- 252 participating sites in 25 countries
- 4 regional coordinating centers
- Opened in 2000; fully accrued in 2003
- Projected completion approximately 2008

STALWART

Study of Aldesleukin with and without Antiretroviral Therapy (STALWART): STALWART is a multicenter, international, open-label, randomized trial comparing impact of cycles of IL-2 +/– peri-cycle ART to no therapy on cell count in ART-naïve HIV-positive patients with CD4$^+$ cell counts >300/mm^3.

- Hypothesis: use of cycles of IL-2 will permit delaying the start of continuous ART in treatment naïve patients
- 480 subjects; 160/subjects/ART
- Primary end-point: change in CD4$^+$ cell count from baseline to week 32

SMART

Strategic Management of Anti-Retroviral Therapy (SMART):

- *Hypothesis.* A drug conservation (DC) strategy that involves episodic use of ART to maintain CD4$^+$ cell count >250/mm^3 will result in a slower rate of progression and fewer toxicities compared with viral suppression (VS) with continuous ART, changed as necessary to maintain suppression.

The SMART study is completed and the findings reinforce the recommendation to avoid use of episodic CD4$^+$ guided ART as used in the SMART study. Data analyses are under way and further studies are needed to fully understand the short-term and long-term consequences of interrupting treatment.

START

Strategic Timing of Anti-Retroviral Therapy (START): START is a multicenter, international, randomized trial comparing initiation of ART at a CD4$^+$ cell count greater than 500 cells/mm^3 (early ART) versus initiation of ART at a CD4$^+$ count of <350 cells/mm^3 (deferred ART) for a composite outcome of AIDS, non-AIDS, and death from any cause.

- *Hypothesis.* Untreated HIV infection is associated with an increased risk of both AIDS and non-AIDS events. Therefore, among asymptomatic participants with a CD4$^+$ count greater than 500 cells/mm^3, immediate use of ART that results in suppression of HIV RNA levels and increases in CD4$^+$ cell counts and potentially other beneficial effects will delay the development of AIDS, non-AIDS, and death from any cause.
- Pilot study of 900 subjects scheduled to begin in 2008.

More information on INSIGHT may be found at http://impaact.s-3.com/.

32.2.7 Microbicide Trials Network

The mission of the Microbicide Trials Network (MTN) is to reduce the sexual transmission of HIV through the development and evaluation of microbicide products, and it will carry out its mission through a strong network of expert scientists and investigators from domestic and international sites. The MTN conducts scientifically rigorous and ethically sound clinical trials that will support licensure of topical microbicide products. The current generation of microbicide candidates may only provide partial protection from HIV infection. Nonetheless, given the dynamics of HIV infection in the developing world, it is likely that even partial protection may translate to significant community benefits for prevention.

Some of the scientific questions that are being addressed through MTN studies include placebo-controlled assessment of the safety and acceptability of candidate microbicide products and potential dosing regimens (e.g., tenofovir gel [daily versus coitally associated use] and Vivagel are currently in such trials); assessment of the acceptability, safety, and efficacy of different prevention strategies (topical microbicide and oral preexposure prophylaxis) in the same population of women using tenovofir gel, oral Truvada, and oral tenofovir disoproxil fumarate (each compared with a matched placebo); new formulation technologies as they become available, such as the vaginal ring; the safety of vaginal microbicides in pregnancy; the safety of vaginal microbicides for rectal use; and the long-term virological sequelae of exposure to reverse transcriptase inhibitor microbicides in subjects who have chronic HIV infection or who are seroconvert during an MTN study. Studies currently under way provide critical infrastructure, expertise, and data to evaluate second-generation products. The depth and breadth of the preclinical pipeline and promising animal model efficacy data provide reason to be optimistic that it is reasonable to expect that a safe and effective microbicide can be identified.

Some examples of MTN studies are given in Tables 32.2 and 32.3.

More information on MTN may be found at http://www.mtnstopshiv.org/.

32.2.8   Non–Clinical Trial Network Studies

The Division of AIDS (DAIDS) sponsors many non–clinical trial network studies or "non-network" studies. Some examples of these include small planning grants, such as R03 grants, or larger R01 or R34 grants, for example. Listed below are examples of programs (i.e., CFARs, CIPRA, and IeDEA) that have been developed from these grants, where not only significant research funding has been invested but also significant DAIDS staff time in order to aid in the success of implementing these initiatives.

32.2.9   Centers for AIDS Research

Since 1988, DAIDS has been funding Centers for AIDS Research (CFARs) grants. The CFARs are a trans-NIH program that is funded by six NIH institutes. They support multidisciplinary environments that promote basic, clinical, behavioral, and translational research in the prevention, detection, and treatment of HIV infections and AIDS (http://www3.niaid.nih.gov/research/cfar/). Major means by which the CFARs accomplish their mission is by (i) strengthening the capacity of HIV/AIDS research in developing countries; (ii) sponsoring training, mentorship, and education; and (iii) stimulating scientific collaboration in interdisciplinary and translational research. To this end, major emphasis is given to collaborating with investigators in the developing countries and by providing logistical, operational, and infrastructure support and small pilot grants for research in developing countries.

The CFAR initiatives have been extended to countries in Africa, Asia, Europe, and the Americas as follows:

- *Africa.* Cameroon, Democratic Republic of Congo, Ethiopia, Ivory Coast, Kenya, Malawi, Mozambique, Rwanda, South Africa, Tanzania, Uganda, Zambia, and Zimbabwe.
- *Asia.* Cambodia, China, India, Thailand, and Vietnam.
- *Central America and the Caribbean.* Belize, Costa Rica, Honduras, Jamaica, Mexico, and St. Kitts.
- *Europe.* Estonia, Romania, Russia, and Ukraine.
- *South America.* Brazil and Peru.

New CFAR developmental pilot projects and supplement awards have been given in the following broad scientific areas: HIV genotypic and viral diversity, predictors of

Table 32.2 MTN trials closed to accrual

Protocol Number	Protocol ID	Protocol Title
MTN-035	10065	Phase II/IIb Safety and Effectiveness Study of the Vaginal Microbicides BufferGel and 0.5% PRO2000/5 Gel (P) for the Prevention of HIV Infection in Women
MTN-035	10145	Phase II Expanded Safety and Acceptability Study of the Vaginal Microbicide 1% Tenofovir Gel

Table 32.3 MTN trials in development

Protocol Number	Protocol ID	Protocol Title
MTN 015	10529	An Observational Cohort Study of Women following HIV-1 Seroconversion in Microbicide Trials
MTN-002	10600	Phase I Study of the Maternal Single-Dose Pharmacokinetics and Placental Transfer of Tenofovir 1% Vaginal Gel among Healthy Term Gravidas
MTN-003	N/A	VOICE Study—Vaginal and Oral Interventions to Control the Epidemic
MTN-005	N/A	Expanded Safety and Acceptability Study of a Non-medicated Placebo Intravaginal Ring
MTN-001	10617	Phase 2 Adherence and Pharmacokinetics Study of Oral and Vaginal Preparations of Tenofovir

virologic failure, HAART adherence, HIV/tuberculosis (TB) co-infection, cellular immunity, neoplasia in HIV-infected women, modeling mobile VCT, behavioral intervention, the potential for medical transmission of HIV, HIV prevention in women, NK cell function, willingness to be vaccinated, neurocognitive deficits and HIV risk behaviors, pharmacokinetics and virologic response to HAART, HIV transmission networks, rapid HIV testing, epidemiology of HIV and HCV among injection drug users, HIV incidence in blood donors, AIDS stigma, SIV pathogenesis in African green monkeys, breast-feeding and HIV, acceptability of male circumcision, and microbicides.

CFAR support has also included training in survey of research techniques, training on ethics, training on observational cohort management, educator and pupil training on HIV/AIDS, and technology transfer to international laboratories.

32.2.10 Comprehensive International Program of Research on AIDS

The Comprehensive International Program of Research on AIDS (CIPRA) initiative was developed in 2001 as part of NIAID's HIV/AIDS global research agenda. CIPRA supported HIV/AIDS research and development efforts at organizations located in eligible resource-poor countries to develop practical, affordable, and acceptable methods to prevent and treat HIV/AIDS in adults and children. CIPRA grant awards were made at three levels: CIPRA R03 Planning and Organizational Grants, CIPRA U01 Exploratory/Developmental Research Grants, and CIPRA U19 Multi-Project Research Grants. More than 30 CIPRA grant awards were made to institutions in more than 20 countries. CIPRA grants were awarded *directly to foreign institutions*.

The major goals of CIPRA were to:

- Provide long-term support for planning and implementing a comprehensive research agenda for the prevention and treatment of HIV/AIDS, including epidemiologic, clinical, and laboratory research on HIV/AIDS.
- Enhance the capability and capacity necessary to conduct research by providing support for continual training of project staff at all levels, as well as support for infrastructure (i.e., facilities, renovations, equipment, training in pharmacy, laboratory methods, and data collection, transmission, and analysis), which are necessary for developing and sustaining ongoing research efforts.

32.2.10.1 CIPRA R03 Planning and Organizational Grants

CIPRA R03 Planning and Organizational Grants provided up to 2 years of support at US$50,000 (direct cost) per year to institutions in nations with very limited HIV/AIDS research experience and capacity for efforts directed at the preparation of an application for one of the larger CIPRA U01 or CIPRA U19 grants. CIPRA R03 Planning and Organizational Grants were awarded in the following countries: Argentina, Brazil, Cambodia, China, Congo, the Dominican Republic, Egypt, Georgia, India, Kenya, Malaysia, Mexico, Mozambique, Peru, Russia, Tanzania, Thailand, Trinidad and Tobago, Vietnam, Zambia, and Zimbabwe.

32.2.10.2 CIPRA U01 Exploratory/Developmental Research Grants

CIPRA U01 Exploratory/Developmental Research Grants provided up to 5 years of support at a maximum total cost of $500,000 per year to develop a comprehensive HIV/AIDS research program in the host country. The U01 supports the implementation of a focused research project, long-term planning, infrastructure development, and continued collaboration and training efforts. CIPRA U01 Exploratory/Developmental Research Grants were awarded in the following countries: Cambodia, Haiti, and Senegal.

Some examples of CIPRA U01 studies include:

- *Cambodia.* CIPRA KH 001 (CAMELIA study): "Cambodian Clinical Research Network for HIV and TB" by the Cambodian Health Committee. The CAMELIA study is to determine if early (2 weeks) versus later (8 weeks) initiation of antiretroviral therapy among those about to begin treatment for tuberculosis affects tuberculosis cure, survival, and relapse and control of HIV in urban and rural settings. This study is cosponsored by the Agence Nationale de Recherches sur le SIDA (ANRS), and much on-site support is provided by Médecins Sans Frontières.
- *Haiti.* CIPRA HT 001: "Haitian Program for Research and Training in HIV/AIDS" by Group for the Study of Kaposi's Sarcoma and Opportunistic Infections (GHESKIO) Centers. This study represents a randomized clinical trial to determine the efficacy of early versus standard antiretroviral therapy in HIV-infected adults with $CD4^+$ T-cell counts between 200 and 350 cells/mm^3.
- *Senegal.* CIPRA SN 001: "A pilot study of safety, effectiveness and adherence of lamivudine/zidovudine plus efavirenz (3TC/ZDV plus EFV) to treat HIV-1 infection in Senegal" by the University of Cheikh Anta Diop de Dakar.

32.2.10.3 CIPRA U19 Multi-Project Research Grants

CIPRA U19 Multi-Project Research Grants provided up to 5 years of renewable support to conduct multiple, coordinated research projects and research support cores focused on developing or implementing preventive and therapeutic interventions for HIV/AIDS, associated opportunistic infections, and tuberculosis in the host country or countries, and continued training efforts to develop the organizational and scientific capability necessary to sustain an ongoing research effort. CIPRA U19 Multi-Project Research Grants were awarded to the following countries: China, Peru, South Africa, and Thailand.

China

Grants were awarded to the National Center for AIDS Prevention and Control in Beijing. The China CIPRA was composed of five inter-related projects and four cores. The overall goal of the China CIPRA grant was to strengthen the existing HIV research infrastructure in China and to build the capacity to conduct multidisciplinary research to explore promising strategies for HIV prevention, treatment, and control.
Some examples of China CIPRA studies include:

- "Epidemiology of HIV-1 infection among residents of former blood donating communities in rural Shanxi Province, China" (National Center for AIDS Prevention and Control)
- "Epidemiology of HIV-1 and other sexually transmitted infections in Honghe Prefecture, Yunnan Province, China" (National Center for AIDS Prevention and Control)
- "A qualitative study for the development of an intervention among HIV-positive former plasma donors (FPDs) in Fuyang, Anhui Province, China" (National Center for AIDS Prevention and Control)
- "A cluster-randomized trial to evaluate the efficacy of a combined individual- and community-based behavioral intervention to improve the quality of life for HIV-positive villagers in Anhui, China" (National Center for AIDS Prevention and Control)
- "Host and viral factors in HIV-1-infected typical progressors and long-term survivors among former blood donors in Anhui Province, China" (National Center for AIDS Prevention and Control)
- "A feasibility study of lamivudine/zidovudine (3TC/ZDV) plus efavirenz (EFV) as initial therapy of HIV-1-infected patients in a rural area of China" (National Center for AIDS Prevention and Control)
- "Development of a novel vaccine against HIV/AIDS in China" (National Center for AIDS Prevention and Control)

More information on the China CIPRA may be found at http://www.ciprancaids.org.cn/old/english/introduction/background/china/china.php.

Peru

Grants were awarded to Association Civil Impacta Salud y Educacion in Lima.
Some examples of CIPRA Peru studies include:

- CIPRA PE 002. "Implementation of a third generation sentinel surveillance approach among men who have sex with men at high risk for HIV type-1 acquisition in the Andean Region" (Asociacion Civil Impacta Salud y Educacion, IMPACTA, Lima, Peru)
- CIPRA PE 003. A Phase II, randomized, double-blind, placebo-controlled trial of acyclovir for suppression of human immunodeficiency virus type 1 (HSV-1) viral load and mucosal shedding in HIV-1, herpes simplex virus type 2 (HSV-2) co-infected women

South Africa

Two CIPRA U19 awards were made in South Africa. One award was made to the University of Natal/CAPRISA in Durban, and the other award was made to the University of Witwaterstrand in Johannesburg.
Some examples of CAPRISA studies include:

- START (CAPRISA 001), "Implementing anti-retroviral therapy in resource constrained settings: a randomized controlled trial to assess the effect of integrated tuberculosis and HIV care on the incidence of AIDS-defining conditions or mortality in participants co-infected with tuberculosis and HIV." A clinical trial to assess the effectiveness of integrated tuberculosis (TB) and HIV care provision through a TB directly observed therapy program with adherence support versus sequential treatment of TB and HIV, by comparing the progression of AIDS-defining illnesses/mortality in TB/HIV co-infected patients (University of Natal). The study is closed to follow-up. More information is available at: http://www.caprisa.org/Projects/start.html.
- CAPRISA. "Viral set point and clinical progression in HIV-1 subtype C infection: the role of immunological and viral factors during acute and early infection" (University of Natal). More information is available at: http://www.caprisa.org/Projects/acute_infection.html.

More information on the CAPRISA may be found at http://www.caprisa.org/.

Other examples of CIPRA South Africa studies include:

- CIPRA ZA 001. "Safeguard the household—a study of HIV antiretroviral therapy treatment strategies appropriate for a resource poor country" (University of Witwatersrand).
- CIPRA ZA 002. "CHER Trial—children with HIV early antiretroviral therapy." This is a Phase III, randomized, open-label trial to evaluate strategies for providing antiretroviral therapy to infants shortly after primary infection in a resource-poor setting (University of Witwatersrand).
- CIPRA ZA 003B. A study of the effects of antiretroviral therapy on rates and transmission of tuberculosis (University of Witwatersrand).
- CIPRA ZA 004. "Evaluation of quantitative and qualitative antibody responses to *Streptococcus pneumoniae* and *Haemophilus influenzae* type B conjugate vaccines in HIV-1 exposed children that are receiving versus those not receiving antiretroviral therapy, as well as among HIV-1 exposed-infected children and HIV-1 unexposed-uninfected children" (University of Witwatersrand).

More information on the CIPRA South Africa project may be found at: http://www.cipra-sa.com/.

Thailand

Grant was awarded to HIV-NAT Thai Red Cross Society in Bangkok.

- CIPRA TH 001. "Pediatric randomized of early versus deferred initiation in Cambodia and Thailand" (PREDICT). An open-label, randomized study to compare antiretroviral therapy (ART) initiation when CD4$^+$ T-cell count is between 15% and 24% and ART initiation when the CD4$^+$ T-cell count falls below 15% in children with HIV infection and moderate immune suppression. This 5-year grant will evaluate HIV treatment strategies in HIV-infected children in Thailand and Cambodia. Researchers from the Thai Red Cross and the international HIV-NAT (HIV Netherlands/Australia /Thailand) group will compare immediate versus delayed antiretroviral therapy for pediatric HIV patients in sites in Thailand and Cambodia. Perinatally acquired HIV infection can result in severe impairment or death. Early treatment with antiretroviral (ARV) drugs may prevent these severe consequences, as well as developmental delays. Experts note, however, that these potential early gains must be measured against the possible loss of therapeutic options due to emergence of drug resistance as well as longer exposure to toxic side effects of the ARVs. Study is enrolling. (Also with CIPRA Thailand, a neurodevelopmental substudy is co-sponsored by NICHD and NIMH.)

More information on the CIPRA Thailand grant may be found at http://www.ciprathailand.org/aboutcipra.html.

32.2.11 International Epidemiologic Databases to Evaluate AIDS

In July 2006, seven regional centers were funded as part of the International Epidemiologic Databases to Evaluate AIDS (IeDEA) initiative. The funded regions include North America, South America/the Caribbean, Australia/Asia, and four regions in Africa (West, Central, East, and Southern Africa). The National Institute of Child Health and Human Development (NICHD) is cofunding this initiative, as several regions have access to data from HIV-infected children.

This initiative will establish international regional centers for collecting and harmonizing data and establishing an international research consortium to address unique and evolving research questions in HIV/AIDS that are currently unanswerable by single cohorts. High-quality data are being collected by researchers throughout the world. This initiative provides a means to establish and implement methodology to effectively pool the collected data—thus providing a cost-effective means of generating large data sets to address the high-priority research questions.

More information on IeDEA may be found at http://www.iedea-hiv.org/.

32.2.12 Male Circumcision

Researchers have noted significant variations in HIV prevalence that seemed, at least in certain African and Asian countries, to be associated with levels of male circumcision in the community. In areas where circumcision is common, HIV prevalence tends to be lower; conversely, areas of higher HIV prevalence overlapped with regions where male circumcision is not commonly practiced.

In December 2006, NIAID announced an early end to two clinical trials of adult male circumcision because an interim review of trial data revealed that medically performed circumcision significantly reduces a man's risk of acquiring HIV through heterosexual intercourse. The trial in Kisumu, Kenya, of 2,784 HIV-negative men showed a 53% reduction in HIV acquisition in circumcised men relative to uncircumcised men, and a trial of 4,996 HIV-negative men in Rakai, Uganda, showed that HIV acquisition was reduced by 48% in circumcised men.

These findings are of great interest to public health policymakers who are developing and implementing comprehensive HIV prevention programs. Male circumcision performed safely in a medical environment complements other HIV prevention strategies and could lessen the burden of HIV/AIDS, especially in countries in sub-Saharan Africa where, according to the 2006 estimates from UNAIDS, 2.8 million new infections occurred in a single year (1,2).

Many studies have suggested that male circumcision plays a role in protecting against HIV acquisition. Whereas the initial benefit will be fewer HIV infections in men, ultimately adult male circumcision could lead to fewer infections in women in those areas of the world where HIV is spread primarily through heterosexual intercourse.

The findings from the African studies may have less impact on the epidemic in the United States for several reasons. In the United States, most men have been circumcised. Also, there is a lower prevalence of HIV. Moreover, most infections among men in the United States are in men who have sex with men, for whom the amount of benefit provided by circumcision is unknown. Nonetheless, the overall findings of the African studies are likely to be broadly relevant regardless of geographic location: a man at sexual risk who is uncircumcised is more likely than a man who is circumcised to become infected with HIV. Still, circumcision is only part of a broader HIV prevention strategy that includes limiting the number of sexual partners and using condoms during intercourse.

In addition to NIAID support, the Kenyan trial was funded by the Canadian Institutes of Health Research and included Kenyan researchers. The Ugandan trial is led by researchers from the Johns Hopkins Bloomberg School of Public Health (Baltimore, Maryland) with additional collaborators from Uganda.

Both trials involved adult, HIV-negative heterosexual male volunteers assigned at random to either intervention (circumcision performed by trained medical professionals in a clinic setting) or no intervention (no circumcision). All participants were extensively counseled in HIV prevention and risk reduction techniques. Both trials reached their enrollment targets by September 2005 and were originally designed to continue follow-up until mid-2007. However, at the regularly scheduled meeting of the NIAID Data and Safety Monitoring Board (DSMB) on December 12, 2006, reviewers assessed the interim data and deemed medically performed circumcision safe and effective in reducing HIV acquisition in both trials. They, therefore recommended the two studies to be halted early. All men who were randomized into the nonintervention arms will now be offered circumcision.

It is critical to emphasize that these clinical trials demonstrated that medical circumcision is safe and effective when the procedure is performed by medically trained professionals and when patients receive appropriate care during the healing period after surgery.

Results of the first randomized clinical trial assessing the protective value of male circumcision against HIV infection, conducted by a team of French and South African researchers in South Africa, were reported in 2005. That trial of more than 3,000 HIV-negative men showed that circumcision reduced the risk of acquiring HIV by 60%. The trial was funded by the French Agence Nationale de Recherches sur le Sida (ANRS) (1) (see http://www.anrs.fr/).

More information on the Kenyan and Ugandan trials of adult male circumcision may be found on the NIAID Questions and Answers document at the following: http://www3.niaid.nih.gov/news/QA/AMC12_QA.htm.

32.2.13 NIAID Collaborative International Research—Nigerian Scholars Program

This program is designed to train Ph.D. students to build Nigerian scientific expertise in medicinal chemistry and drug discovery from medicinal plants. DAIDS and the Division of Intramural Research (DIR) at NIAID are collaborating to support training through a U.S./Nigerian collaborative effort between (i) the DHHS, NIH; (ii) the National Institute of Pharmaceutical Research and Development (NIPRD), Federal Government of Nigeria; and (iii) the University of Ibadan, Nigeria. Students who have matriculated at the University of Ibadan will perform research in Abuja at a renovated teaching laboratory at NIPRD with some travel to the NIH for specialized research training (Division of Intramural Research, NIAID, NIH).

32.2.14 Other International NIAID-Supported Studies

- *Mentored Patient-Oriented Research Career Development Award (K23).* "Concurrent HAART and tuberculosis treatment: drug-to-drug interactions." This study is designed to investigate the interethnic differences in the pharmacokinetic parameters and tolerability of efavirenz and lopinavir/ritonavir before and during concurrent administration with rifampin in HIV/TB co-infected Ghanaian persons, and that in African-American and Caucasian healthy volunteers in the United States (Miriam Hospital, K23-AI-71760).

- *Research on AIDS Co-infections.* "Tuberculosis-related immune reconstitution syndrome in HIV-1-infected South Africans." This clinical research study will assess immune correlates of *immune reconstitution inflammatory syndrome (IRIS)* in TB-co-infected, HIV-positive adults enrolled at the Wits Health Consortium in Johannesburg, South Africa, at clinical presentation, and will identify possible prognostic factors associated with IRIS at antiretroviral therapy initiation (Wistar Institute, AI69996).

- *Novel TB Prevention Regimens for HIV-Infected Adults* [in South Africa]. This study will compare the activity of three novel regimens for the prevention of tuberculosis in a high-risk population using rifapentine (RPT), isoniazid (INH), and rifamycin (RIF) (Johns Hopkins University; R01-AI-048526).

- *International Studies of AIDS-Associated Co-infections (ISAAC)* aimed at establishing a Duke University ISAAC unit in Tanzania. The objectives of the project are to develop critical research infrastructure, to catalyze interactions across ISAAC unit scientific programs, and to foster an independent and sustainable research enterprise within the Kilimanjaro Christian Medical Center (KCMC) [HIV/AIDS Program (Duke University; U01-AI-62563, RFA AI03-036)].

32.2.15 U.S. Military HIV Research Program (USMHRP) Trials Funded by NIAID

In 2005, NIAID and the U.S. Army Medical Research and Materiel Command renewed their Interagency Agreement (IAA) set to address specific tasks related to (i) design and construction of candidate preventive vaccines; (ii) preclinical research and development, including evaluation of candidate vaccines; (iii) pilot lot production; (iv) clinical site development; and (v) Phase I to III human clinical trials for safety, immunogenicity, and efficacy testing.

Some examples of USMHRP/NIAID studies include:

- RV 142. "HIV and malaria cohort study among tea plantation workers and adult dependents in Kericho, Kenya."
- RV 143. "Infectious disease surveillance (HIV, TB, and malaria) and cohort development among urban and rural adults in Mbeya Municipality, Tanzania."
- RV 144. A Phase III trial of Aventis live recombinant vaccine ALVAC-HIV (vCP1521) priming, with VaxGen gp120 B/E (AIDSVAX B/E) boosting in HIV-1-uninfected Thai adults.
- RV 156. A Phase I clinical trial to evaluate the safety and immunogenicity of a multiclade HIV-1 DNA plasmid vaccine, VRC-HIVDNA009-00-VP, in uninfected adult volunteers in Uganda. The RV 156 clinical trial has been funded by NIAID.

- RV 172. A Phase I/II clinical trial to evaluate the safety and immunogenicity of a multiclade HIV-1 DNA plasmid vaccine, VRC-HIVDNA016-00-VP, boosted by a multiclade HIV-1 recombinant adenovirus-5 vector vaccine, VRC-HIVADV014-00-VP, in HIV-1-uninfected adults volunteers in East Africa.

- RV 173. Cohort development for a possible Phase III HIV vaccine trial among the population aged 15–49 of Kayunga District, Uganda.

- South Africa. *PHIDISA I.* "A prospective epidemiologic cohort study of HIV and risk-related co-infections in the SANDF." This study will screen uniformed personnel of the South African National Defense Force (SANDF) and their registered family members for HIV, hepatitis B and C, gonorrhea, syphilis, and chlamydia to determine the incidence and prevalence of these sexually transmitted diseases. It will identify people who may be eligible to participate in clinical trials for preventing or treating HIV disease and will provide information that will be helpful in developing policy and better care for people affected with HIV and other diseases. This study is part of the South Africa–U.S. PHIDISA Programme—a collaboration between the South African Military Health Service (SAMHS) of the SANDF, the U.S. Department of Defense, and the U.S. National Institutes of Health—to help prevent transmission of HIV among South African military and civilian employees and their families. *PHIDISA II.* "Antiretroviral therapy for advanced HIV disease in South Africa." A randomized, open-label, 2×2 factorial study to compare the safety and efficacy of different combination antiretroviral therapy regimens in treating naïve patients with advanced HIV disease and/or CD4$^+$ T-lymphocyte count <200 cells/mm^3. This study will determine how well four different antiretroviral drug therapies work in patients with advanced HIV disease. The trial is part of the South Africa–U.S. PHIDISA Programme HIV collaboration between the South African Military Health Service (SAMHS) of the South African National Defense Force (SANDF), the U.S. Department of Defense, and the U.S. National Institutes of Health to help prevent transmission of HIV among South African military and civilian employees and their families.

32.2.16 Other HIV/AIDS Vaccine Related Work

32.2.16.1 International AIDS Vaccine Initiative

The International AIDS Vaccine Initiative (IAVI) mission is to ensure the development of safe, effective, accessible, preventive HIV vaccines for use throughout the world. IAVI is a global not-for-profit, public-private partnership working to accelerate the development of a vaccine to prevent HIV infection and AIDS (http://www.iavi.org/). Founded in 1996, IAVI is designed to research and develop vaccine candidates, conducts policy analyses, and serves as an advocate for the field with offices in Africa, India, and Europe. IAVI supports a comprehensive approach to HIV and AIDS that balances the expansion and strengthening of existing HIV prevention and treatment programs with targeted investments in new AIDS prevention technologies. As the world's only organization focused solely on the development of an AIDS vaccine, IAVI also works to ensure that a future vaccine will be accessible to all who need it.

The following is an example of IAVI protocols:

- *IAVI V-001*. A Phase I, randomized, placebo-controlled, double-blind clinical trial to evaluate the safety and immunogenicity of a multiclade HIV-1 DNA plasmid vaccine followed by recombinant, multiclade HIV-1 adenoviral vector vaccine or the multiclade HIV-1 adenoviral vector vaccine alone in healthy adult volunteers not infected with HIV-1. Sites of the trial are in Nairobi, Kenya, and Kigali, Rwanda. The IAVI V-001 trial has been cosponsored by NIAID/DAIDS and harmonized with the HVTN 204 study and the USMHRP RV 172 study (see Section 32.2.15).

32.2.17 Partnership for AIDS Vaccine Evaluation

The Partnership for AIDS Vaccine Evaluation (PAVE) is a voluntary consortium of U.S. government agencies and key U.S. government–funded organizations involved in the development and evaluation of HIV/AIDS preventive vaccines and the conduct of HIV vaccine clinical trials.

The goal to develop a safe and effective HIV vaccine is one that no single entity or institution is likely to accomplish on its own. Therefore, PAVE's goal is to achieve better harmony and increased operational and cost efficiencies in HIV vaccine development and in the conduct of HIV vaccine clinical trials, especially Phase III trials, by serving as a forum and clearinghouse for information-sharing and planning. PAVE will also eliminate unnecessary duplication of effort. PAVE is a synergistic partnership that pools intellectual resources and experience to achieve fundamental goals that a number of U.S. government agencies and others share in common. PAVE does not represent a funding organization, and members are expected to support their activities from other governmental or nongovernmental sources.

32.2.17.1 About PAVE 100

NIAID is planning a Phase IIb HIV/AIDS vaccine study (currently referred to as PAVE 100 or The Pave Study) at multiple sites in the United States and internationally, in conjunction with several partner organizations. This will be a Phase IIb test-of-concept, randomized, double-blind, placebo-controlled, international clinical trial to evaluate the efficacy, safety, and immunogenicity of a multiclade HIV-1 DNA plasmid vaccine (VRC-HIVDNA016-00-VP), followed by a multiclade recombinant adenoviral vector vaccine (VRC-HIVADV014-00-VP), in HIV-uninfected persons. The vaccine candidate to be evaluated is being developed by the NIAID's Vaccine Research Center.

No significant safety issues have been identified in Phase I/II trials to date. The upcoming Phase IIb trial will assess the vaccine's efficacy in a larger number of human volunteers, but most likely will not by itself be sufficient for licensure. The best outcome would be a finding that the vaccine offers a high level of protection from infection, or, among those who become infected despite vaccination, results in a large and sustained decrease in viral load, with clinical benefits. Whatever type and level of protection the vaccine may be found to provide, this trial is critically important to help scientists learn how future effective vaccine candidates might be developed and improved.

Locations: Proposed sites are in East Africa, Southern Africa, Latin America, the Caribbean, and the United States (up to 13 countries total), pending approvals from the FDA, the host country, and site regulatory authorities. As of June 2007, documents had not been submitted to all host country regulatory authorities or approved to move forward, so specific countries or sites had not yet been determined. Approximately 3,000 participants in East Africa, 2,500 participants in Southern Africa, and 3,000 participants in the Americas and the Caribbean are expected to take part in the study.

Timing: A phased launch has been planned, starting in the United States in autumn 2007, followed by international sites starting later in 2007 or early 2008. Results are anticipated in late 2011.

Trial Objectives: The study will test whether the vaccine prevents HIV-1 infection and whether vaccination results in decreased levels of HIV-1 in the blood if volunteers later become infected despite vaccination.

Partners:

- Sponsor: Division of AIDS, National Institute of Allergy and Infectious Diseases (NIAID), National Institutes of Health, U.S. Department of Health and Human Services.
- Vaccine Developer: The Dale and Betty Bumpers Vaccine Research Center, NIAID.

The Trial will be conducted by:

- The HIV Vaccine Trials Network (supported by a cooperative agreement with NIAID).
- The International AIDS Vaccine Initiative (partially supported by a cooperative agreement with the U.S. Agency for International Development).
- The U.S. Military HIV Research Program (partially supported by a cooperative agreement with the Henry M. Jackson Foundation for the Advancement of Military Medicine).
- The U.S. Centers for Disease Control and Prevention (decision pending on site development progress).

32.2.17.2 Why the PAVE 100 Study Is Important

New tools for preventing HIV infection are needed. Vaccines have been central in controlling many infectious diseases, and most scientists agree that a vaccine to bring HIV under control is both possible and essential. Despite important advances in antiretroviral therapy, new HIV infections still annually outnumber the people who are able to initiate ART.

Treatment and epidemiologic studies in humans and experiments in animal models led to the hypothesis that vaccination could improve the immune control of viral load in vaccinees who subsequently become HIV-1–infected through natural exposure. This may result in longer disease-free survival, minimize the need for antiretroviral treatment, and diminish a person's ability to transmit the virus to others.

Unless the vaccine is shown to be highly effective in preventing HIV-1 infection, the results from this study alone are unlikely to be sufficient for licensing the vaccine. Study results will enable the sponsor to decide whether the product merits one or more large Phase III trials designed to support licensure. The trial may also provide information about the specific types of immune responses needed to protect from infection or control viral load and thus provide valuable guidance for improved vaccine design and accelerated development.

32.2.18 Center for HIV/AIDS Vaccine Immunology

The Center for HIV/AIDS Vaccine Immunology (CHAVI) is currently one of two implementation projects under the Global HIV Vaccine Enterprise, the other being the recently funded Collaboration for AIDS Vaccine Discovery (CAVD) by grants from the Bill & Melinda Gates Foundation. In July 2005, NIAID awarded the CHAVI grant to a consortium of investigators from Duke University, the Dana-Farber Cancer Institute, Beth Israel Deaconess Medical Center, Oxford University, and the University of Alabama-Birmingham.

CHAVI is designed to test new vaccine strategies to overcome key immunologic roadblocks in HIV vaccine design. These roadblocks include a lack of understanding of the correlates of protective immunity to HIV-1 and a lack of vectors and immunogens that can induce protective, durable immune responses at mucosal sites. CHAVI will study the transmitted virus, and the biological events that occur during transmission. CHAVI will work to define protective innate and adaptive host defenses against HIV in humans and SIV in primates.

The overall goals of CHAVI are to:

1. Determine the viral and immunologic events and host genetic factors associated with HIV transmission, infection, and (partial) containment of virus replication.
2. Develop novel HIV-1 vectors, immunogens, and adjuvants that suppress viral replication and elicit persistent mucosal and/or systemic immune responses.
3. Use SIV infection in primates as a model for HIV infection in humans and determine the factors that lead to mucosal protection from SIV in primates.
4. Test novel HIV-1 vaccine candidates in Phase I clinical trials.

In its third year (2007) since CHAVI was funded, accomplishments included (http://www.chavi.org/modules/chavi_about/index.php?id=1):

- Completing the first genome-wide association study that defined three novel human genes associated with control of HIV viral load
- Sequencing 109 transmitted clade B virus Env proteins by single genome amplification
- Isolating and characterizing the earliest antibody responses after HIV transmission
- Achieving progress toward the development of functional assays of mucosal T and B cells for monitoring HIV vaccine trials
- Beginning enrollment at the majority of CHAVI foreign clinical sites
- Renovating and implementing IT infrastructure at clinical sites
- Recruiting 70 acute HIV-infected patients for the CHAVI 001 protocol
- Implementing non-human primate correlates of immunity studies
- Funding a new Antibodyome program to clone and sequence a large segment of the bone marrow and peripheral blood B cell repertoire in normal and autoimmune disease patients, as well as in acute and chronically HIV-infected subjects

- Acquiring human monoclonal antibodies from acutely infected HIV-1 patients and from autoimmune disease patients to determine their ability to neutralize HIV-1

Accomplishments during the first (2005) and second (2006) year of CHAVI funding (http://www.chavi.org/modules/chavi_about/index.php?id=1) included:

- Establishing its organizational structure
- Establishing clinical trials sites in Africa, the United States, and the United Kingdom
- Writing and implementing a series of observational clinical protocols
- Beginning the study of innate and adaptive cellular and antibody responses in acute HIV infection and exposed and uninfected patients
- Characterizing transmitted viruses and developed the first iteration of the CHAVI HIV-transmitted virus sequence database (1,410 sequences from 72 acquired hemostatic inhibitors (AHI) patients)
- Establishing the EuroCHAVI Genetics Consortium
- Initiating genome-wide HapMap analysis of four separate cohorts for genes that predispose to initial control of HIV viral load

For more information on the progress of CHAVI, see the CHAVI Progress Reports (http://www.chavi.org/modules/chavi_reports/index.php?id=1).

32.2.19 Global HIV Vaccine Enterprise

The Global HIV Vaccine Enterprise (GHVE) is an alliance of independent organizations around the world dedicated to accelerating the development of a preventive HIV vaccine by:

- *Shared scientific plan.* Implementing a strategic plan for HIV vaccine research that spans vaccine discovery, product development and manufacturing, and clinical trials.
- *Increased resources.* Mobilizing significant new funding to achieve the scientific plan.
- *Greater collaboration.* Promoting more efficient, faster ways for researchers to share successes and failures and avoid duplication of efforts.

32.2.20 President's Emergency Plan for AIDS Research

In his State of the Union address on January 28, 2003, President George W. Bush announced the *President's Emergency Plan for AIDS Relief (PEPFAR/Emergency Plan).* The emergency plan is the largest commitment ever by any nation for an international health initiative dedicated to a sin-

gle disease—a 5-year, US$15 billion, multifaceted approach to combating the disease around the world (http://www.pepfar.gov/).

On May 27, 2003, President George W. Bush signed *P.L.108-25,* the *United States Leadership Against Global HIV/AIDS, Tuberculosis, and Malaria Act* of 2003, the legislative authorization for the emergency plan. The United States now leads the world in its level of support for the fight against HIV/AIDS.

The primary implementing departments and agencies of the emergency plan are Department of State (DoS), U.S. Agency for International Development (USAID), Department of Defense (DoD), Department of Commerce (DoC), Department of Labor (DoL), Department of Health and Human Services (HHS), and the Peace Corps.

In fiscal year 2006, 83% of emergency plan partners were local organizations, which support more than 15,000 project sites for prevention, treatment, and care (http://www.pepfar.gov/about/c19785.htm). Furthermore, in 2006, the U.S. Government provided bilateral, regional, and volunteer programs to assist 114 countries in HIV/AIDS prevention, treatment, and care (http://www.pepfar.gov/countries/). As of September 30, 2007, the PEPFAR program had supported antiretroviral treatment for approximately 1,445,500 men, women, and children through bilateral programs in the emergency plan's 15 focus countries in Africa, Asia, and the Caribbean. DAIDS is supporting the work of PEPFAR in Ethiopia, Haiti, Nigeria, Rwanda, South Africa, Uganda, and Zambia (Fig. 32.1).

32.2.20.1 The Role of NIH in PEPFAR Programs

PEPFAR is creating a unique opportunity to study large numbers of patients treated for HIV and TB in the developing world. It is also helping to create health care systems that enable the ethical conduct of HIV research in strategically important developing countries. NIH has a responsibility to provide evidence-based guidance to maximize the impact (and minimize the toxicities) of the use of HIV/TB therapeutics in developing countries.

32.2.20.2 NIAID Intramural Research

The Vaccine Research Center

The Dale and Betty Bumpers Vaccine Research Center (VRC) at the NIH was established to facilitate research in vaccine development.

The VRC is dedicated to improving global human health through the rigorous pursuit of effective vaccines for human diseases. Established by President William J. Clinton as part of an initiative to develop an AIDS vaccine, the VRC is a

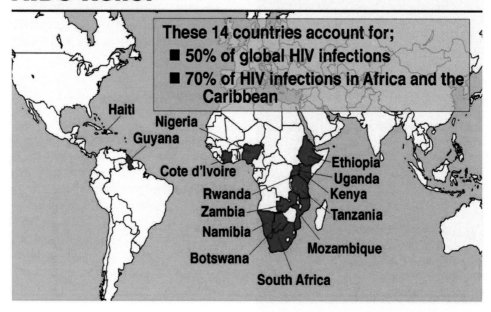

Fig. 32.1 The President's Emergency Plan for AIDS Relief.

unique venture within the NIH intramural research program. Initially spearheaded by the NIAID, the National Cancer Institute, and the NIH Office of AIDS Research, the VRC is now part of the NIAID organization.

The VRC is conducting research that facilitates the development of effective AIDS vaccines. Activities at the center include (i) basic research to establish mechanisms of inducing long-lasting protective immunity against HIV and other pathogens that present special challenges to vaccine development; (ii) the conception, design, and preparation of vaccine candidates for HIV and related viruses; and (iii) laboratory analysis, animal testing, and clinical trials of such candidates. The VRC has begun a comprehensive program of research at the NIH intramural campus and working with scientists in academic, clinical, and industrial laboratories through a program of national and international collaborations. The VRC is actively seeking industrial partners for the development, efficacy testing, and marketing of vaccines and to focus the development of new methodologies and training opportunities that will benefit all HIV vaccine researchers. The potential scientific advances, methodologies, and resources will also provide the basis for research on vaccines for other diseases.

- *Scientists Unveil Piece of HIV Protein That May Be Key to AIDS Vaccine Development*

In a finding that could have profound implications for AIDS vaccine design, researchers led by a team at NIAID have generated an atomic-level picture of a key portion of an HIV surface protein as it looks when bound to an infection-fighting antibody. Unlike much of the constantly mutating virus, this protein component is stable and—more importantly, say the researchers—appears vulnerable to attack from this specific antibody, known as b12, that can broadly neutralize HIV *(3)*. The research team was led by scientists from the NIAID's VRC and included as collaborators other scientists from NIAID and the National Cancer Institute, as well as investigators from the Dana-Farber Cancer Institute, Boston, and The Scripps Research Institute in La Jolla, California (http://www3.niaid.nih.gov/news/ news-releases/2007/B12antibodyimage.htm) (Fig. 32.2)

Some examples of NIAID/VRC Trials:

- *VRC 008.* A Phase I clinical trial of a prime-boost HIV-1 vaccination schedule: multiclade DNA vaccine VRC-HIVDNA016-00-VP, followed by multiclade adenoviral vector vaccine, VRC-HIVADV014-00-VP, in uninfected adult volunteers.
- *VRC 009.* A Phase I clinical trial to evaluate the safety and immunogenicity of a booster dose of a recombinant multiclade HIV-1 adenoviral vector vaccine, VRC-HIVADV014-00-VP, in uninfected subjects who were previously immunized with VRC-HIVDNA009-00-VP in VRC 004 (03-I-0022).
- *VRC 010.* A Phase I clinical trial to evaluate the safety and immunogenicity of a booster dose of a recombinant multiclade HIV-1 adenoviral vector vaccine,

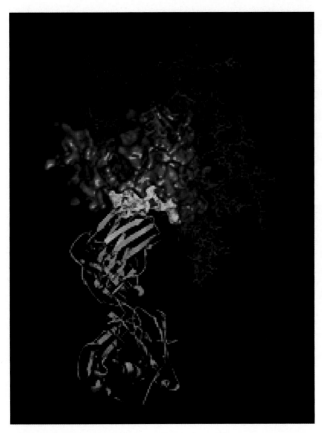

Fig. 32.2 Three-dimensional x-ray crystallographic image showing the broadly neutralizing antibody b12 (green ribbon) in contact with a critical target (yellow) for vaccine development on HIV-1 gp120 (red). (Credit: NIAID.)

VRC-HIVADV014-00-VP, in uninfected subjects who were previously immunized with VRC-HIVDNA016-00-VP in VRC 007.

- *VRC 011.* Intramuscular, subcutaneous, and intradermal administration of an HIV-1 multiclade DNA vaccine, VRC-HIVDNA016-00-VP, and HIV-1 multiclade adenoviral vector vaccine, VRC-HIVADV014-00-VP, in HIV-1-uninfected adult volunteers.

- *VRC 101.* A Phase I clinical trial to evaluate the safety and immunogenicity of a prime-boost HIV-1 vaccination schedule of a six-plasmid multiclade HIV-1 DNA vaccine, VRC-HIVDNA016-00-VP, followed by a recombinant multiclade adenoviral vector HIV vaccine, VRC-HIVADV014-00-VP, in HIV-infected adult volunteers.

32.2.21 Conclusion

NIAID-sponsored researchers have made critical discoveries about the basic biology of HIV and the immune response to HIV infection, which in turn have led to the development of therapies that suppress the growth of the virus in the body. Although much has been learned in recent years, questions remain about the molecular interactions involved in the regulation of HIV expression and replication, why the host immune response fails to control the infection, and how reservoirs of virus persist in the body despite HAART.

NIAID continues to search for more scientific information about how the virus attacks the body and how the body defends itself, which is critical for identifying additional targets for therapeutic interventions and vaccines.

References

1. Williams, B. G., Lloyd-Smith, J. O., Gouws, E., Hankins, C., Getz, W. M., Hargrove, J., de Zoysa, I., Dye, C., and Auvert, B. (2006) The potential impact of male circumcision on HIV in Sub-Saharan Africa, *PLos Med.*, **3**(7), e262.
2. Auvert, B., Taljaard, D., Lagarde, E., Sobngwi-Tambekou, J., Sitta, R., and Puren, A. (2005) Randomized, controlled intervention trial of male circumcision for reduction of HIV infection risk: the ANRS 1265 trial, *PLos Med.*, **2**, e298.
3. Zhou, T., Xu, L., Dey, B., Hessell, A. J., Van Ryk, D., Xiang, S.-H., Yang, X., Zhang, M.-Y., Zwick, M. B., Arthos, J., Burton, D. R., Dimitrov, D. S., Sodroski, J., Wyatt, R., Nabel, G. J., and Kwong, P. D. (2007) Structural definition of a conserved neutralization epitope on HIV-1 gp120, *Nature*, **445**, 732–737.

Chapter 33

HIV/AIDS Epidemiology

Epidemiologic research in HIV/AIDS encompasses research on the biology of HIV and the clinical course of HIV disease in human populations. As such, the findings obtained by this research contribute to a better understanding of the HIV/AIDS disease, from the risk factors that lead from transmission to the development and progression of disease. Epidemiologic research on HIV has, thus far, concentrated on those factors associated with transmission, protection from transmission, and the biology and clinical course of HIV disease. Patterns of use and the efficacy of therapies have also been evaluated in clinical trials and in cohort studies.

Molecular epidemiology to better define the types of viruses circulating in a population will be important in determining the best vaccine candidates.

The dramatic modulation of HIV infection by highly active antiretroviral therapy (HAART) has prompted research into understanding the clinical course of HIV infection in persons using HAART and the very long-term effects of HIV infection and its treatment. Whereas to date there have been no indications of a decrease in the effectiveness of HAART therapy, the development of widespread resistance in circulating virus remains a threat to the current success. Furthermore, the increased age of persons living with HIV raises the possibility that this population of immunocompromised individuals, who have a high prevalence of other disease risk factors, may develop other life-threatening morbidities, such as heart disease or cancer at a younger age than do their HIV-negative peers. In this regard, it is important to note that the risks of death, AIDS, and other diseases increase on episodic antiretroviral therapy (see below).

Despite recent reports of leveling off and even decreases in the prevalence of HIV infection in parts of Africa and Asia, the spread of HIV infection and the AIDS pandemic have continued to rise in 2006, especially in southern Africa (1,2).

Thus, in 2005, an estimated 38.6 million people (range, 33 million to 46 million) worldwide have been living with HIV infection, 4.1 million people (range, 3.4 million to 6.2 million) became newly HIV-infected, and approximately 2.8 million people died of AIDS (2).

The sheer number of newly HIV-infected people has emphasized the utmost importance of efforts to prevent and control the HIV infection. Thus, the individual-level risks for acquisition and transmission of HIV remain at the core of diverse ongoing and emerging HIV/AIDS epidemics in 2006 (1).

Episodic Antiretroviral Therapy. Results from one of the largest HIV/AIDS treatment trials ever conducted have shown that a specific strategy of interrupting antiretroviral therapy more than doubles the risk of AIDS or death from any cause (3). The trial, known as Strategies for Management of Anti-Retroviral Therapies, or SMART, was funded by the National Institute of Allergy and Infectious Diseases (NIAID) and involved 318 clinical sites in 33 countries. The SMART study was coordinated by four international centers: the Medical Research Council Clinical Trials Unit in London; the Copenhagen HIV Program in Denmark; the National Centre in HIV Epidemiology and Clinical Research at the University of New South Wales in Sydney, Australia; and the Terry Beirn Community Programs for Clinical Research on AIDS (CPCRA) in Washington, DC. The statistical and data management center was based at the University of Minnesota in Minneapolis.

In the study, the investigators used two predetermined levels of $CD4^+$ T-cells, the primary immune cell targeted by HIV, to guide them in respectively suspending or restarting the study participants on antiretroviral therapy. As HIV/AIDS has evolved into a chronic disease without a cure, lifelong antiretroviral therapy has become the norm. Lifelong therapy, however, can be difficult to adhere to as well as expensive. For these reasons, there has been a concerted research effort to test treatment interruption strategies that may enhance patients' quality of life and limit adverse drug effects. The experimental strategies vary in their approach to when to interrupt therapy. Some, like SMART, use a specific $CD4^+$ T-cell count as a guide; others schedule regular time periods during which treatment is stopped (e.g., alternating 1 month off and 3 months on).

The SMART study was designed to determine which of two different HIV treatment strategies would result in greater overall clinical benefit. Volunteers with chronic HIV infection—nearly all of whom had taken antiretroviral therapy (ART)—were assigned at random to one of two groups. In the "viral suppression" group, ART was taken on an ongoing basis to suppress HIV viral load; in the "drug conservation" group, participants received episodic ART in an effort to reduce the side effects of the drugs and preserve treatment options. In the latter group, ART was suspended whenever CD4$^+$ T-cell counts were above 350 cells/mm^3, and ART was started only when levels of CD4$^+$ T-cells dropped below 250 cells/mm^3 (http://www.smart-trial.org.). The CD4$^+$ T-cell count thresholds for stopping and starting ART were chosen based on previously reported associations between CD4$^+$ T-cell counts and risks of opportunistic diseases and death.

The results of the SMART trial have provided important new data that will help physicians and their HIV-infected patients make treatment decisions. The study reflects an extraordinary global collaboration among hundreds of dedicated AIDS clinicians and thousands of their patients, all of whom should be commended for their contributions to this pivotal HIV/AIDS treatment study (http://www3.niaid.nih.gov/news/newsreleases/2006/nejmsmart.htm).

The latest U.S. statistics on incidence and prevalence of HIV/AIDS morbidity and mortality can be found on the CDC Web site at http://www.cdc.gov/hiv/stats/hasrlink.htm. The latest global statistics can be found on the UNAIDS Web site at http://www.unaids.org/en/HIV_data/Epidemiology/epi_slides.asp.

33.1 HIV Epidemiology and Transmission Factors: Risks and Risk Contexts

In recent years, researchers have found that the *contexts* in which the HIV pandemic is occurring have became *increasingly diverse (1)*. Thus, individual-level risks for HIV infection, which are at the core of the pandemic, have been powerfully influenced by social, structural, and population-level risks and protections—what might be called *risks contexts* for spread or control of epidemic HIV *(1,4,5)*. These risk contexts have been driven by a host of important factors, including the presence or absence of appropriate prevention tools and services, by enabling or undermining policy environments, by the protections or absence of human rights, by the levels of social tolerance or stigma, and by the civil strife and conflicts *(5–7)*. Even though they are more difficult to study than are individual-level variables, contextual factors may be crucial for understanding why the HIV epidemic has been controlled in some populations/regions and not in others *(1)*.

In several major studies using the case studies approach, increasing contextual heterogeneity was investigated in three

HIV epidemic contexts where the spread of HIV infection was ongoing or accelerating in 2006: (i) the emerging injection drug user (IDU)-driven epidemics across Eastern Europe, Central Asia, and the former Soviet Union; (ii) the emerging epidemic among men who have sex with men (MSM) in developing countries and among minority MSM in the United States; and (iii) the context of ongoing spread in southern Africa *(1)*.

33.1.1 IDU-Driven HIV Epidemics in Eurasia

According to United Nations estimates, IDUs accounted for approximately 10% of all new cases of HIV infection in 2005 but one third of all cases of HIV infection outside sub-Saharan Africa *(2)*. The countries in which the majority of HIV infections were attributed to injection drug use in 2005 included Russia, Ukraine, the Central Asia republics, Iran, China, Indonesia, Nepal, and Vietnam *(2,8,9)*.

Whereas, in general, the risks for HIV infection among IDUs include correlates of needle sharing and lending and borrowing of equipment, the frequency of injection, and the history of incarceration, a number of studies have found that sexual risks for HIV infection may also play an important role in the acquisition of disease in addition to the risks related to injection drug use *(10,11)*. Such "dual-risk" sexual and drug-injection behavior may be of particular importance among adult female IDUs and MSM IDUs *(10,11)*.

Beyond the individual level, the Eurasian HIV epidemics share at least three additional factors: (i) a marked increase in the production and trafficking of narcotics, primarily from Afghanistan, Myanmar, and Laos *(12–14)*; (ii) the widespread lack of evidence-based services for prevention and drug treatment of HIV infection *(12)*; and (iii) restrictive policy environments marked by police harassment, high rates of incarceration, human rights violations, and social stigma *(1)*. For example, opiate analogue substitution therapy still remains illegal in Russia and in much of the former Soviet Union republics *(6)*. One of the most punitive risk contexts is related to incarceration. Recent studies from Thailand, Iran, and Afghanistan have revealed that IDUs who have used drugs while incarcerated were >6 times more likely to become HIV-infected than were IDUs who did not use drugs while incarcerated *(15–17)*.

33.1.2 HIV Infections Among MSM

Since the first recognition of HIV infection and AIDS, it has been clearly demonstrated that in the United States and other developed countries, MSM have been disproportionately affected by the new epidemic. Thus, in 2003, estimates by the CDC have shown that 63% of all new HIV infections in the United States were among MSM *(18)*.

In 2005–2006, a new epidemic trend emerged: high rates of HIV infection among MSM in developing countries that were often not linked to heterosexual prevalence *(1)*. During the period, all reports showed substantial rates increase of HIV infections among MSM, whereas HIV infection rates among the general population (e.g., Senegal, Thailand, Cambodia) remained low and even decreased *(19–24)*. Overall, the prevalence of HIV infection among these men increased from 17.3% in 2003 to 28.3% in 2005 ($p < 0.05$); among the youngest men (aged ≤ 22 years), this prevalence increased from 12.9% to 22.3% ($p < 0.05$) *(1)*. Acquisition risks include—along with unprotected anal intercourse—frequency and number of sexual partners, IDU-related risks, and the use of methamphetamines *(25,26)*.

In many of the developing countries, homosexuality is both illegal and highly stigmatized *(20)*. Accordingly, UNAIDS has stated that vulnerability to HIV has been dramatically increased where sex between men is criminalized *(2)*. Even in countries like India where the existing law has been little enforced, the law legitimized police harassment of MSM and of MSM peer and outreach workers and actively inhibited efforts to prevent HIV infection *(1,27)*.

33.1.3 Generalized HIV/AIDS Epidemic in Southern Africa

In HIV/AIDS epidemic and high-prevalence zones of southern sub-Saharan Africa, there has been little evidence that the epidemic is being controlled *(1)*. Nearly one third of people infected with HIV worldwide live in this region, as do slightly over one half of all HIV-seropositive women aged ≥ 15 years *(2)*. This is in contrast with the lower prevalence and stable or decreasing rates of HIV infection observed across the eastern, western, and Horn regions of Africa (see Table 1 in Ref. *(1)*).

Whereas risk factors for the acquisition and transmission of HIV through heterosexual exposure have been well characterized, their relative importance has varied by location, and the relationships among biological, behavioral, and social risks are incompletely understood *(1)*. An increasing body of evidence suggests that herpes simplex virus-2 infection is a critical factor for infection *(28)*.

Male circumcision has emerged as a relative protective factor against HIV acquisition (see Section 32.2.12 in Chapter 32). Ecologic data regarding male circumcision have been supported by one prospective randomized trial, and its benefit has been confirmed in two others *(29)*. Furthermore, high prevalence of herpes simplex virus-2 infection and a low frequency of male circumcision have been identified in a four-city study of HIV infection in Africa *(30)* as key factors indicating high prevalence of HIV disease.

The use by males of condoms has been recognized as powerful protection against the acquisition and transmission of HIV and other sexually transmitted infections (see HIVNET/HPTN trial in Chapter 32).

Another important issue to be considered as a risk factor for HIV infection is the younger age of initial sexual activity among both male and female adolescents *(31,32)*. Marriages among adolescents have been promoted as protective against HIV infection. However, in many recent studies in southern Africa and beyond, such marriages have been implicated as a risk factor for HIV infection in young women *(33–35)* because of the low use of condoms by husbands with their wives and the high rates of extramarital sex by men *(36,37)*. Although African men and women have not reported a higher number of lifetime sexual partners, the level of concurrent partnerships has been much higher than in other regions of the world *(38)*.

Gender inequalities have been suggested by many as playing a central role, and they may be further exacerbated in environments of conflict and civil strife *(2,39)*.

Social mobility, largely as a result of labor migration patterns, has been another risk factor for the spread of HIV/AIDS in southern Africa. Thus, in 2003 there were nearly 2.5 million legal migrants working in South Africa, of whom the majority came from rural regions of South Africa and the neighboring countries of Lesotho, Botswana, and Mozambique *(40)*. The increased social and labor mobility of migrants, as well as movement of refugees from postconflict regions, have been implicated in the rising rates of HIV infection *(2)*.

33.2 HIV Epidemiology in Children

Most children living with HIV infection have acquired it through transmission of the virus from their mothers. Hence, the number of infants perinatally infected with HIV is directly proportional to the number of HIV-infected women of childbearing age *(41)* (http://womenchildrenhiv.org).

The first reports of children having AIDS appeared in 1982 *(42,43)*. Since those early days of the epidemic, more than 4 million children have died of AIDS-related illnesses *(44)* (http://womenchildrenhiv.org). Thus, in 2005 alone, an estimated 700,000 children were infected with HIV, and approximately 90% of those new infections were transmitted from mother to child *(41,44,45)* (http://womenchildrenhiv.org).

As new infections among women have been rising *(44,45)*, the number of children at risk of perinatal HIV infection has been rising accordingly. At present, women comprise nearly half of the estimated 40 million adults aged 15 to 49 living with HIV worldwide. In the worst affected region, sub-Saharan Africa, alone, close to 60% of HIV-infected adults (13.5 million) are women *(44)*, and 75% to 80% of the 2.3 million children estimated to be living with HIV/AIDS reside in sub-Saharan Africa *(45)*.

33.2.1 *Mother-to-Child HIV Transmission*

Mother-to-child transmission (MTCT) of HIV occurs during pregnancy and labor and after delivery through breast-feeding *(41)* (http://womenchildrenhiv.org) (see Section 32.2.4.1 in Chapter 32). Both terms *perinatal transmission* and *vertical transmission* are being used to describe MTCT, although technically the term *perinatal transmission* does not cover transmission through breast-feeding after the first few days of life *(41)*.

HIV infection during pregnancy and delivery occurs either by a break in the integrity of the placental barrier, the crossing of a mucosal surface after ingestion of contaminated maternal blood during delivery, or the direct transfer of maternal cells into the infant's circulation. Nevertheless, most infants born to HIV-infected mothers are uninfected. In published research, transmission rates in untreated mother-infant pairs vary from 13% in the European Collaborative Study to about 40% in sub-Saharan Africa *(41)* (http://womenchildrenhiv.org). High levels of maternal viremia, low maternal CD4$^+$ T-cell counts, advanced maternal disease, prolonged duration of ruptured membranes, chorioamnionitis, the presence of opportunistic infections, and the absence of elective cesarean section as a mode of delivery have been associated with an increased risk of transmission *(46)*.

Increased risk of HIV transmission through breast-feeding has usually been associated with prolonged breast-feeding, mixed feeding (feeding the child with breast milk as well as replacement feeds), the presence of mastitis, and the mother's HIV infection occurring during or shortly after pregnancy *(47)*. However, in areas where there are safe alternatives to breast-feeding, replacement feeding is strongly encouraged. When this is not possible, the World Health Organization has recommended exclusive breast-feeding *(48)*.

In 1995, after a clinical trial determined that zidovudine was able to reduce perinatal HIV transmission *(49)*, CDC and the American Academy of Pediatrics (AAP) recommended universal voluntary counseling and HIV testing for all pregnant women, to allow for a timely prophylactic use of zidovudine *(50,51)*. In 1999, a study by the Institute of Medicine revealed that the lack of timely HIV diagnosis in pregnant women was the largest contributor to continued perinatal

transmission in the United States *(52)* and recommended universal HIV screening of pregnant women—with notification of the patient and the option of declining the screening (i.e., the opt-out approach).

33.3 Epidemiology of HIV in the United States

In June 1981, the first cases of what was later described as acquired immunodeficiency syndrome (AIDS) in the United States were reported by CDC *(53,54)*.

Although AIDS had not been recognized as a new clinical syndrome until 1981, scientists examining earlier medical data have identified cases that appeared to fit the AIDS surveillance definition as early as the 1950s and 1960s *(55)*. For example, frozen tissue and serum samples were available for one of those possible early AIDS cases, a 15-year-old black male from St. Louis who was hospitalized in 1968 and died of an aggressive, disseminated Kaposi's sarcoma *(56)*. His tissue and serum specimens were HIV-antibody positive on Western blot and antigen-positive on ELISA. This appears to be the first confirmed case of HIV infection in the United States. As the patient had no history of travel out of the country, it is likely that that some other persons in the United States were infected with HIV as long ago as the 1960s, if not earlier *(54)*.

Since 1981, the HIV epidemic has continued to expand in the United States, and at the end of 2003, it was estimated that 1,039,000 to 1,185,000 persons were living with HIV/AIDS, of whom between 24% and 27% were unaware of their infection *(57)*.

During the period 1981–2006, the HIV epidemiology continued to evolve. Major epidemiologic features have included (i) the decrease in the overall incidence of AIDS; (ii) the substantial increase in survival after a diagnosis of AIDS, especially since highly active antiretroviral therapy (HAART) became the standard of care in 1996; and (iii) the continued disparities among racial/ethnic minority populations *(48,58)*.

Although considerable progress has been achieved in reducing the impact of the HIV/AIDS epidemic in the United States, certain populations, especially racial and ethnic minorities, continue to bear a disproportionate burden *(59)*, which can, at least partially, be attributed to late HIV diagnosis and differential access to care *(58,60)*.

The rate of overall decline in the incidence and death from AIDS in the United States in recent years was mostly attributed to widespread use of potent antiretroviral therapy. However, lately the decline has slowed, as problems have emerged such as failing therapies, inadequate access to HIV diagnosis and treatment, and incomplete adherence to complex therapeutic regimens, disproportionately involving minorities, women, adolescents, and IDUs. Furthermore, recent finding among MSM have shown that new HIV infection rates might be increasing, particularly among minority men.

It is estimated that 252,000 to 312,000 individuals in the United States are unaware that they have been infected with HIV and therefore are also unaware of their risk for transmitting the human immunodeficiency virus *(57)*. Thus, analysis of data collected by the National HIV Behavioral Surveillance System, which surveys populations at high risk for HIV infection to assess prevalence and trends in risk behavior, HIV testing, and use of preventive services, has revealed that among MSM surveyed in five U.S. cities, 25% were infected with HIV; and of those, 48% were unaware of their infection *(61)*. Recognizing this fact, CDC, NIAID, and other government agencies are using a comprehensive approach to better understand risk behaviors and barriers preventing persons from getting tested for HIV and accessing medical and preventive services *(61)*. As a result, CDC and the Council of State and Territorial Epidemiologists have recommended that all states and territories conduct confidential, name-based HIV surveillance *(48)*. This integrated surveillance approach will provide the only population-based monitoring of the HIV epidemic in the United States yielding important epidemiologic data to local, state, and federal agencies to improve resource allocation, program planning, and evaluation for HIV-prevention and treatment services *(48)*.

33.3.1 Prevalence and Incidence of HIV Infection in the United States

Trends in the characteristics of AIDS cases provide important information about how the epidemic is evolving over time. In considering these trends, it should also be remembered that the median time from contracting HIV to conversion to AIDS is about 10 years in adults, even without effective treatments—that is to say, in viewing trends in AIDS cases, the observed infection patterns came mostly from a decade earlier *(54)*.

33.3.1.1 Estimating HIV Prevalence

The prevalence of HIV infection has been somewhat easier to obtain than the incidence data. However, because there is no representative national surveillance system for prevalent infections either, estimates of HIV prevalence have been based on (i) the reporting of new HIV infections from states with reporting laws; (ii) a variety of serologic surveys; and (iii) mathematical models that make use of reported AIDS cases *(54)*.

In general, the prevalence of HIV in the United States has been estimated using two different methods:

- Gathering results from serosurveys in different populations and different geographic regions. Next, these results are put together with estimates of the size of the populations at risk, followed by an overall estimate that has synthesized all the data. The drawbacks of this approach include (i) most of the serosurveys are not population-based and are difficult to generalize beyond the venue in which the HIV testing was done; (ii) coverage of the geographic regions and specific subpopulations at risk is not complete; and (iii) the sizes of the populations at risk are not known with any precision—that is, the numbers of homosexual men and injecting drug users in the United States are particularly difficult to estimate *(54)*.

- Estimating prevalence by using "back calculation"—a mathematical model that combines the available data on the numbers of reported AIDS cases and the incubation period distribution of AIDS (the mathematical function that estimates the probability of developing AIDS for each year after HIV infection) to derive how many HIV infections did occur during years past *(62)*. With information on past infections and AIDS cases, current HIV prevalence can be estimated. However, this methodology would require fairly complete surveillance of AIDS cases and an accurate estimate of the incubation period distribution. It is limited by its inability to estimate HIV infections in recent years with any precision. More significantly, the large, and yet largely unmodeled, effect of antiretroviral therapy on the incubation period has rendered back-calculation currently ineffective and requiring an adjustment to the incubation distribution in estimating HIV prevalence. For this reason, back-calculation may no longer be a useful method for estimating HIV prevalence *(54)*.

33.3.1.2 Estimation of HIV Incidence

Although estimates on HIV incidence are more difficult to define than are the prevalence figures, they are more informative about the effects of prevention efforts and the future of the HIV epidemic *(54)*. There are several methodologies currently used to obtain estimates of HIV incidence, including:

- Observing seroconversions by enrolling an HIV-negative population in a longitudinal or cohort study, and testing the participants at regular intervals for new HIV infections, thereby deriving an incidence rate (number of new infections per total number of person-years of follow-up) *(63)*. Although longitudinal studies with incident infections have provided valuable data, they are limited by several factors: the expense of conducting such studies;

the characteristics of the population enrolled; and the consideration that the longer the cohort is followed, the less likely it is that they are still representative of the population from which they were recruited—for example, the individuals at highest risk would be likely to get infected first, and if no new members are recruited to the cohort, it will represent a sample comprising individuals with progressively lower average risk over time *(54)*.

- Estimating HIV incidence by conducting serial cross-sectional surveys in a population *(64)*. This methodology does not estimate HIV incidence directly, but rather indirectly, by estimating the slope of the seroprevalence curve against time if the population being surveyed remains representative over time and if deaths and other losses to follow-up can be considered negligible *(54)*.

- Using the "capture-recapture" method of estimating HIV incidence, which is a variant of the cross-sectional survey approach used to study wildlife populations. It requires the use of a unique identifier, but not necessarily names, of individuals included in repeated surveys, so that the seroconverters among those repeatedly tested can be identified *(54)*.

- Using "back calculation," the same approach used in estimating HIV prevalence *(54)*.

- Estimating HIV incidence by using two HIV enzyme immunoassays: one is a current, highly sensitive test, and the other has been made insensitive ("detuned") in order to identify recent seroconverters from a single cross-sectional sample *(54)*. As the quantity and avidity of antibody in the peripheral blood increases progressively during the first weeks and months after HIV infection, a newly infected person will test positive on the sensitive assay and negative on the less sensitive "detuned" assay. If the average time a newly infected person testing positive on the first test and negative on the second is known, an annualized incidence rate can be extrapolated from the cross-sectional samples *(66)*. One source of variation observed in this method has been the viral subtype (clade) tested. In addition, the average window of time captured by the two assays needs to be determined and validated separately for assays of different manufacture. Furthermore, false-positive seroconversions can occur in individuals with late-stage HIV infection, in which antibody levels decline, and in persons receiving antiretroviral treatment. Despite these limitations, this method has grown in use because it is the only method that would allow an incidence estimate from a single cross-sectional sample *(54,67)*.

- Estimating HIV incidence not *per se* but by using the number of reported AIDS cases in the youngest age range of adult cases (ages 13 to 25) as a surrogate for recent trends in incidence *(68)*. The justification for this approach is that onset of sexual and drug-using risk behavior in the teenage years (or later) would lead to the inference that AIDS cases in this age group will be predominately those with a short incubation time from infection to AIDS and that, therefore, most of the cases will reflect relatively recent infections (e.g., 5 years on average). Although as a crude indicator of recent trends of HIV infection, this approach has some validity, in general, even if 5 years on average would seem not as recent as one would like the data to be *(54)*.

33.3.2 HIV-2 Infection in the United States

The immunodeficiency virus was first isolated in France in 1983 and called first the lymphadenopathy-associated virus (LAV) *(69)*. In 1984, the same virus was isolated by U.S. scientists and designated as human T-lymphotropic virus type III (HTLV-III) *(70)*. Also in 1984, the same virus was isolated again in the United States and published as AIDS-associated retrovirus (ARV) *(71)*. The fact that all three of these designations for the same virus had appeared in the literature prompted the International Committee on the Taxonomy of Viruses in 1986 to select a new designation: human immunodeficiency virus (HIV). However, with the discovery by L. Montagnier's group in late 1986 of the related HIV-2 virus in West Africa, the original HIV virus became HIV-1 *(72)*. Nearly all cases of HIV infection in the United States are due to HIV-1. Reports of HIV-2 infection have been rare, with the first known case of a West African woman identified in 1987 *(54)*. Through June 30, 1995, 62 persons were diagnosed with HIV-2 infection *(62)*. A 1996 serosurvey of 832 patients at a New York hospital serving a community with a high percentage of West African immigrants did not find any HIV-2 infections that were confirmed by Western blot analysis *(73)*. In 1998, the third HIV-2 antibody-positive blood was identified belonging to a native of an HIV-2-endemic country *(74)*. Beginning in 1992, FDA recommended that whole blood and blood components be screened with combination HIV-1/HIV-2 enzyme immunoassays *(75)*.

33.4 NIAID Involvement in Epidemiology Research

In general, NIAID's involvement in epidemiologic research associated with HIV/AIDS is designed to explore the biology of HIV and the clinical course of the human disease, including the risk factors leading to transmission and the development and progression of the disease. Worldwide, NIAID-supported epidemiologic research has also been accelerating in Asia, Africa, and the Caribbean where the populations have been severely affected by the disease. In addition to basic epidemiology, which studies the proportion of populations affected by HIV/AIDS and the rate at which the new infections occur, molecular epidemiology is aimed at better defining the types of viruses circulating in a particular population. The introduction of HAART under the President's Emergency Plan for HIV/AIDS Relief (PEPFAR) program has been initiated, and access to therapy is rapidly expanding in many countries under this program. This has been accompanied by research on the optimal use of therapy in these HIV-infected populations. Optimal therapeutic regimens for HIV may differ in populations affected by other health stressors, such as other infectious diseases and nutritional deficits. Research on the availability, use, and success of HAART in developing economy nations is now under way. Additional research in these settings is being accelerated.

33.4.1 Major HIV/AIDS Programmatic Accomplishment and Developments

- The *Women's Interagency HIV Study (WIHS)* and the *Multicenter AIDS Cohort Study (MACS)* are the two largest observational studies of HIV/AIDS in women and homosexual or bisexual men, respectively, in the United States (http://www3.niaid.nih.gov/news/focuson/hiv/resources/macs_and_wihs.htm). These studies have repeatedly made major contributions to understanding how HIV is spread, how the disease progresses, and how it can best be treated. The research will focus on contemporary questions such as the interactions between HIV infection, aging, and long-term treatment; between HIV and cardiovascular disease; and host genetics and its influence on susceptibility to infection, disease progression, and response to therapy. This year, the MACS completed its 22nd year of research and the WIHS completed its 12th year of research. The four MACS clinical centers are located at Johns Hopkins University, Baltimore, MD; University of Pittsburgh, Pittsburgh, PA; Howard Brown Memorial Clinic/Northwestern University, Chicago, IL; and the University of California at Los Angeles, Los Angeles CA. The six WIHS clinical centers are located at Research Foundation of SUNY, Brooklyn, NY; Montefiore/Bronx Lebanon Hospital, Bronx, NY; Georgetown University, Washington, DC; Cook County Hospital, Chicago, IL; University of California at San Francisco, San Francisco, CA; and the University of Southern California, Los Angeles, CA. The data and statistical management center for both studies is at the Bloomberg School of Public Health at the Johns Hopkins University.
- In July 2006, seven regional centers were funded as part of NIAID's *International Epidemiologic Databases to Evaluate AIDS (IeDEA)* initiative (http://www.iedea-hiv.org/). Funded regional centers include North America, South America/Caribbean, Australia/Asia, and four regions in Africa—West, Central, East, and Southern Africa. These regional centers would provide data from more than 200,000 HIV-infected persons from 38 different countries. Each regional center, in collaboration with multiple independent researchers within its region, has put forth a scientific agenda to address relevant regional HIV research questions. The sources of data to answer these questions include independently funded investigators and clinical networks, domestic and international cohorts, individual clinicians caring for large numbers of HIV-infected persons, and national or local databases. Their proposed research plans include (i) describing the natural history and complications of HIV infection; (ii) the impact of HIV and TB; (iii) evaluating strategies to provide ART to children and adults; (iv) optimizing adherence to HIV treatment; (v) monitoring care and clinical outcomes of ART in adults, children, and pregnant women—particularly treatment toxicities, tuberculosis, other opportunistic infections, immune reconstitution syndrome, hepatitis B co-infection, and viral resistance; (vi) examining the genetic variation of the HIV virus; (vii) evaluating the effectiveness of ART; and (viii) describing the effects of long-term treatment regimens and the effects of aging and malignancy. Although many of these research topics can be and have been addressed by individual cohorts, one strength of the IeDEA initiative is the increase in statistical power gained through combining cohort data. In August 2006, the IeDEA Executive Committee, comprising regional principal investigators and NIAID scientists under the Cooperative Agreement, held their first meeting to develop a scientific agenda for the larger consortium. This required a standardization of data elements from all regional centers, thereby producing not only a higher quality of data but also the identification of standards by which future research could be modeled. Many regions anticipate expanding their coverage during the later years of their 5-year funding. The National Institute of Child Health and Human Development (NICHD) is cofunding this initiative, as several regions have access to data from HIV-infected children.
- Through two funding mechanisms, NIAID is supporting research on the long-term effects of HAART in U.S. populations. The *CFAR Network of Integrated Clinical Systems (CNICS)* project represents an ongoing consolidation of data on an extremely large number of patients in clinical care in centers of excellence across the United States (http://www.cnicsres.ucsd.edu/). This database is designed to standardize and harmonize large numbers of patient records in order to address research questions that cannot be answered at individual clinics. Building upon the platform of CNICS,

the North American IeDEA regional award will further increase the numbers of patients included in the database.

- Data from NIAID-funded cohorts have been used to advance novel statistical methods that account for analytic challenges in observational data. These methods facilitate analyses that address questions on optimal treatment strategies for patients initiating ARV therapies, interrupting therapy, or initiating salvage therapies.

33.5 Recent Scientific Advances

- *Study on the Survival Benefits of AIDS Treatment in the United States.* The results of this study showed the dramatic impact that advances in ART have made in the United States on the long-term survival of HIV-infected patients and those who have developed AIDS. It also emphasized the importance of expanding HIV treatment worldwide, especially in resource-limited countries, and the potential for huge survival benefits in those settings *(76)*.

- *Evaluating the Effectiveness of Highly Active Antiretroviral Therapy by Race/Ethnicity.* The use of HAART has resulted in a dramatic reduction in the clinical progression of HIV infection, as shown by data from the U.S. Military's Tri-Service AIDS Clinical Consortium Natural History Study *(77)*. The multivariable models have evaluated race, pre-HAART and HAART eras, age, gender, and military service. In the large multiracial cohort with equal access to health care, the HIV treatment outcomes by race/ethnicity were similar.

- *Patterns of the Hazard of Death After AIDS Through the Evaluation of Antiretroviral Therapy.* The objective of the study was to characterize changing survival patterns after development of AIDS from 1984 to 2004 when different antiretroviral therapies were being introduced *(78)*. Data from the study have confirmed a sustained beneficial effect of HAART, even in individuals with clinical AIDS and extensive treatment histories, and attenuated concerns about the emergence of resistance. The data also augured that a substantial number of HIV-infected individuals may require care for very long periods

References

1. Beyrer, C. (2007) HIV epidemiology update and transmission factors: risks and risks contexts—16th International AIDS Conference Epidemiology Plenary, *Clin. Infect. Dis.*, **44**, 981–987.
2. UNAIDS. (2006) 2006 Report on the global AIDS epidemic. Geneva: United Nations.
3. El-Sadr, W. M., Lundgren, J. D., Neaton, J. D., et al. (2006) CD4$^+$ count-guided interruption of antiretroviral treatment, *N. Engl. J. Med.*, **355**, 2283–2296.
4. Rhodes, T. and Simic, M. (2005) Transition and the HIV risk environment, *Br. Med. J.*, **331**, 220–223.
5. Cohen, J., Chleifer, R., and Tate, T. (2005) AIDS in Uganda: the human-rights dimension, *Lancet*, **365**, 2075–2076.
6. Malinowska-Sempruch, K., Hoover, J., and Alexandrova, A. (2004) Unintended consequences: drug policies fuel the HIV in Russia and Ukraine. In: *War on Drugs, HIV/AIDS, and Human Rights* (Malinowska-Sempruch, K. and Gallagher, S., eds.), Idea Press, New York, pp. 9–25.
7. Loff, B., Gaze, B., and Fairley, C. (2000) Prostitution, public health, and human rights law, *Lancet*, **356**, 1764.
8. Aceijas, C., Stimson, G. V., Hickman, M., and Rhodes, T. (2004) Global overview of injecting drug use and HIV infection among injecting drug users, *AIDS*, **18**, 2295–2303.
9. Orekhovsky, V., Calzavara, L., Saldanha, V., Yakovler, A., et al. (2002) Determinants and solutions to the IDU/HIV epidemics in Russia: perceptions of focus groups participants, *14th Int. Conf. on AIDS, Barcelona*, July 7–12; 14, abstract TuPeE 183.
10. Beyrer, C., Sripaipan, T., Tovanabutra, S., et al. (2005) High HIV hepatitis C and sexual risks among drug-using men who have sex with men in northern Thailand, *AIDS*, **19**, 1535–1540.
11. Ferreira, A. D., Caiaffa, W. T., Bastos, F. I., and Mingoti, S. A. (2006) Profile of male Brazilian injecting drug users who have sex with men, *Cad. Aude Publica*, **22**, 849–860.
12. Beyrer, C. (2003) Human immunodeficiency virus infection rates and heroin trafficking: fearful symmetries, *Bull. Narc.*, **2**, 400–417.
13. Beyrer, C., Razak, M. H., Lisam, K., Chen, J., Lui, W., and Yu, X. F. (2000) Overland heroin trafficking routes and HIV-1 spread in south and south-east Asia, *AIDS*, **14**, 75–83.
14. United Nations' Office on Drug and Crime (UNODC) (2006) World drug report for 2006. Geneva: United Nations Publications (http://www.unodc.org/unodc/world_drug_report.html).
15. Razak, M. H., Jittiwutikarn, J., Suriyanon, V., et al. (2003) HIV prevalence and risks among injection and noninjection drug users in northern Thailand: need for comprehensive HIV prevention programs, *J. Acquir. Immune Defic. Syndr.*, **33**, 259–266.
16. Zamani, S., Kihara, M., Gouya, M. M., et al. (2005) Prevalence of and factors associated with HIV infection among drug users visiting treatment centers in Tehran, Iran, *AIDS*, **19**(7), 709–716.
17. Todd, C. S., Abed, A., Strathdee, S., Botros, A., Safi, N., and Earhart, K. C. (2006) Prevalence of HIV, viral hepatitis, syphilis, and risk behaviors among injecting drug users in Kabul, Afghanistan, *Program and Abstracts of the 16th International AIDS Conference, Toronto 2006*, abstract TUAC0304.
18. Centers for Disease Control and Prevention (2004) HIV/AIDS surveillance report: 2003. Report no. 15. Atlanta, GA: U.S. Department of Health and Human Services.
19. Tabet, S., Sanchez, J., Lama, J., et al. (2002) HIV, syphilis and heterosexual bridging among Peruvian men who have sex with men, *AIDS*, **16**, 1271–1277.
20. Wade, A. S., Kane, C. T., Diallo, P. A., et al. (2005) HIV infection and sexually transmitted infections among men who have sex with men in Senegal, *AIDS*, **19**, 2133–2140.
21. van Griensven, F., Thanprasertsuk, S., Jommaroeng, R., et al. (2005) Evidence of a previously undocumented epidemic of HIV infection among men who have sex with men in Bangkok, Thailand, *AIDS*, **19**, 521–526.
22. Dandona, L., Dandona, R., Kumar, G. A., Gutierrez, J. P., McPherson, S., and Bertozzi, S. M. (2004) How much attention is needed towards men who sell sex to men for HIV prevention in India? *BMC Public Health*, **6**, 31.
23. Girault, S. P., Saidel, T., Song, S. N., et al. (2004) HIV, STIs, and sexual behaviors among men who have sex with men in Phnom Penh, Cambodia, *AIDS Educ. Prev.*, **16**, 31–44.

24. Action for AIDS. (2006) The enemy within: HIV and STI rates increasing among men who have sex with men (MSM). Singapore; (http://www.afa.org.sg/msm/latest/STI.htm).

25. Koblin, B. A., Husnik, M. J., Colfax, G., et al. (2006) Risk factors for HIV infection among men who have sex with men, *AIDS*, **20**, 731–739.

26. Buchbinder, S. P., Vittinghoff, E., Heagerty, P. J., et al. (2005) Sexual risk, nitrite inhalant use, and lack of circumcision associated with HIV seroconversion in men who have sex with men in the United States, *J. Acquir. Immune Defic. Syndr.*, **39**, 82–89.

27. George, N. (2006) India may scrap gay law over HIV fear, Associated Press, July 26.

28. Corey, L., Wald, A., Celum, C. L., and Quinn, T. C. (2004) The effects of herpes simplex virus-2 on HIV-1 acquisition and transmission: a review of two overlapping epidemics, *J. Acquir. Immune Defic. Syndr.*, **35**, 435–445.

29. Auvert, B., Taljaard, D., Lagarde, E., Sobngwi-Tambekou, J., Sitta, R., and Puren, A. (2005) Randomized, controlled intervention trial of male circumcision for reduction of HIV infection risk: the ANRS 1265 trial, *PLos Med.*, **2**, e298.

30. Auvert, B., Buve, A., Ferry, B., et al. (2001) Ecological and individual level analysis of risk factors for HIV infection in four urban populations in sub-Saharan Africa with different levels of HIV infection, *AIDS*, **15**(Suppl. 4), 15–30.

31. Holmes, K. K., Levine, R., and Weaver, M. (2004) Effectiveness of condoms in preventing sexually transmitted infections, *Bull. WHO*, **82**, 451–461.

32. Pettifor, A. E., van der Straten, A., Dunbar, M. S., Shiboski, S. C., and Padian, N. S. (2004) Early age of first sex: a risk factor for HIV infection among women in Zimbabwe, *AIDS*, **18**, 1435–1442.

33. Clark, S. (2004) Early marriage and HIV risk in sub-Saharan Africa, *Stud. Fam. Plann.*, **35**, 149–160.

34. Xu, S. F., Kilmarx, P. H., Supawitkul, S., et al. (2000) HIV-1 seroprevalence, risk factors, and preventive behaviors among women in northern Thailand, *J. Acquir. Immune Defic. Syndr.*, **25**, 353–359.

35. Bhattacharya, G. (2004) Sociocultural and behavioral contexts of condom use in heterosexual married couples in India: challenges to the HIV prevention program, *Health Educ. Behav.*, **31**, 101–117.

36. Kimuna, S. and Djiamba, Y. (2005) Wealth and extramarital sex among men in Zambia, *Int. Fam. Plan. Perspect.*, **31**, 83–89.

37. Shisana, S. O., Rehle, T., Shimbayi, L. C., et al. (2005) South African national HIV prevalence, HIV incidence, behaviour and communication survey, 2005. Cape Town, South Africa: HSRC Press.

38. Halperin, D. T. and Epstein, H. (2004) Concurrent sexual partnerships help to explain Africa's high HIV prevalence: implications for prevention, *Lancet*, **364**, 4–6.

39. Mills, E. J., Singh, S., Nelson, B. D., and Nachega, J. B. (2006) The impact of conflict on HIV/AIDS in sub-Saharan Africa, *Int. J. STD AIDS*, **17**, 713–717.

40. Lurie, M. N., Williams, B. G., Zuma, K., et al. (2003) The impact of migration on HIV-1 transmission in South Africa: a study of migrant and nonmigrant men and their partners, *Sex. Transm. Dis.*, **30**, 149–156.

41. Global Health Counil. Epidemiology of HIV in children (2002) In: *Women, Children, and HIV: Resources for Prevention and Treatment* (http://www.womenchildrenhiv.org/sources/view.php3?id=336).

42. Ammann, A. J. (1983) Is there an acquired immune deficiency syndrome in infants and children? *Pediatrics*, **72**(3), 430–432.

43. Oleske, J., Minnefor, A., Cooper, R., Jr., Thomas, K., dela Cruz, A., Ahdieh, H., Guerrero, I., Joshi, V. V., and Desposito, F. (1983) Immune deficiency syndrome in children, *JAMA*, **249**(17), 2345–2349.

44. UNAIDS (2005) AIDS epidemic update 2005, UNAIDS Geneva, Switzerland.

45. UNAIDS. (2004) Report on the global AIDS epidemic, UNAIDS Geneva, Switzerland.

46. Magder, L. S., Mofenson, L., Paul, M. E., Zorrilla, C. D., Blattner, W. A., Tuomala, R. E., LaRussa, P., Landesman, S., and Rich, K. C. (2005) Risk factors for in utero and intrapartum transmission of HIV, *J. Acquir. Immune Defic. Syndr.*, **38**(1), 87–95.

47. World Health Organization (2001) New data on the prevention of mother-to-child transmission of HIV and their policy implication: conclusion and recommendation. WHO Technical Consultation on behalf of the UNFPA/UNICEF/WHO/UNAIDS Inter-Agency Task Team on Mother-to-Child Transmission of HIV. Report No. WHO/RHR/01.28.Geneva: World Health Organization, 2001.

48. Schneider, E., Glynn, M. K., Kajese, T., and McKenna, M. T. (2006) Centers for Disease Control. Epidemiology of HIV/AIDS – United States, 1981–2005, *Morb. Mortal. Wkly Rep.*, **55**(21), 589–592.

49. Connor, E. M., Sperling, R. S., Gelber, R., et al. (1994) Reduction of maternal-infant transmission of human immunodeficiency virus type 1 with zidovudine treatment. Pediatric AIDS Clinical Trials Group Protocol 076 Study Group, *N. Engl. J. Med.*, **331**, 1173–1180.

50. Centers for Disease Control (1995) U.S. Public Health Service recommendations for human immunodeficiency virus counseling and voluntary testing for pregnant women, *Morb. Mortal. Wkly Rep.*, **44**(No. RR-7).

51. Provisional Committee on Pediatric AIDS, American Academy of Pediatrics (1995) Perinatal human immunodeficiency virus testing, *Pediatrics*, **95**, 303–307.

52. Institute of Medicine, Committee on Perinatal Transmission of HIV, Commission on Behavioural and Social Sciences and Education (1999) *Reducing the Odds: Preventing Perinatal Transmission of HIV in the United States*, Washington, DC: National Academy Press.

53. Centers for Disease Control and Prevention (1981) *Pneumocystis pneumonia* - Los Angeles, *Morb. Mortal. Wkly Rep.*, **30**, 250–252.

54. Osmond, D. H. (2003) Epidemiology of HIV/AIDS in the United States. HIV InSite Knowledge Base Chapter (http://hivinsite.ucsf.edu/InSite?page=kb-01-03).

55. Huminer, D., Rosenfeld, J. B., and Pitlik, S. D. (1987) AIDS in the pre-AIDS era, *Rev. Infect. Dis.*, **9**(6), 1102–1108.

56. Garry, R. F., Witte, M. H., Gottlieb, A. A., Elvin-Lewis, M., Gottlieb, M. S., Witte, C. L., Alexander, S. S., Cole, W. R., and Drake, W. L., Jr. (1988) Documentation of an AIDS virus infection in the United States in 1968, *J. Am. Med. Assoc.*, **260**(14), 2085–2087.

57. Glynn, M. K. and Rhodes, P. (2005) Estimated HIV prevalence in the United States at the end of 2003, *Proc. 2005 National HIV Prevention Conference, Atlanta, GA, June 14, 2005*, abstract T1-B1101.

58. Fenton, K. A. and Valdiserri, R. O. (2006) Centers for Disease Control. Twenty-five years of HIV/AIDS – United States, 1981–2006, *Morb. Mortal. Wkly Rep.*, **55**(21), 585–589.

59. Centers for Disease Control (2006) Racial/ethnic disparities in diagnoses of HIV/AIDS – 33 states, 2001–2004, *Morb. Mortal. Wkly Rep.*, **55**, 121–125.

60. Gebo, K. A., Fleishman, J. A., Conviser, R., et al. (2005) Racial and gender disparities in receipt of highly active antiretroviral therapy persist in a multistate sample of HIV patients in 2001, *J. Acquir. Immune Defic. Syndr.*, **38**, 96–103.

61. Centers for Disease Control (2005) HIV prevalence, unrecognized infection, and HIV testing among men who have sex with men – five US cities, June 2004–April 2005, *Morb. Mortal. Wkly Rep.*, **54**, 597–601.

62. Centers for Disease Control (1995) HIV-2 infection among blood and plasma donors—United States, June 1992-June 1995, *Morb. Mortal. Wkly Rep.*, **44**(32), 603–606.

63. Winkelstein, W., Jr., Samuel, M., Padian, N. S., Wiley, J. A., Lang, W., Anderson, R. E., and Levy, J. A. (1987) The San Francisco men's Health Study. III. Reduction in human immunodeficiency virus transmission among homosexual/bisexual men, *Am. J. Public Health*, **77**(6), 685–689.

64. Brundage, J. F., Burke, D. S., Gardner, L. I., McNeil, J. G., Goldenbaum, M., Visintine, R., Redfield, R. R., Peterson, M., and Miller, R. N. (1990) Tracking the spread of the HIV infection epidemic among young adults in the United States: results of the first four years of screening among civilian applicants for U.S. military service, *J. Acquir. Immune Defic. Syndr.*, **3**(12), 1168–1180.

65. Moss, A. R., Vranizan, K., Gorter, R., Bacchetti, P., Watters, J., and Osmond, D. (1994) HIV seroconversion in intravenous drug users in San Francisco, *AIDS*, **8**(2), 223–231.

66. Janssen, R. S., Satten, G. A., Stramer, S. L., Rawal, B. D., O'Brien, T. R., Weiblen, B. J., Hecht, F. M., Jack, N., Cleghorn, F. R., Kahn, J. O., Chesney, M. A., and Busch, M. P. (1998) New testing strategy to detect early HIV-1 infection for use in incidence estimates and for clinical and prevention purposes, *J. Am. Med. Assoc.*, **280**(1), 42–48.

67. Schwarcz, S., Kellogg, T., McFarland, W., Louie, B., Kohn, R., Busch, M., Katz, M., Bolan, G., Klausner, J., and Weinstock, H. (2001) Differences in the temporal trends of HIV seroincidence and seroprevalence among sexually transmitted disease clinic patients, 1989–1998: application of the serologic testing algorithm for recent HIV seroconversion, *Am. J. Epidemiol.*, **153**(10), 925–934.

68. Denning, P. H., Jones, J. L., and Ward, J. W. (1997) Recent trends in the HIV epidemic in adolescent and young adult gay and bisexual men, *J. Acquir. Immune Defic. Syndr. Hum Retrovirol.*, **16**(5), 374–379.

69. Barre-Sinoussi, F., Chermann, J. C., Rey, F., Nugeyre, M. T., Chamaret, S., Gruest, J., Dauguet, C., Axler-Blin, C., Vezinet-Brun, F., Rouzioux, C., Rozenbaum, W., and Montagnier, L. (1983) Isolation of a T-lymphotropic retrovirus from a patient at risk for acquired immunodeficiency syndrome (AIDS), *Science*, **220**(4599), 868–871.

70. Gallo, R. C., Salahuddin, S. Z., Popovic, M., Shearer, G. M., Kaplan, M., Haynes, B. F., Palker, T. J., Redfield, R., Oleske, J., Safai, B., et al. (1984) Frequent detection and isolation of cytopathic retroviruses (HTLV-III) from patients with AIDS and at risk for AIDS, *Science*, **224**(4648), 500–503.

71. Levy, J. A., Hoffmann, A. D., Kramer, S. M., Landis, J. A., Shimabukuro, J. M., and Oshiro, L. S. (1984) Isolation of lymphocytopathic retroviruses from San Francisco patients with AIDS, *Science*, **225**(4664), 840–842.

72. Guyader, M., Emerman, M., Sonigo, P., Clavel, F., Montagnier, L., and Alizon, M. (1987) Genome organization and transactivation of the human immunodeficiency virus type 2, *Nature*, **326**(6114), 662–669.

73. Irwin, K. L., Olivo, N., Schable, C., Weber, J. T., Janssen, R., and Ernest, J. (1996) Absence of human immunodeficiency virus type 2 infection among patients in a hospital serving a New York community at high risk for infection. Centers for Disease Control and Prevention/Bronx-Lebanon Hospital Center HIV Serosurvey Team, *Transfusion*, **36**(8), 731–733.

74. Sullivan, M. T., Guido, E. A., Metler, R. P., Schable, C. A., Williams, A. E., and Stramer, S. L. (1998) Identification and characterization of an HIV-2 antibody-positive donor in the United States, *Transfusion*, **38**(2), 189–193.

75. George, J. R., Rayfield, M. A., Phillips, S., Heyward, W. L., Krebs, J. W., Odehouri, K., Soudre, R., De Cock, K. M., and Schochetman, G. (1990) Efficacies of US Food and Drug Administration-licensed HIV-1-screening enzyme immunoassays for detecting antibodies to HIV-2, *AIDS*, **4**(4), 321–326.

76. Walensky, R. P., Paltiel, A. D., Losina, F., Mercincavage, L. M., Schackman, B. R., Sax, P. E., Weinstein, M. C., and Freedberg, K. A. (2006) The survival benefits of AIDS treatment in the United States. *J. Infect. Dis.*, **194**(1), 11–19.

77. Silverberg, M. J., Wegner, S. A., Milazzo, M. J., McKaig, R. G., Williams, C. F., Agan, B. K., Armstrong, A. W., Gange, S. J., Hawkes, C., O'Connell, R. J., Ahuja, S. K., and Dolan, M. J., for the Tri-Service AIDS Clinical Consortium Natural History Study Group (2006) Effectiveness of highly-active antiretroviral therapy by race/ethnicity, *AIDS*, **20**(11), 1531–1538.

78. Schneider, M. F., Gange, S. J., Williams, C. M., Anastos, K., Greenblatt, R. M., Kingsley, L., Detels, R., and Munoz, A. (2005) Patterns of the hazard of death after AIDS through the evolution of antiretroviral therapy, *AIDS*, **19**(17), 2009–2018.

Chapter 34

HIV Therapeutics: Antiretroviral Drugs and Immune-Based Therapies

By providing valuable information about the human immunodeficiency virus (HIV), basic research is one of the cornerstones of the Division of AIDS (DAIDS) therapeutic clinical research efforts. Research supported by DAIDS has defined treatment guidelines for HIV infection and associated opportunistic infections, prophylactic regimens for secondary infections, and biological markers for predicting the effectiveness of therapeutics and disease progression.

Results from clinical trials have demonstrated that highly active antiretroviral therapy (HAART) has been very effective, and even suppresses the HIV viral load to undetectable levels in many HIV-infected individuals. However, even while greatly reducing the mortality, HAART still cannot suppress the virus indefinitely, as the latent virus persists in some tissue reservoirs. In addition, it is still not fully understood how to completely restore the anti-HIV-specific immune function. Also, the long-term consequences of HIV drug resistance are still not defined. Other health problems such as end-organ failure, especially in patients co-infected with hepatitis B and C viruses, and the ever present threat of opportunistic infections are far from being resolved.

Major research goals and objectives for NIAID-supported research in antiretroviral drugs and immune-based therapies include (http://www3.niaid.nih.gov/research/topics/HIV/therapeutics/intro/default.htm):

- Evaluating novel therapeutic strategies and intervention for HIV/AIDS and the complications of therapeutic intervention in all stages of the HIV infection.
- Strengthening the coordination between clinical therapeutics and basic research, with emphasis on the rapid translation of basic research discoveries into clinical practice.
- Continuing to support research toward development of new antiretroviral agents and new HIV targets.
- Assessing the role of immune-based therapies (e.g., IL-2, therapeutic immunogens) in the development of anti-HIV immune responses, control of HIV replication, and complete restoration of immunity.
- Developing and implementing a clinical agenda in regions/countries with limited resources.

- Determining the impact of HAART on disease and preventing HIV transmission.
- Evaluating the effects of viral and host factors, including human genetic factors, on responses to anti-HIV treatment.
- Studying the pathogenesis, natural history, and impact of early treatment intervention strategies in the context of acute HIV-1 infection. In this context, the understanding of the natural mechanisms of defense that succeed and fail upon initial infection will assist in designing further immune-based trials and interventions and will contribute important information to the design of protective vaccines.

34.1 HIV Reverse Transcriptase

The human immunodeficiency virus, a member of the Retroviridae family, has a relatively small, single-stranded, positive sense ribonucleic acid (RNA) genome that contains three small genes (*gag, pol,* and *env*), as well as regulatory (*tat* and *rev*) and accessory (*vif, nef, vpr,* and *vpu*) genes (1).

The virus-encoded deoxyribonucleic acid (DNA) polymerase has been a major target for anti-HIV drug discovery because it produces copies of the viral genome, a key step of HIV replication. The retroviral polymerases are commonly referred to as reverse transcriptases (RTs) because the flow of genetic information is coming from the RNA to the DNA; that is, the opposite direction to that normally specified. Because of its important role in HIV replication, reverse transcriptase has been a major target in research to discover anti-HIV drugs and the subject of intense structural biology studies (1–5).

The reverse transcriptase represents a multifunctional enzyme that functions as RNA-dependent DNA polymerase with two activities: DNA-dependent DNA polymerase, and ribonuclease H (RNase H) (6). After DNA synthesis has been initiated, the conversion of virus genomic RNA into DNA is a multistep process involving enzymatic steps interspersed by a series of strand transfers. The end product of this process is proviral DNA, which is extended relative to the genomic RNA through a duplication of the long-terminal repeat region. Then, the proviral DNA is incorporated into the host genome by HIV integrase (1).

The coding sequence for the reverse transcriptase is located in the *pol* gene, which also contains protease and integrase enzymes. The *pol* gene is then translated as a *gag-pol* fusion protein, followed by the cleavage of the protease as well as other *gag* and *pol* proteins, including RT, from the polyprotein (1).

The recombinant HIV reverse transcriptase can form a homodimer (p66/p51 for HIV-1) that undergoes further HIV protease-catalyzed cleavage of one subunit between residues 440 and 441 (Tyr-Phe), resulting in the removal of the *C*-terminal RNase H domain (p15) and yielding the stable heterodimer (p66/p51), which is the form found in the virion (7).

34.1.1 Crystal Structures of HIV Reverse Transcriptases

Crystal Structures of HIV-1 Reverse Transcriptase. During the past decade, a number of crystal structures of HIV-1 reverse transcriptase have been determined, mainly of the full RT heterodimer but also of some RT domains, including the *C*-terminal HIV-1 RNase (8).

The high number of domains that may increase the flexibility of the protein molecule would make the quality of many of the RT crystals studied relatively poor by showing weak diffractions—often to only medium resolution—making a full and accurate structural refinement difficult to achieve (1). The first crystal structure of HIV-1 RT revealed the basic architecture of the p66/p51 heterodimer (2). It shows the *N*-terminal portion of the p66 to be arranged in a structure that is analogous to an open right hand containing three domains referred to as *fingers*, *palm*, and *thumb*. The connection domain follows the thumb domain and leads finally to the *C*-terminal RNase H domain. One of the most surprising features of this structure has been the radically different arrangement of the four domains within the p51 subunit when compared with the p66 subunit, such as the cleft in p51 being occupied, thereby making this subunit an inactive polymerase (2). Due mostly to the limited resolution of the first RT structures determined, the assignment of secondary structure elements in RT models to date has been varied in the different published reports (2–4).

Crystal Structure of HIV-2 Reverse Transcriptase. HIV-2 is a less-widespread HIV serotype than HIV-1 and is found mostly in West Africa, although some evidence has suggested that it is spreading in Europe and Asia. The

HIV-2 reverse transcriptase also forms a heterodimer—although with different molecular weights than that of HIV-1—reported as either p68/p55 or p68/p58, compared with p66/p51 for HIV-1 (9). The HIV-2 reverse transcriptase has been purified and crystallized (10), and its structure has been determined to 2.35 Å resolution (11). The overall fold of the unliganded HIV-2 RT has been shown to be similar to that of HIV-1 RT, with the thumb domain in a folded-down conformation. In addition, although HIV-2 RT shows approximately 60% sequence identity to HIV RT, it has inherent resistance to most (but not all) non-nucleoside reverse transcriptase inhibitors (NNRTIs). The key aromatic residues of Tyr 181 and Tyr 188 involved in aromatic ring stacking with many inhibitors are changed to aliphatic side chains in HIV-2 (Ile 181 and Leu 188). Comparison of the apo structures of HIV-1 and HIV-2 in the region of the NNRTI site show differences in position for both conserved and unconserved residues that could cause unfavorable inhibitor contacts or destabilization of the pocket. The conformation of Ile 181, compared with Tyr 181 in HIV-1 RT, seems to be an important reason for the inherent drug resistance of HIV-2 RT to NNRTIs. In addition, the less bulky side chains at residues 101 and 138 in HIV-2 RT compared with those of HIV-1 RT have created a pocket that has been occupied by glycerol in the HIV-2 crystal structure (1, 11).

34.2 HIV Reverse Transcriptase Inhibitors: Nucleoside Analogues

The nucleoside analogue acyclovir triphosphate, which acts as a substrate for the herpesvirus-encoded DNA polymerase—leading to incorporation into the primer strand and chain termination, became the starting point in the search for anti-HIV drugs. As a result, a number of nucleoside derivatives were found to be potent inhibitors of HIV RT, and one of them, zidovudine (azidothymidine) triphosphate, has been rapidly approved for treating AIDS patients as a selective inhibitor of HIV reverse transcriptase. Its mechanism of action involves competitive inhibition of the substrate thymidine triphosphate (dTTP), but it can also be incorporated into the primer strand and thereby act as a chain terminator due to the ability of its azido group to occupy the 3′-ribose position (12).

Other nucleoside analogues followed, such as didanosine, zalcitabine, lamivudine, stavudine, and abacavir. Known as nucleoside reverse transcriptase inhibitors (NRTIs), they similarly to zidovudine will also act as RT inhibitors. However, some NRTIs can also inhibit certain cellular DNA polymerases, which is thought to contribute to clinical toxicities, such as neuropathy (13).

34.2.1 Zidovudine, Lamivudine, Abacavir, and Emtricitabine

Zidovudine (Retrovir, ZDV, AZT). AZT is a thymidine analogue (3′-azido-3′-deoxythymidine) *(14)*, first introduced commercially as Retrovir in 1987. In the early studies, ZDV demonstrated clinical and survival benefits alone or in combination with other nucleoside analogues *(15, 16)*. However, these benefits have been of limited durability because of the incomplete virologic suppression and the emergence of resistant HIV-1 strains *(17)*.

Intracellularly, ZDV is converted into its active triphosphate form (ZDV-TP) by anabolic phosphorylation, which acts by competitively inhibiting the use of deoxythymidine triphosphate as an essential substrate for the formation of proviral DNA by the HIV DNA polymerase (reverse transcriptase). In addition, ZDV-TP serves as a DNA chain terminator when incorporated into the proviral DNA chain because the 3′ N-substitution will impede the 5′-3′ phosphodiester linkage necessary for chain elongation. Human cellular DNA polymerases-α and -β were found to be 100 times less susceptible to inhibition by ZDV-TP compared with the retroviral HIV reverse transcriptase *(17)*. However, the human polymerase-γ is inhibited *in vivo* by ZDV concentrations as low as $1.0\,\mu M$. In addition, ZDV inhibits adenine nucleoside translocator-1, which may contribute to the mitochondrial toxicity seen with ZDV *(18)*.

In cell culture drug-combination studies, zidovudine demonstrated synergistic to additive inhibitor activities with other nucleoside reverse transcriptase inhibitors (NRTIs) (zalcitabine, didanosine, lamivudine, and abacavir), non-nucleoside reverse transcriptase inhibitors (NNRTIs) (efavirenz, delavirdine, and nevirapine), protease inhibitors (PIs) (saquinavir, ritonavir, indinavir, nelfinavir, amprenavir, and lopinavir), and interferon-α *(19–24)*. The combination of zidovudine and stavudine (d4T) has shown antagonistic activity in patients receiving the combination by showing progressive declines in the CD4$^+$ T-cell counts with a median of 22 cells/mm^3 below the baseline after 16 weeks; this combination should not be used for treating HIV-1 infections *(25)*. Ribavirin has also antagonized the antiviral activity of ZDV *in vitro* by inhibiting its phosphorylation *(26)*.

Several large studies (the Delta trial, ACTG 175) have demonstrated that zidovudine combined with other nucleoside drugs can provide improved and more durable clinical and survival benefits compared with ZVD alone *(17, 27, 28)*.

The results from a landmark study (PACTG 076) led to the approval of zidovudine to be used in HIV-infected women and their infants to prevent perinatal transmission of HIV *(29)*.

Lamivudine (3TC). 3TC is the negative (−) (*cis*)-enantiomer of 2′-dideoxy-3′-thiacytidine and has shown activity against HIV-1, HIV-2, and hepatitis B virus *(17)*. Structurally, it represents a pyrimidine nucleoside analogue in which the 3′-carbon of the ribose ring of 2′-deoxycytidine has been replaced by a sulfur atom. 3TC has been indicated for treatment of HIV infection *only* in combination with other antiretroviral agents.

Lamivudine requires an initial intracellular phosphorylation to become active (preferentially in resting cells). The mechanism of action of 3TC-triphosphate (3TC-TP) involves inhibition of HIV reverse transcriptase that competes with deoxycytidine triphosphate—an endogenous nucleotide—for binding in the HIV RT-binding site. Insertion of 3TC-TP into the proviral DNA would lead to termination of the DNA chain elongation because 3TC lacks the 3′-hydroxyl group necessary for the 5′ to 3′ linkage required for DNA synthesis *(30)*.

Multiple trials (AVANTI, ACTG 320) have investigated the combinations of 3TC with ZDV or d4T and a protease inhibitor or an NNRTI and demonstrated the potency of these combinations *(31, 32)*. In the AVANTI 2 trial, the median T-cell count increase at week 52 was 177 cells/mm^3 in the triple-drug therapy group and 91 cells/mm^3 in the ZDV plus 3TC group *(31)*. Similarly, results from the ACTG 320 trial have shown a mean T-cell count increase of 121 cells/mm^3 in the triple-drug therapy group compared with 40 cells/mm^3 in the double-drug therapy group *(32)*.

Emtricitabine (FTC, Emtriva, Coviracil). Emtricitabine is an antiretroviral synthetic nucleoside analogue of cytosine *(33)*. Structurally, emtricitabine represents the (−)- enantiomer of [2′,3′-dideoxy-5-fluoro-3′-thiacytidine-(*cis*)-5-fluoro-1-(2-hydroxymethyl)-1,3-oxathiolan-5-yl)cytosine] *(34)*. Emtricitabine differs from lamivudine only by the presence of a fluoro atom at the 5-position of the cytosine ring. Similarly to other nucleoside analogues, emtricitabine is initially phosphorylated by 2′-deoxycytidine kinase *(35)* to emtricitabine 5′-triphosphate (5′-TP), and competition for this enzyme is expected with concomitant intracellular exposure of 5′-TP, lamivudine, and deoxycytidine to compete with the natural substrate, deoxycytidine 5′-TP, for insertion into the growing viral DNA strand *(33)*. Emtricitabine 5′-TP is a weak inhibitor of mammalian DNA polymerases-α, -β, and -ε, and mitochondrial DNA polymerase-γ *(34)*.

In vitro drug combination studies have shown additive-to-synergistic effects of emtricitabine with other NRTIs (abacavir, lamivudine, stavudine, tenofovir, zalcitabine, and zidovudine), as well as NNRTIs (delavirdine, efavirenz, and nevirapine) and protease inhibitors (amprenavir, nelfinavir, ritonavir, and saquinavir) *(34)*.

The major metabolic advantage of emtricitabine has been its complete lack of cytochrome P450 enzyme inhibition (isoforms 1A2, 2A6, 2B6, 2C9, 2C19, 2D6, and 3A4) at supratherapeutic doses, and a lack of uridine-5′-diphosphoglucuronyl transferase inhibition (the enzyme responsible for glucuronidation) *(34)*.

The recommended emtricitabine dosage (as Emtriva) for adults is 200 mg daily, orally *(34)*. Because of its renal clearance, the dosage must be adjusted for renal insufficiency (creatinine clearance; CL_{cr}).

Emtricitabine has demonstrated its antiretroviral efficacy in a number of clinical trials involving both treatment-naïve and treatment-experienced patients *(33)*. Although the cross-resistance between emtricitabine and lamivudine has indicated that emtricitabine has limited usefulness as part of a salvage regimen, the excellent efficacy and tolerability data coupled with the convenience of the fixed-dose combination with tenofovir (Truvada; see below) have suggested that it will play an important role as part of the nucleoside backbone in triple-drug combinations for first-line treatment *(33)*. In 2004, Gilead Sciences and Bristol-Myers Squibb Co. (BMS) entered into an agreement to develop and commercialize a fixed-dose combination tablet containing efavirenz (Sustiva; BMS) and Truvada (Gilead Sciences), which, as a single-tablet daily regimen of emtricitabine-tenofovir-efavirenz, would provide one of the preferred NNRTI-based treatments for use in appropriate patients who are antiretroviral-therapy-naïve *(36)* (http://www.aidsinfo.nih.gov/guidelines/).

Abacavir (ABC, Ziagen). Abacavir [(1*R*)-4-[2-amino-6-(cyclopropylamino)purin-9-yl]-1-cyclopent-2-enyl]methanol)] is a synthetic carbocyclic nucleoside analogue that represents the negative (−)-enantiomer of 2′,3′-dehydro-2′,3′-dideoxyguanosine (carbovir) *(37, 38)*. It has potent and selective inhibitory activity against HIV-1 *(38)*, and, in 1998, ABC was approved by the FDA for use in combination therapy of HIV-1 infections in adults and children age 2 months and older, with the recommendation that it be used as an alternative agent to protease inhibitors or efavirenz (EFV) in combinations with two other NRTIs for the treatment of established HIV infections *(36)*.

Abacavir is anabolized intracellularly into its active triphosphate congener through a unique metabolic pathway using enzymes that do not phosphorylate other NRTIs *(39)*.

As an analogue of deoxy-guanosine-5′-triphosphate, carbovir triphosphate inhibits the HIV-1 reverse transcriptase by competing with the natural substrate, deoxy-guanosine-5′-triphosphate, and by incorporating into the viral DNA. As with the other nucleoside analogues, the lack of 3′-hydroxyl group in the incorporated carbovir triphosphate will prevent the formation of the 5′ to 3′ phosphodiester linkage critical for the viral DNA chain elongation leading to termination of its growth *(17)*.

When used in combination with other HIV-1 inhibitors (zidovudine, lamivudine, didanosine, nevirapine, or amprenavir), ABC has shown *in vitro* synergistic activity in MT4 cells *(40–42)*.

Abacavir is supplied as 300 mg tablets and as an 20 mg/mL oral solution. The recommended daily dose is 600 mg either once daily or in two divided doses for adults, and 8 mg/kg twice daily (up to a maximum dose of 600 mg daily) for adolescent and pediatric patients 3 months to 16 years of age *(17)*.

The use of ABC as part of an initial therapy for antiretroviral-naïve patients is considered attractive from the standpoint of pill burden and potency when combined with a second NRTI and an NNRTI agent *(17)*. Currently, abacavir is recommended as part of an alternative initial regimen containing lamivudine (3TC) and efavirenz (EFV) *(36)*. The use of a three-NRTI regimen consisting of ABC plus ZDV plus 3TC as an initial therapy has been associated with virologic failure and, as such, is recommended for use only in patients in whom an NNRTI and protease inhibitor (PI) cannot be used *(17)*. In addition, the combination of ABC plus tenofovir plus 3TC should not be used as the sole combination at any time, based on the observation of early virologic nonresponse *(43)*.

The "Nucleoside Backbone" Antiretroviral Therapy. The discovery and development of the antiretroviral agents zidovudine (ZDV), lamivudine (3TC), and abacavir (ABC) has resulted in widespread reductions in morbidity and mortality of HIV-1–infected patients. In the evolution from their initial use as monotherapies, followed by their use as combinations together and with other nucleoside congeners, a new antiretroviral *"nucleoside backbone"* therapeutic strategy of triple-combination regimens has emerged. These combination regimens have become some of the most commonly prescribed antiretroviral medications *(17)*. For example, coformulations such as the ZDV plus 3TC (known as COM), abacavir plus lamivudine (Kivexa/Epzicom), and Trizivir (ZDV plus 3TC plus ABC), along with the once-daily dosing formulation of 3TC, have been one of the most beneficial additions to the armamentarium of antiretroviral therapy, with obvious adherence implications. In addition, the capacity to use lamivudine for treatment of HIV-1 and hepatitis B, coupled with its exceptional toxicity profile and ease of dosing, have made 3TC particularly attractive for initial treatment of HIV-1 infections *(17)*.

34.2.2 Didanosine, Zalcitabine, and Stavudine

After the introduction of zidovudine (as Retrovir) in 1987, didanosine (Videx), zalcitabine (Hivid), and stavudine (Zerit) were the next three nucleoside analogues to become commercially available in 1991, 1992, and 1993, respectively.

Didanosine (ddI). Didanosine, which is commercially available as its buffered formulation (Videx), is a delayed-release formulation and was the second antiretroviral compound to be licensed. Because of its acid lability, ddI must be protected from stomach acids by either the enteric coating of the delayed-release formulation (Videx EC) or by the antacid component of the buffered formulations. Unlike other nucleoside analogues, because of its unique acid lability, didanosine quickly undergoes hydrolysis in the gastrointestinal (GI) system to hypoxanthine, an inactive form *(44)*. To prevent its rapid degradation in the acidic environment of the stomach, didanosine is protected by either:

(i) Sheltering the active ingredient by enclosing it within individual enteric-coated beadlets within the capsule (Videx EC). The enteric coating will dissolve, releasing didanosine when the beadlets encounter the higher pH of the small intestine, where absorption of the drug occurs *(45)*.

(ii) With a buffered formulation. Administration of didanosine with antacid will raise the gastric pH, providing protection from degradation by the stomach acids. The antacid is either provided in the dosage form itself (buffered with calcium carbonate and magnesium hydroxide or dibasic sodium phosphate, sodium citrate, and citric acid) or, in the case of Videx Buffered Powder for Oral Solution, the antacid must be admixed by the pharmacist at the time the drug is dispensed. Drug-drug interactions involving didanosine can be divided into two groups: those unique to the antacid buffer, and those caused by didanosine itself. This distinction is important, because interactions caused by the antacid buffer are not encountered when using Videx EC *(45)*.

After its introduction to the clinic, a large, expanded access program was initiated in which more than 21,000 patients received didanosine either under a treatment Investigational New Drug (IND) protocol designed for patients who were intolerant to zidovudine or through an open-label study designed for patients whose conditions were clinically deteriorating despite continued zidovudine therapy. The trials opened for accrual in October 1989 and continued until the drug received FDA approval in October 1991 *(45)*.

Initially introduced for patients failing or intolerant to zidovudine therapy, didanosine is currently indicated for use in combinations with other antiretroviral drugs for treating HIV-1 infections *(44)*. Furthermore, the current U.S. Department of Health and Human Services (DHHS) guidelines have recommended that didanosine may also be used as an alternative two-NRTI backbone in combination with lamivudine or emtricitabine, as part of an initial combination-therapy regimen *(36)* (http://www.aidsinfo.nih.gov/guidelines/).

The dosing of ddI is based on the patient's weight. A daily dose of 400 mg is administered for adults weighing at least 60 kg (132 lb), whereas 250 mg is administered daily for those weighing less than 60 kg *(44)*.

Adverse side effects of didanosine include mitochondrial toxicity, peripheral neuropathy, lactic acidosis, pancreati-

tis, lipodystrophy (fat redistribution syndrome), as well as retinal changes and optic neuritis, and gastrointestinal side effects *(45)*. Current DHHS guidelines recommend against the use of stavudine plus didanosine NRTI backbone regimen because of the high incidence of peripheral neuropathy, pancreatitis, and lactic acidosis, except when no other antiretroviral options exist and the potential benefits outweigh the risks *(36)*.

Zalcitabine (ddC). Zalcitabine is a synthetic pyrimidine nucleoside analogue structurally related to deoxycytidine, in which the 3′-hydroxyl group of the ribose sugar moiety is substituted with hydrogen.

Zalcitabine enters the cell by facilitated diffusion *(46)* and is then converted to its active 5′-triphosphate metabolite (ddCTP) via sequential phosphorylation by cellular enzymes *(47)*. As with the other dideoxynucleosides, the active zalcitabine triphosphate inhibits replication of HIV-1 by both competing with the natural dCTP substrate and by terminating the DNA chain elongation *(45)*. The different DNA polymerases have different degrees of sensitivity *(48)*. Thus, DNA polymerase-α, which is important in DNA synthesis, is relatively resistant to the effects of ddCTP; DNA polymerase-β, which is involved in DNA repair, has intermediate sensitivity to ddCTP. The mitochondrial (mtDNA) polymerase-γ has been the most sensitive, as demonstrated in cultured cell lines *in vitro* *(49–51)*.

Zalcitabine was found to exhibit *in vitro* synergy with zidovudine, stavudine, nelfinavir, recombinant interferon-α, or human leukocyte interferon, as well as several non-nucleoside HIV inhibitors (TIBO, BHAP) *(45)*.

The recommended dosage of zalcitabine in adults is 0.75 mg orally every 8 hours *(52)*. Because of its supratherapeutic dosing-associated teratogenicity in mice and rats, zalcitabine has been classified as a Pregnancy Category C drug. Because safety in human pregnancy has not been established, zalcitabine should be used during pregnancy only when the potential benefit outweighs the potential risk to the fetus (data on file; Hoffmann-La Roche) *(45)*.

The major dose-limiting toxicity of zalcitabine has been a distal sensory peripheral neuropathy of the feet and lower legs (70% of patients receiving doses equal to or greater than 0.01 mg/kg every 4 hours) *(53)*. Other adverse side effects include pancreatitis (a rare but serious complication) and sometimes fatal lactic acidosis syndrome and severe hepatomegaly with steatosis *(52)*.

Large clinical trials have failed to demonstrate any superiority of zalcitabine over other available nucleoside analogues with more favorable toxicity profiles *(45)*. This, coupled with the fact that zalcitabine has been licensed for thrice-daily administration, whereas other available nucleoside and nucleotide drugs have been used in regimens for once- or twice-daily administration, has led to a sharp decline in its use in the developed countries with the licensure of more effective, less toxic, and more convenient antiretroviral agents. As a result, its distribution was halted as of December 31, 2006 (http://www.fda.gov/cder/drug/shortages/Roche_HIVD_MDLetter.pdf) *(45)*.

Stavudine (d4T, Zerit, Zerit XR). Stavudine {1-[5-(hydroxymethyl)-2,5-dihydrofuran-2-yl]-5-methyl-1*H*-pyrimidine-2,4-dione} is a dideoxynucleoside analogue that is introduced either as an immediate-release product (Zerit) or as a once-daily extended-release formulation (Zerit XR) *(45)*.

Stavudine has been indicated for use in combination with other antiretroviral agents for the treatment of HIV-1 infection *(54)*. The current DHHS guidelines have recommended that stavudine may be used as an alternative two-NRTI backbone, in combination with lamivudine or emtricitabine, as part of an initial combination therapy regimen *(36)* (http://www.aidsinfo.nih.gov/guidelines/).

The recommended dose of stavudine is 40 mg twice daily for patients weighing more than 60 kg (132 lb) and 30 mg twice daily for patients weighing less than 60 kg. For pediatric patients, the recommended dose for those weighing less than 30 kg is 1.0 mg/kg per dose administered every 12 hours; pediatric patients weighing at least 30 kg (66 lb) should receive the recommended adult dosage based on their weight *(45)*.

With appropriate dosage adjustment, stavudine may be administered to patients with renal impairment and those undergoing hemodialysis, as well as to patients who had developed peripheral neuropathy *(45)*.

Because both stavudine and zidovudine are thymidine analogues, they undergo triphosphorylation by using the same intracellular thymidine kinases. However, zidovudine is preferentially phosphorylated over stavudine, which will leave the latter not fully phosphorylated in the presence of zidovudine *(55, 56)*. The clinical significance of this stavudine-zidovudine interaction has been demonstrated in clinical trials that showed the inferior antiviral efficacy of the stavudine-zidovudine combination compared with that of other antiretroviral regimens *(25)*. Thus, the intracellular concentrations of stavudine triphosphate were found to be sixfold lower in patients receiving stavudine plus zidovudine compared with that in those receiving stavudine alone. This observation led to the recommendation that stavudine and zidovudine not be used concurrently in clinical practice *(45)*.

There is extensive information available on the antiretroviral efficacy of stavudine primarily concerning its use as part of triple-therapy regimens in line with current treatment guidelines *(45)*. For example, stavudine in combination with another NRTI and a PI (with or without low-dose ritonavir) *(57–62)* or another NRTI and NNRTI *(63, 64)* reduced plasma HIV RNA levels to fewer than 500 copies/mL in 53% to 100% and fewer than 50 copies/mL in 41% to 100% of antiretroviral-naïve patients after 48 to 52 weeks.

Current treatment guidelines for the use of antiretroviral regimens in children have recommended its use with a PI in combination with two NRTIs in both antiretroviral-naïve and antiretroviral-experienced children (http://hivatis.org/guidelines/Pediatric/Dec12_oq/peddec/pdf0 *(45, 65)*. In the latter patient group, the average viral load has been reduced by at least 2 $\log_{10}$ copies/mL from the baseline after 4 to 24 months using stavudine-containing triple regimens *(66)*.

Stavudine's adverse side effects include mitochondrial toxicity (myopathy, neuropathy, cardiomyopathy, lactic acidosis, and pancreatic and/or hepatic failure) *(45)* mainly as the result of its inhibition of human polymerase-γ, which is involved in the replication of mitochondrial DNA (mtDNA) *(67)*. There has been evidence associating lipodystrophy with stavudine treatment (Gilead 903 study) *(45)*.

34.2.3 Dideoxynucleosides Mechanism of Action

As is the case with zidovudine, each of these dideoxynucleoside compounds must first undergo triphosphorylation by intracellular kinases before they compete with the natural nucleoside substrates to abrogate the viral DNA chain elongation *(45)*.

Once triphosphorylated, the dideoxynucleosides, similarly to zidovudine, compete with the natural nucleoside triphosphates for binding to the viral reverse transcriptase in order to integrate into the growing DNA strand and prevent the next endogenous nucleoside triphosphate from continuing to build the DNA chain. Successful inhibition and/or termination of DNA reverse transcription prevents the host cell from becoming infected with the human immunodeficiency virus *(68)*.

The nucleoside analogue chain termination is carried out by the removal or replacement of the natural substrate's 3'-hydroxyl group, where successive nucleosides must attach to the growing chain. In the case of didanosine and zalcitabine, hydrogen would replace the 3'-hydroxyl group, resulting in a dideoxy nucleoside [2',3'-dideoxyinosine (ddI) and 2',3'-dideoxycytidine (ddC), respectively]. The stavudine molecule, which has a double-bond inserted between carbons 2 and 3, would yield a 2',3'-didehydro-3'-deoxythymidine (d4T). Based on this nomenclature, these three compounds are sometimes collectively referred to as the "d" drugs *(45)*.

34.2.4 Resistance to Nucleoside HIV Reverse Transcriptase Inhibitors

The HIV reverse transcriptase converts genomic single-stranded RNA into double-stranded DNA to be integrated in the host DNA. Furthermore, the HIV RT possesses RNA- and DNA-primed DNA polymerase activity, as well as RNase H activity capable of degrading the DNA-RNA intermediates *(69)*.

The DNA elongation exists in equilibrium between a dominant *forward reaction* and a minor *reverse reaction*. The forward reaction is characterized by attack of the 3′-hydroxyl group of the primer on the α-phosphate of the incorporating nucleoside triphosphate (dNTP) to form a phosphodiester bond releasing pyrophosphate. This reaction extends the length of the primer chain by one base, and this process of extending the primer continues until natural completion, or until an incorporated base (such as a nucleoside analogue lacking the 3′-hydroxyl group) forms a bond with the next dNTP to prematurely terminate the chain elongation *(69)*.

The reverse reaction of the RT enzyme involves excision of the terminal nucleoside monophosphate from the primer by coupling with adenosine triphosphate (ATP) or pyrophosphate. If the terminal base is a NRTI, its removal from the terminated primer will unblock the chain so it can continue its extension. This process is referred to as *primer unblocking (69)*.

In general, NRTI resistance mutations cause resistance either by decreasing the incorporation of the NRTIs compared with natural dNTPs (the forward reaction) or by increasing the rate of primer unblocking (the reverse reaction) *(70)*.

Allosteric interference with the incorporation of the nucleoside analogues is considered to be the major mechanism by which mutations M184V, Y115F, Q151M, L74V, V75T, V118I, and K65R cause drug resistance *(71–83)*.

HIV-1 resistance to zidovudine has been associated with the accumulation of specific mutation sites on the HIV-1 *pol* gene that encodes for the reverse transcriptase. The mutations associated with decreased ZDV susceptibility have occurred at amino acid sites 41, 67, 70, 215, and 219, with sites 41, 70, and 215 being the most important for mutations *(84, 85)*. Cross-resistance to multiple nucleoside analogues, including ZDV, didanosine, zalcitabine, and d4T, has been demonstrated with mutation sites 62, 75, 77, 116, and, most notably, 151. The presence of M184V mutation, induced by lamivudine (3TC) and abacavir (ABC), has been shown to induce ZDV hypersusceptibility of the virus and a re-sensitization of ZDV-resistant virus to ZDV *(86, 87)*.

The M184V mutation has been found to reverse the selective advantage ZDV-resistant strains attain in continuing the elongation of the HIV DNA chain and thus would lead to increased ZDV phenotypic susceptibility in the setting of genotypic resistance *(88, 89)*. It has been proposed that HIV-1 resistance to zidovudine results from the selectively decreased binding of ZDV-TP and the increased pyrophosphorolytic cleavage of chain-terminated viral DNA by the mutant RT at physiologic pyrophosphate levels, resulting in a net decrease in chain termination. The increased processivity of viral DNA synthesis may be important to enable facile replication of HIV in the presence of ZDV by compensating for the increased reverse reaction rate *(89)*.

The 3TC monotherapy resulted in a high level of HIV resistance, which was due to a single mutation in codon 184 of the HIV-1 RT gene, in which the methionine had been replaced by either isoleucine or valine *(17)*.

Mutants resistant to zidovudine became phenotypically sensitive *in vitro* by mutation of residue 184 of viral reverse transcriptase to valine, which also induced resistance to 3TC *(90)*. Furthermore, ZDV-3TC coresistance was not observed during extensive *in vitro* selection with both drugs. *In vivo* ZDV-3TC combination therapy resulted in a markedly greater decrease in serum HIV-1 RNA concentrations than did treatment with ZDV alone, even though valine-184 mutants rapidly emerged. Most samples assessed from the combination group remained ZDV-sensitive at 24 weeks of therapy, consistent with *in vitro* mutation studies *(90)*.

Abacavir selects several mutations on the viral reverse transcriptase gene, including M184V, K65R, L74V, and Y115F. In this regard, the M184V mutation alone does not lead to significant ABC resistance. Thus, results from clinical trials have indicated that resistance to abacavir has been associated with the presence of the M184V mutation in combination with at least three thymidine analogue mutations *(91)*. Furthermore, mutations at codons 65, 74, and possibly 184 led to cross-resistance to didanosine (ddI) and ddC. Each of these mutations resulted in a two- to fourfold decrease in susceptibility to abacavir.

Clinical isolates of HIV with reduced *in vitro* susceptibility to zalcitabine have been identified infrequently, in contrast with the high rates of resistance observed with zidovudine and lamivudine. Initially, *in vitro* selection of resistance by passage of virus in the presence of increasing concentrations of zalcitabine identified the key resistance mutation, Lys65Arg, associated with increases in IC_{50} to zalcitabine, didanosine, and lamivudine *(92)*. Viruses containing the K65R mutation, or a second mutation at codon 69 associated with low-level zalcitabine resistance, have been isolated from patients receiving zalcitabine monotherapy or alternating zidovudine therapy *(93–95)*. A third mutation, Met184Val, conferring low-level resistance to zalcitabine and didanosine, and high-level resistance to lamivudine, has been identified from patients on prolonged zalcitabine monotherapy, either alone or with K65R *(96)*. The emergence of resistance to zalcitabine has occurred infrequently during combination therapy *(97)*.

HIV isolates with a reduced susceptibility to stavudine have been both selected *in vitro (98)* and obtained from patients treated with stavudine *(99–101)*. Changes in stavudine sensitivity have usually been associated with the presence of multiresistant phenotypes *(99)*. Studies have shown that prolonged treatment with stavudine can select and/or maintain mutations associated with zidovudine *(101)*.

Nucleoside cross-resistance was first noted in a study of 128 patients who had received zidovudine monotherapy, in which each 10-fold decrease in zidovudine susceptibility was associated with a 2-fold decrease in zalcitabine sensitivity and 2.2-fold decrease in didanosine susceptibility *(102)*. This has been confirmed and more clearly delineated in a recent, large, phenotypic resistance study *(103)*.

34.2.5 Drugs in Development

34.2.5.1 Amdoxovir

Amdoxovir (AMDX, DAPD) [(−)-β-*D*-2,6-diaminopurine dioxolane] is an experimental nucleoside reverse transcriptase inhibitor.

Amdoxovir is currently in Phase I/II clinical development for the treatment of HIV-1. This compound was designed as a prodrug to enhance the oral bioavailability of the active compound, (−)-β-*D*-dioxolane guanosine (DXG). Amdoxovir is deaminated by adenosine deaminase to DXG, which is further metabolized to its 5′-triphosphate (DXG-TP) by host cell enzymes, including deoxyguanosine kinase and high K_m 5′-nucleotidase *(104, 105)*. DXG-TP is a potent alternative substrate inhibitor of the HIV-1 RT. Incorporation of DXG 5′-monophosphate (DXG-MP) into nascent DNA *results in chain termination*. Virus harboring HIV-1 RT mutations associated with resistance to zidovudine (M41L/D67N/K70R/T215Y/K219Q), lamivudine (M184V), abacavir (M41L/D67N, M184V/L210W/T215Y), efavirenz (K103N), and certain multidrug resistance mutations remained sensitive to inhibition by DXG *(106, 107)*. This lack of cross-resistance makes amdoxovir a potential therapeutic agent for patients who have failed the currently available therapies *(104)*.

The primary mutations that confer resistance to DXG are K65R and L74V in the HIV-1 RT *(105, 107, 108)*. The K65R and L74V variants of HIV-1, constructed by site-specific mutagenesis of HIV-1$_{LAI}$, showed a 5.6- and 3.5-fold increase in EC$_{50}$ to DXG, respectively, compared with wild-type HIV-1. In addition, the K65R mutation conferred partial to complete cross-resistance to lamivudine, zalcitabine, didanosine, and {9-[2-(phosphonylmethoxy)ethyl]adenine} *(107, 109)*, whereas L74V is associated with resistance to didanosine and zalcitabine *(110)*.

Two other HIV-1 RT mutations of interest were Q151M and K103N. The Q151M mutation is involved in multiple dideoxynucleoside resistance *(111)*. *In vitro* studies have shown that recombinant viruses with the mutations Q151M

or K65R/Q151M were 9.6-fold and >20-fold less sensitive to DXG. The K103N mutation is associated with resistance to NNRTIs *(112)*. A clinical isolate of HIV that contains the K103N mutation was shown to be hypersensitive to DXG *(105)*. Interestingly, K103N appeared to partially reverse the resistance to DXG conferred by certain mutations *(105)*.

To further understand the molecular mechanism of DXG drug resistance and its lack of cross-resistance toward HIV-1 variants that were resistant to standard nucleoside therapy, the inhibition of DNA synthesis by DXG-TP and incorporation of DXG-MP by wild-type and mutant HIV-1 RTs were investigated *(104)*. Two aspects were evaluated: (i) under the steady-state conditions, the inhibition of HIV-1 RT-catalyzed DNA synthesis by DXG-TP, zidovudine-TP, and lamivudine-TP was studied to assess the overall enzymatic reaction; and (ii) a transient pre–steady-state kinetic approach was used to examine the incorporation of DXG-MP by HIV-1 RTs, which revealed the individual steps involving the binding of DXG-TP and its chemical catalysis. Wild-type HIV-1 RT and a series of mutant enzymes were used in these studies. The mutant RTs employed in the study were found to possess either the single mutations (K65R, L74V, K103N, and Q151M) or combinations of these mutations (K65R/K103N, L74V/K103N, K65R/Q151M, K103N/Q151M, and K65R/K103N/Q151M). AZT-resistant RT (D67N/K70R/T251Y/K219Q) and 3TC-resistant RT (M184V) were also used in this study *(104)*.

Clinical Trials. A study has been carried out to evaluate the pharmacodynamics and safety of escalating doses of Amdoxovir monotherapy in treatment-naïve and treatment-experienced HIV patients over a 15-day period. A primary aim of the study was to assess a dose and a dosing schedule for amdoxovir for use in future studies of the drug *(113)*. Ninety patients with plasma HIV-1 RNA levels between 5,000 and 250,000 copies/mL were randomized to DAPD 25, 100, 200, 300, or 500 mg twice daily or 600 mg once daily monotherapy [antiretroviral therapy (ART)-naïve and ART-experienced] or to add DAPD 300 or 500 mg twice daily to existing ART. After 15 days of dosing, patients were followed for an additional 7 days. Results:

- In ART-naïve patients receiving short-term DAPD monotherapy, a median reduction in plasma HIV-1 RNA of 1.5 log$_{10}$ copies/mL at the highest doses was observed
- In ART-experienced patients, the reduction in viral load observed at each dose was less than that observed in treatment-naïve patients (reduction of 0.7 log$_{10}$ at 500 mg, twice daily)
- The incidence of adverse events was similar across groups, with the majority of adverse events reported as mild or moderate in severity
- Steady-state plasma concentrations of DAPD and dioxolane guanosine followed linear kinetics

Based on these findings, amdoxovir was found to be well tolerated and produced antiviral activity in treatment-naïve and in some treatment-experienced patients. In ART-experienced patients, the antiviral activity was significant in those with no *thymidine-analogue mutations (TAMs)* and higher baseline CD4$^+$ T-cell counts *(113)*.

Two studies have been conducted in which DAPD (500 mg, twice daily) was given to treatment-experienced patients *(114)*. In one of the studies, DAPD was added to a failing regimen, whereas in the other DAPD was given as single drug therapy after a "wash-out" period of no treatment. Six people who added DAPD 500 mg twice daily to their existing treatment had an average viral load drop of 1.9 log. This was superior to the 1.0 log decline seen with DAPD monotherapy *(114)*.

In the DAPD 150 Study, 18 highly treatment-experienced people were given amdoxovir (300 or 500 mg, twice daily) added to their existing regimens (which could be optimized at the discretion of the investigator) *(115)*. At baseline, median viral load was about 25,000 and CD4$^+$ T-count was 338. After 12 weeks, median viral change was −0.9 log with seven patients achieving at least a half log reduction. Ten patients discontinued the study: 2 due to virologic failure, 3 for noncompliance, and 5 due to lens opacities that did not affect vision *(115)*.

34.2.5.2 Apricitabine

Apricitabine (ATC, BCH10618, SPD754, SPD756, AVX754) is an experimental nucleoside reverse transcriptase inhibitor. Structurally, apricitabine represents (−)-2′-deoxy-3′-oxa-4′-thiocytidine.

Although apricitabine has a similar structure to lamivudine and the fluorinated derivative emtricitabine, it has been shown to retain antiretroviral activity against lamivudine-resistant clinical isolates and laboratory strains of HIV-1 *(116)*. Apricitabine also retains a high level of activity against zidovudine-resistant strains; in *in vitro* studies, the addition of up to five thymidine-associated mutations conferred a median reduction in susceptibility of only 1.8-fold *(116)*.

The first stage in the intracellular activation of apricitabine, the formation of apricitabine monophosphate, requires the enzyme deoxycytidine kinase *(117)*, which is also responsible for the phosphorylation of lamivudine and emtricitabine. There is thus potential for pharmacokinetic interactions when these agents are administered concurrently. Coadministration with lamivudine had no significant effect on the plasma and urine pharmacokinetics of apricitabine. However, the formation of apricitabine triphosphate in peripheral blood mononuclear cells was more markedly reduced after the coadministration of apricitabine and lamivudine than after the administration of apricitabine

alone. In contrast, apricitabine had no effect on the plasma pharmacokinetics of lamivudine or on the formation of lamivudine triphosphate in peripheral blood mononuclear cells *(118)*.

Dosing. Daily doses of 400 to 1,600 mg have been studied in early trials. Twice-daily dosing has been selected for further study (http://aidsinfo.nih.gov/DrugsNew/DrugDetailNT.aspx?MenuItem=Drugs&Search=On&int_id=415).

Clinical Trials. Apricitabine was studied in a randomized, double-blind, dose-ranging Phase IIb clinical trial of two doses of ATC (600 or 800 mg ATC, twice daily) compared with lamivudine (taken as 150 mg, twice daily) in treatment-experienced participants with evidence of the M184V mutation. Furthermore, participants were required to be currently taking lamivudine and have a viral load over 2,000 copies/mL and a CD4$^+$ T-cell count greater than 50 cells mm^3. Individuals who were hepatitis B surface antigen-positive, hepatitis C RNA-positive, pregnant, or breast-feeding were excluded. Although the study aimed to enroll 60 participants, only 47 individuals completed 21 days of dosing. Of these, 17 received 600 mg apricitabine and 16 received 800 mg apricitabine, with 14 participants in the control group receiving lamivudine. Results from the trial have shown that patients in both ATC cohorts exceeded the Phase IIb trial primary end-point by a substantial margin *(114)* (http://www.aidsmap.com/en/news/CE4245A3-BE13-438D-BC13-A990A1DE2F50.asp). Mean plasma viral load reduction after 21 days was greater than 0.8 log$_{10}$ in both ATC-treated groups compared with a reduction of less than 0.03 log$_{10}$ in the control group. Nine apricitabine-treated participants achieved a greater than 1.5 log$_{10}$ reduction in plasma viral load; three patients achieved a greater than 2.0 log$_{10}$ drop; and one individual experienced more than a 2.5 log$_{10}$ decline in viral load. However, no details were provided regarding participants' baseline viral load levels. No evidence of mutations resulting in apricitabine resistance was detected in any apricitabine-treated participant during the study, and the press release hinted that the drug may be less fragile than lamivudine or emtricitabine, both of which have a low genetic barrier to resistance. In addition, no details were provided on the background regimens of the participants, and whether or not anyone was effectively responding on apricitabine monotherapy. Apricitabine also appears to be safe in the short-term, with no apricitabine-related serious adverse events observed and no significant incidence of hyperlipasemia (which would indicate pancreatitis) or elevated liver enzymes. After day 21, study participants continued to receive either ATC or lamivudine up to week 24, but have also been able to change their other antiretrovirals. After 24 weeks, open-label ATC has so far been provided to 14 participants for another 24 weeks. A further six individuals have already entered an extension study (AVX-201E) in which they continue to receive apricitabine in addition to other antiretrovirals *(118)* (http://www.aidsmap.com/en/news/CE4245A3-BE13-438D-BC13-A990A1DE2F50.asp).

34.2.5.3 Elvucitabine

Elvucitabine (ACH-126,443, Beta-L-Fd4C), an *L*-cytosine nucleoside analogue, is an experimental nucleoside reverse transcriptase inhibitor that can prevent HIV from entering the nucleus of healthy T cells. This prevents the cells from producing new virus and decreases the amount of virus in the body. Structurally, elvucitabine represents 4-amino-5-fluoro-1-[(2*S*,5*R*)-5-(hydroxymethyl)-2,5-dihydrofuran-2-yl]pyrimidin-2-one.

Elvucitabine, like other dideoxynucleosides (e.g., lamivudine and emtricitabine) in the unnatural *L*-conformation represented by the β-*L*-2′,3′-dideoxy-3′-thiacytidine, have been shown to have good antiviral activity and low mitochondrial toxicity levels *(119–129)*. *However, even with compounds relatively nontoxic to mitochondria, there is a lack of a durable response. This condition can be caused by either the rapid emergence of resistant virus or host changes that cause differences in drug metabolism (130–132). Monotherapy allows the development of resistant strains of virus to occur more readily than in combination therapy (see Section 34.2.4). It is, therefore, necessary for an antiviral compound to work in conjunction with other approved antiviral drugs that have different biochemical determinants of drug resistance. If the compounds are synergistic (or at least additive) with respect to their antiviral activity, but not with respect to their cytotoxic effect on the host cells, improved therapy can be achieved (119).*

Dosing. Dosages of elvucitabine that have been studied include 5 and 10 mg, once daily and 20 mg, once every other day (http://aidsinfo.nih.gov/DrugsNew/DrugDetailNT.aspx?MenuItem=Drugs&Search=On&int_id=385).

Clinical Trials. In a 21-day study, 24 HIV-positive study participants received elvucitabine (ELV) 5 or 10 mg, once daily or 20 mg every 48 hours for 21 days with concomitant Kaletra (400 mg lopinavir/100 mg ritonavir, every 12 hours) treatment *(133)*. The results of the study have demonstrated that:

- ELV was effective and nontoxic at the doses used
- HIV RNA copies decreased 1.8, 1.9, and 2.0 $\log_{10}$ for the 5 mg, once daily, 10 mg, once daily, and 20 mg, every 48 hours cohorts at day 21 versus baseline
- Due to the long ELV half-life ($t_{1/2}$), Kaletra was continued to day 35 for the 2 higher doses
- ELV concentrations at day 28 were 3 times above the IC_{50}

- The continued activity 7 days after stopping ELV supports less frequent dosing (once-weekly or twice-weekly) suggested by the modeling
- There was a trend toward a greater efficacy of the 20 mg every 48 hours cohort
- No patients experienced safety issues or emergence of resistance

The pharmacology of elvucitabine suggested that it may present a better barrier to the development of resistance than do other antiretroviral drugs. The data also showed this may be less affected by adherence issues *(133)*.

Adverse Effects. Along with its desired effects, elvucitabine may cause some unwanted effects. Although not all of these effects are known, serious bone marrow suppression has been reported. Bone marrow suppression caused by elvucitabine appeared to be reversible; production of blood cells returned to normal once taking elvucitabine was stopped. Other side effects include mild rash, mild headache, and gastrointestinal symptoms, including upset stomach and diarrhea. Individuals should tell the clinician if these side effects continue or are bothersome (http://aidsinfo.nih.gov/DrugsNew/DrugDetailNT.aspx?MenuItem=Drugs&Search=On&int_id=385).

34.3 Nucleotide Analogues: Tenofovir DF

Over the years, a number of nucleotide derivatives have shown potent activity against various DNA viruses and retroviruses. Chemically, they represent acyclic nucleoside phosphonates (nucleoside monophosphonates) that have been designed to circumvent the first phosphorylation step necessary for the activation of the nucleoside analogues *(134, 135)*.

To date, three nucleotide analogues have received FDA approval in the United States as antiviral agents: cidofovir, adefovir dipivoxil, and tenofovir disoproxil. Although both tenofovir DF and adefovir dipivoxil have shown activity as RT inhibitors, only tenofovir has received FDA approval for the treatment of HIV-1 infection. The clinical development of adefovir dipivoxil for treating HIV infection was limited by adverse events, especially its renal toxicity (reversible proximal renal tubular dysfunction) *(134)*.

Tenofovir Disoproxil Fumarate (tenofovir DF, Viread, PMPA). Tenofovir DF is the oral prodrug of tenofovir {9-[(*R*)-(2-phosphonylmethoxy)propyl]adenine}, which has been approved for treating HIV-1 infection in combination with other antiretroviral agents.

Designed as a prodrug, tenofovir DF is a lipophilic ester derivative with improved oral bioavailability. After oral administration and adsorption, it is rapidly cleaved by nonspecific carboxylesterases into tenofovir. Once inside the cell, the compound is metabolized by adenylate cyclase to tenofovir monophosphate, and subsequently, by nucleoside diphosphate kinase, to tenofovir diphosphate (PMPApp), the biologically active compound. The antiviral activity of PMPApp is the result of the selective interaction of PMPApp with the viral DNA polymerase *(134)*.

Based on its structural similarity to the natural deoxyadenine triphosphate (dATP), PMPApp may act as both a competitive inhibitor and as an alternative substrate during the DNA polymerase chain reaction, resulting in DNA chain termination *(135)*. The antiviral activity of the unphosphorylated NRTIs (e.g., zidovudine, stavudine, didanosine, lamivudine, and abacavir) may be impeded by their low affinity for cellular nucleoside kinases; however, the nucleotide analogues differ from them in that they may be less dependent on intracellular enzymes for activation *(136)*.

Tenofovir DF Dosage. The dose of tenofovir DF is 300 mg, once daily taken orally, without regard to food. Because tenofovir DF is primarily eliminated through renal excretion, dosing adjustments are recommended. Thus, significantly increased drug exposures have occurred when tenofovir DF has been administered to patients with moderate to severe renal impairment. In such cases, the dosing interval of tenofovir DF should be adjusted in patients with baseline creatinine clearance <50 mL/min. However, because the safety and effectiveness of these recommendations for adjusting the dosing intervals have not been clinically evaluated, clinical response to treatment and renal function should be closely monitored in these patients (http://www.rxlist.com/cgi/generic/viread_ids.htm).

Tenofovir DF Monotherapy. Tenofovir DF has been found active both *in vitro* and *in vivo* against retroviruses *(137)*. The spectrum of its *in vitro* antiretroviral activities include HIV-1, non-B HIV-1 subtypes, and HIV-2, simian immunodeficiency virus, feline immunodeficiency virus, visna-maedi virus in sheep, and murine leukemia and sarcoma viruses *(138–141)*.

Results from a Phase I/II randomized, double-blind, placebo-controlled, dose-escalation study (GS-97-901) in antiretroviral-naïve and antiretroviral-experienced adults with HIV-1 infection and absolute $CD4^+$ T-cell counts of at least 200 cells/mm^3 and plasma HIV-1 RNA levels of at least 10,000 copies/mL have demonstrated a dose-related treatment effect, with patients receiving 300 or 600 mg tenofovir DF once daily showing an overall mean HIV-1 RNA-level reduction of 1.20 and 0.84 $\log_{10}$ copies/mL, respectively, when compared with baseline, whereas placebo recipients experienced a 0.03 $\log_{10}$ copies/mL increase during the same period *(142)*.

Combination Therapy with Tenofovir DF. The role of tenofovir DF in triple-nucleoside analogue RT inhibitor regimens for the treatment of HIV-1 infection has been under-

going extensive investigation *(134)*. Based on preliminary results from two clinical trials (subsequently discontinued), the once-daily triple nucleoside analogue combination of 600 mg abacavir plus 300 mg lamivudine plus 300 mg tenofovir DF seemed to be advantageous relative to potency and tolerability; however, it also showed an unacceptably high rate of virologic failures *(43, 143)*.

In a separate randomized, double-blind, placebo-controlled Phase III study (GS-00-907), 550 antiretroviral-experienced HIV-infected patients received 300 mg tenofovir DF once daily or placebo for 24 weeks in addition to their existing antiretroviral regimen. After week 24, the placebo recipients were allowed to receive tenofovir DF for the remainder of the 48-week study period *(144)*. Through week 24, the mean changes in the plasma HIV RNA levels from the baseline were −0.61 and −0.03 $\log_{10}$ copies/mL in the tenofovir DF and placebo groups, respectively ($p < 0.001$). Through week 48, the prevalence of tenofovir DF recipients with plasma HIV RNA levels of fewer than 400 and fewer than 50 copies/mL were 41% and 18%, respectively, suggesting a sustained response *(144)*.

Tenofovir DF is also available in a mixed-dose combination tablet with emtricitabine (Truvada), which contains 200 mg of emtricitabine and 300 mg of tenofovir disoproxil fumarate (see Section 34.2.1).

Currently, combined with emtricitabine (FTC) and efavirenz (EFV), tenofovir is part of the most recommended U.S. baseline combination (Atripla) (see Section 34.7.5) for the treatment of HIV/AIDS.

Tenofovir DF Toxicity. In general, tenofovir DF was well tolerated by HIV-1–infected patients. The preclinical toxicity of tenofovir DF in animals (rats, dogs, and monkeys), when administered for a minimum of 11 months, has identified the kidneys and bone marrow as potential target organs *(134)*. Specifically, urinary excretion of calcium and phosphorus increased in rats and dogs when tenofovir exposure was 11- and 9-fold higher than standard human exposure, respectively; however, these findings were reversible and were not seen when exposure was increased 3- to 5-fold over standard human exposure.

Decreased bone marrow density and increased parathyroid hormone secretion were observed in animals when dosing was increased 9- to 50-fold over standard human exposure *(134)*.

Resistance to Tenofovir DF. The presence and frequency of genotypic mutations related to tenofovir DF exposure have been examined *in vitro*, and information regarding drug-resistant clinical isolates is accumulating *(134)*.

K65R/N and K70E are key mutations relevant to tenofovir DF (TDF) resistance. Other mutations include M41L, L210W, T215Y, T215C/D/E/S/I/V, the T69 insertion mutation, and the Q151M complex (http://hivdb.stanford.edu/pages/GRIP/TDF.html).

In the presence of TDF, a K65R mutation in the HIV reverse transcriptase has been detected during *in vitro* passage experiments, as well as L228R, W25R, and P272S mutations *(145, 146)*.

K65R is selected *in vitro* when HIV-1 is cultured in the presence of increasing tenofovir DF concentrations *(147)*. It reduces TDF susceptibility about twofold as measured by the PhenoSense assay *(148, 149)*. The clinical significance of K65R-mediated TDF resistance was demonstrated by the rapid virologic failure associated with the emergence of M184V + K65R in patients receiving TDF/3TC/ABC and TDF/3TC/ddI as initial HAART regimen *(70, 150)*.

K65R occurs less commonly in patients receiving TDF/FTC + NVP or EFV, partly because virologic failure is rarer in these patients and partly because virologic failure is often detected at an earlier stage in association with M184V and NNRTI-associated mutations, but not K65R. Although there have been no direct comparative trials, K65R has occurred less commonly with TDF/FTC/EFV than with TDF/3TC/EFV *(151, 152)* possibly because the TDF/FTC coformulation and the longer and comparable half-lives of TDF and FTC reduce the risk for functional mono or dual therapy should adherence to the regimen be suboptimal.

K65R rarely occurs in combination with type I *thymidine analogue mutations (TAMs)* because of a mutual antagonism among these mutations *(153–159)*.

K65N is a rare mutation that has an effect on NRTI susceptibility similar to K65R *(160, 161)*.

K70E is selected in patients with virologic failure on a TDF-containing regimen *(150, 162, 163)*. Like K65R, this mutation usually occurs in viruses lacking TAMs and decreases susceptibility to TDF, ABC, and 3TC *(164, 165)*.

TAMs are selected when TDF is added to a regimen containing ZDV or d4T or when used for treating viruses that already contain TAMs *(166)*. The combination of M41L, L210W, and T215Y reduces TDF susceptibility approximately 4-fold and is associated with a marked decrease in TDF activity when TDF is added to a failing regimen or used as part of a new salvage therapy regimen *(167–169)*. Viruses containing only one or two of these three mutations retain partial susceptibility to TDF *(170)*.

The type II TAMs (D67N, K70R, T215F, K219Q/E) have reduced TDF susceptibility less than that of the type I TAMs *(168, 170)*.

The T215 revertants have been characterized as back mutations that were usually detected in patients primarily infected with a virus containing T215Y or F *(171–175)*. The T215 revertants did not reduce NRTI susceptibility but suggested that T215Y/F may be present *(173)*. Preliminary data suggest that some first-line regimens may be less effective in patients with virus containing a T215 revertant *(176, 177)*.

T69 insertion mutations have occurred in ~1% of treated patients, nearly always in combination with multiple TAMs.

Together, these mutations cause high-level resistance to each of the NRTIs including 3TC, FTC, and TDF *(178–183)*.

The Q151M complex (usually in combination with V75I, F77L, F116Y, Q151M) confers low-level resistance to TDF, 3TC, and FTC, and high-level resistance to each of the remaining NRTIs. In combination with mutations at positions 75, 77, and 116, Q151M conferred intermediate resistance to 3TC, FTC, and TDF, and higher-level resistance to the remaining NRTIs *(179, 182, 184–188)*.

34.4 HIV Reverse Transcriptase Inhibitors: Non-nucleoside Analogues

34.4.1 Nevirapine

Nevirapine is the first non-nucleoside reverse transcriptase inhibitor (NNRTI) approved for use in treating HIV-1–infected patients *(189)*.

Structurally, it is a dipyridodiazepinone derivative that is remarkably specific as an inhibitor of the HIV-1 reverse transcriptase (RT). Thus, even at high concentrations, nevirapine did not inhibit the reverse transcriptase of HIV-2, the simian- and feline immunodeficiency viruses, nor did it inhibit the human DNA polymerases-α, -β, or -γ *(190)*.

As an antiretroviral agent, nevirapine is a noncompetitive inhibitor of deoxyguanosine triphosphate either through allosteric binding to the binary (RT: template-primer) or ternary (RT: template-primer-deoxyguanosine triphosphate) enzyme complex *(191)*, but it did not terminate the viral DNA chain elongation *(192)*.

Nevirapine binds to reverse transcriptase at the tyrosine 181 and tyrosine 188 sites *(193)*. These conserved tyrosine residues of the HIV-1 RT subunit lie in a pocket that is defined by two β-sheets consisting of amino acid residues 100 to 110 and 180 to 190 *(194, 195)*. By binding to this hydrophobic pocket close to the polymerase catalytic site of the reverse transcriptase, nevirapine slows the rate of polymerization catalyzed by the enzyme *(196)*; this hydrophobic pocket binding site is also predictive for where mutations leading to drug resistance would occur *(189)*.

34.4.1.1 Resistance to Nevirapine

Selection for HIV-1 mutants that are resistant to nevirapine occurred rapidly *in vitro (189, 197)*. After a single passage in the presence of low concentrations of the drug, several HIV-1 strains developed a mutation at tyrosine 181 to cysteine (Y181C) that significantly reduced the sensitivity to nevirapine *(198)*. In clinical settings, resistant mutations selected during therapy with nevirapine given alone or in combination with other antiretroviral agents have also emerged rapidly, thereby suggesting that nevirapine has a very low genetic barrier to resistance *(199–207)* (see also Section 34.4.4).

Although there has been a close correlation between genotypic and phenotypic resistance with respect to nevirapine, cross-resistance to other NNRTIs was not absolute *(189)*. For example, whereas the presence of the K103N mutation has been associated with high-level resistance to *all* NNRTIs, the single Y181C mutation *did not always* translate into phenotypic resistance to efavirenz (see Section 34.4.2.1). Thus, nearly one third of the nevirapine-resistance isolates carrying the Y181C mutation in the RT gene remained susceptible to efavirenz, and 14% of those viral isolates have shown only an intermediate level of resistance to efavirenz and delavirdine (both NNRTI drugs). This finding has led some researchers to propose some identifying factors that would favor a response to efavirenz after nevirapine failure *(203–207)*. Similarly, mutations at the G190 position of HIV-1 RT have been observed to increase the sensitivity to delavirdine by 3- to 300-fold *(208)*. Initiation of nevirapine in the absence of zidovudine has favored the emergence of Y181C mutation at the time of the failure, which may preserve efavirenz as a potential component in subsequent regimens *(209)*. Findings such as these have important implications regarding strategies of sequencing antiretroviral regimens, which should be exploited in the design of future clinical trials, despite limited success in exploiting these principles at the present time *(189, 210, 211)*.

34.4.1.2 Clinical Studies

The clinical experience and application of nevirapine for the treatment of HIV-1 infections have been extensively documented *(189, 212, 213)*. As the first NNRTI drug introduced into clinical practice, nevirapine has shown potent activity against HIV-1, manifesting as durable plasma HIV RNA viral load suppression when used in combination with other antiretroviral agents *(189)*. It is currently recommended as an alternative for first-line therapy in the treatment of established HIV infection *(36)* (http://www.aidsinfo.nih.gov/guidelines/). In particular, HIV-infected patients with baseline lipid profile abnormalities in whom a PI-sparing regimen is desired and who have a risk for the CNS adverse side effects of efavirenz would be expected to respond well to nevirapine-containing regimens *(189)*. However, caution should be applied in particular to two adverse effects of nevirapine: rash and hepatotoxicity, especially by patients with preexisting elevations of liver enzyme levels. Hence, close monitoring for further increases in abnormalities in liver function tests (LFTs) is indicated *(189)*.

Nevirapine has been clinically evaluated in three different settings: (i) as a first-line therapy; (ii) as a salvage therapy; and (iii) as an alternative to PIs in virologically suppressed patients experiencing PI-related adverse side effects *(189)*.

First-Line Therapy. Nevirapine-containing regimens conducted in patients who were antiretroviral-naïve can be further divided into three categories *(189)*:

- Early trials that compared dual nucleoside regimens with or without nevirapine *(203, 214, 215)* (the ACTG 241 trial has been unique to the trials reported in that the subjects were not antiretrovirally naïve at baseline)
- PI-sparing regimens *(64, 216–219)*
- Clinical trials that compared PI-sparing with PI-containing regimens *(220–222)*

There have also been several reports describing virologic and immunologic results from the use of nevirapine in non-randomized clinical trials *(223–228)*.

A meta-analysis of the INCAS *(214)* and the ISS047 (http://vh2.boehringer-ingelheim.es:8000/productos/boehringer/vih/inforef/biblio/1998/iss047.html) trials using baseline plasma viral load (pVL) as an indicator of viral load suppression has found an extension of the benefit of nevirapine when added to a dual nucleoside [didanosine/zidovudine (INCAS); or stavudine/lamivudine (ISS047)] regimen in antiretroviral-naïve patients over a wide range of CD4$^+$ T-lymphocyte counts at baseline *(229)*. However, other attempts to correlate the likelihood of achieving an undetectable pVL based on baseline high or low pVL while treating patients with nevirapine triple-drug combination therapy did not support these findings *(220, 225, 230–232)*. Accordingly, results from a subsequent meta-analysis of 30 published and presented studies to investigate the relationship between viral load suppression and baseline pVL, as well as between pVL suppression and baseline CD4$^+$ T-cell count, provided evidence that baseline CD4$^+$ T-cell count was a better predictor of virologic suppression induced by triple-drug combination therapy than was the baseline pVL *(232)*. The same pattern was seen in a subanalysis of trials of nevirapine-containing therapy that identified the baseline factors associated with successful virologic suppression (baseline CD4$^+$ T-cell count, $p = 0.014$ at 6 months; baseline viral load, $p = 0.415$) *(232)*. Ultimately, only prospective clinical trials designed to compare nevirapine-versus PI-containing triple-drug combination therapy regimens, enrolling patients with a range of baseline viral load measurements such as the Atlantic study *(220)*, and other relevant studies *(221)*, will be able to address the important clinical question broached by these retrospective, *ad hoc*, and meta-analytical investigations *(189)*. In addition, studies involving efavirenz have shown equal to superior activity to PI-containing regimens and in subjects with higher viral loads, thus suggesting that active NNRTI therapy can be successful in this setting *(233)*.

Before the 2NN study (http://aids-ed.org/aidsetc?page= croi-10-02), there have been limited data regarding the use of dual NNRTIs *(234, 235)*. Results from these nonrandomized studies suggested that nevirapine and efavirenz in combination with an NRTI was a safe, well-tolerated, and effective regimen in patients who are ART-naïve or ART-experienced.

The 2NN was a four-arm randomized clinical trial that included a dual NNRTI cohort with efavirenz dosing at 800 mg daily *(236)*. Results of the 1,216 ART-naïve subjects randomized to either 400 mg nevirapine once daily, 200 mg nevirapine twice daily, 600 mg efavirenz once daily, or a once-daily combination of 400 mg nevirapine plus 800 mg efavirenz with a backbone regimen of 4dT plus 3TC have been recently published *(237)*. All analyses were performed after 48 weeks of therapy on the intention-to-treat population. The overall data have shown that treatment failure was similar among the single NNRTI arms but was higher in the combination nevirapine plus efavirenz arm, mainly because of more discontinuations of treatment in this arm. The incidence of clinical adverse events did not differ significantly between the single NNRTI arms. Only the incidence of the liver-associated laboratory adverse side effects was significantly different among the arms, with the highest incidence in the once-daily nevirapine arm. The virologic and immunologic efficacy was comparable among all four arms, which led to the conclusion that nevirapine and efavirenz demonstrated equal potency, as did the once-daily versus twice-daily administration of nevirapine. Combination NNRTI therapy was inferior to the other strategies because of the observed increased toxicity in this ART-naïve patient cohort *(237)*.

Salvage Therapy. The role of nevirapine in salvage therapy *(189)* has been investigated in randomized *(238–242)* and nonrandomized *(243, 243–245)* clinical trial settings, as well as in retrospective chart reviews *(223, 224, 227, 246)*.

At the end of a 36-week clinical study, nevirapine in combination with nelfinavir and two NRTIs did provide a significant advantage over nelfinavir plus two NRTIs alone in patients who previously failed PI-containing regimens (pVL <200 copies/mL in 52% vs. 22% of subjects, respectively) without any difference between the two groups in terms of immunologic response *(240)*. This and findings from other studies *(238, 245)* have underscored the hypothesis that a successful salvage therapy will depend on the limited evolution of resistant HIV strains and the need for at least two new agents as part of the salvage regimen to which the patient's HIV strain is sensitive *(247, 248)*.

It was also suggested that the use of nevirapine in the setting of a salvage HIV treatment would succeed when the patients are naïve to NNRTIs and at least one other agent to which the patient's isolate is sensitive as part of the

new regimen *(242)*. Furthermore, potential pharmacokinetic interactions between nevirapine and the other ART medications must also be taken into account beyond baseline HIV-1 isolate sensitivity to each of the agents when devising a new regimen in this setting *(189)*.

HIV Therapy Switch from Protease Inhibitors. A syndrome of peripheral lipodystrophy, hyperlipidemia, and insulin resistance has been observed in HIV-infected patients receiving regimens containing HIV PIs *(249)*. This syndrome, although having uncertain etiology, has been strongly related with PI therapy, NRTI therapy [especially d4T *(250, 251)*], and other unknown risk factors related to HIV infection itself *(189)*. Many of the difficulties of studying this syndrome and, more importantly, devising strategies to correct the consequent abnormalities, have been in developing a case definition for what now appears to be a mixture of several distinct and potentially overlapping fat distribution and metabolism syndromes *(252)*.

Several approaches have been used to correct these metabolic abnormalities associated with long-term antiretroviral therapy, including glucose- or lipid-lowering agents, diet modification, hormonal therapy, and PI-switch strategies, wherein the potentially damaging PI drug is substituted with an NNRTI agent (nevirapine, efavirenz) *(189)*. The last approach has met with the most, albeit occasionally mixed, success *(253–264)*. Nevertheless, using a PI-switching strategy by nevirapine resulted in a better quality of life index compared with continuing the PI, largely because of the new drug regimen was simpler *(249)*. This finding of significantly improved quality of life indices is consistent with other studies reporting this parameter *(265, 266)*.

Furthermore, the risk of losing virologic suppression after substituting nevirapine for the protease inhibitor in a triple-combination therapy regimen is low *(267)*. Nevertheless, caution *must be applied.* Thus, a study prospectively followed 34 patients who were virologically maximally suppressed on a triple-ART regimen, including a protease inhibitor that was subsequently substituted with nevirapine *(258)*. Previous exposure to single- or dual-nucleoside therapy was present in 12 subjects, whereas 22 subjects were naïve to all ART at the time the triple-drug combination regimen was initiated. After a median follow-up of 40 weeks, no subject in the naïve group, versus 41% of the experienced group, developed virologic failure after the nevirapine was substituted ($p = 0.003$) *(258)*.

These findings, though supporting the safety of nevirapine switch studies, add an important caveat of caution that must be observed when substituting nevirapine alone in heavily ART-experienced patients *(189)*. *In view of that, it should be noted that according to current U.S. guidelines (December 1, 2007) (http://aidsinfo.nih.gov/guidelines/ GuidelineDetail.aspx?MenuItem=Guidelines&Search=Off& GuidelineID=7&ClassID=1) (268), efavirenz has to be the preferred NNRTI agent to substitute for a protease inhibitor whenever possible [exceptions: first trimester of pregnancy or in women with high pregnancy potential (i.e., those who are trying to conceive or who are not using effective and consistent contraception)].*

Drug-Drug Interactions. Because nevirapine is metabolized by the cytochrome 450 (CYP450) system and activated by both CYP2B6 and the CYP3A4 isoforms *(269)*, interactions with other antiretroviral agents or medications commonly used in HIV-1–seropositive patients that are also metabolized by the CYP450 system could have important implications for treatment efficacy and adverse drug reactions *(189)*.

The antiretroviral agents that have been studied for their interactions with nevirapine are saquinavir *(270)*, nelfinavir *(271, 272)*, indinavir *(273)*, lopiramide *(274)*, and efavirenz *(236)*. In this regard, recommendations for dosing modifications have been listed in in-text references *(236, 270–274)* and in the HIV Treatment Guidelines by the Centers for Disease Control and Prevention *(36)* (http://www.aidsinfo.nih.gov/guidelines/).

Nevirapine in Pediatric HIV Treatment. Data from several open-label Phase I/II studies and randomized clinical trials, particularly from the Pediatric AIDS Clinical Trials Group (PACTG), have revealed valuable information regarding a broad range of pharmacokinetic, resistance pattern, virologic, immunologic, and safety issues to be considered when using nevirapine in treating HIV-positive children *(189)*. One important consideration is to attain target steady-state nevirapine concentrations (3 to 5 μg/mL) by properly adjusting its dosage for age *(275, 276)*.

Toxicity of Nevirapine. The spectrum and frequency of adverse side effects associated with nevirapine therapy have been extensively documented *(277, 278)*.

Rash is the most frequently observed nevirapine-related adverse event *(277)*. In long-term trials, the majority of rashes in adults were mild, with an incidence of severe rash, such as Stevens-Johnson syndrome (SJS) and toxic epidermal necrolysis (TEN), in 0.3% of patients receiving nevirapine. The highest incidence of rash had occurred in the first 4 weeks of therapy *(277)*.

Although sporadically reported, SJS is a life-threatening complication in patients receiving nevirapine *(279–281)*. A related hypersensitivity condition known as DRESS (drug rash with eosinophilia and systemic symptoms), initially associated with various drugs (allopurinol, sulfonamides, and aromatic anticonvulsants), has also been described with nevirapine use *(282, 283)*. The constellation of manifestations include a generalized maculopapular rash without mucosal involvement that presents as a superficial dermal leukocytoclastic vasculitis and lichenoid reaction on pathology examination, as well as enlarged lymph nodes and hepatosplenomegaly with fever *(189)*.

Nevirapine-associated hepatotoxicity is also a major adverse side effect even though it has been more difficult to characterize than rash *(189)*. Case reports of severe liver damage *(284–289)* have culminated in a series of severe adverse events in previously healthy patients receiving nevirapine in the setting of postexposure prophylaxis *(290, 291)*.

The risk level of nevirapine-associated adverse hepatic events was greater during the first 6 weeks of treatment *(278)*. In one study, the liver damage was characterized by a threefold elevation of the transaminase levels above the baseline determination *(292)*. Clinical hepatitis was reversible when nevirapine was discontinued *(292)*.

At least two possible mechanisms for nevirapine-related hepatotoxicity have been consistent with reported findings *(189)*. The first mechanism is immune-mediated and occurs in conjunction with dermatologic manifestations a few days to weeks after the initiation of nevirapine-containing regimens. This hypersensitivity reaction seems to take place more frequently in patients with healthy immune systems or in HIV-infected patients with high CD4$^+$ T-lymphocyte counts. The occurrence of fulminant hepatitis in patients receiving nevirapine in the setting of postexposure prophylaxis is likely to be mediated by this mechanism *(291)*.

The second mechanism of nevirapine-associated hepatotoxicity has a delayed onset and may represent an intrinsic toxic effect on the hepatocytes. Adverse effects by this mechanism would be expected to occur in patients with underlying liver disease who perhaps have initiated the nevirapine therapy with baseline abnormal transaminase levels leading to hepatic injury likely due to accumulated drug plasma levels *(293, 294)*. However, the metabolism of the parent compound was not found to be affected by the progressive levels of hepatic insufficiency *(295)*.

34.4.2 Efavirenz

Efavirenz (EFV, DMP-266, Sustiva, Stocrin) is a benzoxazin-2-one analogue and the third NNRTI antiretroviral agent to become available after nevirapine and delavirdine *(296)*. Structurally, efavirenz represents the biologically active *S*-enantiomer of 6-chloro-4-(cyclopropylethynyl)-4-(trifluoromethyl)-2,4-dihydro-1*H*-3,1-benzoxazin-2-one; the *R*-(+)-enantiomer is inactive. The drug is poorly soluble in water (<10 μg/mL) *(297)* but is available as a liquid formulation *(298)*.

Efavirenz is a specific inhibitor of the HIV-1 reverse transcriptase, which, unlike NRTIs, does not require intracellular activation to triphosphate. Similarly to all NNRTIs, EFV is inactive against HIV-2 *(296)*. The activity of efavirenz against HIV-1 is at nanomolar concentrations—the K_i (inhibition constant) for wild-type HIV-1 reverse transcriptase is 2.93 nmol/L, and the *in vitro* IC$_{95}$ is at most 1.5 μmol/L against both wild-type virus and viruses possessing a range of single NNRTI-type mutations other than the K103N mutation *(299)*.

In spite of their chemical diversity, efavirenz, like all NNRTIs, acts through the same mechanism by attaching to the HIV-1 reverse transcriptase's NNRTI-binding pocket. The pocket is a hydrophobic, non–substrate-binding domain of the 66-kDa subunit of the HIV-1 reverse transcriptase. Inhibition of RT activity is conferred either by interference with the mobility of the "thumb" subdomain or, most likely, by disruption of the orientation of the conserved aspartic acid side chains that are essential for catalytic activity *(300–302)*.

Significant resistance to individual NNRTIs, which seems to develop quickly, often within a few weeks of initiating therapy, very frequently will involve single point mutations and in many cases would lead to significant cross-resistance to other NNRTIs. Most mutations occurred in the codon groups 98 to 108 and 181 to 190 that encode for the two β-sheets adjacent to the catalytic site of the RT enzyme that form the binding region *(2)*.

34.4.2.1 Resistance to Efavirenz

The most common pathway by which resistance to efavirenz develops is a mutation in the *pol* gene resulting in amino acid substitution affecting the site at which the drug binds to the target enzyme (see also Section 34.4.4). This type of mutation is only beneficial to the virus if the normal function (fitness) of the enzyme is not adversely affected to the point at which continued replication would not be possible *(296)*.

In vitro studies with efavirenz have demonstrated that resistance occurs rapidly. Passage of the immunodeficiency virus in MT-2 cells resulted in mutations V179D, L1991, and Y181C, and after 24 passages there was greater than 1000-fold reduced susceptibility to the drug *(303)*. Secondary mutations, such as V106I, Y108I, Y181H, P225H, and F227L, caused little resistance to efavirenz alone, although they have markedly enhanced *in vitro* resistance when combined with other mutations *(197)*. Other mutations (e.g., L100I, Y188L, and G190S), while conferring higher levels of EFV resistance in laboratory viral constructs, have been observed less frequently *in vivo* than has K103N *(304)*.

The phenotypic susceptibility to efavirenz may seem to be retained with certain primary NNRTI-resistance mutations, such as Y181C. However, the clinical relevance of this apparently retained susceptibility remains unclear *(305)* because continued therapy with an NNRTI drug could rapidly lead to the development of additional mutations,

such as K103N and Y188L. Hence, the recognition that higher-level reduced phenotypic susceptibility (>10-fold) exists to any NNRTI drug (e.g., Y181C) would probably preclude response to any currently available member of this class *(197)*.

The key resistance mutation detected by EFV *in vitro*, and subsequently observed with the drug *in vivo*, is Lys103Asn (K103N) *(306)*. This mutation, which reduces the *in vitro* sensitivity to efavirenz by approximately 18-fold, was found to be present in more than 90% of patients experiencing virologic rebound, becoming a key contributor to the antiviral failure in efavirenz-treated patients *(307, 308)*. Moreover, x-ray crystallographic studies have suggested that K103N mutation seemed to alter the structure of the viral reverse transcriptase at the entrance to the NNRT-binding pocket, thereby slowing the binding rate of all inhibitors of the enzyme and leading to cross-resistance *(309)*.

Further *in vitro* studies have also shown that whereas viruses with K103N or Y188L mutations isolated from patients failing on NNRTI therapy exhibit cross-resistance to all of the currently available NNRTI analogues (EFV, nevirapine, and delavirdine), regardless of the initial selecting agent, some virus isolates from nevirapine- or delavirdine-treatment failures that lacked K103N or Y188L mutations remained sensitive to efavirenz *(310)*.

In another observation, as more patients with non–subtype B viruses begin to receive treatment, the patterns of emergence of drug resistance may be different. For example, in those patients with subtype C virus, the preferred pathway seemed to be the V106M mutation that conferred high-grade cross-resistance to all currently available NNRTI agents *(311)*.

Another interesting aspect of resistance is the possibility that viral isolates may actually become more susceptible to efavirenz than the wild-type strains. This phenomenon, known as *hypersusceptibility* (see Section 34.4.4), was identified in 10.8% of more than 17,000 consecutive plasma samples submitted for phenotypic susceptibility *(296)*.

This phenomenon has been observed more often in NRTI-experienced/NNRI-naïve individuals compared with those naïve to both classes of drugs. The genotypic correlates are complex but largely relate to the number of mutations in the reverse transcriptase gene that resulted from ongoing viral replication in the presence of NRTI drug pressure. More recent data looking at 444 NRTI-experienced/NNRTI-naïve patients has shown that mutations at positions 215, 208, and 1118 were independently associated with NNRTI hypersusceptibility *(312)*. In a small number ($n = 11$) of isolates hypersusceptible to efavirenz, there has been an association with the virologic response to EFV *(313)*, suggesting that this phenomenon may well be of clinical significance in helping to maximize the benefit of efavirenz in salvage or second-line therapy *(296)*.

34.4.2.2 Clinical Studies

Results from clinical studies with efavirenz have strongly supported its use in combination with other antiretroviral agents for initial therapy of HIV infection (296). Additional data have also suggested that EFV may also contribute to the activity of second-line or salvage therapy regimens, as well as to improve the convenience of treatment regimens or after the occurrence of toxicity, by substituting it for protease inhibitors, especially in the setting of maximal virologic suppression (296, 314).

The recommended total daily dose of efavirenz in adults is 600 mg, which in early short-term (12 to 16 weeks) clinical investigations produced superior reductions in viral load compared with those of lower once-daily doses of 200 or 400 mg (315, 316).

First-Line Therapy: Study 006. Study 006, which was a key 48-week investigation for the regulatory approval of efavirenz, compared EFV-containing regimens with a standard-of-care PI-based triple-therapy regimen (3TC, PI, and NNRTI) in ART-naïve patients (233). The results of Study 006 indicated that efavirenz-based triple therapy performed at least similarly in terms of its antiviral efficacy but was better tolerated than was indinavir (IDV)-based therapy. The dual-drug therapy regimen (EFV plus IDV) also performed at least as well as the IDV plus ZDV (zidovudine) plus 3TC (lamivudine) regimen in that 47% of patients in this group at week 48 had a viral load of fewer than 50 copies/mL (233).

Study 006 has been viewed as an important landmark in the evolution of antiretroviral therapy by legitimizing the use of NNRTIs as part of HAART, especially after concerns had been raised regarding the safety of long-term use of PIs (317). Consequently, the established HAART regimen paradigm of two NRTI drugs plus RT has been amended in the HIV/AIDS Treatment Guidelines in the United States and the United Kingdom to recommend that efavirenz may be used as an *alternative* to a PI or a combination of PIs in initial treatment regimens (318–320).

Multiple cohort studies have provided evidence that in clinical practice, EFV-based regimens had been superior to nevirapine in treatment-experienced and treatment-naïve patients (226–228, 321, 322).

In more recent studies [e.g., 2NN study (237)], efavirenz and nevirapine were compared as part of initial therapy. Whereas both drugs have displayed relatively equivalent antiviral efficacy in the randomized study [stavudine with 3TC as a backbone along with nevirapine (once or twice daily), EFV, or both], the combination of nevirapine and efavirenz was significantly more toxic, without added benefit, to be a feasible alternative in this setting (237).

NRTI-Experienced Patients: Study ACTG 364. The ACTG 364 study involved NRTI-experienced patients randomly assigned to receive one or two NRTI agents plus nelfinavir, EFV, or both (323). Both the nelfinavir plus EFV quadruple-therapy regimen and the RFV triple-therapy regimen were statistically superior to the nelfinavir triple-therapy regimen. Although the difference between the nelfinavir plus EFV quadruple-therapy and the EFV triple-therapy groups was not statistically significant compared with the standard assay ($p = 0.09$), the quadruple-therapy regimen was statistically superior to the EFV triple-therapy regimen when the ultrasensitive assay was used ($p = 0.008$). These data have supported a role for efavirenz in second-line regimens even though the suggested use of efavirenz plus a protease inhibitor may be the best approach in NRTI-pretreated patients (296, 323).

Substitution of Efavirenz for Protease Inhibitor: Studies 027 and 049, and the Swiss HIV Cohort Study. Data from an initial small pilot study have indicated that patients with viral loads of fewer than 400 copies/mL and receiving PI-based regimens, when switched to efavirenz continued to maintain virologic control during 48 weeks and exhibited improvement in the clinical appearance of lipodystrophy, as measured by weight gain and reductions in abdominal circumference (324). The preliminary data from this study led to the investigation of substitution of a protease inhibitor with efavirenz in two large randomized studies, 027 and 049, and the Swiss HIV cohort study (296).

The open-label, 48-week studies 027 and 049 evaluated substitution of efavirenz for a protease inhibitor in patients who had achieved suppression of viral load to fewer than 50 copies/mL on a combination of a PI and two NRTI agents administered for mean periods of 23 to 26 months (325). Intent-to-treat (ITT) analysis at 48 weeks has indicated that the viral suppression was maintained in a significantly higher proportion of patients on the EFV-containing regimen versus the PI-containing regimen in both the 029 and 049 studies: 94% versus 74% in study 027 ($p = 0.002$), and 84% versus 73% in study 049 ($p = 0.03$). In both studies, more patients receiving the PI-containing regimen exhibited triglyceride levels greater than 750 mg/dL in comparison with patients receiving the EFV-containing regime (325).

Results from the Swiss HIV Cohort study have shown similar findings (326). This was a matched case-control study in virologically suppressed patients (HIV-1 RNA levels of less than 400 copies/mL), who were switched from a PI-containing regimen to an EFV-containing regimen. After 1 year, the probability of virologic failure was less in patients who switched to efavirenz in comparison with a matched, nonswitched group of patients who remained on their PI-containing regimen (326).

Use of Efavirenz in Children. Evaluation of HAART regimens in HIV-1–infected children yielded less impressive results than that in adults (327, 328).

Drug-Drug Interactions. Because efavirenz is metabolized via the CYP450 system, predominately by the CYP3A4 isoenzyme, it will act both as an inhibitor and inducer of this enzyme and induce its own metabolism *(296)*. Thus, inhibitory effects may predominate during the first weeks of EFV therapy, after which induction may predominate. Consequently, interpretation of pharmacokinetic interaction studies would require considering the timing of coadministration, whether the other drugs were started concomitantly or once an EFV steady-state concentration was established, and whether single doses or multiple doses were administered *(296)*. Results from drug interaction studies with efavirenz *(329–339)*, however, have suggested that relatively few of these pharmacokinetic interactions seemed to require adjusting the dosage.

There may be an interaction with ritonavir that may potentiate the toxicity of ritonavir *(340)*. Although there are no specific guidelines for dosage adjustment, caution should be applied regarding any possible drug-associated toxicity *(296)*.

In addition, administration of saquinavir as the sole protease inhibitor is not recommended because the plasma concentrations of saquinavir have been significantly decreased. However, a triple-combination of efavirenz plus saquinavir plus ritonavir has not been associated with any significant changes in the steady-state concentrations of either saquinavir or ritonavir, and dosage modifications with this triple combination seems unnecessary *(340)*.

When efavirenz is administered with a combination of lopinavir plus ritonavir, an increase in the dosage of the PI combination (from 400/100 mg twice daily to 533/133 mg twice daily) should be considered when reduced susceptibility to lopinavir is clinically suspected, because efavirenz may decrease the plasma concentration of this agent *(341)*.

Toxicity of Efavirenz. Safety data have indicated that the most commonly reported adverse side effects associated with efavirenz have been central nervous system disturbances and skin rashes, both of which generally would occur and resolve during the first month of efavirenz therapy and would only infrequently require discontinuation of therapy *(296)*.

In clinical settings, mild to moderate efavirenz-associated CNS symptoms, including dizziness, sleep disorders, impaired concentration, vivid dreams, and agitation, have been reported in approximately 50% of patients compared with 25% in control groups in comparative trials and have led to discontinuation of therapy in only 2.1% of patients *(339)*. More severe CNS side effects have occurred in about 2% of patients manifesting as severe depression (1.6%), suicidal ideation (0.6%), aggressive behavior (0.4%), paranoid reactions (0.4%), and manic reactions (0.1%). CNS symptoms, which generally begin within the first few days of therapy and have a median duration of 2 to 3 weeks, are not thought to be associated with any known neurotransmitter receptor *(339)*.

Skin rashes associated with efavirenz are mild to moderate maculopapular eruptions that resolve with continuing therapy, but 1.7% of patients have required discontinuation of treatment *(339)*.

34.4.3 Delavirdine

Delavirdine (U-90152S) is a *bis*(heteroaryl)piperazine (BHAP) analogue belonging to a class of specific HIV-1 reverse transcriptase inhibitors discovered by a computer-directed, broad-based screening of compounds *(342)*. Structurally, delavirdine represents *N*-[2-[4-[3-(1-methylethylamino)pyridin-2-yl]piperazin-1-yl]carbonyl-1*H*-indol-5-yl]methanesulfonamide. A number of other congeners were synthesized to enhance both selectivity and activity. Indole substitution for the aryl group resulted in greatly enhanced activity, leading to the identification of atevirdine (U-87201).

No inhibition of HIV-2 by delavirdine has been observed at concentrations up to 10 μM *(343)*, nor was there any inhibition of HIV-1 ribonuclease H activity *(344)*. Furthermore, delavirdine did not inhibit mitochondrial DNA polymerase-γ *(345)*.

Studies on the mechanism of action have revealed that delavirdine, like other BHAP compounds, did not bind to the nucleic acid binding site of the reverse transcriptase enzyme, but rather inhibited its function in an allosteric manner *(342)*. This allosteric binding resulted in a stable conformational change in the polymerase site of the 66-kDa molecular weight subunit of the enzyme, restricting its flexibility and rendering it inactive *(2)*. Further studies have demonstrated that contrary to other NNRTI agents, the binding of delavirdine to the enzyme has been stabilized through a number of hydrophobic interactions with the proline residue at codon 236, which may explain its somewhat unique resistance pattern *(346)*. Kinetic studies have shown that the BHAP analogues seemed to impair an event occurring *after* the formation of the enzyme:substrate complex, which involved either inhibition of the phosphoester bond formation or translocation of the enzyme after the formation of the ester bond *(347)*. Consistent with these different modes of action, *in vitro* evaluations repeatedly show synergistic activity with zidovudine *(342, 348)*.

34.4.3.1 Resistance to Delavirdine

As with all NNRTI agents, delavirdine rapidly selects for drug-resistant isolates when used as monotherapy *(197, 349)*. *In vitro*, delavirdine selects for the P236L mutant, which rarely occurs *in vivo* *(349)*.

Results from the ACTG 260 clinical trial have shown that high-grade resistance to delavirdine emerged in 93% of patients within 8 weeks *(350, 394)*. Interestingly, the P236L mutation known to confer enhanced susceptibility to other NNRTIs occurred in less than 10% of patients. In a fitness study, the P236L mutant was shown to be less fit than the K103N mutant, which may partially explain the infrequent occurrence of this mutant *in vivo (351, 420)* (see Section 34.4.4).

Delavirdine resistance is also associated with cross-resistance to other NNRTI agents. Thus, in a study of delavirdine administered as monotherapy, phenotypic resistance was found in 28 of 30 patients within 8 weeks, with K103N and Y181C being the most common mutations. By comparison, P236L, which confers delavirdine resistance, but hypersusceptibility to nevirapine and efavirenz (see Section 34.4.4), was seen in less than 10% of the 30 patients studied *(351)*.

34.4.3.2 Clinical Studies

Although the established dose of delavirdine is 400 mg twice daily, from both clinical and pharmacokinetic perspectives a number of studies have supported the administration of 600 mg twice daily *(349)*.

In the context of HAART, several clinical trials have evaluated the benefit of having delavirdine as part of three-drug combinations *(349)*. For example, ACTG 261—a Phase II, randomized, double-blind, multicenter trial—has compared triple-combinations consisting of delavirdine plus zidovudine plus didanosine with two-drug combinations of these drugs *(352)*. Overall, the median baseline CD4$^+$ T-cell count was 295 cells/mm^3 and the plasma viral level was 28,000 copies/mL. In the triple-drug arm, a transient 1.25 log$_{10}$ copies/mL decrease in plasma viral load was observed at week 4, with 26% of patients having plasma viral load measures of fewer than 200 copies/mL at week 12, a proportion that was relatively well maintained to week 48 *(352)*.

Another clinical study, Protocol 0021 Part II, was designed as a double-blind, placebo-controlled, randomized trial in the United States and Canada from 1996 to 1998 *(353)*. Treatment-naïve patients were randomized to receive zidovudine plus delavirdine, zidovudine plus lamivudine, or the combination of all three drugs (zidovudine plus lamivudine plus delavirdine). At week 52, the mean decrease in the plasma viral load in the triple-combination group was 2.1 log$_{10}$ copies/mL, with 59% of the enrolled patients having values of fewer than 50 copies/mL at that time point. These results have paralleled those obtained from clinical studies conducted in the Italy, The Netherlands, Canada, and Australia Study (INCAS), a protocol evaluating nevirapine in a similar trial *(214)*. Results from Study 13C conducted in

Europe and South America were also similar—at 1 year, the mean decrease in plasma viral load was 1.8 log$_{10}$ copies/mL in patients taking the triple therapy, with 40% of them having values of fewer than 50 copies/mL *(354)*.

A number of controlled studies have also been conducted to evaluate the positive effect of delavirdine—as part of different antiretroviral combinations—on the circulating levels of various protease inhibitors (indinavir, nelfinavir, saquinavir) *(349, 355–360)*. In this regard, in cases of more advanced HIV disease, the effect of delavirdine has been studied—as part of more complex regimens—to enhance the activity of protease inhibitors *(349)*. Thus, in a small study of stavudine plus saquinavir, either delavirdine or ritonavir was used as an agent to increase the blood levels of saquinavir (with a control arm in which nelfinavir was used as the third drug) *(361)*. Results after 6 months of treatment showed that the virologic suppression was superior in the patients taking ritonavir (-0.71 log$_{10}$ copies/mL) compared with those taking delavirdine (-0.29 log$_{10}$ copies/mL); in fact, there did not seem to be any benefit of delavirdine over nelfinavir.

There has been increased attention on the use of delavirdine in salvage therapy *(349)*. In one study, patients who had experienced a virologic breakthrough taking a PI-based regimen but were naïve to NNRTI agents were treated with a regimen consisting of two NRTI drugs plus delavirdine (600 mg twice daily) plus indinavir (800 mg twice daily), taken with food *(362)*. Because the treatment-limiting toxicity was significant, 43% of the patients had discontinued therapy within the first 2 weeks, largely because of gastrointestinal tolerance. The results from the remaining patients demonstrated that even if one considers an intent-to-treat (ITT) analysis, 35% of the subjects initially starting the regimen showed a maximal response—a result that is comparable with that of ACTG 359, in which a much more complex regimen was applied *(349)*. Another study conducted along the same lines has shown similar results *(363)*. Hence, it seems that the greatest benefit of delavirdine may remain in the setting of a salvage therapy. In this setting, the viral isolates will often carry multiple resistance mutations, and the added advantage of boosting the circulating levels of the protease inhibitors with delavirdine may make the difference between a borderline success and a borderline failure *(349)*.

Whereas a number of options are currently available for the use of delavirdine in initial HAART regimens, the amount of data is limited on the short- and long-term potency of delavirdine-based regimens in this setting *(349)*. In addition, even if more information is available, it is unclear how much delavirdine would be used because, in contrast with delavirdine, other NNRTI drugs can be administered only once a day. However, one can also argue that delavirdine could be used in those patients who cannot take either efavirenz or nevirapine because of toxicity and/or a desire to avoid protease inhibitors. Such patients may include intravenous drug users who could be at an increased risk of hepatic toxicity (due to intercurrent hepatitis C infection) and who may also experience drug interactions with efavirenz and/or nevirapine when receiving methadone *(349)*.

Overall, in second-line therapy, the use of delavirdine has been easier to rationalize based on results from clinical trials such as ACTG 359. That is to say, because of issues of cross-resistance, it is likely that delavirdine will not be effective in patients having experienced a virologic breakthrough on an initial NNRTI agent. If a PI is used, it could be argued that an NNRTI drug should be used in the design of the triple-class regimen. If this is the case, the pharmacokinetic interactions of delavirdine with the PI agents can be used to create a more effective regimen than could be put forward using the other NNRTI agents *(349)*.

Drug-Drug Interactions. The drug-drug interactions of delavirdine have been summarized *(364)* and presented in a continuously updated format at: www.hiv-druginteractions.org. Upon coadministration, delavirdine increased the circulating levels of amprenavir, indinavir, nelfinavir, ritonavir, and saquinavir *(365)*. However, nelfinavir also caused a significant reduction in the peak delavirdine levels as well as a less significant reduction in total drug exposure *(365)*. Hence, the efficacy of a delavirdine-nelfinavir combination would have to be carefully evaluated in clinical trials before its use could be recommended in practice *(349)*.

Although no specific drug interactions have been extensively studied with nucleoside analogues, delavirdine cannot be administered simultaneously with the older formulation of didanosine, because the latter agent has been formulated with a buffer that would raise the gastric pH and delay the absorption of delavirdine *(366)*. Although the effect of enteric-coated didanosine on delavirdine absorption has not been studied, its lack of interaction with indinavir and ketoconazole *(367)* would suggest that the levels of delavirdine are unlikely to be affected by the simultaneous administration of enteric-coated didanosine.

Although interactions of delavirdine with other NNRTI agents could be expected, there have never been any relevant studies because the role (if any) of the combination of delavirdine with either efavirenz or nevirapine in antiretroviral therapy has never been defined *(349)*.

Toxicity. The most common side effects of delavirdine reported in patients enrolled in clinical settings included headache, fatigue, gastrointestinal disturbances, and rash (in more than one third of patients) *(349, 363)*.

Rash usually starts 1 to 2 weeks after the beginning of therapy and presents initially with maculopapular eruptions, especially in subjects with more advanced HIV disease. In approximately 85% of cases, the rash will resolve within 2 weeks. In one study, only one case of mild Stevens-Johnson syndrome (with no long-term sequelae) was reported *(368)*.

One intriguing question to address has been whether a rash resulting from therapy with one NNRTI agent can be successfully resolved with another drug from the same class. A study involving patients taking either delavirdine or nevirapine has shown that overall, 27% of the patients developed a rash that required therapy to be interrupted *(369)*. The results have shown that rash recurred in as many patients re-initiating therapy with the same agent as those patients who crossed over to the other drug, and this outcome suggested that there is probably little value in attempting to re-initiate therapy with other drugs from the same class compared with re-initiating therapy with the same drug, unless there is an absolutely compelling reason to use NNRTI agents in the regimen *(349)*.

Combined data from a number of clinical trials have failed to demonstrate that, compared with nevirapine and efavirenz, there had been any significant association between any form of hepatic toxicity and the use of delavirdine *(370–372)*.

A small study of seven women who became pregnant while receiving delavirdine as part of a clinical trial showed that three patients had ectopic pregnancies, one delivered an infant with a small muscular ventricular septal defect, and three had normal pregnancies *(373)*. In light of these results (along with limited data from animal experiments suggesting teratogenicity), delavirdine should be avoided in pregnancy *(349)*.

34.4.4 Resistance to Non-nucleoside HIV Reverse Transcriptase Inhibitors

The prevalence of resistance to non-nucleoside reverse transcriptase inhibitors has been increasing as the number of patients who have been treated with this class of antiretroviral agents has grown in recent years *(197)*. However, compared with other classes of antiretroviral agents, the resistance to NNRTI drugs has occurred more frequently and presents itself as a serious limitation to their use (see also Sections 34.4.1.1, 34.4.2.1, and 34.4.3.1).

Defining resistance to NNRTI agents is straightforward with both genotype and phenotype assays. In general, primary resistance mutations often confer high-level (>30-fold) phenotype resistance, so that genotype and phenotype assays yield concordant resistance interpretations. However, occasional mutations associated with NNRTI resistance do not confer phenotypic resistance *(374, 375)*.

The resistance profile of NNRTI agents involves a non-competitive binding to the p66 subunit of the HIV RT in a hydrophobic pocket near the active site (see Section 34.1.1). X-ray crystallographic studies of the RT complex with nevirapine *(2)* revealed that the drug lies on top of a hairpin motif that contains aspartic acid at positions 185 and 186, thus allowing the tyrosine at positions 181 and 188 to come in contact with nevirapine. This may partially explain why the Y181C mutation will confer resistance to nevirapine. Furthermore, the nevirapine binding may also indirectly affect the conformation of aspartic acid residues at the active site, or the binding may also prohibit movement of different domains of the protein in relation to each other, thus inhibiting the function of the RT enzyme *(2)*.

There are several single-point mutations that have been associated with significant decreases in the susceptibility to NNRTI agents, as well as several combinations of mutations that have further reduced susceptibility *(197)*.

The most widely recognized NNRTI-resistance mutation is K103N. It confers resistance to all three (nevirapine, efavirenz, and delavirdine) NNRTI drugs. The NNRTIs bind the RT enzyme at a site distinct from the active site, generally between codons 100 to 110 and 180 to 190 *(2)*. To the contrary, the NRTIs bind at the active site. Because of the difference in binding sites of the two drug classes, there is a little overlap in the mutations that confer NRTI and NNRTI resistance. One exception may be Q145M mutation. Q145M may be responsible for drug recognition and processing and has been shown to confer resistance to both NNRTI and NRTI agents *(376)*.

Mutations at other sites of the RT enzyme, such as Y318F, may also confer resistance to NNRTI drugs. When site-directed mutants containing only the Y318F mutation were constructed, significant resistance to delavirdine (41-fold decrease in susceptibility) has been observed along with less than a threefold decrease in susceptibility to nevirapine or efavirenz. However, in clinical isolates, the presence of Y318F when Y181C mutation was also present conferred an additional 3.3-fold increase in resistance to efavirenz. Furthermore, when Y318F was present with K103N mutation, there was a marked increase in resistance—from 15-fold for K103N alone to 43-fold when both mutations were present *(377, 378)*.

Detecting which mutations confer resistance to specific drugs should be made more difficult because mutations selected by serial passage of virus with subinhibitory drug concentration *in vitro* may be different from those observed *in vivo*. There are different hypotheses to explain this phenomenon, one of which is *viral fitness*. The mutations selected for *in vitro* may confer significant fitness disadvantages limiting their emergence *in vivo*. Furthermore, certain mechanisms of resistance may provide a marked fitness disadvantage *in vivo* that is not seen *in vitro* because of the absence of host interactions in the *in vitro* model *(197)*.

Cross-Resistance. The cross-resistance among the NNRTI agents is broad, and after treatment failure of one NNRTI, the likelihood of another one retaining antiviral activity is low, thereby largely preventing the sequential use of this class of drugs *(197)*. The cross-resistance is mainly associated with

the K103N mutation, which is among the most common mutations arising in this class of antiretroviral agents. Other mutations, such as Y181C, confer resistance to delavirdine and nevirapine, but only low-level reduced phenotypic susceptibility to efavirenz.

The cross-resistance of the three NNRTIs currently available can be explained by their binding to the same site of the HIV reverse transcriptase, and a mutation altering the binding properties of one of these drugs will also affect the other two members of the class *(197)*. Moreover, *in vitro* studies have shown that a newly found mutation after NNRTI therapy seemed to stimulate viral replication in the presence of other NNRTIs. Thus, in a small study of four patients, the M230L mutation observed either alone or in combination with other known NNRTI-resistant mutations seemed to markedly reduce the susceptibility of all NNRTIs (>250-fold decreased susceptibility) *(379)*. Interestingly, the virus isolated from three of the four patients had 50% to 100% greater levels of replication in the presence of NNRTI than in the absence of these drugs.

Transmission of NNRTI-Resistant Virus in Treatment-Naïve Patients. Transmitted NNRTI resistance is a well-documented phenomenon that is becoming a major problem in HIV therapy, with high-level resistance defined as a 10-fold decrease in susceptibility of the virus to a particular antiretroviral drug *(197)*. When studied in a retrospective cohort of patients infected with HIV-1 between 1999 and 2000, the rate of high-level phenotypic NNRTI resistance has been estimated at 7.1% *(380)*. Although this high prevalence of resistance is not observed in every population studied, it is nevertheless cause for concern, especially when given the broad cross-resistance among the NNRTI agents *(197)*.

If the trend of increasing transmission of NNRTI resistance continues, the empiric use of these drugs may become problematic if resistance testing is not performed. In this regard, one could argue that in untreated, therapy-naïve patients, in the absence of selective drug pressure, the virus may revert to wild-type, and a routine resistance test may not be able to detect transmitted resistant viral subpopulations *(197)*. Emerging data *(381, 382)*, however, contradict this conventional wisdom by suggesting that it may be possible to use resistance assays in treatment-naïve patients, even when it is not clear when transmission of resistance did occur.

There is also evidence to suggest that drug resistance is detectable in chronically infected but antiretroviral-naïve patients by testing, using the *Visible Genetics* algorithm *(383)*. The K103N and Y181C mutations were the most frequent NNRTI-resistance mutations *(384)*.

Resistance and Viral Fitness. Viral fitness (also referred to as *replication capacity*) refers to the ability of the virus to replicate and cause disease. Because viral fitness is generally assessed in tissue culture systems, its relevance to the clinical situation may be difficult to fully establish. At the same time, inferences about the relative fitness or replication competence of different types of viruses can often be derived from clinical trial data and particularly from determinations of levels of plasma viremia (http://www.cmeonhiv.com/pub/viral.fitness.php).

In tissue culture, the ability of any given strain of HIV to replicate may be somewhat dependent on the types of cells that are used for viral propagation in the first place; for example, certain cell types may display greater or lesser degrees of receptiveness for given viral strains. In some cases, this may be a reflection of the use of coreceptors by a particular viral subtype and, therefore, the determinants of fitness can be varied and can include considerations of coreceptor usage. Drug resistance–conferring mutations have also been shown to affect viral fitness, and many have argued that any individual resistance-conferring mutation must, by definition, be one that impairs fitness, because otherwise, these mutated varieties should appear in the absence of treatment as wild type. However, this interpretation may be overly simplistic because it fails to take into account how individual mutations may affect one another to alter viral phenotype (http://www.cmeonhiv.com/pub/viral.fitness.php).

Research on HIV/AIDS has uncovered new evidence that points to the "fitness" of the human immunodeficiency virus as a primary factor in explaining different patterns of resistance to drugs that treat the disease. This research may also help to explain why some antiviral drugs lead to the development of drug-resistant HIV even when they represent a very small part of the patient's antiretroviral regimen. *In general, incomplete adherence by patients to their antiretroviral therapy may cause HIV to mutate and become resistant to the effects of the medications, while the medications that were consumed, in turn, caused the newly resistant virus to become less fit.*

The effect of various NNRTI mutations on viral fitness has been evaluated in several trials *(197)*. In one such study *(385)*, site-directed mutagenesis was used to construct viruses with NNRTI-resistance mutations. The replication capacities and phenotypic susceptibilities of the constructs were then compared with those of wild-type virus. The following commonly occurring mutations had no effect on viral replication capacity: K103N, Y181C/I, Y188C/H/L, and G190A. Several other mutations (V106A, G190C/S, P225H, M230L, and P236L) conferred substantial reduction in viral fitness. Double mutants had varying degrees of altered replication capacity, indicating that the replication capacity of virus with more than one NNRTI mutation cannot be predicted based on the replication capacity of single mutants *(385)*. However, the accumulation of multiple mutations has been shown to cause a significant reduction in fitness *(386)*.

Because virus with NNRTI-resistance mutations may persist long after the NNRTI-selective drug pressure is removed, whether these mutations cause fitness impairment still remains controversial *(197)*. Whereas several common mutations (K103N, Y181C, and Y188C/H/L) did not reduce viral fitness, other mutations did confer a significant loss of fitness. Another study evaluated the replication capacity (fitness) of the P236L mutation that occurs *in vitro*, but infrequently *in vivo*, in the presence of delavirdine *(349–351)*. Conversely, the K103N mutation occurs more frequently during delavirdine therapy, leading to the hypothesis that virus with the K103N mutation is more "fit" than virus with the P236L mutation *(351)*. On the other hand, the P236L mutant demonstrated decreased rates of ribonuclease H cleavage that were presumed to be the cause of the differential fitness. Differential rates of ribonuclease H cleavage were also observed in another study demonstrating that a virus harboring the V179D mutation was more fit than one with the Y181C mutation, which in turn was more fit than the one with the V106 mutation *(387)*. However, whether the reductions in fitness caused by NNRTI-resistant mutations have any significant clinical consequences has not yet been determined *(197)*.

Hypersusceptibility. Recent studies based on phenotypic susceptibility have revealed that some virus isolates have increased susceptibility to NNRTI agents showing IC_{50} values lower than those of the reference (wild-type) virus *(197)*. This phenomenon has been termed *hypersusceptibility.*

In a large analysis of 17,000 sequentially received plasma samples, specimens were analyzed for both phenotypic and genotypic resistance *(388)*. Hypersusceptibility (defined as FC <0.4) to efavirenz, delavirdine, and nevirapine) have been detected in 10.8%, 10.7%, and 8% of the specimens, respectively, and was most common in NNRTI-naïve/NRTI-experienced patients. Mutations at several sites in the reverse transcriptase were significantly associated with NNRTI hypersusceptibility, predominately at codons 41, 44, 67, 69, 74, 75, 118, 184, 210, and 219 *(388)*.

34.4.5 Drugs in Development

34.4.5.1 Etravirine

Etravirine (TMC-125, R165335, Intelence) is a NNRTI that was approved by the FDA in January 2008. Structurally, etravirine represents 4-{[6-amino-5-bromo-2-((4-cyanophenyl) amino) -4-pyrimidinyl]oxy}-3,5-dimethyl-benzonitrile.

It is the first NNRTI to demonstrate antiviral activity in patients with NNRTI-resistant virus. Etravirine will be sold under the trade name Intelence. Etravirine is indicated for use in combination with other antiretroviral agents for the treatment of HIV-1 infection in antiretroviral treatment–experienced adult patients who have evidence of viral replication and HIV-1 strains resistant to a NNRTI and other antiretroviral agents. FDA granted this accelerated approval based on the viral load and CD4 data from a 24-week treatment of 1,203 adults in two randomized, double-blind, placebo-controlled trials (DUET-1 and -2 studies) conducted in clinically advanced, antiretroviral treatment–experienced adults with evidence of resistance to NNRTI(s) and PIs (see below).

Mechanism of Action. Etravirine and related anti-AIDS drug candidates can bind the reverse transcriptase in multiple conformations and thereby escape the effects of drug-resistance mutations *(389)*. Structural studies showed that etravirine and other diarylpyrimidine (DAPY) analogues *(390)* can adapt to changes in the NNRTI-binding pocket in several ways: (i) DAPY analogues can bind in at least two conformationally distinct modes; (ii) within a given binding mode, torsional flexibility ("wiggling") of DAPY analogues permits access to numerous conformational variants; and (iii) the compact design of the DAPY analogues permits significant repositioning and reorientation (translation and rotation) within the pocket ("jiggling"). Such adaptations appear to be critical for potency against wild-type and a wide range of drug-resistant mutant HIV-1 reverse transcriptases. Exploitation of favorable components of an inhibitor's conformational flexibility (such as torsional flexibility about strategically located chemical bonds) can be a powerful drug design concept, especially for designing drugs that will be effective against rapidly mutating targets *(389, 391)*.

Dosing and Administration. Etravirine is administered orally. In clinical trials, 100 and 200 mg capsules of TMC-125 have been tested in dosages of 400, 800, and 1,200 mg, twice daily; 900 mg, twice daily; and 1,600 mg, twice daily. New tablet formulations have been developed in an effort to increase AUC and C_{max} while reducing pill burden. The new 100 mg tablet provides better bioavailability and reduced pill burden; when administered as two tablets twice daily, its exposure is comparable with that of 800 mg twice-daily dosages used in early studies (http://aidsinfo.nih. gov/DrugsNew/DrugDetailT.aspx?int_id=398).

Drug Resistance. TMC-125 was designed by Belgian scientists to reduce drug resistance, partly by making a flexible molecule that can fit in the active pocket of HIV's reverse transcriptase in different ways, even when the shape of that pocket changes because of viral mutations that would defeat other drugs *(389)*. TMC-125 has garnered attention because of its activity against NNRTI-resistant HIV strains *(392)*. *In vitro*, TMC-125 has equipotent activity against wild-type HIV and NNRTI-resistant variants that encode L100I, K103N, Y181C, Y188L, and G190A/S mutations *(393)*.

Drug-Drug Interactions. Studies have been conducted to determine the drug interactions between etravirine and ritonavir-boosted tipranavir (TPV/r). When TMC-125 was coadministered with TPV/r, exposure to TMC-125 (AUC) was decreased by 76%. TPV and ritonavir exposures increased 18% and 23%, respectively, when these drugs were taken concurrently with twice-daily 800 mg TMC-125. Given the clinical relevance of these drug interactions, coadministration of TMC-125 and TPV/r is not recommended *(394)*.

In some small studies in healthy volunteers, when twice-daily 200 mg TMC-125 and twice-daily ritonavir-boosted darunavir (darunavir/r) 600 mg/100 mg were coadministered, changes to darunavir's pharmacokinetics were not clinically relevant. Although the serum concentration of TMC-125 decreased by 37% compared with that of twice-daily 100 mg TMC-125, the decrease was not considered clinically relevant. However, serum concentration of darunavir/r increased when given with twice-daily 200 mg TMC-125 (at a magnitude greater than when given with twice-daily 100 mg TMC-125); this finding indicated that twice-daily 200 mg TMC-125 exhibited the best clinical exposure, and current Phase III trials have been using this dosing scheme *(395)*.

When TMC-125 was coadministered with lopinavir/ ritonavir or with tenofovir disoproxil fumarate, the AUC and initial plasma concentration of TMC-125 were significantly decreased. However, no relationships between these pharmacokinetic changes and laboratory or other adverse events have been observed (http://aidsinfo.nih.gov/ DrugsNew/DrugDetailT.aspx?int_id=398).

TMC-125 has been studied in combination with the integrase inhibitor raltegravir (also active against treatment-resistant HIV mutants) in 19 healthy participants. Raltegravir at 400 mg twice-daily for 4 days had no significant effect on TMC-125 exposure or plasma concentrations. TMC-125 modestly decreased raltegravir AUC and C_{max}, but no dosage adjustment during coadministration appears necessary *(396)*.

Results from a study to evaluate the effect of coadministration of elvitegravir/ritonavir and etravirine on the pharmacokinetics of elvitegravir and etravirine, and to evaluate the safety and tolerability of short-term administration of elvitegravir/ritonavir and etravirine alone and in combination, have shown lack of clinically relevant drug-drug interactions *(397)*.

Clinical Trials and Adverse Effects. Several studies of TMC-125 in HIV-infected patients have shown promising antiviral activity, especially against HIV that has already developed resistance to other NNRTI drugs.

DUET-1 and DUET-2 are identically designed, ongoing Phase III, double-blind, randomized trials of etravirine versus placebo, both in combination with an optimized background regimen containing the protease inhibitor combination darunavir/ritonavir, with or without enfuvirtide *(398–401)*. The combined intent-to-treat population included 1,203 patients. Most (89%) were men, 70% were Caucasian, 58% had CDC stage C HIV disease, the median HIV RNA level was 4.8 $\log_{10}$ copies/mL, and the median

CD4$^+$ T-cell count was 105 cells/mm^3. At baseline, participants had documented NNRTI resistance-associated mutations (RAMs) and at least three primary protease inhibitor resistance mutations. About 25% started enfuvirtide for the first time, but about 17% had no fully active background drugs in addition to etravirine. The results have shown that etravirine was consistently superior to placebo with respect to:

- Confirmed viral load <50 copies/mL (59% vs. 41%; $p < 0.0001$)
- Viral load <400 copies/mL (74% vs. 53%; $p < 0.0001$)
- Mean reduction in viral load (2.38 vs. 1.69 log$_{10}$ copies/mL; $p < 0.0001$)
- Mean CD4 cell increase (86 vs. 67 cells/mm^3; $p < 0.0001$)
- 45% of patients with no other fully active drugs in their regimen achieved a viral load below 50 copies/mL
- Response rate increased with more active background drugs
- There was a trend toward reduced numbers of AIDS-defining illnesses and deaths in the etravirine arm
- 13 baseline reverse transcriptase mutations (etravirine RAMs), usually present with additional NNRTI RAMs, were associated with decreased response to etravirine
- A larger number of etravirine RAMs was associated with reduced responses to etravirine, with the largest impact among the 15% of patients with 3 or more etravirine RAMs
- 75% of the patients with no etravirine RAMs achieved a viral load below 50 copies/mL
- The K103N mutation, which confers resistance to nevirapine and efavirenz, was not associated with resistance to etravirine
- Adverse events and laboratory data, including blood lipids and liver enzymes, were generally similar in the etravirine and placebo arms
- Most adverse events were mild to moderate (grade 1 or 2) and seldom led to discontinuation of treatment (6% with etravirine vs. 5% with placebo)
- The most common adverse events were skin rash (17% vs. 9%), diarrhea (15% vs. 20%), and nausea (14% vs. 11%)
- The nature, severity, and incidence of central nervous system adverse events (15% vs. 19%) and psychiatric adverse events (13% vs. 15%) were similar in the etravirine and placebo arms
- Rashes in the etravirine arm were

  ○ Usually self-limited and grade 1 or 2 (only 1.3% with grade 3, none with grade 4)
  ○ Occurred during the first 1 to 2 weeks after starting the drug
  ○ Were more common in women
  ○ Had no apparent association with CD4$^+$ T-cell count

  ○ Usually resolved if treatment continued
  ○ The reason 2.2% discontinued

Based on these findings, it has been concluded at week 24 that in treatment-experienced patients with documented NNRTI resistance, etravirine showed statistically superior virologic and immunologic responses vs. placebo, and both groups showed a similar tolerability profile *(398–401)*.

In the ongoing, Phase III DUET-1 and -2 trials conducted in treatment-resistant, HIV-infected patients, TMC-125 appeared safe and well tolerated at week 24 analyses. The most common adverse events occurring in both trials, and rarely requiring discontinuation of treatment, were diarrhea (although less frequent in the treatment arm), nausea, and mild to moderate rash of any type. Grade 3 or 4 adverse events or laboratory changes were comparable in the treatment and control arms *(399)*.

A Phase II, 48-week clinical trial (TMC-125-C223) enrolled 199 HIV-positive patients who had failed regimens containing NNRTIs and protease inhibitors in the past. The study volunteers were randomized to one of two etravirine doses (400 or 800 mg, twice daily) plus an "optimized background regimen" (OBR) consisting of available HIV medications. These patients were compared with an "active control" group, in which patients put together the best possible regimen using approved HIV medications. By week 48, approximately 39 of the 40 (98%) patients in the active control group had discontinued their selected treatment, mostly due to rebounding viral loads. In both etravirine groups, rebounds in viral load were only seen in 9% of the patients. Patients in the active control group remained on their selected treatment regimen for an average of 18 weeks, compared with an average of 48 weeks in the etravirine groups *(400–402)*.

34.4.5.2 Rilpivirine

Rilpivirine (TMC-278, R278474) is an experimental NNRTI currently being developed. It has not yet been evaluated by the FDA for use in treating HIV disease.

Structurally, rilpivirine represents 4-{[4-[[4-[(1*E*)-2-cyanoethenyl]-2,6-dimethylphenyl] amino]-2-pyrimidinyl] amino}benzonitrile *(403)*.

Preclinical and Clinical Studies. In studies to data, rilpivirine has demonstrated potent and sustained anti-HIV activity in treatment-naïve patients.

The primary objective of the ongoing TMC-278-C204 Phase IIb trial has been to determine the best TMC-278 dose to be used in future trials of rilpivirine. The primary end-point was the proportion of patients with confirmed viral load <50 copies/mL [(time to loss of virologic response (TLOVR) definition, noncompleter = failure] at 48 weeks *(404)*. The study involved 368 treatment-naïve HIV patients receiving three different once-daily doses of

TMC-278 (25, 75, or 150 mg) compared with efavirenz (600 mg, once daily). Both drugs were used in combination with zidovudine/lamivudine or tenofovir/emtricitabine. TMC-278 demonstrated potent and sustained viral suppression over 48 weeks similar to that of efavirenz. In addition, the drug has shown a lower incidence of rash and lipid effects (cholesterol/triglycerides). Finally, compared with efavirenz, TMC-278 had a substantially lower incidence of central nervous system (CNS) disorders, affecting 33% of those receiving TMC-278 compared with 53% of those receiving efavirenz *(404)*.

During the ongoing TMC-278-C204 trial, the metabolic profiles—fasting lipid levels, blood glucose, and insulin sensitivity—were assessed and compared among subjects taking rilpivirine or efavirenz *(405)*. The results have shown no significant differences in the metabolic parameters between the different rilpivirine dose groups. The mean increases from baseline in total cholesterol, low-density lipoprotein (LDL, or "bad") cholesterol, and triglycerides were significantly lower among patients taking rilpivirine (all dose groups combined) compared with those taking efavirenz. The protective high-density lipoprotein (HDL, or "good") cholesterol also increased less in the rilpivirine group compared with the efavirenz group (+5 vs. +12 mg/dL). Overall, higher total cholesterol, LDL cholesterol, and triglycerides were observed with efavirenz than with TMC-278 *(405)*.

34.4.5.3 (+)-Calanolide A

(+)-Calanolide A (NSC-675451), a pyranocoumarin derivative, is a new, experimental NNRTI and a synthetic version of a compound found in nature. The compound was isolated from extracts from the latex produced by a tree [*Calophyllum lanigerum* var. *austrocoriaceum* (N10907, Q66O2389)] native to the tropical rainforest of Sarawak, Malaysia. Because the plant source is relatively rare, a chemical version was synthesized.

Structurally, (+)-calanolide A represents 1*H*,3*H*-thiazolo [3,4- a]benzimidazole *(406–414)*. The total syntheses of optically active (+)-calanolide A *(415)* was accomplished in 1996, and the racemic (±)-calanolide in 1993 *(416)*.

The safety and pharmacokinetics of (+)-calanolide A was examined in four successive single-dose cohorts (200, 400, 600, and 800 mg) in healthy, HIV-negative volunteers. In this initial Phase I study, the toxicity of (+)-calanolide A was minimal in the 47 subjects treated. Dizziness, taste perversion, headache, eructation (better known as burping or belching), and nausea were the most frequently reported adverse events. These events were not all judged to be related to the study medication nor were they dose-related. In general, levels of (+)-calanolide A in human plasma were higher than would have been predicted from animal studies, yet the safety profile remained benign. Overall, the study demonstrated the safety and favorable pharmacokinetic profile of single doses of (+)-calanolide A in healthy, HIV-negative individuals *(417)*.

(+)-Calanolide A is currently being evaluated in clinical trials in the United States. (+)-Calanolide A, the congeners costatolide and dihydrocostatolide, and (+)-12-oxo(+)-calanolide A were evaluated in combination with a variety of mechanically diverse inhibitors of HIV replication to define the efficacy and cellular toxicity of potential clinical drug combinations. These assays should be useful in prioritizing the use of different combination drug strategies in a clinical setting. The calanolides exhibited synergistic antiviral interactions with other nucleoside and non-nucleoside reverse transcriptase inhibitors and protease inhibitors. Additive interactions were also observed when the calanolides were used with representative compounds from each of these classes of inhibitors. No evidence of either combination toxicity or antagonistic antiviral activity was detected with any of the tested compounds. The combination antiviral efficacy of three-drug combinations involving the calanolides, and the efficacy of two- and three-drug combinations using a (+)-calanolide A-resistant challenge virus (bearing the T139I amino acid change in the reverse transcriptase), was also evaluated *in vitro*. These assays suggest that the best combination of agents based on *in vitro* anti-HIV assay results would include the calanolides in combination with lamivudine and nelfinavir, as this was the only three-drug combination exhibiting a significant level of synergy. Combination assays with the (+)-calanolide A–resistant strain yielded identical results as seen with the wild-type virus, although the concentration of the calanolides had to be increased *(418)*.

34.5 HIV Protease

The assembly of infectious virions is dependent on the action of (i) an aspartyl protease encoded by the viral *pol* gene and responsible for cleavage of the gag and gag-pol precursors into mature proteins *(419, 420)*; and (ii) cellular *N*-protein myristoyl transferase (NMT), which adds myristic acid to the *N*-terminus of gag, gag-pol, and nef viral polyprotein precursors *(421)*.

The HIV-1 protease (HIV PR) is a dimeric enzyme composed of two identical polypeptide chains that associate with twofold symmetry. The x-ray crystal structure of the HIV-1 protease has been resolved by numerous laboratories around the world, with atomic coordinates becoming available mainly through the Atomic Data Bank *(422)*.

The general topology of the HIV-1 protease monomer is similar to that of a single domain in pepsin-like aspartic proteases; the main difference is that the dimer interface of the

HIV-1 protease is made up of four short strands, rather than the six long strands present in pepsins. The second half of the HIV-1 protease molecule is topologically related to the first half by an approximate intramolecular twofold axis *(422)*.

In one study, the crystal structure of a covalently tethered dimer of HIV-1 protease has been determined to 1.8Å *(423)*. The tethered dimer:inhibitor complex was shown to be identical in nearly every respect to the complex of the same inhibitor with the wild-type dimeric molecule, except for the linker region. It has been suggested that the tethered dimer may be a useful surrogate enzyme for studying the effects of single-site mutations on substrate and inhibitor binding as well as on enzyme asymmetry, and for simulating independent mutational drift of the two domains, which has been proposed to have led to the evolution of modern day, single-chain aspartic proteinases *(423)*.

The HIV-1 protease is unusual in that it is a dimer made of two identical subunits, but with *only one active site*, which is C_2 symmetric in the absence of any ligands other than water *(422)*. In this regard, dimerization of the HIV protease is an essential step in the replication of the virus. The active enzyme is a homodimer, held together in large part by 8 residues in each monomer that form a 4-stranded B-sheet. The homodimers of this 99-amino-acid protein have the aspartyl protease activity that is typical of retroviral proteases; monomers are enzymatically inactive *(424)*.

The HIV-1 protease targets are amino acid sequences in the gag and gag-pol polyproteins, which must be cleaved before nascent viral particles (virions) can mature *(419, 425–429)*. Cleavage of the gag polyprotein produces three large proteins (p24, p17, and p7) that contribute to the structure of the virion and to RNA packaging, and three smaller proteins (p6, p2, and p1) of uncertain function *(429)*. Although mammalian cells contain aspartyl proteases, none efficiently cleaves the gag polyprotein *(430, 431)*. Three of the HIV-cleavage sites are phenylalanine-proline or tyrosine-proline bonds, which are unusual sites of attack for mammalian proteases *(432)*.

The proteolytic cleavage of the gag polyprotein would result in morphologic changes in the virion and condensation of the nucleoprotein core *(425)*. The protease is packaged into virions, and the cleavage events it catalyzes would occur simultaneously with or soon after the budding of the virion from the surface of an infected cell *(433)*. Proviral DNA lacking functional proteases would produce immature, noninfectious viral particles *(428)*.

34.6 HIV Protease Inhibitors

As a result of cloning and purification of the HIV protease, the development of rapid enzyme assays *(434–440)*, elucidation of the HIV protease structure, and the development of

potent and selective peptide-based inhibitors of HIV protease have been accomplished *(441–447)*.

Currently, all FDA-approved protease inhibitors are structurally related molecules that are based on amino acid sequences recognized and cleaved in HIV proteins. Most contain a synthetic moiety of the phenylalanine-proline sequence at positions 167 and 168 of the gag-pol polyprotein that is cleaved by the protease *(432)*.

Potential problems with the use of peptide-based drugs include degradation by proteolytic enzymes and rapid elimination by the liver, leading to a short duration of action, and poor bioavailability when taken orally. To circumvent their proteolytic degradation, chemical modifications of the peptide-based drug molecules are usually necessary. One such avenue to exploit is to use the C_2 symmetry of the protease enzyme and try to design novel protease inhibitors with C_2 symmetry *(448, 449)*, but with "less peptide-like" molecules, by retaining the two peptide *N*-termini and eliminating the *C*-terminus *(447, 450)*.

Specific inhibition of the myristoylation of HIV proteins by myristate analogues has also been pursued. Thus, heteroatom-substituted analogues of myristate were reported to inhibit the replication of HIV-1 in acutely infected CD4$^+$ H9 cells at concentrations that were not toxic to uninfected cultured cells *(451)*. The blockade of myristoylation was associated with a dramatic reduction in the rate of proteolytic processing of the polyprotein precursor by viral protease, probably resulting from the inability of the gag and gag-pol precursor to associate with the plasma membrane (http://www.thebody.com/content/art6626.html).

34.6.1 Mechanism of Action

The mechanism of action of the HIV protease inhibitors involves preventing the cleavage of gag and gag-pol protein precursors in both acutely and chronically infected cells and arresting maturation and thereby blocking the infectivity of the nascent virions *(431, 441)*. That is to say, because these antiretroviral agents cannot affect cells that are already harboring integrated DNA, their mechanism of action is focused on preventing subsequent waves of infection caused by both HIV-1 and HIV-2 *(425)*.

Specifically, the protease inhibitors act by blocking the HIV aspartyl protease, a viral enzyme that cleaves the HIV gag and gag-pol polyprotein backbone at nine specific cleavage sites to produce shorter, functional proteins *(452)*. Three of the nine cleavage reactions occur between a phenylalanine or a tyrosine and a proline. By contrast, none of the known mammalian endopeptidases cleaves before the proline. For this reason, most HIV protease inhibitor drugs have been designed *to mimic the phenylalanine-proline peptide bond and to have no (or weak) activity against human aspartyl proteases (441)*. This confers a remarkable specificity of action to the HIV protease inhibitors, and with short-term treatment these agents have shown only mild adverse toxicity and side effects *(453)*.

Because all of the currently available HIV protease inhibitors are metabolized by cytochrome P450 enzymes, mainly the 3A4 isoform *(454–456)*, they can interact with both inhibitors and inducers of cytochrome P450 drug-metabolizing enzymes *(457)*. However, of more concern is the effect of concurrent therapy with P450 inducers, such as rifampin and rifabutin, which can accelerate the clearance of HIV protease inhibitors and reduce their plasma concentrations. The latter can directly affect the therapeutic efficacy of the protease inhibitors and facilitate the development of drug resistance *(425)*.

34.6.2 Metabolic Disorders

The currently available protease inhibitors have been associated with the development of *peripheral lipodystrophy syndrome*—a group of metabolic disorders including hyperlipidemia *(458)*, glucose intolerance, and abnormal fat distribution (buffalo hump) *(459, 460)* (see also Section 34.4.1.2).

The peripheral lipodystrophy syndrome is manifested by (i) fat wasting in the face, arms, and legs; (ii) fat accumulation in the abdomen, dorsocervical region, and/or the breasts (women only); and (iii) hyperlipidemia, hypercholesterolemia, and insulin resistance *(459)*. A review of 15 observational studies and case reports have shown that the incidence of peripheral lipodystrophy syndrome increased with time of exposure to protease inhibitors, with >60% incidence seen after 1 year of continuous treatment *(459)*.

It is thought that protease inhibitors cause the syndrome by impairing the conversion of retinoic acid into *cis*-9-retinoic acid leading to impaired peripheral fat storage, sequestration of body fat to central adipocytes, and hyperlipidemia, as well as by inhibiting the low-density lipoprotein receptor-related protein (LPR), thus preventing postprandial chylomicron clearance and further contributing to hyperlipidemia *(459)*.

Although the central fat accumulation, hyperlipidemia, and insulin resistance manifestations may reverse after the protease inhibitor therapy is discontinued, it is not clear whether a complete normalization of fat-wasted body regions would be possible *(459)*.

Results from *in vitro* studies have suggested that more than one pathway may be involved in the development of the lipodystrophy syndrome and that pathways may differ among protease inhibitors as well *(459)*.

Mitochondria, the key energy-generating organelles in the cell, are unique in having their own DNA (a double-stranded circular genome of about 16,000 bases). There is a separate enzyme, polymerase-γ, present inside the cell that replicates mitochondrial DNA. *NRTIs can affect the function of this enzyme and this may lead to depletion of mitochondrial DNA or changes in its functions (461)*. Human hepatoma HepG2 cell lines were studied *in vitro* for 25 days to assess the long-term mitochondrial toxicity of NRTIs using clinically relevant concentrations of NRTIs (C_{max}, one third C_{max}, and 10 times C_{max}), both singly and in combination *(462)*. Cell growth, lactate production, intracellular lipids, mtDNA, and the expression of the mitochondrial DNA (mtDNA)-encoded cytochrome c oxidase subunit II (COX II) were measured every 5 days. *In order of toxicity, zalcitabine (ddC), didanosine (ddI), and stavudine (d4T) administered singly were most often associated with mtDNA and COX II depletion.* They were also associated with cytotoxicity and an increase in lactate and intracellular lipid levels. Significantly, didanosine and stavudine exposure did not reach steady-state levels of mtDNA depletion even after 25 days. Three dual-NRTI combinations were tested. Compared with either NRTI alone, combining ddC with d4T increased cytotoxicity and lactate production and depleted mtDNA. Combining 3TC with ZDV also significantly increased cytotoxicity and no cells survived after day 15 *(462)*.

In particular, dideoxy-NRTIs appear to have the greatest effects on mitochondrial DNA by affecting the mitochondria-encoded enzymes in the oxidative phosphorylation pathway, causing the cell to be more dependent on the lactate-generating, anaerobic, cytosolic metabolism of pyruvate. Failure of oxidative phosphorylation means that acid (H^+) generated by the hydrolysis of ATP will no longer be consumed, leading to acidosis *(462)*.

34.6.3 Anti-inflammatory, Antiangiogenic, and Antitumor Activities

The long-term treatment of HIV-infected patients with PI-containing HAART has been shown to be associated with adverse side effects, including hyperbilirubinemia, insulin resistance, hyper- or hypolipidemia, fat body redistribution, osteopenia, and osteoporosis *(460)*.

However, a reduced incidence and an increased regression of AIDS-associated tumors, including Kaposi's sarcoma (KS) and some types of non–Hodgkin's lymphomas (NHLs), namely cerebral and immunoblastic lymphomas, have been described since the introduction of PI-containing HAART compared with the pre-HAART era *(463–467)*. The exact mechanism(s) of these effects, which appear to involve metabolic pathways, tissue remodeling processes, and immunologic responses is still not clear. However, a number of studies have helped to shed some light on identifying specific non-antiretroviral activities of the protease inhibitors, which may explain their effect during HAART, affecting glucose transporter GLUT4, bilirubin UDP-glucuronosyltransferase, apolipoprotein B degradation and secretion, and enzymes involved in the function and differentiation of adipocytes, osteoclasts, or osteoblasts *(468–471)*.

Protease inhibitors may also exert activities that, overall, may have beneficial effects on the progression of HIV disease and increase the therapeutic efficacy of HAART. For example, they can inhibit or stimulate the survival and activation of peripheral blood mononuclear cells, T cells, or endothelial cells *(472–474)*. In addition, protease inhibitors inhibit the production of inflammatory cytokines and modulate the presentation of antigens and T-cell responses *(474–476)*. Thus, ritonavir has recently been shown to inhibit the expression of adhesion molecules and the production or release of inflammatory cytokines or chemokines, including the tumor necrosis factor (TNF)-α, interleukin (IL)-6, or IL-8 by endothelial cells *(474)*. Moreover, owing to their capability of inhibiting maturation and function of dendritic cells, protease inhibitors may even prevent T-cell priming *(477)*.

Kaposi's Sarcoma. The capacity of protease inhibitors to reduce the incidence or cause regression of Kaposi's sarcoma and non–Hodgkin's lymphomas still remains to be fully determined. Kaposi's sarcoma is an angioproliferative disease characterized by infiltration of inflammatory cells, intense and aberrant angiogenesis, edema, and growth of spindle cells of endothelia or monocytic cell origin *(464, 478, 479)*. As a result, inflammatory cytokines are known to induce the production of basic fibroblast growth factor (bFGF) and vascular endothelial growth factor (VEGF). Both bFGF and VEGF are potent angiogenic factors that are highly expressed in Kaposi's sarcoma and promote the formation of Kaposi's sarcoma lesions *(464, 478, 479)* and can induce the development of Kaposi's sarcoma lesions even in the absence of T-cell responses and viral infections. These data may explain why regression of Kaposi's sarcoma with HAART has been, in some cases, unrelated to HIV suppression or immune reconstitution *(464)*.

Owing to their anti-inflammatory, immunomodulating, and retroviral activities, the HIV protease inhibitors may affect the development of Kaposi's sarcoma in several ways. These may include (i) the inhibition of HIV replication and the consequent production and release of the HIV Tat protein, a Kaposi's sarcoma progression factor *(478, 479)*; (ii) blocking by the protease inhibitors of the production of inflammatory cytokines by HIV-1–infected or activated T cells, and thereby suppressing both the production of angiogenic factors (bFGF, VEGF) and reactivation of human herpes virus-8 (HHV-8), which are both triggered by the inflamma-

tory cytokines *(478–480)*; (iii) although no direct inhibitory effects of the protease inhibitors have been detected on the HHV-8 replication or gene expression *(480)*, treatment with these antiretroviral agents may clear HHV-8 from tissues and circulation by restoring the protective immune responses to the virus *(479, 481)*; and (iv) some protease inhibitors (e.g., ritonavir) did inhibit the NF-κB transcriptional activation induced in an immortalized Kaposi's sarcoma cell line by TNF-α, Tat, or HHV-8 *(474)*.

34.6.4 Clinical Studies

Monotherapy. The HIV protease inhibitors rapidly and profoundly reduce the viral load, as seen by the decline in plasma HIV RNA concentrations within few days after the initiation of therapy *(425, 480, 481)*. Thus, monotherapy with indinavir, nelfinavir, or ritonavir reduced the plasma HIV RNA concentrations by a factor of 100 to 1,000 in 4 to 12 weeks *(482, 483)*. Moreover, reductions in the viral load have been paralleled by mean increases in the CD4$^+$ T-cell counts of 100 to 150 cells/mm^3 *(482–485)*.

As with other antiretroviral drug classes, no single regimen containing protease inhibitors is currently considered preferable to any other in terms of antiviral or immunologic efficacy *(486–489)*. Each protease inhibitor has advantages and disadvantages with regard to issues such as ease of administration, tolerability, adherence, drug interactions, and resistance profile. Careful consideration of these factors in relation to the individual patient's history (e.g., disease status, antiretroviral treatment history, concomitant disease, and drug intake) is required when determining which drug to use *(487, 488, 490)*.

A number of studies have directly related the magnitude and duration of the reduction in the viral load with PI monotherapy to the dose and the dose regimen *(425)*. For example, in a study of indinavir, daily doses of less than 2.4 g caused only a short-lived suppression of the viral load *(491)*. In the case of ritonavir, although twice-daily doses of 300, 400, 500, or 600 mg resulted in equivalent initial reductions in the viral load, only the 600 mg dose caused a sustained suppression of the viral load and a sustained increase in the CD4$^+$ T-cell counts *(482, 483)*. The dose-response effects of nelfinavir and amprenavir were similar *(492, 493)*. Because of the poor oral bioavailability of saquinavir in its older formulation (Invirase), only daily doses of 3.6 to 7.2 g have been able to reduce the viral load to levels approaching those achieved with indinavir, nelfinavir, or ritonavir *(494)*.

Monotherapy with HIV protease inhibitors is no longer recommended, because the duration of the antiretroviral response is usually limited because of drug resistance (495).

Combination Therapy. The use of protease inhibitors in HAART for the treatment of HIV disease has been highly efficient, leading to decrease in hospital admissions and fewer opportunistic infections as the result of sustained decrease in viral load *(496–503)*. Phase III clinical trials have evaluated the administration of HIV protease inhibitors in combinations with nucleoside and non-nucleoside reverse transcriptase inhibitor drugs *(425)*.

With the significant number of antiretroviral agents currently approved for clinical use, a variety of two-, three-, and even four-drug combinations to treat HIV/AIDS have found their way in the clinic *(425)*. For example, a combination of two protease inhibitors has been shown to suppress the viral load in patients who have not previously received protease inhibitors—the combination of ritonavir (400 mg, twice daily) and saquinavir (400 mg, twice daily) was tolerated by most patients and reduced the plasma viral load to a level of less than 500 copies/mL for more than 16 weeks *(504, 505)*. These results were similar to those of studies using either drug in combination with nucleoside analogues. However, the effects of combination therapy with ritonavir and saquinavir have been less impressive in patients in whom prior therapy with a protease inhibitor had failed *(425)*.

Nonetheless, despite the positive results achieved with HAART, nonadherence, treatment with suboptimal regimens, and inherent viral resistance all contribute to treatment failures *(425)* (see Section 34.7).

Resistance to Protease Inhibitors. The limited duration of the anti-HIV response that occurs in most patients treated with protease inhibitor monotherapy has been associated with the appearance of drug-resistant virus *(506, 507)*. The major amino acid mutations (G48V, L90M) leading to clinical resistance have been mapped *(508)*.

A substitution of phenylalanine for valine at position 82 was identified as the initial mutation associated with resistance to indinavir and ritonavir, an aspartate-to-asparagine mutation at position 30 resulted in initial resistance to nelfinavir, and mutations in glycine at position 48 and leucine at position 90 resulted in initial resistance to saquinavir *(508)*.

When, in general, initial single amino acid mutations may yield only a slight change (by less than a factor of 5) in drug sensitivity, secondary mutation will accumulate in the virus that can lead to a high level of drug resistance *(506–508)*. In this regard, the HIV protease can tolerate a significant amount of mutations—at least one third of its 99 amino acids can deviate from the wild-type sequence without the enzyme altering its function *(506, 507)*. Patients who developed resistance to protease inhibitors have shown their plasma viral loads and CD4$^+$ T-cell counts returning back to pretreatment values, indicating that the resistant mutants are virulent *(506, 507, 509, 510)*.

Prolonged treatment with one protease inhibitor can lead to the emergence of virus with both primary and secondary mutations that can be also resistant to other protease inhibitors that the patient has never received *(425)*. One such case of *cross-resistance* has been observed after monotherapy with indinavir *(511)* and ritonavir *(507)*, which resulted in resistance to other protease inhibitors—once the patient has resistant virus, it is retained even after the treatment is stopped *(425)*.

In patients with indinavir-resistant virus who discontinued monotherapy with indinavir and then received indinavir combined with nucleoside analogues, an initial small reduction in the viral load was followed by an increase within 4 weeks. The failure of this treatment has been associated with the rapid re-emergence of indinavir-resistant virus *(510)*.

In some cases, the development of virus resistant to protease inhibitors may be a function of the plasma drug concentrations—drug regimens that maintained high plasma concentrations may be more effective in preventing the emergence of resistant virus than regimens with lower plasma concentrations *(425)*. Results from several studies indicated that higher drug doses, with higher plasma concentrations, were associated with a more prolonged antiretroviral response and presumably a lower propensity for the development of drug-resistant virus *(482, 483, 491–493)*.

The currently recommended regimens for ritonavir, indinavir, and nelfinavir result in plasma concentrations greater than or equal to the concentration required to reduce virus production by 90% (IC$_{90}$) throughout an average dosing interval *(512)*. *Because drug resistance may be a consequence of suboptimal plasma drug concentrations, strict adherence to recommended regimens should be strongly encouraged* (see also Section 34.7.3). In addition, *because of the problem of cross-resistance, a switch from one protease inhibitor to another should take place, preferably before high-level resistance to the initial drug has occurred* *(425)*.

Combining a potent protease inhibitor with a different class of retroviral agents appeared to prevent the emergence of resistance to either class of drugs *(513)*. Occasional lapses in compliance may also be less dangerous in patients taking combinations of antiretroviral agents because of the ability of one type of drug to suppress the replication of virus resistant to the other type of drug *(425)*.

34.6.5 Saquinavir

Saquinavir (Invirase, Fortovase) was the first protease inhibitor (and the sixth antiretroviral) approved by the FDA in 1995 as Invirase (saquinavir mesylate, SQV-HGC), a poorly absorbed hard-gel capsule that quickly led to viral resistance in many of the pioneer patients. A second formulation, Fortovase (saquinavir, SQV-SGC), a soft-gel capsule reformulated with improved bioavailability, was approved in 1997.

The production of Fortovase was discontinued in 2006 in favor of Invirase boosted with ritonavir to increase the bioavailability of saquinavir (http://rocheusea.com/product/FTVDearDoctorFINAL.pdf).

Structurally, saquinavir represents N-{1-benzyl-2-hydroxy-3-[3-(*tert*-butylcarbamoyl) -1,2,3,4,4a,5,6,7,8,8a-decahydroisoquinolin-2-yl]-propyl}-2-quinolin-2-ylcarbonylamino-butanediamide. Saquinavir is a protease inhibitor that prevents the enzyme from cleaving viral protein molecules into smaller fragments. The protease activity is vital for both the replication of HIV within the cell and for the release of mature viral particles from an infected cell. Saquinavir inhibits both HIV-1 and HIV-2 proteases.

Treatment guidelines of the U.S. Department of Health and Human Services have designated the ritonavir-boosted saquinavir as an "acceptable" antiretroviral component for initial treatment of HIV infection when preferred or alternative components cannot be used. Furthermore, the guidelines have classified unboosted saquinavir as "not recommended" (http://AIDSinfo.nih.gov).

Bioavailability and Drug Interactions. Saquinavir, in the Invirase formulation, has low and variable bioavailability when administered alone. In contrast, the Fortovase formulation at the standard dosage delivers approximately eightfold more active drug than Invirase, also at the standard dosage *(514)*.

In clinical settings, the oral bioavailability of saquinavir in both formulations significantly increases when patients also receive another protease inhibitor, ritonavir. For patients, this represents a major benefit, because they can take less saquinavir while maintaining sufficient saquinavir blood plasma levels to efficiently suppress the replication of HIV *(515, 516)*.

A plausible mechanism of action, although not directly established, may involve the potent ability of ritonavir (at subtherapeutic doses) to inhibit the cytochrome P450 (CYP) 3A4 isozyme. Normally, this enzyme metabolizes saquinavir to an inactive form, but with ritonavir inhibiting CYT 3A4, the saquinavir blood plasma levels increase considerably. Furthermore, ritonavir inhibits multidrug transporters, although much less *(515)*. In addition, unlike other protease inhibitors, the absorption of saquinavir seems to also be improved by omeprasole *(517)*.

Observations from several drug interaction studies that have been completed indicated that drug interactions with the saquinavir soft-gel formulation may not be predictive for Invirase (http://rxlist.com/cgi/generic/saquin_ad.htm). In addition, because ritonavir is coadministered as part of boosted saquinavir regimens, drug interactions associated with this agent should be taken into consideration.

In general, because saquinavir affects both CYP 3A4 and the P-glycoprotein (a substrate for saquinavir), that may also modify the pharmacokinetics of other drugs that are substrates for CYP 3A4 or the P-glycoprotein, and vice versa (http://rxlist.com/cgi/generic/saquin_ad.htm). In this regard, ritonavir, nelfinavir, and ketoconazole each inhibit CYP 3A4 activity and increase saquinavir levels, whereas efavirenz and rifampin induce CYP 3A4, thereby decreasing saquinavir levels *(518–520)*. A drug-induced hepatitis with marked elevation of transaminase levels has been observed in a study involving healthy volunteers receiving rifampin in combination with ritonavir/saquinavir *(520)*.

Dosing. The recommended dose of invirase for adults is five 200 mg capsules (twice daily) plus ritonavir (100 mg, twice daily), taken within 2 hours of a meal *(521)*.

The recommended dose of Fortovase for adults is six 200 mg capsules (three times a day) plus one 100 mg capsule of ritonavir (twice daily), taken within 2 hours of a meal. Fortovase must be stored in the refrigerator at 2°C to 3°C (36°F to 46°F) *(521)*.

Saquinavir-Boosted Regimens. In combination with other protease inhibitors, particularly with a "low-dose" ritonavir, the oral bioavailability of saquinavir (as either a hard-gel capsule or soft-gel capsule formulation) is markedly increased, thus allowing for reduced dosing frequency and/or dosage *(514, 515)*. It is thought that the beneficial effect of ritonavir is the result of its ability to change the saquinavir metabolism rather than inhibiting the P-glycoprotein *(522)*.

In clinical trials of PI-naïve and PI-experienced HIV-infected patients, twice-daily and once-daily boosted saquinavir regimens were well tolerated and beneficial by lowering the viral load and increasing the $CD4^+$ T-cell counts *(515)*. The largest clinical trials have been multicenter, randomized comparisons of twice-daily boosted saquinavir versus twice-daily boosted indinavir ($MaxC_{min\,1}$) or lopinavir ($MaxC_{min\,2}$) regimens. In the $MaxC_{min\,1}$ study, more than 90% of patients in both groups had an undetectable viral load (<400 copies/mL) after 48 weeks of therapy in the on-treatment analysis. However, viral suppression was achieved in significantly more saquinavir than indinavir recipients in the intention-to-treat analysis, which appeared to be due to the significantly greater percentage of patients in the indinavir group who switched from randomized therapy because of adverse events *(515)*. Interim 24-week data from the $MaxC_{min\,2}$ study indicated that 90% of patients in both groups combined had plasma HIV RNA levels of <400 copies/mL *(515)*.

A study on the efficacy of a combination comprising once-daily, low-dose ritonavir-boosted saquinavir (SQV) plus two NRTI agents in pregnant women was prospectively evaluated, ensuring a SQV minimum concentration (C_{min}) of at least 100 ng/mL or higher, with a therapeutic drug monitoring strategy *(516)*. The saquinavir levels were in excess of the target C_{min} in 43 of 46 (93.4%) episodes in which the end of pregnancy was reached on 1,200/100 mg daily; the dosage was increased to 1,600/100 mg in the remaining 3 episodes to achieve the target levels. No cases of vertical transmission of HIV were observed. The pharmacokinetics, efficacy, and tolerability of this regimen have suggested that once-daily low-dose boosted saquinavir may be considered as an appropriate option in PI-naïve or limited-PI-experienced HIV-infected pregnant women *(516)*.

Toxicity. The most frequent adverse side effects of saquinavir in either formulation include mild gastrointestinal symptoms, such as diarrhea, nausea, loose stools, and abdominal discomfort. Invirase is better tolerated than Fortovase (which is more likely to cause diarrhea and abdominal pain) *(521)*.

Saquinavir may also cause skin reactions, liver failure, seizures, and failure of the pancreas (pancreatitis) (http://rxlist.com/cgi/generic/saquin_ad.htm).

Like other protease inhibitors, saquinavir can cause or contribute to abnormal fat distribution characterized by an enlarged belly, thinning of the face, arms, and legs (lipodystrophy) (see also Section 34.6.2). In most cases, this is also accompanied by elevated cholesterol levels, elevated triglyceride levels, and even a tendency to develop diabetes (http://www.hivinfo.us/saquinavir.html).

34.6.6 Indinavir

Indinavir (Crixivan) is a protease inhibitor used in HAART to treat HIV infection and AIDS. The FDA approved indinavir in 1996 as its sulfate salt, making it the eighth approved antiretroviral drug. Indinavir was much more powerful than any prior antiretroviral drugs; using it with dual NRTIs set the standard for treatment of HIV/AIDS and raised the bar on the design and introduction of subsequent antiretroviral drugs. Protease inhibitors changed the very nature of the AIDS epidemic from one of a terminal illness to a somewhat manageable one.

Increasingly, indinavir is being replaced by newer drugs that are more convenient to take and less likely to promote resistant virus, such as lopinavir or atazanavir.

Structurally, indinavir represents 1-{2-hydroxy-4-[(2-hydroxy-2,3-dihydro-1*H*-inden-1-yl)carbamoyl] -5-phenyl-pentyl}-4- (pyridin-3-ylmethyl) -*N-tert*-butyl-piperazine-2-carboxamide.

Dosing. Indinavir is a protease inhibitor licensed for the treatment of HIV infection in combination with other antiretroviral agents at a dose of 800 mg three times daily taken without food *(523)*. In recent years, however, there has been an overwhelming trend toward combining protease inhibitors with low doses of ritonavir to take advantage of the capacity of this agent to inhibit the cytochrome P450–mediated metabolism of protease inhibitors, thereby allowing for dosing regardless of food intake in twice-daily,

and in some instances once-daily, dosing schedules *(524)*. Clinical experience with indinavir has demonstrated that it has a relatively narrow therapeutic window and is frequently associated with nephrotoxicity, which may manifest as a syndrome of renal colic, tubulo-interstitial nephritis, or even acute renal failure, as well as with chronic elevations in serum creatinine *(525–529)*. Therefore, patients experiencing nephrotoxicity on a regimen containing indinavir were safely maintained on indinavir by means of therapeutic drug monitoring. Parameters of renal function improved but did not return to baseline values, at least in the short term *(523)*.

Drug Resistance. Isolates of HIV-1 with reduced susceptibility to the drug have been recovered from some patients treated with indinavir. The viral resistance was correlated with the accumulation of mutations that resulted in the expression of amino acid substitutions in the viral protease. Eleven amino acid positions (L10I/V/R, K20I/M/R, L24I, M46I/l, L63V, A71T/V, V82A/F/T, I84V, and L90M), at which substitutions were associated with resistance, have been identified. Resistance has been mediated by the coexpression of multiple and variable substitutions at these positions, with no single substitution being either necessary or sufficient for measurable resistance. In general, higher levels of indinavir resistance have been associated with the coexpression of greater numbers of substitutions, although their individual effects varied and have not been additive. However, at least three amino acid substitutions must be present for phenotypic resistance to indinavir to reach measurable levels. In addition, mutations in the p7/p1 and p1/p6 gag cleavage sites were observed in some indinavir-resistant HIV-1 isolates (http://www.rxlist.com/cgi/generic/indinavir_cp.htm).

Compared with other protease inhibitors, indinavir resistance appears to be less predictable. There is preferential selection for mutations at positions 82 (valine to alanine, V82A) and 84 (isoleucine to valine, I84V) *(530, 531)*. However, mutations involving at least 11 different sites can occur in a sporadic pattern *(532)*. It may be that a low number of mutations might decrease susceptibility to indinavir slightly, but when the number of mutations accumulate, a high-level resistance will develop *(531)*. In clinical trials, resistant strains emerged after about 6 months of monotherapy in almost half the patients *(533, 534)*. In early dose-ranging studies, lower doses of indinavir were inadequate, as shown by a rapid return to baseline after initial reductions in viral load *(535)*. This failed response could not be reversed by increasing doses reflecting the presence of viral mutants.

Resistance mutations selected by indinavir frequently confer or contribute to resistance against other protease inhibitors. Different mutations are associated with cross-resistance to different drugs. For example, the M46I mutation is associated with cross-resistance to ritonavir, nelfinavir, and amprenavir (but not to saquinavir); V82A,F,T,S alone is associated with cross-resistance to ritonavir, but in combination with other mutations also confers resistance to nelfinavir, amprenavir, and saquinavir; and the I84V mutation contributes to resistance to all available protease inhibitors. Although no single one of these mutations is associated with full resistance to lopinavir or tipranavir, each contributes partial resistance, and the presence of several mutations together can confer resistance. Response to ritonavir is unlikely in the setting of resistance to indinavir (http://hivinsite.ucsf.edu/InSite?page=ar-03-03). Thus, evaluation of results of zidovudine-experienced patients for whom treatment with indinavir, lamivudine, and zidovudine failed because of indinavir-resistant minority variants has shown that of 10 patients with plasma HIV-1 RNA suppression and subsequent rebound, 6 patients without primary indinavir-resistance mutations underwent clonal analysis. One patient had evidence of V82A mutation in 9 of 30 clones at week 24, with no increase at week 40. The dominant week-40 82V-M184V clones had changes at protease codons 62 to 64, compared with all clones at week 24 and minority clones at week 40. Resistance to indinavir can emerge during treatment failure in nucleoside-experienced patients but may be missed by routine sequence analysis. Selection for indinavir-resistant variants in treatment with indinavir, lamivudine, and zidovudine may occur slowly, depending on the genetic context in which they arise. Genotypic or phenotypic testing may be useful in predicting the likelihood of response to other protease inhibitors after the failure of regimens containing indinavir (536).

Clinical Trials. Indinavir, as monotherapy or in combination with reverse transcriptase inhibitors, has markedly reduced viral RNA concentrations and increased CD4$^+$ T-cell counts (http://www.rxlist.com/cgi/generic/indinav.htm).

A 2-year follow-up study of patients treated with indinavir monotherapy (800 mg, every 8 hours) for 48 weeks, followed by the addition of a reverse transcriptase inhibitor for 48 weeks, reported a substantial increase in CD4$^+$ T-cell count and suppression of viral RNA concentrations below detectable limits (>500 copies/mL) in 22% of patients evaluated at 96 weeks (537).

Since the introduction of protease inhibitors in HIV treatment, HAART is usually given as a combination of three drugs. *In the past few years, long-term side effects, particularly mitochondrial toxicity of NRTIs, were recognized as a cumulative risk for patients on long-term HAART.* One approach to lowering the potential side-effects could be to reduce the number of drugs after initial induction with HAART (538). Previous attempts to switch to indinavir monotherapy after induction with a three-drug regimen failed (539). However, the high inhibitory efficacy of currently used ritonavir-boosted protease inhibitors makes these compounds potential candidates for efficient mono-maintenance

therapy (540). If effective, such a simplified treatment would not only limit side-effects but would also reduce costs and results in more acceptable treatment regimens with improved adherence. In one such study, the feasibility of a 48-week maintenance therapy with ritonavir-boosted indinavir in 12 HIV-infected patients was evaluated (538). All patients maintained viral suppression (<50 copies/mL) throughout the study (one dropout after week 32) and opted to continue on this monotherapy thereafter. The dosage of ritonavir was either 100 or 200 mg, twice daily, and the doses of indinavir ranged from 400 mg (twice daily) to 800 mg (twice daily). Individual patient dosages were determined based on therapeutic drug monitoring—the goal was to maintain indinavir C$_{min}$ levels between 500 and 200 nmol/L. At week 48, there were no cases of virologic failure. Moreover, no changes in fat distribution patterns were detectable using a dual-energy x-ray absorptiometry scan.

In addition to indinavir monotherapy, further follow-up studies have shown promising results for a double therapy with zidovudine and lamivudine, and triple therapy with indinavir, zidovudine, and lamivudine (541). Thus, viral RNA concentrations were measured for each group at 48 weeks: 6 (86%) of 7 patients from the triple-therapy group, 5 (56%) of 9 from the monotherapy group, and 0 to 8 from the double-therapy group had viral RNA concentrations below the detectable limits of the assay (500 copies/mL) (485).

The benefit of an indinavir dose increase (1,000 mg, twice daily) to compensate the enzymatic induction by nevirapine (200 mg, twice daily), was evaluated over 72 weeks with regard to virologic response and adverse effects in HIV-1–infected patients (541). The study compared nevirapine versus lamivudine in combination with indinavir and stavudine. The results showed a significant association between the number of indinavir-related adverse events occurring after week 24 and the indinavir C$_{min}$ ($p = 0.03$), whereas there was no relationship with indinavir C$_{max}$ ($p = 0.33$). These and other results from the study have provided further evidence that early therapeutic drug monitoring of indinavir and nevirapine might anticipate a drug-drug interaction, as well as predict the virologic response and prevent the occurrence of adverse events (541).

Ritonavir-Boosted Indinavir. The combination of efavirenz and indinavir given with nucleoside analogues has demonstrated a potent and durable antiretroviral effect in nucleoside-experienced patients (542). The same combination of efavirenz and indinavir when given in the absence of nucleoside analogues has shown efficacy similar to that achieved with the regimen of indinavir, zidovudine, and lamivudine (543).

However, the addition of efavirenz (600 mg, once daily) to an indinavir/ritonavir combination (800/100 mg, twice daily) resulted in significant decreases in the indinavir levels in healthy volunteers (544). Although such a combination has the potential to be a potent, compact antiretroviral regimen that should be easy to adhere to, drug interactions among these three drugs may alter the pharmacokinetic properties of indinavir, ritonavir, or efavirenz, potentially resulting in subtherapeutic drug levels. These pharmacokinetic findings have yet to be confirmed in HIV-1–infected patients, and it may be that differences may exist between subjects infected with HIV-1 and healthy volunteers not infected with HIV-1 with respect to the pharmacokinetics of these antiretroviral drugs. To shed more light on this, a study was conducted to investigate the 12-hour pharmacokinetic profiles for indinavir/ritonavir and efavirenz in HIV-infected subjects *(545)*. The results of the study showed that despite the known pharmacokinetic interaction between efavirenz (600 mg, once daily) and indinavir/ritonavir (800/100 mg, twice daily), there were adequate minimum concentrations of both indinavir and efavirenz for treatment-naïve patients *(545)*.

NRTIs, particularly stavudine and zidovudine, can cause loss of fat from under the skin (*lipoatrophy*). This is thought to be due to NRTIs *damaging the mitochondria within the fat cells*—the subcellular bodies that produce energy by breaking down food molecules. To establish whether using a treatment regimen that does not include NRTI drugs can ameliorate lipoatrophy, in a study conducted by the HIV Netherlands-Australia-Thailand Collaboration Group, a cohort of patients experiencing failure of various combinations of NRTI analogues were switched to a nucleoside-sparing regimen of ritonavir-boosted indinavir (800 mg of ritonavir and 100 mg of indinavir, twice daily) and efavirenz (600 mg, every day) *(546)*. After the switch, recovery of virologic control was observed, which in the majority of patients was associated with clinically modest but statistically significant increases in peripheral and visceral fat as well as in mitochondrial nucleic acid content. *However, these improvements in fat loss (lipoatrophy) were accompanied by a substantial deterioration in the overall metabolic profile (blood fat, cholesterol, and sugar levels), which may dispose patients to accelerated cardiovascular disease (547, 548).* These observations suggested that the various aspects of toxicity associated with combination antiretroviral therapy may be relatively independent phenomena that have explanatory mechanisms dependent on either the different classes of antiretrovirals or, seemingly more likely, on specific agents within these classes. Antiretroviral combinations employing protease inhibitors that display minimal lipid or glycemic effects (particularly atazanavir or saquinavir) or NRTIs that demonstrate *less intrinsic toxicity to mitochondria* are attractive for the design of future studies that may avoid or ameliorate the complication of lipoatrophy and adverse metabolic changes (see also Section 34.4.1.2).

Drug-Drug Interactions. Indinavir should not be used with atazanavir due to possible severe hyperbilirubinemia (see Section 34.6.10). In addition, nevirapine, efavirenz, and rifabutin may lower indinavir levels (http://hivmanagement.org/indinavir.html).

When studied in healthy volunteers, St. John's wort reduced the area under the curve of indinavir by a mean of 57% and decreased the extrapolated 8-hour trough by 81%. A reduction in indinavir exposure of this magnitude could lead to the development of drug resistance and treatment failure *(549)*.

Toxicity. Nephrolithiasis/urolithiasis is one of the most serious toxicities observed after treatment with indinavir *(525–529, 550–555)*. If symptoms or signs of nephrolithiasis/urolithiasis occur (including flank pain, with or without hematuria or microscopic hematuria) temporary interruption (e.g., 1 to 3 days) or discontinuation of therapy may have to be considered. The cumulative frequency of nephrolithiasis has been substantially higher in pediatric patients (29%) compared with that in adult patients (12.4%; range across individual trials, 4.7% to 34.4%). Although the cumulative frequency of nephrolithiasis events increased with increasing exposure to indinavir, the risk over time remained relatively constant. In some cases, nephrolithiasis/urolithiasis has been associated with renal insufficiency or acute renal failure and pyelonephritis, with or without bacteremia. Hyperbilirubinemia and nephrolithiasis/urolithiasis have occurred more frequently at daily doses exceeding 2.4 g compared with doses ≤2.4 g daily (http://www.rxlist.com/cgi/generic/indinav.htm).

Long-term therapy with indinavir has also been associated with renal atrophy *(538, 553)*, and in one case hypertension had predated the renal atrophy by 6 months *(553)*. After the detection of renal injury, hypertension has been considered a secondary manifestation due to renal parenchymal disease *(546, 548, 553)*. Although the mechanism of renal atrophy associated with indinavir is still not completely understood, chronic renal inflammation as a result of "crystal pyelonephritis" has been suggested as one possible mechanism *(556)*.

Because approximately 20% of the administered dose of indinavir is excreted in the urine *(557)*, the wide spectrum of urinary tract disorders with potentially serious complications caused by crystalluria and kidney stones are due to the low solubility of the indinavir crystals *(551, 552)*. An elevated pH with a reduced excretion of citric acid contributes to the low urinary solubility of indinavir—its solubility exceeds 0.1 mg/mL only at pH values below 5.0 *(558)*. Cornerstones of treatment and prevention are *increased fluid intake* and possibly *urinary acidification (551, 552)*.

Other serious toxicity included increased spontaneous bleeding in patients with hemophilia, acute hemolytic anemia, and hepatitis/hepatic failure that may occasionally result in death (http://www.rxlist.com/cgi/generic/indinav.htm).

Hyperglycemia manifested as new-onset diabetes mellitus and exacerbation of preexisting diabetes mellitus have been reported during postmarketing surveillance of HIV-infected patients receiving protease inhibitor therapy (http://www.rxlist.com/cgi/generic/indinav.htm).

As with other protease inhibitors, body fat redistribution/accumulation (lipodystrophy) has also been associated with indinavir therapy (http://AIDSinfo.nih.gov).

34.6.7 Nelfinavir

Nelfinavir mesylate (Viracept, AG1343) is a potent and orally bioavailable human immunodeficiency virus HIV-1 protease inhibitor ($K_i = 2$ nM) and is being widely prescribed in combination with HIV reverse transcriptase inhibitors for treating HIV infection. Nelfinavir mesylate contains the castor oil derivative Cremophor EL. Structurally, nelfinavir represents 2-[2-hydroxy-3-(3-hydroxy-2-methyl-benzoyl) amino-4-phenylsulfanyl-butyl]-N-tert-butyl-1,2,3,4, 4a,5,6,7,8,8a-decahydroisoquinoline-3-carboxamide. It was the fourth protease inhibitor approved by the the FDA for therapeutic use in 1997. However, nelfinavir never secured a large market share, and newer protease inhibitors are generally preferred for first-line therapy in HIV/AIDS (559, 560).

Dosing. The recommended dosage for adults is either 1,250 mg twice daily or 750 mg, three times a day, taken with food. Initiation of nelfinavir therapy in pediatric patients is not recommended by the FDA, although in pediatric patients who are already on nelfinavir-containing regimens, treatment may continue (http://hivinsite.ucsf.edu/InSite?page=ar-03-04).

Clinical Trials. The results of a number of clinical trials of nelfinavir-containing regimens have shown potent suppression of viral load in previously untreated individuals. Regimens containing nelfinavir have also been studied in treatment-experienced individuals (561–565).

Nelfinavir is an inhibitor of cytochrome P450 3A (CYP3A). Coadministration with nelfinavir may, therefore, cause clinically significant alterations in serum levels of several drugs, including other protease inhibitors, certain benzodiazepines, oral contraceptives, and ergot derivatives. Because nelfinavir is also metabolized in part by CYP3A, drugs that affect this enzyme system, such as ketoconazole, rifampin, and rifabutin, that may affect nelfinavir levels as well. Information on drug interactions should be consulted, as dose adjustments are frequently required, and some combinations are clearly contraindicated (http://hivinsite.ucsf.edu/InSite?page=ar-03-04).

Treatment guidelines of the U.S. Department of Health and Human Services do not include nelfinavir as a "preferred" or "alternative" component for initial treatment of HIV infection. Instead, they designate it as "acceptable" for use if preferred or alternative components are contraindicated (http://AIDSinfo.nih.gov).

Failure of a regimen containing nelfinavir may decrease the likelihood that subsequent regimens containing protease inhibitors will succeed. However, there is evidence that changing to a regimen containing ritonavir and another protease inhibitor (e.g., saquinavir) may achieve long-term suppression of viral load after failure of an initial nelfinavir-containing regimen (566).

Nelfinavir has been studied as a component of subsequent therapies. In patients with nucleoside analogue experience, combinations containing nelfinavir and efavirenz were effective at suppressing viral load (567).

Nelfinavir combined with saquinavir and nucleoside analogues has been studied in patients without prior protease inhibitor use and compares favorably with regimens containing one protease inhibitor (568). In patients with virologic relapse on indinavir-containing regimens, regimens containing nelfinavir-efavirenz-abacavir-adefovir were effective in the short term, especially if the viral load was <15,000 copies/mL at the time of the switching (569).

Drug Resistance. Resistance to nelfinavir is associated with the selection of one or more of several resistance mutations. Resistance mutations selected by nelfinavir may or may not confer or contribute to resistance to other protease inhibitors. The commonly selected D30N mutation does not appear to be associated with resistance to other drugs, whereas the L90M mutation, which is less commonly selected by nelfinavir, confers or contributes to resistance to all other protease inhibitors. Genotypic or phenotypic testing may be useful in predicting the likelihood of response to other protease inhibitors after failure of regimens containing nelfinavir.

In a study designed to explore the phenotypic resistance profile, fitness, and virus replicative capacity of HIV-1 subtype B and C proteases carrying nelfinavir-resistance mutations, the phenotypic contribution of mutation D30N to nelfinavir resistance was nearly identical between subtype B and C clones, although their replicative capacity was significantly different. The subtype C (D30N mutation) could only arise from transfected cell supernatant after accumulation of N83T mutation or in the presence of the N88D compensatory mutation. Both B and C virus with the L90M substitution, nevertheless, presented comparable values of EC_{50} for nelfinavir with higher replicate capacity and fitness *in vitro (570).*

Toxicity and Factors Affecting Adherence to Treatment. The most common and dose-limiting symptomatic side effect of nelfinavir is diarrhea, which usually can be controlled with nonprescription antidiarrheal or antimotility agents (491, 571, 572). As with other protease inhibitors, nelfinavir may cause dyslipidemia and abnormalities of body fat distribution.

It is important to assess the patient's motivation and discuss possible side effects and strategies for managing them before initiating treatment with a protease inhibitor.

In June 2007, high levels of ethyl methanesulfonate (EMS), a chemical used during the making of nelfinavir, were detected in European-made nelfinavir by the European manufacturer Roche Ltd. The U.S. manufacturer Pfizer released a statement in September 2007 to inform clinicians that some amounts of EMS had been detected in nelfinavir manufactured in the United States. EMS may cause cancer in humans; in animals, EMS has caused birth defects and cancer.

European-made nelfinavir was recalled in June 2007 by the European Union because of too-high levels of EMS. The amount of EMS in U.S.-made nelfinavir was much lower than that found in European-made nelfinavir and at this time, the FDA considers the risk of stopping nelfinavir therapy resulting from a recall to be greater than the risks of taking U.S.-made nelfinavir. The FDA and Pfizer are continuing to study EMS levels in U.S.-made nelfinavir to make sure the product does not contain an unacceptable amount of EMS.

Nelfinavir has been studied in patients taking the drug during pregnancy; it is classified as an FDA Pregnancy Category B drug. The FDA advises that children and pregnant women taking anti-HIV medications for the first time not be prescribed nelfinavir-containing regimens. As a precaution, pregnant women currently taking nelfinavir as part of an HIV treatment regimen should be given alternative therapy. All other HIV-infected patients currently taking nelfinavir-containing regimens should continue taking nelfinavir (http://aidsinfo.nih.gov/DrugsNew/DrugDetailNT.aspx?MenuItem=Drugs&Search=On&int_id=263).

34.6.8 Ritonavir

Ritonavir (Norvir) is another protease inhibitor approved by the FDA in 1996 as the seventh antiretroviral drug in the United States. Structurally, ritonavir represents 1,3-thiazol-5-ylmethyl{3-hydroxy-5-{3-methyl-2- [methyl-[(2-propan-2-yl-1,3-thiazol-4-yl)methyl] carbamoyl] amino-butanoyl}amino-1,6-diphenyl-hexan-2-yl}aminoformate.

Dosing. Ritonavir is now rarely used for its own antiviral activity but remains widely used as a booster of other protease inhibitors. This discovery, which has drastically reduced the adverse effects and improved the efficacy of the protease inhibitors and HAART, is due to ritonavir's ability to inhibit cytochrome p450 3A4 (314).

When ritonavir is used as the primary protease inhibitor, not as a booster of the other protease inhibitor in the regimen, the standard dose of ritonavir is six 100 mg capsules (600 mg) every 12 hours, although there are some data that indicate that four 100 mg capsules (400 mg) every 12 hours have also been effective. When given as a protease inhibitor booster, the dosing may range from 100 to 400 mg, twice daily or, if used as a part of a once-daily regimen, 100 to 200 mg, once daily. Though ritonavir is rarely used as the only protease inhibitor, and is generally used for protease inhibitor boosting, the decision regarding which dose of the drug to use should be made by a clinician with experience in treating HIV infection (http://www.hivandhepatitis.com/hiv_and_aids/norvir_dosage.html).

For pediatric use, ritonavir is not FDA approved for infants ≤1 month; for children age 1 month to 12 years old: 350 to 400 mg/m^2 (twice daily; maximum 600 mg). For pediatric use, ritonavir should start at 250 mg/m^2 twice daily, increasing by 50 mg/m^2 every 2 to 3 days until full dosage is reached. For children over 12 years old, adult dosing is recommended (http://hivinsite.ucsf.edu/InSite?page=ar-03-02).

Ritonavir should be taken with food. It is a FDA Pregnancy Category B drug.

Drug Resistance. Key mutations that conferred ritonavir resistance are I84V and V82A/V *(573)*. Another mutation at codon 54 has also been observed. These mutations were associated with repeated cessations of antiretroviral treatment. No lipodystrophy was observed *(573)*.

Resistance mutations selected by ritonavir frequently confer or contribute to resistance against other protease inhibitors. Different mutations are associated with cross-resistance to different drugs. For example, the M46I mutation is associated with cross-resistance to indinavir, nelfinavir, and fosamprenavir (but not to saquinavir); the V82A,F,T,S mutation alone is associated with cross-resistance to indinavir, but in combination with other mutations also confers resistance to nelfinavir, fosamprenavir, and saquinavir; and I84V contributes to resistance to all available protease inhibitors. Although no single one of these mutations is associated with full resistance to lopinavir, each contributes partial resistance, and the presence of several mutations together can confer resistance. Response to indinavir is unlikely in the setting of resistance to ritonavir. Genotypic or phenotypic testing may be useful in predicting the likelihood of response to other protease inhibitors after failure of a regimen containing ritonavir (http://hivinsite.ucsf.edu/InSite?page=ar-03-02).

It has long been assumed that the evolution of HIV-1 is best described by deterministic evolutionary models because of the large population size. Recently, however, it was suggested that the *effective population size* (N_e) (see Section 27.1.4 in Chapter 27) may be rather small, thereby allowing chance to influence evolution, a situation best described by a stochastic evolutionary model *(574, 575)*. To gain experimental evidence supporting one of the evolutionary models, how the development of resistance to ritonavir affected the evolution of the *env* gene has been investigated in a small group of patients *(576)*. Here, sequential serum samples from five patients treated with ritonavir were used to analyze the protease gene and the V3 domain of the *env* gene. Multiple reverse transcription–PCR products were cloned, sequenced, and used to construct phylogenetic trees and to calculate the genetic variation and N_e. Genotypic resistance to ritonavir developed in all five patients, but each patient displayed a unique combination of mutations, indicating a stochastic element in the development of ritonavir resistance. Furthermore, development of resistance induced clear bottle-neck effects in the *env* gene. The mean intrasample genetic variation, which ranged from 1.2% to 5.7% before treatment, decreased significantly ($p < 0.025$) during treatment. In agreement with these findings, N_e was estimated to be very small (500 to 15,000) compared with the total number of HIV-1 RNA copies *(576)*.

Clinical Trials. The clinical efficacy of ritonavir has been evaluated as monotherapy and in combination with several other antiretroviral agents *(577–581)*. Unlike saquinavir, ritonavir has shown excellent bioavailability and seemed to be effective in both antiretroviral-naïve and antiretroviral-experienced patients.

More than 1,000 patients have been evaluated in Study M94-247 by adding ritonavir or a placebo to the patient's current antiretroviral therapy. In the retonavir group, results have shown reduced concentrations of viral RNA by 0.6 $\log_{10}$ at week 28, as well as a statistically significant improvement in disease progression and overall mortality (50%) *(577)*.

A clinical trial of ritonavir in combination with zidovudine and lamivudine in patients with symptomatic primary infection resulted in reduced viral RNA concentrations below detectable limits (400 copies/mL) in 9 of 13 patients as of week 12 *(578)*. An open-label trial conducted in France using ritonavir monotherapy for 12 weeks and then adding stavudine and didanosine reduced viral RNA concentrations in 7 patients (41%) to below the detectable limit (200 copies/mL) *(579)*.

Ritonavir-Boosting Regimens (see Sections 34.6.5 and 34.6.6). Ritonavir is a potent inhibitor of cytochrome P4503A4 that strongly increases bioavailability of other protease inhibitors. In this regard, the safety and antiretroviral efficacy of a combination of ritonavir-sequinavir in patients pretreated and receiving continued treatment with zidovudine and lamivudine (who were protease inhibitor naïve and who had a CD4 T-cell counts below 200/mm^3) has been assessed *(573)*. In this 48-week pilot study, all patients received 600 mg ritonavir and 400 mg saquinavir, twice daily. Administration of zidovudine and lamivudine was continued without a change in previous doses. Viral load, CD4 T-cell count, and the emergence of resistance to the two protease inhibitors were evaluated repeatedly up to week 48. Overall, the study results have indicated that ritonavir and saquinavir in combination were quite well tolerated and induced a high and sustained antiretroviral efficacy. A four-drug combination that includes these two protease inhibitors should be considered as a first line of treatment in patients with low CD4$^+$ T-cell counts *(573)*.

A prospective, randomized, open-label, controlled 24-week study has been carried out to evaluate the long-term pharmacokinetics and safety of adding ritonavir 100 mg twice daily to a nelfinavir 1,250 mg twice daily regimen in HIV-1-infected patients *(582)*. The concentrations of both nelfinavir and especially its metabolite M8 increased when low-dose ritonavir was added to a nelfinavir-containing regimen. The combination seems to be safe, and the nelfinavir/ritonavir regimen could be an option in patients with low nelfinavir-plus-M8 concentrations *(582)*.

Drug-Drug Interactions. Ritonavir is a potent inhibitor of cytochrome p450 3A (CYP3A) and CYP2D6, as well as an inducer of other hepatic enzyme systems. Coadministration with ritonavir therefore causes clinically significant alterations in serum levels not only of other antiretroviral agents but also of a variety of drugs including certain calcium channel blockers, cholesterol-lowering agents, antiarrhythmics, sedative-hypnotics, erectile dysfunction agents, oral contraceptives, recreational substances, and others. Information on drug interactions should be consulted, as dose adjustments are frequently required, and some combinations are clearly contraindicated. However, because of its strong inhibitory effect on CYP3A, ritonavir at doses below the normal therapeutic dosage has been frequently combined with other protease inhibitors to achieve therapeutic levels of the second protease inhibitor while reducing either the number of pills required or the dosing frequency, or both.

Coadministration of low-dose ritonavir may also be used to compensate for drug interactions that tend to decrease levels of a protease inhibitor metabolized by CYP3A (for example, in the case of fosamprenavir combined with efavirenz) (http://hivinsite.ucsf.edu/InSite?page=ar-03-02).

Toxicity. Nausea, vomiting, and abdominal pain during the first weeks of therapy are the manifested adverse events of ritonavir, especially during the first weeks of therapy *(583)*.

Ritonavir also causes circumoral paresthesia (a morbid or perverted sensation) in up to 25% of patients, and, less commonly, paresthesia of the arms and legs *(583)*. Though the reason is unclear, these symptoms resolve during continued treatment and have not been severe enough to cause therapy to be discontinued *(583)*.

One puzzling side effect of ritonavir is hyperglycemia in up to 5% of patients. Serum triglyceride concentrations can exceed 1,000 mg/dL (11 mmol/L) *(583)*. It appears that it directly inhibits the GLUT4 insulin-regulated transporter, keeping glucose from entering fat and muscle cells. Though this side effect has not been accompanied by complications such as pancreatitis, it can still lead to insulin resistance and cause problems for type 1 diabetics *(583)*. Ritonavir, like all protease inhibitors currently in the clinic, can lead to fat redistribution and glucose intolerance.

34.6.9 Amprenavir

Amprenavir (Agenerase) was approved by the FDA in 1999 for twice-a-day dosing instead of needing to be taken every 8 hours. Structurally, amprenavir represents tetrahydrofuran-3-yl{3-[(4-aminophenyl)sulfonyl-(2-methylpropyl) amino]-1-benzyl-2-hydroxy-propyl}aminomethanoate.

The convenient dosing of amprenavir came at a price, however, as the dose required for treatment, 1.2 g, is delivered in eight very large gel capsules. Production of amprenavir was discontinued by the manufacturer on December 31, 2004.

A prodrug version of amprenavir called *fosamprenavir* is now available. Marketed as fosamprevir calcium (Lexiva), it was approved by the FDA in 2003. The chemical structure of fosamprenavir is [(2R,3S)-1-[(4-aminophenyl)sulfonyl-(2-methylpropyl)amino] -3-{[(3S)-oxolan-3-yl]oxycarbonylamino}-4-phenyl-butan-2-yl]oxyphosphonic acid (see 34.6.9.1).

The human body metabolizes fosamprenavir to form amprenavir, which is the active ingredient. That metabolization increases the duration of amprenavir's bioavailability, making fosamprenavir a slow-release version of amprenavir and thus reducing the number of pills required in comparison with standard amprenavir.

Dosing. Amprenavir comes in soft-gel capsule and oral solution forms and is taken by mouth. Both may be taken with or without food but should not be taken with high-fat foods. Because both forms contain vitamin E, patients who are taking either form of amprenavir should not take vitamin E supplements. Individuals who are taking the oral solution form should not drink alcohol (http://aidsinfo.nih.gov/DrugsNew/DrugDetailNT.aspx?int_id=0258).

The recommended dose of amprenavir is based on age, weight, and the formulation. Individuals 4 to 12 years old, or 13 to 16 years old and weighing less than 50 kg, should receive 22.5 mg/kg twice daily or 17 mg/kg three times daily of the oral solution; or 20 mg/kg twice daily or 15 mg/kg three times daily of the capsules. Individuals 13 to 16 years old who weigh 50 kg or more and individuals older than 16 years of age should receive 1.4 g twice daily of the oral solution or 1,200 mg twice daily of the capsules. The maximum daily dose is 2.8 g. The amprenavir capsules and solution are not interchangeable milligram for milligram (http://www.medicinenet.com/amprenavir/article.htm). The oral solution should only be used when it is not possible to administer the capsules (http://aidsinfo.nih.gov/DrugsNew/DrugDetailNT.aspx?int_id=0258).

Drug Resistance. HIV-1 isolates with a decreased susceptibility to amprenavir have been selected *in vitro* and obtained from patients treated with amprenavir (http://www.rxlist.com/cgi/generic/ampren.htm). Genotypic analysis of isolates from amprenavir-treated patients showed mutations in the HIV-1 protease gene, resulting in amino acid substitutions primarily at positions V32I, M46I/L, I47V, I50V, I54L/M, and I84V, as well as mutations in the p7/p1 and p1/p6 gag cleavage sites. Phenotypic analysis of HIV-1 isolates from 21 NRTI-experienced and PI-naïve patients treated with amprenavir in combination with NRTIs for 16 to 48 weeks identified isolates from 15 patients who exhibited a 4- to 17-fold decrease in susceptibility to amprenavir *in vitro* compared with wild-type virus. Clinical isolates that exhibited a decrease in susceptibility to amprenavir harbored one or more amprenavir-associated mutations. The clinical relevance of the genotypic and phenotypic changes associated with amprenavir therapy is under evaluation (http://www.rxlist.com/cgi/generic/ampren.htm).

Varying degrees of HIV-1 cross-resistance among protease inhibitors have been observed. Five of 15 amprenavir-resistant isolates exhibited 4- to 8-fold decreases in susceptibility to ritonavir. However, amprenavir-resistant isolates were susceptible to either indinavir or saquinavir (http://www.rxlist.com/cgi/generic/ampren.htm).

Clinical Trials. The clinical efficacy of amprenavir as part of antiretroviral combinations therapy has been investigated in a number of studies *(486, 584–594).*

Triple therapy with amprenavir, lamivudine, and zidovudine was significantly more effective than double therapy with lamivudine plus zidovudine (plus placebo) in a double-blind multicenter Phase III trial in 221 antiretroviral-naïve patients *(595).* Patients experiencing virologic failure after 16 weeks could switch to non-blind amprenavir-containing therapy. The proportion of patients with viral load of <400 copies/mL after 48 weeks was significantly higher with amprenavir than with the placebo, according to both intent-to-treat (41% vs. 3%) and as-treated (93% vs. 42%) analyses.

Quadruple therapy with amprenavir, abacavir, lamivudine, and zidovudine (dosages not reported; the two last drugs were given as combined formulation) produced a marked reduction in viral load and a statistically significant increase from baseline in CD4$^+$ T-count in 98 treatment-naïve patients with primary HIV infection, according to a preliminary report of interim data from the noncomparative QUEST trial (median follow-up 28 weeks) *(596).* The median reduction in viral load was 5.1 log$_{10}$ copies/mL (baseline = 5.2 log$_{10}$ copies/mL, reported as both mean and median) and the mean increase in CD4$^+$ T-count was 249 cells/μL from a mean baseline of 490 cells/μL ($p < 0.0001$) (type of analysis not reported). Kaplan-Meyer estimates for the percentage of patients with HIV RNA <50 and <5 copies/mL at 36 weeks were 87% and 58%, respectively.

In a substudy of the QUEST trial *(597)*, HIV RNA was detected in seminal fluid from only 2 of 22 patients (9.5%) treated for 48 weeks, compared with 30 of 32 patients (94%) at baseline (level of detail (LOD) 50 copies/mL; median baseline HIV RNA level in seminal fluid was 4.23 $\log_{10}$ copies/mL). Preliminary 64-week data from a subsequent randomized, non-blind trial suggest that the amprenavir-containing quadruple regimen used in the QUEST study produced a higher rate of adverse events and withdrawals than did standard PI-based triple therapy but is superior to the latter for those patients remaining on treatment *(598)*. The primary analysis revealed that the time to treatment failure based on virologic and toxicity end-points was significantly shorter for patients receiving the amprenavir/abacavir/lamivudine/zidovudine regimen than for those receiving nelfinavir/lamivudine/zidovudine ($p = 0.017$; no further quantitative data reported). This finding resulted from more adverse events and withdrawals with quadruple therapy (quantitative data not reported). Only 41% of 150 quadruple therapy recipients were eligible for the as-treated analysis, compared with 61% of 152 triple therapy patients; however, within this group, more quadruple than triple therapy recipients achieved plasma viral load ≤120 copies/mL (87% vs. 70%; $p = 0.016$) *(486)*.

Triple therapy with amprenavir plus lamivudine and zidovudine showed virologic efficacy in two comparative trials enrolling both treatment-naïve and treatment-experienced patients (the median reduction in viral load, as assessed by intent-to-treat analysis, was ≈2 $\log_{10}$ copies/mL at 12 weeks in both) *(599, 600)*. As expected, triple therapy with amprenavir, lamivudine, and zidovudine was more effective than amprenavir monotherapy (viral load reduction 2.16 vs. 0.91 $\log_{10}$ copies/mL) in 92 antiretroviral-naïve or antiretroviral-experienced patients *(599)*. A planned interim intent-to-treat analysis after 12 weeks of double-blind treatment indicated a 2.4-fold greater median reduction in HIV RNA level and a 2.8-fold greater proportion of patients with viral load <500 copies/mL in the triple therapy group compared with the monotherapy group. A substudy of this trial showed that viral load in semen was below the limit of detection (400 copies/mL) in most men receiving amprenavir monotherapy or triple therapy *(601)*. Thirty patients were evaluable for seminal viral load at baseline and during treatment, with a further 5 evaluable only at baseline. At the first follow-up (8 to 20 weeks), 14 of 19 men receiving amprenavir monotherapy and 9 of 11 receiving amprenavir, lamivudine, and zidovudine had seminal viral load of <400 copies/mL (viral load in the two remaining patients in the triple therapy group was reduced by >1 $\log_{10}$ copies/mL). In contrast, only 7 of 23 (monotherapy) and 4 of 14 (triple therapy) evaluable baseline samples had HIV RNA of <400 copies/mL. *The data for monotherapy represent the first demonstration of viral suppression with a protease inhibitor in the male genital tract (601).*

Triple or quadruple therapy with amprenavir plus NRTIs has shown variable efficacy in children and adolescents; moderate efficacy was seen in protease inhibitor-naïve patients, whereas such treatment had limited efficacy in PI-experienced patients *(486)*. Thus, amprenavir plus two NRTIs had moderate but durable efficacy in PI-naïve patients but limited efficacy in PI-experienced patients when given to 228 antiretroviral-naïve and antiretroviral-experienced children and adolescents *(602)*. Patients aged 2 to 19 years received the non-blind treatment for 48 weeks as part of the Phase III trial. The amprenavir dosage was 1,200 mg or 20 mg/kg, twice daily (capsules; $n = 117$) or 22.5 mg/kg, twice daily (oral solution; $n = 140$).

Fosamprenavir-ritonavir, twice daily in treatment-naïve patients provided similar antiviral efficacy, safety, tolerability, and emergence of resistance as lopinavir-ritonavir, each in combination with abacavir/lamivudine. A head-to-head study with lopinavir showed the two drugs to have comparable potency, but patients on fosamprenavir tended to have a higher serum cholesterol level. Fosamprenavir's main advantage over lopinavir is that it is cheaper *(584)* (see 34.6.9.1).

Drug-Drug Interactions. St. John's wort and rifampin decrease the concentration of amprenavir in the body, and this could reduce the effectiveness of amprenavir. Amprenavir may also decrease the effectiveness of oral contraceptives.

In addition, amprenavir oral solution should not be administered with disulfiram (Antabuse), metronidazole, or alcohol. Administration of the solution with these agents could cause severe side effects because of the substantial amount of propylene glycol in the oral solution.

Administration of amprenavir and didanosine or antacids should be separated by 1 hour (http://www.medicinenet.com/amprenavir/article.htm).

Toxicity. The most frequent adverse events of amprenavir have been headache, weakness, diarrhea, nausea, and stomach pain. Amprenavir may also cause severe skin reactions and breakdown of red blood cells. The propylene glycol in the oral solution can cause seizures, stupor, increased heart rate, metabolic disturbance, and kidney failure.

Like other protease inhibitors, use of amprenavir may be associated with redistribution or accumulation of body fat, increased cholesterol, and worsening of diabetes (http://aidsinfo.nih.gov/DrugsNew/DrugDetailNT.aspx?int_id=0258).

34.6.9.1 Fosamprenavir

Fosamprenavir (Lexiva, Telzir) was approved by the FDA in October 2003 for use in adults with HIV infection (http://hivinsite.ucsf.edu/InSite?page=ar-03-08). In 2007, it was approved for treatment of children 2 years of age and older. Fosamprenavir is a prodrug of amprenavir. As of

October 2007, fosamprenavir is the only amprenavir product available in the United States.

The FDA approval was based on three Phase III studies—two in previously untreated patients and one in patients with prior protease inhibitor treatment. An open-label study compared fosamprenavir (without ritonavir boosting) with nelfinavir, each given twice daily with abacavir plus lamivudine in previously untreated patients. At 48 weeks, higher rates of virologic suppression and CD4$^+$ T-lymphocyte increase were seen in the fosamprenavir treatment arm *(603)*. A second open-label study in previously untreated patients compared a once-daily combination of fosamprenavir plus ritonavir with standard-dose nelfinavir, each in combination with twice-daily abacavir plus lamivudine. Similar rates of virologic suppression and CD4$^+$ T-cells increase were observed in the two groups *(604)*.

In patients with prior virologic failure on one or two regimens containing a protease inhibitor, two combinations of ritonavir-boosted fosamprenavir were compared with lopinavir/ritonavir (Kaletra). Each regimen included two active nucleoside analogues. Through week 48, similar rates of virologic suppression and CD4$^+$ T-cells increase were seen in the twice-daily fosamprenavir plus ritonavir group and in the lopinavir/ritonavir group; higher rates of virologic failure were seen in the third treatment group, in which fosamprenavir plus ritonavir was given once daily *(605, 606)*.

Dosing. Because of superior pharmacokinetic profile and lack of resistance with failure, it has been recommended that fosamprenavir (700 mg, twice daily) is taken with ritonavir (100 mg, twice daily) with or without food; or fosamprenavir (1,400 mg, twice daily) with or without food; or fosamprenavir (1,400 mg) plus ritonavir (100 to 200 mg), once daily with or without food (once daily dosing for PI-naïve patients only).

When taken in combination with efavirenz, the following dosing regimens have been recommended: fosamprenavir (700 mg, twice daily) plus ritonavir (100 mg, twice daily) plus efavirenz (600 mg, at bedtime); or fosamprenavir (1,400 mg, once daily) plus ritonavir (300 mg, once daily) plus efavirenz (600 mg at bedtime) (http://www. hopkins-hivguide.org/drug/antiretrovirals/protease_inhibitor/ fosamprenavir.html).

Clinical Use. As with other antiretrovirals, *fosamprenavir should be used only in combination regimens.* Amprenavir, the active metabolite of fosamprenavir, is metabolized by the cytochrome p450 3A4 (CYP3A4) isoenzyme and may alter the concentrations of other drugs metabolized by this pathway, including rifabutin, hormonal contraceptives, ergot derivatives, certain benzodiazepines, antiarrhythmics, lipid-lowering agents, and others. Similarly, drugs or herbal preparations that induce or inhibit the action of this isoenzyme may cause therapeutically significant alterations in amprenavir levels. For example, rifampin induces CYP3A4 and markedly decreases amprenavir levels (http://hivinsite.ucsf.edu/InSite?page=ar-03-08).

Fosamprenavir has not been thoroughly studied in combinations with other protease inhibitors and non-nucleoside reverse transcriptase inhibitors; in most cases, precise information on dosing in combination with other antiretrovirals is lacking. Coadministration of fosamprenavir with lopinavir/ritonavir causes reductions in levels of both amprenavir and lopinavir; it appears that this adverse interaction cannot be overcome by increasing ritonavir levels *(607, 608)*.

Coadministration of amprenavir with tipranavir plus ritonavir causes a decrease in amprenavir levels; the same effect would be expected to occur with fosamprenavir *(609)*. Coadministration of fosamprenavir with efavirenz has been shown to decrease amprenavir levels, but boosting with sufficient doses of ritonavir may maintain therapeutic amprenavir levels in the presence of efavirenz *(610)*.

Information on drug interactions should be consulted, as dose adjustments are frequently required and some combinations are contraindicated (http://hivinsite. ucsf.edu/InSite?page=ar-03-08).

Use in Initial Versus Subsequent Therapy. Treatment guidelines of the U.S. Department of Health and Human Services designate ritonavir-boosted fosamprenavir as a "preferred" component for initial treatment of HIV infection. They also include unboosted fosamprenavir as an "alternative" component *(314)*.

When used in initial therapy, fosamprenavir appeared to compare favorably with nelfinavir, either when used as a single protease inhibitor or when boosted with ritonavir. In one Phase III study of twice-daily fosamprenavir/abacavir/ lamivudine versus nelfinavir/abacavir/lamivudine, similar rates of viral suppression were seen through 48 weeks [by intent-to-treat analysis, viral load <50 copies/mL in 55% of fosamprenavir recipients and 41% of nelfinavir recipients; 95% confidence interval (CI): 2%, 28%]. In patients with baseline viral loads >100,000 copies/mL, the fosamprenavir arm appeared to achieve higher rates of viral suppression, to <400 copies/mL. Median CD4$^+$ T-cell counts increases were 201 to 216 cells/μL *(603)*.

In the second comparison of fosamprenavir and nelfinavir in initial therapy, a once-daily combination of fosamprenavir boosted with low-dose ritonavir was used. Patients in both arms were also given twice-daily abacavir and lamivudine. Through week 48, by intent-to-treat analysis, comparable rates of viral suppression to <50 copies/mL were seen in the fosamprenavir/ritonavir group (55%) and the nelfinavir group (53%) (95% CI: 6%, 10%). In patients with baseline viral load >500,000 copies/mL, higher rates of viral suppression to <400 copies/mL were seen in the fosamprenavir + ritonavir group (73% vs. 53%). Median CD4$^+$ T-cell counts increases were similar in the two groups (approximately 205 cells/μL) *(604)*.

In a study comparing ritonavir-boosted fosamprenavir with lopinavir/ritonavir in initial therapy, each boosted protease inhibitor was given twice daily in combination with once-daily abacavir/lamivudine. At 48 weeks, by intent-to-treat analysis, the proportion of subjects with viral suppression to <50 copies/mL was 66% in the fosamprenavir/ritonavir group and 65% in the lopinavir/ritonavir group. The CD4$^+$ T-count increases were 176 cells/μL and 191 cells/μL, respectively (611).

In patients with prior virologic failure on one or two protease inhibitors, a Phase III study compared two regimens containing fosamprenavir/ritonavir (a twice-daily combination and a once-daily combination) with fixed-dose lopinavir/ritonavir, each in combination with two active nucleoside analogues (dosed twice daily). At 48 weeks, similar rates of viral suppression to <400 copies/mL were seen in the fosamprenavir/ritonavir twice-daily group and the lopinavir/ritonavir group (58% and 61%, respectively; 95% CI for the difference: 16.6 to 10.1), with comparable CD4$^+$ T-cell counts increases of approximately 85 cells/μL. In the once-daily fosamprenavir/ritonavir arm, patients had lower rates of viral suppression: 50% achieved HIV-1 RNA <400 copies/mL (506, 605, 612).

Drug Resistance. Resistance to fosamprenavir is associated with the selection of one or more of several resistance mutations (http://hivinsite.ucsf.edu/InSite?page=ar-03-08).

Mutations selected by fosamprenavir were also characteristic of amprenavir resistance and included I50V, I54L/M, V32I, I47V, and M46I. These mutations did not appear to confer significant cross-resistance to other protease inhibitors. It appeared that resistance to fosamprenavir may develop more readily during treatment with unboosted fosamprenavir than during treatment containing ritonavir-boosted fosamprenavir (613).

Results from clinical studies were needed to elucidate fosamprenavir resistance and its implications for subsequent therapy. Genotypic or phenotypic testing may be useful in predicting the likelihood of response to other protease inhibitors after regimens containing fosamprenavir have failed.

Few data are available regarding the efficacy of fosamprenavir in individuals with HIV that is resistant to other protease inhibitors. Genotypic or phenotypic testing may be useful in predicting the likelihood of response to fosamprenavir after failure of regimens containing other antiretrovirals, but further clinical studies are needed to clarify this question (http://hivinsite.ucsf.edu/InSite?page=ar-03-08).

34.6.10 Atazanavir

Atazanavir (Reyataz, BMS 232632) is a novel azapeptide protease inhibitor that was approved in 2003 by both the FDA and the European Medicine Agency (EMEA) for the treatment of HIV infection (614). Structurally, atazanavir represents methyl N-{(1S)-1-[[[(2S,3S)-2-hydroxy-3-[[(2S)-2-(methoxycarbonylamino)-3,3-dimethylbutanoyl]amino]-4-phenyl-butyl]-[(4-pyridin-2-ylphenyl)methyl]amino]carbamoyl]-2,2-dimethyl-propyl}carbamate. x-ray studies of an enzyme-azapeptide complex were crucial for its design and synthesis (615).

Atazanavir is the first protease inhibitor approved for once-daily dosing, and it also appears to be less likely to cause lipodystrophy and elevated cholesterol, as well as gastrointestinal symptoms, as side effects. It may also not be cross-resistant with other protease inhibitors. When boosted with ritonavir, it is of equivalent potency to lopinavir for use in salvage therapy in patients with a degree of drug resistance; although boosting with ritonavir eliminates the metabolic advantages of atazanavir.

In 2006, the FDA approved a new formulation of atazanavir (300 mg capsules) to be taken as part of combination drug therapy. This formulation should reduce pill burden, as one 300 mg capsule may replace two 150 mg capsules (614).

Dosing. For antiretroviral-naïve patients, the recommended dose of atazanavir is 400 mg (two 200 mg capsules) once daily. The recommended dose of atazanavir in antiretroviral-experienced patients is 300 mg (two 150 mg capsules) taken with ritonavir 100 mg once daily with food.

When coadministered with efavirenz, it is recommended that atazanavir (300 mg) and ritonavir (100 mg) be given with efavirenz 600 mg (all as a single daily dose). When coadministered with tenofovir, it is recommended that atazanavir (300 mg) be given with ritonavir (100 mg) and tenofovir (300 mg), all in a single daily dose with food. Atazanavir taken without ritonavir is not recommended for treatment-experienced patients who have previously failed other treatment regimens. The dose of atazanavir should be adjusted when atazanavir is given with certain other anti-HIV medications and H2-receptor antagonists.

For patients with hepatic impairment, a dose reduction to 300 mg once a day should be considered for moderate hepatic insufficiency (Child-Pugh class B) (http://aidsinfo.nih.gov/DrugsNew/DrugDetailNT.aspx?MenuItem=Drugs&Search=On&int_id=314).

Drug Resistance. Drug-resistant variants were selected with the *in vitro* passage of HIV in the presence of atazanavir (616). Genotype and phenotype analysis of three different HIV strains indicated that an N88S substitution appeared in two of three strains (one in combination with an I50L substitution), and an I84V appeared in the third strain. After drug selection, mutations at the protease cleavage site were also observed (614).

Analysis of 943 PI-susceptible and PI-resistant clinical isolates identified a strong correlation between the presence of amino acid changes at specific residues (10I/V/F, 20R/M/I, 24I, 33I/F/V, 36I/L/V, 46I/L/V, 46I/L, 48V, 54V/L, 63P, 71V/T/I, 73C/S/T/A, 82A/F/S/T, 84V, and 90M) and decreased susceptibility to atazanavir. Whereas no single substitution or combination of substitutions was predictive of resistance to atazanavir, the presence of five or more of these substitutions correlated strongly with the loss of susceptibility to atazanavir *(617)*.

Clinical isolates obtained from previously PI-naïve patients manifesting virologic failure while receiving atazanavir-containing antiretroviral therapy have shown a unique I50L substitution. This substitution is regarded as the signature mutation for atazanavir resistance *(614)*. Furthermore, the I50L mutation has emerged in a variety of different backgrounds and was accompanied by A71 V, K45R, and /or G73S mutations.

Comparison of viruses bearing the I50L mutation with those bearing the I50V mutation did not reveal specific resistance to atazanavir and amprenavir, respectively, and there was no evidence of cross-resistance *(618)*. However, in PI-experienced patients, atazanavir displayed high cross-resistance compared with lopinavir or amprenavir in the presence of resistance to other protease inhibitors—which could be partially reversed with enhanced drug exposure due to ritonavir boosting *(619)*.

Drug-Drug Interactions. Atazanavir is a moderate CYP 3A inhibitor and may interact with other antiretroviral agents *(614)*:

- Atazanavir should be taken more than 2 hours before or 1 hour after buffered didanosine tablets to avoid interactions in absorption resulting from the effects on gastric pH of the buffering agent. Atazanavir requires an acidic environment to be absorbed.
- When efavirenz is administered with atazanavir, ritonavir-boosted atazanavir is recommended to compensate for the reduction in atazanavir levels produced by efavirenz *(620)*. Preliminary results have indicated that amprenavir could be boosted with atazanavir without the need of ritonavir enhancement *(621)*.
- Tenofovir should be combined with atazanavir (300 mg) and ritonavir (100 mg) because of a decrease in atazanavir concentrations when taken with tenofovir only (without ritonavir boosting) *(622)*.
- Atazanavir should not be used in combination with indinavir because of the potential increase in bilirubin levels *(623)*.

Clinical Trials. A number of clinical trials *(624–631)* in both antiretroviral-naïve and antiretroviral-experienced patients have been conducted to evaluate the efficacy of atazanavir as monotherapy and as part of HAART *(614)*.

A Phase II dose-ranging clinical trial in antiretroviral-naïve patients compared the anti-HIV efficacy of atazanavir at three different dosages (200, 400, and 500 mg, once daily) with nelfinavir (750 mg, twice daily) in monotherapy for 2 weeks, and from that point on, in combination with didanosine and stavudine *(624)*. Results after 48 weeks of treatment showed that the proportion of patients with HIV viral load of <400 copies/mL (56% to 64%) and <50 copies/mL (28% to 42%) was similar in the different treatment arms. Whereas the patients receiving atazanavir did not experience a change in lipid profile, those in the nelfinavir arm had an increase in total cholesterol, fasting LDL cholesterol, and fasting triglycerides *(624)*.

A dose-ranging, randomized clinical trial in antiretroviral-naïve patients compared two different doses of atazanavir (400 and 600 mg, once daily) with nelfinavir (1.25 g, twice daily), plus stavudine and lamivudine *(625)*. The 467 randomized subjects had comparable baseline characteristics across treatments. With atazanavir (given at 400 mg and 600 mg) and nelfinavir, the respective mean changes in HIV-1 RNA ($\log_{10}$ copies/mL) from baseline to 48 weeks were −2.51, −2.58, −2.31; HIV-1 RNA <400 copies/mL [intent-to-treat population (ITT), noncompletion = failure (NC = F)], 64%, 67%, 53%, respectively; HIV-1 RNA <50 copies/mL (ITT NC = F), 35%, 36%, 34%, respectively. Adverse events were similar across treatments with the exception of diarrhea (more frequent with nelfinavir) and jaundice (more frequent with atazanavir). Mean changes from baseline to 48 weeks were fasting LDL cholesterol +5.2%, +7.1%, and +23.2% (at 56 weeks) and fasting triglycerides (48 weeks) +7.2%, +7.6%, and +49.5% in the atazanavir 400 mg, 600 mg, and nelfinavir groups, respectively ($p < 0.01$, atazanavir vs. nelfinavir). The atazanavir dose of 600 mg was chosen in terms of activity and tolerance *(625)*.

Another randomized, double-dummy, active-controlled, two-arm study compared the efficacy and safety of atazanavir (400 mg) with efavirenz, each in combination with zidovudine and lamivudine, as initial therapy for HIV infection *(626)*. At week 48, the proportion of patients with an HIV viral load of <400 copies/mL was 70% in the atazanavir arm and 64% in the efavirenz arm ($p = 0.11$), and the proportion of patients with <50 copies/mL at 48 weeks was 32% and 37%, respectively ($p = 0.14$). From the results of this study, it seems that atanazavir is as efficacious and well tolerated as efavirenz. However, the rates of virologic suppression, at least in the efavirenz arm, were lower than those previously reported *(627)*.

A study conducted in heavily pretreated HAART patients with viral failure compared the efficacy of two doses of atanazavir (400 and 600 mg) plus saquinavir (1.2 g) with saquinavir (400 mg) plus ritonavir (400 mg), and two nucleoside analogues *(628)*. The combination of atazanavir and saquinavir was safe and well tolerated and had comparable efficacy to ritonavir/saquinavir with only small lipid changes.

The antiretroviral efficacy, metabolite changes, and safety of atazanavir (400 mg) were compared with those of lopinavir/ritonavir in combination with two nucleoside reverse transcriptase inhibitors in patients who experienced virologic failure on a PI-based regimen *(629)*. The proportion of patients with an HIV RNA level of <400 copies/mL at week 24 was 77% in the lopinavir/ritonavir arm and 59% in the atazanavir arm. Furthermore, whereas the virologic efficacy of the atazanavir arm was lower [estimated difference between atazanavir and lopinavir/ritonavir = 0.90 (95% CI, 0.09 to 0.51)], patients in that arm experienced only minor increases in lipid levels compared with that in the lopinavir/ritonavir arm *(629)*.

A randomized clinical trial was conducted in patients who failed two or more HAART regimens containing at least one PI, NRTI, and NNRTI *(630)*. The patients were divided into three different treatment arms: atazanavir/ritonavir (300/100 mg daily), atazanavir/saquinavir (400/1,200 mg daily), and lopinavir/ritonavir (400/100 mg, twice daily), with each of these arms combined with tenofovir (300 mg daily) and one NRTI. At week 48, the proportion of patients with an HIV RNA level of <400 copies/mL was 56%, 38%, and 58%, respectively [estimated difference between atazanavir/ritonavir and lopinavir: −1.9 (95% CI, −14.3 to 10.6)]. The analysis of the atazanavir/saquinavir arm was not continued after week 48 because of inferior results in an interim analysis conducted at week 24, likely due to the interaction between tenofovir and atazanavir without ritonavir boosting. At week 96, 72% of the patients who remained in the study had an HIV RNA load of <50 copies/mL both on the atazanavir/ritonavir and lopinavir/ritonavir arms (on-treatment analysis). When compared, the atazanavir/ritonavir combination showed efficacy similar to that of lopinavir/ritonavir [estimated difference between atazanavir/ritonavir and lopinavir: −0.7 (95% CI, −12.0, 14.7)], in addition to demonstrating also a more favorable lipid profile than lopinavir/ritonavir, as lipid levels decreased on atazanavir-containing regimens and increased or remained stable on the lopinavir/ritonavir arm. Furthermore, the atazanavir/ritonavir arm showed superior gastrointestinal tolerability *(630)*.

In a rollover study of patients who were previously on a nelfinavir-containing regimen *(625)* (see above), switching to atazanavir resulted in maintaining the viral suppression and reversion of the nelfinavir-related lipid abnormalities *(614)*.

Toxicity. The rate of discontinuation due to adverse events has been low in clinical trials studying atazanavir-containing regimens *(614)*. In general, the drug has little impact on the lipid metabolism, and despite causing elevation in unconjugated bilirubin levels, significant liver toxicity has been extremely infrequent. However, atazanavir has shown cardiac toxicity at high plasma concentrations when the PR interval [(the time (in seconds) from the beginning of the P wave (onset of atrial depolarization) is prolonged to the beginning of the QRS complex (onset of ventricular depolarization)] *(614)*.

Compared with other currently approved retroviral agents (nelfinavir, efavirenz, saquinavir/ ritonavir, lopinavir/ ritonavir), atazanavir has shown a better lipid profile (fasting LDL, fasting triglycerides) *(624, 628–630, 632, 633)*.

Clinical data have demonstrated a lower effect of atazanavir on the glucose metabolism than that of other protease inhibitors *(633)*, which seems to be related to the lack of inhibition of the glucose transporter GLUT4 *(634)*. A study conducted in HIV-negative, healthy subjects suggested that atazanavir had a negligible effect on insulin sensitivity, whereas lopinavir/ritonavir induced insulin resistance *(635)*.

The incidence of lipodystrophy caused by atazanavir has been low in antiretroviral-naïve patients (<10%) and when it did occur, it was grade 1 or 2 *(624–626)*. It should be noted that in many of these trials, the treatment regimens contained didanosine or stavudine, which have been associated with higher risk of lipodystrophy *(635)*. In addition, there has been a report of three patients who, after being switched to atazanavir from another protease inhibitor, had experienced a rapid regression of dorsocervical and abdominal fat accumulation *(636)*.

Elevation of total and indirect bilirubin (hyperbilirubinemia) has been commonly observed in patients taking atazanavir—as many as 35% to 47% of patients have experienced an increase in the total bilirubin level (>2.6 times the upper limit of normal; grade 3 or 4 hyperbilirubinemia), and 7% of patients have presented with clinical apparent jaundice or scleral icteris *(614)*. Nevertheless, jaundice did not lead to discontinuation of treatment. The hyperbilirubinemia, which usually is well tolerated and is similar to that observed with indinavir *(637)*, is generally not accompanied by elevated liver enzymes when compared with other protease inhibitors *(638)*. It is thought to be related to inhibition of the uridine diphosphate-glucoronyl transferase enzyme. The pathophysiology of hyperbilirubinemia is similar to that of Gilbert's syndrome, which occurs in about 8% of the population.

Patients with chronic hepatitis C infection did not experience atazanavir-induced hyperbilirubinemia to a higher degree *(629, 630)*.

Although atazanavir is not considered directly nephrotoxic despite recent reports of urinary stones *(639–641)*, a recent report has described a patient in whom direct nephrotoxic effects of atazanavir appeared to develop *(642)*.

34.6.11 Lopinavir/Kaletra

Lopinavir (ABT-378) is an antiretroviral drug that is currently marketed as Kaletra, a coformulation with a subtherapeutic dose of ritonavir, as a component of combination therapy to treat HIV/AIDS. As of 2006, lopinavir/ritonavir forms part of the preferred combination for first-line therapy recommended by the U.S. Department of Health and Human Services (http://AIDSinfo.nih.gov).

Structurally, lopinavir represents (2S)-N-[(2S,4S,5S)-5-{[2-(2,6-dimethylphenoxy)acetyl]amino-4-hydroxy-1,6-diphenyl-hexan-2-yl]-3-methyl-2-(2-oxo-1,3-diazinan-1-yl) butanamide.

Lopinavir was developed in an attempt to improve on the HIV resistance and serum protein-binding properties of another earlier protease inhibitor, ritonavir *(643)*. When administered alone, lopinavir has insufficient bioavailability. However, like several other HIV protease inhibitors, its blood levels have been greatly increased by low doses of ritonavir, a potent inhibitor of cytochrome P450 3A4 *(644)*. Hence, a strategy was developed of coadministering lopinavir with subtherapeutic doses of ritonavir, leading to marketing of lopinavir *only as a coformulation with ritonavir*. It is the first multidrug capsule to contain a drug not available individually.

Lopinavir/ritonavir (Kaletra) was approved by the FDA in 2000 and in Europe in 2001.

Lopinavir/Ritonavir (Kaletra). Lopinavir/ritonavir is a fixed combination of two HIV protease inhibitors. Currently, the fixed combination of lopinavir and ritonavir and two NRTIs is one of several preferred regimens for initial antiretroviral therapy in HIV-positive adults who are treatment-naïve. In 2006, the capsule formulation of Kaletra was phased out in favor of a new tablet formulation. The tablet form of lopinavir/ritonavir offers distinct advantages over the capsule formulation, including a lower pill burden, no required dose adjustments for concomitant use of certain NNRTIs in treatment-naïve patients, and easier storage requirements (http://www.hivandhepatitis.com/hiv_and_aids/kaletra_1.html).

Dosing and Administration. Lopinavir/ritonavir is dosed orally in the following forms: film-coated tablets containing lopinavir 200 mg and ritonavir 50 mg; oral solution containing lopinavir 80 mg/mL and ritonavir 20 mg/mL; and soft gelatin capsules containing lopinavir 133.3 mg and ritonavir 33.3 mg *(645)* (http://aidsinfo.nih.gov/other/factsheet.aspx; http://www.hivandhepatitis.com/hiv_and_aids/kaletra_1.html #dos).

The recommended dosage of lopinavir/ritonavir in antiretroviral-naïve and antiretroviral-experienced adults and adolescents is 400 mg/100 mg, twice daily, and the recommended dosage in children is 100 mg/25 mg to 400 mg/100 mg, twice daily based on body surface area *(646)* or weight *(647, 648)*; further guidance on pediatric dosages is available in the manufacturer's prescribing information *(646–648)*.

Whereas once-daily lopinavir/ritonavir 800 mg/200 mg may be administered in antiretroviral-naïve patients *(649–651)*, it is not recommended in antiretroviral-experienced patients. *Because of pharmacokinetic drug interactions in patients receiving concomitant efavirenz, nelfinavir, nevirapine, or amprenavir, the use of these drugs is contraindicated in patients receiving once-daily lopinavir/ritonavir (646–648)*. When these drugs or fosamprenavir are coadministered with twice-daily lopinavir/ritonavir, the lopinavir/ritonavir dosage should be increased to 533 mg/133 mg with the capsules or oral solution, or to 600 mg/150 mg with the tablets in adults and adolescents *(646–648)*, or according to body weight in children *(647, 648)*.

Lopinavir/ritonavir capsules and oral solution should be administered with food to ensure maximal absorption *(646, 648)*.

Because lopinavir/ritonavir may cause increases in serum lipid concentrations, it is recommended that total cholesterol and triglyceride levels be tested when lopinavir/ritonavir treatment is initiated and during therapy, and pancreatitis should be considered in patients with elevated lipid concentrations *(646–648)*.

Therapeutic drug monitoring is recommended in children receiving the oral capsule coformulation to ensure optimal exposure to lopinavir *(646)*.

Drug-Drug Interactions. Lopinavir/ritonavir induces glucuronidation and has the potential to reduce plasma concentrations of zidovudine or abacavir if these drugs are taken concurrently. The clinical significance of this potential drug interaction is unknown.

When taken concurrently, lopinavir/ritonavir increases tenofovir (Viread) concentrations; the mechanism of this interaction is unknown. Patients taking both lopinavir/ritonavir and tenofovir should be monitored for tenofovir-associated adverse events. An increased rate of adverse events has also been observed when fosamprenavir is coadministered with lopinavir/ritonavir. Appropriate doses of both drugs with respect to safety have not been established (http://www.hivandhepatitis.com/hiv_and_aids/kaletra_1.html#dos).

Lopinavir/ritonavir is contraindicated for use in patients with severe hepatic impairment *(646)* and is contraindicated or not recommended for use in conjunction with other drugs that depend on the CYP3A isoenzyme for metabolism *(646–648)*. In addition to several protease inhibitors, other CYP3A-associated drugs include antihistamines (astemizole, terfenadine), ergot derivatives (dihydroergotamine, ergonovine, ergotamine, methylergonovine), the gastrointestinal motility agent cisapride, the neuroleptic pimozide, and sedatives (midazolam, triazolam). Concurrent use of any of these drugs with lopinavir/ritonavir is contraindicated because of the potential for serious and/or life-threatening reactions, such as cardiac arrhythmias, prolonged or increased sedation, or respiratory depression. Lopinavir/ritonavir has also been shown *in vivo* to induce its own metabolism and to increase the biotransformation of some drugs metabolized by cytochrome P450 enzymes and by glucuronidation.

Lopinavir concentrations decrease in patients concurrently taking efavirenz, nevirapine, amprenavir, or nelfinavir, because these drugs induce CYP3A; increased dosage of lopinavir/ritonavir may be required (http://www. hivandhepatitis.com/hiv_and_aids/kaletra_1.html#dos).

The concurrent use of St. John's wort and rifampicin is contraindicated in the European Union *(646)* and not recommended in the United States *(647, 648)* because of potential pharmacokinetic drug interactions with lopinavir/ritonavir. The manufacturer's prescribing information should be consulted for further information on dosages, warnings, precautions, and contraindications *(646–650)*.

Use of rifampin with lopinavir/ritonavir is also contraindicated, as it may lead to the loss of virologic response and possible resistance to lopinavir/ritonavir, other protease inhibitors, or any other coadministered antiretroviral agents.

The Norvir (ritonavir) and Kaletra (lopinavir/ritonavir) package inserts (product labeling) were recently updated to include information regarding interactions with fluticasone (a synthetic corticosteroid, the active component of Flonase Nasal Spray) and trazodone (Desyrel, a non-tricyclic antidepressant). In addition, alfuzosin [an alpha-blocker used to increase the flow of urine in people with *benign prostatic hypertrophy (BPH)*] was added to the contraindications section of the Norvir package insert.

Drug Resistance. The pattern of primary (active-site) mutations associated with resistance to the lopinavir/ ritonavir coformulation has not been determined in ART-naïve patients with HIV infection *(647)*. There was no evidence of clinical resistance to lopinavir in viral isolates from antiretroviral-naïve adults in three clinical studies *(651–654)* who received lopinavir/ritonavir 400 mg/100 mg twice daily for up to 7 years *(655–658)* or 800 mg/200 mg once daily for up to 96 weeks *(659)*, or in isolates from antiretroviral-naïve or PI-naïve children who received lopinavir/ritonavir for 48 weeks in a clinical trial *(660)*. Development of primary resistance mutations in antiretroviral-naïve adult patients occurred in 45% of nelfinavir recipients but was absent in lopinavir/ritonavir recipients ($p < 0.001$) *(657)*. Isolates with secondary mutations retained susceptibility similar to wild-type HIV *(657, 658)*.

In vitro resistance to lopinavir in PI-experienced patients in whom treatment had failed is associated with 11 substitution mutations in the protease gene (L10F/I/R/V, K20M/R, L24I, M46I/L, F53L, I54L/T/V, L63P, A71I/L/T/V, V82A/F/T, I84V, and L90M) *(661)*. Lopinavir-related mutations developed in approximately one third of antiretroviral-experienced adults and adolescents in three clinical trials *(662)*, with the most common mutations occurring

at M46I/L, I54V, and V82A. Mutations associated with lopinavir resistance developed during treatment in most (17 of 22) antiretroviral-naïve and antiretroviral-experienced children with virologic failure in the French ATU (Autorisation Temporaire d'Utilisation) Program (an extension of the Expanded Access Programme [EAP], in which potentially life-saving medications are made available to patients prior to approval) *(663)*.

The number of lopinavir-associated mutations at baseline is significantly associated with virologic response in antiretroviral-experienced adults *(662, 664, 665)* and children *(663)* according to data from clinical trials and the EAP or ATU. Significantly more adults with ≤5 lopinavir-associated mutations at baseline achieved a virologic response (>1 $\log_{10}$ decrease in plasma HIV RNA and/or plasma HIV RNA <500 copies/mL) at 6 months in the EAP program (88% vs. 48%; $p < 0.001$ vs. patients with >5 mutations) *(665)*. PI-naïve or PI-experienced children with HIV infection in the ATU program with ≥4 lopinavir-associated mutations at baseline were significantly more likely to experience virologic failure (plasma HIV RNA >400 copies/mL) than were children with <4 mutations at baseline ($p = 0.0001$) *(663)*.

The incidence of cross-resistance to other protease inhibitors associated with lopinavir/ritonavir treatment appears to be low *(657, 662)*. Protease mutations at positions 54 and 82, which are associated with cross-resistance to multiple protease inhibitors *(666)*, were among the most frequently occurring *de novo* resistance mutations reported with lopinavir/ritonavir in clinical trials *(662)*. Mutations associated with lopinavir resistance, including V32I, M46I/L, I47V, I50V, and I54M, are also associated with atazanavir resistance and may confer cross-resistance between the two agents *(667)*. There was no association between the virologic response to lopinavir/ritonavir-based treatment and the presence of the D30N mutation, which confers resistance to nelfinavir, in a cohort of 456 antiretroviral-experienced patients who received lopinavir/ritonavir as salvage therapy for 12 months *(668)*.

Clinical Trials. One-hundred-ninety antiretroviral-naïve subjects with plasma HIV-1 RNA level of >1,000 copies/mL and any CD4$^+$ T-cell count were randomized to lopinavir/ritonavir at a dose of 800/200 mg administered once daily ($n = 115$) or lopinavir/ritonavir at a dose of 400/100 mg administered twice daily ($n = 75$). Subjects also received tenofovir disoproxil fumarate (TDF) at a dose of 300 mg and emtricitabine (FTC) at a dose of 200 mg administered once daily *(651)*. The results have shown that the virologic responses of the subjects through 48 weeks were comparable; 70% (once daily) and 64% (twice daily) achieved an HIV-1 RNA level <50 copies/mL (by intent-to-treat, noncompleter = failure analysis). No subject demonstrated LPV or TDF resistance, but three subjects (two in the once-daily group, one in the twice-daily group) demonstrated FTC resistance. Mean increases in CD4$^+$ T-counts were similar. Diarrhea (16% in the once-daily group, 5% in the twice-daily group; $p = 0.036$) was the most common moderate or severe drug-related adverse event in the study. Overall, through 48 weeks, a once-daily regimen of lopinavir/ritonavir plus tenofovir plus emtricitabine appeared to have similar virologic and immunologic responses in antiretroviral-naïve subjects as the same regimen with lopinavir/ritonavir administered twice daily. Both regimens were relatively well tolerated, and no LPV or TDF resistance has been observed (651).

A randomized, open-label, multicenter, comparative trial was conducted to evaluate the safety and noninferiority and to explore the efficacy of administration, of once-daily versus twice-daily lopinavir/ritonavir (LPV/r) in antiretroviral-naïve HIV-1–infected adults (669). Sixteen patients who started lopinavir-ritonavir (LPV/RTV; 400/100 mg, twice daily) and atazanavir (ATV; 300 mg, once daily) were enrolled in the study group (arm A). The lopinavir pharmacokinetics was compared with those of two historical groups: arm B, 15 patients who received LPV/RTV (400/100 mg, twice daily); and arm C, 25 patients who received LPV/RTV/saquinavir(SQV) (400/100/1,000 mg, twice daily). Atazanavir pharmacokinetics were compared with those of 15 consecutive patients who received ATV and RTV (300/100 mg, once daily) (arm D). Drug concentrations were measured by HPLC. The results showed that LPV concentrations were significantly higher in arm A than in arms B and C. Treatment was not discontinued in any patient because of adverse effects. At 24 weeks, viral load was <50 copies/mL in 13 of 16 patients. The combination of atazanavir and lopinavir/ritonavir provided high plasma concentrations of both drugs, which seemed to be appropriate for patients with multiple prior therapeutic failures, yielding good tolerability and substantial antiviral efficacy (669).

Lopinavir/ritonavir is approved for treatment of HIV-infected children at a dosage regimen of 230/57.5 mg/m^2, twice daily. However, once-daily administration could increase convenience and patients' adherence to the regimen. One study was conducted to evaluate whether inhibitory concentrations are maintained in plasma after lopinavir/ritonavir is administered once daily (670). The results of the study suggested that lopinavir/ritonavir once daily may be a suitable regimen for antiretroviral-naïve children. However, due to the high interindividual variability and low concentrations in some patients, therapeutic drug monitoring may be necessary to ensure that concentrations are adequate to inhibit viral replication. A formal clinical study of lopinavir/ritonavir once daily in treatment-naïve children is warranted (670).

Toxicity. Pancreatitis has been observed in patients receiving lopinavir/ritonavir, including those who developed marked triglyceride elevations; in some cases, fatal-

ities have occurred. Although a causal relationship with lopinavir/ritonavir has not been established, marked triglyceride elevation is a risk factor in the development of pancreatitis. Patients with advanced HIV disease may also be at increased risk of elevated triglycerides and pancreatitis, and patients with a history of pancreatitis may be at increased risk for recurrence during lopinavir/ritonavir therapy. Pancreatitis should be considered if clinical symptoms suggestive of pancreatitis occur, including nausea, vomiting, abdominal pain, or abnormal laboratory values such as increased serum lipase or amylase. Patients who exhibit these signs or symptoms should be evaluated, and lopinavir/ritonavir or other antiretroviral therapy should be suspended (http://www. hivandhepatitis.com/hiv_and_aids/kaletra_1.html#dos).

Although there is clear evidence that effective antiretroviral therapy can result in beneficial immune reconstitution in patients with advanced HIV disease, some patients who have initiated antiretroviral therapy may also experience exuberant inflammatory responses to opportunistic pathogens, which can lead to troublesome immune reconstitution disease syndromes. The *immune reconstitution syndrome (IRS)* has been reported in patients treated with combination antiretroviral therapy, including lopinavir/ritonavir (671). Thus, during the initial phase of lopinavir/ritonavir-containing combination antiretroviral therapy, patients whose immune systems have responded may develop an inflammatory response to indolent or residual opportunistic infections (such as *Mycobacterium avium* infection, cytomegalovirus, *Pneumocystis jirovecii* pneumonia, or tuberculosis), which may necessitate further evaluation and treatment.

New-onset diabetes mellitus, exacerbation of preexisting diabetes mellitus, and hyperglycemia have been reported during postmarketing surveillance of HIV-infected patients receiving protease inhibitor therapy. Some patients required either initiation or dose adjustments of insulin or oral hypoglycemia agents for treatment of these events; in some cases, diabetic ketoacidosis has occurred. In those patients who discontinued PI therapy, hyperglycemia persisted in some cases. Because these events have been reported voluntarily during clinical practice, estimates of frequency cannot be made and a causal relationship between PI therapy and these events has not been established (http://www. hivandhepatitis.com/hiv_and_aids/kaletra_1.html#dos).

Other clinically observed adverse effects include body fat redistribution and accumulation, increased bleeding in patients with hemophilia type A and B, lipid elevations, and exacerbation of existing hepatitis or other liver disease.

Other adverse effects seen with the use of lopinavir/ritonavir (lopinavir/r) include diabetes mellitus or hyperglycemia, pancreatitis, bradyarrhythmias, diarrhea, nausea, abdominal pain, abnormal stools, asthenia, headache, insomnia, pain, rash, vomiting, and redistribution of body fat. In one study, the incidence of diarrhea was greater in patients taking lopinavir/ritonavir once daily than for those taking it twice daily (http://www.hivandhepatitis. com/hiv_and_aids/kaletra_1.html#dos).

34.6.12 Tipranavir

Tipranavir (PNU-140690, TPV, Aptivus), which is to be coadministered with ritonavir, was approved by the FDA in 2005 for use with other antiretroviral agents in the treatment of HIV infection in adults (672). It is the first in a new class of nonpeptidic HIV-1 protease inhibitors and is active against HIV-1 strains that are resistant to other protease inhibitors. Structurally, tipranavir represents N-[3-{1(R)-(5,6-dihydro-4-hydroxy-2-oxo-6(R)-phenethyl-6-propyl-2H-pyran-3-yl)propyl}phenyl]-5-trifluoromethylpyridine-2-sulfonamide (673).

Dosing and Administration. Tipranavir is available in 250 mg soft-gel capsules and is taken with ritonavir. The recommended dose of tipranavir for adults is 500 mg (two 250 mg capsules) taken with ritonavir 200 mg twice daily. Recommended doses for children are currently being studied in clinical trials. Some patients may benefit from different doses of tipranavir. Tipranavir and ritonavir are always taken with food. It is very important to take tipranavir with food to prevent it from irritating the stomach and bowels (http://www.aidsinfo.nih.gov/DrugsNew/DrugDetailNT. aspx?MenuItem=Drugs&Search=On&int_id=351).

Drug Resistance. Tipranavir resistance *in vitro* develops slowly. The selection of resistance in wild-type virus in the presence of increasing tipranavir concentrations has been evaluated (674). In one study, the virus was passaged in the presence of tipranavir over various concentrations (400 nmol/L to 20 μmol/L) for a 9-month period (675). L33F and I84V mutations were the first to emerge, and viruses grown in the presence of 20 μmol/L tipranavir contained up to 11 mutations. Tipranavir-resistant virus selected *in vitro* had decreased susceptibility to all PIs except saquinavir (675).

The accumulation of at least six mutations appears to be necessary to reduce HIV susceptibility to tipranavir. A reconstructed mutant virus containing at least six mutations in the protease gene exhibited a 14-fold reduced susceptibility to tipranavir; these mutations included I13V, V32I, L33F, K45I, V82L, and I84V (675). Similar results were seen in another *in vitro* study, where the presence of six mutations, including L33F, V82L, and I84V in the protease gene, was necessary to confer high-level resistance (defined as >10-fold) to tipranavir (676).

BI 1182.2 was a Phase II, open-label study comparing low-dose tipranavir/ritonavir 500 mg/100 mg, twice daily, with high-dose tipranavir/ritonavir 1,000 mg/100 mg, twice

daily, in multiple-PI-experienced, NNRTI-naïve patients receiving at least two new NRTIs. HIV-1 clinical isolates from 35 of 41 (85.4%) patients at baseline demonstrated susceptibility to tipranavir, defined as <4-fold change in IC_{50} (677). Resistance to tipranavir, defined as >10-fold change in IC_{50}, was detected in only one patient at baseline. Treatment emerging mutations at codons L33 and V82 were found in four of six patients who had reduced susceptibility to tipranavir at the end of treatment (678).

BI 1182.4 was also a Phase II, open-label study that compared tipranavir/ritonavir 500 mg/100 mg and tipranavir/ritonavir 1,250 mg/100 mg, twice daily, with saquinavir/ritonavir 400 mg/400 mg, twice daily, in single-PI-experienced patients receiving at least two new NRTIs. The protease inhibitor experience in the majority of patients was limited to nelfinavir (679). Clinical HIV-1 isolates from 73 of 74 single-PI-experienced patients were susceptible to tipranavir at baseline. Susceptibility of isolates to other protease inhibitors, including amprenavir, indinavir, nelfinavir, ritonavir, and saquinavir, were also evaluated. Isolates containing ≤5 protease gene mutations remained susceptible to all protease inhibitors, 6 to 10 mutations demonstrated reduced susceptibility to nelfinavir only, and 11 to 20 mutations exhibited cross-resistance to other protease inhibitors (679).

Similar results were found when data from these two studies were pooled (680, 681). A total of 106 of 114 (94%) patients with one to two PI-regimen experience entered with susceptibility to tipranavir (tipranavir IC_{50} <2-fold increase), and 16 to 20 protease mutations at baseline were necessary to see reduced tipranavir susceptibility. Virus suppression occurred in the majority of single-PI-experienced patients at 24 weeks (BI 1,182.2) and in those failing multiple protease inhibitors at 48 weeks (BI 1,182.4) and was not related to the number of baseline protease gene mutations. Evaluation of treatment-emergent resistance mutations indicated that key mutations at codons 33, 82, and 84 were the most frequently occurring mutations and were associated with reduced susceptibility to tipranavir (681).

BI 1,182.52 was a randomized, double-blind trial evaluating tipranavir/ritonavir 500 mg/100 mg, tipranavir/ritonavir 500 mg/200 mg, or tipranavir/ritonavir 750 mg/200 mg, twice daily, combined with optimized background therapy in 216 triple-class-experienced patients whose protease inhibitor regimens had failed at least twice (682). Patients with ≥1 primary but not more than one key mutation at 82L/T, 84V, or 90M were included. Study results revealed that tipranavir/ritonavir dose and the number of baseline protease inhibitor resistance mutations influenced treatment outcomes. After 2 weeks of therapy, decline in HIV viral load was less substantial for those subjects with >2 baseline key protease inhibitor resistance mutations. Subjects with two key mutations receiving the tipranavir/ritonavir

500 mg/200 mg dose experienced the greatest median decrease in HIV RNA (1.4 $\log_{10}$ copies/mL). Antiviral activity results in conjunction with pharmacokinetic and safety data from this study supported the selection of the tipranavir/ritonavir 500 mg/200 mg dose for further evaluation in the Phase III studies [RESIST (randomized evaluation of strategic intervention in multidrug-resistant patients with tipranavir 1 and 2] (683). The results further suggested that tipranavir-resistant virus had decreased susceptibility to amprenavir, atazanavir, indinavir, lopinavir, nelfinavir, and ritonavir, while sensitivity to saquinavir remained (683).

Drug-Drug Interactions. Tipranavir is a potent P-glycoprotein (P-gp) inducer, and this may result in significant drug-drug interactions with P-gp substrates. *In vivo* studies confirmed *in vitro* results (i.e., tipranavir is a substrate of CYP3A4 isoenzymes), and doses ranging from 250 to 1,250 mg given twice daily have been shown to induce the CYP3A4 system (684). Enzyme induction by tipranavir, however, is overcome by the enzyme inhibitory effect of low-dose ritonavir when these two agents are coadministered (685). Thus, a 200 mg dose of ritonavir provides consistent CYP3A4 enzyme inhibition and significantly improves the tipranavir pharmacokinetics.

Animal studies report glucuronidation as the major mechanism of tipranavir clearance, with the potential for tipranavir to induce glucuronidation (686).

The use of tipranavir/ritonavir in combination with antiretrovirals and other drugs that are substrates, inducers, or inhibitors of CYP3A4 and/or glucuronidation increases the potential for drug-drug interactions. Although evaluations of tipranavir drug interactions have been conducted primarily in healthy volunteers, these data provide insight into the possibility of interactions in HIV-infected patients (674).

Several studies have examined tipranavir drug interactions with other antiretroviral agents (NRTIs and NNRTIs), whereas only one study has evaluated the interaction between tipranavir/ritonavir and other protease inhibitors (674). In this regard, although NRTI intracellular concentrations may be a better predictor of drug efficacy (687), examination of NRTI plasma concentrations may provide insight into potential drug-drug interactions. Furthermore, zidovudine and abacavir are metabolized via hepatic glucuronidation, which is induced by tipranavir (688, 689). The NNRTIs efavirenz and nevirapine are substrates and inducers of CYP3A4 (690, 691). Because tipranavir also induces CYP3A4, the question is whether the inhibitory effects of ritonavir will overcome the induction effects of tipranavir and efavirenz or nevirapine (if used) on the CYP enzyme system (674). In addition, the use of ritonavir-boosted dual protease inhibitor therapy has increased substantially over the past several years, and some of these combinations (e.g., fosamprenavir, lopinavir, and ritonavir) have produced unexpected negative drug interaction results (692).

Interactions between tipranavir/ritonavir 500 mg/100 mg or tipranavir/ritonavir 750 mg/200 mg and either zidovudine, tenofovir, or enteric-coated (EC) didanosine were evaluated in HIV-negative volunteers (693). Steady-state pharmacokinetic parameters were determined after 14 days of therapy with zidovudine, tenofovir, and didanosine. Tipranavir/ritonavir at both doses reduced zidovudine C_{max} and AUC from 0 to 6 hours (AUC_6) by approximately 60% and 40%, respectively. There was no significant effect of zidovudine on the pharmacokinetics of tipranavir. Tipranavir/ritonavir decreased tenofovir C_{max} in a dose-dependent manner but had no effect on the extent of absorption or exposure of tenofovir. Tenofovir caused a small reduction in tipranavir concentrations (17% at tipranavir/ritonavir 500 mg/100 mg, 11% at tipranavir/ritonavir 750 mg/200 mg), but these changes were not considered to be clinically significant. Although no interaction was noted between tipranavir/ritonavir and didanosine, the obtained data did suggest that these antiretroviral drugs should be administered 2 hours apart because of a potential interaction between the self-emulsifying drug delivery systems (SEDDS) formulation of tipranavir and the didanosine EC outer coat (693). No dose adjustments are required when combining tipranavir/ritonavir with tenofovir, didanosine, or efavirenz (694).

Tipranavir/ritonavir had no significant effect on efavirenz pharmacokinetics in HIV-negative volunteers (693). However, tipranavir-^{12}C decreased 42% at a dose of tipranavir/ritonavir 500 mg/100 mg in the presence of efavirenz (600 mg). Tipranavir-^{12}C, C_{max} and AUC from 0 to 24 hours (AUC_{24}) increased approximately 40%, 60%, and 30%, respectively, when administered at tipranavir/ritonavir 750 mg/200 mg in the presence of efavirenz (600 mg). These results have suggested that 200 mg ritonavir was sufficient to overcome the induction effects of efavirenz (693).

A randomized, open-label, parallel-group study was performed in healthy volunteers to assess the interaction between tipranavir and nevirapine (695). The overall results of the study indicated that nevirapine can be administered with tipranavir and low-dose ritonavir without the need for dose adjustments.

A similar antiretroviral-tipranavir drug interaction study was performed in 208 HIV-infected patients receiving stable HAART, including NRTIs with or without an NNRTI for 12 weeks (696). Tipranavir/ritonavir 1,250 mg/100 mg, tipranavir/ritonavir 750 mg/100 mg, or tipranavir/ritonavir 250 mg/200 mg administered twice daily were evaluated in patients receiving one of seven HAART regimens, including zidovudine plus lamivudine plus efavirenz or nevirapine, stavudine plus lamivudine plus efavirenz or nevirapine, stavudine plus didanosine plus efavirenz or nevirapine, and zidovudine plus lamivudine plus abacavir. Pharmacokinetic sampling was performed on day 1 of HAART therapy and

21 days after the addition of tipranavir/ritonavir. Mean ratios of nevirapine C_{min} (day 22) and efavirenz C_{min} (day 23) versus baseline showed no significant interaction and did not differ relative to tipranavir/ritonavir doses studied. Different doses of tipranavir had no clinically significant effect on the plasma concentrations of lamivudine, stavudine, or didanosine. Plasma concentrations of zidovudine and abacavir were reduced 31% to 43%. Because zidovudine and abacavir are phosphorylated intracellularly to their active moiety, studies evaluating intracellular concentrations of these drugs in the presence of tipranavir/ritonavir need further evaluation before a definitive statement about a dose adjustment can be made (674).

The pharmacokinetics of tipranavir/ritonavir 500 mg/ 200 mg twice daily alone or in combination with saquinavir, amprenavir, or lopinavir were evaluated in HIV-infected patients participating in a Phase II tipranavir trial (697). Patients were randomized to receive an optimal background regimen in combination with either tipranavir/ritonavir 500 mg/200 mg twice daily (n=66), lopinavir/ritonavir 400 mg/100 mg twice daily (n=79), amprenavir/ritonavir 600 mg/100 mg twice daily (n=76), or saquinavir/ritonavir 1,000 mg/100 mg twice daily (n=75). Two weeks after therapy was initiated, tipranavir/ritonavir 500 mg/100 mg was added to the regimen of those patients receiving lopinavir, amprenavir, or saquinavir (final ritonavir dose, 200 mg in all arms). As mentioned earlier, the net effect of tipranavir/ritonavir on P-gp is induction. The protease inhibitors evaluated in this study are dual substrates of CYP3A and P-gp and are subject to high intestinal first-pass effect. They may also potentially induce CYP3A. It is possible that the intestinal CYP3A system and P-gp functionally work together in reducing the oral bioavailability of drugs. Thus, the net interplay between intestinal CYP3A, P-gp, and the protease inhibitors may have decreased their systemic exposure when coadministered with tipranavir/ritonavir. The overall results from this study clearly indicate that tipranavir/ritonavir should not be administered concurrently with these protease inhibitors (697).

Clinical Studies. Tipranavir received FDA approval for use in combination with ritonavir in adults with HIV infection. It is intended to be used as part of combination therapy in patients who have HIV strains that are resistant to multiple other protease inhibitors and who have ongoing viral replication while taking antiretroviral therapy. The guidelines of the U.S. Department of Health and Human Services designate tipranavir as "not recommended" for initial treatment of HIV infection (http://www.aidsinfo.nih.gov/guidelines/).

Tipranavir has not been assessed in initial therapy; studies are under way. Currently, tipranavir (coadministered with ritonavir) is approved for use in subsequent therapy in patients with viral resistance to multiple protease inhibitors (http://hivinsite.ucsf.edu/InSite?page=ar-03-09).

In patients with advanced HIV disease, extensive prior exposure to at least three classes of antiretrovirals, and evidence of resistance to protease inhibitors, two Phase III studies compared tipranavir/ritonavir with several other ritonavir-boosted protease inhibitors, each in combination with a background regimen. By intent-to-treat analysis, the combined tipranavir groups had higher rates of virologic response (34% vs. 15%), viral suppression to <400 copies/mL (30% vs. 14%), and viral suppression to <50 copies/mL (23% vs. 10%) at 48 weeks (698,699). These differences were statistically significant ($p < 0.0001$). The inclusion of enfuvirtide in the antiretroviral regimen significantly improved the rates of virologic response in the tipranavir groups (HIV RNA <400 copies/mL 43% vs. 27% of tipranavir recipients treated with and without enfuvirtide, respectively; $p < 0.0001$). The tipranavir groups also had greater increases in CD4$^+$ T-cell counts than did the comparator groups: 48 cells/μL versus 21 cells/μL ($p < 0.0001$) (698,699).

The RESIST (randomized evaluation of strategic intervention in multidrug-resistant patients with tipranavir) trials are randomized, controlled, open-label, Phase III trials designed to study tipranavir combined with ritonavir versus a group of ritonavir-boosted protease inhibitors. The RESIST clinical trial program is one of the largest study programs undertaken with an investigational antiretroviral agent in patients previously treated with three classes of antiretrovirals, with Phase II and III data from more than 1,400 patients taking the 500 mg/200 mg dose of tipranavir/ritonavir. RESIST-1 was conducted in the United States and Australia, and RESIST-2 was carried out in Europe and Latin America. These trials were designed to compare the safety and effectiveness of twice-daily, 500 mg tipranavir boosted by 200 mg ritonavir twice daily versus the standard of care, comparator protease inhibitor also boosted with ritonavir. An analysis of the RESIST trials shows that ritonavir-boosted tipranavir, used as part of combination antiretroviral therapy, provided a potent and durable treatment response in highly treatment-experienced female patients through 48 weeks of treatment (698–703) (http://www.natap.org/2005/EACS/eacs_8.htm; http://bbs.thebody.com/content/treat/art14781.html; http://www.prnewswire.com/cgi-bin/stories.pl?ACCT=104&STORY=/www/story/02-09-2006/0004278726&EDATE=).

However, in June 2006, a 558-person study of ritonavir-boosted tipranavir in treatment-naïve patients (Study 1182.33) was discontinued due to poorer than expected efficacy and concerns about liver toxicity.

A study arm using tipranavir plus 200 mg ritonavir (the dose currently approved for treatment-experienced individuals) was stopped in February 2006 after patients had similar virologic response at 48 weeks, but they were more likely to develop elevated liver enzymes compared with patients taking lopinavir/ritonavir (Kaletra).

Also in 2006, the U.S. Data and Safety Monitoring Board recommended halting the study arm receiving tipranavir plus 100 mg ritonavir because patients were less likely to achieve undetectable HIV viral load after 60 weeks than were those taking lopinavir/ritonavir (http://www.hivandhepatitis.com/recent/2006/ad1/070706_b.html).

Toxicity. In June 2006, the FDA issued a warning stating that patients taking tipranavir/ritonavir medication had appeared to be at greater risk of developing *intracranial hemorrhage*. The warning followed an analysis of data showing that 13 of 6,840 patients taking ritonavir-boosted tipranavir in clinical trials experienced intracranial hemorrhage; 1 patient experienced 2 hemorrhages, and 8 died. Several of these individuals had other medical conditions or were receiving other drugs that might have contributed to the bleeding. It has been strongly recommended that caution be applied when prescribing tipranavir/ritonavir to patients who may be at risk for bleeding due to trauma, surgery, or other medical conditions or who are taking medications, such as antiplatelet agents or anticoagulants, that may increase the risk of bleeding (www.fda.gov/medwatch/safety/2006/Aptivus-tipranavir_DHCP.pdf; www.fda.gov/medwatch/safety/2006/Aptivus_PI.pdf).

In preclinical studies, tipranavir inhibited human platelet aggregation (clotting) *in vitro*. It also caused impaired coagulation in mice and fatal bleeding at high doses, but this effect was not seen in dogs (http://www.hivandhepatitis.com/recent/2006/ad1/070706_b.html).

34.6.13 Darunavir

Darunavir (Prezista) was approved by the FDA in 2006. Several ongoing Phase III trials have shown the darunavir/ritonavir combination to be highly efficient and superior to lopinavir/ritonavir (Kaletra) as first-line therapy *(704–706)*. Structurally, darunavir represents [(1*R*,5*S*,6*R*)-2,8-dioxabicyclo[3.3.0]oct-6-yl]*N*-[(2*S*,3*R*)-4-[(4-aminophenyl)sulfonyl-(2-methylpropyl)amino]-3-hydroxy-1-phenyl-butan-2-yl]carbamate.

Dosage and Administration. The recommended daily dose of darunavir is 600 mg (two 300 mg tablets) taken orally with ritonavir (Norvir) 100 mg twice daily with food. Darunavir and ritonavir doses of 400/100 mg to 800/100 mg have been studied in clinical trials. The FDA-approved darunavir and ritonavir dosage of 600/100 mg twice daily is the dose that has been chosen for continued study (http://www.hivandhepatitis.com/hiv_and_aids/prezista_1.html).

Note: If a patient happened to miss a dose of darunavir/ritonavir by more than 6 hours, he or she should be told to wait and then take the next dose of darunavir/ritonavir at the regularly scheduled time. If the patient misses a dose by less than 6 hours, he or she should be told to take darunavir/ritonavir immediately and then take the next dose at the regularly scheduled time. If a dose of darunavir/ritonavir is skipped, the patient should not double the next dose. Patients should not take more or less than the prescribed dose of darunavir or ritonavir at any one time (http://www.hivandhepatitis.com/hiv_and_aids/prezista_1.html).

Drug Resistance. In vitro studies of darunavir/ritonavir have shown the emergence of a number of protease mutations. However, the resistance profile of darunavir in human subjects has not been characterized fully. Results from studies of darunavir in antiretroviral-naïve patients (now under way) are needed to identify darunavir resistance in initial therapy and to assess its implications for subsequent treatment. In patients with multiple preexisting mutations associated with resistance to protease inhibitors, emergent protease mutations included V32I, L33F, I47V, I54L, G73S, and L89V *(707, 708)*. In *in vitro* studies, viral isolates resistant to darunavir also were resistant to all other available protease inhibitors with the exception of tipranavir; some viruses remained susceptible to tipranavir *(707, 708)*. Clinical correlations for these observations are not available.

During the TMC-114-C213 and TMC-114-C202 clinical trials (see below), all subjects demonstrated at least one primary protease inhibitor resistance mutation (D30N, M46I/L, G48V, I50L/V, V82A/F/S/T, I84V, L90M) at patient screening *(706, 708, 709)* (http://www.centerwatch.com/patient/drugs/dru902.html).

Although no single mutation has been found to confer high-level resistance to darunavir, resistance mutations selected by other protease inhibitors can contribute to darunavir resistance. A number of protease mutations, including V11I, V32I, L33F, I47V, I50V, I54L/M, G73S, L76V, I84V, and L89V, are associated with decreased virologic response to darunavir. In addition, the total number of primary protease mutations is associated with diminished response to darunavir. If seven or more protease resistance mutations are present at baseline, the probability of darunavir + ritonavir treatment failure increases significantly *(707–709)*.

Drug-Drug Interactions. Coadministration of darunavir/ritonavir with efavirenz (Sustiva) caused a decrease in darunavir AUC [the *area under the curve (AUC)* is the area under the curve in a plot of concentration of drug in plasma against time] by 13% and minimum serum concentrations (C_{min}) by 31%, whereas the AUC and C_{min} of efavirenz increased by 21% and 17%, respectively. The clinical significance has not been established; however, this combination of drugs should be used with caution *(710)* (http://www.hivandhepatitis.com/hiv_and_aids/prezista_1.html).

Because didanosine (Videx) must be administered on an empty stomach, didanosine should be administered 1 hour before or 2 hours after darunavir and ritonavir dosing with food. Coadministration of darunavir/ritonavir with indinavir (Crixivan) resulted in a serum concentration increase in both darunavir and indinavir. The appropriate dose of indinavir in combination with darunavir and ritonavir has not been established (http://www.hivandhepatitis.com/hiv_and_aids/prezista_1.html).

Coadministration of darunavir with lopinavir/ritonavir (Kaletra) resulted in a 53% decrease in darunavir AUC. Coadministration of darunavir/ritonavir with saquinavir (Invirase) resulted in a 26% decrease in darunavir AUC. Hence, coadministration of these drugs with darunavir is not recommended (http://www.hivandhepatitis.com/hiv_and_aids/prezista_1.html).

Both darunavir and ritonavir are inhibitors of CYP3A. Coadministration of darunavir and ritonavir with protease inhibitor drugs primarily metabolized by CYP3A may result in increased plasma concentrations of such drugs, which could increase or prolong their therapeutic effect and adverse effects. In this regard, carbamazepine, phenobarbital, phenytoin, and rifampin, which are inducers of CYP450 enzymes, should not be used in combination with darunavir and ritonavir because they may interfere with the optimal plasma concentrations of darunavir/ritonavir. St. John's wort should also not be used concomitantly with darunavir and ritonavir. Coadministration of these drugs may cause significant decreases in darunavir plasma concentrations and a loss of darunavir's therapeutic effect (http://www.hivandhepatitis.com/hiv_and_aids/prezista_1.html).

Concomitant administration of darunavir/ritonavir with phosphodiesterase type 5 (PDE-5) inhibitors, including sildenafil, vardenafil, and tadalafil, should be done with caution. PDE-5 inhibitor dosing should not exceed the doses indicated by the manufacturer. Furthermore, darunavir/ritonavir with the selective serotonin reuptake inhibitors (SSRIs) sertraline and paroxetine should be taken concomitantly with caution. The recommended approach is a careful dose titration of the SSRI based on a clinical assessment of response to the antidepressant. In addition, patients on a stable dose of sertraline and paroxetine who start treatment with darunavir and ritonavir should be monitored for antidepressant response (http://www.hivandhepatitis.com/hiv_and_aids/prezista_1.html).

Clinical Trials. A randomized, open-label, controlled, Phase IIA clinical trial at 15 sites in Europe with 50 HIV-1–infected patients who had taken multiple protease inhibitors was conducted to evaluate antiviral activity, tolerability, and safety of darunavir boosted with low-dose ritonavir *(711)*. At entry, protease inhibitors in nonsuppressive regimens were replaced with darunavir/ritonavir (300 mg/100 mg or 600 mg/100 mg twice daily, or 900 mg/100 mg once daily)

or left unchanged for 14 days. The time-averaged difference (DAVG) in HIV-1 RNA from baseline, change in HIV-1 RNA from baseline, proportions achieving plasma HIV-1 RNA <400 copies/mL and ≥ 0.5 and ≥ 1.0 $\log_{10}$ copies/mL reductions in HIV-1 RNA, and safety were all assessed. The results showed that the DAVG responses in all darunavir/ritonavir groups (range, -0.56 to -0.81 $\log_{10}$ copies/mL) were significantly greater ($p < 0.001$) than in the controls (-0.03 $\log_{10}$ copies/mL). Median change at day 14 was -1.38 and $+0.02$ $\log_{10}$ copies/mL for all darunavir/ritonavir groups and the control group, respectively. A reduction of ≥ 0.5 and ≥ 1.0 $\log_{10}$ copies/mL was attained by 97% and 76% of patients, respectively, in all darunavir/ritonavir groups and by 25% and 17%, respectively, in the control group. HIV-1 RNA <400 copies/mL at any time during treatment was achieved by 40% in the darunavir/ritonavir groups and 8% in the control group. Most common reported adverse events were gastrointestinal and central nervous system disorders (mild to moderate severity). No dose relationship was observed. Biochemical, hematologic, and electrocardiographic parameters showed no significant changes. The overall results demonstrated a potent antiretroviral effect of the darunavir/ritonavir combination over 14 days in multiple-PI-experienced patients and was generally well tolerated *(711)*.

Trials TMC-114-C213 and TMC-114-C202. The accelerated approval of darunavir for the treatment of HIV-1 infections was based on 24-week data from a pair of ongoing, randomized Phase IIb trials (TMC-114-C213 and TMC-114-C202; POWER 1 and 2 Studies), which were ongoing at the time of approval *(712)* (http://www.clinicaltrials.gov/ct/show/NCT00081588;jsessionid=9A719C00C3CD8D44E0DF3C1F988B3EC5?order=2). Both trials investigated the efficacy of darunavir in antiretroviral treatment–experienced HIV-1–infected adult subjects. Subjects in both studies received 600 mg darunavir plus 100 mg ritonavir twice daily plus an *optimized background regimen (OBR)*, including at least two NRTIs with or without enfuvirtide, or a control regimen consisting of an investigator-selected protease inhibitor regimen plus OBR. The 24-week data set included 318 subjects in TMC-114-C213 and 319 subjects in TMC-114-C202 who had completed 24 weeks of treatment or discontinued earlier. Pooled data from the two studies indicated that 69.5% of subjects receiving the darunavir regimen achieved virologic response, as measured by a reduction of HIV-1 RNA of at least 1.0 $\log_{10}$ from baseline at week 24, compared with a 21.0% reduction for the control regimen. Mean change from baseline was -1.89 $\log_{10}$ copies/mL for darunavir versus -0.48 $\log_{10}$ copies/mL for control. In addition, 63% of subjects achieved HIV-1 RNA levels <400 copies/mL, and 45.0% achieved levels <50 copies/mL at week 24, versus 19% and 12.1% for control, respectively; 26.0% of subjects failed to sufficiently respond to treatment on the darunavir regimen versus 71%

for control. Increase from baseline in mean CD4$^+$ T-cell counts were greater for darunavir (92 cells/mm^3) than for control (17 cells/mm^3) (712).

Trials TMC-114-C215 and TMC-114-C208. Additional data supporting the approval of darunavir were obtained from a pair of nonrandomized clinical trials (TMC-114-C215 and TMC-114-C208; POWER 3 Study) (713). These data included 24-week results from 246 subjects receiving the 600 mg darunavir/100 mg ritonavir twice-daily regimen. Furthermore, the data indicated that 65% of subjects achieved a reduction in HIV-1 RNA of at least 1.0 log$_{10}$, 57% achieved levels <400 copies/mL, and 40% achieved levels <50 copies/mL, compared with baseline; mean reduction was 1.65 log$_{10}$ copies/mL. Mean CD4$^+$ T-cell counts increased by 80 cells/mm^3 from baseline at week 20 (713).

The TITAN Study. The TITAN (TMC-114/r in treatment-experienced patients naïve to lopinavir) study is an ongoing, international, randomized, controlled, open-label, 96-week Phase III trial that is being conducted at 159 medical centers in 26 countries (704). Treatment-experienced, lopinavir-naïve, HIV-1–infected patients (viral load (VL) >1,000 copies/mL) on stable HAART or off treatment for ≥12 weeks were randomized to receive darunavir/lopinavir 600 mg/100 mg twice daily or lopinavir/ritonavir 400 mg/100 mg twice daily plus optimized background regimen (OBR; ≥2 NRTIs/NNRTIs). The primary end-point of the trial was noninferiority of darunavir/ritonavir to lopinavir/ritonavir in confirmed virologic response (VL <400copies/mL, TLOVR; the FDA's algorithm "TLOVR" means time to loss of virologic response) at 48 weeks. In case of noninferiority, darunavir/ritonavir superiority was a secondary end-point. The secondary analysis results of the TITAN study after 48 weeks have suggested that the virologic response to darunavir/ritonavir was superior to that of lopinavir/ritonavir (704).

Toxicity. The safety assessment of darunavir has been based on all safety data from the TMC-114-C213 and TMC-114-C202 clinical studies and the TMC-114-C215/C208 analysis reported with the recommended dose of darunavir/ritonavir 600 mg/100 mg twice daily in the 458 subjects who initiated treatment with the recommended dose (*de novo* subjects) (712, 713). In the TMC-114-C213 and TMC-114-C202 studies, the mean exposure in weeks for subjects in the darunavir/ritonavir 600 mg/100 mg twice-daily arm and comparator protease inhibitor arm was 63.5 and 31.5, respectively. The mean exposure in weeks for subjects in the TMC-114-C215/C208 analysis was 23.9.

The most common treatment-emergent adverse events (>10%) reported in the *de novo* subjects, regardless of causality or frequency, were diarrhea, nausea, headache, and nasopharyngitis (712, 713). For subjects in the darunavir/ritonavir 600 mg/100 mg twice-daily arm and the comparator protease inhibitor arm in the pooled analysis for

the TMC-114-C213 and TMC-114-C202 studies, diarrhea was reported in 19.8% and 28.2%, nausea in 18.3% and 12.9%, headache in 15.3% and 20.2%, and nasopharyngitis in 13.7% and 10.5% of subjects, respectively. In the randomized trials, rates of discontinuation of therapy due to adverse events were 9% in subjects receiving darunavir/ritonavir and 5% in subjects in the comparator protease inhibitor arm (712).

Severe side effects of darunavir may include severe allergic reactions (rash, hives, difficulty breathing, tightness in the chest, or swelling of the mouth, face, lips, or tongue), changes in the amount of urine produced, chest pain, confusion, fast heartbeat, fever, chills, or persistent sore throat, rapid breathing, red, swollen, or blistered skin, severe headache or dizziness, unusual bleeding or bruising, unusual drowsiness, unusual swelling of the arms or legs, and unusual thirst (http://www.drugs.com/sfx/prezista-side-effects.html).

34.7 Fixed-Dose Combinations

34.7.1 Truvada

Emtricitabine is also available in a mixed-dose combination tablet with tenofovir disoproxil fumarate (Truvada), which contains 200 mg emtricitabine and 300 mg tenofovir disoproxil fumarate. Truvada is administered as one tablet every day for patients with a calculated creatinine clearance (calcCL$_{cr}$) of 50 mL/min or greater. The dosing interval should be lengthened to every 48 hours in patients with calcCL$_{cr}$ between 30 and 49 mL/min. Truvada is not recommended for use in patients with calcCL$_{cr}$ of less than 30 mL/min or in patients on hemodialysis (33).

34.7.2 Trizivir

Trizivir is the only three-drug fixed-dose coformulation of antiretroviral medication and was approved for use in adults and adolescent weighing more than 40 kg in November 2000. Each Trizivir tablet contains 300 mg abacavir, 150 mg lamivudine, and 300 mg zidovudine. A single Trizivir tablet is bioequivalent to one 300 mg abacavir tablet, one 150 mg lamivudine tablet, and one 300 mg zidovudine tablet after single-dose administration to 24 fasting healthy subjects (714). The recommended oral dose of Trizivir is one tablet twice daily. Because it is a fixed-dose tablet, Trizivir should not be prescribed to patients requiring dosage adjustment, such as those with creatinine clearance of less than 50 mL/min or those experiencing dose-limiting adverse side effects (17).

Toxicity. The Trizivir-related toxicity of most concern is hypersensitivity to abacavir. This is an idiosyncratic drug reaction that occurs in 5% of individuals treated with this drug *(715)*. Discontinuing the drug usually resolves the symptoms promptly. Rechallenge with abacavir can result in more severe symptoms and death *(716, 717)*. Because of this, abacavir should not be given to individuals who have had a prior hypersensitivity reaction. A clinical diagnosis is necessary to identify abacavir hypersensitivity. There are no laboratory parameters that identify abacavir hypersensitivity. Although it can be difficult to distinguish abacavir hypersensitivity from other febrile illness, the complexity of symptoms make it possible to identify this illness. In a case-controlled study of patients with abacavir hypersensitivity and culture-proved influenza, abacavir hypersensitivity was strongly associated with fever, rash, and gastrointestinal symptoms, and influenza was strongly associated with fever and respiratory symptoms without gastrointestinal symptoms *(718)*.

Lactic acidosis has been associated with all nucleoside analogues including abacavir, lamivudine, and zidovudine. Most of the case reports have occurred in patients treated with zidovudine, although more recent reports have implicated stavudine. This is an uncommon complication, occurring in <1% of patients treated with these medications. Lactic acidosis is often associated with hepatic steatosis and has been fatal. The cause of *lactic acidosis syndrome* is thought to be inhibition of mitochondrial DNA synthesis by the nucleoside analogues. This, in turn, leads to anaerobic glycolysis and accumulation of lactate. Of the components of Trizivir, lamivudine has the greatest affinity to mitochondrial DNA *(719, 720)*. In most cases, nucleoside-induced lactic acidosis has been seen in women. Risk factors include obesity and prolonged nucleoside exposure.

Trizivir is associated with bone marrow suppression, primarily due to the zidovudine component, although abacavir has been associated with neutropenia *(721)*. Zidovudine is associated with neutropenia, thrombocytopenia, and anemia. Paradoxically, these parameters may improve in patients with advanced HIV disease because suppression of viral replication reverses the suppressive effects of HIV-1. However, care should be taken when administering this medication to individuals with severe bone marrow suppression, as these parameters can worsen with therapy. Combination of Trizivir with other agents, such as ganciclovir and other cytotoxic agents, can cause severe anemia. The use of erythropoietin can ameliorate these affects in some cases.

Drug Resistance. Antiretroviral resistance has been observed in viral isolates from patients treated with Trizivir and its components *(722–724)*. Resistance to the zidovudine component of this combination typically occurs through the accumulation of *nucleoside-associated mutations (NAMs)*. The accumulation of NAMs can also confer cross-resistance to other nucleoside analogues, particularly stavudine. Lamivudine has a unique resistance profile. Abacavir has unique mutations associated with the emergence of resistance, but accumulation of NAMs can also lead to decreased susceptibility to abacavir *(725)*.

There is concern that clinical failure to Trizivir will result in broad cross-resistance to nucleoside analogues. Clinical trial data suggest that this can be avoided by careful monitoring of patients *(722)*. Subjects in the CNA3005 study who failed Trizivir initially developed resistance to lamivudine and then to zidovudine and abacavir. The median time from lamivudine resistance to the development of resistance to the other components of Trizivir was almost 6 months. Thus, by closely monitoring HIV-1 plasma RNA and then testing resistance early, the antiretroviral regimen can be changed to avoid further emergence of resistance. In studies with efavirenz and Trizivir, a fairly consistent pattern emerges: most subjects with the wild-type virus failed. In those viral isolates that show resistance-associated mutations, the most common was K103N alone, which confers resistance to efavirenz; followed in order of frequency by M184V (which confers resistance to lamivudine); a combination of the two; then NAMs. Mutations that conferred resistance to abacavir or tenofovir (L74V and K65R, respectively) were uncommon.

34.7.3 Combivir

Combivir is a fixed-dose combination of two NRTI drugs: 300 mg Retrovir (AZT, zidovudine) and 150 mg Epivir (3TC, lamivudine) approved by the FDA in 1997 for treating HIV disease.

Study 934 is an ongoing international open-label Phase III trial in which treatment-naïve patients were randomly assigned to receive either once-daily tenofovir DF plus emtricitabine plus efavirenz or else twice-daily Combivir plus efavirenz. The first regimen includes the three drugs in the newly approved Atripla fixed-dose combination tablet. Data from 144-week treatment has indicated a few possible efficacy and safety advantages of Truvada over Combivir *(726)*. Study 934 enrolled 517 HIV-positive patients starting HIV treatment for the first time. The 48-week data from the study *(727)* found that 80% of patients in the Truvada group had HIV RNA viral loads below 50 copies/mL (undetectable), compared with 70% in the Combivir group *(728)*. After 144 weeks of treatment, 71% of Truvada/efavirenz patients compared with 58% of Combivir/efavirenz patients achieved and maintained viral loads of less than 400 copies/mL. The difference between the two groups was statistically significant. Using the more sensitive viral load assay, which measures levels down to 50 copies/mL, 64% of patients taking Truvada and 56% of patients taking Combivir had undetectable viral loads. This difference was just shy of statistical significance, meaning that both drugs remain comparable with respect to HIV RNA viral load reductions below 50 copies/mL (729). Among patients who stopped responding to their assigned treatment regimen, fewer patients taking Truvada—compared with those taking Combivir—did so because of resistance to their emtricitabine (in Truvada) or lamivudine (in Combivir), both of which are hobbled by the M184V mutation in HIV's reverse transcriptase gene. In the Truvada group, two patients developed the mutation, compared with 10 patients in the Combivir group (729).

As for CD4$^+$ T-cell count increases, patients in the Truvada group had significantly higher levels at weeks 48 and 96 of the study. By week 144, there was still a noticeable difference between the two groups—a 312-cell increase in the Truvada group versus a 271-cell increase in the Combivir group—but the comparison was no longer statistically significant (729). Other results of Study 934 have also shown that after 96 weeks of treatment, discontinuation of study medications due to side effects was significantly higher among Combivir patients (11%) than among those receiving Truvada (5%). The most common side effect–related reasons for discontinuing treatment were anemia (14% in the Combivir group vs. 0% in the Truvada group) and rash (1% vs. 4%, respectively) (729).

The SWEET study is a Phase III clinical trial evaluating virologically suppressed patients with HIV who switched from treatment with twice-daily Combivir (lamivudine/zidovudine) to treatment with the once-daily Truvada (emtricitabine and tenofovir disoproxil fumarate) as part of their combination drug therapy. In the SWEET (simplification with easier emtricitabine and tenofovir) study, patients who switched from Combivir to Truvada, both in combination with once-daily Sustiva (efavirenz), experienced improvements in a number of treatment-related side effects (http://biz.yahoo.com/bw/071029/20071029005478.html?.v=1).

Patients in both study arms maintained virologic suppression at 48 weeks. In the SWEET study, 234 patients who had undetectable viral loads while taking efavirenz plus Combivir were randomized to either continue on that regimen or substitute the Combivir with the Truvada combination. Twenty-four weeks after switching—the midpoint of the study—89.7% in the Combivir group and 94% in the Truvada groups maintained viral loads below 50 copies/mL, with no statistically significant difference between the two arms. There were, however, *statistically significant improvements in hemoglobin, total cholesterol, and triglyceride levels, all in favor of Truvada* (711).

A study comparing the antiviral response with abacavir/Combivir to indinavir/Combivir in therapy-naïve adults

at 48 weeks (Study CNA3005) has shown the antiviral effect of both combinations to be similar in the HIV therapy of treatment-naïve patients (730).

In June 2006, the FDA approved safety labeling revisions for lamivudine/zidovudine tablets (Combivir) to warn of the potential risk for hepatic decompensation associated with concomitant use of interferon-α. The warning was based on reports of hepatic decompensation (some fatal) in patients co-infected with HIV and hepatitis C virus (HCV) who were receiving combination antiretroviral therapy for HIV and interferon-α with or without ribavirin. The FDA noted that although *in vitro* studies have shown that ribavirin can reduce the phosphorylation of pyrimidine nucleoside analogues, such as lamivudine and zidovudine, no evidence of a pharmacokinetic or pharmacodynamic interaction (i.e., loss of virologic suppression) was observed with their concurrent administration in HIV-HCV co-infected patients. Patients receiving interferon-α with or without ribavirin in addition to lamivudine/zidovudine should be closely monitored for treatment-associated toxicities, especially hepatic decompensation, neutropenia, and anemia (http://www.medscape.com/viewarticle/545855).

Discontinuation of lamivudine/zidovudine therapy should be considered as medically appropriate. Also, dose reduction or discontinuation of interferon-α, ribavirin, or both should also be considered if worsening clinical toxicities are observed, including hepatic decompensation (e.g., Childs-Pugh score >6; this value is used to assess the prognosis of chronic liver disease). The FDA also warned of the risk for immune reconstitution syndrome in patients receiving combination antiretroviral therapy, including lamivudine and lamivudine/zidovudine. Patients whose immune system responds during the initial phase of treatment may develop an inflammatory response to indolent or residual opportunistic infections, such as *Mycobacterium avium* infection, cytomegalovirus, *Pneumocystis jiroveci* pneumonia, and tuberculosis (http://www.medscape.com/viewarticle/545855).

34.7.4 Epzicom

Abacavir sulfate (600 mg) and lamivudine (300 mg), two reverse transcriptase inhibitors that have been used for years to treat HIV infection, are available as Epzicom. Epzicom, which was approved by the FDA in 2004, is prescribed as once-daily tablet. In Europe, Epzicom is marketed under the trade name Kivexa.

In clinical practice, abacavir and lamivudine have been administered separately twice daily as a dual-nucleoside backbone for PI-based (731, 732) and NNRTI-based (733, 734) HAART regimens. Epzicom (a fixed-dose combination of abacavir and lamivudine administered once daily) as a component of combination antiretroviral therapy has the benefit of simplifying a regimen already used in clinical practice and may provide further adherence and efficacy advantages *(735, 736)*.

Dosing and Administration. Epzicom is a tablet taken once a day. It can be taken with or without food. Epzicom should not be taken at the same time as Emtriva or Truvada (containing Viread and Emtriva). This is because the Epivir in Epzicom is very similar to Emtriva, and it is not believed that combining these two anti-HIV drugs will make a regimen any more effective against the virus.

Clinical Trials. The open-label BICOMBO study included 335 participants in Spain with viral loads of less than 200 cells/mm^3 who were receiving regimens containing 3TC (lamivudine, Epivir) *(737)*. Baseline characteristics were similar in the two arms. About 75% were men, the median age was 43 years, the median baseline CD4$^+$ T-cell count was about 500 cells/mm^3, and about one third were co-infected with hepatitis C virus. Patients were randomly assigned to switch their current NRTIs to either Truvada or Epzicom while staying on the same NNRTI or PI. (Some subjects changed from individual drugs to the corresponding combination tablet, e.g., from separate emtricitabine plus tenofovir to Truvada.) Subjects were not screened in advance for abacavir hypersensitivity. The results of the study showed that after 48 weeks: (i) significantly more patients in the Epzicom arm experienced treatment failure compared with that in the Truvada arm (19% vs. 13%); (ii) the rates of virologic failure were low in both arms: 2.4% of those taking Epzicom and none of those taking Truvada; (iii) the CD4$^+$ T-cell counts increased more in the Epzicom arm (+44 T-cells/mm^3) than in the Truvada arm (−3 T-cells/mm^3); (iv) about twice as many patients in the Epzicom arm discontinued treatment early due to adverse events compared with that in the Truvada arm (10.2% vs. 5.4%). In the Epzicom arm, 9 subjects had suspected abacavir hypersensitivity reactions; and (v) patients taking Truvada had lower fasting triglyceride, total cholesterol, and LDL cholesterol levels, but also had lower levels of HDL cholesterol *(737)*. The overall conclusion was that switching the NRTI component of an existing suppressive regimen to Epzicom was not inferior to Truvada in terms of virologic efficacy, but not in terms of overall effectiveness of treatment.

The difference, however, was mainly driven by the Epzicom interruptions due to suspected abacavir hypersensitivity. These data suggest that prescreening patients using the new *HLA-B*5071 genetic test* [the PREDICT-1 Study *(738–740)*] might help select a subgroup of individuals who could benefit as much from Epzicom as from Truvada.

Toxicity. An important side effect of Epzicom is sometimes severe hypersensitivity reaction (see also Section 34.7.2). Approximately 5% of patients who take abacavir, one of the two medications in Epzicom, are allergic to it. This can be serious and generally requires that Epzicom be stopped, and that Epzicom or abacavir should not be taken again. A hypersensitivity reaction usually appears during the second week of therapy, but it can take as long as 6 weeks to notice any symptoms. The most common symptoms are fever and rash, followed by headaches, stomach upset, feeling sick or tired, sore throat, cough, and shortness of breath. These symptoms usually get worse over time.

Lactic acidosis, which can be fatal, and severe liver problems have been reported (see Section 34.7.2) (http://aidsinfo. nih.gov/DrugsNew/DrugDetailNT.aspx?MenuItem=Drugs &Search=On&int_id=407).

In August 2006, the FDA approved a safety warning for abacavir sulfate/lamivudine tablets (Epzicom) to warn of the potential risk for hepatic decompensation associated with concomitant use of interferon-α. The warning was based on reports of hepatic decompensation (some fatal) in patients co-infected with HIV and hepatitis C virus (HCV) who were receiving combination antiretroviral therapy for HIV and interferon-α with or without ribavirin. The FDA noted that although *in vitro* studies have shown that ribavirin can reduce the phosphorylation of pyrimidine nucleoside analogues, such as lamivudine, no evidence of a pharmacokinetic or pharmacodynamic interaction (i.e., loss of virologic suppression) was observed with their concurrent administration in HIV-HCV co-infected patients.

Patients receiving interferon-α with or without ribavirin in addition to abacavir/lamivudine should be closely monitored for treatment-associated toxicities, especially hepatic decompensation, neutropenia, and anemia.

Discontinuation of abacavir/lamivudine therapy should be considered as medically appropriate. Also, dose reduction or discontinuation of interferon-α, ribavirin, or both should also be considered if worsening clinical toxicities are observed, including hepatic decompensation (e.g., Childs-Pugh score >6). The FDA also warned of the risk for immune reconstitution syndrome in patients receiving combination antiretroviral therapy, including abacavir/lamivudine. Patients whose immune system responds during the initial phase of treatment may develop an inflammatory response to indolent or residual opportunistic infections, such as *Mycobacterium avium* infection, cytomegalovirus, *Pneumocystis jiroveci* pneumonia, and tuberculosis (http://www.medscape. com/viewarticle/547861).

34.7.5 Atripla

Atripla is a complete regimen in a single, once-daily, fixed-dose combination tablet that contains efavirenz 600 mg, emtricitabine 200 mg, and tenofovir disoproxil fumarate

300 mg. Current treatment guidelines recommend this triple combination for initial therapy because of its excellent potency, tolerability, and favorable safety profile. Individually, these agents have long half-lives that allow for once-daily dosing and may provide a pharmacologic bridge for the occasional missed dose. Although several options for once-daily regimens are available, comparative clinical trials are still in progress. However, patient characteristics vary greatly, and there is no "one size fits all" regimen that is optimal for all individuals. Therefore, it is important to consider that other once-daily regimens are also available and include protease inhibitors and/or other dual-nucleoside reverse transcriptase inhibitor combinations. These combinations offer potential advantages and disadvantages with respect to tolerability, long-term complications, and drug-drug interaction profiles, as well as distinctive drug resistance patterns during episodes of treatment failure *(741)*.

Long-term resistance data for efavirenz/emtricitabine/tenofovir DF is available. In Study 934, a total of 41 patients (14 in the tenofovir DF/emtricitabine group vs. 27 in the zidovudine/lamivudine group) met criteria for treatment failure and had genotypic data for drug resistance available after 96 weeks of therapy *(742)*. For those receiving tenofovir DF/emtricitabine, efavirenz resistance mutations were most common ($n = 10$), followed by the M184V/I mutation, which occurred simultaneously with efavirenz mutations in two individuals. Of note, no patient developed the K65R mutation. In contrast, 8 of 299 (2.7%) patients developed a K65R mutation after 3 years of therapy in Study 903, which evaluated lamivudine (instead of emtricitabine) combined with efavirenz and tenofovir DF *(743)*.

34.8 Viral Entry/Fusion Inhibitors

Individual HIV-1 isolates vary markedly in their tropisms for infecting different CD4-positive target cell types. Some isolates (macrophage-tropic) infect macrophages but not continuous T-lymphocyte cell lines, whereas others (T-cell line-tropic) display the opposite preference. It has been shown that the cytotropisms of different HIV variants were due to the inherent fusion specificities of the corresponding Envs, which in turn result from the ability of each Env to use distinct "fusion cofactors" that are differentially expressed on various CD4-positive cell types *(744)*. Using a novel functional cDNA screening method, a fusion cofactor for T-cell line-tropic isolates has been identified and designated as "fusin" (CXCR4). Subsequently, another cofactor, CCR5 [chemokine (C-C motif) receptor 5], which functions preferentially for macrophage-tropic variants, has also been identified. Both cofactors are members of the chemokine receptor family of G protein–coupled receptors. Primary HIV-1

isolates from diverse genetic subtypes were found to function with CCR5 and/or fusin (and in some cases with other chemokine receptors). Further studies have determined that signaling through G proteins is not required for fusion cofactor activity. Fusin and CCR5 expression are regulated differently upon T-cell activation, suggesting implications for HIV replication *in vivo*. Of particular interest are findings indicating that genetic alterations in the fusion cofactors can directly influence susceptibility to HIV infection and possibly rates of disease progression in infected persons *(744)*.

A number of inflammatory CC-chemokines, including MIP-1α and MIP-1β, RANTES, MCP-2, and HCC-1, act as CCR5 agonists, whereas MCP-3 is a natural antagonist of the receptor *(745, 746)*. CCR5 is mainly expressed in memory T cells, macrophages, and immature dendritic cells, and is upregulated by proinflammatory cytokines. It is coupled to the Gi class of heterotrimeric G proteins and inhibits cAMP production, stimulates Ca^{2+} release, and activates PI3-kinase and MAP kinases, as well as other tyrosine kinase cascades. A mutant allele of CCR5, CCR5 delta 32, is frequent in populations of European origin and encodes a nonfunctional truncated protein that is not transported to the cell surface. Homozygotes for the delta 32 allele exhibit a strong, although incomplete, resistance to HIV infection, whereas heterozygotes display delayed progression to AIDS. Many other alleles, affecting the primary structure of CCR5 or its promoter, have been described, some of which lead to nonfunctional receptors or otherwise influence AIDS progression. CCR5 is considered a drug target in the field of HIV but also in a growing number of inflammatory diseases. Modified chemokines, monoclonal antibodies, and small chemical antagonists, as well as a number of gene therapy approaches, have been developed in this framework *(746)*.

CCR5 is located on chromosome 3 on the short (p) arm at position 21. It is likely that CCR5 plays a role in inflammatory responses to infection, although its exact role in normal immune function is unclear *(745)*.

HIV uses CCR5 or another protein, CXCR4, as a coreceptor to enter its target cells. Several chemokine receptors can function as viral coreceptors, but CCR5 is likely the most physiologically important coreceptor during natural infection. The normal ligands for this receptor, RANTES, MIP-1β, and MIP-1α, are able to suppress HIV-1 infection *in vitro*. In individuals infected with HIV, CCR5-using viruses are the predominant species isolated during the early stages of viral infection, suggesting that these viruses may have a selective advantage during transmission or the acute phase of disease. Moreover, at least half of all infected individuals harbor only CCR5-using viruses throughout the course of infection *(746)*.

A number of new experimental HIV drugs have been designed to interfere with the interaction between CCR5 and HIV, including PRO140, Vicriviroc, Aplaviroc (GW-873140), and Maraviroc (UK-427857). A potential problem with this approach is that, although CCR5 is the major coreceptor by which HIV infects cells, it is not the only such coreceptor. It is possible that under selective pressure, HIV will evolve to use another coreceptor. However, examination of viral resistance to AD101, molecular antagonist of CCR5, indicated that resistant viruses did not switch to another coreceptor (CXCR4) but persisted in using CCR5, either by binding to alternative domains of CCR5 or by binding to the receptor at a higher affinity.

CCR5-Δ32 (CCR5-D32, CCR5 delta 32) is a genetic variant of CCR5 *(747, 748)*, resulting from a deletion mutation of a gene that has a specific impact on the function of T cells. CCR5-Δ32 is widely dispersed throughout northern Europe and in individuals of European descent. It has been hypothesized that this allele was favored by natural selection during the Black Death, or during smallpox outbreaks, which is unlikely, given that the frequency of CCR5-Δ32 in Bronze Age samples is similar to that seen today *(749)*. The allele has a negative effect upon T-cell function but appears to protect against smallpox, plague, and HIV. Individuals with the Δ32 allele of CCR5 are healthy, suggesting that CCR5 is largely dispensable. However, CCR5 plays a role in mediating resistance to West Nile virus infection in humans, as CCR5-Δ32-defective individuals are enriched in cohorts of West Nile virus–symptomatic patients *(750)*, indicating that all of the functions of CCR5 may not be compensated by other receptors. Though CCR5 has multiple variants in its coding region, the deletion of a 32-bp segment results in a nonfunctional receptor, thus preventing HIV R5 entry; two copies of this allele provide strong protection against HIV infection *(751)*. This allele is found in 5% to 14% of Europeans but is rare in people from Africa and Asia *(752)*. Multiple studies of HIV-infected persons have shown that the presence of one copy of this allele delays progression to the condition of AIDS by about 2 years. CCR5-Δ32 decreases the number of CCR5 proteins on the outside of the CD4 cell, which can have a large effect on the progression rates of HIV disease. It is possible that a person with the CCR5-Δ32 receptor allele will not be infected with HIV R5 strains *(751)*.

34.8.1 Enfuvirtide

Enfuvirtide (Fuzeon, T-20) is the first antiretroviral agent that acts by inhibiting the fusion of HIV-1 with CD4$^+$ T-cells. It was approved by the FDA in 2003.

Enfuvirtide represents a linear 36-amino-acid synthetic peptide, in which the *N*-terminus is acetylated and the *C*-terminus is a carboxamide. It is composed of naturally occurring *L*-amino acid residues. The empirical formula of enfuvirtide is $C_{204}H_{301}N_{51}O_{64}$, and the molecular weight is 4,492. Enfuvirtide has the following primary amino acid sequence: CH$_3$CO-Tyr-Thr-Ser-Leu-Ile-His-Ser-Leu-Ile-Glu-Glu-Ser-Gln-Asn-Gln-Gln-Glu-Lys-Asn-Glu-Gln-Glu-Leu-Leu-Glu-Leu-Asp-Lys-Trp-Ala-Ser-Leu-Trp-Asn-Trp-Phe-NH$_2$.

Enfuvirtide is a white to off-white amorphous solid. It has negligible solubility in pure water, but the solubility increases in aqueous buffers (pH 7.5) to 85 to 142 g/100 mL.

Mechanism of Action. Enfuvirtide interferes with the entry of HIV-1 into cells by inhibiting fusion of viral and cellular membranes. Enfuvirtide binds to the first heptad-repeat (HR1) in the gp41 subunit of the viral envelope glycoprotein and prevents the conformational changes required for the fusion of viral and cellular membranes.

The HIV entry into cells is mediated by the viral envelope glycoprotein, which comprises noncovalently associated surface (gp120) and transmembrane (gp41) subunits *(753)*. The gp120 is primarily involved in recognizing cellular receptors, whereas gp41 directly mediates membrane fusion. When peptides isolated from the gp41 *N*- and *C*-peptide regions (*N*- and *C*-peptides) are mixed in solution, they form a six-helix bundle, which represents the postfusion gp41 structure *(754–756)*. Three *N*-peptides form a central parallel trimeric coiled-coil (*N*-trimer) surrounded by three antiparallel helical *C*-peptides that nestle into long grooves between neighboring *N*-peptides. The importance of this structure is indicated by the dominant negative inhibition of HIV entry by *N*- and *C*-peptides *(757)*.

The available inhibitory and structural data support a working model of HIV membrane fusion *(753, 757)*. Initially, gp120 interacts with cellular CD4 and a chemokine coreceptor (typically CXCR4 or CCR5), causing large conformational changes in gp120 that propagate to gp41 via the gp120–gp41 interface. The gp41 then undergoes a dramatic structural rearrangement that exposes its *N*-terminal fusion peptide, which embeds in the target cell membrane. At this stage of fusion, gp41 adopts an extended "prehairpin intermediate" conformation that bridges both viral and cellular membranes and exposes its *N*-trimer region. This intermediate is relatively long lived (minutes) *(757–759)* but ultimately collapses as the *N*- and *C*-peptide regions of each gp41 monomer associate to form a hairpin structure. Three such hairpins (trimer-of-hairpins) form the six-helix bundle, which forces the viral and cellular membranes into tight apposition, inducing membrane fusion *(753)*.

According to this model, any inhibitor that binds to the *N*-trimer and prevents hairpin formation will inhibit viral entry. This prediction has been well supported by the discovery of numerous peptide, protein, and small-molecule inhibitors that bind the *N*-trimer *(760)*. A particularly interesting feature of the *N*-trimer is the deep hydrophobic "pocket" formed by the *N*-peptide's 17 *C*-terminal residues. This pocket has several enticing features as an inhibitory target, including (i) a very highly conserved sequence *(754,*

761, 762); (ii) an essential role in viral entry *(763);* (iii) a compact binding site that is vulnerable to inhibition by small molecules or short peptides; and (iv) the availability of several designed peptides that authentically mimic the pocket structure (e.g., IQN17, IZN17, 5-helix, and $N_{CCG}N13$) *(761, 762, 764, 765).*

To date, enfuvirtide is the only currently approved HIV-1 entry inhibitor that binds to the *N*-trimer but not the pocket region *(766, 767).*

Dosing and Administration. Enfuvirtide for injection is a white to off-white, sterile, lyophilized powder. Each single-use vial contains 108 mg of enfuvirtide for the delivery of 90 mg. Prior to subcutaneous administration, the contents of the vial are reconstituted with 1.1 mL of Sterile Water for Injection, giving a volume of approximately 1.2 mL to provide the delivery of 1.0 mL of the solution. Each 1.0 mL of the reconstituted solution contains approximately 90 mg enfuvirtide with approximate amounts of the following excipients: 22.55 mg mannitol, 2.39 mg sodium carbonate (anhydrous), and sodium hydroxide and hydrochloric acid for pH adjustment as needed. The reconstituted solution has an approximate pH of 9.0.

The recommended dose of enfuvirtide in adult patients is 90 mg (1.0 mL) twice daily injected subcutaneously into the upper arm, anterior thigh, or abdomen. Each injection should be given at a site different from the preceding injection site, and only where there is no current injection site reaction from an earlier dose. Enfuvirtide should not be injected into moles, scar tissue, bruises, or the navel (http://www.rxlist.com/cgi/generic/fuzeon_ids.htm).

No data are available to establish a dose recommendation of enfuvirtide in pediatric patients below age 6. In pediatric patients 6 years through 16 years of age, the recommended dosage of enfuvirtide is 2.0 mg/kg twice daily up to a maximum dose of 90 mg twice daily injected subcutaneously into the upper arm, anterior thigh, or abdomen. The dosing guidelines for enfuvirtide should be based on body weight. Body weight should be monitored periodically and the enfuvirtide dose adjusted accordingly (http://www.rxlist.com/cgi/generic/fuzeon.htm).

An analysis of the correlation between the severity of injection site reactions and the amount of subcutaneous fat has shown that the increased peripheral fat is associated with a decreased incidence of grade 3 or 4 *injection-site reactions (ISRs) (768).*

Adverse events associated with the use of the Biojector 2000 needle-free device for administering enfuvirtide have included nerve pain (neuralgia and/or paresthesia) lasting up to 6 months associated with administration at anatomic sites where large nerves course close to the skin, bruising, and hematomas. Patients receiving anticoagulants or persons with hemophilia or other coagulation disorders may have a higher risk of postinjection bleeding (http://www.thebody.com/content/treat/art39833.html).

Drug Resistance. HIV-1 isolates with reduced susceptibility to enfuvirtide have been selected *in vitro.* Genotypic analysis of the *in vitro*–selected resistant isolates showed mutations that resulted in amino acid substitutions at the enfuvirtide binding HR1 domain positions 36 to 38 of the HIV-1 envelope glycoprotein gp41. Phenotypic analysis of site-directed mutants in positions 36 to 38 in an HIV-1 molecular clone showed a 5-fold to 684-fold decrease in susceptibility to enfuvirtide (http://www.rxlist.com/cgi/generic/fuzeon.htm).

In clinical trials, HIV-1 isolates with reduced susceptibility to enfuvirtide have been recovered from subjects failing an enfuvirtide-containing regimen. Posttreatment HIV-1 virus from 277 subjects experiencing protocol-defined virologic failure at 48 weeks exhibited a median decrease in susceptibility to enfuvirtide of 33.4-fold (range, 0.4 to 6,318-fold) relative to their respective baseline virus. Of these, 249 had decreases in susceptibility to enfuvirtide greater than 4-fold, and all but 3 of those 249 exhibited genotypic changes in the codons encoding gp41 HR1 domain amino acids 36 to 45. Substitutions in this region were observed with decreasing frequency at amino acid positions 38, 43, 36, 40, 42, and 45 (http://www.rxlist.com/cgi/generic/fuzeon.htm).

HIV-1 clinical isolates resistant to NRTIs, NNRTIs, and PIs were susceptible to enfuvirtide in cell culture (http://www.rxlist.com/cgi/generic/fuzeon.htm).

Clinical Trials. Enfuvirtide in combination with other antiretroviral agents is indicated for treating HIV-1 infection in treatment-experienced patients with evidence of HIV-1 replication despite ongoing antiretroviral therapy. Enfuvirtide exhibited additive to synergistic effects in cell culture assays when combined with individual members of various antiretroviral classes, including lamivudine, zidovudine, indinavir, nelfinavir, and efavirenz.

Results from an open-label, randomized, multiple dose, two-period crossover study have shown that the administration of enfuvirtide 180 mg once-daily resulted in bioequivalence compared with twice-daily 90 mg of the drug based on AUC with a similar short-term safety profile but a trend toward a weaker antiretroviral effect *(769).* However, larger and longer-term studies are needed to determine whether 180 mg once daily is an effective dosing alternative for enfuvirtide.

The BLQ (below the level of quantification) study is a prospective, open-label, 24-week, single-arm, multicenter, cohort study conducted in the United States and Australia. The trial was designed to explore the impact of baseline variables—including darunavir phenotypic sensitivity (prior drug resistance)—on virologic responses in highly treatment-experienced patients receiving regimens containing enfuvirtide and darunavir/ritonavir. Interim results from the BLQ study have shown that almost two thirds (64%) of three-class treatment-experienced patients achieved undetectable HIV viral loads (<50 copies/mL) at 24 weeks. In addition, baseline sensitivity to darunavir did not appear to influence patient response *(770)*.

T20-310 was a multicenter, open-label, nonrandomized, noncomparative study to assess the safety and efficacy of enfuvirtide in children *(771)*. A total of 52 treatment-experienced pediatric HIV patients (3 to 16 years old) received 2.0 mg/kg (maximum 90 mg) twice-daily subcutaneous enfuvirtide for 48 weeks, along with optimized background therapy. Enfuvirtide was generally well tolerated, and no new patterns of adverse events compared with those seen in adults were observed. Mild-to-moderate injection-site reactions were the most common adverse event. Among those participants on treatment for 48 weeks, the median HIV RNA decrease from baseline was 1.17 $\log_{10}$ copies/mL ($n = 32$). The median $CD4^+$ T-cell increase from baseline was 106 cells/mm^3, and the median CD4 percentage increase was 4.7 ($n = 25$). Seventeen (32.7%) children achieved a viral load decrease of at least 1.0 $\log_{10}$ copies/mL and 11 (21.2%) children achieved an HIV RNA level below 400 copies/mL. Whereas the virologic and immunologic treatment responses were substantially better for children (<11 years) than for adolescents, the steady-state mean enfuvirtide C_{trough} levels were stable over 24 weeks with no differences between children and adolescents. The overall results of the study have suggested that enfuvirtide is an effective treatment for children and adolescents with HIV infection receiving optimized background therapy and has a favorable safety profile *(771)*.

Toxicity. Enfuvirtide is the only antiretroviral administered by infusion. With the long-term use of enfuvirtide ISRs and needle fatigue develop in 98% of patients. The severity of ISRs is for the most part mild to moderate, including itching, swelling, redness, pain or tenderness, hardened skin or bumps; other symptoms are headache and fever. Bumps ("nodules") developed more frequently and severely in areas of high muscle mass (stomach, legs), often hurting during movement *(772)*.

Recently, the Biojector B2000 was introduced as an alternative needle-free gas-powered injection system for subcutaneous administration of enfuvirtide *(753, 773)*. Although B2006 reduced the incidence of ISRs, some patients experienced long-lasting nerve pain, bruising, and bleeding below the skin, which led to its withdrawal (http://www.aidsmap.com/en/news/B4036654-5524-4B09-9A26-FAAF5B1B22DA.asp).

34.8.2 Maraviroc

Maraviroc (Selzentry, Celsentri, UK-427,857) is a CCR5-blocking entry inhibitor that was approved by the FDA in August 2007. Maraviroc received accelerated approval from FDA for use in treating adults with CCR5-tropic HIV-1 infection who have HIV strains that are resistant to multiple other antiretroviral agents and who have ongoing viral replication while receiving antiretroviral therapy. Maraviroc is the first agent in the class of chemokine coreceptor antagonists to be approved by the FDA. It binds to CCR5, one of two possible coreceptors used by HIV to enter $CD4^+$ T-cells, thus blocking entry of CCR5-tropic HIV into these cells.

Maraviroc has not yet been approved for patients with drug-sensitive HIV strains, such as those starting antiretroviral therapy for the first time. In countries other than the United States, maraviroc will be approved and sold under the brand name Celsentri.

Structurally, maraviroc represents 4-difluoro-*N*-{(1*S*)-3-[3-(3-isopropylmethyl-4*H*-1,2,4-triazol-4-yl)-8-azabicyclo[3.2.1]oct-8-yl]-1-phenylpropyl}cyclohexanecarboxamide.

Mechanism of Action. Maraviroc acts by binding to a protein on the membrane of CD4 T-cells called CCR5. Once it does this, HIV cannot successfully attach itself to the surface of CD4 cells and is thus prevented from infecting healthy cells.

A critical step in cellular entry by HIV-1 is the binding of the viral envelope protein gp120 to chemokine receptors on the surface of immune cells *(774–778)*. The CC-chemokine receptors CCR5 and CXCR4 are the major coreceptors for R5 and X4 virus strains, respectively *(779, 780)*.

CCR5 is the coreceptor used by macrophage-tropic viruses, whereas CXCR4 is predominately used by T-lymphocyte–tropic variants *(781, 782)*. The CCR5-tropic variant of the virus is common in earlier HIV infection, whereas viruses adapted to use the CXCR4 receptor gradually become dominant as HIV infection progresses. *Maraviroc did not display efficacy against CXCR4-tropic or mixed- or dual-tropic virus in Phase II efficacy studies* (http://aidsinfo.nih.gov/DrugsNew/DrugDetailT.aspx?int_id=408). By inhibiting these coreceptors, chemokine receptor antagonists impede the release of gp41 from its metastable conformation within the HIV-1 envelope, thereby blocking the fusion between the viral and the cellular membranes *(782)*.

In the search for new antiretroviral agents, the CCR5 receptor has been the target of anti-HIV-1 strategies for disrupting the interaction with the HIV-1 envelope protein gp120. Studies suggest that gp120 binds preferentially to the *N*-terminus of CCR5 *(783)* and that the second extracellular region is mostly responsible for the binding of the endogenous chemokine peptides *(784)*. The two domains are not clearly separated, because some single-point mutations in the *N*-terminus can also abolish the binding of chemokines *(785)*. HIV-1 and chemokines mainly interact with the extracellular regions of CCR5, whereas small synthetic ligands mostly bind to residues of the transmembrane region *(774, 786)*.

Using a computational approach, a comprehensive model of CCR5 that elucidates the binding of small ligands, and its sensitivity to mutations for the binding of chemokines and the coat protein gp120 of HIV-1, has been developed. The computational approach has sought to enhance homology-modeling techniques with *ab initio* simulations and knowledge-based information to generate structural models that are then corroborated by comparison with additional data *(774)*.

Clinical Trials. Maraviroc has been shown to be safe and well tolerated in almost all of the human volunteers who have received it *(787–789)*.

Initial studies in patients with CCR5-tropic viruses showed that oral doses of maraviroc could lead to significant reductions in viral load *(790)*, providing support for the evaluation of maraviroc in large-scale clinical trials. Moreover, early trials *(791)* have demonstrated remarkable, sustained drops in viral load for the short time that patients were on medication, with declines in viral load over an approximate 10-day period of treatment. Although viral rebound was observed after the drug was discontinued, such findings are consistent with other trials that have monitored the effects of very short courses of antiviral drugs.

Recently, however, there has been data on one patient who had apparently suffered hepatotoxicity while on maraviroc *(792)* (www.hivforum.org/uploads/CCR5/RT%202/Maraviroc.pdf). It is a cause of concern that hepatotoxicity might be a class effect for this category of drugs because another CCR5 inhibitor (aplaviroc) has shown serious hepatotoxicity during clinical trials *(793–795)* and its development had to be halted. Clinical trials with a third CCR5 inhibitor, vicriviroc, were also suspended because of concern for potential hepatotoxicity *(795)* (http://www.hivandhepatitis.com/recent/ad/102805_b.html).

The FDA approval of maraviroc has been based on the results of one completed clinical trial, A4001029, and two ongoing clinical trials, A4001027 (MOTIVATE-1) and A4001028 (MOTIVATE-2) (maraviroc plus optimized therapy in viremic antiretroviral treatment-experienced patients).

Study A4001029 is an exploratory, randomized, double-blind, multicenter trial that was designed to determine the safety and efficacy of maraviroc in subjects infected with dual/mixed coreceptor-tropic HIV-1 *(787)*. Subjects were randomized in a 1:1:1 ratio to maraviroc once daily, maraviroc twice daily, or placebo. Maraviroc treatment was not associated with increased risk of infection or progression of HIV disease, nor was it associated with a significant decrease in HIV-1 RNA viral loads compared with the placebo. In addition, no adverse effect was noted on CD4+ T-cell count *(787)*.

The A4001027 (MOTIVATE-1) and A4001028 (MOTIVATE-2) studies are ongoing, double-blind, randomized, placebo-controlled, multicenter studies that have enrolled approximately 1,000 subjects infected with CCR5-tropic HIV-1 *(788, 789)*. All subjects received an optimized background therapy (OBT) consisting of three to six antiretroviral agents (excluding low-dose ritonavir). They were then randomized 2:2:1 to maraviroc 300 mg once daily, maraviroc 300 mg twice daily, or placebo. Pooled analysis at 24 weeks revealed the percentage of subjects with a mean change from baseline to week 24 in HIV-1 RNA viral loads ($\log_{10}$ copies/mL) to <400 copies/mL was 60.8% in the maraviroc group versus 27.8% for the placebo. The percentage of subjects with a mean change from baseline to week 24 in HIV-1 RNA viral loads ($\log_{10}$ copies/mL) to <50 copies/mL was 45.3% in the maraviroc arm compared with 23.0% in the placebo arm. The mean changes in plasma HIV-1 RNA viral loads from baseline to week 24 was −1.96 $\log_{10}$ copies/mL for subjects receiving maraviroc plus OBT compared with −0.99 $\log_{10}$ copies/mL for subjects receiving OBT only. The mean increase in CD4+ T-counts was higher on maraviroc twice daily plus OBT (106.3 cells/mm^3) than on placebo plus OBT (57.4 cells/mm^3) *(788, 789)*.

A Phase III, multicenter, randomized, double-blind, comparative trial was conducted to compare the safety and efficacy of maraviroc (MVC) versus efavirenz (EFV), both administered with Combivir (CBV) in antiretroviral-naïve patients with only CCR5-tropic HIV-1 infection *(796)*. The results of the study have shown that compared with efavirenz, maraviroc failed to meet the noninferiority threshold with respect to the proportion of subjects who reached suppressed plasma HIV-1 RNA levels to below 50 copies per mL *(796)*. One possible reason for the slightly higher rate of virologic failure in the maraviroc arm is that low levels of CXCR4-using virus may have gone undetected by standard testing, with subsequent emergence of dual/mixed (DM) or X4 virus and virologic failure in some recipients of the maraviroc-containing regimen. Improvements to the sensitivity of the currently available tropism test could reduce the number of patients with undetected D/M or X4 virus *(797)*.

34.8.3 Vicriviroc

Vicriviroc (SCH-D, or SCH 417690) is a piperazine derivative under development as CCR5 antagonist. Structurally, it represents 1-[(4,6-dimethyl-5-pyrimi-dinyl)carbonyl]-4-[4-[2-methoxy-1(*R*)-4-(trifluoromethyl)phenyl]ethyl-3(*S*)-methyl-1-piperazinyl]-4-methyl-piperidine.

Vicriviroc has demonstrated synergistic anti-HIV activity in combination with drugs from all other classes of approved antiretrovirals. Competition binding assays revealed that vicriviroc binds with higher affinity to the CCR5 coreceptor.

Functional assays, including inhibition of calcium flux, guanosine $5'$-[^{35}S]triphosphate exchange, and chemotaxis, confirmed that vicriviroc acts as a receptor antagonist by inhibiting signaling of CCR5 by chemokines (798).

Mechanism of Action. To characterize the interaction of vicriviroc with CCR5 more completely, a series of receptor binding and functional activity studies were performed (798). In three different functional assays, chemotaxis, calcium flux, and GTPS binding, vicriviroc potently inhibited the activation of CCR5 by its natural ligands, RANTES, MIP-1α, and MIP-1β, with activity in the low-nanomolar range. Vicriviroc alone did not activate the receptor in any of the functional assays, thus demonstrating that it is a pure receptor antagonist (798).

Clinical Trials. The antiviral activity, pharmacokinetic properties, and safety of vicriviroc as monotherapy has been studied in HIV-infected patients in an ascending, multiple-dose, placebo-controlled study randomized within the treatment group (799). Forty-eight HIV-infected individuals were enrolled sequentially to dose groups of vicriviroc—10, 25, and 50 mg twice a day—and were randomly assigned within the group to receive the drug or placebo (16 total patients/group) for 14 days. Significant reductions from baseline HIV RNA viral loads after 14 days were achieved in all active treatment groups. Suppression of viral RNA persisted 2 to 3 days beyond the end of treatment. Reductions of 1.0 log$_{10}$ HIV RNA or greater were achieved in 45%, 77%, and 82% of patients in the three groups, respectively. Eighteen percent, 46%, and 45% of subjects achieved declines of 1.5 log$_{10}$ or greater in HIV RNA in the three groups, respectively. Vicriviroc was rapidly absorbed, with a half-life of 28 to 33 hours, supporting once-daily dosing. Vicriviroc was well tolerated in all dose groups. The frequencies of adverse events were similar in the vicriviroc and placebo groups: 72% and 62%, respectively. The most frequently reported adverse events included headache, pharyngitis, nausea, and abdominal pain, which were not dose related. Whereas all doses were well tolerated and produced significant declines in plasma HIV RNA, total oral daily doses of 50 or 100 mg vicriviroc monotherapy for 14 days appeared to provide the most potent antiviral effect in this study (799).

Vicriviroc demonstrated durable antiretroviral activity and CD4 response in treatment-experienced HIV-1–infected subjects at 48 weeks (ACTG 5211) (800). In a follow-up 2-year study, the treatment-experienced patients who successfully completed the ACTG 5211 trial participated in a roll-over, multicenter, open-label study (801). The patients received 15 mg of vicriviroc in addition to previously optimized background therapy (OBT) that included a ritonavir-boosted protease inhibitor. Of 79 subjects entering the study, 54 had at least 12 months exposure to vicriviroc. Data available for 39 subjects (data still pending for 15 ongoing subjects) has shown that vicriviroc (15 mg dose) plus OBT was generally well tolerated and provided potent and durable antiretroviral activity. These results represent data for the longest follow-up period available for a CCR5-containing regimen to date (801).

Vicriviroc is not only a CCR5 antagonist, but it is also a potent inhibitor of chemokine binding and receptor signaling, which could have immunomodulatory effects. The immunologic profiles of HIV-infected subjects after vicriviroc treatment, in particular, to assess its effect on peripheral lymphocyte populations has recently been evaluated (802). Complete differential blood counts, including absolute CD4 and %CD4, were measured in 282 HIV-infected subjects enrolled in 4 independent trials in which patients received a range of vicriviroc doses for 2 to 48 weeks, either as monotherapy or in combination with an optimized background or Combivir. Results have shown that baseline differential blood counts and absolute and %CD4 were similar across studies. There was no clinically significant impact on white blood cells, lymphocytes, or neutrophils during follow-up. As expected in antiretroviral (ARV)-treated patients, there was a substantial and sustained improvement in CD4$^+$ T-cell counts with vicriviroc; this was greater than that seen with the control. There was no apparent increase in infections with vicia cryptic virus (VCV) relative to control (802).

In 2005, upon the recommendation of the Data Safety Monitoring Board (DSMB), the Phase II trial of the CCR5 HIV entry inhibitor vicriviroc in treatment-naïve HIV patients was terminated. DSMB recommended halting the trial after observing virologic rebound in some naïve patients in the vicriviroc-containing arm of the study versus the Combivir-plus-Sustiva control arm. The decision to stop the vicriviroc Phase II trial was not based on hepatotoxicity (as has been the case with aplaviroc, another CCR5 antagonist) or on other safety-related issues in patients receiving vicriviroc in the study or in another Phase II study in treatment-experienced patients, but rather on the observance of loss of virologic suppression by some patients in the vicriviroc arm. The study of the drug in the treatment-experienced patients is continuing (http://www.hivandhepatitis.com/recent/ad/102805_b.html).

34.9 Integrase Inhibitors

In order for HIV to successfully take over a CD4 cell's machinery so that it can produce new viruses, HIV RNA is converted into DNA by the reverse transcriptase enzyme. (Nucleotide/nucleoside reverse transcriptase inhibitors can block this process.) After the "reverse transcription" of RNA into DNA is complete, HIV DNA must then be incorporated into the CD4 cell's DNA. This is known as integration. As their name implies, integrase inhibitors work by blocking this process.

The integrase inhibitors may offer a great deal of hope for HIV-positive patients, especially those who have developed HIV resistance to drugs that target HIV's two other major enzymes, reverse transcriptase and protease. As for integrase inhibitors, a fundamental innovative step was the introduction of the *keto-enol acids* [often referred to as "diketo acids" (DKAs)]. Although these compounds show a keto-enol tautomery, they are γ-keto α-enol acids in their biologically active form.

HIV-1 integrase is a 32-kDa enzyme composed of three domains: the catalytic core domain (CCD), and the *C*- and *N*-terminal domains. The CCD is thought to be responsible for the reaction(s) catalyzed by the enzyme. It seems that all three domains cooperate for the diversity of the functions catalyzed by the integrase, in that recombinant molecules consisting of the isolated CCD only catalyze the disintegration reaction *(803, 804)*.

The crystal structures of the three integrase domains have been solved separately *(805–807)*. The catalytic domain spans residues 50 to 212 and is highly conserved among retroviruses *(805)*. A total of three highly conserved amino acids (D64, D116, and E152) constitute the catalytic triad. Metal ions (possibly two) coordinate the three principal catalytic residues and are thought to be important for interactions with DNA. Similarities of the CCD structure with other nucleic acid–binding molecules have been described *(803, 804)*.

Approximately 40 to 100 integrase molecules are packaged within each HIV particle. The primary role of integrase is to catalyze the insertion of the viral cDNA into the genome of infected cells, although integrase can also act as a cofactor for reverse transcription *(808, 809)*. Integration is required for the virus to replicate, because transcription of the viral genome and the production of viral proteins require that the viral cDNA be fully integrated into a host chromosome *(810)*. After reverse transcription, the viral cDNA is primed for integration in the cytoplasm by integrase-mediated trimming of the 3′-ends of the viral DNA. This step is referred to as *3′-processing*. It requires both fully functional integrase and the integrity of the last 10 to 20 base pairs at both ends of the viral cDNA. The 3′-processing consists of the endonucleolytic cleavage of the 3′-ends of the viral DNA. This cleavage occurs immediately 3′ to a conserved CA dinucleotide motif. Alterations of this sequence prevent integrase from catalyzing the 3′-processing. This reaction generates CA-3′-hydroxyl DNA ends, which are the reactive intermediates required for the *strand transfer (804)*.

After 3′-processing, integrase remains bound to the viral cDNA as a multimeric complex that bridges both ends of the viral DNA within intracellular particles called *preintegration complexes* (PICs). Isolated PICs contain both viral and cellular proteins in addition to the integrase-DNA complexes. The viral proteins reverse transcriptase (RT), matrix (Ma), nucleocapsid (Nc), and Vpr can contribute to the transport of PICs through the nuclear envelope. Some cellular proteins packaged within PICs can bind to integrase *(811)* and stimulate the enzymatic activities of integrase. Two cellular proteins, *high-mobility group protein A1* [HMGA1, also known as HMG1(Y)] and the *barrier to autointegration factor* (BAF), regulate the integration by binding to DNA directly. HMGA1 stimulates integrase activity *(812, 813)*, and BAF stimulates the intermolecular integration and suppresses autointegration *(811)*. By contrast with other lentiviruses, such as the oncoretroviruses murine Moloney virus and Rous sarcoma virus, which require mitotic nuclear-envelope breakdown to access the chromosomes of infected cells, HIV-1 PICs are able to cross the nuclear envelope. The karyophilic property of the PICs enables HIV to replicate in nonproliferative cells, such as macrophages *(814)*.

Once in the nucleus, integrase catalyzes the insertion of the viral cDNA ends into host chromosomes. This "*strand transfer*" reaction consists of the ligation of the viral 3′-OH DNA ends (generated by 3′-processing) to the 5′-DNA phosphate of a host chromosome. The integrase can also catalyze the reverse reaction, referred to as *disintegration (815)*. Physiologic integration requires the concerted joining of both ends of the viral cDNA on opposite DNA strands of the target (*acceptor DNA*) host chromosome with a canonical five-base-pair stagger. The five-base stagger indicates that each viral cDNA end attacks the chromosomal DNA across its major groove. Completion of integration requires ligation of the 5′-end of the viral DNA. This last step of integration can only take place after trimming of the last two nucleotides at the proviral DNA 5′-ends and extension (gap filling) from the 3′-OH end of the genomic DNA. It is likely that cellular enzymes/pathways are involved in this 5′-processing, although their identity remains uncertain *(803, 816, 817)*.

Polymorphisms in Integrase. Several studies have been carried out to analyze the importance of preexisting integrase mutations in integrase-naïve patients. Although the range of natural polymorphisms seems very extensive, they do not seem to be related to reduced susceptibility to diketo acid compounds or to a higher risk of treatment failure, in either naïve-or treatment-experienced patients *(818–820)*.

An analysis of 1,250 integrase inhibitor–naïve isolates from the Los Alamos database has identified 41 mutations at 30 positions in the integrase *(818)*. The most prevalent variants were V201I (in 80%) and V72I (46%). Fifteen mutations occurred at >5% frequency in different HIV subtypes. Other common mutations were identified at codons 74, 97, 125, 154, 163, and 206. However, some of the between-clade differences led to the conclusion that susceptible-to-integrase inhibitors may vary by subtypes and that this should be examined in future *in vitro* models *(818)*.

Data looking at the prevalence of naturally occurring integrase polymorphisms amplified from the RT-RNase-H-IN region in 47 patient samples and 89 clones have indicated that the most common polymorphisms were V72I (in 41 patients but also 77 isolates) and V201I (in 33 patients and 48 clones) and included L74M/I, T97A, V151I, K156N, 165I, I203M, T206S, and S230R/N, though none were associated with significant fold-changes. There had been no differences between HIV subtype, or between RTI-sensitive and -resistant isolates *(819)*.

Studies focused on gene sequences for the whole sequence of reverse transcriptase and integrase (1 to 320 residues) from 448 patients with HIV-1 subtype B (134 naïve and 314 experienced) have shown that the protein sequences in integrase were unaltered at 62% and 67% of codons in naïve and experienced patients, respectively. However 24/37 integrase mutations were not found in either naïve or reverse transcriptase inhibitor–treated patients. The eight position changes showing >5% variability were I72V, T125A/V, M154I, K156N, V165I, V201I, T206S, and S230N *(820)*. Furthermore, some mutations were present significantly more frequently in treated compared with naïve patients: M154I (21% vs. 6%, $p < 0.001$), V165I (13% vs. 6%, $p = 0.022$), M185L (6% vs. 0%, $p = 0.003$). Significantly, M185L was positively associated with V165I in the integrase and F227L and T215Y in the reverse transcriptase. I72V occurred more frequently in untreated patients and was positively associated with the protective R83K mutation in the reverse transcriptase and negatively associated with D67G and M184V mutations in the reverse transcriptase ($p < 0.03$). The overall conclusion from the study results is that the association found between selected integrase and reverse transcriptase mutations supported the hypothesis of a tight interaction of these two proteins and suggested the importance of integrase-sequencing for reverse transcriptase–experienced patients prior to starting integrase-based regimens *(820)*.

Integrase Inhibitors Sensitivity to HIV-2. A study on the phenotypic sensitivity of raltegravir and elvitegravir in isolates from 19 integrase-naïve patients infected with HIV-2 (9 with subtype A; 9 with subtype B; and one with subtype H) has shown that the HIV-2 integrase gene differed from HIV-1 at 133/288 codons, including some that have been described as integrase-resistant sites for HIV-1 *(821)*. However, the IC_{50} mean values were similar between the HIV-2 and HIV-1 reference strains, including two isolates with MDR Q151M mutation in the reverse transcriptase. Despite overall amino acid polymorphism of 31%, this did not alter phenotypic susceptibility of HIV-2 to either raltegravir or elvitegravir.

34.9.1 Raltegravir

Raltegravir (MK-0518, Isentress) is the first drug belonging to the new class of integrase inhibitors to be approved. It was approved by the FDA in October 2007. Raltegravir has been approved for treatment-experienced patients who have HIV strains that are resistant to multiple antiretroviral drugs. It is not yet approved for people with drug-sensitive HIV strains, such as those starting antiretroviral therapy for the first time.

Raltegravir acts by inhibiting the insertion of HIV DNA into human DNA by the integrase enzyme. Inhibiting integrase from performing its essential function limits the *ability of the virus to replicate and infect new cells.*

Structurally, raltegravir represents *N*-[2-(4-(4-fluoro-benzylcarbamoyl)-5-hydroxy-1-methyl-6-oxo-1, 6-dihydro-pyrimidin-2-yl)propan-2-yl]-5-methyl-1, 3, 4-oxadiazole-2-carboxamide.

Mechanism of Action. Raltegravir, and other integrase inhibitors, are often termed *strand transfer inhibitors.* This refers to the process of DNA strand transfer from the viral genome to the host genome. Raltegravir inhibits the catalytic activity of HIV-1 integrase. The inhibition of integrase prevents the covalent insertion, or integration, of unintegrated linear HIV-1 DNA into the host cell's genome, thereby preventing the HIV-1 provirus from forming. The provirus is required to direct the production of progeny virus. Raltegravir did not significantly inhibit human phosphoryltransferases, including DNA polymerases-α, -β, and -γ.

Dosing and Administration. The recommended dosage of raltegravir for adults is 400 mg twice a day. Doses of 200, 400, and 600 mg have been studied in clinical trials (http://www.aidsinfo.nih.gov/DrugsNew/DrugDetailNT.aspx?MenuItem=Drugs&Search=On&int_id=420).

Drug Resistance. One caution regarding the otherwise impressive results available on raltegravir is that it appeared to have a low genetic barrier to resistance *(822, 823)*. Thus, results from a Phase II dose-finding study demonstrated that 35 of 38 patients randomized to either 200, 400, or 600 mg raltegravir or placebo in addition to optimized background therapy showed mutations in integrase *(822)*.

Two distinct pathways were also identified in *in vitro* studies—either via N155H ($n = 14$) or Q148H/R/K ($n = 20$)—which reduced raltegravir susceptibility by 10- and 25-fold, respectively. One patient developed the Y143R mutation. Secondary mutations found with N155H included L74M, E92Q, T97A, Y143H, V515I, G163R, and D232N; and with the Q148H/R/K mutation included L74M, E138A/K, and G140S/A. All secondary mutations led to increased resistance. Fold changes in IC_{50} were greatest in patients whose virus developed the 148 mutation pathway, with secondary mutations increasing from 10-fold (Q148H) to more than 500-fold (Q148H plus G140S, and Q148K plus E138A plus G140A) *(822)*. There was no dose-related relationship with the pattern of these mutations. Impact on fold-change of other integrase inhibitors indicated cross-resistance to elvitegravir *(822)*.

Another study has reported resistance patterns from four highly treatment-experienced patients who received raltegravir as part of a rescue therapy *(823)*.

Baseline viral load ranged from 4.3 to 5.5 logs. Two patients had a genotypic sensitivity score (GSS) of 0 and two patients had a GSS of 1. Resistance mutations at failure included Q140S + Q148H, which occurred at the same time; N155H; E92Q and E157Q with viral load returning to pretreatment levels by week 8 to 24 as these mutations were detected, with a loss of 7- to 14-fold drug sensitivity *(823)*.

It is thought that selection of only one mutation that led to failure in these patients emphasized the low genetic barrier to resistance and highlights that raltegravir should only be used with other active drugs in the antiretroviral regimen (http://www.i-base.info/htb/v8/htb8-6-7/Integrase.html.

Clinical Trials. The approval of raltegravir was based on the twin BENCHMRK studies (Phase III), which included about 700 treatment-experienced patients with documented drug resistance in North and South America, Europe, and Asia *(824, 825)*. These studies demonstrated that at 16 to 24 weeks, participants who took raltegravir plus optimized background therapy (OBT) were about twice as likely to achieve a viral load below 50 copies/mL than were those taking OBT plus placebo (61% to 62% vs. 33% to 36%, respectively). CD4 cell gains were also larger in the raltegravir arm (85 vs. about 35 cells/mm^3). Raltegravir worked best in patients who started another active antiretroviral drug at the same time *(824, 825)*.

Longer-term data from an earlier Phase II trial *(826)* showed that raltegravir continued to be effective after 48 weeks, with 64% of patients taking the 400 mg dose having a viral load below 50 copies/mL, and CD4 counts increased by 110 cells/mm^3. Among a subset of patients followed for up to 72 weeks, about 70% maintained a viral load below 400 copies/mL.

Raltegravir was well tolerated overall, with less than 2% of study participants in the BENCHMRK studies discontinuing therapy due to adverse events. The most common side effects were nausea, diarrhea, headache, fever, and skin rash. Patients taking raltegravir were more likely to have elevated blood levels of creatine kinase, an enzyme associated with muscle damage. Although early data indicated that more people in the raltegravir arms developed cancer, this appears to be attributable to an unusually low rate of cancer in the placebo groups, and the rates evened out with longer follow-up.

To assess the safety and efficacy of raltegravir when added to optimized background regimens in HIV-infected patients, HIV-infected patients with HIV-1 RNA viral load greater than 5,000 copies per mL, CD4$^+$ T-cell counts greater than 50 cells per mL, and documented genotypic and phenotypic resistance to at least one NRTI, one NNRTI, and one PI were randomly assigned to receive raltegravir (200, 400, or 600 mg) or placebo orally twice daily in a multicenter, triple-blind, dose-ranging, randomized trial (NCT00105157) *(826, 827)*. The primary end-points were change in viral load

from baseline at week 24 and safety. Analyses were done on a modified intention-to-treat basis. *Raltegravir at all doses showed a safety profile much the same as that of the placebo; there were no dose-related toxicities (827).*

Results from another recent study have shown that raltegravir worked as well as efavirenz in treatment-naïve patients after 48 weeks. However, raltegravir has not yet been approved for such individuals. Studies with raltegravir in HIV-positive children are currently under way. Raltegravir has not been tested in pregnant women *(828)*.

A multicenter, double-blind, randomized, placebo-controlled two-part study, with the first part using raltegravir in 1 of 4 doses (100, 200, 400, and 600 mg) versus placebo (randomized 1:1:1:1:1) given twice daily for 10 days of short-term monotherapy has shown potent antiretroviral activity. The drug was generally well tolerated at all doses *(829)*.

Three double-blind, randomized, placebo-controlled, pharmacokinetic, safety, and tolerability studies were conducted as follows: (i) single-dose escalation study (10 to 1,600 mg); (ii) multiple-dose escalation study (100 to 800 mg every 12 hours × 10 days), and (iii) single-dose female study (400 mg) *(830)*. Raltegravir was rapidly absorbed, with a terminal half-life ($t_{1/2}$) ~7 to 12 hours. Approximately 7% to 14% of raltegravir was excreted unchanged in urine. Raltegravir has been generally well tolerated at doses of up to 1,600 mg/day given for up to 10 days and exhibits a pharmacokinetic profile supportive of twice-daily dosing with multiple doses of 100 mg and greater, achieving trough levels >33 nM *(830)*.

A multicenter, triple-blind, dose-ranging study has been conducted to assess the safety and efficacy of raltegravir when added to optimized background regimens in HIV-infected patients *(831)*. HIV-infected patients eligible for this study had HIV-1 RNA viral load higher than 5,000 copies/mL, CD4$^+$ T-cell counts of >50 cells/µL, and documented genotypic and phenotypic resistance to at least one NRTI, one NNRTI, and one PI. The main outcome measures were change in viral load from baseline at week 24, and safety; analysis was by modified intention-to-treat. Of 179 patients eligible for randomization, 44 patients were randomized to oral treatment twice daily with raltegravir 200 mg, 45 to raltegravir 400 mg, 45 to raltegravir 600 mg, and 45 to placebo. One patient in the 200 mg group did not receive treatment and was therefore excluded from analysis. Median duration of previous antiretroviral treatment was 9.9 years (range, 0.4 to 17.3 years), and mean baseline viral load was 4.7 ± 0.5 log$_{10}$ copies/mL. Of 4 patients who discontinued because of adverse events, 3 (2%) were in the raltegravir groups and 1 (2%) was in the placebo group. Of 41 patients who discontinued because of lack of efficacy, 14 (11%) were in the raltegravir groups and 27 (60%) were in the placebo group. Mean change in viral load from baseline at week 24 was −1.80 (95% confidence interval (CI), −2.10 to −1.50) $\log_{10}$ copies/mL in the 200 mg group, −1.87 (95% CI, −2.16 to −1.58) $\log_{10}$ copies/mL in the 400 mg group, −1.84 (95% CI, −2.10 to −1.58) $\log_{10}$ copies/mL in the 600 mg group, and −0.35 (95% CI, −0.61 to −0.09) $\log_{10}$ copies/mL in the placebo group. At all doses, raltegravir had a safety profile similar to that of the placebo, with no dose-related toxicities *(831, 832)*.

Toxicity. The safety assessment of raltegravir in treatment-experienced subjects is based on the pooled safety data from the randomized, double-blind, placebo-controlled trials, BENCHMRK 1 and BENCHMRK 2 (Protocols 018 and 019) *(824, 825)*, and the randomized, double-blind, placebo-controlled, dose-ranging trial Protocol 005 in antiretroviral treatment-experienced HIV-infected adult subjects reported using the recommended dose of raltegravir 400 mg twice daily in combination with optimized background therapy (OBT) in 507 subjects, in comparison with 282 subjects taking placebo in combination with OBT. During the double-blind treatment, the total follow-up was 332.2 patient-years in the raltegravir 400 mg twice-daily group and 150.2 patient-years in the placebo group. The following adverse events were observed: gastrointestinal disorders (diarrhea, nausea), headache, and pyrexia (http://www.rxlist.com/cgi/generic/isentress_ad.htm).

The following serious drug-related reactions were reported in the clinical studies under Protocols P005, P018, and P019: hypersensitivity (it was seen in two patients; therapy was interrupted and upon rechallenge the subjects were able to resume the drug), anemia, neutropenia, myocardial infarction, gastritis, hepatitis, herpes simplex, toxic nephropathy, renal failure, chronic renal failure, and renal tubular necrosis (http://www.rxlist.com/cgi/generic/isentress_ad.htm).

During the initial phase of treatment, patients responding to antiretroviral therapy may develop an inflammatory response to indolent or residual opportunistic infections (such as *Mycobacterium avium* complex, cytomegalovirus, *Pneumocystis jiroveci* pneumonia, *Mycobacterium tuberculosis*, or reactivation of varicella zoster virus), which may necessitate further evaluation and treatment (http://www.rxlist.com/cgi/generic/isentress_wcp.htm).

Caution should be used when coadministering raltegravir with strong inducers of uridine diphosphate glucuronosyltransferase (UGT) 1A1 (e.g., rifampin) because of reduced plasma concentrations of raltegravir (http://www.rxlist.com/cgi/generic/isentress_wcp.htm).

34.9.2 Elvitegravir

Elvitegravir (GS 9137, JTK-303) is an experimental integrase inhibitor that is currently being developed. It is intended to be used in clinical practice in combination with other antiretroviral agents.

Structurally, elvitegravir represents 6-(3-chloro-2-fluorobenzyl)-1-[(2S)-1-hydroxy-3-methylbutan-2-yl]-7-methoxy-4-oxo-1,4-dihydroquinoline-3-carboxylic acid. Elvitegravir is a low-molecular-weight, highly selective integrase inhibitor that shares the core structure of the quinolone antibiotics.

Clinical Trials. The results of a double-blind, randomized, placebo-controlled monotherapy study *(833)* to evaluate the safety, tolerability, and antiviral activity of elvitegravir in HIV-infected treatment-naïve and treatment-experienced individuals were presented in 2006. The study evaluated elvitegravir with different administration schemes: 200 to 800 mg twice daily; 800 mg once daily; and 50 mg twice daily, boosted with coadministration of ritonavir 100 mg (ritonavir boosting can significantly improve pharmacokinetics of antiretrovirals metabolized by CYP3A4). At study entry, patients were not receiving antiretroviral therapy. The best results were obtained in those individuals treated with the highest dosages of elvitegravir alone and boosted with ritonavir 50 mg once daily. In these groups, decreases in viral load (amounting to ∼ 2 $\log_{10}$ viral RNA copies/mL) were significantly greater than in placebo. There were no discontinuations or serious adverse events in the groups receiving GS-9137. All adverse events were grade 1 or 2 in severity, resolved during treatment, and were not associated with GS-9137 dosing *(833)*.

Clinically, elvitegravir is most effective against HIV when patients use it in combination with the injectable entry inhibitor, enfuvirtide, and other active drugs, including ritonavir-boosted protease inhibitors *(834)*. This ongoing randomized and partially-blind Phase II study demonstrated that treatment-experienced HIV patients given 125-mg elvitegravir once daily, boosted with ritonavir, had a superior average change in HIV RNA at week 24 (DAVG24) versus that in a boosted comparator protease inhibitor (CPI) arm *(834)*.

A new analysis of the data revealed more detail concerning resistance and the influence on outcomes of OBT *(835)*. The patients received NRTIs (with or without enfuvirtide) with either a boosted comparator protease inhibitor or boosted elvitegravir 20, 50, or 125-mg. Protease inhibitors were permitted after week 8. Patients in the 125-mg elvitegravir/ritonavir arm were analyzed for their viral load responses by activity of the OBT *(835)*. The DAVG24 for elvitegravir/ritonavir 125-mg subjects with newly added enfuvirtide ($n = 19$) was −2.6 $\log_{10}$ copies/mL, compared with −1.6 $\log_{10}$ copies/mL for boosted CPI subjects with newly added enfuvirtide ($n = 12$; $p = 0.03$). Furthermore, only two elvitegravir/ritonavir 125-mg patients added protease inhibitor prior to week 16; at week 16, 74% (14 of 19) of elvitegravir/ritonavir 125-mg subjects with new enfuvirtide had HIV RNA <50 copies/mL compared with 25% (3 of 12) of boosted CPI subjects with new enfuvirtide

(ITT, M = F; $p = 0.012$). Finally, elvitegravir/ritonavir 125-mg subjects who added a protease inhibitor ($n = 23$) had an additional mean change in HIV RNA of $-1.1 \log_{10}$ copies/mL over a median of >16 weeks after adding a protease inhibitor *(835)*.

The antiviral activity of elvitegravir in combinations with approved antiretroviral drugs [and with the investigational NNRTI etravirine (TMC-125)] has been studied *in vitro (836)*. A range of drug concentrations were tested in a matrix format for each drug combination with elvitegravir. All approved NRTIs (except ddC), NNRTIs including TMC-125 but excluding delavirdine, PIs, and the entry/fusion inhibitor enfuvirtide were tested in combination with elvitegravir. A control for antiviral antagonism, d4T (Zerit) plus ribavirin, was also tested. MT-2 cells were preinfected with HIV-1 III_B (MOI, 0.001), added to the drug combinations, and incubated for 5 days under standard conditions. Data were reported as the mean synergy volume ($\text{nM}^2.\%$) at the 95% confidence interval. The overall results have shown additive to synergistic interactions with all approved antiretroviral drugs *(836)*. For example, for the seven NRTIs tested, mean synergy volume scores ranged from 12.07 to 97.57 $\text{nM}^2.\%$ (additive to moderate synergy); for the three NNRTIs tested (efavirenz, nevirapine, and etravirine), the mean synergy volume scores ranged from 35.89 to 80.34 $\text{nM}^2.\%$ (minor to moderate synergy); for the nine PIs tested, the mean synergy volume scores ranged from 13.84 to 48.97 $\text{nM}^2.\%$ (additive to minor synergy). For enfuvirtide, the combination with elvitegravir resulted in a mean synergy volume score of 26.28 $\text{nM}^2.\%$ (minor synergy). In contrast, d4T combined with ribavirin showed strong evidence of antagonism (mean synergy volume $-480.93 \text{nM}^2.\%$). Based on these results, *in vitro* combination studies of elvitegravir with approved antiretroviral drugs and etravirine demonstrated additive to moderately synergistic interactions with no evidence of antiviral antagonism between elvitegravir and any antiretroviral drug observed *(836)*.

Drug Resistance. A study conducted to provide more insight into elvitegravir resistance has reported the emergence of an initial T66I mutation and subsequently additional mutations *(837)*. Site-directed mutant viruses carrying the T66I mutation showed reduced susceptibility to elvitegravir, but remained susceptible to other integrase inhibitors, including raltegravir. In contrast, site-directed mutant viruses with E92Q mutation demonstrated both resistance to elvitegravir and evidence of cross-resistance to raltegravir. Overall, the integrase inhibitor mutants remained fully susceptible to ART drugs of other classes *(837)*.

34.10 Maturation Inhibitors

Because of the large number of potential therapeutic targets, HIV assembly and budding have long been a focus of drug development efforts. HIV-1 assembly is driven largely by the gag precursor protein Pr55^{gag} *(838)*. After synthesis, Pr55^{gag} is transported to the plasma membrane where virus assembly occurs *(839, 840)*. Through a complex combination of gag-lipid, gag-gag, and gag-RNA interactions, a multimeric budding structure forms at the inner leaflet of the plasma membrane. The budding virus particle is ultimately released from the cell surface in a process that is promoted by an interaction between the late domain in the p6 region of gag *(841, 842)* and host proteins, most notably the endosomal sorting factor TSG101 *(tumor susceptibility gene 101) (843)*. Concomitant with the release of the particle, the viral protease cleaves Pr55^{gag} and $\text{Pr160}^{\text{gag-pol}}$. These processing events generate the mature gag proteins matrix (MA), capsid (CA), nucleocapsid, and p6, two small gag spacer peptides (SP1 and SP2), and the mature pol-encoded enzymes PR, RT, and integrase. Gag and gag-pol cleavage trigger a structural rearrangement, termed *maturation*, during which the immature particle transitions to a mature virion characterized by an electron-dense, conical core *(838)*.

The efficiencies with which the viral protease cleaves its target sequences vary widely, resulting in a highly ordered gag and gag-pol processing cascade *(844–846)*. The sequential nature of gag processing can be disrupted by altering the amino acid sequence at cleavage sites within gag *(847–849)*, and even partial inhibition of gag processing profoundly impairs the maturation and infectivity of the virus *(850)*. Mutating key residues in the p6 late domain *(841,842,851)* or inhibiting the interaction between p6 and TSG101 *(852,853)*, also delays gag processing and increases levels of the gag cleavage intermediates p25 (CA-SP1) and p41 (MA-CA) in virions. It has also been reported that deletions in the dimer initiation site of the viral genomic RNA led to an accumulation of p25 and a defect in virus maturation *(838, 854, 855)*.

34.10.1 Bevirimat

Bevirimat (PA-457) is the first HIV-1 maturation inhibitor to enter clinical testing *(856)*. The drug interferes with the virus' replication by blocking cleavage of the HIV gag protein, which results in the production of defective virus particles that cannot infect new cells.

Structurally, PA-457 represents 3-O-($3'$,$3'$-dimethylsuccinyl) betulinic acid. It has been developed by activity-directed derivatization of betulinic acid, which was originally identified as a weak inhibitor (therapeutic index <5) of HIV-1 replication in a mechanism-blind screening assay *(857, 858)*.

Bevirimat was found to exhibit a high degree of potency against both prototypic and clinical HIV-1 isolates and, importantly, *retains its potent antiviral activity against a panel of viruses resistant to the three classes of approved drugs targeting the viral protease and reverse transcriptase.*

Although bevirimat has demonstrated promising antiviral activity in clinical trials, it has been difficult to develop a formulation that will deliver an adequate concentration of the drug, leading to increasing doses in the ongoing studies.

Mechanism of Action. In a study using a series of *in vitro* experiments, it was established that PA-457 did not target the activities of the HIV-1 protease and reverse transcriptase *(838)*. Consistent with a previous report *(859)*, PA-457 blocked replication of HIV-1 at a late step in the virus' life cycle. However, unlike that earlier work *(859)*, it was determined that the PA-457 did not reduce the efficiency of virus particle release; rather, it induced a defect in the Gag processing. Specifically, the cleavage of the CA precursor (p25) to mature CA (p24) was disrupted. Finally, by isolating and characterizing a PA-457–resistant isolate, it was demonstrated that the determinants of activity mapped the p25 to p24 cleavage site. These observations demonstrate that PA-457 acts through a novel target to inhibit virus replication by disrupting conversion of p25 to p24, resulting in the formation of defective, noninfectious virus particles *(838)*.

Preclinical and Clinical Studies. Bevirimat has been studied at doses of 25 to 600 mg and is taken once daily in clinical trials *(860)*.

In a placebo-controlled, double-blind study, 33 HIV patients were given PA-457 orally once daily for 10 days (placebo, 25, 50, 100, or 200 mg). Study participants had ≥ 200 CD4$^+$ T-cells/mm^3, HIV RNA viral load of 5,000 to 250,000 copies/mL, and were ARV-naïve or ≥ 12 weeks without therapy *(861)*. The results have shown that the 100 mg and 200 mg doses yielded significant reductions in HIV RNA viral load compared with placebo. Median reductions observed on day 11 were 0.03, 0.05, −0.17, −0.48, and −1.03 log$_{10}$ for the placebo, 25, 50, 100, and 200 mg doses, respectively. Patients in the 100 mg and 200 mg dose groups with baseline viral loads <5 log$_{10}$ had median reductions on day 11 of −0.56, and −1.52, respectively. Genotypic data, available for 21 of the 33 patients, have shown no evidence of development of resistance to PA-457. All doses were generally safe and well tolerated with no grade 3/4 laboratory abnormalities. All adverse experiences were mild to moderate. One serious adverse event, of moderate severity, was described as possibly related to treatment in a patient with a 5-year history of poorly controlled hypertension and transient findings of a possible lacunar cerebrovascular accident (CVA) *(861)*.

A 300 mg, once-daily oral solution dose of bevirimat has a potent anti-HIV effect and is well tolerated, according to the results of the product's latest Phase IIb study (http://www. fdanews.com/ newsletter/ article?articleId = 100310&issueId=10919).

Compound PA1050040 (PA-040). PA-040 has recently been reported as a second-generation maturation inhibitor agent displaying a better pharmacologic profile than that of bevirimat *(685)* (http://goliath.ecnext.com/coms2/gi_0199-6081478/Panacos-Files-IND-for-Second.html). PA-040 has shown a reduced serum protein binding compared with that of PA-457, as well as a unique resistance pattern, while retaining bevirimat's advantageous metabolic characteristics that minimize the potential for drug-drug interactions. Similar to bevirimat, PA-040 inhibited the conversion of p25 (CA-SP1) to p25 (CA) disrupting the CA-SP1 cleavage and blocking the release of mature CA protein, yielding noninfectious virions. Furthermore, PA-040 retained activity against wild-type L363M, a bevirimat-resistant isolate, as well as against other isolates resistant to approved antiretroviral agents (http://www.ashm.org.au/news/182/11/).

In laboratory studies, the effect of PA-040 on HIV-1 gag processing was assessed using Western blot assays. Standard viral inhibition assays were also performed. *In vitro* assays were conducted to determine the compound's cytotoxicity. Serum shift experiments were used to assess the effects of human serum protein binding on PA-040 activity. Non-clinical pharmacology studies evaluated PA-040's *in vitro* metabolic profile and investigated the compound's pharmacokinetics in rats. In particular:

- PA-040 specifically blocked p25 to p24 processing, similar to bevirimat
- PA-040 had a mean IC$_{50}$ (50% inhibitory concentration) of 14.9 nM against HIV-1 prototypic and primary isolates
- PA-040 had a median *in vitro* CC$_{50}$ (50% cytotoxicity) of >50 μM
- PA-040 maintained potency against a panel of HIV-1 isolates resistant to the four classes of approved antiretroviral drugs (NRTIs, NNRTIs, PIs, and the fusion inhibitor enfuvirtide)
- PA-040 retained wild-type activity against the bevirimat-resistant gag mutant, L363M, but had reduced activity against another bevirimat-resistant mutant, A364V
- PA-040 exhibited approximately eightfold lower human serum protein binding compared with that of bevirimat
- PA-040 was glucuronidated *in vitro* by UGT1A1, 1A3, 1A4, and 1A8 and had minimal interaction with the CYP450 enzymes, suggesting it will have minimal interactions with other anti-HIV drugs
- PA-040 was orally bioavailable in rats with a half-life of 3 hours

Overall, the reduced serum protein binding of PA-040 compared with that of bevirimat may yield greater potency *in vivo*. In addition, PA-040 had a distinct *in vitro* resistance profile, and like bevirimat, PA-040 maintained advantageous metabolic characteristics that may reduce the potential for metabolic drug-drug interactions *(685)*.

34.11 HAART: Triple Highly Active Antiretroviral Combinations

The ultimate goal in the era of highly active antiretroviral therapy (HAART) has always been to achieve both substantial and sustained suppression of viral replication in all cellular and body compartments *(296, 318, 319)*. Thus, in one U.S. study of 1,255 patients in the early years of HAART, mortality declined from 29.4 per 100 person-years in the first quarter of 1995 to 8.8 per 100 person-years in the second quarter of 1997 *(862)*. A Canadian-based, population-based cohort study also confirmed that patients initially treated with a triple-antiretroviral regimen had a 2.37-fold lower risk of morbidity and death after 12 months than that of patients receiving double nucleoside analogue therapy in the pre-HAART era *(863)*.

The clinical value of triple combinations of antiretroviral therapy has been established as a result of a number of large, randomized, controlled clinical trials showing—compared with single- and double-agent therapies—improved survival and marked reduction in the risk of adverse clinical events and/or death resulting from disease progression. Thus, *initiating treatment with a triple-combination consisting of three antiretroviral agents (a protease inhibitor or a non-nucleoside reverse transcriptase inhibitor plus two nucleoside reverse transcriptase inhibitors) is now considered the standard of care for the clinical management of HIV disease.* Yet a significant proportion of treatment-naïve patients may still fail to achieve optimal treatment responses with this triple-combination therapy. Many researchers have considered, therefore, that although the initial treatment of HIV-infected patients using a triple combination should be planned so that it does not compromise initial activity, a second-line or salvage therapy option must also be available *(296)* for patients who fail to achieve or maintain optimal virologic responses.

Another aspect to consider when using triple combinations has been the recognition of the metabolic toxicities (peripheral lipodystrophy syndrome, hyperlipidemia, and insulin resistance) associated with the prolonged use of PIs *(249)*. Concerns over the metabolic abnormalities caused by PIs have caused a reevaluation of the risk of using them, particularly in early disease *(678)*. Until recently, the PI drugs were the preferred third agent to combine with two NNRTIs because of their established antiretroviral potency in both treatment-naïve and treatment-experienced patients. However, these concerns have led some clinicians to provide equipotent but better tolerated therapy by using *PI-sparing regimens* instead, in which the PI drug is substituted with a NNRTI. Some of the advantages of the NNRTI agents can be summarized, as follows *(296)*:

- More convenient, patient-friendly dosage regimens (once or twice daily)
- Fewer pills per day
- No established long-term metabolic disturbances (e.g., lipodystrophy, diabetes, or renal dysfunction)
- Transient initial toxicities that do not generally overlap with or potentiate those associated with the use of NRTI
- The option of maintaining PIs for second-line therapy
- Fewer potentially serious drug interactions, such as those associated with ritonavir boosting

For example, data on the durability of the response, the virologic response in the nonplasma (the so-called sanctuary sites, such as the lymph nodes), and changes in the immune functions have suggested that some NNRTI drugs, such as efavirenz, would produce similar (or even better) benefits to those observed with the protease inhibitors *(296)*.

However, recent reports have suggested the potential for long-term toxicity with HAART *(864, 865)*, a consideration that may outweigh any benefit that HAART therapy may confer in certain populations *(866)*. In this regard, outside of certain populations (pregnant women and persons with acute HIV infection), it is now recommended that the initiation of triple-combination therapy be delayed until there is clear evidence of progression of immune disease, as ascertained by a $CD4^+$ T-cell count of fewer than 350 cells/mm^3 and a plasma viral load greater than 30,000 copies/mL *(867)*. It has also been suggested that disease progression and death are mostly limited to persons who wait until their $CD4^+$ T-cell counts are fewer than 200 cells/mm^3 before starting treatment *(868)*.

In the same vein, concerns about metabolic toxicities and the pursuit of better-tolerated and more convenient dose regimens have resulted in the investigation of a number of PI agents that can be effectively administered once daily with as few as two tablets *(869, 870)*.

Statistical Analysis of Clinical Data. Data from clinical studies are analyzed mainly by using three statistical techniques: (i) intent-to-treat (ITT); (ii) ITT, last observation carried forward; and (iii) observed or on-treatment analysis *(296)*. Each of these analyses will provide different information regarding the clinical outcome.

The ITT analysis is the most conservative type because it includes all patients who entered the study, and missing data are treated as representing failure. ITT also tends to underestimate the treatment effect in practice *(296)*.

By contrast, with the ITT, last observation carried forward analysis, the missing data are handled by assigning the value recorded at the last patient visit *(296)*.

The third statistical technique, the observed or on-treatment analysis, is the most common way of presenting clinical data. It provides results only for patients for whom follow-up data are available; missing values are disregarded. Thus, the denominator for this type of analysis may not be the same as the number of patients who originally entered the study. Observed or on-treatment analysis tends to overestimate the treatment effect in practice by ignoring patients who are unable to take therapy or who change therapy because of an insufficient response, but it is a good reflection of the efficacy of a particular approach in those who actually take it *(296)*.

34.11.1 Immunologic Response to HAART

A significant amount of evidence has substantiated the importance of the CD4$^+$ T-cell count as an independent prognostic indicator for progression of HIV disease *(871)*, and in clinical settings, together with the plasma RNA levels, changes in the CD4$^+$ T-cell count levels are considered as key surrogate markers of disease progression. In this context, it is notable that PI-based HAART can rapidly increase the CD4$^+$ T-cell count early in the treatment of both therapy-naïve and therapy-experienced patients and can sustain gains in CD4$^+$ T-cell counts in a durable manner *(871)*.

Four mechanisms have been suggested to explain this rapid increase in the CD4$^+$ T-cell count: CD4$^+$ T-cell redistribution from the lymphatic tissues; increased CD4$^+$ T-cell production; reduction of apoptotic CD4$^+$ T-cells; and the recovery of hematopoietic activity in the bone marrow *(871)*. These four mechanisms are not mutually exclusive, and all of them may play a role in the regeneration of CD4$^+$ T-cells.

CD4$^+$ T-Cell Redistribution. Considering all possible mechanisms for the rapid increase in the CD4$^+$ T-cell count that accompanies the decline in plasma viral load when HAART is initiated, the lymphocyte redistribution from lymphatic tissues may be the most important *(872)*. The redistribution would most likely arise from the resolution of the immune activation state that had previously sequestered the T cells within the lymphoid tissues, rather than the generation of "new" T cells in all anatomic compartments *(871)*.

Increased CD4$^+$ T-Cell Production. Although the thymic function declines with age, a measurable level of thymic activity is maintained throughout adult life. During HIV disease, a measurable decrease in the thymic function is observed in both peripheral blood and lymphoid tissues. However, a rapid and sustained increase in the thymic output has been observed as reflected in the increase in CD4$^+$ T-cells after initiation of HAART *(871)*.

Reduction of Apoptotic CD4$^+$ T-Cells. The effects of HAART on T-cell apoptosis in distinct T-cell subsets in peripheral blood were investigated during a 6-month follow-up study of HIV-infected patients *(873)*. The rapid and sustained increase in both naïve and memory CD4$^+$ and CD8$^+$ T-cells in response to HAART was associated with a significant decrease in apoptotic CD4$^+$ and CD8$^+$ T-cells. These findings have supported the notion that viral suppression can help reduce T-cell abnormalities that cause high levels of CD4$^+$ apoptosis in HIV-infected patients, and this may contribute to the immunologic reconstitution observed during HAART *(871)*.

Data from another study has suggested a different pathway for T-cell apoptosis, which did not require viral replication but was dependent on Fas or activation of CD95 *(874)*.

Recovery of Hematopoietic Activity in Bone Marrow. HIV infection is known to suppress the *in vitro* growth of hematopoietic stem cells in the bone marrow from which CD4 cell progenitors are derived *(875)*. Although the mechanism(s) responsible for the suppression of bone marrow in HIV-infected patients are still not very well understood, it is postulated that a decreased number of hematopoietic stem cells or a defective modulation of stem cell growth may cause the hematologic abnormalities *(876)*. In spite of this, immunologic reconstitution through the increased production of long-term, culture-initiating cells has been reported in HAART-treated patients *(871)*.

34.11.2 Pathophysiologic Consequences

Despite potential problems of resistance, triple-drug antiretroviral combinations have a number of beneficial pathophysiologic consequences *(425)*. For example, in addition to increasing the overall CD4$^+$ T-cell count, the triple combination therapies may also increase the naïve and memory T-cell counts, enhance lymphoproliferative responses, and reduce the plasma concentrations of harmful cytokines, such as the tumor necrosis factor-α *(877)*. Results from studies with small number of patients with recent seroconversion have shown antiretroviral combination regimens to be able to forestall the loss of HIV-specific CD4$^+$ T-lymphocyte responses that characterizes the natural history of this disease *(878)*.

Unfortunately, however, triple-combination regimens containing protease inhibitors may not correct deficiencies in the T-cell repertoire already induced by HIV, and lost lymphocyte clones may not be replaced *(425, 879)*. These observations may explain why infections caused by opportunistic pathogens, such as cytomegalovirus, have developed in some patients during the late stage of AIDS, even though their CD4$^+$ T-cell counts have increased from less than 50 to more than 200 cells/mm^3 while they were still receiving highly active regimens containing protease inhibitors *(880, 881)*.

In spite of the prolonged suppression of HIV viremia observed in large numbers of patients, HAART has not yet led to the cure of HIV infection. Patients with undetectable plasma viral loads and greatly reduced numbers of viral particles in the lymph nodes and peripheral blood cells still had detectable amount of proviral DNA in the cells that was capable of replication *(882–884)* even after 6 to12 months of HAART *(885, 886)*.

Eradication of HIV with the current combination regimens may be impossible even after 3 to 5 years of continuous treatment *(887, 888)*. In this regard, *adherence to HAART* is fast becoming extremely important. Thus, results from patients with undetectable viral loads who have been receiving indinavir combined with zidovudine and lamivudine have shown that those who stopped taking one or two of the drugs after 3 to 6 months of therapy had relapses up to six times as often as those who continued to take all three drugs *(889, 890)*.

34.11.3 Factors Influencing Response to HAART

$CD4^+$ *T-Cells Decline*. The CD4 responses generally correlate with the suppression of viral load *(871)* but conflicting results are not unusual *(891–893)* and have been observed in both treatment-naïve and treatment-experienced patients *(891)*. Thus, in a prospective cohort study of 2,236 patients, 36.3% had a discordant response after 6 months of HAART; 17.3% had a virologic response (plasma viral load reduction of over $1.0 \log_{10}$ copies/mL) but no immunologic response, and 19% had an immunologic ($CD4^+$ T-cell count increase >50 cells/mm^3) but no virologic response *(891)*.

Several possible reasons have been postulated to explain the presence of low $CD4^+$ T-cell counts in patients with HIV disease despite effective virologic suppression with HAART *(871)*. One such hypothesis has been to explain the observed discordance by lymphatic toxicity of the antiretroviral agents (e.g., didanosine) *(894–896)*. In other investigations, a deficiency in the regeneration of central $CD4^+$ T-cells *(897)*, excessive apoptosis *(636)*, and reduced expression of cytokines such as IL-7Rα *(898)* have been implicated in the low-level regeneration of the $CD4^+$ T-cells.

Drug Absorption and Treatment Adherence. There have been strong indications that drug absorption and treatment adherence have influenced the response of HIV-infected patients to HAART *(233, 726, 889, 890, 899–902)*.

Antiretroviral agents have different food restrictions that affect their absorption in the gut; for example, lopinavir and atazanavir must be taken with food, whereas efavirenz must be taken on an empty stomach. If food restrictions are not followed, this would affect drug plasma concentrations and subsequently the degree to which antiretroviral drugs would penetrate the blood-brain barrier *(871)*.

Hence, strong adherence to treatment (≥85%) to unboosted HAART has been recommended in order to achieve virologic suppression (plasma virologic load of less than 400 copies/mL) and increased $CD4^+$ T-cell count *(726, 899, 900)*. Results from some studies have suggested that the same effect may also be achieved with only moderate adherence (at least 54%) to NNRTI-containing regimens *(899, 900)*—probably due to the antiretroviral potency of NNRTIs, their convenient administration (once daily), and tolerability *(233, 901)*. Regardless, it should be noted that these studies *(726, 899, 900)* have used different methods to measure adherence, and the best method to assess adherence to antiretroviral regimens is still unknown *(902)*.

34.12 Recent Scientific Advances

- *Episodic CD4-Guided Use of ART: Results of the SMART Study*. This study was initiated to clarify whether it is best to reserve antiretroviral therapy (ART) for cases where the $CD4^+$ T-cell counts are low and patients are immunocompromised, or whether continuous treatment that keeps the viral burden as low as possible is better. Results have shown that, compared with continuous therapy, the use of ART has been associated with multiple risks including metabolic and cardiovascular complications, waning adherence, and HIV resistance *(903–906)*.

- *Phase II Study of the Safety and Efficacy of Vicriviroc in HIV-Infected Treatment-Experienced Patients (ACTG 5211)*. This study, which was a double-blind, randomized, 48-week Phase II trial designed to evaluate the virologic activity of vicriviroc (a CCR5 receptor antagonist) in 118 treatment-experienced HIV-positive patients with R5-tropic virus (Monogram assay) HIV-1 RNA (viral load), have shown that the drug demonstrated potent 14-day virologic suppression, and after optimization of the background antiretroviral drugs, it sustained its antiretroviral activity over 24 weeks. However, the relationship of vicriviroc to malignancy remained uncertain *(907)*.

- *A Prospective, Randomized, Phase III Trial of NRTI- and NNRTI-Sparing Regimens for Initial Treatment of HIV-1 Infection (ACTG 5142)*. This randomized, open-label, prospective trial compared three class-sparing regimens for naïve subjects: lopinavir/ritonavir (LPV/r) plus efavirenz (EFV) (L/E) versus LPV/r plus 2NRTI (lopinavir; soft gel, twice-daily) versus EFV plus 2NRTI (EFV). The study, which was designed to detect differences in the rates of virologic failure and regimen completion, has demonstrated that compared with a regimen of EFV plus 2NRTI, the LPV plus 2NRTI regimen tended to have shorter time to virologic failure and regimen completion. The NRTI-sparing regimen of L/E had similar efficacy and safety as EFV plus 2NRTI. In the subsequent substudy (ACTG 5152s), the effects of all three ART regimens were compared for their effects on vascular reactivity *(908)*. ART containing PIs has been associated with increased cardiac risk due to endothelial dysfunction in small experimental studies and with increased cardiovascular risk in large observational studies. NRTIs and NNRTIs have also been associated with increased cardiovascular risk. Results from the preliminary analysis of substudy ACTG 5152s have shown that ART has rapidly improved impaired endothelial functions in treatment-naïve HIV-infected patients with the benefits being similar for all three ART regimens. In addition, all tested regimens improved vascular reactivity *(909)*.

- *Long-Term Clinical and Immunologic Outcomes Are Similar in HIV-Infected Persons Randomized to NNRTI versus PI versus NNRTI plus PI-Based Antiretroviral Regimens as Initial Therapy: Results of the CPCRA 058 FIRST Study.* The FIRST (flexible initial retrovirus suppressive therapies) study was design to compare the relative benefits of starting previously untreated HIV-infected patients on regimens that include two classes of drugs: a PI (or a NNRTI) plus a NTRI, or all three classes of drugs. The results of the study have demonstrated that the 3-class strategy was not superior to a 2-class strategy for immunologic or clinical outcomes and was associated with more treatment-limiting toxicity. The two 2-class strategies (NNRTI and PIs) of initial antiretroviral therapy were equivalent when compared using a composite outcome based on decline in CD4$^+$ T-cell count, an AIDS-defining event, or death after a median follow-up of 5 years. Consistent with earlier finding, the (2-class) NNRTI strategy provided better and more sustained virologic suppression compared with the (2-class) PIs strategy. Furthermore, a regimen combining two classes (either an NNRTI or a PI with an NRTI) was more beneficial than a regimen combining the three classes as an initial treatment strategy for long-term antiretroviral management of treatment-naïve HIV-infected individuals *(910)*.

- *A Prospective, Open-Label, Pilot Trial of Regimen Simplification to Atazanavir/Ritonavir Alone as Maintenance Antiretroviral Therapy After Sustained Virologic Suppression (ACTG 5201).* The trial was designed to evaluate the therapeutic effect of a combination of atazanavir and ritonavir as maintenance therapy *(911)*. The combination was attractive because of the low pill burden, the once-daily dosing, safety, and the unique resistance profile. The data from the trial suggested that a simplified maintenance therapy with atazanavir/ritonavir alone can sustain virologic suppression and may also be beneficial as a maintenance therapy for some treatment-experienced patients.

- *Efavirenz (EFV)-Based Regimens Are Potent in Treatment-Naïve Subjects—Across a Wide Range of Pretreatment HIV-1 RNA (VL) and CD4$^+$ T-Cell Counts:*

3-Year Results from ACTG 5095. This randomized study, with 3 years median follow-up, has compared viral load (VL) and CD4$^+$ T-cell responses in treatment-naïve patients receiving regimens containing EFV with two or three NRTIs, and assessed whether adding a third NRTI improved responses in any subgroup *(912)*. The overall data suggested that regimens containing EFV and two NRTIs may be virologically potent for a wide range of patient populations, including those with low-pretreatment CD4$^+$ T-cell counts and high VL.

References

1. Stammers, D. K. and Ren, J. (2006) Structural studies on HIV reverse transcriptase related to drug discovery. In: *Reverse Transcriptase Inhibitors in HIV/AIDS Therapy* (Skowron, G. and Ogden, R., eds.), Humana Press, Totowa, NJ, pp. 1–32.
2. Kohlstaedt, L. A., Wang, J., Friedman, J. M., Rice, P. A., and Steitz, T. A. (1992) Crystal structure at 3.5 Å resolution of HIV-1 reverse transcriptase complexed with an inhibitor, *Science*, **256**, 1783–1790.
3. Jacobo-Molina, A., Ding, J. P., Nanni, R. G., et al. (1993) Crystal structure of human immunodeficiency virus type 1 reverse transcriptase complexed with double-stranded DNA at 3.0 Å resolution shows bent DNA, *Proc. Natl. Acad. Sci. U.S.A.*, **90**, 6320–6324.
4. Ren, J., Esnouf, R., Garman, E., et al. (1995) High resolution structures of HIV-1 RT from four RT-inhibitor complexes, *Nat. Struct. Biol.*, **2**, 293–302.
5. Rodgers, D. W., Gamblin, S. J., Harris, B. A., et al. (1995) The structure of unliganded reverse transcriptase from the human immunodeficiency virus type 1, *Proc. Natl. Acad. Sci. U.S.A.*, **92**, 1222–1226.
6. Goff, S. P. (1990) Retroviral reverse transcriptase: synthesis, structure, and function, *J. Acquir. Immune Defic. Syndr.*, **3**, 817–831.
7. De Marzo Veronese, F., Copeland, T. D., De Vico, A. L., et al. (1986) Characterization of highly immunogenic p66/p51 as the reverse transcriptase of HTLV-III/LAV, *Science*, **231**, 1289–1291.
8. Davies II, J. F., Hostomska, Z., Hostomsky, Z., Jordan, S. R., and Matthews, D. A. (1991) Crystal structure of the ribonuclease H domain of HIV-1 reverse transcriptase, *Science*, **252**, 88–95.
9. Fan, N., Rank, K. B., Poppe, S. M., Tarpley, W. G., and Sharma, S. K. (1996) Characterization of the p68/p58 heterodimer of human immunodeficiency virus type 2 reverse transcriptase, *Biochemistry*, **35**(6), 1911–1917.
10. Bird, L. E., Chamberlain, P. P., Stewart-Jones, G., Ren, J., Stuart, D. I., and Stammers, D. K. (2003) Cloning, expression, purification and crystallization of HIV-2 reverse transcriptase, *Protein Expr. Purif.*, **27**, 8–12.
11. Ren, J., Bird, L. E., Chamberlain, P. P., Stewart-Jones, G. B., Stuart, D. I., and Stammers, D. K. (2002) Structure of HIV-2 reverse transcriptase at 2.35 Å resolution and the mechanism of resistance to non-nucleoside inhibitors, *Proc. Natl. Acad. Sci. U.S.A.*, **99**, 14410–14415.
12. Goody, R. S., Muller, B., and Restle, T. (1991) Factors contributing to the inhibition of HIV reverse transcriptase by chain-terminating nucleosides in vivo, *FEBS Lett.*, **291**, 1–5.
13. LeLacheur, S. F. and Simon, G. L. (1991) Exacerbation of dideoxycitidine-induced neuropathy with dideoxyinosine, *J. Acquir. Immune Defic. Syndr.*, **4**(5), 538–539.

14. Zemlicka, J., Freisler, J. V., Gasser, R., and Horwitz, J. P. (1973) Nucleosides XVI. The synthesis of 2′, 3′-dideoxy-3′,4′-didehydronucleosides, *J. Org. Chem.*, **38**, 990.

15. Dube, S., Pragnell, I., Kluge, N., Gaedicke, G., Steinheider, G., and Ostertag, W. (1975) Induction of endogenous and of spleen-forming viruses during diethylsulfoxide-induced differentiation of mouse erythroleukemia cells transformed by spleen focus-forming virus, *Proc. Natl. Acad. Sci. U.S.A.*, **72**, 1863–1867.

16. Mitsuya, H., Weinhold, J., Furman, P., et al. (1985) 3′-Azido-3′-deoxythymidine (BW A509U), *Proc. Natl. Acad. Sci. U.S.A.*, **82**, 7096–7100.

17. Carten, M. and Kessler, H. (2006) Zidovidine, lamivudine, and abacavir. In: *Reverse Transcriptase Inhibitors in HIV/AIDS Therapy* (Scowron, G. and Ogden, R, eds.) Humana Press, Totowa, NJ, pp. 33–76.

18. Birkus, G., Hitchcock, M., and Cihlar, T. (2002) Assessment of mitochondrial toxicity in human cells treated with tenofovir: comparison with other nucleoside reverse transcriptase inhibitors, *Antimicrob. Agents Chemother.*, **46**, 716–723.

19. Hayashi, S., Fine, R. L., Chou, T. C., et al. (1990) In vitro inhibition of the infectivity and replication of human immunodeficiency virus type 1 by combination of antiretroviral 2′, 3′-dideoxynucleosides and virus-binding inhibitors, *Antimicrob. Agents Chemother.*, **34**, 82–88.

20. Dornsife, R. E., St. Clair, M. H., Huang, A. T., et al. (1991) Anti-human immunodeficiency virus synergism by zidovudine (3′-azidothymidine) and didanosine (dideoxyinosine) contrasts with their additive inhibition or normal human marrow progenitor cells, *Antimicrob. Agents Chemother.*, **35**, 322–328.

21. Eron, J. J., Jr., Johnson, V. A., Merrill, D. P., et al. (1992) Synergistic inhibition of replication of human immunodeficiency virus type 1, including that of a zidovudine-resistant isolate, by zidovudine and 2′, 3′-dideoxycytidine in vitro, *Antimicrob. Agents Chemother.*, **36**, 1559–1562.

22. Merrill, D. P., Moonis, M., Chou, T.-C., and Hirsch, M. S. (1996) Lamivudine (3TC) or stavudine (d4T) in two- and three-drug combinations against HIV-1 replication in vitro, *J. Infect. Dis.*, **173**, 355–364.

23. Richman, D., Rosenthal, A. S., Skoog, M., et al. (1991) BI-RG-587 is active against zidovudine-resistant human immunodeficiency virus type 1 and synergistic with zidovudine, *Antimicrob. Agents Chemother.*, **35**, 305–308.

24. Johnson, V. A., Merrill, D. P., Chou, T.-C., and Hirsch, M. S. (1992) Human immunodeficiency virus type 1 (HIV-1) inhibitory interactions between protease inhibitor Ro 31-8959 and zidovudine, 2′,3′-dideoxycytidine, or recombinant interferon-α against zidovudine-sensitive or -resistant HIV-1 in vitro, *J. Infect. Dis.*, **166**, 1143–1146.

25. Havlir, D., Tierney, C., Friedland, G., et al. (2000) In vivo antagonism with zidovudine plus stavudine combination therapy, *J. Infect. Dis.*, **182**, 321–325.

26. Vogt, M. W., Hartshorn, K. L., Furman, P. A., et al. (1987) Ribavirin antagonizes the effect of azidothymidine on HIV replication, *Science*, **235**, 1376–1379.

27. Darbyshire, J. H. and Aboulker, J.-P. (1996) Delta: a randomized double-blind controlled trial comparing combinations of zidovudine plus didanosine or zalcitabine with zidovudine alone in HIV-infected individuals, *Lancet*, **348**, 2–5.

28. Hammer, S. M., Katzenstein, D. A., Hughes, M. D., et al. for the AIDS Clinical Trial Group Study 175 Study Team (1996) A trial comparing nucleoside monotherapy with combination therapy in HIV-infected adults with CD4 cell counts from 200 to 500 per cubic millimeter, *N. Engl. J. Med.*, **335**, 1081–1089.

29. Connor, E. M., Sperling, R. S., Gelbert, R., et al. (1994) Reduction of maternal-infant transmission of human immunodeficiency virus type 1 with zidovudine treatment, *N. Engl. J. Med.*, **331**(18), 1173–1180.

30. Yarchoan, R., Mitsuya, H., Myers, C., and Broder, S. (1989) Clinical pharmacology of 3′-azido-2′,3′-dideoxythymidine (zidovudine) and related dideoxynucleosides, *N. Engl. J. Med.*, **321**(11), 726–738.

31. The AVANTI Study Group (2000) AVANTI 2: a randomized, double-blind trial to evaluate the efficacy and safety of zidovudine plus lamivudine versus zidovudine plus lamivudine plus indinavir in HIV-infected antiretroviral-naïve patients, *AIDS*, **14**, 367–373.

32. Hammer, S. M., Squires, K. E., Hughes, M. D., et al. for the AIDS Clinical Trials Group 320 Study Team (1997) A controlled trial of two nucleoside analogues plus indinavir in persons with human immunodeficiency virus infection and CD4 cell counts of 200 per cubic milliliter or less, *N. Engl. J. Med.*, **337**, 725–732.

33. Skowron, G., Bratberg, J., and Pauwels, R. (2006) Emtricitabine. In: *Reverse Transcriptase Inhibitors of HIV/AIDS Therapy* (Skowron, G. and Ogden, R., eds.), Humana Press, Totowa, NJ, pp. 133–156.

34. Gilead Sciences (2004) Emtriva (Emtricitabine) product information, Gilead Sciences, Foster City, CA.

35. Shewach, D. S., Liotta, D. C., and Schinazi, R. F. (1993) Affinity of the antiviral enantiomers of oxathiolane cytosine nucleosides for human 2′-deoxycytidine kinase, *Biochem. Pharmacol.*, **45**(7), 1540–1543.

36. Panel on Clinical Practices for Treatment of HIV Infection (2005) Guidelines for the use of antiretroviral agents in HIV-infected adults and adolescents, October 6. U.S. Department of Health and Human Services, Washington, DC.

37. Daluge, S. M., Good, S. S., Faletto, M. B., et al. (1997) 159U89, a novel carbocyclic nucleoside analog with potent, selective anti-human immunodeficiency virus activity, *Antimicrob. Agents Chemother.*, **41**, 1082–1093.

38. Vince, R., Hua, M., Brownell, J., et al. (1988) Potent and selective activity of a new carbocyclic nucleoside analog (carbovir: NSC 614846) against human immunodeficiency virus in vitro, *Biochem. Biophys. Res. Commun.*, **156**, 1046–1053.

39. Faletto, M. B., Miller, W. H., Garvey, E. P., St. Clair, M. H., Daluge, S. M., and Good, S. S. (1997) Unique intracellular activation of the potent anti-human immunodeficiency virus agent 159U89, *Antimicrob. Agents Chemother.*, **41**(5), 1099–1107.

40. Carter, S. G., Kessler, J. A., and Rankin, C. D. (1990) Activities of (−)-carbovir and 3′-azido-3′-deoxythymidine against human immunodeficiency virus in vitro, *Antimicrob. Agents Chemother.*, **34**(6), 1297–1300.

41. Tisdale, M., Alnadaf, T., and Cousens, D. (1997) Combination of mutations in human immunodeficiency virus type 1 reverse transcriptase required for resistance to the carbocyclic nucleoside 1592U89, *Antimicrob. Agents Chemother.*, **41**, 1094–1098.

42. St. Clair, M. H., Millard, J., Rooney, J., et al. (1996) In vitro antiviral activity of 41W94 (VX-478) in combination with other antiretroviral agent, *Antivir. Res.*, **29**(1), 53–56.

43. Gallant, J. E., Rodriguez, A., Weinberg, W., et al. (2003) Early non-response to tenofovir DF + abacavir and lamivudine in a randomized trial compared to efavirenz+abacavir+lamivudine: ESS 30009 an unplanned interim analysis, *43th Interscience Conference on Antimicrobial Agents and Chemotherapy, Chicago, IL*, September 14–17 [abstract H-1722a].

44. Bristol-Myers Squibb Company (2004) Videx and Videx EC delayed-release capsules enteric-coated beadlets product information, Bristol-Myers Squibb Company, Princeton, NJ.

45. Skowron, G., Chowdhry, S., and Stevens, M. R. (2006) Stavudine, didanosine, and zalcitabine. In: *Reverse Transcriptase Inhibitors in HIV/AIDS Therapy* (Skowron, G. and Ogden R., eds.), Humana Press, Totowa, NJ, pp. 77–132.

46. Plagemann, P. G., Wohlhueter, R. M., and Woffendin, C. (1988) Nucleoside and nucleobase transport in animal cells, *Biochem. Biophys. Acta*, **947**(3), 405–443.

47. Cooney, D. A., Dalal, M., Mitsuya, H., et al. (1986) Initial studies on the cellular pharmacology of 2′,3′-dideoxycytidine, an inhibitor of HTLV-III infectivity, *Biochem. Pharmacol.*, **35**(13), 2065–2068.

48. Starnes, M. C. and Cheng, Y. C. (1987) Cellular metabolism of 2′,3′-dideoxycytidine, a compound active against human immunodeficiency virus in vitro, *J. Biol. Chem.*, **262**(3), 988–991.

49. Faraj, A., Fowler, D. A., Bridges, E. G., and Sommadossi, J. P. (1994) Effects of 2′,3′-dideoxynucleosides on proliferation and differentiation of human pluripotent progenitors in liquid culture and their effects on mitochondrial DNA synthesis, *Antimicrob. Agents Chemother.*, **38**(5), 924–930.

50. Keilbaugh, S. A., Hobbs, G. A., and Simpson, M. V. (1993) Anti-human immunodeficiency virus type 1 therapy and peripheral neuropathy: prevention of 2′,3′-dideoxycytidine toxicity in PC12 cells, a neuronal model, by uridine and pyruvate, *Mol. Pharmacol.*, **44**(4), 702–706.

51. Medina, D. J., Tsai, C. H., Hsiung, G. D., and Cheng, Y. C. (1994) Comparison of mitochondrial morphology, mitochondrial DNA content, and cell viability in cultured cells treated with three anti-human immunodeficiency virus dideoxynucleosides, *Antimicrob. Agents Chemother.*, **38**(8), 1824–1828.

52. Roche Laboratories (2002) HIVID (Zalcitabine) product information, Roche Laboratories, Nutley, NJ.

53. Merigan, T. C., Skowron, G., Bozzette, S. A., et al. (1989) Circulating p24 antigen levels and responses to dideoxycytidine in human immunodeficiency virus (HIV) infections. A phase I and II study, *Ann. Intern. Med.*, **110**(3), 189–194.

54. Bristol-Myers Squibb Company (2002) Zerit® (Stavudine) product information, Bristol-Myers Squibb Company, Princeton, NJ.

55. Ho, H. T. and Hitchcock, M. J. (1989) Cellular pharmacology of 2′,3′-dideoxy-2′,3′-didehydrothymidine, a nucleoside analog active against human immunodeficiency virus, *Antimicrob. Agents Chemother.*, **33**(6), 844–849.

56. Hoggard, P. G., Kewn, S., Barry, M. G., Khoo, S. H., and Back, D. J. (1997) Effects of drugs on 2′,3′-dideoxy-2′,3′-didehydrothymidine phosphorylation in vitro, *Antimicrob. Agents Chemother.*, **41**(6), 1231–1236.

57. Squires, K. E., Gulick, R., Tebas, P., et al. (2000) A comparison of stavudine plus lamivudine versus zidovudine plus lamivudine in combination with indinavir in antiretroviral naïve individuals with HIV infection: selection of thymidine analog regimen therapy (START I), *AIDS*, **24**(11), 1591–1600.

58. Eron, J. J., Jr., Murphy, R. L., Peterson, D., et al. (2000) A comparison of stavudine, didanosine and indinavir with zidovudine, lamivudine and indinavir for the initial treatment of HIV-1 infected individuals: selection of thymidine analog regimen therapy (START II), *AIDS*, **14**(11), 1601–1610.

59. Carr, A., Chuah, J., Hudson, J., et al. (2000) A randomized, open-label comparison of three highly active antiretroviral therapy regimens including two nucleoside analogues and indinavir for previously untreated HIV-1 infection: the OzCombo 1 study, *AIDS*, **14**(9), 1171–1180.

60. Murphy, R. L., Brun, S., Hicks, C., et al. (2001) ABT-378/ritonavir plus stavudine and lamivudine for the treatment of antiretroviral-naïve adults with HIV-1 infection: 48-week results, *AIDS*, **15**(1), F1–F9.

61. Robbins, G. K., De Gruttola, V., Shafer, R. W., et al. (2003) Comparison of sequential three-drug regimens as initial therapy for HIV-1 infection, *N. Engl. J. Med.*, **349**(24), 2293–2303.

62. Siegfried, N. L., Van Deventer, P. J. U., Mahomed, F. A., and Rutherford, G. W. (2006) Stavudine, lamivudine and nevirapine combination therapy for treatment of HIV infection and AIDS in adults, *Cochrane Database of Systematic Reviews* 2006, Issue 2. Art. No.: CD004535. DOI: 10.1002/14651858.CD004535.pub2.

63. Gallant, J. E., Staszewski, S., Pozniak, A. L., et al. (2004) Efficacy and safety of tenofovir DF vs. stavudine in combination therapy in antiretroviral-naïve patients: a 3-year randomized trial, *J. Am. Med. Assoc.*, **292**(2), 191–201.

64. French, M., Amin, J., Roth, N., et al. (2002) Randomized, open-label, comparative trial to evaluate the efficacy and safety of three antiretroviral drug combinations including two nucleoside analogues and nevirapine for previously untreated HIV-1 infection: the OzCombo 2 study, *HIV Clin. Trials*, **3**(3), 177–185.

65. Working Group on Antiretroviral Therapy and Medical Management of HIV-Infected Children (2003) Guidelines for the use of antiretroviral agents in pediatric HIV infection. Bethesda (MD): U.S. Department of Health and Human services, December 14, 2003.

66. Monpoux, F., Sirvent, N., Cottalorda, J., Mariani, R., and Lefèbvre, J. C. (1997) Stavudine, lamivudine and indinavir in children with advanced HIV-1 infection: preliminary experience, *AIDS*, **11**(12), 1523–1525.

67. Kakuda, T. N. (2000) Pharmacology of nucleoside and nucleotide reverse transcriptase inhibitor-induced mitochondrial toxicity, *Clin. Ther.*, **22**(6), 685–708.

68. Mitsuya, H. and Broder, S. (1986) Inhibition of the in vitro infectivity and cytopathic effect of human T-lymphotropic virus type III/lymphodenopathy-associated virus (HTLV-III/LAV) by 2′,3′-dideoxynucleosides, *Proc. Natl. Acad. Sci. U.S.A.*, **83**(6), 1911–1915.

69. Shulman, N. and Winters, M. (2006) Resistance to nucleoside and nucleotide reverse transcriptase inhibitors. In: *Reverse Transcriptase Inhibitors in HIV/AIDS Therapy* (Skowron, G. and Ogden, R., eds.), Humana Press, Totowa, NJ, pp. 179–207.

70. Gallant, J. E., Rodriguez, A. E., Weinberg, W. G., et al. (2005) Early virologic nonresponse to tenofovir, abacavir, and lamivudine in HIV-infected antiretroviral-naive subjects, *J. Infect. Dis.*, **192**, 1921–1930.

71. Huang, H., Chopra, R., Verdine, G. L., and Harrison, S. C. (1998) Structure of a covalently trapped catalytic complex of HIV-1 reverse transcriptase: implications for drug resistance, *Science*, **282**(5394), 1669–1675.

72. Sarafianos, S. G., Das, K., Clark, A. D., et al. (1999) Lamivudine (3TC) resistance in HIV-1 reverse transcriptase involves steric hindrance with beta-branched amino acids, *Proc. Natl. Acad. Sci. U.S.A.*, **96**(18), 10027–10032.

73. Gao, H. Q., Boyer, P. L., Sarafianos, S. G., Arnold, E., and Hughes, S. H. (2000) The role of steric hindrance in 3TC resistance of human immunodeficiency virus type-1 reverse transcriptase, *J. Mol. Biol.*, **300**(2), 403–418.

74. Lennerstrand, J., Hertogs, K., Stammers, D. K., and Larder, B. A. (2001) Correlation between viral resistance to zidovudine and resistance at the reverse transcriptase level for a panel of immunodeficiency virus type 1 mutants, *J. Virol.*, **75**(15), 7202–7205.

75. Deval, J., Selmi, B., Boretto, J., et al. (2002) The molecular mechanism of multidrug resistance by the q151m human immunodeficiency virus type 1 reverse transcriptase and its suppression using alpha-boranophosphate nucleotide analogues, *J. Biol. Chem.*, **277**(44), 42097–42104.

76. Kaushik, N., Talele, T. T., Pandey, P. K., Harris, D., Yadav, P. N., and Pandey, V. N. (2000) Role of glutamine 151 of human immunodeficiency virus type-1 reverse transcriptase in substrate selection as assessed by site-directed mutagenesis, *Biochemistry*, **39**(11), 2912–2920.

77. Ray, A. S., Basavapathruni, A., and Anderson, K. S. (2002) Mechanistic studies to understand the progressive development of resistance in human immunodeficiency virus type 1 reverse transcriptase to abacavir, *J. Biol. Chem.*, **277**(43), 40479–40490.

78. Martin, J. L., Wilson, J. E., Haynes, R. L., and Furman, P. A. (1993) Mechanism of resistance of human immunodeficiency virus type 1 to 2′,3′-dideoxyinosine, *Proc. Natl. Acad. Sci. U.S.A.*, **90**(13), 6135–6139.

79. Lennerstrand, J., Stammers, D. K., and Larder, B. A. (2001) Biochemical mechanism of human immunodeficiency virus type 1 reverse transcriptase resistance to stavudine, *Antimicrob. Agents Chemother.*, **45**(7), 2144–2146.

80. Selmi, B., Boretto, J., Sarfati, S. R., Guerreiro, C., and Canard, B. (2001) Mechanism-based suppression of dideoxynucleotide resistance by K65R human immunodeficiency virus reverse transcriptase using an alpha-boranophosphate nucleoside analogue, *J. Biol. Chem.*, **276**(51), 48466–48472.

81. Sluis-Cremer, N., Arion, D., Kaushik, N., Lim, H., and Parniak, M. A. (2000) Mutational analysis of Lys65 of HIV-1 reverse transcriptase, *Biochem. J.*, **348**(Part 1), 77–82.

82. White, K. L., Margot, N. A., Chen, S., et al. (2004) The HIV-1 K65R RT mutant utilizes a combination of decreased incorporation and decreased excision to evade NRTI, *11th Conference on Retroviruses and Opportunistic Infections, San Francisco, CA*, February 8–11 [abstract 55].

83. Girouard, M., Diallo, K., Marchand, B., Suzanne, M., and Gotte, M. (2003) Mutations E44D and V118I in the reverse transcriptase of HIV-1 play distinct mechanistic roles in dual resistance to AZT and 3TC, *J. Biol. Chem.*, **278**(36), 34403–34410.

84. Richman, D. D., Guatelli, J. C., Grimes, J., Tsiatis, A., and Gingeras, T. (1991) Detection of mutations associated with zidovudine resistance in human immunodeficiency virus by use of the polymerase chain reaction, *J. Infect. Dis.*, **164**(6), 1075–1081.

85. Boucher, C., O'Sullivan, E., Mulder, J., et al. (1992) Ordered appearance of zidovudine resistance mutations during treatment of 18 human immunodeficiency virus-positive patients, *J. Infect. Dis.*, **165**(1), 105–110.

86. Masquelier, B., Descamps, D., Carriere, I., et al. (1999) Zidovudine resensitization and dual HIV-1 resistance to zidovudine and lamivudine in the delta lamivudine roll-over study, *Antivir. Ther.*, **4**, 69–77.

87. Naeger, L. K., Margot, N. A., and Miller, R. D. (2001) Increased drug susceptibility of HIV-1 reverse transcriptase mutants containing M184V and zidovudine-associated mutations: analysis of enzyme processivity, chain-terminator removal and viral replication, *Antivir. Ther.*, **6**, 115–126.

88. Meyer, P. R., Matsuura, S. E., Mian, A. M., So, A. G., and Scott, W. A. (1999) A mechanism of AZT resistance: an increase in nucleotide-dependent primer unblocking by mutant HIV-1 reverse transcriptase, *Moll. Cell*, **4**, 35–43.

89. Arion, D., Kaushik, N., McCormick, S., et al. (1998) Phenotypic mechanism of HIV-1 resistance to 3′-azido-3′-deoxythymidine (AZT): increased polymerization processivity and enhanced sensitivity to pyrophosphate of the mutant viral reverse transcriptase, *Biochemistry*, **37**, 15908–15917.

90. Larder, B. A., Kemp, S. D., and Harrigan, P. R. (1995) Potential mechanism for sustained antiretroviral efficacy of AZT-3TC combination therapy, *Science*, **269**, 696–699.

91. Tisdale, M., Alnadaf, T., and Cousens, D. (1997) Combination of mutations in human immunodeficiency virus type 1 reverse transcriptase required for resistance to the carbocyclic nucleoside 1592U89, *Antimicrob. Agents Chemother.*, **41**, 1094–1098.

92. Zhang, D., Caliendo, A. M., Eron, J. J., et al. (1994) Resistance to 2′,3′-dideoxycytidine conferred by a mutation in codon 65 of the human immunodeficiency virus type 1 reverse transcriptase, *Antimicrob. Agents Chemother.*, **38**(2), 282–287.

93. Shirasaka, T., Yarchoan, R., O'Brien, M. C., et al. (1993) Changes in drug sensitivity of human immunodeficiency virus type 1 during therapy with azidothymidine, dideoxycytidine, and dideoxyinosine: an in vitro comparative study, *Proc. Natl. Acad. Sci. U.S.A.*, **90**(2), 562–566.

94. Fitzgibbon, J. E., Howell, R. M., Haberzettl, C. A., Sperber, S. J., Kim, H., and Dubin, D. T. (1993) Human immunodeficiency virus type 1 pol gene mutations which cause decreased susceptibility to 2′,3′-dideoxycytidine, *Antimicrob. Agents Chemother.*, **36**(1), 153–157.

95. Wainberg, M. A., Gu, Z., Gao, Q., et al. (1993) Clinical correlates and molecular basis of HIV drug resistance, *J. Acquir. Immune Defic. Syndr.*, **6**(Suppl. 1), S36–S46.

96. Shirasaka, T., Kavlick, M. F., Ueno, T., et al. (1995) Emergence of human immunodeficiency virus type 1 variants with resistance to multiple dideoxynucleosides in patients receiving therapy with dideoxynucleosides, *Proc. Natl. Acad. Sci. U.S.A.*, **92**(6), 2398–2402.

97. Craig, C. and Moyle, G. (1997) The development of resistance of HIV-1 to zalcitabine, *AIDS*, **11**(3), 271–279.

98. Bossi, P., Yvon, A., Mouroux, M., Huraux, J. M., Agut, H., and Calvez, V. (1998) Mutations in the human immunodeficiency virus type 1 reverse transcriptase gene observed in stavudine and didanosine strains obtained by in vitro passages, *Res. Virol.*, **149**(6), 355–361.

99. Lin, P. F., Gonzalez, C. J., Griffith, B., et al. (1999) Stavudine resistance: an update on susceptibility following prolonged therapy, *Antivir. Ther.*, **4**(1), 21–28.

100. Coakley, E. P., Gillis, J. M., and Hammer, S. M. (2000) Phenotypic and genotypic resistance patterns of HIV-1 isolates derived from individuals treated with didanosine and stavudine, *AIDS*, **14**(2), F9–F15.

101. Deminie, C. A., Bechtold, C. M., Riccardi, K., et al. (1998) Clinical HIV-1 isolates remain sensitive to stavudine following prolonged therapy, *AIDS*, **12**(1), 110–112.

102. Mayers, D. L., Japour, A. J., Arduino, J. M., Hammer, M. S., et al. (1994) Dideoxynucleoside resistance emerges with prolonged zidovudine monotherapy. The RV43 Study Group, *Antimicrob. Agents Chemother.*, **38**(2), 307–314.

103. Whitcomb, J. M., Huang, W., Limoli, K., et al. (2002) Hypersusceptibility to non-nucleoside reverse transcriptase inhibitors in HIV-1: clinical, phenotypic and genotypic correlates, *AIDS*, **16**(15), F41–F47.

104. Jeffrey, J. L., Feng, J. Y., Qi, C. C. R., Anderson, K. S., and Furman, P. A. (2003) Dioxolane guanosine 5′-triphosphate, an alternative substrate inhibitor of wild-type and mutant HIV-1 reverse transcriptase: steady state and pre-steady state kinetic analyses, *J. Biol. Chem.*, **278**(21), 18971–18979.

105. Mewshaw, J. P., Myrick, F. T., Wakefield, D. A., Hooper, B. J., Harris, J. L., McCreedy, B., and Borroto-Esoda, K. (2002) Dioxolane guanosine, the active form of the prodrug diaminopurine dioxolane, is a potent inhibitor of drug-resistant HIV-1 isolates from patients for whom standard nucleoside therapy fails, *AIDS*, **29**, 11–20.

106. Gu, Z., Wainberg, M. A., Nguyen-Ba, N., L'Heureux, L., de Muys, J.-M., Bowlin, T. L., and Rando, R. F. (1999) Mechanism of action and in vitro activity of 1′,3′-dioxolanylpurine nucleoside analogues against sensitive and drug-resistant human immunodeficiency virus type 1 variants, *Antimicrob. Agents Chemother.*, **43**, 2376–2382.

107. Bazmi, H. Z., Hammond, J. L., Cavalcanti, S. C. H., Chu, C. K., Schinazi, R. F., and Mellors, J. W. (2000) In vitro selection of mutations in the human immunodeficiency virus type 1 reverse transcriptase that decrease susceptibility to (−)-β-D-dioxolane-guanosine and suppress resistance to 3′-azido-3′-deoxythymidine, *Antimicrob. Agents Chemother.*, **44**, 1783–1788.

108. Mellors, J. W., Bazmi, H., Chu, C. K., and Schinazi, R. F. (1996) K65R mutation in HIV-1 reverse transcriptase causes resistance

to (−)-b-D-dioxolane-guanosine and reverses AZT resistance, *5th International Workshop on HIV Drug Resistance, Whistler, Canada*, July 3–6 [abstract 7].

109. Gu, Z., Gao, Q., Fang, H., Salomon, H., Parniak, M. A., Goldberg, E., Cameron, J., and Wainberg, M. A. (1994) Identification of a mutation at codon 65 in the IKKK motif of reverse transcriptase that encodes human immunodeficiency virus resistance to 2′,3′-dideoxycytidine and 2′,3′-dideoxy-3′-thiacytidine, *Antimicrob. Agents Chemother.*, **38**, 275–281.

110. St. Clair, M. H., Martin, J. L., Tudor-Williams, G., Bach, M. C., Vavro, C. L., King, D. M., Kellam, P., Kemp, S. D., and Larder, B. A. (1991) Resistance to ddI and sensitivity to AZT induced by a mutation in HIV-1 reverse transcriptase, *Science*, **253**, 1557–1559.

111. Shirasaka, T., Kavlick, M. F., Ueno, T., Gao, W. Y., Kojima, E., Alcaide, M. L., Chokekijchai, S., Roy, B. M., Arnold, E., and Yarchoan, R. (1995) Emergence of human immunodeficiency virus type 1 variants with resistance to multiple dideoxynucleosides in patients receiving therapy with dideoxynucleosides, *Proc. Natl. Acad. Sci. U.S.A.*, **92**, 2398–2402.

112. Bacheler, L. T. (1999) Resistance to non-nucleoside inhibitors of HIV-1 reverse transcriptase, *Drug Resistance Update*, **2**(1), 56–67.

113. Avexa Press Release (2007) Avexa reports positive Phase IIb result: ATC shows superior activity, Avexa Melbourne, Australia.

114. Eron, J. J., Kessler, H., Thompson, M., et al. (2000) Clinical HIV suppression after short term monotherapy with DAPD, *40th Interscience Conference on Antimicrobial Agents and Chemotherapy, Toronto*, September 17–20 [abstract 690].

115. Thompson, M., Richmond, G., Kessler, H., et al. (2003) Preliminary results of dosing of amdoxovir in treatment-experienced patients, *10th Conference on Retroviruses and Opportunistic Infections, Boston*, February 10–14 [abstract 554].

116. Holdich, T., Shiveley, L. A., and Sawyer, J. (2007) Effect of lamivudine on the plasma and intracellular pharmacokinetics of apricitabine, a novel nucleoside reverse transcriptase inhibitor, in healthy volunteers, *Antimicrob. Agents Chemother.*, **51**(8), 2943–2947.

117. Bethell, R. C., Lie, Y. S., and Parkin, N. T. (2005) In vitro activity of SPD754, a new deoxycytidine nucleoside reverse transcriptase inhibitor (NRTI), against 215 HIV-1 isolates resistant to other NRTIs, *Antivir. Chem. Chemother.*, **16**, 295–302.

118. de Muys, J. M., Gourdeau, H., Nguyen-Ba, N., Taylor, D. L., Ahmed, P. S., Mansour, T., Locas, C., Richard, N., Wainberg, M. A., and Rando, R. F. (1999) Anti-human immunodeficiency virus type 1 activity, intracellular metabolism, and pharmacokinetic evaluation of 2′-deoxy-3′-oxa-4′-thiocytidine, *Antimicrob. Agents Chemother.*, **43**, 1835–1844.

119. Dutschman, G. E., Grill, S. P., Gullen, E. A., et al. (2004) Novel 4′-substituted stavudine analog with improved anti-human immunodeficiency virus activity and decreased cytotoxicity, *Antimicrob. Agents Chemother.*, **48**(5), 1640–1646.

120. Bridges, E. G., Dutschman, G. E., Gullen, E. A., and Cheng, Y.-C. (1996) Favorable interaction of β_L(-) nucleoside analogues with clinically approved anti-HIV nucleoside analogues for the treatment of human immunodeficiency virus, *Biochem. Pharmacol.*, **51**, 731–736.

121. Coates, J. A., Cammack, N., Jenkinson, H. J., Mutton, I. M., Pearson, B. A., Storer, R., Cameron, J. M., and Penn, C. R. (1992) The separated enantiomers of 2′-deoxy-3′-thiacytidine (BCH 189) both inhibit human immunodeficiency virus replication in vitro, *Antimicrob. Agents Chemother.*, **36**, 202–205.

122. Doong, S. L., Tsai, C. H., Schinazi, R. F., Liotta, D. C., and Cheng, Y.-C. (1991) Inhibition of the replication of hepatitis B virus in vitro by 2′,3′-dideoxy-3′-thiacytidine and related analogues, *Proc. Natl. Acad. Sci. U.S.A.*, **88**, 8495–8499.

123. Dutschman, G. E., Bridges, E. G., Liu, S.-H., Gullen, E., Guo, X., Kukhanova, M., and Cheng, Y.-C. (1998) Metabolism of 2′,3′-dideoxy-2′,3′-didehydro-β_L(-)-5-fluorocytidine and its activity in combination with clinically approved anti-human immunodeficiency virus β_D(+) nucleoside analogs in vitro, *Antimicrob. Agents Chemother.*, **42**, 1799–1804.

124. Lin, T. S., Luo, M. Z., Liu, M. C., Pai, S. B., Dutschman, G. E., and Cheng, Y.-C. (1994) Antiviral activity of 2′,3′-dideoxy-beta-L-5-fluorocytidine (beta-L-FddC) and 2′,3′-dideoxy-beta-L-cytidine (beta-L-ddC) against hepatitis B virus and human immunodeficiency virus type 1 in vitro, *Biochem. Pharmacol.*, **47**, 171–174.

125. Lin, T. S., Luo, M. Z., Liu, M. C., Pai, S. B., Dutschman, G. E., and Cheng, Y.-C. (1994) Synthesis and biological evaluation of 2′,3′-dideoxy-L-pyrimidine nucleosides as potential antiviral agents against human immunodeficiency virus (HIV) and hepatitis B virus (HBV), *J. Med. Chem.*, **37**, 798–803.

126. Lin, T. S., Luo, M. Z., Liu, M. C., Zhu, Y. L., Gullen, E., Dutschman, G. E., and Cheng, Y.-C. (1996) Design and synthesis of 2′,3′-dideoxy-2′,3′-didehydro-beta-L-cytidine (beta-L-d4C) and 2′,3′-dideoxy 2′,3′-didehydro-beta-L-5-fluorocytidine (beta-L-Fd4C), two exceptionally potent inhibitors of human hepatitis B virus (HBV) and potent inhibitors of human immunodeficiency virus (HIV) in vitro, *J. Med. Chem.*, **9**, 1757–1759.

127. Gosselin, G., Schinazi, R. F., Sommadossi, J.-P., Mathé, C., Bergogne, M.-C., Aubertin, A.-M., Kirn, A., and Imbach, J.-L. (1994) Anti-human immunodeficiency virus activities of the β-*L*-enantiomer of 2′,3′-dideoxycytidine and its 5-fluoro derivative in vitro, *Antimicrob. Agents Chemother.*, **38**, 1292–1297.

128. Schinazi, R. F., Chu, C. K., Peck, A., McMillan, A., et al. (1992) Activities of the four optical isomers of 2′,3′-dideoxy-3′-thiacytidine (BCH-189) against human immunodeficiency virus type 1 in human lymphocytes, *Antimicrob. Agents Chemother.*, **36**, 672–676.

129. Coates, J. A., Cammack, N., Jenkinson, H. J., Jowett, A. J., et al. (1992) (−)-2′-Deoxy-3′-thiacytidine is a potent, highly selective inhibitor of human immunodeficiency virus type 1 and type 2 replication in vitro, *Antimicrob. Agents Chemother.*, **36**, 733–739.

130. De Clercq, E. (1994) HIV resistance to reverse transcriptase inhibitors, *Biochem. Pharmacol.*, **47**, 155–169.

131. Larder, B. A. (1995) Viral resistance and the selection of antiretroviral combinations, *J. Acquir. Immune Defic. Syndr. Hum. Retrovirol.*, **10**(Suppl. 1), S28-S33.

132. Richman, D. D. (1993) Resistance of clinical isolates of human immunodeficiency virus to antiretroviral agents, *Antimicrob. Agents Chemother.*, **37**, 1207–1213.

133. Colucci, P., Pottage, J., Robison, H., et al. (2005) The different clinical pharmacology of elvucitabine (beta-L-Fd4C) enables the drug to be given in a safe and effective manner with innovative drug dosing, *45th Interscience Conference on Antimicrobial Agents and Chemotherapy, Washington, D.C.*, December 16–19 [abstract LB-27].

134. Hoesley, C. J. (2006) Nucleotide analogs. In: *Reverse Transcriptase Inhibitors in HIV/AIDS Therapy* (Scowron, G. and Ogden, R., eds.), Humana Press, Totowa, NJ, pp. 157–178.

135. Naesens, I., Snocek, R., Andrei, G., et al. (1997) HPMC (cidofovir), PMEA (adefovir), and related acyclic nucleoside phosphonate analogues: a review of their pharmacology and clinical potential in the treatment of viral infections, *Antivir. Chem. Chemother.*, **8**, 1–23.

136. Balzarini, J. and De Clerq, E. (1991) 5-Phosphoribosyl-1-pyrophosphate synthetase converts the acyclic nucleoside phosphonates 9-(3-hydroxy-2-phosphonylmethoxypropyl)adenine and 9-(2-phosphonylmethoxyethyl)adenine directly to their antivirally active phosphate derivatives, *J. Biol. Chem.*, **266**, 8686–8689.

137. Srinivas, R., Robbins, B., Connelly, M., Gong, Y. F., et al. (1993) Metabolism and in vitro antiretroviral activities of bis(pivaloyloxymethyl) prodrugs of acyclic nucleoside phosphonates, *Antimicrob. Agents Chemother.*, **37**(10), 2247–2250.

138. De Clerq, E. (1997) Acyclic nucleoside phosphonates in the chemotherapy of DNA virus and retrovirus infections, *Intervirology*, **40**, 295–303.

139. Hartmann, K., Balzarini, J., Higgins, J, et al. (1994) In vitro activity of acyclic nucleoside phosphonate derivatives against feline immunodeficiency virus in Crandall feline kidney cells and feline peripheral blood lymphocytes, *Antivir. Chem. Chemother.*, **5**, 13–18.

140. Thormar, H., Balzarini, J., Holý, A., et al. (1993) Inhibition of visna virus replication by 2′,3′-dideoxynucleosides and acyclic nucleoside phosphonate analogs, *Antimicrob. Agents Chemother.*, **37**, 2540–2544.

141. Haesens, L., Balzarini, J., Rosenberg, I., Holý, A., et al. (1989) 9-(2-Phosphonylmethoxyethyl)-2,6-diaminopurine (PMEDAP): a novel agent with anti-human immunodeficiency virus activity in vitro and potent anti-moloney murine sarcoma virus activity in vivo, *Eur. J. Clin. Microbiol.*, **8**, 1043–1047.

142. Barditch-Crovo, P., Deeks, S., Collier, A., et al. (2001) Phase I/II trial of the pharmacokinetics, safety, and antiretroviral activity of tenofovir disoproxil fumarate in human immunodeficiency virus-infected adults, *Antimicrob. Agents Chemother.*, **45**, 2733–2739.

143. Farthing, C., Khanlou, H., and Yeh, V. (2003) Early virologic failure in a pilot study evaluating the efficacy of abacavir, lamivudine, and tenofovir in the treatment of naïve HIV-infected patients, *2nd International AIDS Society Conference on HIV Pathogenesis and Treatment, Paris, France*, July 13–16 [abstract 43].

144. Squires, K., Pozniak, A., Pierone, G., et al. (2003) Tenofovir disoproxil fumarate in nucleoside-resistant HIV-1 infection: a randomized trial, *Ann. Intern. Med.*, **139**, 313–320.

145. Gu, Z., Gao, I., Fang, H., et al. (1994) Identification of a mutation at codon 65 in the JKKK motif of reverse transcriptase that encodes resistance to 2′,3′-dideoxycytidine and 2′,3′-dideoxythiacytidine, *Antimicrob. Agents Chemother.*, **38**, 275–281.

146. Gu, Z., Salomon, H., Cherrington, J., et al. (1995) K65R mutation of human immunodeficiency virus type 1 reverse transcriptose encodes cross-resistance to 9-(2-phosphonylmethoxyethyl)adenine, *Antimicrob. Agents Chemother.*, **39**, 1888–1891.

147. Wainberg, M. A., Miller, M. D., Quan, Y., et al. (1999) In vitro selection and characterization of HIV-1 with reduced susceptibility to PMPA, *Antivir. Ther.*, **4**, 87–94.

148. Rhee, S. Y., Taylor, J., Wadhera, G., et al. (2006) Genotypic predictors of human immunodeficiency virus type 1 drug resistance, *Proc. Natl. Acad. Sci. U.S.A.*, **103**, 17355–17360.

149. Whitcomb, J. M., Parkin, N. T., Chappey, C., Hellmann, N. S., and Petropoulos, C. J. (2003) Broad nucleoside reverse-transcriptase inhibitor cross-resistance in human immunodeficiency virus type 1 clinical isolates, *J. Infect. Dis.*, **188**, 992–1000.

150. Delaunay, C., Brun-Vezinet, F., Landman, R., et al. (2005) Comparative selection of the K65R and M184V/I mutations in human immunodeficiency virus type 1-infected patients enrolled in a trial of first-line triple-nucleoside analog therapy (Tonus IMEA 021), *J. Virol.*, **79**, 9572–9578.

151. Gallant, J. E., DeJesus, E., Arribas, J. R., et al. (2006) Tenofovir DF, emtricitabine, and efavirenz vs. zidovudine, lamivudine, and efavirenz for HIV, *N. Engl. J. Med.*, **354**, 251–260.

152. Gallant, J. E., Staszewski, S., Pozniak, A. L., et al. (2004) Efficacy and safety of tenofovir DF vs. stavudine in combination therapy in antiretroviral-naive patients: a 3-year randomized trial, *J. Am. Med. Assoc.*, **292**, 191–201.

153. McColl, D. J., Margot, N. A., Wulfsohn, M., et al. (2004) Patterns of resistance emerging in HIV-1 from antiretroviral-experienced patients undergoing intensification therapy with tenofovir disoproxil fumarate, *J. Acquir. Immune Defic. Syndr.*, **37**, 1340–1350.

154. Parikh, U. M., Bacheler, L., Koontz, D., and Mellors, J. W. (2006) The K65R mutation in human immunodeficiency virus type 1 reverse transcriptase exhibits bidirectional phenotypic antagonism with thymidine analog mutations, *J. Virol.*, **80**, 4971–4977.

155. Parikh, U. M., Barnas, D. C., Faruki, H., and Mellors, J. W. (2006) Antagonism between the HIV-1 reverse-transcriptase mutation K65R and thymidine-analogue mutations at the genomic level, *J. Infect. Dis.*, **194**, 651–660.

156. Parikh, U. M., Koontz, D. L., Chu, C. K., Schinazi, R. F., and Mellors, J. W. (2005) In vitro activity of structurally diverse nucleoside analogs against human immunodeficiency virus type 1 with the K65R mutation in reverse transcriptase, *Antimicrob. Agents Chemother.*, **49**, 1139–1144.

157. Trotta, M. P., Bonfigli, S., Ceccherini-Silberstein, F., Bellagamba, R., et al. (2006) Clinical and genotypic correlates of mutation K65R in HIV-infected patients failing regimens not including tenofovir, *J. Med. Virol.*, **78**, 535–541.

158. White, K. L., Margot, N. A., Ly, J. K., et al. (2005) A combination of decreased NRTI incorporation and decreased excision determines the resistance profile of HIV-1 K65R RT, *AIDS*, **19**, 1751–1760.

159. Wirden, M., Marcelin, A. G., Simon, A., et al. (2005) Resistance mutations before and after tenofovir regimen failure in HIV-1 infected patients, *J. Med. Virol.*, **76**, 297–301.

160. Margot, N. A., Waters, J. M., and Miller, M. D. (2006) In vitro HIV-1 resistance selections with combinations of tenofovir and emtricitabine or abacavir and lamivudine, *Antimicrob. Agents Chemother.*, **50**, 4087–4095.

161. Ross, L. L., Dretler, R., Gerondelis, P., Rouse, E. G., Lim, M. L., and Lanier, E. R. (2006) A rare HIV reverse transcriptase mutation, K65N, confers reduced susceptibility to tenofovir, lamivudine and didanosine, *AIDS*, **20**, 787–789.

162. Delaugerre, C., Roudiere, L., Peytavin, G., et al. (2005) Selection of a rare resistance profile in an HIV-1-infected patient exhibiting a failure to an antiretroviral regimen including tenofovir DF, *J. Clin. Virol.*, **32**, 241–244.

163. Van Houtte, M., Staes, M., Geretti, A., Patterry, T., and Bacheler, L. (2006) NRTI resistance associated with the RT mutation K70E in HIV-1, *XV International HIV Drug Resistance Workshop, Sitges, Spain*, June 13–17.

164. Ross, L., Gerondelis, P., Liao, Q., et al., (2005) Selection of the HIV-1 reverse transcriptase mutation K70E in antiretroviral-naive subjects treated with tenofovir/abacavir/lamivudine therapy, *XIV International HIV Drug Resistance Workshop, Quebec City, Canada*, June 7–11 [abstract S102].

165. Sluis-Cremer, N., Sheen, S. W., Zelina, S., et al. (2007) Molecular mechanism by which K70E in HIV-1 reverse transcriptase confers resistance to nucleoside reverse transcriptase inhibitors, *Antimicrob. Agents Chemother.*, **51**(10), 48–53.

166. Margot, N. A., Isaacson, E., McGowan, I., Cheng, A., and Miller, M. D. (2003) Extended treatment with tenofovir disoproxil fumarate in treatment-experienced HIV-1-infected patients: genotypic, phenotypic, and rebound analyses, *J. Acquir. Immune Defic. Syndr.*, **33**, 15–21.

167. Masquelier, B., Tamalet, C., Montes, B., et al. (2004) Genotypic determinants of the virological response to tenofovir disoproxil fumarate in nucleoside reverse transcriptase inhibitor-experienced patients, *Antivir. Ther.*, **9**, 315–323.

168. Miller, M. D., Margot, N., Lu, B., et al. (2004) Genotypic and phenotypic predictors of the magnitude of response to tenofovir disoproxil fumarate treatment in antiretroviral-experienced patients, *J. Infect. Dis.*, **189**, 837–846.

169. Squires, K., Pozniak, A. L., Pierone, Jr., G., et al. (2003) Tenofovir disoproxil fumarate in nucleoside-resistant HIV-1 infection: a randomized trial, *Ann. Intern. Med.*, **139**, 313–320.

170. Barrios, A., de Mendoza, C., Martin-Carbonero, L., et al. (2003) Role of baseline human immunodeficiency virus genotype as a predictor of viral response to tenofovir in heavily pretreated patients, *J. Clin. Microbiol.*, **41**, 4421–4423.

171. Chappey, C., Wrin, T., Deeks, S., and Petropoulos, C. (2003) Evolution of amino acid 215 in HIV-1 reverse transcriptase in response to intermittent drug selection, *XII International HIV Drug Resistance Workshop, Los Cabos, Mexico*, June 10–14 [abstract 32].

172. de Ronde, A., van Dooren, M., van Der Hoek, L., et al. (2001) Establishment of new transmissible and drug-sensitive human immunodeficiency virus type 1 wild types due to transmission of nucleoside analogue-resistant virus, *J. Virol.*, **75**, 595–602.

173. Garcia-Lerma, J. G., Nidtha, S., Blumoff, K., Weinstock, H., and Heneine, W. (2001) Increased ability for selection of zidovudine resistance in a distinct class of wild-type HIV-1 from drug-naive persons, *Proc. Natl. Acad. Sci. U.S.A.*, **98**, 13907–13912.

174. Goudsmit, J., de Ronde, A., de Rooij, E., and de Boer, R. (1997) Broad spectrum of in vivo fitness of human immunodeficiency virus type 1 subpopulations differing at reverse transcriptase codons 41 and 215, *J. Virol.*, **71**, 4479–4484.

175. Yerly, S., Rakik, A., De Loes, S. K., et al. (1998) Switch to unusual amino acids at codon 215 of the human immunodeficiency virus type 1 reverse transcriptase gene in seroconvertors infected with zidovudine-resistant variants, *J. Virol.*, **72**, 3520–3523.

176. Van Laethem, K., De Munter, P., Schrooten, Y., et al. (2007) No response to first-line tenofovir + lamivudine + efavirenz despite optimization according to baseline resistance testing: impact of resistant minority variants on efficacy of low genetic barrier drugs, *J. Clin. Virol.*, **39**, 43–47.

177. Violin, M., Cozzi-Lepri, A., Velleca, R., et al. (2004) Risk of failure in patients with 215 HIV-1 revertants starting their first thymidine analog-containing highly active antiretroviral therapy, *AIDS*, **18**, 227–235.

178. Cases-Gonzalez, C. E., Franco, S., Martinez, M. A., and Menendez-Arias, L. (2006) Mutational patterns associated with the 69 insertion complex in multi-drug-resistant HIV-1 reverse transcriptase that confer increased excision activity and high-level resistance to zidovudine, *J. Mol. Biol.*, **365**(2), 298–309.

179. Clevenbergh, P., Kirstetter, M., Liotier, J. Y., et al. (2002) Long-term virological outcome in patients infected with multi-nucleoside analogue-resistant HIV-1, *Antivir. Ther.*, **7**, 305–308.

180. de Jong, J. J., Goudsmit, J., Lukashov, V. V., et al. (1999) Insertion of two amino acids combined with changes in reverse transcriptase containing tyrosine-215 of HIV-1 resistant to multiple nucleoside analogs, *AIDS*, **13**, 75–80.

181. Eggink, D., Huigen, M. C., Boucher, C. A., et al. (2007) Insertions in the beta3-beta4 loop of reverse transcriptase of human immunodeficiency virus type 1 and their mechanism of action, influence on drug susceptibility and viral replication capacity, *Antivir. Res.*, **75**, 93–103.

182. Gallego, O., de Mendoza, C., Labarga, P., et al. (2003) Long-term outcome of HIV-infected patients with multinucleoside-resistant genotypes, *HIV Clin. Trials*, **4**, 372–381.

183. Kew, Y., Olsen, L. R., Japour, A. J., and Prasad, V. R. (1998) Insertions into the beta3-beta4 hairpin loop of HIV-1 reverse transcriptase reveal a role for fingers subdomain in processive polymerization, *J. Biol. Chem.*, **273**, 7529–7537.

184. Deval, J., Selmi, B., Boretto, J., et al. (2002) The molecular mechanism of multidrug resistance by the Q151M human immunodefi-

ciency virus type 1 reverse transcriptase and its suppression using alpha-boranophosphate nucleotide analogues, *J. Biol. Chem.*, **277**, 42097–42104.

185. Feng, J. Y., Myrick, F. T., Margot, N. A., et al. (2006) Virologic and enzymatic studies revealing the mechanism of K65R- and Q151M-associated HIV-1 drug resistance towards emtricitabine and lamivudine, *Nucleosides Nucleotides Nucleic Acids*, **25**, 89–107.

186. Garcia-Lerma, J. G., Gerrish, P. J., Wright, A. C., Qari, S. H., and Heneine, W. (2000) Evidence of a role for the Q151L mutation and the viral background in development of multiple dideoxynucleoside-resistant human immunodeficiency virus type 1, *J. Virol.*, **74**, 9339–9346.

187. Iversen, A. K., Shafer, R. W., Wehrly, K., et al. (1996) Multidrug-resistant human immunodeficiency virus type 1 strains resulting from combination antiretroviral therapy, *J. Virol.*, **70**, 1086–1090.

188. Matsumi, S., Kosalaraksa, P., Tsang, H., et al. (2003) Pathways for the emergence of multi-dideoxynucleoside-resistant HIV-1 variants, *AIDS*, **17**, 1127–1137.

189. Asmuth, D. and Pollard, R. (2006) Nevirapine. In: *Reverse Transcriptase Inhibitors in HIV/AIDS Therapy* (Skowron, G. and Ogden R., eds.), Humana Press, Totowa, NJ, pp. 303–344.

190. Merluzzi, V. J., Hargrave, K. D., Labadia, M., et al. (1993) Inhibition of HIV-1 replication by a nonnucleoside reverse transcriptase inhibitor, *Science*, **250**(4986), 1411–1413.

191. Koup, R. A., Merluzzi, V. J., Hargrave, K. D., et al. (1991) Inhibition of human immunodeficiency virus type 1 (HIV-1) replication by the dipyridodiazepinone BI-RG-587, *J. Infect. Dis.*, **163**(5), 966–970.

192. Gu, Z., Quan, Y., Li, Z., Arts, E. J., and Wainberg, M. A. (1995) Effects of non-nucleoside inhibitors of human immunodeficiency virus type 1 in cell-free recombinant reverse transcriptase assays, *J. Biol. Chem.*, **270**(52), 31046–31051.

193. Grob, P. M., Wu, J. C., Cohen, K. A., et al. (1992) Nonnucleoside inhibitors of HIV-1 reverse transcriptase: nevirapine as a prototype drug, *AIDS Res. Hum. Retroviruses*, **8**(2), 145–152.

194. Shih, C. K., Rose, J. M., Hansen, G. L., Wu, J. C., Bacolla, A., and Griffin, J. A. (1991) Chimeric human immunodeficiency virus type 1/type 2 reverse transcriptases display reversed sensitivity to nonnucleoside analog inhibitors, *Proc. Natl. Acad. Sci. U.S.A.*, **88**(21), 9878–9882.

195. Wu, J. C., Warren, T. C., Adams, J., et al. (1991) A novel dipyridodiazepinone inhibitor of HIV-1 reverse transcriptase acts through a nonsubstrate binding site, *Biochemistry*, **30**(8), 2022–2026.

196. Spence, R. A., Kati, W. M., Anderson, K. S., and Johnson, K. A. (1995) Mechanism of inhibition of HIV-1 reverse transcriptase by nonnucleoside inhibitors, *Science*, **267**(5200), 988–993.

197. Asfour, F. R. and Haubrich, R. (2006) Resistance to non-nucleoside reverse transcriptase inhibitors. In: *Reverse Transcriptase Inhibitors in HIV/AIDS Therapy* (Skowron, G. and Ogden, R., eds.), Humana Press, Totowa, NJ, pp. 401–424.

198. Richman, D., Shih, C. K., Lowy, I., et al. (1991) Human immunodeficiency virus type 1 mutants resistant to nonnucleoside inhibitors of reverse transcriptase arise in tissue culture, *Proc. Natl. Acad. Sci. U.S.A.*, **88**(24), 11241–11245.

199. De Clercq, E. (1998) The role of non-nucleoside reverse transcriptase inhibitors (NNRTs) in the therapy of HIV-1 infection, *Antivir. Res.*, **38**(3), 153–179.

200. Cheeseman, S. H., Havlir, D., McLaughlin, M. M., et al. (1995) Phase I/II evaluation of nevirapine alone and in combination with zidovudine for infection with human immunodeficiency virus, *J. Acquir. Immune Defic. Syndr. Hum. Retrovirol.*, **8**(2), 141–151.

201. Guay, L. A., Musoke, P., Fleming, T., et al. (1999) Intrapartum and neonatal sungle-dose nevirapine compared with zidovudine for prevention of mother-to-child transmission of HIV-1 in Kampala, Uganda: HIVNET 012 randomised trial, *Lancet*, **354**(9181), 795–802.

202. de Jong, M. D., Vella, S., Carr, A., et al. (1997) High-dose nevirapine in previously untreated human immunodeficiency virus type 1-infected persons does not result in sustained suppression of viral replication, *J. Infect. Dis.*, **175**(4), 966–970.

203. D'Aquila, R. T., Hughes, M. D., Johnson, V. A., et al. (1996) Nevirapine, zidovudine, and didanosine compared with zidovudine and didanosine in patients with HIV-1 infection. A randomized, double-blind, placebo-controlled trial. National Institute of Allergy and Infectious Diseases AIDS Clinical Trials Group Protocol 241 Investigators, *Ann. Intern. Med.*, **124**(12), 1019–1030.

204. Baldanti, F., Paolucci, S., Maga, G., et al. (2003) Nevirapine-selected mutations Y181I/C of HIV-1 reverse transcriptase confer cross-resistance to stavudine, *AIDS*, **17**(10), 1568–1570.

205. Gilbert, P. B., Hanna, G. J., De Gruttola, V., et al. (2000) Comparative analysis of HIV type 1 genotypic resistance across antiretroviral trial treatment regimens, *AIDS Res. Hum. Retroviruses*, **16**(14), 1325–1336.

206. Casado, J. L., Hertogs, K., Ruiz, L., et al. (2000) Non-nucleoside reverse transcriptase inhibitor resistance among patients failing a nevirapine plus protease inhibitor-containing regimen, *AIDS*, **14**(2), F1–F7.

207. Briones, C., Soriano, V., Dona, C., Barreiro, P., and Gonzalez-Lahoz, J. (2000) Can early failure with nevirapine be rescued with efavirenz? *J. Acquir. Immune Defic. Syndr.*, **24**(1), 76–78.

208. Huang, W., Gamarnik, A., Limoli, K., Petropoulos, C. J., and Whitcomb, J. M. (2003) Amino acid substitutions at position 190 of human immunodeficiency virus type 1 reverse transcriptase increase susceptibility to delavirdine and impair virus replication, *J. Virol.*, **77**(2), 1512–1523.

209. MacArthur, R. D., Kosmyna, J. M., Crane, L. R., and Kovari, L. (1999) The presence or absence of zidovudine in a nevirapine-containing antiretroviral regimen determines which of two nevirapine-limiting mutations occurs on virologic failure, *39th Interscience Conference on Antimicrobial Agents and Chemotherapy, San Francisco, CA*, September 26–28 [abstract 1171].

210. Antoniou, T. and Tseng, A. L. (2002) Interactions between recreational drugs and antiretroviral agents, *Ann. Pharmacother.*, **36**(10), 1598–1613.

211. Casado, J. L., Moreno, A., Hertogs, K., Dronda, F., and Moreno, S. (2002) Extent and importance of cross-resistance to efaverenz after nevirapine failure, *AIDS Res. Hum. Retroviruses*, **18**(11), 771–775.

212. Harris, M. and Montaner, J. S. (2000) Clinical uses of non-nucleoside reverse transcriptase inhibitors, *Rev. Med. Virol.*, **10**(4), 217–229.

213. Podzamczer, D. and Fumero, E. (2001) The role of nevirapine in the treatment of HIV-1 disease, *Expert Opin. Pharmacother.*, **2**(12), 2065–2078.

214. Montaner, J. S., Reiss, P., Cooper, D., et al. (1998) A randomized, double-blind trial comparing combinations of nevirapine, didanosine, and zidovudine for HIV-infected patients: the INCAS Trial. Italy, The Netherlands, Canada, and Australia Study, *J. Am. Med. Assoc.*, **279**(12), 930–937.

215. Floridia, M., Bucciardini, R., Ricciardulli, D., et al. (1999) A randomized, double-blind trial on the use of a triple combination including nevirapine, a nonnucleoside reverse transcriptase HIV inhibitor, in antiretroviral-naïve patients with advance disease, *J. Acquir. Immune Defic. Syndr. Hum. Retrovirol.*, **20**(1), 11–19.

216. Garcia, F., Knobel, H., Sambeat, M. A., et al. (2000) Comparison of twice-daily stavudine plus once- or twice-daily didanosine and nevirapine in early stages of HIV infection: the scan study, *AIDS*, **14**(16), 2485–2494.

217. Raffi, F., Reliquet, V., Ferre, V., et al. (2000) The VIRGO study: nevirapine, didanosine and stavudine combination therapy in antiretroviral-naïve HIV-1-infected adults, *Antivir. Ther.*, **5**(4), 267–272.

218. Nunez, M., Soriano, V., Martin-Carbonero, L., et al. (2002) SENC (Spanish efavirenz vs. nevirapine comparison) trial: a randomized, open-label study in HIV-infected naïve individuals, *HIV Clin. Trials*, **3**(3), 186–194.

219. Allan, P. S., Arumainayagam, J., Harindra, V., et al. (2003) Sustained efficacy of nevirapine in combination with two nucleoside analogues in the treatment of HIV-infected patients: a 48-week retrospective multicenter study, *HIV Clin. Trials*, **4**(4), 248–251.

220. Giardiola, J. M., Domingo, P., Gurgui, M., and Vazquez, G. (2000) An open-label, randomized comparative study of stavudine (d4T) + didanosine (ddI) + indinavir versus d4T + ddI + nevirapine (NVP) in treatment of HIV-infected naïve patients, *40th Interscience Conference on Antimicrobial Agents and Chemotherapy, Toronto, Canada*, September 17–20 [abstract 539].

221. van Leeuwen, R., Katlama, C., Murphy, R. L., et al. (2003) A randomized trial to study first-line combination therapy with or without a protease inhibitor in HIV-1-infected patients, *AIDS*, **17**(7), 987–999.

222. Podzamczer, D., Ferrer, E., Consiglio, E., et al. (2002) A randomized clinical trial comparing nelfinavir or nevirapine associated to zidovudine/lamivudine in HIV-infected naïve patients (the Combine Study), *Antivir. Ther.*, **7**(2), 81–90.

223. Wit, F. W. (2000) Experience with nevirapine in previously treated HIV-1-infected individuals, *Antivir. Ther.*, **5**(4), 257–266.

224. Easterbrook, P. J., Newson, R., Ives, N., Pereira, S., Moyle, G., and Gazzard, B. G. (2001) Comparison of virologic, immunologic, and clinical response to five different initial protease inhibitor-containing and nevirapine-containing regimens, *J. Acquir. Immune Defic. Syndr.*, **27**(4), 350–264.

225. Sabin, C. A., Fisher, M., Churchill, D., et al. (2001) Long-term follow-up of antiretroviral-naïve HIV-positive patients treated with nevirapine, *J. Acquir. Immune Defic. Syndr.*, **26**(5), 462–465.

226. Matthews, G. V., Sabin, C. A., Mandalia, S., et al. (2002) Virological suppression at 6 months is related to choice of initial regimen in antiretroviral-naïve patients: a cohort study, *AIDS*, **16**(1), 53–61.

227. Phillips, A. N., Pradier, C., Lazzarin, A., et al. (2001) Viral load outcome of non-nucleoside reverse transcriptase inhibitor regimens for 2203 mainly antiretroviral-experienced patients, *AIDS*, **15**(18), 2385–2395.

228. Cozzi-Lepri, A., Phillips, A. N., d'Arminio, M. A., et al. (2002) Virologic and immunologic response to regimens containing nevirapine or efavirenz in combination with 2 nucleoside analogues in the Italian Cohort Naïve Antiretrovirals (I.Co.N.A.) study, *J. Infect. Dis.*, **185**(8), 1063–1069.

229. Raboud, J. M., Rae, S., Vella, S., et al. (1999) Meta-analysis of two randomized controlled trials comparing combined zidovudine and didanosine therapy with combined zidovudine, didanosine, and nevirapine therapy in patients with HIV, INCAS study team, *J. Acquir. Immune Defic. Syndr.*, **22**(3), 260–266.

230. Raffi, F., Reliquet, V., Podzamczer, D., and Pollard, R. B. (2001) Efficacy of nevirapine-based HAART in HIV-1-infected treatment-naïve persons with high and low baseline viral loads, *HIV Clin. Trials*, **2**(4), 317–322.

231. Yozviak, J. L., Doerfler, R. E., and Woodward, W. C. (2001) Effectiveness and tolerability of nevirapine, stavudine, and lamivudine in clinical practice, *HIV Clin. Trials*, **2**(6), 474–476.

232. Skowron, G., Street, J. C., and Obee, E. M. (2001) CD4(+) cell count, not viral load, correlates with virologic suppression induced by potent antiretroviral therapy, *J. Acquir. Immune Defic. Syndr.*, **28**(4), 313–319.

233. Staszewski, S., Morales-Ramirez, J., Tashima, K. T., et al. (1999) Efavirenz plus zidovudine and lamivudine, efavirenz plus indinavir, and indinavir plus zidovudine and lamivudine in the treatment of HIV-1 infection in adults. Study 006 Team, *N. Engl. J. Med.*, **341**(25), 1865–1873.

234. Jordan, W. C., Jefferson, R., Yemofio, F., et al. (2000) Nevirapine + efavirenz + didanosine: a very simple, safe, and effective once-daily regimen, *XIIIth International AIDS Conference, Durban, South Africa*, July 9–14 [abstract TuPeB3207].

235. Olivieri, J. (2002) Nevirapine + efavirenz based salvage therapy in heavily pretreated HIV infected patients, *Sex. Transm. Infect.*, **78**(1), 72–73.

236. Veldkamp, A. I., Harris, M., Montaner, J. S., et al. (2001) The steady-state pharmacokinetics of efavirenz and nevirapine when used in combination in human immunodeficiency virus type 1-infected persons, *J. Infect. Dis.*, **184**(1), 37–42.

237. van Leth, F., Phanuphak, P., Ruxrungtham, K., et al. (2004) Comparison of the first-line antiretroviral therapy with regimens including nevirapine, efavirenz, or both drugs, plus stavudine and lamivudine: a randomized open-label trial, the 2NN Study, *Lancet*, **363**(9417), 1253–1263.

238. Deeks, S. G., Hellmann, N. S., Grant, R. M., et al. (1999) Novel four-drug salvage treatment regimens after failure of a human immunodeficiency virus type 1 protease inhibitor-containing regimen: antiviral activity and correlation of baseline phenotypic drug susceptibility with virologic outcome, *J. Infect. Dis.*, **179**(6), 1375–1381.

239. Manfredi, R. and Chiodo, F. (2001) Limits of deep salvage antiretroviral therapy with nelfinavir plus either efavirenz or nevirapine, in highly pre-treated patients with HIV disease, *Int. J. Antimicrob. Agents*, **17**(6), 511–516.

240. Jensen-Fangel, S., Thomsen, H. F., Larsen, L., Black, F. T., and Obel, N. (2001) The effect of nevirapine in combination with nelfinavir in heavily pretreated HIV-1-infected patients: a prospective, open-label, controlled, randomized study, *J. Acquir. Immune Defic. Syndr.*, **27**(2), 124–129.

241. Perez-Molina, J. A., Perez, N. R., Miralles, P., et al. (2001) Nelfinavir plus nevirapine plus two NRTIs as salvage therapy for HIV-infected patients receiving long-term retroviral treatment, *HIV Clin. Trials*, **2**(1), 1–5.

242. Benson, C. A., Deeks, S. G., Brun, S. C., et al. (2002) Safety and antiviral activity at 48 weeks of lopinavir/ritonavir plus nevirapine and 2 nucleoside reverse-transcriptase inhibitors in human immunodeficiency virus type 1-infected protease inhibitor-experienced patients, *J. Infect. Dis.*, **185**(5), 599–607.

243. Harris, M., Durakovic, C., Rae, S., et al. (1998) A pilot study of nevirapine, indinavir, and lamivudine among patients with advanced human immunodeficiency virus disease who have had failure of combination nucleoside therapy, *J. Infect. Dis.*, **177**(6), 1514–1520.

244. Casado, J. L., Dronda, F., Hertogs, K., et al. (2001) Efficacy, tolerance, and pharmacokinetics of the combination of stavudine, nevirapine, nelfinavir, and saquinavir as salvage regimen after ritonavir or indinavir failure, *AIDS Res. Hum. Retroviruses*, **17**(2), 93–98.

245. Gulick, R. M., Smeaton, L. M., D'Aquila, R. T., et al. (2001) Indinavir, nevirapine, stavudine, and lamivudine for human immunodeficiency virus-infected, amprenavir-experienced subjects: AIDS Clinical Trials Group protocol 373, *J. Infect. Dis.*, **183**(5), 715–721.

246. Sullivan, A. K., Nelson, M. R., Shaw, A., et al. (2000) Efficacy of a nelfinavir- and nevirapine-containing salvage regimen, *HIV Clin. Trials*, **1**(1), 7–12.

247. Parkin, N. T., Deeks, S. G., Wrin, M. T., et al. (2000) Loss of antiretroviral drug susceptibility at low viral load during early virological failure in treatment-experienced patients, *AIDS*, **14**(18), 2877–2887.

248. Lorenzi, P., Opravil, M., Hirschel, B., et al. (1999) Impact of drug resistance mutations on virologic response to salvage therapy. Swiss HIV Cohort Study, *AIDS*, **13**(2), F17–F21.

249. Carr, A., Samaras, K., Burton, S., et al. (1998) A syndrome of peripheral lipodystrophy, hyperlipidaemia and insulin resistance in patients receiving HIV protease inhibitors, *AIDS*, **12**(7), F51–F58.

250. Mauss, S., Corzillius, M., Wolf, E., et al. (2002) Risk factors for the HIV-associated lipodystrophy syndrome in a closed cohort of patients after 3 years of antiretroviral treatment, *HIV Med.*, **3**(1), 49–55.

251. Amin, J., Moore, A., Carr, A., et al. (2003) Combined analysis of two years follow-up from two open-label randomized trials comparing efficacy of three nucleoside reverse transcriptase inhibitor backbones for previously untreated HIV-1 infection: OzCombo 1 and 2, *HIV Clin. Trials*, **4**(4), 252–261.

252. Shevitz, A., Wanke, C. A., Falutz, J., and Kotler, D. P. (2001) Clinical perspectives on HIV-associated lipodystrophy syndrome: an update, *AIDS*, **15**(15), 1917–1930.

253. Martinez, E., Conget, I., Lozano, L., Casamitjana, R., and Gatell, J. M. (1999) Reversion of metabolic abnormalities after switching from HIV-1 protease inhibitors to nevirapine, *AIDS*, **13**(7), 805–810.

254. Barreiro, P., Soriano, V., Blanco, F., Casimiro, C., de la Cruz, J. J., and Gonzalez-Lahoz, J. (2000) Risks and benefits of replacing protease inhibitors by nevirapine in HIV-infected subjects under long-term successful triple combination therapy, *AIDS*, **14**(7), 807–812.

255. De Lucca, A., Baldini, F., Cingolani, A., et al. (2000) Benefits and risks of switching from protease inhibitors to nevirapine with stable background therapy in patients with low or undetectable viral load: a multicentre study, *AIDS*, **14**(11), 1655–1656.

256. Carr, A., Hudson, J., Chuah, J., et al. (2001) HIV protease inhibitor substitution in patients with lipodystrophy: a randomized, controlled, open-label, multicentre study, *AIDS*, **15**(14), 1811–1822.

257. Gonzalez de Requena, D., Nunez, M., Jimenez-Nacher, I., and Soriano, V. (2002) Liver toxicity caused by nevirapine, *AIDS*, **16**(2), 290–291.

258. Ruiz, L., Negredo, E., Domingo, P., et al. (2001) Antiretroviral treatment simplification with nevirapine in protease inhibitor-experienced patients with HIV-associated lipodystrophy: 1-year prospective follow-up of a multicenter, randomized, controlled study, *J. Acquir. Immune Defic. Syndr.*, **27**(3), 229–236.

259. Masquelier, B., Neau, D., Chene, G., et al. (2001) Mechanism of virologic failure after substitution of a protease inhibitor by nevirapine in patients with suppressed plasma HIV-1 RNA, *J. Acquir. Immune Defic. Syndr.*, **28**(4), 309–312.

260. Domingo-P., Matias-Guiu, X., Pujol, R. M., et al. (2001) Switching to nevirapine decreases insulin levels but does not improve subcutaneous adipocyte apoptosis in patients with highly active antiretroviral therapy-associated lipodystrophy, *J. Infect. Dis.*, **184**(9), 1197–1201.

261. Negredo, E., Cruz, L., Paredes, R., et al. (2002) Virological, immunological, and clinical impact of switching from protease inhibitors to nevirapine or to efavirenz in patients with human immunodeficiency virus infection and long-lasting viral suppression, *Clin. Infect. Dis.*, **34**(4), 504–510.

262. Dieleman, J. P., Sturkenboom, M. C., Wit, F. W., et al. (2002) Low risk of treatment failure after substitution of nevirapine for protease inhibitors among human immunodeficiency virus-infected patients with virus suppression, *J. Infect. Dis.*, **185**(9), 1261–1268.

263. Negredo, E., Ribalta, J., Paredes, R., et al. (2002) Reversal of atherogenic lipoprotein profile in HIV-1 infected patients with lipodystrophy after replacing protease inhibitors by nevirapine, *AIDS*, **16**(10), 1383–1389.

264. Barreiro, P., Camino, N., De Julian, R., Gonzalez-Lahoz, J., and Soriano, V. (2003) Replacement of protease inhibitors by nevirapine or efavirenz in simplification and rescue interventions: which works better? *HIV Clin. Trials*, **4**(4), 244–247.

265. Bucciardini, R., Wu, A. W., Floridia, M., et al. (2000) Quality of life outcomes of combination zidovudine-didanosine-nevirapine and zidovudine-didanosine for antiretroviral-naïve advanced HIV-infected patients, *AIDS*, **14**(16), 2567–2574.

266. Conway, B. (2000) Initial therapy with protease inhibitor-sparing regimens: evaluation of nevirapine and delavirdine, *Clin. Infect. Dis.*, **30**(Suppl. 2), S130-S134.

267. Murphy, R. L. and Smith, W. J. (2002) Switch studies: a review, *HIV Med.*, **3**(2), 146–155.

268. Gathe, J. C., Jr., Ive, P., Wood, R., et al. (2004) SOLO: 48-week efficacy and safety comparison of once-daily fosamprenavir/ritonavir versus twice-daily nelfinavir in naïve HIV-1-infected patients, *AIDS*, **18**(11), 1529–1537.

269. Erickson, D. A., Mather, G., Trager, W. F., Levy, R. H., and Keirns, J. J. (1999) Characterization of the in vitro biotransformation of HIV-1 reverse transcriptase inhibitor nevirapine by human hepatic cytochrome P-450, *Drug Metab. Dispos.*, **27**(12), 1488–1495.

270. Sahai, J., Cameron, W., Salgo, M., et al. (1997) Drug interaction study between saquinavir and nevirapine, *4th Conference on Retroviruses and Opportunistic Infections, Washington, D.C.*, January 22–26 [abstract 496].

271. Merry, C., Barry, M. G., Mulcahy, F., et al., (1998) The pharmacokinetics of combination therapy with nelfinavir plus nevirapine, *AIDS*, **12**(10), 1163–1167.

272. Skowron, G., Leoung, G., Kerr, B., et al. (1998) Lack of pharmacokinetic interaction between nelfinavir and nevirapine, *AIDS*, **12**(10), 1243–1244.

273. Murphy, R. L., Sommadossi, J. P., Lamson, M., Hall, D. B., Hall, D. B., Myers, M., and Dusek, A. (1999) Antiviral effect and pharmacokinetic interaction between nevirapine and indinavir in persons infected with human immunoderficiency virus type 1, *J. Infect. Dis.*, **179**(1), 1116–1123.

274. Lal, R., Hsu, A., Bertz, R., et al. (1999) Evaluation of the pharmacokinetics of the concurrent administration of ABT-378/ritonavir and nevirapine, *7th European Conference on the Clinical Aspects and Treatment of HIV-Infection, Lisbon, Portugal*, October 23–27 [abstract 782].

275. Luzuriaga, K., Bryson, Y., McSherry, G., et al. (1996) Pharmacokinetics, safety, and activity of nevirapine in human immunodeficiency virus type 1-infected children, *J. Infect. Dis.*, **174**(4), 713–721.

276. Verweel, G., Sharland, M., Lyall, H., et al. (2003) Nevirapine use in HIV-1-infected children, *AIDS*, **17**(11), 1639–1647.

277. Pollard, R. B., Robinson, P., and Dransfield, K. (1998) Safety profile of nevirapine, a nonnucleoside reverse transcriptase inhibitor for the treatment of human immunodeficiency virus infection, *Clin. Ther.*, **20**(6), 1071–1092.

278. Stern, J., Lanes, S., Love, J., Robinson, P., Imperiale, M., and Mayers, D. (2003) Hepatic safety of nevirapine: results of the Boehringer Ingelheim Viramune®Hepatic Safety Project, *XIV International AIDS Conference, Barcelona, Spain*, July 7–12 [abstract LBOR15].

279. Warren, K. J., Boxwell, D. E., Kim, N. Y., and Drolet, B. A. (1998) Nevirapine-associated Stevens-Johnson syndrome, *Lancet*, **351**(9102), 567.

280. Dodi, F., Alessandrini, A., Camera, M., Gaffuri, L., Morandi, N., and Pagano, G. (2002) Stevens-Johnson syndrome in HIV patients treated with nevirapine: two case reports, *AIDS*, **16**(8), 1197–1198.

281. Fagot, J. P., Mockenhaupt, M., Bouwes-Bavinck, J. N., Naldi, L., Viboud, C., and Roujeau, J. C. (2001) Nevirapine and the risk of Stevens-Johnson syndrome or toxic epidermal necrolysis, *AIDS*, **15**(14), 1843–1848.

282. Bourezane, Y., Salard, D., Hoen, B., Vandel, S., Drobacheff, C., and Laurent, R. (1998) DRESS (drug rash with eosinophilia and systemic symptoms) syndrome associated with nevirapine therapy, *Clin. Infect. Dis.*, **27**(5), 1321–1322.

283. Lanzafame, M., Rovere, P., De Checchi, G., Trevenzoli, M., Turazzini, M., and Parrinello, A. (2001) Hypersensitivity syndrome (DRESS) and meningoencephalitis associated with nevirapine therapy, *Scand. J. Infect. Dis.*, **33**(6), 475–476.

284. Cattelan, A. M., Erne, E., Salatino, A., et al. (1999) Severe hepatic failure related to nevirapine treatment, *Clin. Infect. Dis.*, **29**(2), 455–456.

285. Jarrousse, B., Cohen, P., Berlureau, P., Bentata, M., Mahr, A., and Guillevin, L. (1999) Nevirapine induced fulminant hepatitis: presentation of case and analysis of risk factors, *7th European Conference on the Clinical Aspects and Treatment of HIV-Infection, Lisbon, Portugal*, October 23–27 [abstract 1009].

286. Mateu, S., Gurgui, M., Sambeat, M. A., et al. (1999) Cholestatic hepatitis by nevirapine: report of five cases, *7th European Conference on the Clinical Aspects and Treatment of HIV-Infection, Lisbon, Portugal*, October 23–27 [abstract 1080].

287. Clarke, S., Harrington, P., Condon, C., Kelleher, D., Smith, O. P., and Mulcahy, F. (2000) Late onset hepatitis and prolonged deterioration in hepatic function associated with nevirapine therapy, *Int. J. STD AIDS*, **11**(5), 336–337.

288. Nunez, M., Lana, R., Mendoza, J. L., Martin-Carbonero, L., and Soriano, V. (2001) Risk factors for severe hepatic injury after introduction of highly active antiretroviral therapy, *J. Acquir. Immune Defic. Syndr.*, **27**(5), 426–431.

289. Prakash, M., Poredy, V., Tiyyagura, L., and Bonacini, M. (2001) Jaundice and hepatocellular damage associated with nevirapine therapy, *Am. J. Gastroenterol.*, **96**(5), 1571–1574.

290. Johnson, S., Baraboutis, J. G., Sha, B. E., Proia, L. A., and Kessler, H. A. (2000) Adverse effects associated with use of nevirapine in HIV postexposure prophylaxis for 2 health care workers, *J. Am. Med. Assoc.*, **284**(21), 2722–2723.

291. Benn, P. D., Mercey, D. E., Brink, N., Scott, G., and Williams, I. G. (2001) Prophylaxis with a nevirapine-containing triple regimen after exposure to HIV-1, *Lancet*, **367**(9257), 687–688.

292. Martinez, E., Blanco, J. L., Arnaiz, J. A., et al. (2001) Hepatotoxicity in HIV-1-infected patients receiving nevirapine-containing antiretroviral therapy, *AIDS*, **15**(10), 1261–1268.

293. Gonzalez de Requena, D., Nunez, M., Jimenez-Nacher, I., and Soriano, V. (2002) Liver toxicity caused by nevirapine, *AIDS*, **16**(2), 290–291.

294. Veldkamp, A. I., Meenhorst, P. L., Mulder, J. W., and Beijnen, J. H. (2001) HAART, or just mini-HAART? *J. Acquir. Defic. Syndr.*, **28**(5), 495–496.

295. Lamson, M., Robinson, P., McDonough, M., Hutman, H. W., MacGregor, T., and Nusrat, R. (2000) The effects of underlying renal or hepatic dysfunction on the pharmacokinetics of nevirapine, *XIII International AIDS Conference, Durban, South Africa*, July 9–14 [abstract TuPeB3301].

296. Moyle, G. J. and Conway, B. (2006) Efavirenz. In: *Reverse Transcriptase Inhibitors in HIV/AIDS Therapy* (Skowron, G. and Ogden, R., eds.), Humana Press, Totowa, NJ, pp. 345–373.

297. Rabel, S. R., Maurin, M. B., Rowe, S. M., and Hussain, M. (1996) Determination of the pKa and pH-solubility behavior of an ionizable cyclic carbamate, (S)-(−)-6-chloro-4-(cyclopropylethynyl)-4-(trifluoromethyl)-2,4-dihydro-1H-3,1-benzoxazin-2-one (MDP 266), *Pharm. Dev. Technol.*, **1**, 91–95.

298. Starr, S. E., Fletcher, C. V., Spector, S. A., et al., and the PACTG 382 Study Team, for the Pediatric AIDS Clinical Trials Group (2002) Efavirenz liquid formulation in human immunodeficiency virus-infected children, *Pediatr. Infect. Dis.*, **21**, 659–663.

299. Young, S. D., Britcher, S. F., Tran, L. O., et al. (1995) L-743,726 (DMP-266): a novel, highly potent non-nucleoside inhibitor of the human immunodeficiency virus type 1 reverse transcriptase, *Antimicrob. Agents Chemother.*, **39**, 2602–2605.

300. Erickson, J. W. and Burt, S. K. (1996) Structural mechanisms of HIV drug resistance, *Ann. Rev. Pharmacol. Toxicol.*, **36**, 545–571.

301. D'Aquila, R. T. (1994) HIV-1 drug resistance: molecular pathogenesis and laboratory monitoring, *Clin. Lab. Med.*, **14**, 393–423.

302. Arnold, E., Ding, J., Hughes, S. H., and Hostomsky, Z. (1995) Structures of DNA and RNA polymerases and their interactions with nucleic acid substrates, *Curr. Opin. Struct. Biol.*, **5**, 27–38.

303. Winslow, D. L., Garber, S., Reid, C., et al. (1996) Selection conditions affect the evolution of specific mutations in the reverse transcriptase gene associated with resistance to DMP 266, *AIDS*, **10**(11), 1205–1209.

304. Jeffrey, S., Baker, D., Tritch, R., Rizzo, C., Logue, K., and Bacheler, L. (1998) A resistance and cross-resistance profile for Sustiva (efavirenz, DMP 266), *5th Conference on Retroviruses and Opportunistic Infections, Chicago, IL*, February 1–5 [abstract 702].

305. Bacheler, L. T., Anton, E. D., Kudish, P., et al. (2000) Human immunodeficiency virus type 1 mutations selected in patients failing efavirenz combination therapy, *Antimicrob. Agents Chemother.*, **44**(9), 2475–2484.

306. Jeffrey, S., Corbett, J., and Bacheler, L. (1999) In vitro NNRTI resistance of recombinant HIV carrying mutations observed in efavirenz treatment failures, *6th Conference on Retroviruses and Opportunistic Infections, Chicago, IL*, January 31–February 4 [abstract 110].

307. Bacheler, L. T., Anton, E., Jeffrey, S., George, H., Hollis, G., Abremski, K., and the Sustiva Resistance Study Team (1998) RT gene mutations associated with resistance to efavirenz, *2nd International Workshop on HIV Drug Resistance and Treatment Strategies, Lake Maggiore, Italy*, June 24–27 [abstract 19].

308. Bacheler, L., George, H., Hollis, G., Abremski, K., and the Sustiva Resistance Study Team (1998) Resistance to efavirenz (Sustiva) in vivo, *5th Conference on Retroviruses and Opportunistic Infections, Chicago, IL*, February 1–5 [abstract 703].

309. Hsiou, Y., Ding, J., Das, K., et al. (2001) The Lys103Asn mutation of HIV-1 RT: a novel mechanism of drug resistance, *J. Mol. Biol.*, **309**, 437–445.

310. Bacheler, L., Jeffrey, S., Hanna, G., et al. (2001) Genotypic correlates of phenotypic resistance to efavirenz in virus isolates from patients failing nonnucleoside reverse transcriptase inhibitor therapy, *J. Virol.*, **75**, 4999–5008.

311. Brenner, B., Turner, D., Oliveira, M., et al. (2003) A V106M mutation in HIV-1 clade C viruses exposed to efavirenz confers cross-resistance to non-nucleoside reverse transcriptase inhibitors, *AIDS*, **17**, F1–F5.

312. Shulman, N. S., Bosch, R. J., Mellors, J. W., Albrecht, M. A., and Katzenstein, D. A. (2004) Genetic correlates of efavirenz hypersusceptibility, *AIDS*, **18**(13), 1781–1785.

313. Shulman, N., Zolopa, A. R., Passaro, D., et al. (2001) Phenotypic hypersusceptibility to non-nucleoside reverse transcriptase inhibitors in treatment-experienced HIV-infected patients: impact on virological response to efavirenz-based therapy, *AIDS*, **15**, 1125–1132.

314. AIDSinfo (2007) U.S. Department of Health and Human Services: Guidelines for the Use of Antiretroviral Agents in HIV-1-Infected Adults and Adolescents—December 1, 2007 (http://aidsinfo.nih.gov/guidelines/GuidelineDetail.aspx?MenuItem=Guidelines& Search=Off&GuidelineID=7& ClassID=1).

315. Mayers, D., Jemsek, J., Eyster, E., et al., for the Efavirenz Clinical Development Team and the DMP 266-044 Study Team (1998) A double-blind, placebo-controlled study to assess the safety, tolerability and antiviral activity of efavirenz (EFV, Sustiva, DMP 266) in combination with open-label zidovudine (ZDV) and lamivudine (3TC) in HIV-1 infected patients [DMP 266-004], *12th World AIDS Conference, Geneva, Switzerland*, June 28–July 3 [abstract 22340].

316. Haas, D. W., Seeking, D., Cooper, R., et al., for the Efavirenz Clinical Development Team and the DMP 266-044 Study Team (1998) A Phase II double-blind, placebo-controlled, dose-ranging study to assess the antiretroviral activity and safety of efavirenz (RFV, Sustiva, DMP 266) in combination with open-label zidovudine (ZDV) and lamivudine (3TC) at 36 weeks [DMP 266-005], *12th World AIDS Conference, Geneva, Switzerland*, June 28–July 3 [abstract 22334].

317. Moyle, G. J. (2000) Considerations in the choice of protease inhibitor-sparing regimens in initial therapy for HIV-1 infection, *Curr. Opin. Infect. Dis.*, **13**, 19–25.

318. BHIVA Writing Committee (2001) British HIV Association (BHIVA) guidelines for the treatment of HIV-infected adults with antiretroviral therapy, *HIV Med.*, **2**, 276–313.

319. Yeni, P. G., Hammer, S. M., Carpenter, C. C., et al. (2002) Antiretroviral treatment for adult HIV infection in 2002: updated recommendations of the International AIDS Society-USA Panel, *J. Am. Med. Assoc.*, **288**, 222–235.

320. Department of Health and Human Services (DHHS) (2005) Guidelines for the Use of Antiretroviral Agents in HIV-Infected Adults and Adolescents (http://aidsinfo.nih.gov/guidelines/).

321. Moyle, G. J., Wilkins, E., Leen, C., Cheesbrough, A., Reynolds, B., and Gazzard, B. G. (2000) Salvage therapy with abacavir plus efavirenz or nevirapine in HIV-1-infected persons with previous nucleoside analogue and protease inhibitor use, *AIDS*, **14**, 1453–1454.

322. Keiser, P., Nassar, N., White, C., Koen, G., and Moreno, S. (2001) Comparison of efavirenz-containing regimens to nevirapine-containing regimens in antiretroviral-naive HIV infected patients: a cohort study, *8th European Conference on Clinical Aspects and Treatment of HIV Infection, Athens, Greece*, October 28–31 [abstract].

323. Albrecht, M. A., Borsch, R. J., Liou, S. H., and Katzenstein, D. (2002) ACTG 364: efficacy of nelfinavir (NFV) and/or efavirenz (AFV) in combination with new NRTIs in nucleoside experienced subjects: week-144 study, *9th Conference on Retroviruses and Opportunistic Infections, Seattle, Washington*, February 24–28 [abstract 425-W].

324. Moyle, G., Baldwin, C., Mandalia, S., Comitis, S., Burn, P., and Gazzard, B. (2001) Changes in metabolic parameters and body shape after replacement of protease inhibitor with efavirenz in virologically controlled HIV-1-positive persons: single-arm observational cohort, *J. Acquir. Immune Defic. Syndr.*, **28**, 399–401.

325. Katlama, C., Rachilis, A., Staszewski, S., and the Study 027 and 049 Teams (2001) Better virologic suppression after substitution of protease inhibitors with efavirenz in patients with unquantifiable viral loads, *8th European Conference on Clinical Aspects and Treatment of HIV Infection, Athens, Greece*, October 28–31 [abstract].

326. Hirschel, B., Flepp, M., Bucher, H. C., et al., and the Swiss HIV Cohort (2002) Switching from protease inhibitors to efavirenz: differences in efficacy and tolerance among risk groups: a case-control study from the Swiss HIV Cohort, *AIDS*, **16**, 381–385.

327. Starr, S. E., Fletcher, C. V., Spector, S. A., et al., for the Pediatric AIDS Clinical Trials Group 382 Team (1999) Combination therapy with efavirenz, nelfinavir, and nucleoside reverse-transcriptase inhibitors in children with human immunodeficiency virus type 1, *N. Engl. J. Med.*, **341**, 1874–1881.

328. McComsey, G., Alvarez, A., Joseph, J., Rathore, P., and Lederman, M. (2001) Is simplification of HAART safe in HIV-infected children? First pediatric swith study, *5th Conference on Retroviruses and Opportunistic Infections, Chicago, IL*, February 4–8 [abstract 679].

329. Bacheler, L. T., Anton, E., Baker, D., et al. (1997) Impact of mutation, plasma protein binding and pharmacokinetics on clinical efficacy of the HIV-1 non nucleoside reverse transcriptase inhibitor, DMP 266, *37th Interscience Conference on Antimicrobial Agents and Chemotherapy, Toronto, Canada*, September 28–October 1 [abstract I-115].

330. Joshi, A., Fiske, W. D., Benedek, I. H., White, S. J., Joseph, J. L., and Kornhauser, D. M. (1998) Lack of pharmacokinetic interaction between efavirenz (DMP 266) and ethinyl estradiol in healthy volunteers, *5th Conference on Retroviruses and OpportunisticInfections, Chicago, IL*, February 4–8 [abstract 348].

331. Graul, A., Rabasseda, X., and Castaner, J. (1998) Efavirenz, *Drugs Future*, **23**, 133–141.

332. Mayers, D., Riddler, S., Stein, D., Bach, M., Havlir, D., and Kahn, J. (1996) A double blind pilot study to evaluate the antiviral activity, tolerability and pharmacokinetics of DMP 266 alone and in combination with indinavir, *36th Interscience Conference on Antimicrobial Agents and Chemotherapy, New Orleans, LA*, September 15–18 [abstract LB8a].

333. Fiske, W. D., Benedek, I. H., Joseph, J. L., et al. (1998) Pharmacokinetics of efavirenz (EFV) and ritonavir (RTV) after multiple oral doses in healthy volunteers, *12th World AIDS Conference, Geneva, Switzerland*, June 28–July 3 [abstract 42269].

334. Benedek, I. H., Joshi, A., Fiske, W. D., et al. (1998) Pharmacokinetic interaction between efavirenz (EFV) and rifampin (RIF) in healthy volunteers, *12th World AIDS Conference, Geneva, Switzerland*, June 28–July 3 [abstract 42280].

335. Benedek, I. H., Joshi, A., Fiske, W. D., et al. (1998) Pharmacokinetic (PK) interaction studies with efavirenz (EFV) and the macrolide antibiotics azitromycin (AZM) and clarithromycin (CLR), *5th Conference on Retroviruses and Opportunistic Infections, Chicago, IL*, February 4–8 [abstract 347].

336. Fiske, W. D., Benedek, I. H., White, S. J., Joseph, J. L., and Kornhauser, D. M. (1997) Pharmacokinetic interaction between DMP 266 and nelfinavir mesylate (NFV) in healthy volunteers, *37th Interscience Conference on Antimicrobial Agents and Chemotherapy, Toronto, Canada*, September 28–October 1 [abstract I-174].

337. Fiske, W. D., Mayers, D., Wagner, K., et al. and the DMP 266 Development Team (1997) Pharmacokinetics of DMP 266 and indinavir multiple oral doses in HIV-1 infected individuals, *4th Conference on Retroviruses and Opportunistic Infections, Washington, D.C.*, January 22–26 [abstract].

338. Fiske, W. D., Benedek, I. H., Joshi, A. S., Joseph, J. L., and Kornhauser, D. M. (1998) Summary of pharmacokinetic drug interactions studies with efavirenz, *36th Annual Meeting of the Infectious Disease Society of America, Denver, CO*, November 12–15 [abstract 460].

339. Bristol-Myers Squibb Company (2002) Sustiva package insert, Bristol-Myers Squibb Co., Princeton, NJ.

340. Hendrix, C. W., Fiske, W. D., Fuchs, E. J., et al. (2000) Pharmacokinetics of the triple combination of saquinavir, ritonavir and efavirenz in HIV positive patients, *7th Conference on Retroviruses and Opportunistic Infections, San Francisco, CA*, January 30–February 2 [abstract].

341. Abbott Laboratories (2008) Kaletra package insert, Abbott Laboratories, North Chicago, IL.

342. Romero, D. L., Busso, M., Tan, C. K., et al. (1991) Nonnucleoside reverse transcriptase inhibitors that potently and specifically block human immunodeficiency virus type 1 replication, *Proc. Natl. Acad. Sci. U.S.A.*, **88**, 8806–8810.

343. Busso, M., Mian, A. M., Hahn, E. F., and Resnick, L. (1988) Nucleotide dimers suppress HIV expression in vitro, *AIDS Res. Hum. Retroviruses*, **4**, 449–455.

344. Tan, C. K., Zhang, J., Li, Z. Y., Tarpley, W. G., Downey, K. M., and So, A. G. (1991) Functional characterization of RNA-dependent DNA polymerase and RNase H activities of a recombinant HIV reverse transcriptase, *Biochemistry*, **30**, 2651–2655.

345. Freimuth, W. W. (1996) Delavurdine mesylate, a potent non-nucleoside HIV-1 reverse transcriptase inhibitor, *Adv. Exp. Med. Biol.*, **394**, 279–289.

346. Esnouf, R. M., Ren, J., Hopkins, A. L., et al. (1997) Unique features in the structure of the complex between HIV-1 reverse transcriptase and the bis(heteroaryl)piperazine (BHAP) U-90152 explain resistance mutations for this nonnucleoside inhibitor, *Proc. Natl. Acad. Sci. U.S.A.*, **94**, 3984–3989.

347. Althaus, I. W., Chou, J. J., Gonzales, A. J., et al. (1994) Kinetic studies with the non-nucleoside human immunodeficiency virus type-1 reverse transcriptase inhibitor U-90152S, *Biochem. Pharmacol.*, **47**, 2017–2028.

348. Dueweke, T. J., Poppe, S. M., Romero, D. L., et al. (1993) U-90152, a potent inhibitor of human immunodeficiency virus type 1 replication, *Antimicrob. Agents Chemother.*, **37**, 1127–1131.

349. Conway, B. (2006) Delavirdine. In: *Reverse Transcriptase Inhibitors in HIV/AIDS Therapy* (Skowron, G. and Ogde, R., eds.), Humana Press, Totowa, NJ, pp. 375–400.

350. Demeter, L. M., Shafer, R. W., Meehan, P. M., et al. (2000) Delavirdine susceptibilities and associated reverse transcriptase mutations in human immunodeficiency virus type 1 isolates from patients in a phase I/I trial of delavirdine monotherapy (ACTG 260), *Antimicrob. Agents Chemother.*, **44**, 794–797.

351. Gerondelis, P., Archer, R. H., Palaniappan, C., et al. (1999) The P236L delavirdine-resistant human immunodeficiency virus type 1 mutant is replication defective and demonstrates alterations in both RNA 5'-end and DNA 3'-end-directed RNase H activities, *J. Virol.*, **73**(7), 5803–5813.

352. Friedland, G. H., Pollard, R., Griffith, B., et al. (1999) Efficacy and safety of delavirdine mesylate with zidovudine and didanosine compared with two-drug combinations of these agents in persons with HIV disease with CD4 counts of 100 to 500 cells/mm3 (ACTG 261). ACTG 261 Team, *J. Acquir. Immune Defic. Syndr.*, **21**, 281–292.

353. Conway, B. (2000) Initial therapy with protease inhibitor-sparing regimens: evaluation of nevirapine and delavirdine, *Clin. Infect. Dis.*, **30**(Suppl. 2), S130–S134.

354. Wood, R., Hawkins, D. A., Moyle, G., De Cain, W., Ingrosso, A., and Greenwald, C. (1999) Second placebo-controlled study in naïve individuals confirms the role of delavirdine in highly active antiretroviral, protease-sparing treatment, *6th Conference on Retroviruses and Opportunistic Infections, Chicago, IL*, January 31–February 4 [abstract 624].

355. Kuritzkes, D. R., Bassett, R. L., Johnson, V. A., et al. (2000) Continued lamivudine versus delavirdine in combination with indinavir and zidovudine or stavudine in lamivudine-experienced patients: results of Adult AIDS Clinical Trials Group Protocol 370, *AIDS*, **14**, 1553–1561.

356. Smith, G. H., Boulassel, M. R., Klein, M, et al., (2004) Virologic and immunologic response to a boosted double-protease inhibitor-based therapy in highly pretreated HIV-1 infected patients, *HIV Clin. Trials*, **6**, 63–72.

357. Gatell, J., Kuritzkes, D., and Green, S. (1999) Twice daily dosing of delavirdine in combination with nelfinavir, didanosine, and stavudine results in significant decreases in viral burden, *39th Interscience Conference on Antimicrobial Agents and Chemotherapy, San Francisco, CA*, September 26–29 [abstract 520].

358. Conway, B., Chu, A., Tran, T., et al., for the 0081 Study Group (2001) A pilot study of combinations of delavirdine (DLV), zidovudine (ZDV), lamivudine (3TC), and saquinavir-SGC (Fortovase®, FTV) as initial antiretroviral therapy: virologic and pharmacokinetic considerations, *8th Conference on Retroviruses and Opportunistic Infections, Chicago, IL*, February 4–8 [abstract 331].

359. Eron, J., Chu, A., Petersen, C., et al. (2001) 48 week efficacy of triple drug HAART containing delavirdine and reduced dose indinavir is comparable to HAART containing full dose indinavir, *1st IAS Conference on HIVPathogenesis and Treatment, Buenos Aires, Argentina*, July 8–11 [abstract 232].

360. Bellman, P. C. (1998) Clinical experience with adding delavirdine to combination therapy in patients in whom multiple antiretroviral treatment including protease inhibitors has failed, *AIDS*, **12**, 1333–1340.

361. Smith, D., Hales, G., Roth, N., et al. (2001) A randomized trial of nelfinavir, ritonavir, or delavirdine in combination with saquinavir-SGC and stavudine in treatment-experienced HIV-1-infected patients, *HIV Clin. Trials*, **2**, 97–107.

362. Blanco, J. L., Mallolas, J., Sarasa, M., et al. (2000) A pilot study of a twice daily (BID) combination of indinavir/delavirdine plus two nucleoside analogues for salvage therapy in HIV-1 infected patients, *40th Interscience Conference on Antimicrobial Agents and Chemotherapy, Toronto, Canada*, September 17–20 [abstract 1543].

363. Baril, J. G., Lefebvre, E. A., Lalonde, R. G., Shafran, S. D., and Conway, B. (2003) Nelfinavir and non-nucleoside reverse transcriptase inhibitor-based salvage regimens in heavily HIV pretreated patients, *Can. J. Infect. Dis.*, **14**, 201–205.

364. Tran, J. Q., Gerber, J. G., and Kerr, B. M. (2001) Delavirdine: clinical pharmacokinetics and drug interactions, *Clin. Pharmacokinet.*, **40**, 207–226.

365. Cox, S. R., Schneck, D. W., Herman, B. D., et al. (1998) Delavirdine (DLV) and nelfinavir (NFV): a pharmacokinetic (PK) drug-drug interaction study in healthy adult volunteers, *5th Conferences on Retroviruses and Opportunistic Infections, Chicago, IL*, February 1–5 [abstract 345].

366. Morse, G. D., Fischl, M. A., Shelton, M. J., et al. (1997) Single-dose pharmacokinetics of delavirdine mesylate and didanosine in patients with human immunodeficiency virus infection, *Antimicrob. Agents Chemother.*, **41**, 169–174.

367. Voorman, R. L., Maio, S. M., Hauer, M. J., Sanders, P. E., Payne, M. A., and Ackland, M. J. (1998) Metabolism of delavirdine, a human immunodeficiency virus type 1 reverse transcriptase inhibitor, by microsomal cytochrome P450 in humans, rats, and other species: probable involvement of CYP2D6 and CYP3A, *Drug Metab. Dispos.*, **26**, 631–639.

368. Freimuth, W. W. (1996) Delavirdine mesylate, a potent nonnucleoside HIV-1 reverse transcriptase inhibitor, *Adv. Exp. Med. Biol.*, **394**, 279–289.

369. Gangar, M., Arias, G., O'Brian, J. G., and Kemper, C. A. (2000) Frequency of cutaneous reactions on rechallenge with nevirapine and delavirdine, *Ann. Pharmacother.*, **34**, 839–842.

370. Para, M., Slater, L., Daly, P., et al. (1999) Delavirdine in combination therapy has a favorable liver safety profile in HIV-1 patients, *39th Interscience Conference on Antimicrobial Agents and Chemotherapy, San Francisco*, September 26–29 [abstract 331].

371. Reisler, R., Liou, S., Servoos, J., et al. (2001) Incidence of hepatotoxicity and mortality in 21 adult antiretroviral treatment trials, *1st IAS Conference on HIV Pathogenesis and Treatment, Buenos Aires*, July 8–11 [abstract 43].

372. Palmon, R., Koo, B. C., Shoultz, D. A., and Dieterich, D. T. (2002) Lack of hepatotoxicity associated with nonnucleoside reverse transcriptase inhibitors, *J. Acquir. Immune Defic. Syndr.*, **29**, 340–345.

373. Scott, L. J. and Perry, C. M. (2000) Delavirdine: a review of its use in HIV infection, *Drugs*, **60**, 1411–1444.

374. Clevenbergh, P., Cua, E., Dam, E., et al. (2002) Prevalence of nonnucleoside reverse transcriptase inhibitor (NNRTI) resistance-associated mutations and polymorphisms in NNRTI-naïve HIV-infected patients, *HIV Clin. Trials*, **3**(1), 36–44.

375. Nissley, D. V., Church, J. D., Guay, L. A., et al. (2006) Phenotypic NNRTI resistance and genetic diversity in drug-naive individuals, *XV International HIV Drug Resistance Workshop, Sitges, Spain*, June 13–17, abstract 138.

376. Paolucci, S., Baldani, F., Tinelli, M., et al. (2002) Q145M, a novel HIV-1 reverse transcriptase mutation conferring resistance to nucleoside and nonnucleoside reverse transcriptase inhibitors, *Antivir. Ther.*, **7**(2), S35.

377. Harrigan, P. R., Salim, M., Stammers, D. K., et al. (2002) A mutation in the 3′ region of the human immunodeficiency virus type 1 reverse transcriptase (Y318F) associated with non-nucleoside reverse transcriptase inhibitor resistance, *J. Virol.*, **76**(13), 6836–6840.

378. Kemp, S., Salim, M., Stammers, D., Wynhoven, B., Larder, B., and Harrigan, P. R. (2001) A mutation in HIV-1 RT at codon 318 (Y to F) confers high level NNRTI resistance in clinical samples, *41th Interscience Conference on Antimicrobial Agents and Chemotherapy, Chicago, IL*, December 16–19 [abstract 1762].

379. Huang, W., Parkin, N. T., Lie, Y. S., et al. (2000) A novel HIV-1 RT mutation (M230L) confers NNRTI resistance and dose-dependent stimulation of replication, *Antivir. Ther.*, **5**(Suppl. 3), S24–S25.

380. Little, S. J., Holte, S., Routy, J. P., et al. (2002) Antiretroviral-drug resistance among patients recently infected with HIV, *N. Engl. J. Med.*, **347**(6), 385–394.

381. Pilon, R., Sandstrom, P., Burchell, A., et al. (2002) Transmitted HIV-1 reverse transcriptase inhibitor resistance mutation stability in ART-naïve recent seroconverters: results of the polaris HIV seroconversion study, *XIV International AIDS Conference, Barcelona*, July 7–12 [abstract TuPeB4611].

382. Imrie, A., Carr, A., Duncombe, C., et al. (1996) Primary infection with zidovudine-resistant human immunodeficient virus type 1 does not adversely affect outcome at 1 year. Sydney Primary HIV Infection Study group, *J. Infect. Dis.*, **174**(1), 195–198.

383. Conant, M., Brown, S., Cohen, C., et al. (1999) An epidemiological prospective survey assessing the prevalence of HIV-1 drug resistance in 230 HIV-1-positive antiretroviral naïve patients from the USA, *39th Interscience Conference on Antimicrobial Agents and Chemotherapy, San Francisco, CA*, September 26–29 [abstract 443].

384. Becker, M. I., Haubrich, R., Wesselman, C. W., et al. (2002) HIV-1 genotypic resistance in treatment-naïve subjects enrolled in an observational trial (GAIN), *Antivir. Ther.*, **7**(Suppl. 2), S134.

385. Huang, W., Wrin, T., Gamarnik, A., Beauchaine, J., Whitcomb, J. M., and Petropoulos, C. J. (2002) Reverse transcriptase mutations that confer non-nucleoside reverse transcriptase inhibitor resistance may also impair replication capacity, *Antivir. Ther.*, **7**(Suppl. 2), S60.

386. Soderberg, K., Thompson, M., and Alexander, L. (2002) Impaired in vitro fitness of nevirapine resistant HIV-1 mutants, *9th Conference on Retroviruses and Opportunistic Infections, Seattle WA*, February 24–28 [abstract 577].

387. Archer, R. H., Dykes, C., Gerondeles, P., et al. (2000) Mutants of human immunodeficiency virus type 1 (HIV-1) reverse transcriptase resistant to nonnucleoside reverse transcriptase inhibitors demonstrate altered rates of RNase H cleavage that correlate with HIV-1 replication fitness in cell culture, *J. Virol.*, **74**(18), 8390–8401.

388. Whitcomb, J. M., Huang, W., Limoli, K., et al. (2002) Hypersusceptibility to non-nucleoside reverse transcriptase inhibitors in HIV-1: clinical, phenotypic and genotypic correlates, *AIDS*, **16**(15), F41–F47.

389. Das, K., Clark, A. D., Jr., Lewi, P. J., Heeres, J., et al. (2004) Roles of conformational and positional adaptability in structure-based design of TMC125-R165335 (etravirine) and related non-nucleoside reverse transcriptase inhibitors that are highly potent and effective against wild-type and drug-resistant HIV-1 variants, *J. Med. Chem.*, **47**(10), 2550–2560.

390. Ludovici, D. W., De Corte, B. L., Kukla, M. J., Ye, H., et al. (2001) Evolution of anti-HIV drug candidates. Part 3: diarylpyrimidine (DAPY) analogues, *Biorg. Med. Chem. Lett.*, **11**(17), 2235–2239.

391. Lewi, P. J., de Jonge, M., Daeyaert, F., Koymans, L., et al. (2003) On the detection of multiple-binding modes of ligands to proteins, from biological, structural, and modeling data, *J. Comput. Aided Mol. Des.*, **17**(2–4), 129–134.

392. Grossman, H. A., Hicks, C., Nadler, J., et al. (2005) Efficacy and tolerability of Tmc125 in HIV patients with NNRTI and PI resistance at 24 weeks: Tmc125-c223, *45th Interscience Conference of Antimicrobial Agents and Chemotherapy, Washington, D.C.*, December 16–19 [abstract H-416c].

393. Medscape—The continuing promise of TMC125, a second-generation NNRTI (http://www.medscape.com/viewarticle/429091).

394. Schöller, M., Kraft, M., Hoetelmans, R., et al. (2006) Significant decrease in TMC125 exposures when co-administered with tipranavir boosted with ritonavir in healthy subjects, *13th Conference on Retroviruses and Opportunistic Infections, Denver, CO*, February 5–8 [abstract 583].

395. Kukuda, T., M. Schöller-Gyüre, M., Peeters, M., Woodfall, B., et al. (2006) Pharmacokinetic interaction study with TMC125 and TMC114/RTV in HIV-negative volunteers, *16th International AIDS Conference, Toronto, Canada*, August 13–18 [abstract TuPe0086].

396. Anderson, M. S., Kakuda, T. N., Miller, J. L., et al. (2007) Pharmacokinetic evaluation of non-nucleoside reverse transcriptase inhibitor (NNRTI) TMC125 and integrase inhibitor (InSTI) raltegravir (RAL) in healthy subjects, *4th International AIDS Society (IAS) Conference on HIV Pathogenesis, Treatment and Prevention, Sydney, Australia*, July 22–25 [abstract TUPDB02].

397. Ramanathan, S., West, S., Kakuda, T. N., et al. (2007) Lack of clinically relevant drug interaction between ritonavir-boosted elvitegravir and TMC 125, *47th Interscience Conference on Antimicrobial Agents and Chemotherapy, Chicago, IL*, September 17–20 [abstract H-1407].

398. Mills, A., Cahn, P., Grinsztejn, B., et al. (2007) DUET-1: 24 week results of a phase III randomised double-blind trial to evaluate the efficacy and safety of TMC125 versus placebo in 612 treatment-experienced HIV-1 infected patients, *4th International AIDS Society (IAS) Conference on HIV Pathogenesis, Treatment, and Prevention, Sydney, Australia*, July 22–25 [abstract (late-breaker) WeSS204:1].

399. Katlama, C., Campbell, T., Clotet, B., et al. (2007) DUET-2: 24 week results of a phase III randomised double-blind trial to eval-

uate the efficacy and safety of TMC125 versus placebo in 591 treatment-experienced HIV-1 infected patients, *4th International AIDS Society (IAS) Conference on HIV Pathogenesis, Treatment, and Prevention, Sydney, Australia*, July 22–25 [abstract (late-breaker) WeSS204:2].

400. Madruga, J. V., Cahn, P., Grinsztejn, B., et al. on behalf of the DUET-1 Study Group (2007) Efficacy and safety of TMC125 (etravirine) in treatment-experienced HIV-1-infected patients in DUET-1: 24-week results from a randomised, double-blind, placebo-controlled trial, *Lancet*, **370**(9581), 29–38.

401. Lazzarin, A., Campbell, T., Clotet, B., et al. on behalf of the DUET-2 Study Group (2007) Efficacy and safety of TMC125 (etravirine) in treatment-experienced HIV-1-infected patients in DUET-2: 24-week results from a randomised, double-blind, placebo-controlled trial, *Lancet*, **370**(9581), 39–48.

402. Cohen, C., Steinhart, C. R., and Ward, D. J. (2006) Efficacy and safety results at 48 weeks with the novel NNRTI, TMC125, and impact of baseline resistance on the virologic response in study TMC125-C223, *XVIth International AIDS Conference, Toronto, Canada*, August 13–18 [abstract TUPE0061].

403. Jansen, P. A. J., Lewi, P. J., Arnold, E., et al. (2005) In search of a novel anti-HIV drug: multidisciplinary coordination in the discovery of 4-[[4-[[4-[(1E)-2-cyanoethenyl]-2,6-dimethylphenyl]amino]-2-pyrimidinyl]amino]benzonitrile (R278474, rilpivirine), *J. Med. Chem.*, **48**(6), 1901–1909.

404. Pozniak, A., Morales-Ramirez, J., Mohapi, L., et al. (2007) 48-week primary analysis of trial TMC278-C204: TMC278 demonstrates potent and sustained efficacy in ART-naïve patients, *14th Conference of Retroviruses and Opportunistic Infections, Los Angeles, CA*, February 25–28 [abstract 144LB].

405. Ruxrungtham, K., Bellos, N., Morales-Ramirez, J., et al. (2007) The metabolic profile of TMC278, an investigational non-nucleoside reverse transcriptase inhibitor (NNRTI), *4th International AIDS Society Conference on HIV Pathogenesis, Treatment, and Prevention, Sydney. Australia*, July 22–25 [abstract TUAB105].

406. Kashman, Y., Gustafson, K. R., Fuller, R. W., et al. (1992) The calanolides, a novel HIV-inhibitory class of coumarin derivatives from the tropical rainforest tree, *Calophyllum lanigerum, J. Med. Chem.*, **35**, 2735–2743.

407. Boyer, P. L., Currens, M. J., McMahon, J. B., Boyd, M. R., and Hughes, S. H. J. (1993) Analysis of nonnucleoside drug-resistant variants of human immunodeficiency virus type 1 reverse transcriptase, *Virology*, **67**, 2412–2420.

408. Hizi, A., Tal, R., Shaharabany, M., Currens, M. J., Boyd, M. R., Hughes, S. B., and McMahon, J. B. (1993) Specific inhibition of the reverse transcriptase of human immunodeficiency virus type 1 and the chimeric enzymes of human immunodeficiency virus type 1 and type 2 by nonnucleoside inhibitors, *Antimicrob. Agents Ther.*, **37**, 1037–1042.

409. Cardellina, J. H., II, Bokesch, H. R., McKee, T. C., and Boyd, M. R. (1995) Resolution and comparative anti-HIV evaluation of the enantiomers of calanolides A and B, *BioMed. Chem. Lett.*, **5**, 1011–1014.

410. Galinis, D. L., Fuller, R. W., McKee, T. C., Cardellina, J. H., II, Gulakowski, R. J., McMahon, J. B., and Boyd, M. R. (1996) Structure-activity modifications of the HIV-1 inhibitors (+)-calanolide A and (−)-calanolide B, *J. Med. Chem.*, **39**, 4507–4510.

411. Currens, M. J., Gulakowski, R. J., Mariner, J. M., Moran, R. A., Buckheit, R. W., et al. (1996) Antiviral activity and mechanism of action of calanolide A against the human immunodeficiency virus type-1, *J. Pharmacol. Exp. Ther.*, **279**, 645–651.

412. Currens, M. J., Mariner, J. M., McMahon, J. B., and Boyd, M. R. (1996) Kinetic analysis of inhibition of human immunodeficiency

virus type-1 reverse transcriptase by calanolide A, *J. Pharmacol. Exp. Ther.*, **279**, 652–661.

413. McKee, T. C., Covington, C. D., Fuller, R. W., et al. (1998) Pyranocoumarins from tropical species of the genus Calophyllum: a chemotaxonomic study of extracts in the National Cancer Institute collection, *J. Nat. Prod.*, **61**, 1252–1256.

414. Kashman, Y., Gustafson, K. R., Fuller, R. W., et al. (1992) The calanolides, a novel HIV-inhibitory class of coumarin derivatives from the tropical rainforest tree, *Calophyllum lanigerum, J. Med. Chem.*, **35**(15), 2735–2743.

415. Khilevich, A., Mar, A., Flavin, M. T., Rizzo, J. D., et al. (1996) Synthesis of (+)-calanolide A, an anti-HIV agent, via enzyme-catalyzed resolution of the aldol products, *Tetrahedron: Asymmetry*, 7(11), 3315–3326.

416. Chenera, B., West, M. L., Finkelstein, J. A., and Dreyer, G. B. (1993) Total synthesis of (+)-calanolide A, a non-nucleoside inhibitor of HIV reverse transcriptase, *J. Org. Chem.*, **58**, 5605–5606.

417. Creagh, T., Ruckle, J. L., Tolbert, D. T., Giltner, J., Eiznhamer, D. A., Dutta, B., Flavin, M. T., and Xu, Z.-Q. (2001) Safety and pharmacokinetics of single doses of (+)-calanolide A, a novel, naturally occurring nonnucleoside reverse transcriptase inhibitor, in healthy, human immunodeficiency virus-negative human subjects, *Antimicrob. Agents Chemother.*, **45**(5), 1379–1386.

418. Buckheit, R. W., Jr., Russell, J. D., Xu, Z. Q., and Flavin, M. (2000) Anti-HIV-1 activity of calanolides used in combination with other mechanistically diverse inhibitors of HIV-1 replication, *Antivir. Chem. Chemother.*, **11**(5), 321–327.

419. Kohl, N. R., Emini, E. A., Schleif, W. A., et al. (1988) Active human immunodeficiency virus protease is required for viral infectivity, *Proc. Natl. Acad. Sci. U.S.A.*, **85**, 4686–4690.

420. Peng, C., Ho, B. K., Chang, T. W., and Chang, N. T. (1989) Role of human immunodeficiency virus type 1-specific protease in core protein maturation and viral infectivity, *J. Virol.*, **63**, 2550.

421. Gottlinger, H. G., Sodroski, J. G., and Haseltine, W. A. (1989) Role of the capsid precursor processing and myristoylation in morphogenesis and infectivity of human immunodeficiency virus type 1, *Proc. Natl. Acad. Sci. U.S.A.*, **86**, 5781–5789.

422. Wlodawer, A. and Erickson, J. W. (1993) Structure-based inhibitors of HIV-1 protease, *Rev. Biochem.*, **62**, 543–585.

423. Bhat, T. N., Baldwin, E. T., Liu, B., Cheng, Y.-S. E., and Erickson, J. W. (1994) Crystal structure of a tethered dimer of HIV-1 proteinase complexed with an inhibitor, *Nat. Struct. Biol.*, **1**, 552–556.

424. Pearl, L. H. and Taylor, W. R. (1987) A structural model for the retroviral proteases, *Nature*, **329**, 351–354.

425. Flexner, C. (1998) HIV-protease inhibitors, *N. Engl. J. Med.*, **338**(18), 1281–1291.

426. Kramer, R. A., Schaber, M. D., Skalka, A. M., Ganguly, K., Wong-Staal, F., and Reddy, E. P. (1986) HTLV-III gag protein is processed in yeast cells by the virus pol-protease, *Science*, **231**, 1580–1584.

427. Graves, M. C., Lim, J. J., Heimer, E. P., and Kramer, R. A. (1988) An 11-kDa form of human immunodeficiency virus protease expressed in Escherichia coli is sufficient for enzymatic activity, *Proc. Natl. Acad. Sci. U.S.A.*, **85**, 2449–2453.

428. Le Grice, S. F. J., Mills, J., and Mous, J. (1988) Active site mutagenesis of the AIDS virus protease and its alleviation by trans complementation, *EMBO J.*, **7**, 2547–2553.

429. Henderson, L. E., Bowers, M. A., Sowder, R. C., II, et al. (1992) Gag proteins of the highly replicative MN strain of human immunodeficiency virus type 1: posttranslational modifications, proteolytic processings, and complete amino acid sequences, *J. Virol.*, **66**, 1856–1865.

430. Flexner, C., Broyles, S. S., Earl, P., Chakrabarti, S., and Moss. B. (1988) Characterization of human immunodeficiency virus gag/pol gene products expressed by recombinant vaccinia viruses, *Virology*, **166**, 339–349.

431. Karacostas, V., Nagashima, K., Gonda, M. A., and Moss, B. (1989) Human immunodeficiency virus-like particles produced by a vaccinia virus expression vector, *Proc. Natl. Acad. Sci. U.S.A.*, **86**, 8964–8967.

432. Debouk, C. (1992) The HIV-1 protease as a therapeutic target for AIDS, *AIDS Res. Hum. Retroviruses*, **8**, 153–164.

433. Overton, H. A., McMillan, D. J., Gridley, S. J., Brenner, J., Redshaw, S., and Mills, J. S. (1990) Effect of two novel inhibitors of the human immunodeficiency virus protease on the maturation of the HIV gag and gag-pol polyproteins, *Virology*, **179**, 508–511.

434. Tomaszek, T. A., Magaard, V. W., Bryan, H. G., Moore, M. L., and Meek, T. D. (1990) Chromophoric peptide substrates for the spectrophotometric assay of HIV-1 protease, *Biochem. Biophys. Res. Commun.*, **168**, 274–280.

435. Hyland, L. J., Dayton, B. D., Moore, M. L., Shu, A. Y., Heys, J. R., and Meek, T. D. (1990) A radiometric assay for HIV-1 protease, *Anal. Biochem.*, **188**, 408.

436. Phylip, L. H., Richards, A. D., Kay, J., et al. (1990) Hydrolysis of synthetic chromogenic substrates by HIV-1 and HIV-2 proteinases, *Biochem. Biophys. Res. Commun.*, **171**, 439.

437. Tamburini, P. P., Dreyer, R. N., Hansen, J., et al. (1990) A fluorometric assay for HIV-protease activity using high-performance liquid chromatography, *Anal. Biochem.*, **186**, 363.

438. Richards, A. D., Phylip, L. H., Farmeri, W. G., et al. (1990) Sensitive, soluble chromogenic substrates for HIV-1 proteinase, *J. Biol. Chem.*, **265**, 7733–7736.

439. Matayoshi, E. D., Wang, G. T., Krafft, G. A., and Erickson, J. (1990) Novel fluorogenic substrates for assaying retroviral proteases by resonance energy transfer, *Science*, **247**, 954–958.

440. Billich, A. and Winkler, G. (1990) Colorimetric assay of HIV-1 proteinase suitable for high-capacity screening, *Peptide Res.*, **3**, 274.

441. Roberts, N. A., Martin, J. A., Kinchington, D., et al. (1990) Rational design of peptide-based HIV proteinase inhibitors, *Science*, **248**, 358–361.

442. Meek, T. D., Lambert, D. M., Dreyer, G. B., et al. (1990) Inhibition of HIV-1 protease in infected T-lymphocytes by synthetic peptide analogues, *Nature*, **343**, 90–92.

443. Rich, D. H., Green, J., Toth, M. V., Marshall, G. R., and Kent, S. B. (1990) Hydroxyethylamine analogues of the p17/p24 substrate cleavage site are tight-binding inhibitors of HIV protease, *J. Med. Chem.*, **33**, 1285–1288.

444. McQuade, T. J., Tomasselli, A. G., Liu, L., et al. (1990) A synthetic HIV protease inhibitor with antiviral activity arrests HIV-like particle maturation, *Science*, **247**, 454–456.

445. Ashorn, P., McQuade, T. J., Thaisrivongs, S., Tomasselli, A. G., Tarpley, W. G., and Moss, B. (1990) An inhibitor of the protease blocks maturation of human and simian immunodeficiency viruses and spread of infection, *Proc. Natl. Acad. Sci U.S.A.*, **87**, 7472–7476.

446. Dreyer, G. B., Metcalf, B. W., Tomaszek, T. A., et al. (1989) Inhibition of human immunodeficiency virus 1 protease in vitro: rational design of substrate analogue inhibitors, *Proc. Natl. Acad. Sci. U.S.A.*, **86**, 9752–9755.

447. Kempf, D. J., Norbeck, D. W., Codavoli, L., et al. (1990) Structure-based, C2 symmetric inhibitors of HIV protease, *J. Med. Chem.*, **33**, 2687–2689.

448. Chrusciel, R. A. and Romines, K. R. (1997) Recent developments in HIV protease inhibitor research, *Exp. Opin. Ther. Patents*, **7**(2), 111–121.

449. Lea, A. P. and Faulds, D. (1996) Ritonavir, *Drugs*, **52**(4), 541–546.

450. Erickson, J., Neidhart, D. J., Vandrie, J., et al. (1990), Design, activity and 2.8 Å crystal structure of a C2 symmetric inhibitor complexed to HIV-1 protease, *Science*, **249**, 527–533.

451. Bryant, M. L., Heuckeroth, R. O., Kimata, J. T., Ratner, L., and Gordon, J. I. (1989) Replication of human immunodeficiency virus 1 and moloney murine leukemia virus is inhibited by different heteroatom-containing analogs of myristic acid, *Proc. Natl. Acad. Sci. U.S.A.*, **86**, 8655–8659.

452. Monini, P., Sgarari, C., Barillari, G., and Ensoli, B. (2003) HIV protease inhibitors: antiretroviral agents with anti-inflammatory, anti-angiogenic and anti-tumor activity, *J. Antimicrob. Chemother.*, **51**, 207–211.

453. Deeks, S. G., Smith, M., Holodniy, M., and Kahn, J. O. (1997) HIV-1 protease inhibitors. A review for clinicians, *J. Am. Med. Assoc.*, **277**(2), 145–153.

454. Fitzimmons, M. E. and Collins, J. M. (1997) Selective biotransformation of the human immunodeficiency virus protease inhibitor saquinavir by human small-intestinal cytochrome P4503A4; potential contribution to high first-pass metabolism, *Drug Metab. Dispos.*, **25**, 256–266.

455. Kumar, G. N., Rodrigues, A. D., Buko, A. M., and Denissen, J. F. (1996) Cytochrome (ABT-538) in human liver microsomes, *J. Pharmacol. Ther.*, **277**, 423–431 [erratum: *J. Pharmacol. Ther.*, **281**, 1506, (1997)].

456. Chiba, M., Hensleigh, M., Nishime, J. A., Balani, S. K., and Lin, J. H. (1996) Role of cytochrome P450 3A4 in human metabolism of MK-639, a potent human immunodeficiency virus protease inhibitor, *Drug Metab. Dispos.*, **24**, 307–314.

457. Piscitelli, S. C., Flexner, C., Minor, J. R., Polis, M. A., and Masur, H. (1996) Drug interactions in patients infected with human immunodeficiency virus, *Clin. Infect. Dis.*, **23**, 685–693.

458. Roberts, A. D., Muesing, A., Parenti, D. M., Hsia, J., Wasserman, A. G., and Simon, G. L. (1999) Alteration of serum lipids and lipoproteins with indinavir in HIV-infected patients, *Clin. Infect. Dis.*, **29**, 441–443.

459. Graham, N. M. (2000) Metabolic disorders among HIV-infected patients treated with protease inhibitors: a review, *J. Acquir. Immune Defic. Syndr.*, **25**(Suppl. 1), S4–S11.

460. Powderly, W. G. (2002) Long-term exposure to lifelong therapies, *J. Acquir. Immune Defic. Syndr.*, **29**(Suppl. 1), S28–S40.

461. White, A. J. (2001) Mitochondrial toxicity and HIV disease, *Sex. Transm. Infect.*, **77**, 158–173.

462. Walker, U. A., Setzer, B., and Venhoff, N. (2002) Increased long-term mitochondrial toxicity in combinations of nucleoside analogue reverse-transcriptase inhibitors, *AIDS*, **16**(16), 2165–2173.

463. Boshoff, C. and Weiss, R. (2002) AIDS-related malignancies, *Nat. Rev. Cancer*, **2**, 373–382.

464. Sgadari, C., Barillari, G., Toschi, E., Carlei, D., Bacigalupo, I., Baccarini, S., et al. (2002) HIV protease inhibitors are potent anti-angiogenic molecules and promote regression of Kaposi sarcoma, *Nat. Med.*, **8**, 225–232.

465. International Collaboration on HIV and Cancer (2000) Highly active antiretroviral therapy and incidence of cancer in human immunodeficiency virus-infected adults, *J. Natl. Cancer Inst.*, **92**, 1823–1830.

466. Cattelan, A. M., Calabro, M. L., Aversa, S. M., Zanchetta, M., Meneghetti, F., De Rossi, A., et al. (1999) Regression of AIDS-related Kaposi's sarcoma following antiretroviral therapy with protease inhibitors: biological correlates of clinical outcome, *Eur. J. Cancer*, **35**, 1809–1815.

467. Fischle, M. A., Richman, D. D., Grieco, M. H., Gottlieb, M. S., Volberding, P. A., Laskin, O. L., et al. (1987) The efficacy of azidothymidine (AZT) in the treatment of patients with AIDS and AIDS-related complex, *N. Engl. J. Med.*, **317**, 185–191.

468. Zucker, S. D., Qin, X., Rouster, S. D., Yu, F., Green, R. M., Keshavan, P., et al. (2001) Mechanism of indinavir-induced hyperbilirubinemia, *Proc. Natl. Acad. Sci. U.S.A.*, **98**, 12671–12676.

469. Liang, J. S., Distler, O., Cooper, D. A., Jamil, H., Deckelbaum, R. J., Ginsberg, H. N., et al. (2001) HIV protease inhibitors protect apolipoprotein B from degradation by the proteasome: a potential mechanism for protease inhibitor-induced hyperlipidemia, *Nat. Med.*, **7**, 1327–1331.

470. Murata, H., Hruz, P. W., and Mueckler, M. (2002) Indinavir inhibits the glucose transporter isoform Glut4 at physiologic concentrations, *AIDS*, **16**, 859–863.

471. Jain, R. G. and Lenhard, J. M. (2002) Select HIV protease inhibitors alter bone and fat metabolism ex vivo, *J. Biochem. Chem.*, **277**, 19247–19250.

472. Phenix, B. N., Lum, J. J., Nie, Z., Sanchez-Dardon, J., and Badley, A. D. (2001) Antiapoptotic mechanism of HIV protease inhibitors: preventing mitochondrial transmembrane potential loss, *Blood*, **98**, 1078–1085.

473. Chavan, S., Kodoth, S., Pahwa, R., and Pahwa, S. (2001) The HIV protease inhibitor indinavir inhibits cell-cycle progression in vitro in lymphocytes of HIV-infected and uninfected individuals, *Blood*, **98**, 383–389.

474. Pati, S., Pelser, C. B., Dufraine, J., Bryant, J. L., Reitz, M. S., and Weichold, F. F. (2002) Antitumorigenic effects of HIV protease inhibitor ritonavir: inhibition of Kaposi sarcoma, *Blood*, **99**, 3771–3779.

475. Andre, P., Groettrup, M., Klenerman, P., de Giuli, R., Booth, B. L., Jr., Cerundolo, V., et al. (1998) An inhibitor of HIV-1 protease modulates proteasome activity, antigen presentation, and T cell responses, *Proc. Natl. Acad. Sci. U.S.A.*, **95**, 13120–13124.

476. Tovo, P. A. (2000) Highly active antiretroviral therapy inhibits cytokine production in HIV-uninfected subjects, *AIDS*, **14**, 743–744.

477. Gruber, A., Wheat, J. C., Kuhen, K. L., Looney, D. J., and Wong-Staal, F. (2001) Differential effects of HIV-1 protease inhibitors on dendritic cell immunophenotype and function, *J. Biol. Chem.*, **276**, 47840–47843.

478. Ensoli, B., Gendelman, R., Markham, P., Fiorelli, V., Colombini, S., Raffeld, M., et al. (1994) Synergy between basic fibroblast growth factor and HIV-1 Tat protein in induction of Kaposi's sarcoma, *Nature*, **371**, 674–680.

479. Ensoli, B., Sturzl, M., and Monini, P. (2001) Reactivation and role of HHV-8 in Kaposi's sarcoma initiation, *Adv. Cancer Res.*, **81**, 161–200.

480. Wei, X., Ghosh, S. K., Taylor, M. E., et al. (1995) Viral dynamics in human immunodeficiency virus type 1 infection, *Nature*, **373**, 117–122.

481. Ho, D. D., Neumann, A. U., Perelson, A. S., Chen, W., Leonard, J. M., and Markowitz, M. (1995) Rapid turnover of plasma virions and CD4 lymphocytes in HIV-1 infection, *Nature*, **373**, 123–126.

482. Danner, S. A., Carr, A., Leonard, J. M., et al. (1995) A short-term study of the safety, pharmacokinetics, and efficacy of ritonavir, an inhibitor of HIV-1 protease, *N. Engl. J. Med.*, **333**, 1528–1533.

483. Markowitz, M., Saag, M., Powderly, W. G., et al. (1995) A preliminary study of ritonavir, an inhibitor of HIV-1 protease, to treat HIV-1 infection, *N. Engl. J. Med.*, **333**, 1534–1539.

484. Hammer, S. M., Squires, K. E., Hughes, M. D., et al. (1997) A controlled trial of two nucleoside analogues plus indinavir in persons with human immunodeficiency virus infection and CD4 cell counts of 200 per cubic millimeter or less, *N. Engl. J. Med.*, **337**, 725–733.

485. Gulick, R. M., Mellors, J. W., Havlir, D., et al. (1997) Treatment with indinavir, zidovudine, and lamivudine in adults with human

immunodeficiency virus infection and prior antiretroviral activity, *N. Engl. J. Med.*, **337**, 734–739.

486. Noble, S. and Goa, K. L. (2000) Amprenavir: a review of its potential in patients with HIV infection [drug evaluation], *Drugs*, **60**(6), 1383–1410.

487. Carpenter, C. C. J., Cooper, D. A., Fischl, M. A., et al. (2000) Antiretroviral therapy in adults: updated recommendations of the International AIDS Society-USA Panel, *J. Am. Med. Assoc.*, **283**(3), 381–390.

488. BHIVA Writing Committee on Behalf of the BHIVA Executive Committee. (2000) British HIV Association (BHIVA) guidelines for the treatment of HIV-infected adults with antiretroviral therapy [online]. British HIV Association (http://www.aidsmap.com/bhiva/bhivagd1299.htm).

489. Moyle, G. J. and Gazzard, B. G. (1999) A risk-benefit assessment of HIV protease inhibitors, *Drug Safety*, **20**, 299–321.

490. Panel on Clinical Practices for Treatment of HIV Infection (2000) Guidelines for the use of antiretroviral agents in HIV-infected adults and adolescents [online]. U.S. Department of Health and Human Services (http://www.hivatis.org/guidelines/ adult/text/).

491. Steigbigel, R. T., Berry, P., Mellors, J., et al. (1996) Efficacy and safety of the HIV protease inhibitor indinavir sulfate (MK 639) at escalating doses, *3rd Conference on Retroviruses and Opportunistic Infections, Washington, D.C.*, January 28–February 1 [abstract 146].

492. Moyle, G. L., Youle, M., Higgs, C., et al. (1996) Extended follow-up of the safety and activity of Agouron's HIV protease inhibitor AG1343 (Viracept) in virological responders from the UK phase I/II dose finding study, *11th International Conference on AIDS, Vancouver, British Columbia*, July 7–12 [abstract Mo.B.173].

493. Schooley, R. T. (1996) Preliminary data on the safety and antiviral efficacy of the novel protease inhibitor 141W94 in HIV-infected patients with 150 to 400 CD4+ cells/mm3, *36th Interscience Conference on Antimicrobial Agents and Chemotherapy, New Orleans, LA*, September 15–18 [addendum: abstract].

494. Schapiro, J. M., Winters, M. A., Stewart, F., et al. (1996) The effect of high-dose saquinavir on viral load and CD4+ T-cell counts in HIV-infected patients, *Ann. Intern. Med.*, **124**, 1039–1050.

495. Condra, J. H., Schleif, W. A., Blahy, O. M., et al. (1995) In vivo emergence of HIV-1 variants resistant to multiple protease inhibitors, *Nature*, **374**, 569–571.

496. Murphy, R., El-Sader, W., Cheung, T., et al. (1998) Impact of protease inhibitor containing regimens on the risk of developing opportunistic infections and mortality in the CPCRA 034/ACTG 277 study, *5th Conference on Retroviruses and Opportunistic Infections, Chicago, IL*, February 1–5 [abstract 181].

497. Moore, R. D., Keruly, J. C., and Chaisson, R. E. (1998) Decline in CMV and other opportunistic diseases with combination antiretroviral therapy, *5th Conference on Retroviruses and Opportunistic Infections, Chicago, IL*, February 1–5 [abstract 184].

498. McCollum, M., Klaus, B., La Rue, R., et al. (1998) HAART reduced overall costs of HIV care at DVAMC, *5th Conference on Retroviruses and Opportunistic Infections, Chicago, IL*, February 1–5 [abstract 200].

499. Keisher, P., Kvanh, M., Turner, D., et al. (1998) Decreased hospital utilization and costs are associated with protease inhibitor therapy but not nucleoside therapy, *5th Conference on Retroviruses and Opportunistic Infections, Chicago, IL*, February 1–5 [abstract 204].

500. Paul, S., Ziecheck, W., Gilgert, H. M., et al. (1998) Impact of HAART on rates and types of hospitalization at a New York City hospital, *5th Conference on Retroviruses and Opportunistic Infections, Chicago, IL*, February 1–5 [abstract 205].

501. Bermudes, R. A., Toerner, J. G., Mathews, W. C., et al. (1997) The effect of initiating protease inhibitor therapy on hospitalization rates and the quality of life in HIV+ patients, *37th Interscience Conference on Antimicrobial Agents and Chemotherapy, Toronto, Canada*, September 28–October 1 [abstract I-182].

502. Hogg, R. S., Heath, K. V., Yip, B., et al. (1997) Improved survival among HIV-infected individuals: the potential impact of newer antiretroviral therapy strategies, *37th Interscience Conference on Antimicrobial Agents and Chemotherapy, Toronto, Canada*, September 28–October 1 [abstract I-198].

503. Palella, F. J., Delaney, K. M., Moorman, A. C., et al. (1998) Declining morbidity and mortality among patients with advanced human immunodeficiency virus infection, *N. Engl. J. Med.*, **338**, 853–860.

504. Cohen, C., Sun, E., Cameron, W., et al (1996) Ritonavir-saquinavir combination treatment in HIV-infected patients, *36th Interscience Conference on Antimicrobial Agents and Chemotherapy, New Orleans, LA*, September 15–18 [abstract Th.b.934].

505. Cameron, D. W., Japour, A. J., Xu, A., et al. (1999) Ritonavir and saquinavir combination therapy for the treatment of HIV infection, *AIDS*, **13**(2), 213–224.

506. Condra, J. H., Schleif, W. A., Blahy, O. M., et al. (1995), In vivo emergence of HIV-1 variants resistant to multiple protease inhibitors, *Nature*, **374**, 569–571.

507. Molla, M., Korneyeva, M., Gao, Q., et al. (1996) Ordered accumulation of mutations in HIV protease confers resistance to ritonavir, *Nat. Med.*, **2**, 760–766.

508. Schinazi, R. F., Larder, B. A., and Mellors, J. W. (1996) Mutations in retroviral genes associated with drug resistance, *Int. Antiviral News*, **4**, 95–107.

509. Schapiro, J. M., Winters, M. A., Vierra, M., et al. (1996) Causes of long-term efficacy and/or drug failure in protease inhibitor monotherapy, *11th International Conference on AIDS, Vancouver, B.C.*, July 7–12 [abstract Mo.B.414].

510. Romano, L., Venturi, G., Giomi, S., Pippi, L., Valensin, P. E., and Zazzi, M. (2002) Development and resistance to protease inhibitors in HIV-1—infected adults under triple-drug therapy in clinical practice, *J. Med. Virol.*, **66**(2), 143–150.

511. el-Farrash, M. A., Kuroda, M. J., Kitazaki, T., et al. (1994) Generation and characterization of a human immunodeficiency virus type 1 (HIV-1) mutant resistant to an HIV-1 protease inhibitor, *J. Virol.*, **68**, 233–239.

512. Flexner, C. (1996) Pharmacokinetics and pharmacodynamics of HIV protease inhibitors, *Infect. Med.*, **13**(Suppl.), F16–F23.

513. Condra, J. H., Holder, D. J., Schleif, W. A., et al. (1996) Bi-directional inhibition of HIV-1 drug resistance selection by combination therapy with indinavir and reverse transcriptase inhibitors, *11th International Conference on AIDS, Vancouver, B.C.*, July 7–12 [abstract Th.B.932].

514. Figgitt, D. P. and Plosker, G. L. (2000) Saquinavir soft-gel capsule: an updated review of its use in the management of HIV infection, *Drugs*, **60**(2), 481–516.

515. Plosker, G. L. and Scott, L. J. (2003) Saquinavir: a review of its use in boosted regimens for treating HIV infection, *Drugs*, **63**(12), 1299–1324.

516. Lopez-Cortes, L. F., Ruiz-Valderas, R., Rivero, A., Camacho, A., Marquez-Solero, M., Santos, J., Rodriguez-Banos, J., and Ocampo, A. (2007) Efficacy of low-dose boosted saquinavir once daily plus nucleoside reverse transcriptase inhibitors in pregnant HIV-1-infected women with a therapeutic drug monitoring strategy, *Ther. Drug Monit.*, **29**(2), 171–176.

517. Winston, A., Back, D., Fletcher, C., et al. (2006) Effect of omeprasole on the pharmacokinetics of saquinavir-500 mg formulation with ritonavir in healthy male and female volunteers, *AIDS*, **20**(10), 1401–1406.

518. Collazos, J., Martínez, E., Mayo, J., and Blanco, M.-S. (2000) Effect of ketoconazole on plasma concentrations of saquinavir, *J. Antimicrob. Chemother.*, 46, 151–153.

519. Hendrix, C. W., Fiske, W. D., Fuchs, E. J., Redpath, E. C., Stevenson, D. L., Benedek, I. H., and Kornhauser, D. M. (2000) Pharmacokinetics of the triple combination of saquinavir, ritonavir, and efavirenz in HIV-positive patients, *7th Conference on Retroviruses and Opportunistic Infections, San Francisco, CA*, January 30–February 2 [abstract 79].

520. Roche Laboratories (2005) Important drug interaction warning: drug-induced hepatitis with marked transaminase elevation has been observed in healthy volunteers receiving rifampin 600 mg once daily in combination with ritonavir 100 mg/saquinavir 100 mg twice daily (ritonavir boosted saquinavir), Roche Laboratories, Nutley, NJ.

521. Roche Laboratories (1997) FortovaseTM (saquinavir) soft gelatin capsules. Product information (http://www.rocheusa.com/products/invirase/).

522. Huisman, M. T., Smit, J. W., Wiltshire, H. R., et al. (2001) P-glycoprotein limits oral availability, brain, and fetal penetration of saquinavir even with high doses of ritonavir, *Mol. Pharmacol.*, 59(4), 806–813.

523. Boyd, M. A., Siangphoe, U., Ruxrungtham, K., Reiss, P., Apicha Mahanonthar, A., et al. (2006) The use of pharmacokinetically guided indinavir dose reductions in the management of indinavir-associated renal toxicity, *J. Antimicrob. Chemother.*, 7(6), 1161–1167.

524. Kempf, D. J., Marsh, K. C., Kumar, G., et al. (1997) Pharmacokinetic enhancement of inhibitors of the human immunodeficiency virus protease by coadministration with ritonavir, *Antimicrob. Agents Chemother.*, 41, 654–660.

525. Gulick, R. M., Meibohm, A., Havlir, D., et al. (2003) Six-year follow-up of HIV-1-infected adults in a clinical trial of antiretroviral therapy with indinavir, zidovudine, and lamivudine, *AIDS*, 17, 2345–2349.

526. Kopp, J. B., Miller, K. D., Mican, J. A., et al. (1997) Crystalluria and urinary tract abnormalities associated with indinavir, *Ann. Intern. Med.*, 127, 119–125.

527. Boubaker, K., Sudre, P., Bally, F., et al. (1998) Changes in renal function associated with indinavir, *AIDS*, 12, F249–F54.

528. Berns, J. S., Cohen, R. M., Silverman, M., et al. (1997) Acute renal failure due to indinavir crystalluria and nephrolithiasis: report of two cases, *Am. J. Kidney Dis.*, 30, 558–560.

529. Vigano, A., Rombola, G., Barbiano di Belgioioso, G., et al. (1998) Subtle occurrence of indinavir-induced acute renal insufficiency, *AIDS*, 12, 954–955.

530. Kohl, N. E., Emini, E. A., Schleif, W. A., et al. (1988) Active human immunodeficiency virus protease is required for viral infectivity, *Proc. Natl. Acad. Sci. U.S.A.*, 85, 4686–4690.

531. Condra, J. H., Gabryelski, W. A., Blahy, O. M., et al. (1996) In vivo evolution of resistance to the HIV-1 protease inhibitor indinavir, *3rd Conference on Retroviruses and Opportunistic Infections, Washington, D.C.*, January 28–February 1, [abstract 88].

532. Mellors, J., Steigbigel, R., Gulick, R., et al. (1995) Antiretroviral activity of the oral protease inhibitor, MK-639, in p24-antigenemic, HIV-1 infected patients with < 500 CD4/mm^3, *35th Interscience Conference on Antimicrobial Agents and Chemotherapy, San Francisco, CA*, September 17–20 [abstract 235].

533. Vacca, J. P., Dorsey, B. D., Schleif, W. A., et al. (1994) L-735,524: an orally bioavailable human immunodeficiency virus type 1 protease inhibitor, *Proc. Natl. Acad. Sci. U.S.A.*, 91, 4096–4100.

534. Condra, J. H., Schleif, W. A., Blahy, O. M., et al. (1995) In vivo emergence of HIV-1 variants resistant to multiple protease inhibitors, *Nature*, 374, 569–571.

535. Roberts, N. A., Race, E., Tomlinson, P., Gilbert, S., and Duncan, I. B. (1995) Resistance and cross resistance issues: studies with saquinavir, *35th Interscience Conference on Antimicrobial Agents and Chemotherapy, San Francisco, CA*, September 17–20 [abstract 254].

536. Dykes, C., Najjar, J., Bosch, R. J., Wantman, M., et al. (2004) Detection of drug-resistant minority variants of HIV-1 during virologic failure of indinavir, lamivudine, and zidovudine, *J. Infect. Dis.*, 189, 1091–1096.

537. Stein, D., Drusano, G., Steigbigel, R., et al. (1997) Two year follow-up of patients treated with indinavir 800 mg q8h, *4th Conference on Retroviruses and Opportunistic Infections, Washington, D.C.*, January 22–26 [abstract 195].

538. Hupfer, M., Wagels, T., Kahlert, C., Bueche, D., Fierz, W., Walker, U., and Vernazza, P. (2004) Ritonavir boosted indinavir treatment as a simplified maintenance "mono"-therapy for HIV infection, *AIDS*, 18(6), 955–957.

539. Havlir, D. V., Marschner, I. C., Hirsch, M. S., Collier, A. C., Tebas, P., Bassett, R. L., et al. (1998) Maintenance antiretroviral therapies in HIV-infected subjects with undetectable plasma HIV RNA after triple-drug therapy, *N. Engl. J. Med.*, 39, 1261–1268.

540. Moyle, G. (2000) Use of HIV protease inhibitors as pharmacoenhancers, *AIDS Reader*, 11, 87–98.

541. Peytavin, G., Flandre, P., Morand-Joubert, L., Lamotte, C., Launay, O., Gerard, L., Izard, S., Levy, C., Joly, V., Aboulker, J. P., Farinotti, R., and Yeni, P. (2003) Efficacy and safety related to indinavir and nevirapine plasma concentrations in a randomized controlled trial comparing indinavir and nevirapine versus indinavir containing regimen in HIV-1 infected patients (Trianon-ANRS081 Study), *Antivir. Ther.*, 8(Suppl. 1), abstract 842.

542. Haas, D. W., Fessel, W. J., Delapenha, R. A., et al. (2001) Therapy with efavirenz plus indinavir in patients with extensive prior nucleoside reverse-transcriptase inhibitor experience: a randomized, double-blind, placebo-controlled trial, *J. Infect. Dis.*, 18, 392–400.

543. Staszewski, S., Morales-Ramirez, J., Tashima, K. T., et al. (1999) Efavirenz plus zidovudine and lamivudine, efavirenz plus indinavir, and indinavir plus zidovudine and lamivudine in the treatment of HIV-1 infection in adults, *N. Engl. J. Med.*, 34, 1865–1873.

544. Aarnoutse, R. E., Grintjes, K. J. T., Telgt, D., et al. (2002) The influence of efavirenz on the pharmacokinetics of a twice daily indinavir/ritonavir (800/100 mg) combination in healthy volunteers, *Clin. Pharmacol. Ther.*, 71, 57–67.

545. Boyd, M. A., Aarnoutse, R. E., Ruxrungtham, K., Stek, M., van Heeswijk, R. P. G., Lange, J. M. A., Cooper, D. A., Phanuphak, P., and Burger, D. M. (2000) Pharmacokinetics of indinavir/ritonavir (88/100 mg) in combination with efavirenz (600 mg) in HIV-1-infected subjects, *J. Acquir. Immune Defic. Syndr.*, 34(2), 134–139.

546. Boyd, M. A., Carr, A., Ruxrungtham, K., Srasuebkul, P., Bien, D., Law, M., Wangsuphachart, S., Krisanachinda, A., et al. (2004) Changes in body composition and mitochondrial nucleic acid content in patients switched from failed nucleoside analogue therapy to ritonavir-boosted indinavir and efavirenz, *J. Infect. Dis.*, 194, 642–650.

547. Cattelan, A. M., Trevenzoli, M., Naso, A., Meneghetti, F., and Cadrobbi, P. (2000) Severe hypertension and renal atrophy associated with indinavir, *Clin. Infect. Dis.*, 30, 619–621.

548. Cattelan, A. M., Trevenzoli, M., Sasset, L., Rinaldi, L., Balasso, V., and Cadrobbi, P. (2001) Indinavir and systemic hypertension [Research Letters], *AIDS*, 15(6), 805–807.

549. Piscitelli, S. C., Burstein, A. H., Chaitt, D., Alfaro, R. M., and Falloon, J. (2000) Indinavir concentrations and St. John's

wort, *Lancet*, **355**(9203), 547–548 [erratum: *Lancet*, **357**(9263), **1210** (2001)].

550. Dieleman, J., Gyssens, I. C., van der Ende, M. E., de Marie, S., and Burger, D. M. (1998) Urologic complaints in relation to indinavir plasma levels in HIV-infected patients, *XIIth Conference on AIDS, Geneva, Switzerland*, June 28–July 3 [abstract 12372]

551. Familaro, G., Di Toro, S., Moretti, S., and De Simone, C. (2000) Symptomatic crystalluria associated with indinavir, *Ann. Pharmacother.*, **34**(12), 1414–1418.

552. Trainor, L. D., Steinberg, J. P., Austin, G. W., and Solomon, H. M. (1998) Indinavir crystalluria: identification of patients at increased risk of developing nephrotoxicity, *Arch. Pathol. Lab. Med.*, **122**, 256–259.

553. Kohan, A. D., Armenakas, N. A., and Fracchia, J. A. (1999) Indinavir urolithiasis: an emerging cause of renal colic in patients with human immunodeficiency virus, *J. Urol.*, **161**(6), 1765–1768.

554. Brodie, S. B., Keller, J. K., Ewenstein, B. M., et al. (1998) Variation in incidence of indinavir-associated nephrolithiasis among HIV-positive patients, *AIDS*, **12**, 2433–2437.

555. Tashima, K. T., Horowitz, J. D., and Rosen, S. (1997) Indinavir nephropathy, *N. Eng. J. Med.*, **336**, 138–140.

556. Hanabusa, H., Tagami, H., and Hataya, H. (1999) Renal atrophy associated with long-term treatment with indinavir, *N. Engl. J. Med.*, **340**, 392–393.

557. Balani, S. K., Ariso, B. H., and Mathai, L. (1995) Metabolites of L-735,524, a potent HIV-1 protease inhibitor, in human urine, *Drug Metab. Dispos.*, **23**, 266–270.

558. Lin, J. H., Chen, I.-W., Vastag, K. J., et al. (2005) pH-dependent oral absorption of L-735,524, a potent HIV protease inhibitor, in rats and dogs, *Drug Metab. Dispos.*, **23**, 730–735.

559. Pai, V. B. and Nahata, M. C. (1999) Nelfinavir mesylate: a protease inhibitor, *Ann. Pharmacother.*, **33**, 325–339.

560. Bardsley-Elliot, A. and Plosker, G. L. (2000) Nelfinavir: an update on its use in HIV infection, *Drugs*, **59**, 581–620.

561. Gathe, J., Jr., Burkhardt, B., Hawley, P., et al. (1996) A randomized phase II study of viracept, a novel HIV protease inhibitor, used in combination with stavudine (d4T) vs. stavudine (d4T) alone, *XIth International Conference on AIDS, Vancouver, British Columbia*, July 7–12 [abstract Mo.B.413].

562. Pedneault, L., Elion, R., Adler, M., et al. (1997) Stavudine (d4T), didanosine (ddI), and nelfinavir combination therapy in HIV-infected subjects: antiviral effect and safety in an ongoing pilot study, *4th Conference on Retroviruses and Opportunistic Infections, Washington, D.C.*, January 22–26 [abstract 241].

563. Conant, M., Markowitz, M., Hurley, A., et al. (1996) A randomized phase II dose range-finding study of the HIV protease inhibitor viracept as monotherapy in HIV-positive patients, *XIth International Conference on AIDS, Vancouver, British Columbia*, July 7–12 [abstract Tu.B.2129].

564. Markowitz, M., Cao, Y., Hurley, A., et al. (1996) Triple therapy with AZT an 3TC in combination with nelfinavir mesylate in 12 antiretroviral-naïve subjects chronically infected with HIV-1, *XIth International Conference on AIDS, Vancouver, British Columbia*, July 7–12 [abstract LB.B.6031].

565. Saag, M., Knowles, M., Chang, Y., et al. (1997) Durable effect of viracept (nelfinavir mesylate, NFV) in triple combination therapy, *37th Interscience Conference on Antimicrobial Agents and Chemotherapy, Toronto, Canada*, September 28–October 1 [abstract I-101].

566. Tebas, P., Patick, A., Kane, E. M., Klebert, M. K., Simpson, J. H., et al. (1999) Virologic responses to a ritonavir-saquinavir-containing regimen in patients who had previously failed nelfinavir, *AIDS*, **13**, F23–F28.

567. Albrecht, M. A., Bosch, R. J., Hammer, S. M., Liou, S. H., Kessler, H., Para, M. F., Eron, J., Valdez, H., Dehlinger, M.,

Katzenstein, D. A., and the AIDS Clinical Trials Group 364 Study Team (2001) Nelfinavir, efavirenz, or both after the failure of nucleoside treatment of HIV infection, *N. Engl. J. Med.*, **345**(6), 398–407.

568. Moyle, G., Pozniak, A., Opravil, M., Clumeck, N., DelFraissy, J. F., Johnson, M., Pelgrom, J., Reynes, J., Vittecoq, D., DeLora, P., Salgo, M., and Duff, F. (2000) The SPICE study: 48-week activity of combinations of saquinavir soft gelatin and nelfinavir with and without nucleoside analogues. Study of Protease Inhibitor Combinations in Europe, *J. Acquir. Immune Defic. Syndr.*, **23**(2), 128–137.

569. Hammer, S. M., Bassett, R., Squires, K. E., Fischl, M. A., Demeter, L. M., Currier, J. S., Mellors, J. W., Morse, G. D., Eron, J. J., Santana, J. L., DeGruttola, V. and the ACTG 372B/D Study Team (2003) A randomized trial of nelfinavir and abacavir in combination with efavirenz and adefovir dipivoxil in HIV-1-infected persons with virological failure receiving indinavir, *Antivir. Ther.*, **8**(6), 507–518.

570. Gonzalez-Olivieri, L. M., Brindeiro, R., Soares, M., Pereira, H., Santana, R., Abreu, C., and Tanuri, A. (2004) Impact of nelfinavir-resistance mutations on the human immunodeficiency virus type 1 with subtype B and C proteases, *XVth International Conference on AIDS, Bangkok, Thailand*, July 11–16 [abstract WePeB5704].

571. Agouron Pharmaceuticals (1997) Viracept (nelfinavir mesylate) tablets and oral powder product monograph (package insert), Agouron Pharmaceuticals, La Jolla, CA.

572. Gathe, J., Burkhardt, B., Hawley, P., et al. (1996) A randomized phase II study of viracept, a novel HIV protease inhibitor, used in combination with stavudine vs. stavudine alone, *11th International Conference on AIDS, Vancouver, British Columbia*, July 7–12 [abstract Mo.B. 413].

573. Michelet, C., Bellissant, E., Ruffault, A., et al. (1999) Safety and efficacy of ritonavir and saquinavir in combination with zidovudine and lamivudine, *Clin. Pharmacol. Ther.*, **65**, 661–671.

574. Domingo, E., Escarmis, C., Sevilla, N., et al. (1996) Basic concepts in RNA virus evolution, *FASEB J.*, **10**, 859–864.

575. Coffin, J. M. (1992) Genetic diversity and evolution of retroviruses, *Curr. Top. Microbiol. Immunol.*, **176**, 143–164

576. Nijhuis, M., Boucher, C. A. B., Schipper, P., Leitner, T., Schuurman, R., and Albert, J. (1998) Stochastic processes strongly influence HIV-1 evolution during suboptimal protease-inhibitor therapy, *Proc. Natl. Acad. Sci. U.S.A.*, **95**(24), 14441–14446.

577. Abbott Pharmaceuticals (1999) Norvir (ritonavir) package insert. Abbott Pharmaceuticals, Abbott Park, IL.

578. Hoen, B., Harzic, M., Fleury, H. F., et al. (1997) ARNS053 trial of zidovudine (ZDV), lamivudine (3TC), and ritonavir combination in patients with symptomatic primary HIV-1 infection: preliminary results, *4th Conference on Retroviruses and Opportunistic Infections, Washington, D.C.*, January 22–26 [abstract 232].

579. Saimot, A. G., Landman, R., Damond, F., et al. (1997) Ritonavir, stavudine (d4T), didanosine (ddI) as triple combination treatment in antiretroviral-naïve patients, *4th Conference on Retroviruses and Opportunistic Infections, Washington, D.C.*, January 22–26 [abstract 246].

580. Markowitz, M., Saag, M., Powderly, W. G., et al. (1995) Preliminary study of ritonavir, an inhibitor of HIV-1 protease, to treat HIV-1 infection, *N. Engl. J. Med.*, **328**, 1534–1539.

581. Danner, S. A., Carr, A., Leonard, J. M., et al. (1995) A short-term study of the safety, pharmacokinetics, and efficacy of ritonavir, an inhibitor of HIV-1 protease, *N. Engl. J. Med.*, **328**, 1528–1533.

582. Justesen, U. S., Hansen, I. M., Andersen, A. B., et al. (2005) The long-term pharmacokinetics and safety of adding low-dose ritonavir to a nelfinavir 1250 mg twice-daily regimen in HIV-infected patients, *HIV Medicine*, **6**, 334–340.

583. Abbott Laboratories (1997) Norvir (ritonavir) capsule product monograph (package insert), Abbott Laboratories, North Chicago, IL.

584. Eron, J., Jr., Yeni, P., Gathe, J., Jr., et al. (2006) The KLEAN study of fosamprenavir-ritonavir versus lopinavir-ritonavir, each in combination with abacavir-lamivudine, for initial treatment of HIV infection over 48 weeks: a randomised non-inferiority trial, *Lancet*, **368**, 476–482.

585. De Pasquale, M. P., Murphy, R., Kuritzkes, D., Martinez-Picado, J., Sommadossi, J. P., Gulick, R., Smeaton, L., DeGruttola, V., Caliendo, A. M., Sutton, L., Savara, A., and D'Aquila, R. T. (1998) Resistance during early virologic rebound on amprenavir plus zidovudine plus lamivudine triple therapy or amprenavir monotherapy in ACTG 347, *Antivir. Ther.*, **3**(Suppl. 1), 50–51 [abstract 71].

586. Descamps, D., Masquelier, B., Mamet, J. P., Calvez, C., Ruffault, A., Telles, F., Goetschel, A., Girard, P. M., Brun-Vezinet, F., and Costagliola, D. (2001) A genotypic sensitivity score for amprenavir based genotype at baseline and virological response, *Antivir. Ther.*, **6**, 103.

587. Falloon, J., Piscitelli, S., Vogel, S., Sadler, B., Mitsuya, H., Kavlick, M. F., Yoshimura, K., Rogers, M., LaFon, S., Manion, D. J., Lane, H. C., and Masur, H. (2000) Combination therapy with amprenavir, abacavir, and efavirenz in human immunodeficiency virus (HIV)-infected patients failing a protease-inhibitor regimen: pharmacokinetic drug interactions and antiviral activity, *Clin. Infect. Dis.*, **30**, 313–318.

588. Klein, A., Maguire, M., Paterson, D., Nacci, P., Mustafa, N., Yeo, J., Snowden, W., and Kleim, J. P. (2000) Virological response to amprenavir combination therapy in PI-experienced paediatric patients: association with distinct baseline HIV-1 protease variants—study PROAB3004, *Antivir. Ther.*, **5**(Suppl. 2), 4 [abstract].

589. Maguire, M., MacManus, S., Griffin, P., Guinea, C., Harris, W., Richard, N., Wolfram, J., Tisdale, M., Snowden, W., and Klein, J.-P. (2001) Interaction of HIV-1 protease and gag gene mutations in response to amprenavir-selective pressure exerted in amprenavir-treated subjects—contribution of gag p6 changes L449F and P453L, *Antivir. Ther.*, **6**, 48.

590. Murphy, R. L., Gulick, R. M., DeGruttola, V., D'Aquila, R. T., Eron, J. J., Sommadossi, J. P., Currier, J. S., Smeaton, L., Frank, I., Caliendo, A. M., Gerber, J. G., Tung, R., and Kuritzkes, D. R. (1999) Treatment with amprenavir alone or amprenavir with zidovudine and lamivudine in adults with human immunodeficiency virus infection. AIDS Clinical Trials Group 347 Study Team, *J. Infect. Dis.*, **179**, 808–816.

591. Prado, J. G., Wrin, T., Beauchaine, J., Ruiz, L., Petropoulos, C., Clotet, B., D'Aquila, R., and Martinez-Picado, J. (2001) Lopinavir resistance of amprenavir-selected, replication-impaired mutants of HIV-1, *Antivir. Ther.*, **6**, 51.

592. Schmidt, B., Korn, K., Moschik, B., Paatz, B., Uberla, K., and Walter, H. (2000) Low level of cross-resistance to amprenavir (141W94) in samples from patients pretreated with other protease inhibitors, *Antimicrob. Agents Chemother.*, **44**, 3213–3216.

593. Snowden, W., Shortino, D., Klein, A., Harris, W., Manohitharajah, V., Elston, R., Tisdale, M., and Maguire, M. (2000) Development of amprenavir resistance in NRTI-experienced patients: alternative mechanisms and correlation with baseline resistance to concomitant NRTIs, *Antivir. Ther.*, **5**(Suppl. 3), 84 [abstract 108].

594. Ziermann, R., Limoli, K., Das, K., Arnold, E., Petropoulos, C. J., and Parkin, N. T. (2000) A mutation in human immunodeficiency virus type 1 protease, N88S, that causes in vitro hypersensitivity to amprenavir, *J. Virol.*, **74**, 4414–4419.

595. Goodgame, J., Hanson. C., Vafidis, I., et al. (1999) Amprenavir (141W94, APV)/3TC/ZDV exerts durable antiviral activity in HIV-1 infected antiretroviral therapy-naïve subjects through 48 weeks of therapy, *39th Interscience Conference on Antimicrobial Agents and Chemotherapy, San Francisco, CA*, September 26–29 [abstract 509].

596. Cooper, D., Perrin, L., Kinloch, S., et al. (2000) Intervention with quadruple HAART [Combivir (COM)/abacavir (ABC)/amprenavir (APV)] intervention during primary HIV-1 infection (PHI) is associated with rapid viraemia clearance and decrease of immune activation, *7th Conference on Retroviruses and Opportunistic Infections, San Francisco, CA*, January 30–February 2 [abstract/poster 552].

597. Vernazza, P., Perrin, L., Vora, S., et al. (2000) Increased seminal shedding of HIV during primary infection augments the need for earlier diagnosis and intervention, *7th Conference on Retroviruses and Opportunistic Infections, San Francisco, CA*, January 30–February 2 [abstract/poster 564].

598. Eron, J., Junod, P., Becker, S., et al. (2000) NZT4002: 64 week analysis of combivir (COM)-based triple and quadruple therapy in antiretroviral-naive, HIV-1 infected subjects, *13th International AIDS Conference, Durban, South Africa*, July 9–14 [abstract no. WeOrB608].

599. Murphy, R. L., Gulick, R. M., De Gruttola, V., et al. (1999) Treatment with amprenavir alone or amprenavir with zidovudine and lamivudine in adults with human immunodeficiency virus infection, *J. Infect. Dis.*, **179**, 808–816.

600. Haubrich, R., Thompson, M., Schooley, R., et al. (1999) A phase II safety and efficacy study of amprenavir in combination with zidovudine and lamivudine in HIV-infected patients with limited antiretroviral experience, *AIDS*, **13**(17), 2411–2420.

601. Eron, J. J., Jr., Smeaton, L. M., Fiscus, S. A., et al. (2000) The effects of protease inhibitor therapy on human immunodeficiency virus type 1 levels in semen (AIDS Clinical Trials Group Protocol 850), *J. Infect. Dis.*, **181**, 1622–1628.

602. Church, J, Rathore M, Rubio T., et al. (2000) A phase III study of amprenavir (APV, AgeneraseTM) in protease-inhibitor naïve and experienced HIV-infected children and adolescents, *7th Conference on Retroviruses and Opportunistic Infections, San Francisco, CA*, January 30–February 2 [abstract/poster 693].

603. Rodriguez-French, A., Boghossian, J., Gray, G. E., et al. (2004) The NEAT study: a 48-week open-label study to compare the antiviral efficacy and safety of GW433908 versus nelfinavir in antiretroviral therapy-naïve HIV-1-infected patients, *J. Acquir. Immune Defic. Syndr.*, **35**(1), 22–32.

604. Gathe, J. C., Jr., Ive, P., Wood, R., et al. (2004) SOLO: 48-week efficacy and safety comparison of once-daily fosamprenavir/ritonavir versus twice-daily nelfinavir in naive HIV-1-infected patients, *AIDS*, **18**(11), 1529–1537.

605. Vertex (2003) Press release: Vertex reports preliminary 48-week data from Phase III study of 433908, an investigational HIV protease inhibitor (http://www.vpharm.com/ Pressreleases2003/pr072403.html).

606. DeJesus, E., LaMarca, A., Sension, M., Beltran, C., and Yeni, P. (2003) The Context Study: efficacy and safety of GW433908/RTV in PI-experienced subjects with virological failure (24 week results), *10th Conference on Retroviruses and Opportunistic Infections, Boston, MA*, February 10–14 [abstract 178].

607. Corbett, A. H., Davidson, L., Park, J. J., et al. (2004) Dose separation strategies to overcome the pharmacokinetic interaction of a triple protease inhibitor regimen containing fosamprenavir, lopinavir, and ritonavir, *11th Conference on Retroviruses and Opportunistic Infections, San Francisco, CA*, Feburary 8–11 [abstract 611].

608. Kashuba, A. D., Tierney, C., Downey, G. F., et al. (2005) Combining fosamprenavir with lopinavir/ritonavir substantially reduces amprenavir and lopinavir exposure: ACTG protocol A5143, *AIDS*, **19**(2), 145–152.

609. Walmsley, S., Leith, J., Katlama, C., et al. (2004) Pharmacokinetics and safety of tipranavir/ritonavir (TPV/r) alone and in combination with saquinavir (SQV), amprenavir (APV), or lopinavir (LPV): interim analysis of BI1182.51, *XVth International AIDS Conference, Bangkok, Thailand*, July 11–16 [abstract WeOrB1236].

610. Wire, M. B., Ballow, C., Preston, S. L., et al. (2004) Pharmacokinetics and safety of GW433908 and ritonavir, with and without efavirenz, in healthy volunteers, *AIDS*, **18**(6), 897–907.

611. Eron, J., Jr., Yeni, P., Gathe, J., Jr., et al. (2006) KLEAN study team. The KLEAN study of fosamprenavir-ritonavir versus lopinavir-ritonavir, each in combination with abacavir-lamivudine, for initial treatment of HIV infection over 48 weeks: a randomized non-inferiority trial, *Lancet*, **368**(9534), 476–482

612. Elston, R. C., Yates, P., Tisdale, M., et al. (2004) GW433908 (908)/ritonavir (r): 48 week results in PI-experienced subjects: a retrospective analysis of virological response based on baseline genotype and phenotype, *XVth International AIDS Conference, Bangkok, Thailand*, July 11–16 [abstract MoOrB1055].

613. MacManus, S., Yates, P. J., Elston, R. C., et al. (2004) GW433908/ritonavir once daily in antiretroviral therapy-naïve HIV-infected patients: absence of protease resistance at 48 weeks, *AIDS*, **518**(4), 651–655.

614. Fuster, D. and Clotet, B. (2005) Review of atazanavir: a novel HIV protease inhibitor, *Expert Opin. Pharmacother.*, **6**(9), 1565–1572.

615. Whiterel, G. (2001) BMS-232632 (Novartis/Bristol-Meyers Squibb), *Curr. Opin. Investig. Drugs*, **2**, 340–347.

616. Gong, Y. F., Robinson, B. S., Rose, R. E., et al. (2000) In vitro resistance profile of the human immunodeficiency virus type-1 protease inhibitor BMS-232632, *Antimicrob. Agents Chemother.*, **44**, 2319–2326.

617. Colonno, R. J., Thiry, A., Limoli, K., and Parkin, N. (2003) Activities of atazanavir (BMS-232632) against a large panel of human immunodeficiency virus type 1 clinical isolates resistant to one or more approved protease inhibitors, *Antimicrob. Agents Chemother.*, **47**, 1324–1333.

618. Colonno, R., Rose, R., McLaren, C., Thiry, A., Parkin, N., and Friborg, J. (2004) Identification of I50L as the signature atazanavir (ATV)-resistance mutation in treatment-naïve HIV-1-infected patients receiving ATV-containing regimens, *J. Infect. Dis.*, **189**, 1802–1810.

619. Schnell, T., Schmidt, B., Moschik, G., et al. (2003) Distinct cross-resistance profiles of the new protease inhibitors amprenavir, lopinavir, and atazanavir in a panel of clinical samples, *AIDS*, **17**, 1258–1261.

620. Tackett, D., Child, M., Agarwall, S., et al. (2003) Atazanavir: a summary of two pharmacokinetics drug interaction studies in healthy subjects, *10th Conference on Retroviruses and Opportunistic Infections, Boston, MA*, February 10–14 [abstract 543].

621. Guffanty, M., De Pascalis, C. R., Seminari, E., et al. (2003) Pharmacokinetics of amprenavir given once or twice a day when combined with atazanavir in heavily pretreated HIV-positive patients, *AIDS*, **17**, 2669–2671.

622. Taburet, A. M., Piketty, C., Chazallon, C., et al. (2004) Interactions between atazanavir-ritonavir and tenofovir in heavily pretreated human immunodeficiency virus-infected patients, *Antimicrob. Agents Chemother.*, **48**, 2031–2096.

623. Bristol-Myers Squibb Company. (2003) Reyataz™ (atazanavir) full prescribing information, Bristol-Myers Squibb Company, Princeton, NJ.

624. Sanne, I., Piliero, P., Squires, K., Thiry, A., and Schnittman, S. (2003) Results of a Phase II clinical trial at 48 weeks (AI424–007): a dose ranging, safety, and efficacy comparative trial of atazanavir at three doses in combination with didanosine and stavudine in antiretroviral-naïve subjects, *J. Acquir. Immune Defic. Syndr.*, **32**, 18–29.

625. Murphy, R. L., Sanne, I., Canh, P., et al. (2003) Dose-ranging, randomized, clinical trial of atazanavir with lamivudine and stavudine in antiretroviral-naïve subjects: 48-week results, *AIDS*, **17**, 2603–2614.

626. Squires, K., Lazzarin, A., and Gatell, J. M. (2004) Comparison of once-daily atazanavir with efavirenz, each in combination with fixed-dose zidovudine and lamivudine, as initial therapy for patients infected with HIV, *J. Acquir. Immune Defic. Syndr.*, **36**, 1011–1019.

627. Staszewski, S., Morales-Ramirez, J., Tashima, K. T., et al. (1999) Efavirenz plus zidovudine and lamivudine, efavirenz plus indinavir, and indinavir plus zidovudine and lamivudine in the treatment of HIV-1 infection in adults, *N. Engl. J. Med.*, **341**, 1865–1873.

628. Haas, D. W., Zala, C., Schrader, S., et al. (2003) Therapy with atazanavir plus saquinavir in patients failing highly active antiretroviral therapy: a randomized comparative pilot trial, *AIDS*, **17**, 1339–1349.

629. Nieto-Cisneros, L., Zala, C., Fessel, W. J., et al. (2003) BMS AI424–043: antiviral efficacy, metabolic changes and safety of ATV versus LPV/RTV in combination with 2 NRTIs in patients who have experienced virology failure with prior PI-containing regimens: 24 wk results, *2nd IAS Conference on HIV Pathogenesis and Treatment, Paris, France*, July 13–16 [abstract 117].

630. Johnson, M., De Jesus, E., Grinsztejn, B., et al. (2004) Long-term efficacy and durability of atazanavir (ATV) with ritonavir (RTV) or saquinavir (SQV) versus lopinavir/ritonavir (LPV/RTV) in HIV—infected patients with multiple virologic failures: 96-week results from a randomized, open-label trial BMS AI424-045, *7th International Congress on Drug Therapy in HIV Infection*, Glagow, UK, November 14–18 [abstract PL 14.4].

631. Wood, R., Phanuphak, P., Cahn, P., et al. (2004) Long-term efficacy and safety of atazanavir with stavudine and lamivudine in patients previously treated with nelfinavir or atazanavir, *J. Acquir. Immune Defic. Syndr.*, **36**, 684–692.

632. Agarwala, S., Eley, T., Villegas, C., et al. (2005) Pharmacokinetic effect of famotidine on atazanavir with and without ritonavir in healthy subjects, *6th International Workshop on Clinical Pharmacology of HIV Therapy, Quebec City, Canada*, April 28–30 [abstract 11].

633. Jemsek, J. G., Arathoon, E., Arlotti, M., et al. (2003) Atazanavir and efavirenz, each combined with fixed-dose zidovudine and lamivudine, have similar effects on body fat distribution in antiretroviral-naïve patients: 48-weeks results from the metabolic substudy of BMS AI423-034, *Antivir. Ther.*, **8**, L13.

634. Wang, S., Mulvey, R., Elosua, C., Flint, O. P., and Parker, P. A. (2003) Association of HIV-protease inhibitors with insulin resistance is related to potency of inhibition of GLUT4 and GLUT1 activity in adipocytes and miocytes, *Antivir. Ther.*, **8**, L36.

635. Carr, A., Miller, J., Law, M., and Cooper, D. A. (2000) A syndrome of lipoatrophy, lactic acidaemia and liver dysfunction associated with HIV nucleoside analogue therapy: contribution to protease inhibitor-related lipodystrophy syndrome, *AIDS*, **14**, F25–F32.

636. Haerter, G., Manfras, B. J., Mueller, M., Kern, P., and Trein, A. (2004) Regression of lipodystrophy in HIV-infected patients under therapy with the new protease inhibitor atazanavir, *AIDS*, **18**, 952–955.

637. Zucker, S. D., Qin, X., Rouster, S. D., Yu, F., Green, R. M., Keshavan, P., Feinberg, J., and Sherman, K. E. (2001) Mechanism of indinavir-induced hyperbilirubinemia, *Proc. Natl. Acad. Sci. U.S.A.*, **98**(22), 12671–12676.

638. Sulkowski, M. S. (2004) Drug-induced liver injury associated with antiretroviral therapy that include HIV-1 protease inhibitors, *Clin. Infect. Dis.*, **38**(Suppl. 2), S90–S97.

639. Chang, H. R. and Pella, P. M. (2006) Atazanavir urolithiasis, *N. Engl. J. Med.*, **355**, 2158–2159.

640. Pacanowski, J., Poirier, J. M., Petit, I., Meynard, J. L., and Girard, P. M. (2006) Atazanavir urinary stones in an HIV-infected patient, *AIDS*, **20**, 2131.

641. Anderson, P. L., Lichtenstein, K. A., Gerig, N. E., Kiser, J. J., and Bushman, L. R. (2007) Atazanavir-containing renal calculi in an HIV-infected patient, *AIDS*, **21**, 1060–1062.

642. Izzedine, H., M'rad, M. B., Bardier, A., Daudon, M., and Salmon, D. (2007) Atazanavir crystal nephropathy, *AIDS*, **21**(17), 2357–2358.

643. Sham, H. L., Kempf, D. J., Molla, A., et al. (1998) ABT-378, a highly potent inhibitor of the human immunodeficiency virus protease, *Antimicrob. Agents Chemother.*, **42**(12), 3218–3224.

644. Cvetkovic, R. S. and Goa, K. L. (2003) Lopinavir/ritonavir: a review of its use in the management of HIV infection, *Drugs*, **63**(8), 769–802.

645. Oldfield, V. and Plosker, G. L. (2006) Lopenavir/ritronavir: a review of its use in the management of HIV infection, *Drugs*, **66**(9), 1275–1299.

646. Abbott Laboratories Ltd. Kaletra®(lopinavir/ritonavir) soft capsules: summary of product characteristics [online] (http://emc.medicines.org).

647. Abbott Laboratories. Kaletra®(lopinavir/ritonavir) tablets and oral solution. Prescribing information [online] (http://www.kaletra.com).

648. Abbott Laboratories. Kaletra®(lopinavir/ritonavir) capsules and oral solution. Product label information [online] (http://www.kaletra.com).

649. Eron, J., Feinberg, J., Kessler, H. A., et al. (2004) Once-daily versus twice-daily lopinavir/ritonavir in antiretroviral-naive HIV-positive patients: a 48-week randomized clinical trial, *J. Infect. Dis.*, **189**(2), 265–272.

650. Bertz, R., Foit, C., Ye, X., et al. (2002) Pharmacokinetics of once-daily vs. twice-daily Kaletra®(lopinavir/ritonavir) in HIV+ subjects, *9th Conference on Retroviruses and Opportunistic Infections, Seattle, WA*, February 24–28 [abstract 126].

651. Johnson, A., Gathe, J. C., Jr., Podzamczer, D., et al. (2006) A once-daily lopinavir/ritonavir-based regimen provides noninferior antiviral activity compared with a twice-daily regimen, *J. Acquir. Immune Defic. Syndr.*, **43**(2), 153–160.

652. Murphy, R. L., Brun, S., Hicks, C., et al. (2001) ABT-378/ritonavir plus stavudine and lamivudine for the treatment of antiretroviral-naive adults with HIV-1 infection: 48-week results, *AIDS*, **15**(1), F1–F9.

653. Molina, J. M., Wilkins, A., Domingo, P., et al. (2005) Once-daily vs. twice-daily lopinavir/ritonavir in antiretroviral-naive patients: 96-week results, *3rd International AIDS Society Conference on HIV Pathogenesis and Treatment, Rio de Janeiro, Brazil*, July 24–27 [abstract WePe12.3C12 plus poster].

654. King, M. S., Bernstein, B. M., Walmsley, S. L., et al. (2004) Baseline HIV-1 RNA level and CD4 cell count predict time to loss of virologic response to nelfinavir, but not lopinavir/ritonavir, in antiretroviral therapy-naive patients, *J. Infect. Dis.*, **190**(2), 280–284.

655. Murphy, R., Da Silva, B., McMillan, F., et al. (2005) Seven year follow-up of a lopinavir/ritonavir-based regimen in antiretroviral-naive subjects, *10th European AIDS Conference, Dublin, Ireland*, November 17–20 [abstract PE7.9/3 plus poster].

656. Hicks, C., da Silva, B., Benson, C., et al. (2004) Extensive resistance testing during 5 years of lopinavir/ritonavir treatment in antiretroviral-naive HIV infected patients: results from study m97-720, *15th International AIDS Conference, Bangkok, Thailand*, July 11–16 [abstract WeOrB1291 plus oral presentation].

657. Kempf, D. J., King, M. S., Bernstein, B., et al. (2004) Incidence of resistance in a double-blind study comparing lopinavir/ritonavir plus stavudine and lamivudine to nelfinavir plus stavudine and lamivudine, *J. Infect. Dis.*, **189**(1), 51–60.

658. King, M., Lipman, B., Molla, A., et al. (2005) Assessing the potential for protease inhibitor cross-resistance in antiretroviral-naive patients experiencing viral rebound on a lopinavir/ritonavir-based regimen, *3rd European HIV Drug Resistance Workshop, Athens, Greece*, March 30–April 1 [abstract 9.9 plus poster].

659. Molina, J. M., Gathe, J., Lim, P. L., et al. (2004) Comprehensive resistance testing in antiretroviral naive patients treated with once-daily lopinavir/ritonavir plus tenofovir and emtricitabine: 48-week results from study 418, *15th International AIDS Conference, Bangkok, Thailand*, July 11–16 [abstract no. WePeB5701 plus poster].

660. Saez-Llorens, X., Violari, A., Deetz, C. O., et al. (2003) Forty-eight-week evaluation of lopinavir/ritonavir, a new protease inhibitor, in human immunodeficiency virus-infected children, *Pediatr. Infect. Dis. J.*, **22**, 216–223.

661. Kempf, D. J., Isaacson, J. D., King, M. S., et al. (2001) Identification of genotypic changes in human immunodeficiency virus protease that correlate with reduced susceptibility to the protease inhibitor lopinavir among viral isolates from protease inhibitor-experienced patients, *J. Virol.*, **75**(16), 7462–7469.

662. Mo, H., King, M. S., King, K., et al. (2005) Selection of resistance in protease inhibitor-experienced, human immunodeficiency virus type 1-infected subjects failing lopinavir- and ritonavir-based therapy: mutation patterns and baseline correlates, *J. Virol.*, **79**(6), 3329–3338.

663. Delaugerre, C., Teglas, J. P., Treluyer, J. M., et al. (2004) Predictive factors of virologic success in HIV-1-infected children treated with lopinavir/ritonavir, *J. Acquir. Immune Defic. Syndr.*, **37**(2), 1269–1275.

664. Kempf, D. J., Isaacson, J. D., King, M. S., et al. (2002) Analysis of the virologic response with respect to baseline viral phenotype and genotype in protease inhibitor-experienced HIV-1-infected patients receiving lopinavir/ritonavir, *Antivir. Ther.*, **7**(3), 165–174.

665. de Mendoza, C., Martin-Carbonero, L., Barreiro, P., et al. (2002) Salvage treatment with lopinavir/ritonavir (Kaletra), *HIV Clin. Trials*, **3**(4), 304–309.

666. Yusa, K. and Harada, S. (2004) Acquisition of multi-PI (protease inhibitor) resistance in HIV-1 in vivo and in vitro, *Curr. Pharm. Design*, **10**, 4055–4064.

667. Parkin, N. T., Chappey, C., and Petropoulos, C. J. (2003) Improving lopinavir genotype algorithm through phenotype correlations: novel mutation patterns and amprenavir cross-resistance, *AIDS*, **17**, 955–961.

668. Loutfy, M. R., Raboud, J. M., Walmsley, S. L., et al. (2004) Predictive value of HIV-1 protease genotype and virtual phenotype on the virological response to lopinavir/ritonavir-containing salvage regimens, *Antivir. Ther.*, **4**, 595–602.

669. Ribera, E., Azuaje, C., Lopez, R. M., et al. (2006) Atazanavir and lopinavir/ritonavir: pharmacokinetics, safety and efficacy of a promising double-boosted protease inhibitor regimen, *AIDS*, **20**(8), 1131–1139.

670. Rosso, R., Di Biagio, A., Dentone, C., et al. (2006) Lopinavir/ritonavir exposure in treatment-naive HIV-infected children following twice or once daily administration, *J. Antimicrob. Chemother.*, **57**(6), 1168–1171.

671. Connick, E., Lederman, M. M., Kotzin, B. L., Spritzler, J., Kuritzkes, D. R., St. Clair, M., Sevin, A. D., Fox, L., Chiozzi, M. H., Leonard, J. M., Rousseau, F., D'Arc Roe, J., Martinez, A., Kessler, H., and Landay, A. (2000) Immune reconstitution in the first year of potent antiretroviral therapy and its relationship to virologic response, *J. Infect. Dis.*, **181**, 358–863.

672. Thaisrivongs, S. and Strohbach, J. W., (1999) Structure-based discovery of tipranavir disodium (PNU-140690E): a potent, orally bioavailable, nonpeptidic HIV protease inhibitor, *Biopolymers*, **51**(1), 51–58.

673. Turner, S. R., Strohbach, J. W., Tommasi, R. A., Aristoff, P. A., et al. (1998) Tipranavir (PNU-140690): a potent, orally bioavailable nonpeptidic HIV protease inhibitor of the 5,6-dihydro-4-hydroxy-2-pyrone sulfonamide class, *J. Med. Chem.*, **41**(18), 3467–3476.

674. King, J. R. and Acosta, E. (2006) Tipranavir: a novel nonpeptidic protease inhibitor of HIV, *Clin. Pharmacokinet.*, **45**(7), 665–682.

675. Chong, K. T. and Pagano, P. J. (1997) In vitro combination of PNU-140690, a human immunodeficiency virus type 1 protease inhibitor, with ritonavir against ritonavir-sensitive and -resistant clinical isolates, *Antimicrob. Agents Chemother.*, **41**, 2367–2373.

676. Doyon, L., Tremblay, S., Wardrop, E., et al. (2003) Characterization of HIV-1 isolates showing decreased susceptibility to tipranavir and their inhibition by tipranavir containing drug mixtures, *12th International HIV Drug Resistance Workshop, Cabo San Lucas, Mexico*, June 10–14 [abstract].

677. Schwartz, R., Kazanjian, P., Slater, L., et al. (2002) Resistance to tipranavir is uncommon in a randomized trial of tipranavir/ritonavir (TPV/RTV) in multiple PI-failure patients (BI 1182.2), *9th Conference on Retroviruses and Opportunistic Infections, Seattle, WA*, February 24–28 [poster 562 T].

678. Moyle, G. J. and Gazzard, B. G. (1999) A risk-benefit assessment of HIV protease inhibitors, *Drug Safety*, **20**, 299–321.

679. Jayaweera, D., Slater, L., Haas, D., et al. (2002) Susceptibility profile of tipranavir at baseline and subsequent virologic response in a cohort of patients with single-protease inhibitor failure, *2nd International HIV Workshop on Management of Treatment-Experienced Patients, San Diego, CA*, September 26–27 [poster P5].

680. McCallister, S., Neubacher, D., Verblest, W., et al. (2002) Resistance profile of tipranavir (TPV) in patients with single- or multiple-protease inhibitor (PI) failure, *HIV DART 2002: Frontiers in Drug Development for Antiretroviral Therapies, Naples, FL*, December 15–19 [abstract].

681. Hall, D., McCallister, S., Neubacher, D., et al. (2003) Characterization of treatment-emergent resistance mutations in two phase II studies of tipranavir (TPV), *12th International HIV Drug Resistance Workshop, Cabo San Lucas, Mexico*, June 10–14 [poster 13].

682. Gathe, J., Kohlbrenner, V. M., Pierone, G., et al. (2003) Tipranavir/ritonavir (TPV/r) demonstrates potent efficacy in multiple protease inhibitor (PI)-experienced patients: BI 1182.52, *10th Conference on Retroviruses and Opportunistic Infections, Boston, MA*, February 10–14 [presentation 179].

683. McCallister, S., Kohlbrenner, V., Villacian, J., et al. (2004) 24-week combined analysis of the TPV RESIST studies of 1483 treatment-experienced patients given either tipranavir/ritonavir (TPV/r) or an optimized standard of care regimen using 1 of 4 RTV-boosted comparator PIs (CPI/r), *HIV DART 2004: Frontiers in Drug Development for Antiretroviral Therapies, Montego Bay, Jamaica*, December 12–16 [abstract 060].

684. McCallister, S., Sabo, J. P., Mayers, D. L., et al. (2002) An open-label, steady-state investigation of the pharmacokinetics (PK) of tipranavir (TPV) and ritonavir (RTV) and their effects on cytochrome P-450 (3A4) activity in normal, healthy volunteers

(BI 1182.5), *9th Conference on Retroviruses and Opportunistic Infections, Seatlle, WA*, February 24–28 [poster 434W].

685. Kilgore, N., Reddick, M., Zuiderhof, M., et al. (2007) Characterization of PA1050040, a second generation HIV-1 maturation inhibitor, *4th International AIDS Society (IAS) Conference on HIV Pathogenesis, Treatment and Prevention, Sydney, Australia*, July 22–25 [abstract MOPDX05].

686. Phillips, L., Borin, M. T., Hopkins, N. K., et al. (2000) The pharmacokinetics of nucleoside reverse transcriptase inhibitors when coadministered with the HIV protease inhibitor tipranavir in HIV-1 infected patients, *7th Conference on Retroviruses and Opportunistic Infections, San Francisco, CA*, January 30–February 4 [poster 81].

687. Fletcher, C. V., Kawle, S. P., Kakuda, T. N., et al. (2000) Zidovudine triphosphate and lamivudine triphosphate concentration-response relationships in HIV-infected persons, *AIDS*, **14**, 2137–2144.

688. GlaxoSmithKline (2003) Retrovir (zidovudine) [package insert]. GlaxoSmithKline, Research Triangle Park, NC.

689. GlaxoSmithKline (2004) Ziagen (abacavir) [package insert]. GlaxoSmithKline, Research Triangle Park, NC.

690. Bristol-Myers Squibb (2005) Sustiva (efavirenz) [package insert]. Bristol-Myers Squibb, Princeton, NJ.

691. Boehringer Ingelheim (2005) Viramune (nevirapine) [package insert]. Boehringer Ingelheim, Ridgefield, CT.

692. Kashuba, A. D., Tierney, C., Downey, G. F., et al. (2005) Combining fosamprenavir with lopinavir/ritonavir substantially reduces amprenavir and lopinavir exposure: ACTG protocol A5143 results, *AIDS*, **19**, 145–152.

693. Roszko, P. J., Curry, K., Brazina, B., et al. (2003) Standard doses of efavirenz (EFV), zidovudine (ZDV), tenofovir (TDF), and didanosine (ddI) may be given with tipranavir/ritonavir (TPV/r), *2nd International AIDS Society (IAS) Conference on HIV Pathogenesis and Treatment, Paris, France*, July 13–16 [poster 865].

694. Boehringer Ingelheim (2005) Aptivus (tipranavir) [package insert]. Boehringer Ingelheim, Ridgefield, CT.

695. Sabo, J., MacGregor, T., Lamson, M., et al. (2001) Pharmacokinetics of tipranavir and nevirapine, *10th Annual Canadian Conference on HIV/AIDS Research, Toronto, Canada*, May 31–June 3 [poster 249P].

696. Goebel, F. D., Sabo, J. P., MacGregor, T. R., et al. (2202) Pharmacokinetic drug interaction screen of three doses of tipranavir/ritonavir (TPV/r) in HIV-infected patients on stable highly active antiretroviral therapy (HAART), *HIV DART 2002: Frontiers in Drug Development for Antiretroviral Therapies, Naples, FL*, December 15–19 [abstract].

697. Curry, K., Samuels, C., Leith, J., et al. (2004) Pharmacokinetics and safety of tipranavir/ritonavir (TPV/r) alone or in combination with saquinavir (SQV), amprenavir (APV), or lopinavir (LPV): interim analysis of BI 1182.51, *5th International Workshop on Clinical Pharmacology of HIV Therapy, Rome, Italy*, April 1–3 [poster 5.1].

698. Hicks, C. (2004) RESIST-1: A phase 3, randomized, controlled, open-label, multicenter trial comparing tipranavir/ritonavir (TPV/r) to an optimized comparator protease inhibitor/r (CPI/r) regimen in antiretroviral (ARV) experienced patients: 24-week data, *44th Interscience Conference on Antimicrobial Agents and Chemotherapy, Washington, D.C.*, October 30–November 2 [abstract H-1137a].

699. Hicks, C. B., Cahn, P., Cooper, D. A., Walmsley, S. L., Katlama, C., Clotet, B., Lazzarin, A., Johnson, M. A., Neubacher, D., Mayers, D., Valdez, H., and on behalf of the RESIST Investigator Group (2006) Durable efficacy of tipranavir-ritonavir in combination with an optimised background regimen of antiretroviral drugs for treatment-experienced HIV-1-infected patients at 48 weeks in the randomized evaluation of strategic intervention

in multi-drug resistant patients with tipranavir (RESIST) studies: an analysis of combined data from two randomised open-label trials, *Lancet*, **368**(9534), 466–475.

700. Cahn, P. (2004) 24-Week data from RESIST 2: phase 3 of the efficacy and safety of either tipranavir/ritonavir (TRV/r) or an optimized ritonavir (RTV)-boosted standard-of-care (SOC) comparator PI (CPI) in a large randomized multicenter trial in treatment-experienced HIV+ patients, *7th International Congress on Drug Therapy in HIV Infection, Glasgow, UK*, November 14–18 [abstract PL 14.3].

701. Katlama, C., Walmsley, S., Hicks, C., Cahn, P., Neubacher, D., and Villacian, J., for the RESIST Investigator Group (2006) Tipranavir achieves twice the rate of treatment response and prolongs durability of response vs comparator PI in ART-experienced patients, independent of baseline CD4 cell count or viral load: week 48 RESIST 1 and 2 combined analyses, *13th Conference on Retroviruses and Opportunistic Infections, Denver, CO*, February 5–8.

702. Farthing, C., Ward, D., Hicks, C., Johnson, M., Cauda, R., and Cahn, P. (2007) *46th Interscience Conference on Antimicrobial Agents and Chemotherapy, San Francisco, CA*, September 27–30, [abstract. H-1385].

703. Gazzard, B., Antinori, A., and Cheli, C. (2006) Combined analysis of RESIST 96 week data: durability and efficacy of tipranavir/r in treatment experienced patients, *8th International Congress on Drug Therapy in HIV Infection, Glasgow, UK*, November 12–16 [abstract P23].

704. Madruga, J. V., Berger, D., McMurchie, M., and the TITAN Study Group (2007) Efficacy and safety of darunavir-ritonavir compared with that of lopinavir-ritonavir at 48 weeks in treatment-experienced, HIV-infected patients in TITAN: a randomised controlled phase III trial, *Lancet*, **370**(9581), 49–58.

705. Surleraux, D. L., Tahri, A., Verschueren, W. G., Pille, G. M., de Kock, H. A., et al. (2005) Discovery and selection of TMC114, a next generation HIV-1 protease inhibitors, *J. Med. Chem.*, **48**(6), 1813–1822.

706. Kovalevsky, A. Y., Tie, Y., Liu, F., Boross, P. I., Wang, Y. F., et al. (2006) Effectiveness of nonpeptide clinical inhibitor TMC-114 on HIV-1 protease with highly drug resistant mutations D30N, I50V, and L90M, *J. Med. Chem.*, **49**(4), 1379–1387.

707. Tibotec Therapeutics (2006) Darunavir [package insert], Tibotec Therapeutics, East Bridgewater, NJ.

708. De Meyer, S., Hill, A., De Baere, I., et al. (2006) Effect of baseline susceptibility and on-treatment mutations on TMC114 and control PI efficacy: preliminary analysis of data from PI-experienced patients from POWER 1 and POWER 2, *13th Conference on Retroviruses and Opportunistic Infections, Denver, CO*, February 5–9 [abstract 157].

709. De Meyer, S., Vangeneugden, T., Lefebvre, E., van Marck, H., Azijn, H., De Baere, I., van Baelen, B., and de Béthune, M. P. (2006) Response to TMC114 is based on genotypic/phenotypic resistance: POWER 1/2/3 pooled analysis, *8th International Congress on Drug Therapy in HIV Infection, Glasgow, UK*, November 12–16 [poster 196].

710. Sekar, V. J., De Pauw, M., Mariën, K., et al. (2007) Pharmacokinetic interaction between TMC114/r and efavirenz in healthy volunteers, *Antivir. Ther.*, **12**(4), 509–514.

711. Arasteh, K., Clumeck, N., Pozniak, A., Lazzarin, A., De Meyer, S., Muller, H., Peeters, M., Rinehart, A., and Lefebvre, E. (2005) TMC114-C207 Study Team: TMC114/ritonavir substitution for protease inhibitor(s) in a non-suppressive antiretroviral regimen: a 14-day proof-of-principle trial, *AIDS*, **19**(9), 943–947.

712. De Meyer, S., Azijn, H., Surleraux, D., Jochmans, D., Tahri, A., Pauwels, R., Wigerinck, P., and de Bethune, M. P. (2005) TMC114, a novel human immunodeficiency virus type 1 protease inhibitor active against protease inhibitor-resistant viruses,

including a broad range of clinical isolates, *Antimicrob. Agents Chemother.*, 49(6), 2314–2321.

713. Molina, J. M., Cohen, C., Katlama, C., Grinsztejn, B., Timerman, A., Pedro, R., De Meyer, S., de Béthune, M. -P., Vangeneugden, T., and Lefebvre, E. (2006) TMC114/r in treatment-experienced HIV patients in POWER 3: 24-week efficacy and safety analysis, *XVIth International AIDS Conference, Toronto, Canada*, August 13–18 [poster TUPE 0060].

714. Cremieux, A. C., Gillotin, C., Demarles, D., Yuen, G. J., Raffi, F., and the AZ110002 Study Group (2001) A comparison of the steady-state pharmacokinetics and safety of abacavir, lamivudine, and zidovudine taken as a triple combination tablet and as abacavir plus a lamivudine-zidovudine double combination tablet by HIV-1-infected adults, *Pharmacotherapy*, **21**, 424–430

715. Shapiro, M., Ward, K. M., and Stern, J. J. (2001) A near-fatal hypersensitivity reaction to abacavir: case report and literature review, *AIDS Read*, **11**(4), 222–226.

716. Frissen, P. H., De Vries, J., Weigel, H. M., and Brinkman, K. (2001) Severe anaphylactic shock after rechallenge with abacavir without preceding hypersensitivity, *AIDS*, **15**(2), 289.

717. Escaut, L., Liotier, J. Y., Albengres, E., Cheminot, N., and Vittecoq, D. (1999) Abacavir rechallenge has to be avoided in case of hypersensitivity reaction, *AIDS*, **13**(11), 1419–1420.

718. Staszewski, S., Keiser, P., Montaner, J., et al. (2001) Abacavir-lamivudine-zidovudine versus indinavir-lamivudine-zidovudine in antiretroviral-naive HIV-infected adults: a randomized equivalence trial, *J. AM. Med. Assoc.*, **285**(9), 1155–1163.

719. Kakuda, T. N. (2000) Pharmacology of nucleoside and nucleotide reverse transcriptase inhibitor-induced mitochondrial toxicity, *Clin. Ther.*, **22**(6), 685–708.

720. Jonhson, A. A., Ray, A. S., Hanes, J., et al. (2001) Toxicity of antiviral nucleoside analogs and the human mitochondrial DNA polymerase, *J. Biol. Chem.*, **276**(44), 40847–40857.

721. Tikhomirov, V., Namek, K., and Hindes, R. (1999) Agranulocytosis induced by abacavir, *AIDS*, **13**(11), 1420–1421.

722. Lanier, E. R., Ait-Khaled, M., Scott, J., et al. (2004) Antiviral efficacy of abacavir in antiretroviral therapy-experienced adults harbouring HIV-1 with specific patterns of resistance to nucleoside reverse transcriptase inhibitors, *Antivir. Ther.*, **9**(1), 37–45.

723. Latham, V., Stebbing, J., Mandalia, S., et al. (2005) Adherence to trizivir and tenofovir as a simplified salvage regimen is associated with suppression of viraemia and a decreased cholesterol, *J. Antimicrob. Chemother.*, **56**(1), 186–189.

724. Sosa, N., Hill-Zabala, C., DeJesus, E., et al. (2005) Abacavir and lamivudine fixed-dose combination tablet once daily compared with abacavir and lamivudine twice daily in HIV-infected patients over 48 weeks (ESS30008, SEAL), *J. Acquir. Immune Defic. Syndr.*, **40**(4), 422–427.

725. Fallon, J., Ait-Khaled, M., Thomas, D. A., et al. (2002) HIV-1 genotype and phenotype correlate with virological response to abacavir, amprenavir and efavirenz in treatment-experienced patients, *AIDS*, **16**(3), 387–396.

726. Paterson, D. L., Swindells, S., Mohr, J., et al. (2000) Adherence to protease inhibitor therapy and outcomes in patients with HIV infection, *Ann. Intern. Med.*, **133**, 21–30.

727. Moyle, G., Fisher, M., Reilly, G., et al. (2007) A randomized comparison of continued zidovudine plus lamivudine BID (Combivir, CBV) versus switching to tenofovir DF plus emtricitabine (Truvada, TVD), each plus efavirenz (EFV), in stable HIV-infected persons: results of a planned 24-week analysis, *4th International AIDS Society (IAS) Conference on HIV Pathogenesis, Treatment and Prevention, Sydney, Australia*, July 22–25 [abstract WEPEB028].

728. Gallant, J. E., DeJesus, E., Arribas, J. R., et al., for Study 934 Group (2006) Tenofovir DF, emtricitabine, and efavirenz vs.

zidovudine, lamivudine, and efavirenz for HIV, *N. Engl. J. Med.*, **354**, 251–260.

729. Arribas, J., Pozniak, A., Gallant, J., et al. (2007) Three-year safety and efficacy of emtricitabine (FT)/tenofovir DF (TDF) and efavirenz (EFV) compared to fixed dose zidovudine/lamivudine (CBV) in antiretroviral treatment-naïve patients, *4th International AIDS Society (IAS) Conference on HIV Pathogenesis, Treatment and Prevention, Sydney*, July 22–25 [abstract WEPEB029].

730. Staszewski, S., Keiser, P., Gathe, J., Haas, D., Montaner, J., et al. (1999) Comparison of antiviral response with abacavir/combivir to indinavir/combivir in therapy-naive adults at 48 weeks (CN3005), *47th Interscience Conference on Antimicrobial Agents and Chemotherapy, San Francisco, CA*, September 26–29 [abstract no. 505].

731. Rodriguez-French, A., Boghossian, J., Gray, G. E., et al. (2004) The NEAT Study: a 48-week open-label study to compare the antiviral efficacy and safety of GW433908 versus nelfinavir in antiretroviral therapy-naive HIV-1-infected patients, *J. Acquir. Immune Defic. Syndr.*, **35**, 22–32.

732. Gathe, J., Ive, P., Wood, R., et al. (2004) SOLO: 48-week efficacy and safety comparison of once-daily fosamprenavir/ritonavir versus twice-daily nelfinavir in naïve HIV-1-infected patients, *AIDS*, **18**, 1529–1537.

733. Gazzard, B., DeJesus, E., Cahn, P., et al. (2003) Abacavir (ABC) once daily (OAD) plus lamivudine (3TC) OAD in combination with efavirenz (EFV) OAD is well-tolerated and effective in the treatment of antiretroviral therapy (ART) naïve adults with HIV-1 infection (Zodiac Study: CNA30021), *43rd Interscience Conference on Antimicrobial Agents and Chemotherapy, Chicago, IL*, September 14–17 [abstract H1722b].

734. DeJesus, E., Herrera, G., Teofilo, E., et al., for the CNA30024 Study Team (2004) Abacavir versus zidovudine combined with lamivudine and efavirenz for the treatment of antiretroviral-naïve HIV-infected adults, *Clin. Infect. Dis.*, **39**, 38–46.

735. Sosa, N., Hill-Zabala, C., DeJesus, E., Herrera, G., Florance, A., Watson, M., Vavro, C., and Shaefer, M. (2005) Abacavir and lamivudine fixed-dose combination tablet once daily compared with abacavir and lamivudine twice daily in HIV-infected patients over 48 weeks, *J. Acquir. Immune Defic. Syndr.*, **40**(4), 422–427.

736. Kubota, M., Cohen, C., Scribner, A., et al. (2006) Short-term safety and tolerability of ABC/3TC administered once-daily (QD) compared with the separate components administered twice-daily (BID): results from ESS101822 (ALOHA), *46th Interscience Conference on Antimicrobial Agents and Chemotherapy, San Francisco*, September 27–30 [poster H-1904].

737. Martinez, E., Arranz, J. A., Podzamczer, D., et al. (2007) Efficacy and safety of NRTIs switch to tenofovir plus emtricitabine (Truvada) vs. abacavir plus lamivudine (Kivexa) in patients with virologic suppression receiving a lamivudine containing HAART: the BICOMBO study, *4th International AIDS Society (IAS) Conference on HIV Pathogenesis, Treatment and Prevention, Sydney, Australia*, July 22–25 [abstract WESS102].

738. Mallal, S., Phillips, E., Carosi, G., et al. (2007) PREDICT-1: a novel randomised prospective study to determine the clinical utility of HLA-B*5701 screening to reduce abacavir hypersensitivity in HIV-1 infected subjects (study CNA106030), *4th International AIDS Society (IAS) Conference on HIV Pathogenesis, Treatment, and Prevention. Sydney, Australia*, July 22–25 [abstract WESS101].

739. Trottier, B., Thomas, R., Nguyen, V. K., et al. (2007) How effectively HLA screening can reduce the early discontinuation of abacavir in real life? *4th International AIDS Society (IAS) Conference on HIV Pathogenesis, Treatment, and Prevention, Sydney, Australia*, July 22–25 [abstract MOAB103].

740. Saag, M., Balu, R., Brachman, P., et al. (2007) High sensitivity of HLA-B*5701 in whites and blacks in immunologically-confirmed cases of abacavir hypersensitivity (ABC HSR), *4th International AIDS Society (IAS) Conference on HIV Pathogenesis, Treatment, and Prevention, Sydney, Australia*, July 22–25 [abstract WEAB305].

741. Goicoechea, M. and Best, B. (2007) Efavirenz/emtricitabine/tenofovir disoproxil fumarate fixed-dose combination: first-line therapy for all? *Expert Opin. Pharmacother.*, **8**(3), 371–382.

742. Pozniak, A. L., Gallant, J. E., DeJesus, E., et al. (2006) Tenofovir disoproxil fumarate, emtricitabine, and efavirenz versus fixed-dose zidovudine/lamivudine and efavirenz in antiretroviral-naive patients: virologic, immunologic, and morphologic changes—a 96-week analysis, *J. Acquir. Immune Defic. Syndr.*, **4**, 535–540.

743. Gallant, J. E., Staszewski, S., Pozniak, A. L. et al. (2004) Efficacy and safety of tenofovir DF versus stavudine in combination therapy in antiretroviral-naive patients: a 3-year randomized trial, *J. Am. Med. Assoc.*, **292**, 191–201.

744. Berger, E. A. (1997) HIV entry and tropism: when one receptor is not enough, *4th Conference on Retroviruses and Opportunistic Infections, Washington, D.C.*, January 22–26, [abstract S7].

745. Fox, J. and Pease, J. E. (2005) The molecular and cellular biology of CC chemokines and their receptors, *Curr. Topics Membr.*, **55**, 73–102.

746. Blanpain, C., Libert, F., Vassart, G., and Parmentier M. (2002) CCR5 and HIV infection, *Receptor Channels*, **8**(1), 19–31.

747. Galvani, A. and Slatkin, M. (2003) Evaluating plague and smallpox as historical selective pressures for the CCR5-Δ32 HIV-resistance allele, *Proc. Natl. Acad. Sci. U.S.A.*, **100**(25), 15276–15279.

748. Stephens, J., Reich, D. E., Goldstein, D. B., et al. (1998) Dating the origin of the CCR5-delta32 AIDS-resistance allele by the coalescence of haplotypes, *Am. J. Hum. Genet.*, **62**(6), 1507–1515.

749. Hedrick, P. W. and Verrelli, B. C. (2006) "Ground truth" for selection on CCR5-Δ32, *Trends in Genet.*, **22**(6), 293–296.

750. Glass, W. G., McDermott, D. H., and Lim, J. K. (2006) CCR5 deficiency increases risk of symptomatic West Nile virus infection, *J. Exp. Med.*, **203**(1), 35–40.

751. Duncan, S. R., Scott, S., and Duncan, C. J. (2005) Reappraisal of the historical selective pressures for the CCR5-Δ32 mutation, *J. Med. Genet.*, **42**, 205–208.

752. Sabeti, P. C., Walsh, E., Schaffner, S. F., et al. (2005), The case for selection at CCR5-Delta32, *PLoS Biology*, **3**(11), e378.

753. Welch, B. D., VanDemark, A. P., Heroux, A., Hill, C. P, and Kay, M. S. (2007) Potent D-peptide inhibitors of HIV-1 entry, *Proc. Natl. Acad. Sci. U.S.A.*, **104**(43), 16828–16833.

754. Chan, D. C., Fass, D., Berger, J. M., and Kim, P. S. (1997) Core structure of gp41 from the HIV envelope glycoprotein, *Cell*, **89**, 263–273.

755. Weissenhorn, W., Dessen, A., Harrison, S. C., Skehel, J. J., and Wiley, D. C. (1997) Atomic structure of the ectodomain from HIV-1 gp41, *Nature*, **387**, 426–430.

756. Tan, K., Liu, J., Wang, J., Shen, S., and Lu, M. (1997) Atomic structure of a thermostable subdomain of HIV-1 gp41, *Proc. Natl. Acad. Sci. U.S.A.*, **94**, 12303–12308.

757. Eckert, D. M. and Kim, P. S. (2001) Mechanisms of viral membrane fusion and its inhibition, *Annu. Rev. Biochem.*, **70**, 777–810.

758. Chan, D. C. and Kim, P. S. (1998) HIV Entry and its inhibition, *Cell*, **93**, 681–684.

759. Furuta, R. A., Wild, C. T., Weng, Y., and Weiss, C. D. (1998) Capture of an early fusion-active conformation of HIV-1 gp41, *Nat. Struct. Biol.*, **5**, 276–279.

760. Root, M. J. and Steger, H. K. (2004) HIV-1 gp41 as a target for viral entry inhibition, *Curr. Pharm. Des.*, **10**, 1805–1825.

761. Eckert, D. M., Malashkevich, V. N., Hong, L, H., Carr, P, A., and Kim, P. S. (1999) Inhibiting HIV-1 entry: discovery of D-peptide inhibitors that target the gp41 coiled-coil pocket, *Cell*, **99**, 103–115.

762. Root, M. J., Kay, M. S., and Kim, P. S. (2001) Protein design of an HIV-1 entry inhibitor, *Science*, **291**, 884–888.

763. Chan, D. C., Chutkowski, C. T., and Kim, P. S. (1998) Evidence that a prominent cavity in the coiled coil of HIV type 1 gp41 is an attractive drug target, *Proc. Natl. Acad. Sci. U.S.A.*, **95**, 15613–15617.

764. Louis, J. M., Bewley, C. A., and Clore, G. M. (2001) Design and properties of NCCG-gp41, a chimeric gp41 molecule with nanomolar HIV fusion inhibitory activity, *J. Biol. Chem.*, **276**, 29485–29489.

765. Eckert, D. M. and Kim, P. S. (2001) Design of potent inhibitors of HIV-1 entry from the gp41 N-peptide region, *Proc. Natl. Acad. Sci. U.S.A.*, **98**, 11187–11192.

766. Wild, C. T., Shugars, D. C., Greenwell, T. K., McDanal, C. B., and Matthews, T. J. (1994) Peptides corresponding to a predictive α-helical domain of human immunodeficiency virus type 1 gp41 are potent inhibitors of virus infection, *Proc. Natl. Acad. Sci. U.S.A.*, **91**, 9770–9774.

767. Rimsky, L. T., Shugars, D. C., and Matthews, T. J. (1998) Determinants of human immunodeficiency virus type 1 resistance to gp41-derived inhibitory peptides, *J. Virol.*, **72**, 986–993.

768. Cooper, D., on behalf of the Alliance Investigator Group (2005) An analysis of the correlation between the severity of injection site reactions and the amount of subcutaneous fat in the Alliance cohort, *12th Conference on Retroviruses and Opportunistic Infections, Boston, MA*, February 22–25 [poster 838].

769. Thompson, M., DeJesus, E., Richmond, G., et al. (2006) Pharmacokinetics, pharmacodynamics and safety of once-daily versus twice-daily dosing with enfuvirtide in HIV-infected subjects, *AIDS*, **20**(3), 397–404.

770. DeJesus, E., Zolopa, A., Farthing, C., et al. (2007) Response to darunavir/ritonavir (DRV/r) combined with enfuvirtide (ENF)-containing ARV in triple-class experienced patients was not predicted by baseline darunavir (DRV) sensitivity or viral tropism (VT): the BLQ study preliminary results, *4th International AIDS Society (IAS) Conference on HIV Pathogenesis, Treatment and Prevention, Sydney, Australia*, July 22–25 [poster WEPEB039].

771. Wiznia, A., Church, A., Emmanuel, P., and the T20-310 Study Group (2007) Safety and efficacy of enfuvirtide for 48 weeks as part of an optimized antiretroviral regimen in pediatric human immunodeficiency virus 1-infected patients, *Pediatr. Infect. Dis. J.*, **26**(9), 799–805.

772. Tschida, S., Zappa, A., and Godwin, M. (2006) An ongoing nonrandomized large prospective evaluation of alternative injection devices (Biojector B2000, standard needles/syringes, or insulin needles/syringes) for enfuvirtide in a national community-based specialty pharmacy, *XVIth International AIDS Conference, Toronto, Canada*, August 13–18 [poster TUPE0147].

773. Harris, M., Joy, R., Larsen, G.,Valyi, M., Walker, E., et al. (2006) Enfuvirtide plasma levels and injection site reactions using a needle-free gas-powered injection system (Biojector), *AIDS*, **20**(5), 719–723.

774. Paterlini, M. G. (2002) Structure modeling of the chemokine receptor CCR5: implications for ligand binding and selectivity, *Biophys. J.*, **83**(6), 3012–3031.

775. Hoffman, T. L., LaBranche, C. C., Zhang, W., Canziani, G., Robinson, J., Chaiken, I., Hoxie, J. A., and Doms, R. W. (1999) Stable exposure of the coreceptor-binding site in a CD4-independent HIV-1 envelope protein, *Proc. Natl. Acad. Sci. U.S.A.*, **96**, 6359–6364.

776. Kolchinsky, P., Mirzabekov, T., Farzan, M., Kiprilov, E., Cayabyab, M., Mooney, L. J., Choe, H., and Sodroski, J. (1999) Adaptation of a CCR5-using, primary human immunodeficiency virus type 1 isolate for CD4-independent replication, *J. Virol.*, **73**, 8120–8126.

777. Rizzuto, C. D., Wyatt, R., Hernandez-Ramos, N., Sun, Y., Kwong, P. D., Hendrickson, W. A., and Sodroski, J. (1998) A conserved HIV gp120 glycoprotein structure involved in chemokine receptor binding, *Science*, **280**, 1949–1953.

778. Wu, L., Gerard, N. P., Wyatt, R., Choe, H., Parolin, C., Ruffing, N., et al. (1996) CD4-induced interaction of primary HIV-1 gp120 glycoproteins with the chemokine receptor CCR-5, *Nature*, **384**, 179–183.

779. Berger, E. A., Doms, R. W., Fenyo, E. M., Korber, B. T., Littman, D. R., et al. (1998) A new classification for HIV-1, *Nature*, **391**, 240.

780. Robertson, D. L., Anderson, J. P., Bradac, J. A., Carr, J. K., Foley, B., et al. (2000) HIV-1 nomenclature proposal, *Science*, **288**, 55–56.

781. Lucas, A. D., Gaudieri, S., Rauch, A., et al. (2005) Cellular tropism of HIV-1 mediated and constrained by coreceptor dependencies, *J. Vir. Entry*, **1**, 17–27.

782. Clotet, B. (2007) CCR5 Inhibitors: promising yet challenging, *J. Infect. Dis.*, **196**, 178–180.

783. Dragic, T., Trkola, A., Lin, S. W., Nagashima, K. A., Kajumo, F., Zhao, L., et al. (1998) Amino-terminal substitutions in the CCR5 coreceptor impair gp120 binding and human immunodeficiency virus type 1 entry, *J. Virol.*, **72**, 279–285.

784. Samson, M., LaRosa, G., Libert, F., Paindavoine, P., Detheux, M., Vassart, G., and Parmentier, M. (1997) The second extracellular loop of CCR5 is the major determinant of ligand specificity, *J. Biol. Chem.*, **272**, 24934–24941.

785. Blanpain, C., Doranz, B. J., Vakili, J., Rucker, J., Govaerts, C., Baik, S. S., et al. (1999) Multiple charged and aromatic residues in CCR5 amino-terminal domain are involved in high affinity binding of both chemokines and HIV-1 Env protein, *J. Biol. Chem.*, **274**, 34719–34727.

786. Dragic, T., Trkola, A., Thompson, D. A., Cormier, E. G., Kajumo, F. A., et al. (2000) A binding pocket for a small molecule inhibitor of HIV-1 entry within the transmembrane helices of CCR5, *Proc. Natl. Acad. Sci. U.S.A.*, **97**, 5639–5644.

787. Mayer, H., van der Ryst, E., Saag, M., et al. (2006) Safety and efficacy of maraviroc (MVC), a novel CCR5 antagonist, when used in combination with optimized background therapy (OBT) for the treatment of antiretroviral-experienced subjects infected with dual/mixed-tropic HIV-1: 24-week results of a Phase 2b exploratory trial, *XVI International AIDS Conference, Toronto, Canada*, August 13–18 [abstract THLB0215].

788. Lalezari, J., Goodrich, J., DeJesus, E., Lampiris, H., Gulick, R., et al. on behalf of the MOTIVATE 1 Study Group. (2007) Efficacy and safety of maraviroc plus optimized background therapy in viremic, ART-experienced patients infected with CCR5-tropic HIV-1: 24-week results of Phase 2b/3 studies, *14th Conference on Retroviruses and Opportunistic Infections, Los Angeles, CA*, February 25–28 [presentation 104bLB].

789. Nelson, M., Fätkenheuer, G., Konourina, I., Lazzarin, A., Clumeck, N., Horban, A., et al., on behalf of the MOTIVATE 2 Study Group (2007) Efficacy and safety of maraviroc plus optimized background therapy in viremic, ART-experienced patients infected with CCR5-tropic HIV-1: 24-week results of Phase 2b/3 studies, *14th Conference on Retroviruses and Opportunistic Infections, Los Angeles, CA*, February 25–28 [presentation 104aLB].

790. Fätkenheuer, G., Pozniak, A. L., Johnson, M. A., et al. (2005) Efficacy of short-term monotherapy with maraviroc, a new

CCR5 antagonist, in patients infected with HIV-1, *Nat. Med.* **11**, 1170–1172.

791. McHale, M., Abel, S., Russell, D., et al. (2005) Overview of Phase I and 2a safety and efficacy data of maraviroc (UK-427,857), *3rd International AIDS Society (IAS) Conference on the HIV Pathogenesis and Treatment, Rio de Janeiro, Brazil*, July 24–27 [abstract TuOa0204].

792. Tsibris, A. M. and Kuritzkes, D. R. (2007) Chemokine antagonists as therapeutics: focus on HIV-1, *Annu. Rev. Med.*, **58**, 445–459.

793. GlaxoSmithKline (2005) Statement to HIV patient community: information from GlaxoSmithKline on changes to studies of investigational CCR5 entry inhibitor aplaviroc (GW873140), GlaxoSmithKline, Research Triangle Park, NC.

794. Steel, H. M. (2005) Special presentation on aplaviroc-related hepatotoxicity, *10th European AIDS Conference, Dublin, Ireland*, November 17–20 [abstract].

795. Temesdgen, Z., Warnke, D., and Kasten, M. J. (2006) Current status of antiretroviral therapy, *Expert Opin. Chemother.*, **7**(12), 1541–1554.

796. Saag, M., Ive, P., Heers, J., et al. (2007) A multicenter, randomized, double-blind, comparative trial of a novel CCR5 antagonist, maraviroc versus efavirenz, both in combination with Combivir (zidovudine [ZDV]/lamivudine [3TC]), for the treatment of antiretroviral naive subjects infected with R5 HIV-1: week 48 results of the MERIT study, *4th International AIDS Society (IAS) Conference on HIV Pathogeneis, Treatment and Prevention, Sydney, Australia*, July 22–25 [abstract WESS104].

797. Reeves, J. D., Han, D., Liu, Y., et al. (2007) Enhancements to the Trofile HIV coreceptor tropism assay enable reliable detection of CXCR4-using subpopulations at less than 1%, *47th Interscience Conference on Antimicrobial Agents and Chemotherapy, Chicago, IL*, September 17–20 [abstract H-1026].

798. Strizki, J. M., Tremblay, C., Xu, S., et al. (2005) Discovery and characterization of vicriviroc (SCH 417690), a CCR5 antagonist with potent activity against human immunodeficiency virus type 1, *Antimicrob. Agents Chemother.*, **49**(12), 4911–4919.

799. Schurmann, D., Fätkenheuer, G., Reynes, J. (2007) Antiviral activity, pharmacokinetics and safety of vicriviroc, an oral CCR5 antagonist, during 14-day monotherapy in HIV-infected adults, *AIDS*, **21**(10), 1293–1299.

800. Gulick, R., Su, Z., Flexner, C., Hughes, M. (2007) ACTG 5211: phase II study of the safety and efficacy of vicriviroc (VCV) in HIV-infected treatment-experienced subjects: 48 week results, *4th International AIDS Conference (IAS) on Pathogenesis, Treatment and Prevention, Sydney, Australia*, July 22–25 [abstract 1623].

801. Gulick, R., Haas, D., Collier, A. C., Lennox, J., Parker, C., and Greaves, W. (2007) Two-year follow-up of treatment-experienced patients on vicriviroc (VCV), *47th Interscience Conference on Antimicrobial Agents and Chemotherapy, Chicago, IL*, September 17–20 [abstract H-1030].

802. Fätkenheuer, G., Hoffmann, C., Sansone-Parsons, A., Greaves, W., and Dunkle, L. (2007) CD4 lymphocyte and leukocyte response to vicriviroc (VCV) in 282 HIV-infected treatment-naive and experienced subjects: pooled data from 4 randomized clinical trials, *47th Interscience Conference on Antimicrobial Agents and Chemotherapy, Chicago, IL*, October 25–27 [abstract H-1031].

803. Savarino, A. (2006) A historical sketch of the discovery and development of HIV-1 integrase inhibitors, *Expert Opin. Investig. Drugs*, **15**(12), 1507–1522.

804. Pommier, Y., Johnson, A. A., and Marchand, C. (2005) Integrase inhibitors to treat HIV/AIDS, *Nat. Rev. Drug Discov.*, **4**(3), 236–248.

805. Goldgur, Y., Craigie, R., Cohen, R., et al. (1999) Structure of the HIV-1 integrase catalytic domain complexed with an inhibitor: a platform for antiviral drug design, *Proc. Natl. Acad. Sci. U.S.A.*, **96**(23), 13040–13043.

806. Wang, J. Y., Ling, H., Yang, W., et al., (2001) Structure of a two-domain fragment of HIV-1 integrase: implications for domain organization in the intact protein, *EMBO J.*, **20**(24), 7333–7343.

807. Chen, J. C. H., Krucinski, J., Miercke, W., et al. (2000) Crystal structure of the HIV-1 integrase catalytic core and C-terminal domains: a model for viral DNA binding, *Proc. Natl. Acad. Sci. U.S.A.*, **97**(15), 8233–8238.

808. Tsurutani, N., Kubo, M., Maeda, Y., et al. (2000) Identification of critical amino acid residues in human immunodeficiency virus type 1 IN required for efficient proviral DNA formation at steps prior to integration in dividing and nondividing cells, *J. Virol.*, **74**, 4795–4806.

809. Zhu, K., Dobard, C., and Chow, S. A. (2004) Requirement for integrase during reverse transcription of human immunodeficiency virus type 1 and the effect of cysteine mutations of integrase on its interactions with reverse transcriptase, *J. Virol.*, **78**, 5045–5055.

810. Brown, P. O. (1998) Integration. In: *Retroviruses* (Coffin, J. M., Hughes, S. H., and Varmus, H. E., eds.), Cold Spring Harbor Press, Cold Spring Harbor, NY, pp. 161–203.

811. Turlure, F., Devroe, E., Silver, P. A., and Engelman, A. (2004) Human cell proteins and human immunodeficiency virus DNA integration, *Front. Biosci.*, **9**, 3187–3208.

812. Hindmarsh, P., Ridky, T., Reeves, R., Andrake, M., Skalka, A. M., and Leis, J. (1999) HMG protein family members stimulate human immunodeficiency virus type 1 and avian sarcoma virus concerted DNA integration in vitro, *J. Virol.*, **73**, 2994–3003.

813. Farnet, C. and Bushman, F. D. (1997) HIV-1 cDNA integration: requirement of HMG I (Y) protein for function of preintegration complexes in vitro, *Cell*, **88**, 483–492.

814. Bukrinsky, M. I., Sharova, N., Dempsey, M. P., Stanwick, T. L., Bukrinskaya, A. G., Haggerty, S., and Stevenson, M. (1992) Active nuclear import of human immunodeficiency virus type 1 preintegration complexes, *Proc. Natl. Acad. Sci. U.S.A.*, **89**, 6580–6584.

815. Chow, S. A., Vincent, K. A., Ellison, V., and Brown, P. O. (1992) Reversal of integration and DNA splicing mediated by integrase of human immunodeficiency virus, *Science*, **255**, 723–726.

816. Yoder, K. E. and Bushman, F. D. (2000) Repair of gaps in retroviral DNA integration intermediates, *J. Virol.*, **74**, 11191–11200.

817. Daniel, R., Greger, J. G., Katz, R. A., Taganov, K., et al. (2004) Evidence that stable retroviral transduction and cell survival following DNA integration depend on components of the nonhomologous end joining repair pathway, *J. Virol.*, **78**, 8573–8581.

818. Myers, R. E. and Pillay, D. (2007) HIV-1 integrase sequence variation and covariation, *Antivir. Ther.*, **12**, S65.

819. Van Baelen, K., Clynhens, M., Rondelez, E., et al. (2007) Low level of baseline resistance to integrase inhibitors L731,988 and L870,810 in randomly selected subtype B and non-B HIV-1 strains, *Antivir. Ther.*, **12**, S7.

820. Ceccherini-Silberstein, F., Malet, I., Perno, C. F., et al. (2007) Specific mutations related to HIV-1 integrase inhibitors are associated with reverse transcriptase mutations in HAART-treated patients, *Antivir. Ther.*, **12**, S6.

821. Roquebert, B., Dmaond, F., Descamps, D., et al. (2007) Polymorphism of HIV-2 integrase gene and in vitro phenotypic susceptibility of HIV-2 clinical isolates to integrase inhibitors: raltegravir and elvitegravir, *Antivir. Ther.*, **12**, S92.

822. Hazuda, D. J., Miller, M. D., Hguyen, B. Y., et al. (2007) Resistance to the HIV-integrase inhibitor raltegravir: analysis of protocol 005, a Phase II study in patients with triple-class resistant HIV-1 infection, *Antivir. Ther.*, **12**(5), S10.

823. Malet, I., Delelis, O., Calvez, V., et al. (2007) Biochemical characterizations of the effect of mutations selected in HIV-1

integrase gene associated with failure to raltegravir (MK-0518), *Antivir. Ther.*, **12**(5), S9.

824. Cooper, D., Gatell, J., Rockstroh, J., et al. (2007) Results from BENCHMRK-1, a phase III study evaluating the efficacy and safety of MK-0518, a novel HIV-1 integrase inhibitor, in patients with triple-class resistant virus, *14th Conference on Retroviruses and Opportunistic Infections, Los Angeles, CA*, February 25–28 [abstract 105aLB].

825. Steigbigel, R., Kumar, P., Eron, J., et al. (2007) Results from BENCHMRK-2, a phase III study evaluating the efficacy and safety of MK-0518, a novel HIV-1 integrase inhibitor, in patients with triple-class resistant virus, *14th Conference on Retroviruses and Opportunistic Infections, Los Angeles, CA*, February 25–28 [abstract 105bLB].

826. Grinsztejn, B., Nguyen, B., Katlama, C., et al. (2007) 48 week efficacy and safety of MK-0518, a novel HIV-1 integrase inhibitor, in patients with triple-class resistant virus, *47th Interscience Conference on Antimicrobial Agents and Chemotherapy. Chicago, IL*, September 17–20 [abstract H-713].

827. Grinsztejn, B., Nguyen, B., Katlama, C., et al. (2007) Safety and efficacy of the HIV-1 integrase inhibitor raltegravir (MK-0518) in treatment-experienced patients with multidrug-resistant virus: a phase II randomised controlled trial, *Lancet*, **369**(9569), 1261–1269.

828. Markowitz, M., Nguyen, B. Y., Gotuzzo, E., et al. (2007) Rapid and durable antiretroviral effect of the HIV-1 integrase inhibitor raltegravir as part of combination therapy in treatment-naive patients: results of a 48-week controlled study, *J. Acquir. Immune Defic. Syndr.*, **46**(2), 125–133.

829. Markowitz, M., Morales-Ramirez, J. O., Nguyen, B-Y., et al. (2006) Antiretroviral activity, pharmacokinetics, and tolerability of MK-0518, a novel inhibitor of HIV-1 integrase, dosed as monotherapy for 10 days in treatment-naive HIV-1-infected individuals, *J. Acquir. Immune Defic. Syndr.*, **43**(5), 509–515.

830. Iwamoto, M., Wenning, L. A., Petry, A. S., et al. (2007) Safety, tolerability, and pharmacokinetics of raltegravir after single and multiple doses in healthy subjects, *Clin. Pharmacol. Ther.*, **83**(2), 293–299.

831. Cahn, P. and Sued, O. (2007) Raltegravir: a new antiretroviral class for salvage therapy, *Lancet*, **369**, 1235–1236.

832. Grinsztejn, B., Nguyen, B., Katlama, C., et al. (2007) Safety and efficacy of the HIV-1 integrase inhibitor raltegravir (MK-0518) in treatment-experienced patients with multidrug-resistant virus: a phase II randomised controlled trial, *Lancet*, **369**(9569), 1261–1269.

833. DeJesus, E., Berger, D., Markowitz, M., et al. (2006) The HIV integrase inhibitor GS-9137 (JTK-303) exhibits potent antiviral activity in treatment-naive and experienced patients, *13th Conference on Retroviruses and Opportunistic Infections, Denver, CO*, February 5–8 [abstract 159LB].

834. Zolopa, A. R., Mullen, M., Berger, D., et al. (2007) The HIV integrase inhibitor GS-9137 demonstrates potent ARV activity in treatment-experienced patients, *14th Conference on Retroviruses and Opportunistic Infections, Los Angeles, CA*, February 25–28, [oral presentation/abstract 143LB].

835. Zolopa, A. R., Lampiris, H., Blick, G., et al (2007) The HIV integrase inhibitor elvitegravir (EVG/r) has potent and durable activity in treatment-experienced patients with active optimized background therapy (OBT), *47th Interscience Conference on Antimicrobial Agents and Chemotherapy, Chicago, IL*, September 17–20 [oral presentation/abstract H-714].

836. Ledford, R., Margot, N., Miller, M., et al. (2007) Elvitegravir (GS-9137/JTK-303), an HIV-1 integrase inhibitor, has additive to synergistic interactions with other antiretroviral drugs in vitro, *4th International AIDS Society (IAS) Conference on Pathogenesis, Treatment and Prevention, Sydney, Australia*, July 22–25 [abstract/poster MOPEA052].

837. Jones, G., Ledford, R., Yu, F., et al. (2007) Resistance profile of HIV-1 mutants in vitro selected by the HIV-1 integrase inhibitor, GS-9137 (JTK-303), *14th Conference on Retroviruses and Opportunistic Infections, Los Angeles, CA*, February 25–28 [poster 627].

838. Li, F., Goila-Gaur, R., Salzwedel, K., Kilgore, N. R., Reddick, M., et al. (2003) PA-457: a potent HIV inhibitor that disrupts core condensation by targeting a late step in Gag processing, *Proc. Natl. Acad. Sci. U.S.A.*, **100**(23), 13555–13560.

839. Swanstrom, R. and Wills, J. W. (1997) Synthesis, assembly, and processing of viral proteins. In: *Retroviruses* (Weiss, R., Teich, N., Varmus, H., and Coffin, J. M., eds.), Cold Spring Harbor Laboratory Press, Plainview, NY, pp. 263–334.

840. Freed, E. O. (1998) HIV-1 gag proteins: diverse functions in the virus life cycle, *Virology*, **251**, 1–15.

841. Gottlinger, H. G., Dorfman, T., Sodroski, J. G., and Haseltine, W. A. (1991) Effect of mutations affecting the p6 gag protein on human immunodeficiency virus particle release, *Proc. Natl. Acad. Sci. U.S.A.*, **88**, 3195–3199.

842. Huang, M., Orenstein, J. M., Martin, M. A., and Freed, E. O. (1995) p6Gag is required for particle production from full-length human immunodeficiency virus type 1 molecular clones expressing protease, *J. Virol.*, **69**, 6810–6818.

843. Freed, E. O. (2002) Viral late domains, *J. Virol.*, **76**, 4679–4687.

844. Kräusslich, H. G., Schneider, H., Zybarth, G., Carter, C. A., and Wimmer, E. (1988) Processing of in vitro-synthesized gag precursor proteins of human immunodeficiency virus (HIV) type 1 by HIV proteinase generated in *Escherichia coli, J. Virol.*, **62**, 4393–4397.

845. Mervis, R. J., Ahmad, N., Lillehoj, E. P., Raum, M. G., Salazar, F. H., Chan, H. W., and Venkatesan, S. (1988) The gag gene products of human immunodeficiency virus type 1: alignment within the gag open reading frame, identification of posttranslational modifications, and evidence for alternative gag precursors, *J. Virol.*, **62**, 3993–4002.

846. Erickson-Viitanen, S., Manfredi, J., Viitanen, P., Tribe, D. E., Tritch, R., Hutchison, C. A., Loeb, D. D., and Swanstrom, R. (1989) Cleavage of HIV-1 gag polyprotein synthesized in vitro: sequential cleavage by the viral protease, *AIDS Res. Hum. Retroviruses*, **5**, 577–591.

847. Kräusslich, H. G., Facke, M., Heuser, A. M., Konvalinka, J., and Zentgraf, H. (1995) The spacer peptide between human immunodeficiency virus capsid and nucleocapsid proteins is essential for ordered assembly and viral infectivity, *J. Virol.*, **69**, 3407–3419.

848. Wiegers, K., Rutter, G., Kottler, H., Tessmer, U., Hohenberg, H., and Kräusslich H. G. (1998) Sequential steps in human immunodeficiency virus particle maturation revealed by alterations of individual Gag polyprotein cleavage sites, *J. Virol.*, **72**, 2846–2854.

849. Accola, M. A., Höglund, S., and Göttlinger, H. G. (1998) A putative α-helical structure which overlaps the capsid-p2 boundary in the human immunodeficiency virus type 1 Gag precursor is crucial for viral particle assembly, *J. Virol.*, **72**, 2072–2078.

850. Kaplan, A. H., Zack, J. A., Knigge, M., Paul, D. A., Kempf, D. J., Norbeck, D. W., and Swanstrom, R. (1993) Partial inhibition of the human immunodeficiency virus type 1 protease results in aberrant virus assembly and the formation of noninfectious particles, *J. Virol.* **67**, 4050–4055.

851. Demirov, D. G., Orenstein, J. M., and Freed, E. O. (2002) The late domain of human immunodeficiency virus type 1 p6 promotes virus release in a cell type-dependent manner, *J. Virol.*, **76**, 105–117.

852. Garrus, J. E., von Schwedler, U. K., Pornillos, O. W., Morham, S. G., Zavitz, K. H., Wang, H. E., Wettstein, D. A., Stray, K. M., Cote, M., Rich, R. L., et al. (2001) Tsg101 and the vacuolar

protein sorting pathway are essential for HIV-1 budding, *Cell*, **107**, 55–65.

853. Demirov, D. G., Ono, A., Orenstein, J. M., and Freed, E. O. (2002) Overexpression of the N-terminal domain of TSG101 inhibits HIV-1 budding by blocking late domain function, *Proc. Natl. Acad. Sci. U.S.A.*, **99**, 955–960.

854. Liang, C., Rong, L., Laughrea, M., Kleiman, L., and Wainberg, M. A. (1998) Compensatory point mutations in the human immunodeficiency virus type 1 Gag region that are distal from deletion mutations in the dimerization initiation site can restore viral replication, *J. Virol.*, **72**, 6629–6636.

855. Liang, C., Rong, L., Cherry, E., Kleiman, L., Laughrea, M., and Wainberg, M. A. (1999) Deletion mutagenesis within the dimerization initiation site of human immunodeficiency virus type 1 results in delayed processing of the p2 peptide from precursor proteins, *J. Virol.*, **73**, 6147–6151.

856. PR Newswire. (2004) Panacos Pharmaceuticals' HIV Drug Candidate, PA-457, exhibits potent anti-HIV activity following a single dose in HIV-infected patients. Press release, November 23 (http://www.pressurebiosciences.com/news_releases/article-157.html).

857. Fujioka, T., Kashiwada, Y., Kilkuskie, R. E., Cosentino, L. M., Ballas, L. M., Jiang, J. B., Janzen, W. P., Chen, I. S., and Lee, K. H. (1994) Anti-AIDS agents. 11. Betulinic acid and platanic acid as anti-HIV principles from *Syzigium claviflorum*, and the anti-HIV activity of structurally related triterpenoids, *J. Nat. Prod.*, **57**, 243–247.

858. Kashiwada, Y., Hashimoto, F., Cosentino, L. M., Chen, C. H., Garrett, P. E., and Lee, K. H. (1996) Betulinic acid and dihydrobetulinic acid derivatives as potent anti-HIV agents, *J. Med. Chem.*, **39**, 1016–1017.

859. Kanamoto, T., Kashiwada, Y., Kanbara, K., Gotoh, K., Yoshimori, M., Goto, T., Sano, K., and Nakashima, H. (2001) Anti-human immunodeficiency virus activity of YK-FH312 (a betulinic acid derivative), a novel compound blocking viral maturation, *Antimicrob. Agents Chemother.*, **45**, 1225–1230.

860. Martin, D. E., Blum, R., Wilton, J., et al. (2007) Safety and pharmacokinetics of bevirimat (PA-457), a novel inhibitor of human immunodeficiency virus maturation, in healthy volunteers, *Antimicrob. Agents Chemother.*, **51**(9), 3063–3066.

861. Beatty, G., Lalezari, J., Eron, J., et al. (2005) Safety and antiviral activity of PA-457, the first-in-class maturation inhibitor, in a 10-day monotherapy study in HIV-1 infected patients, *45th Interscience Conference on Antimicrobial Agents and Chemotherapy, Washington, D.C.*, December 16–19 [abstract H-416d; abstract LB-27].

862. Palella, F. J., Jr., Delaney, K. M., Moorman, A. C., et al (1998) Declining morbidity and mortality among patients with advanced human immunodeficiency virus infection. HIV Outpatient Study Investigators, *N. Engl. J. Med.*, **338**, 853–860.

863. Hogg, R. S., Yip, B., Kully, C., et al. (1999) Improved survival among HIV-infected patients after initiation of triple-drug antiretroviral regimens, *Can. Med. Assoc. J.*, **160**, 695–665.

864. Moyle, G. and Carr, A. (2002) HIV-associated lipodystrophy, metabolic complications, and antiretroviral toxicities, *HIV Clin. Trials*, **3**, 89–98.

865. Grinspoon, S. and Carr, A. (2005) Cardiovascular risk and body-fat abnormalities in HIV-infected adults, *N. Engl. J. Med.*, **352**, 48–62.

866. Conway, B. (2006) Delavirdine. In: *Reverse Transcriptase Inhibitors in HIV/AIDS Therapy* (Skowron, G. and Ogde, R., eds.), Humana Press, Totowa, NJ, pp. 375–400.

867. Yeni, P. G., Hammer, S. M., Hirsch, M. S., et al. (2004) Treatment of adult HIV infection: 2004 recommendation of the International AIDS Society-USA Panel, *J. Am. Med. Assoc.*, **292**, 251–265.

868. Wood, E., Hogg, R. S., Harrigan, P. R., and Montaner, J. S. (2005) When to initiate antiretroviral therapy in HIV-1-infected adults: a review for clinicians and patients, *Lancet Infect. Dis.*, **5**, 407–414.

869. Busti, A. J., Hall, R. G., and Margolis, D. M. (2004) Atazanavir for the treatment of human immunodeficiency virus infection, *Pharmacotherapy*, **24**, 1732–1747.

870. Eron, J. J., Feinberg, J., Kessler, H. A., et al. (2004) Once-daily versus twice-daily lopinavir/ritonavir in antiretroviral-naïve HIV-positive patients: a 48-week randomized clinical trial, *J. Infect. Dis.*, **189**, 265–272.

871. Wainberg, M. A. and Clotet, B. (2007) Immunologic response to protease inhibitor-based highly active antiretroviral therapy: a review, *AIDS Patient Care and STDs*, **21**(9), 609–620.

872. Bucy, R. P., Hockett, R. D., Derdeyn, C. A., et al. (1999) Initial increase in blood CD4(+) lymphocytes after HIV antiretroviral therapy reflects redistribution from lymphoid tissues, *J. Clin. Microbiol.*, **103**, 1391–1398.

873. Ensoli, F., Fiorelli, V., Alario, C., et al. (2000) Decreased T cell apoptosis and T cell recovery during highly active antiretroviral therapy (HAART), *Clin. Imunol.*, **97**, 9–20.

874. Estaquier, J., Lelievre, J. D., Petit, F., et al. (2002) Effects of antiretroviral drugs on human immunodeficiency virus type 1-induced CD4(+) T-cell death, *J. Virol.*, **76**, 5966–5973.

875. Steinberg, H. N., Crumpacker, C. S., and Chatis, P. A. (1991) In vitro suppression of normal human bone marrow progenitor cells by human immunodeficiency virus, *J. Virol.*, **65**, 1765–1769.

876. Isgro, A., Mezzaroma, I., Aiuti, A., et al. (2000) Recovery of hematopoietic activity in bone marrow from human immunodeficiency virus type 1-infected patients during highly active antiretroviral therapy, *AIDS Res. Hum. Retroviruses*, **16**, 1471–1479.

877. Lederman, M., Connick, E., Landay, A, et al. (1997) Partial immune reconstitution after 12 weeks of HAART (AZT, 3TC, ritonavir): preliminary results of ACTG 315, *4th Conference on Retroviruses and Opportunistic Infections, Washington, D.C.*, January 22–26 [abstract LB13].

878. Rosenberg, E. S., Billingsley, J. M., Caliendo, A. M., et al. (1997) Vigorous HIV-1-specific CD4+ T cell responses associated with control of viremia, *Science*, **27**, 1447–1450.

879. Connors, M., Kovacs, J. A., Krevat, S., et al. (1997) HIV infection induces changes in CD4+ T-cell phenotype and depletions within the CD4+ T-cell repertoire that are not immediately restored by antiviral or immune-based therapies, *Nat. Med.*, **3**, 533–540.

880. Jacobson, M. A., Kramer, F., Pavan, P. R., Owens, S., and Pollard, R. (1997) Failure of highly active antiretroviral therapy (HAART) to prevent CMV retinitis despite marked CD4 count increase, *4th Conference on Retroviruses and Opportunistic Infections, Washington, D.C.*, January 22–26 [abstract 353].

881. Gilquin, J., Piketty, C., Thomas, V., Gonzales-Canali, G., Kazatchine, M. D. (1997) Acute CMV infection in AIDS patients receiving combination therapy involving protease inhibitors, *4th Conference on Retroviruses and Opportunistic Infections, Washington, D.C.*, January 22–26 [abstract 354].

882. Finzi, D., Hermankova, M., Pierson, T., et al. (1997) Identification of a reservoir for HIV-1 in patients on highly active antiretroviral therapy, *Science*, **278**, 1295–1300.

883. Wong, J. K., Hezareh, M., Gunthard, H. F., et al. (1997) Recovery of replication-competent HIV despite prolonged suppression of plasma viremia, *Science*, **278**, 1291–1295.

884. Chun, T. W., Stuyver, L., Mizell, S. B., et al. (1997) Presence of an inducible HIV-1 latent reservoir during highly active antiretroviral therapy, *Proc. Natl. Acad. Sci. U.S.A.*, **94**, 13193–13197.

885. Cavert, W., Staskus, K., Zupancic, M., et al. (1997) Quantitative in situ hybridization measurement of HIV-1 RNA clearance kinetics from lymphoid tissue cellular compartments during triple-drug therapy, *4th Conference on Retroviruses and Opportunistic Infections, Washington, D.C.*, January 22–26 [abstract LB9].

886. Wong, J. K., Gunthard, H. F., Havlir, D. V., et al. (1997) Reduction of HIV-1 in blood and lymph nodes following potent antiretroviral therapy and the virologic correlates of treatment failure, *Proc. Natl. Acad. Sci. U.S.A.*, **94**, 12574–12579.

887. Chun, T. W., Carruth, L., Finzi, D., et al. (1997) Quantification of latent tissue reservoirs and total body viral load in HIV-1 infection, *Nature*, **387**, 183–188.

888. Perelson, A. S., Essunger, P., Cao, Y., et al. (1997) Decay characteristics of HIV-1-infected compartments during combination therapy, *Nature*, **387**, 188–191.

889. Havlir, D. V., Hirsch, M., Collier, A., et al. (1998) Randomized trial of indinavir (IDV) vs. zidovudine (ZDV)/lamivudine (3TC) vs. IDV/ZDV/3TC maintenance therapy after induction IDV/ADV/3TC therapy, *5th Conference on Retroviruses and Opportunistic Infections, Chicago, IL*, February 1–5; 225 [abstract LB16].

890. Raffi, F., Pialoux, G., Brun-Vezinet, F., et al. (1998) Results of TRILEGE trial, a comparison of three maintenance regimens for HIV infected adults receiving induction therapy with zidovudine (ZDV), lamivudine (3TC), and indinavir (IDV), *5th Conference on Retroviruses and Opportunistic Infections, Chicago, IL*, February 1–5; 225 [abstract LB15].

891. Grabar, S., Le Moing, V., Goujard, C., et al. (2000) Clinical outcome of patients with HIV-1 infection accorfing to immunologic and virologic response after 6 months of highly active antiretroviral therapy, *Ann. Intern. Med.*, **133**, 401–410.

892. Piketty, C., Castiel, P., Belec, L., et al. (1998) Discrepant responses to triple combination antiretroviral therapy in advanced HIV disease, *AIDS*, 12, 745–750.

893. Piketty, C., Weiss, L., Thomas, F., et al. (2001) Long-term clinical outcome of human immunodeficiency virus-infected patients with discordant immunologic and virologic responses to a protease inhibitor-containing regimen, *J. Infect. Dis.*, **183**, 1328–1335.

894. Negredo, E., Molto, J., Burger, D., et al. (2004) Unexpected CD4 cell count decline in patients receiving didanosine and tenofovir-based regimens despite undetectable viral load, *AIDS*, **18**, 459–463.

895. Negredo, E., Bonjoch, A., Paredes, R., et al. (2005) Compromised immunologic recovery in treatment-experienced patients with HIV infection receiving both tenofovir disoproxil fumarate and didanosine in the TORO studies, *Clin. Infect. Dis.*, **41**, 901–905.

896. Pruvost, A., Negredo, E., Benech, H., et al. (2005) Measurement of intracellular didanosine and tenofovir phosphorylated metabolites and possible interaction of the two drugs in human immunodeficiency virus-infected patients, *Antimicrob. Agents Chemother.*, **49**, 1907–1914.

897. Benveniste, O., Flahault, A., Rollot, F., et al. (2005) Mechanisms involved in the low-level regeneration of CD4+ cells in HIV-1-infected patients receiving highly active antiretroviral therapy who have prolonged undetectable plasma viral loads, *J. Infect. Dis.*, **191**, 1670–1679.

898. Marziali, M., De Santis, W., Carello, R., et al. (2006) T-cell homeostasis alteration in HIV-1 infected subjects with low CD4+ T-cell count despite undetectable virus load during HAART, *AIDS*, **20**, 2033–2041.

899. Maggiolo, F., Ravasio, L., Ripamonti, D., et al. (2005) Similar adherence rates favor different virologic outcomes for patients treated with nonnucleoside analogues or protease inhibitors, *Clin. Infect. Dis.*, **40**, 158–163.

900. Bangsberg, D. R. (2006) Less than 90% adherence to nonnucleoside reverse-transcriptase inhibitor therapy can lead to viral suppression, *Clin. Infect. Dis.*, **43**, 939–941.

901. Robbins, G. K., De Gruttola, V., Shafer, R. W., et al. (2003) Comparison of sequential three-drug regimens as initial therapy for HIV-1 infection, *N. Engl. J. Med.*, **349**, 2293–2303.

902. Gulick, R. M. (2006) Adherence to antiretroviral therapy: how much is enough? *Clin. Infect. Dis.*, **43**, 942–944.

903. El-Sadr, W. and Neaton, J., for the SMART Study Group (2006) Episodic CD4-guided use of ART is inferior to continuous therapy: results of the SMART Study, *13th Conference on Retroviruses and Opportunistic Infections, Denver, CO*, February 5–8 [abstract 106LB].

904. Lundgren, J. D., for the SMART Study Group (2006) Progression of HIV-related disease or death (POD) in the randomized SMART Study: why was the risk of POD greater in the CD4-guided [(Re)-initiate ART at CD4<250 cells/μL] drug conservation (DC) vs. the virological suppression (VS) arm? *XVIth International Conference on AIDS, Toronto, Canada*, August 13–16 [abstract WEAB0203].

905. Burman, W., for the SMART Study Group (2006) The effect of episodic CD4-guided antiretroviral therapy on quality of life: results of the quality of life substudy of SMART, *XVIth International Conference on AIDS, Toronto, Canada*, August 13–18 [abstract 18588].

906. El-Sadr, W. M., Lundgren, J. D., Neaton, J. D., et al. (2006) CD4+ count-guided interruption of antiretroviral treatment, *N. Engl. J. Med.*, **355**, 2283–2296.

907. Gulick, R., Su, Z., Flexner, C., Hughes, M., Skolnik, P., Godfrey, C., Greaves, W., Wilkin, T., Gross, R., Coakley, E., Zolopa, A., Hirsch, M., and Kuritzkes, D., for the ACTG 5211 Study Team (2006) ACTG 5211: Phase II study of the safety and efficacy of vicriviroc in HIV-infected treatment-experienced subjects, *XVIth International Conference on AIDS, Toronto, Canada*, August 13–18 [abstract THLB0217].

908. Ridler, S. A., Haubrich, R., DiRienzo, G., Peeples, L., Powderly, W. G., Klingman, K. L., Garren, K. W., George, T., Rooney, J. F., Brizz, B., Havlir, D., and Mellors, J. W., for the AIDS Clinical Trials Group 5142 Study Team (2006) A prospective, randomized, Phase III trial of NRTI-, PI-, and NNRTI-sparing regimens for initial treatment of HIV-1 infection, *XVIth International AIDS Conference, Toronto, Canada*, August 13–18 [abstract THLB0204].

909. Torriani, F. J., Parker, R. A., Murphy, R. L., Fichtenbaum, C. J., Currier, J. S., Dubé, M. P., Squires, K. E., Gerschenson, M., Komarow, L., Cotter, B. R., Mitchell, C. K., and Stein, J. H., for the ACTG 5152s Team (2005) A5152s a substudy of A5142: antiretroviral therapy improves endothelial function in individuals with human immunodeficiency virus infection: a prospective, randomized multicenter trial (Adult AIDS Clinical Trials Group Study), *American Heart Association Scientific Session, Dallas, TX*, November 11–13 [abstract PS5].

910. MacArthur, R. D., Novak, R. M., Peng, G., Chen, L., Xiang, Y., Kozal, M. J., van den Berg-Wolf, M., Henely, C., Huppler-Hullsiek, K., Schmetter, B., and Dehlinger, M., for the CPCRA 058 Study Team and the Terry Beirn Community Programs For Clinical Research on AIDS (CPCRA) (2006) Long-term clinical and immunologic outcomes are similar in HIV-infected persons randomized to NNRTI versus PI versus NNRTI + PI-based antiretroviral regimens as initial therapy: results of the CPCRA 058 FIRST Study, *XVIth International Conference on AIDS, Toronto, Canada*, August 13–18 [abstract TUAB01].

911. Swindells, S., DiRienzo, G., Wilkin, T., Fletcher, C. V., Margolis, D. M., Thal, G. D., Godfrey, C., Bastow, B., Ray, M. G.,

Wang, H., Coombs, R. W., McKinnon, J., and Mellors, J. W., for the AIDS Clinical Trials Group 5201 Study Team (2006) A prospective, open-label, pilot trial of regimen simplification to atazanavir/ritonavir alone as maintenance antiretroviral therapy after sustained virologic suppresion, *J. Am. Med. Assoc.*, **296**(7), 806–814.

912. Ribaudo, H., Kuritzkes, D., Lalama, C., Schouten, J., Schackman, B., Gullick, R., AIDS Clinical Trials Group (2006) Efavirenz (EFV)-based regimens are potent in treatment-naïve subjects across a wide range of pre-treatment HIV-1 RNA (VL) and CD4 cell counts: 3-year results from ACTG 5095, *XVIth International Conference on AIDS, Toronto, Canada*, August 13–18 [abstract THLB0211].

Chapter 35

Vaccine Development

To control the alarming spread of HIV, a vital need exists for developing an effective vaccine that would prevent individuals from becoming infected. In the context of NIAID-supported HIV vaccine research, identifying new vaccine concepts is the first step in the discovery and development of new vaccines. Basic research in HIV pathogenesis, immunology, virology, and development of animal models will form the basis for the identification of new vaccine concepts and will guide approaches for testing the most promising candidates in both domestic and international clinical trials (http://www3.niaid.nih.gov/research/topics/HIV/vaccines/).

A desirable HIV vaccine to control the global spread of AIDS must be (i) simple to administer; (ii) inexpensive; (iii) capable of inducing long-lasting immunity; and (iv) effective against all HIV subtypes.

Although developing an HIV/AIDS vaccine remains one of NIAID's highest priorities, it presents a formidable scientific challenge to the scientific community (1). The support for HIV vaccine development by NIAID is channeled through:

- Fundamental basic research—the discovery phase
- Preclinical screening and development of predictive animal models
- Product development and manufacturing
- Clinical research

Over the years, HIV vaccine research has progressed from an early focus on HIV surface antigens, particularly the envelope protein and the role of neutralizing antibodies, to increased attention to cytotoxic T-lymphocytes (CTLs) in HIV immunity. Many novel approaches to elicit anti-HIV neutralizing antibodies and CTLs are now under investigation (http://www3.niaid.nih.gov/research/topics/HIV/vaccines/).

Goals. Major goals and objectives in the NIAID-supported program on HIV vaccine development have targeted both preclinical and clinical research as follows (http://www3.niaid.nih.gov/research/topics/HIV/vaccines/):

Preclinical Research and Development

- Identify and develop promising vaccine candidates in *predictive* animal models that induce (i) broadly neutralizing antibodies; (ii) a consistent and high level of cytotoxic T-lymphocytes; and (iii) strong mucosal immune responses.
- Evaluate the candidates for immunogenicity, safety, and efficacy in animal models.
- Produce products with the most promise, including those that may not have adequate industry support under good manufacturing conditions, and move those products through the Investigational New Drug (IND) approval process.
- Develop and test new adjuvants and cytokines that will increase the magnitude and duration of the immune response when formulated with or given in conjunction with candidate AIDS vaccines.
- Foster studies on the genetic variability of the virus and of the host at international sites that are currently conducting or will conduct HIV vaccine clinical trials.

Vaccine Clinical Research

- Identify a safe and effective HIV vaccine through the conduct of all phases of the clinical trials by (i) harmonizing protocols to facilitate and promote the evaluation in humans of a broad range of promising HIV vaccine candidates with *different designs*, and whenever possible conducting studies with common protocols, reagents, and assays to permit meaningful comparisons of various approaches, products, doses, and routes of administration; (ii) ensuring the safety of volunteers during trials; and (iii) ensuring compliance with regulatory agency requirements.
- Advance knowledge of protective immunity by developing and improving laboratory assays of vaccine-induced human immune responses.
- Collaborate with governmental and nongovernmental agencies that conduct HIV vaccine research through interagency agreements (IAAs) for domestic and international research to ensure that the best researchers vigorously

pursue the best approaches worldwide and thereby expedite the identification of an effective HIV vaccine.

- Develop and implement mechanisms to timely monitor safety data from volunteers in HIV vaccine trials, and provide the Food and Drug Administration (FDA), on time, with final reports that evaluate vaccine safety.
- Improve the capacity of the HIV Vaccine Trials Network (HVTN) to carry out a comprehensive HIV vaccine research agenda, including the conduct of domestic and international clinical trials of the most promising HIV vaccine candidates.
- Accelerate the evaluation of candidate HIV vaccines worldwide through collaborative efforts with the International AIDS Vaccine Initiative (IAVI) at sites receiving IAVI intellectual and financial support.
- Foster early and continued collaboration with the industry in the clinical development of candidate HIV/AIDS vaccines.
- Develop the necessary infrastructure and collaborations with other institutions to conduct vaccine trials according to the highest scientific and ethical standards, and focus on studies leading to the selection of appropriate endpoints to be considered in vaccine trials.
- Develop novel strategies to test HIV vaccines in efficacy trials that address the multiple challenges of preventing infection, slowing disease progression, and diminishing the transmissibility of HIV infection to uninfected persons.

35.1 Vaccine Clinical Trials

NIAID is supporting a number of vaccine trials around the world with a variety of organizations, centers, partnerships, and programs, as follows:

- *The Dale and Betty Bumpers Vaccine Research Center (VRC).* The VRC at the NIAID was established to facilitate research in vaccine development. The VRC is dedicated to improving global human health through the rigorous pursuit of effective vaccines for human diseases (http://www.niaid.nih.gov/vrc/).
- *HIV Vaccine Trials Network (HVTN).* Formed in 1999 by NIAID, the HVTN is an international collaboration of scientists and educators searching for an effective and safe HIV vaccine. The HVTN's mission is to facilitate the process of testing preventive vaccines against HIV/AIDS. The HVTN conducts all phases of clinical trials, from evaluating experimental vaccines for safety and the ability to stimulate immune responses, to testing a vaccine's efficacy. The HVTN is conducting its research through multicenter clinical trials in a global network of domestic and international sites. Organized by committee and scientific

discipline, the investigators develop, discuss, implement, analyze, and prioritize both vaccine design concepts and studies. Protocols are developed by HVTN investigators and include partnerships between vaccine developers, clinical experts, and biostatisticians. The HVTN works closely with NIAID staff in initiating, conducting, funding, and coordinating all vaccine development processes (http://www.hvtn.org/).

- *Partnership for AIDS Vaccine Evaluation (PAVE).* PAVE is a voluntary consortium of U.S. government agencies and U.S. government-funded organizations involved in HIV vaccine research. Members of PAVE include the NIH, the HVTN, the Dale and Betty Bumpers Vaccine Research Center, the U.S. Military HIV Research Program, and the Centers of Disease Control and Prevention (CDC) (http://www.hivpave.org/).
- *Center for HIV/AIDS Vaccine Immunology (CHAVI).* CHAVI was established by NIAID as part of the Global HIV/AIDS Vaccine Enterprise. It aims to elucidate basic science questions and conduct early-phase clinical trials of HIV vaccine candidates at clinical sites around the world (http://www.chavi.org/).
- *The U.S. Military HIV Research Program (USMHRP).* Established in 1985 to protect troops entering endemic HIV areas, this program brings together scientists from the U.S. Army, Navy, and the Air Force. NIAID jointly plans and executes HIV/AIDS research projects with the USMHRP through an interagency agreement (http://www.hivresearch.org/).
- *Global HIV Vaccine Enterprise.* This is a virtual consortium of organizations committed to developing a preventive HIV/AIDS vaccine as well implementing shared scientific plans, mobilizing resources, and improving worldwide collaborations (http://www.hivvaccineenterprise.org/about/index.html).
- *International AIDS Vaccine Initiative (IAVI).* IAVI was founded in 1996 to speed discovery of an HIV vaccine. It partners with private companies, academic institutions, and government agencies, such as NIH, worldwide (http://www.iavi.org/).

A list of all federally funded vaccine trials can be accessed at http://www.AIDSinfo.gov.

35.2 Vaccine Discovery and Development/Clinical Research

In the context of HIV/AIDS vaccine discovery and development, identifying new vaccine concepts is of utmost importance. Basic research in the fields of HIV pathogenesis, microbiology, immunology, virology, and development of animal models creates the cornerstone for the development of new HIV/AIDS vaccines. In the majority of patients, such vaccines are expected to (i) induce broadly neutralizing antibody; (ii) consistently generate high levels of CTLs; and (iii) produce strong mucosal immune responses. In addition, the development and testing of new adjuvants and cytokines will increase the magnitude and duration of the humoral and/or cellular immune response when formulated with or given in conjunction with candidate HIV/AIDS vaccines (http://www3.niaid.nih.gov/research/topics/HIV/vaccines/research/clinical/).

35.2.1 HIV Vaccine Strategies

Although the current antiretroviral drug therapy has proved successful at reducing patient viral loads, most HIV-infected individuals will never benefit from these therapeutic agents. The overwhelming number of all new HIV infections occurs in developing countries where adequate financial resources are not available to allow for easy access to drugs. Even in wealthy, industrialized nations, where antiretroviral drugs are available, poor drug tolerance, poor adherence to treatment, and emerging drug-resistant viral strains make long-term responsiveness to antiretroviral therapy far from certain. Moreover, once patients are removed from drug therapy, their viral loads increase to levels equivalent to those detected before treatment. This is likely a result of reactivation of latent virus. Successful containment of the AIDS pandemic will ultimately require an effective vaccination strategy designed to prevent HIV infection (http://www.brown.edu/Courses/Bio_160/Projects1999/hiv/vacstrat.html).

Major impediments to developing a successful vaccine include the constant variability of the virus (within the individual) through mutation and recombination, multiple virus subtypes, the inability of most known specificities of anti-HIV antibodies to consistently neutralize primary HIV isolates, and the lack of full understanding of the correlates of immunity. Given the unique biology of HIV and its interactions with the immune system, it is not surprising that traditional strategies for vaccination are not proving useful in protecting against HIV infection. Live attenuated virus, inactivated virus, and recombinant protein strategies for vaccination safely protect against a variety of viral pathogens in humans. However, these strategies are not likely to be useful for vaccinating against HIV (1–5).

35.2.1.1 Immune Control of HIV Replication

HIV differs from viruses for which successful vaccines have been developed in that it is controlled predominately by a cellular rather than a humoral immune response (2). Diverse evidence supports the importance of the cellular immune response in HIV containment (1). CD8$^+$ T-lymphocytes can inhibit the replication of HIV in CD4$^+$ T-lymphocytes *in vitro*, probably through direct cytotoxicity and the production of soluble factors including beta chemokines (6, 7).

The CD8$^+$ CTLs, key effectors of cellular immunity, recognize viral peptides bound to major histocompatibility complex (MHC) molecules on the surface of virus-infected cells (8). Numerous studies support the importance of T-cell–mediated immune responses in the early and subsequent control of both HIV infection in humans and simian immunodeficiency virus (SIV) infection in non-human primates (9, 10). CTLs can kill or suppress cells infected with HIV in the laboratory (11), and the emergence of these lymphocytes has correlated with early containment of viremia (12). The qualitative nature of CD8$^+$ T-cell responses may be critical in the control of HIV infection (13), even though they do not clear HIV reservoirs completely (1).

The clinical status of infected individuals is associated with the level of virus-specific CD8$^+$ CTLs in their peripheral blood; high levels are predictive of good clinical status (14). The early containment of HIV replication in acutely infected individuals coincides with the emergence of an HIV-specific CTL response (15). The most direct evidence for the importance of CD8$^+$ T-lymphocytes in controlling HIV replication comes from studies in monkeys (16). These studies have convincingly demonstrated the importance of CD8$^+$ CTLs in controlling HIV replication and thereby suggest that an effective HIV vaccine should elicit high-frequency CTL responses (2).

The extraordinary rate of mutation of HIV has a profound impact on immune control of viral replication (1, 2). Recent studies have demonstrated that HIV continually accrues mutations that enable it to escape recognition by neutralizing antibodies in chronically infected individuals (17, 18). However, to date there is no evidence of an association between this process and the abrupt clinical deterioration in infected subjects. Mutations have also been shown to result in a loss of HIV and SIV recognition by CTL in both acutely and chronically infected individuals (19, 20). In many of the documented instances of viral escape from CTL recognition, this escape phenomenon has been associated with an abrupt increase in viral replication and decrease in immune function in the infected individuals. Thus, the phenomenon of viral mutation away from recognition by antibodies and CTL is considered to be a central reason why the immune system eventually fails to contain HIV replication (2).

T-Cell Vaccines. Animal models of HIV infection have proved to be very valuable in exploring the mechanisms by which vaccines that induce primarily T-cell responses might have an effect on viral infection and disease (1). Immunization of non-human primates with vaccines that induced primarily T-cell responses resulted in weakening of the initial burst of viremia, a reduction in virus levels at the set point, a decrease in the total virus produced during the early stage of infection, or a combination of these changes *(21–23)*. Disease progression was delayed in many of these animals, and the delay correlated with the level of vaccine-induced T-cell responses. Immunization with one candidate vaccine preserved memory CD4$^+$T-cells throughout the body, and this preservation was associated with an improved long-term outcome *(21, 24)*. The peak viral levels were reduced by a factor of approximately 10 and peak levels of infected memory CD4$^+$ T-cells by approximately 75%. A reduction of only one-half log of viral RNA resulted in a slowed disease progression. If natural-history and animal-model studies prove to be predictive, persons who receive T-cell vaccines before infection might remain disease-free for a prolonged period, and antiretroviral therapy, which can be burdensome and have serious side effects over time, might be delayed *(1, 25)*. However, one complicating factor is that the T-cell–mediated control of infection may not prove to be complete. The disease has eventually progressed in some immunized and protected macaques, probably as a result of changes in critical T-cell epitopes that enabled the virus to escape immune recognition *(26)*.

35.2.1.2 Vaccine Types

Currently, a number of concepts for HIV vaccine strategies are actively being investigated. They are mostly being developed as single-approach vaccines, but it may ultimately be determined that the most effective immunization strategy will be to combine more than one approach. The majority of vaccine efforts to date have been focused on the envelope glycoprotein, gp160, or its cleavage product gp120, which forms the outer spike projection of the virion. In 1987, NIAID initiated the first clinical trial of an HIV vaccine, a gp160 subunit vaccine candidate, and since then more than 40 clinical trials of various vaccine strategies have been implemented worldwide to find an effective vaccine (http://www.brown.edu/Courses/Bio_160/Projects1999/hiv/vacstrat.html).

The types of experimental HIV vaccines currently under consideration include *(3)* (http://www.hvtn.org/science/strategies.html):

(i) *Peptide Vaccines.* The peptide vaccines are made of tiny pieces of proteins from the HIV virus.

(ii) *Recombinant Subunit Protein Vaccines.* These vaccines are made of bigger pieces of proteins that are on the surface of the HIV virus. Examples of recombinant subunit proteins are gp120, gp140, or gp160 produced by genetic engineering. Some of the risks associated with attenuated or killed whole organism vaccines can be avoided by using specific macromolecules derived

from the pathogen. Theoretically, the gene encoding any immunogenic protein can be isolated and cloned into bacterial, yeast, or mammalian cells using recombinant DNA technology. The expressed protein is purified and used in combination with immune enhancers as the vaccine. Such a subunit vaccine was first proposed for the hepatitis B vaccine. One disadvantage of subunit vaccines, like the whole-killed pathogen, is that the primary response is antibody-mediated, with very little induction of cell-mediated activity. Despite the limited immune response, there are several ongoing Phase III trials (United States and Thailand) of this type of vaccine for HIV using the structural envelope protein gp120. Data from two recently concluded efficacy trials of these vaccines in the United States and Thailand show no evidence of protection against HIV infection *(27)*. These disappointing results bolster the argument for moving forward in the future with scientifically defensible HIV vaccine strategies *(2)*.

(iii) *Live Vector Vaccines.* These vaccines contain non-HIV viruses or bacteria engineered to carry genes encoding HIV proteins. It is possible to introduce HIV genes into attenuated viruses or bacteria. The attenuated organism serves as a vector, replicating within host cells and expressing the proteins that are capable of inducing HIV-specific immune responses without causing disease. Several organisms that have being examined for vector vaccines include vaccinia virus, canarypox virus, adenovirus, and *Salmonella*. Clinical trials have shown that this type of vaccine is capable of inducing cell-mediated as well as antibody-mediated immunity. Many vaccines used today, such as the smallpox vaccine, use this approach. Currently, there is a well-documented clinical trial under way in Uganda, which is using attenuated canarypox virus to deliver HIV genes to uninfected individuals (http://www.iavi.org/newpage/sdemand.html).

(iv) *DNA Vaccines.* These vaccines contain copies of a small number of HIV genes that are inserted into pieces of DNA called plasmids. The HIV genes will produce proteins very similar to the ones from real HIV. Using this recently developed vaccine concept, plasmid DNA, encoding a viral antigen, is injected directly into the muscle of the recipient, where it is used to produce HIV proteins. The encoded protein that is expressed has been shown to elicit a CTL response, but only a weak antibody response, to the viral antigen. This type of vaccine may be suited for worldwide use, as it has the potential to be inexpensive, stable, and easy to transport relative to other vaccines. There are HIV DNA vaccines in current clinical trials against clade B.

(v) *Vaccine Combinations.* The combinations use two HIV vaccines, one after another, to create a stronger immune response. This vaccine type is often referred to as *prime-boost strategy*. The prime-boost strategy has been developed with the intent to strengthen both the humoral and cellular immune responses to vaccination by combining a cell-stimulating vaccine such as recombinant plasmid DNA or a live recombinant vectored vaccine with a subunit vaccine, especially one based on envelope proteins (gp120, gp140, or gp41) *(3)*. There is no strong evidence, however, that such a dual vaccination regimen results in a significantly higher antibody or T-cell response. For any prime-boost strategy to be commercially feasible, the combined regimen needs to demonstrate significantly greater efficacy over single-modality vaccines in order to balance the increased costs and complexities associated with developing two vaccines, including potential regulatory and licensing problems, as well as logistical hurdles with the delivery of the vaccines in the field *(3)*.

(vi) *Virus-like Particle Vaccines (Pseudovirion Vaccines).* These are noninfectious HIV look-alike vaccines that have one or more, but not all, HIV proteins.

(vii) *Fusion Proteins and Peptides.* Multiepitopic combinations of peptides, fusion proteins, and long lipopeptides are at an early stage of clinical development, either alone or in prime-boost combinations with live vector-based recombinant vaccines *(3)*. Vaccine constructs that express a series of minimal epitopes arranged in a string-like fashion have been explored as a potential strategy to generate diverse CTL responses and bypass the natural hierarchy of epitope bias *(28, 29)*. Multi-epitope DNA immunogens can, efficiently prime for broadly reactive CTL responses *(30–32)* but do not necessarily overcome hierarchies of epitope dominance *(33)*. One multiepitope DNA vaccine is currently undergoing a Phase I trial in the United States and Peru and will be followed by booster immunization with a multi-epitope recombinant fusion protein *(3)*.

Induction of persistent HIV gag-specific CD8$^+$ CTL responses was evaluated in a Phase I trial involving immunization with a fusion protein comprising the HIV p24 gag protein and detoxified *Bacillus anthracis* lethal factor to target antigen-presenting cells *(34)*.

Synthetic lipopeptides containing MHC class I–restricted T-cell epitopes were found to induce strong CD8$^+$ T-cell responses against HIV in mice, non-human primates, and humans without additional adjuvant *(35–38)*. Lipopeptides with sequences corresponding with that of CTL epitope-rich regions in the HIV-1 gag and nef proteins were tested in Phase I trials and were shown to induce strong, multiepitopic CD4$^+$ and CD8$^+$ T-cell responses *(3)*. Parallel Phase II trials were started in 2004 in the United States and in France under the sponsorship of NIAID and ANRS, respectively, to study the efficiency of lipopeptides as priming or boosting immunogens, but the trials had to be interrupted due to the occurrence of a severe neurologic side effect in one of the U.S. volunteers. The trial now has resumed in France *(3)*.

Several vaccines that induce primarily T-cell responses are currently in Phase I and Phase II clinical trials (see Table 1 in Ref. *1*) *(9, 39)*. A recombinant canarypox vector combined with a gp120 boost is being evaluated in about 16,000 subjects in a community-based Phase III trial in Thailand *(1)*. A recombinant, nonreplicating adenovirus vector is in two Phase IIb trials involving populations at high risk for HIV infection. There is skepticism that either of these vaccines will be effective in the prevention of HIV infection. The canarypox vector–gp120 combination did not induce broadly neutralizing antibodies, whereas the adenovirus vector expressed only internal viral proteins that were recognized by the immune system only after productive infection (see Section 35.3). However, these trials are expected to also evaluate whether immunization will affect the early viral load in subjects who become infected with HIV despite repeated counseling. Modeling studies have suggested that even a vaccine that does not provide adequate protection against infection might alter the course of the epidemic *(39)*. It should also be noted that immune responses to the HIV genes that were inserted into the adenovirus vector may be affected by prior immunity to adenovirus *(9, 40, 41)*.

35.2.1.3 Principles of HIV Vaccine Development

Given the unique biology of HIV and its interactions with the immune system, it is not surprising that traditional strategies for vaccination are not proving useful in protecting against HIV infection. Live attenuated virus, inactivated virus, and recombinant protein strategies for vaccination safely protect against a variety of viral pathogens in humans. However, these strategies are not likely to be useful for vaccinating against HIV *(2)*.

Many viruses can be mutated through tissue culture passage such that they remain infectious but lose their pathogenic potential *(2)*. Such pathogenically attenuated viruses have provided safe and effective protection against smallpox, measles, and polio. Data in monkeys indicated that this strategy protects against simian immunodeficiency virus (SIV) infection *(42)*. Large deletions made in certain of the nonstructural genes of SIV resulted in the virtual elimination of early pathogenic consequences of SIV infection in adult monkeys. Moreover, the monkeys infected with these gene-deleted viruses were protected from subsequent infection with pathogenic SIV. However, adult monkeys infected with these pathogenically attenuated viruses were found to develop disease with a delayed onset, and newborn monkeys developed disease soon after infection *(43)*. Similarly, a cohort of humans who received a blood product infected with an HIV isolate that had a large genetic deletion were at first reported to be free of disease. Later, however, these individuals did develop AIDS *(44)*. Thus, accumulating experience has raised serious questions concerning the safety of this vaccine modality for HIV, and there is little enthusiasm among investigators at the present time for pursuing this vaccine approach for AIDS *(2)*.

In light of the limitations of traditional vaccine strategies for preventing HIV infections, investigators have been exploring novel approaches. The most promising of these are the use of plasmid DNA and live recombinant vectors *(2)*.

It has been shown that intramuscular inoculation of a plasmid encoding a viral gene under the control of a potent promoter elicits both antibody and cell-mediated immune responses in laboratory animals *(45)*. This vaccine modality is a safe and effective means of eliciting CTL responses in non-human primates *(46)*. Although plasmid DNAs have been less immunogenic in early-phase clinical testing in humans than in laboratory animals, a number of changes in plasmid DNA constructs have been shown to increase their immunogenicity. These changes include altering the nucleotides of the viral genes to optimize the ability of the plasmids to produce viral proteins in mammalian cells and altering the regulatory elements in the plasmids *(2)*.

Live recombinant microorganisms are also being evaluated as potential HIV vaccines *(2)*. Genes of HIV and SIV can be engineered into microorganisms that have proved safe and effective as live attenuated vaccines, such as the smallpox vaccine virus vaccinia or the tuberculosis vaccine Bacille Calmette-Guérin (BCG) *(47,48)*. As these engineered viruses and bacteria replicate in the inoculated individual, immunity is developed to both the vector and the HIV gene product. Importantly, because these are live, replicating organisms, both humoral and cellular immune responses are generated in vaccine recipients *(2)*.

The best studied of the live vectors are the poxviruses. Although vaccinia virus might be an effective vector for HIV genes, safety issues preclude its use as an HIV vaccine *(2)*. Vaccinia virus was reported to disseminate and cause fatal encephalitis in an immunosuppressed HIV-infected individual *(49)*. There is a well-founded concern that if a worldwide HIV eradication effort were mounted, a recombinant vaccinia virus vaccine would cause fatal disease in undiagnosed immunosuppressed individuals in areas where HIV infection is endemic *(2)*. Therefore, most work using poxviruses as vectors for HIV immunization has been done with viruses that undergo an abortive replication cycle in human cells. These viruses, which include modified vaccinia Ankara (MVA) and the avian poxviruses canarypox and fowlpox (FPV), can produce sufficient HIV protein during an abortive

cycle of replication to initiate both humoral and cellular anti-HIV immune responses *(2)*. These recombinant vectors have proved immunogenic in non-human primates *(50,51)*. A trial in Thailand is assessing the efficacy of a recombinant canarypox vaccine delivered with a recombinant HIV envelope protein, although its immunogenicity has been quite disappointing in human trials to date *(52)*. Early-phase human clinical trials with recombinant MVA and FPV HIV constructs are ongoing *(2)*.

Initial studies with recombinant adenovirus vectors have been particularly promising *(53)*. Adenovirus serotype 5, made replication-incompetent by deletion of its E1 and/or E3 gene(s), has proved highly immunogenic as a vector for HIV gene products in small laboratory animals and non-human primates *(54)*. Studies are demonstrating that recombinant adenovirus can elicit HIV-specific T-cell immune responses in human volunteers *(2)*. A problem with this vaccine approach, however, is the emerging evidence that preexisting immunity to the vector significantly decreases the immunogenicity of these constructs *(55)* (see Section 35.3). Several strategies are being explored to circumvent this problem. Vaccination with plasmid DNA constructs before boosting with recombinant adenovirus is being evaluated as a means of augmenting vaccine-elicited immunity in individuals with preexisting antibody responses to adenovirus serotype 5 *(56)*. Work is also ongoing to explore the immunogenicity of rare-serotype human adenoviruses and chimpanzee adenoviruses as HIV vaccine vectors; the reasoning is that the properties of these viruses as vectors should resemble those of serotype 5 adenovirus, but human populations should not have significant preexisting immunity to these viruses *(2)*.

Other live recombinant vectors are also being explored as potential HIV vaccine modalities. These include single-strand RNA alphaviruses (Semliki forest virus and Venezuelan equine encephalitis virus) and the parvovirus adeno-associated virus. The pathogenically attenuated mycobacterium Bacille Calmette-Guérin is also being evaluated as an HIV vector in preclinical and early-phase human testing *(2)*.

Although plasmid DNA and recombinant live vector strategies can elicit cellular immune responses, the development of a vaccine that induces broadly neutralizing antibodies remains a high research priority *(1)*. The existence of broadly neutralizing monoclonal antibodies provides hope that an immunogen that reliably induces protective antibodies can be designed. The creation of such a protein immunogen is, however, a challenge that is very difficult to resolve *(2)*.

Numerous approaches using various immunogens are currently under investigation but have yet to yield more than incremental improvements over gp120 (see Table 2 in Ref. *1*). Although a protein immunogen can be designed to elicit an antibody that neutralizes a single HIV isolate, that antibody is unlikely to neutralize a significant number of other HIV isolates due to their extreme genetic diversity. Because regions of the envelope that are genetically conserved appear to be shielded from access to antibodies by highly variable loop structures and sugars, envelope proteins with variable loops and glycosylation sites deleted are being evaluated as immunogens *(57, 58)*. New data on the structure of native virions has indicated that the envelope glycoprotein exists as a trimer *(59)*. Therefore, trimeric envelope immunogens are being assessed for their ability to elicit broadly neutralizing antibodies. Because monoclonal antibodies have been generated that can neutralize a wide spectrum of HIV isolates, there is reason to assume that it will ultimately be possible to configure an immunogen that can elicit a broadly neutralizing antibody response *(60, 61)*.

The recent observation that two broadly reactive monoclonal antibodies to the HIV envelope are polyspecific and react with phospholipids such as cardiolipin suggests that some species of HIV antibodies, like autoimmune antibodies, may be controlled by B-cell tolerance mechanisms *(62–64)*. Innovative adjuvants or immunogens might be capable of circumventing tolerance pathways and inducing more broadly reactive antibodies. Ensuring the safety of such approaches will be critical. In addition, understanding and counteracting the mechanisms responsible for the delay in the appearance of neutralizing antibodies may lead to more rapid and effective immune responses. Finally, a thorough analysis of the sequence of transmitted viruses and the structures of their envelopes may yield clues to help guide vaccine design *(1)*.

Research on innate immunity could influence the design of future HIV vaccines. Innate immune responses occur early and, unlike adaptive responses, are neither antigen-specific nor durable. Natural killer cells are cytolytic cells that are key mediators of innate immunity and the first responders to viral infection *(65)*. Natural killer cells also secrete cytokines and chemokines that help drive virus-specific adaptive immune responses. The recent report of a form of adaptive immunity that is independent of T cells and B cells and is mediated by natural killer cells is the first observation of innate immune memory in a higher vertebrate (the mouse) *(66)*. Improving the understanding of how innate immunity is turned on and off could lead to strategies that augment innate responses or make them more durable. Immune responses that more effectively slow or blunt the primary stage of HIV infection might increase the window of opportunity for clearing HIV before latent reservoirs become established. An improved understanding of the role of Toll-like receptors in triggering innate immune-response pathways could also suggest approaches to augmenting induced immune responses *(67)*.

Design of Protective HIV Vaccines. The design of protective HIV vaccines is currently based on two general ideas *(5)*. One is a "minimalistic" approach, using only two HIV proteins (a regulatory and a structural protein). The other

approach aims at "imitating" a live-attenuated vaccine using as many HIV genes as necessary ("maximalistic" approach). In both general approaches, different technical methods will be tested to achieve a protective immune response. "Protective immunity" is primarily defined as protection against "infection" but also as protection against "disease development" in case of the failure of protection against infection *(5)*. Thus, both protective mechanisms should be evaluated with the proposed vaccines.

The "minimalistic" approach is based on the fact that the primary target cells for HIV in mucosal tissues, the Langerhans cells, as well as other dendritic cell types, need further contact with specific T cells to initiate a full infection cycle *(68)*. Like other cell types characterized by low HIV replication capacity, these cells also seem to predominately express early regulatory proteins like Tat and Nef. Tat and Nef, on the one hand, induce the expression of cytokines and chemokines in the infected cells, activating further gene expression, and on the other hand are, as extracellular proteins, chemoattractants for HIV target cells, which they activate to facilitate and increase virus infection. These extracellular proteins are also efficiently taken up by target cells where they activate and/or facilitate virus replication directly or indirectly. Thus, to interfere with this local process in the mucosa, the following immune responses are necessary: (i) strong CTL responses against early proteins like Tat and/or Nef to eliminate the first infected cells; (ii) specific neutralizing antibodies against the activities of extracellular Tat and/or Nef to block their role in facilitating further virus transmission and replication in new HIV target cells; and (iii) broadly neutralizing antibodies against HIV to prevent the transfer of the virus from the first to the next generation of infected cells *(5)*.

The aim of the "minimalistic" approach is, therefore, to design a vaccine that elicits T-cell responses and neutralizing antibodies against Tat or Nef, as well as neutralizing antibodies against Env. The Tat/Env vaccine will be administered as a protein/protein vaccine regimen with adjuvant, whereas the Nef/Env vaccine will be based on a modified vaccinia Ankara virus vector/protein approach *(5)*.

The target of the "maximalistic" approach is a vaccine that can provide the same protection mechanism as that inherent to a "live-attenuated vaccine." Technically, this could be achieved by the use of multiple HIV genes rather than live virus. Because currently it is not completely understood how protection is provided by a live-attenuated virus, it will be necessary to include in the vaccine all possible HIV genes known to be antigenic and to induce both broad T-cell responses, as well as antibody responses. The two technical approaches are to provide the vaccine either in a "flexible" way as a mixture of single DNAs together with immunostimulatory genes or as a single DNA vector containing all the necessary genes/epitopes *(5)*.

In general, candidate vaccines that induce relevant immune responses in more than 50% of the trial participants (preferably, at multiple time points) will be considered for further studies in Phase II trials (5). In particular, the key elements for being selected for use in a prophylactic vaccine for adults at risk of infection will be (i) the ability to induce cross-reactive cellular immune responses and/or cross-reactive neutralizing antibodies against circulating strains in the country where the Phase II trial will be conducted; (ii) the ability to induce CD4$^+$ T-helper cell activity and memory functions for HIV-specific cytotoxic CD8$^+$ T-cells, providing a potential barrier that will limit the initial spread of virus or virus-infected cells (5).

For vaccines to be used in HIV-positive individuals, the selection criteria include the induction of CD4$^+$ and CD8$^+$ T-cell immunity (expansion of the epitope repertoire or favorable changes in the antigen-specific T-cell phenotypes) against HIV-specific antigens (Gag, Nef, Tat, RT, and Env) recognized during infection (5).

The use of more rigorous, standardized, and quantitative enzyme-linked immunospot (Elispot) assays restricted to a single-day stimulation period did generate confidence in the results of ongoing HIV vaccine clinical trials that would help comparing results involving recombinant adenovirus type 5 (Ad5), selected DNA vaccines, and poxviral and adeno-associated virus, among other recombinant HIV vaccine platforms (4). Based on these studies, a hierarchy has been established supporting the concept that Ad5 vectors appear to be the most potent current vaccine strategy for inducing anti-HIV CTL responses in humans. Specific recombinant DNA platforms appear to be in second place regarding their cellular immune potency, but with improvement, they could be within striking distance of the Ad5 platform (4). In addition, results from the Vaccine Research Center at the National Institute of Allergy and Infectious Diseases suggest that the two modalities together appear complementary in humans (see Section 35.3).

Among the most novel and anticipated recombinant viral platforms, the recombinant vesicular stomatitis virus (VSV) vector system represents a top new candidate platform (4).

- *HIV Vaccine Approach: Tat Plus ΔV2 Env.* The rationale for this vaccine concept is to combine the Tat early regulatory viral antigen with the surface glycoprotein Env (5). The trimeric ΔV2 Env immunogen was designed to expose cryptic conserved sites for neutralization, and Tat protein will serve as both an antigen and an immunoactivator. Expected immune responses are specific antibody production and induction of CD4$^+$ helper activity and CD8$^+$ cytotoxic activity. Immune responses to these two antigens have the potential to act synergistically to prevent or to reduce entry of the virus via anti-Env responses and spread of the virus via anti-Tat

or anti-Env responses. In addition to safety and feasibility, the criteria for advancement beyond Phase I of this approach will be the observation that the combined Tat plus ΔV2 Env vaccine is showing an increase in the potency and/or breadth of the immune responses compared with the single vaccine alone. The minimum criteria for Env-specific responses will be the measurement of neutralizing antibodies against the vaccine strain and Env-specific CD4$^+$ T-cell responses in at least 50% of the trial participants. The minimum criteria for Tat will be specific antibody production and induction of CD4$^+$ and CD8$^+$ responses in at least 50% of the trial participants. The potency and breadth of virus neutralization will be measured against a well-characterized panel of subtype B strains. The potency and breadth of Tat antibody and T-cell responses will be measured by ELISA, Elispot, and peptide epitope mapping, respectively, using standardized procedures (5).

- *HIV Vaccine Approach: Nef Plus ΔV2 Env.* The major scientific rationale for this vaccine concept is to combine the early regulatory gene *nef*, in order to induce primarily anti-Nef cellular immunity, with the structural protein Env to elicit humoral immunity (5). The ΔV2 Env will expose cryptic sites for antibody neutralization. This approach would also seek to achieve immunity against both early and late phases of the virus replication cycle. In addition to safety and feasibility, a criterion for advancing this approach beyond Phase I will be observing that the combined Nef plus Env vaccine shows an increase in the potency and/or breadth of the immune responses compared with each antigen applied alone. The minimum criterion for Env-specific responses will be the induction of neutralizing antibodies against the vaccine strain in at least 50% of the trial participants. The potency and breadth of virus neutralization will be measured against a panel of subtype B primary strains. The minimum criteria for Nef will be CD4$^+$ and CD8$^+$ T-cell responses in at least 50% of the trial participants as well as Nef chemotaxis-neutralizing antibody (5).

- *HIV Vaccine Approach: Multi-HIV Antigens/Epitopes.* This DNA-based vaccine is a combination of full-length genes encoding the regulatory proteins Nef, Tat, and Rev, genes encoding the Gag products p17 and p24, and DNA encoding for more than 20 T-helper and cytotoxic epitopes from Pol, Protease, and Env (A, B, C, and FGH clade) antigens (5). It is designed to induce CD4$^+$ help and CD8$^+$ cytotoxicity, and the inclusion of the granulocyte macrophage colony-stimulating factor (GM-CSF) adjuvant will warrant high neutralizing antibody titers. The delivery by Biojector will increase the efficacy of dendritic cell targeting. The minimum criteria for going forward will be the induction of CD4$^+$ and CD8$^+$ T-cell responses to more than one viral antigen and the presence of neutralizing antibodies in at least 50% of the trial participants *(5)*.

- *HIV Vaccine Approach: HIV Multigene.* The vaccine includes in a DNA plasmid: the regulatory antigens nef, tat, and rev, the structural antigen gag, and 20 predicted epitopes for env and reverse transcriptase *(5)*. The plasmid localizes in the nucleus for increased transcription and has a prolonged half-life. It will induce CTLs against the encoded HIV antigens, and delivery devices (i.e., gene gun or the like) aimed at reducing the dose of DNA will be used. The minimum criteria for advancement will be the induction of CD4$^+$ and CD8$^+$ T-cell responses to more than one viral antigen and the presence of neutralizing antibodies in at least 50% of the trial participants *(5)*.

- *HIV Vaccine Approach: ALVAC vCP205.* In February 1999, NIAID announced the first HIV vaccine trial to be held in Africa. It was a small Phase I trial, known as HIVNET 007, conducted in Uganda by the Joint Clinical Research Center and the Ugandan Virus Research Institute (http://www.iavi.org/newpage/sdemand.html). The vaccine, referred to as ALVAC vCP205, consists of a weakened canarypox virus carrying three HIV genes derived from clade B virus. Because the HIV genes will be presented to the immune system by the live canarypox virus, both humoral and cell-mediated responses are expected to be elicited. The vaccine has already been tested on 800 volunteers in the United States and France with no reports of serious side effects. The Ugandan trial involved 40 healthy volunteers aged 18 to 40 who were at low risk of contracting HIV. Volunteers had received four injections over a period of 6 months (20 volunteers received HIV vaccine; 10 served as controls receiving a similar experimental canarypox vaccine for rabies virus; and 10 received placebo injections). The recipients' immune response to HIV was monitored over a 2-year period by *in vitro* analysis, and no volunteers had been intentionally exposed to HIV. The HIV vaccine trial in Uganda has been met with some skepticism. The vaccine is composed of HIV genes derived from clade B, which is predominately found in the United States and in Europe. Because clades A and D are predominately found in Uganda, critics have asked why genes from these clades were not incorporated in the HIV vaccine tested in Uganda. Researchers defend the Ugandan trial, explaining it as a way to determine if cross-clade immunogenicity will be achieved with this vaccine. Recent evidence revealed that cytotoxic T cells, derived from individuals naturally infected with clades A and D, can recognize clade B isolates in the laboratory. However, laboratory isolates tested *in vitro* often behave very differently than do primary isolates within a human host. Global eradication of HIV will require researchers to focus on developing a vaccine that will elicit effective immune responses against all known clades of HIV.

- *HIV Vaccine Approach: Multiple HIV Subtypes.* A novel vaccine targeted to multiple HIV subtypes found worldwide has moved into the second phase of clinical testing (www.hvtn.org). The first Phase II study (HVTN 204), which is broadly relevant to the global HIV/AIDS pandemic, will involve a total of 480 participants at sites in Africa, North America, South America, and the Caribbean to test the safety and immune response to the vaccine. The unique vaccine, which combines synthetically modified elements of four HIV genes found in subtypes A, B, and C of the virus—the subtypes commonly found in Africa, the Americas, Europe, and parts of Asia—has been developed in the Vaccine Research Center at NIAID. These subtypes represent about 85% of HIV infections worldwide. The rationale has been to develop a prime-boost strategy using a multiclade DNA plasmid vaccine for the prime vaccinations and a recombinant adenoviral vector vaccine (rAd5) for the booster vaccination. Phase I/II studies testing this VRC 6-plasmid DNA/rAd5 boost product are ongoing.

The HVTN 204 trial is being coordinated with two other planned clinical studies, an unprecedented collaboration among researchers in three clinical trial networks and NIAID. The International AIDS Vaccine Initiative plans to conduct a Phase I study of the VRC vaccine at sites in Kenya and Rwanda, and the U.S. Military HIV Research Program plans Phase I and II studies at sites in Uganda, Kenya, and Tanzania; the studies are contingent on these countries granting the appropriate regulatory and ethical approvals. The three harmonized trials will be testing a "prime-boost" strategy composed of two vaccine components given at different times. Both contain synthetic versions of four HIV genes: gag, pol, nef, and env. The gag, pol, and nef genes come from HIV subtype B, the primary virus found in Europe and North America. Env, the fourth gene, codes for an HIV coat protein that allows the virus to recognize and attach to human cells. The vaccine incorporates modified env genes from subtypes A and C, most common in Africa and parts of Asia, as well as subtype B. The two vaccine components differ in how the genes are packaged. One contains only the naked gene fragments, which cannot reconstitute into an infectious virus. The other uses a weakened type of respiratory virus known as adenovirus as a vector to shuttle the noninfectious gene fragments into the body. Adenoviruses cause upper respiratory tract illness, such as the common cold. However, because the vaccine contains only HIV gene fragments housed in an adenovirus that cannot replicate, study participants cannot become infected with HIV or get a respiratory infection from the vaccine.

The geographic diversity of participants allows the researchers to evaluate whether the immune responses generated to the vaccine vary according to the amount of prior exposure to adenovirus, as measured by pre-existing levels of adenovirus antibodies. Africans, for example, generally have had greater exposure to adenovirus than have people living in North America. The participants, divided into two groups, will receive four injections spread out over a period of 6 months. One group will receive three injections of the naked DNA component followed by a booster injection of the adenoviral vector component. The second group will receive four injections of a placebo vaccine consisting of sterile saltwater. Because the study is "double blind," neither the participants nor the researchers will know whether a volunteer is receiving the study vaccine or the placebo until the end of the trial (http://www3.niaid. nih.gov/news/newsreleases/2005/globalvax.htm).

35.2.2 Major Scientific Advances

- *Hexon-Chimeric Adenovirus Serotype 5 Vectors Circumvent Preexisting Antivector Immunity.* Whereas recombinant, replication-incompetent adenovirus serotype 5 (rAd5) vector-based HIV-1 vaccines have proved highly immunogenic in preclinical studies, such vaccines would likely be limited by the high prevalence of preexisting anti-Ad5 immunity in human populations. To circumvent anti-Ad5 immunity, novel chimeric rAd5 vectors have been constructed in which the seven short hypervariable regions (HVRs) on the surface of the Ad5 hexon protein were replaced with the corresponding HVRs from the rare adenovirus serotype Ad48 *(69).*

- *A Group M Consensus Envelope Glycoprotein Induces Antibodies That Neutralize Subsets of Subtype B and C HIV-1 Primary Viruses.* Although HIV-1 subtype C is the most common HIV-1 group M subtype in Africa as well in many regions of Asia, present HIV-1 vaccine candidate immunogens have not been able to induce potent and broadly neutralizing antibodies against subtype C primary isolates. However, recent research data have shown that using a centralized gene strategy to address HIV-1 diversity has allowed for the generation of a group M consensus envelope gene with shortened consensus variable loops (CON-S) for comparative studies with wild-type (WT) Env immunogens. Furthermore, the consensus HIV-1 group M CON-S Env elicited cross-subtype neutralizing antibodies of similar or greater breadth and titer than did the WT Env's tested, thus indicating the utility of a centralized gene strategy *(70).*

- *Relative Dominance of Gag p24-Specific Cytotoxic T-Lymphocytes Is Associated with HIV Control.* Data from untreated, clade B HIV-1–infected subjects have demonstrated that the proportion of gag-specific, and in particular p24-reactive, CTL responses among the total virus-specific CTL activity is associated with the individual's $CD4^+$ T-cell counts and viral loads. The results point toward a dominant role of gag-specific immunity in effectively controlling the HIV infection, thereby providing important guidance for HIV vaccine development *(71).*

- *Nature of Nonfunctional Envelope Proteins on the Surface of the Human Immunodeficiency Virus.* HIV-1 neutralizing antibodies are thought to be distinguished from the non-neutralizing antibodies by their ability to recognize functional gp120/gp41 envelope glycoprotein (Env) trimers. However, the antibody responses induced by natural HIV-1 infection or by tested-to-date vaccine candidates consist largely of non-neutralizing antibodies. The surprising paradox that non-neutralizing antibodies can specifically capture HIV-1 has been explained by recent evidence of the existence on the viral surfaces of Env of nonfunctional forms (gp120/gp41 monomers and gp120-depleted gp41 stumps) to which non-neutralizing antibodies can bind *(72).* It has been postulated that the existence of such nonfunctional forms of Env on the viral surfaces serve to divert the antibody response. This diversion and the resulting generation of non-neutralizing antibodies provide another mechanism helping HIV to evade neutralization.

- *Molecularly Cloned SHIV-1157ipd3N4: A Highly Replication-Competent, Mucosally Transmissible R5 Simian-Human Immunodeficiency Virus Encoding HIV Clade C env.* Because HIV-1 clade C causes more than 50% of all HIV infections worldwide and an estimated 90% of all transmissions occur mucosally with R5 strains, a pathogenic R5 simian-human immunodeficiency virus (SHIV) encoding HIV clade C *env* would be highly desirable for evaluating candidate HIV vaccines in non-human primates. To this end, SHIV-1157i, a molecular clone *env*, has been generated *(73).* In parallel, genomic DNA from the blood donor was amplified to generate the late proviral clone SHIV-1157ipd3. The latter proves to be a highly replication-competent, mucosally transmissible R5 SHIV that represents a valuable tool to test candidate HIV vaccines targeting the HIV-1 clade C Env *(73).*

- *Simian Immunodeficiency Virus (SIV) Envelope Quasispecies Transmission and Evolution in Infant Rhesus Macaques After Oral Challenge with Uncloned SIV-mac251: Increased Diversity Is Associated with Neutralizing Antibodies and Improved Survival in Previously Immunized Animals.* Immunization of infant rhesus macaques with either modified vaccinia Ankara

(MVA) virus vaccine expressing SIV *gag, pol,* and *env* or live-attenuated SIVmac1A11 vaccine resulted in lower viremia and longer survival compared with that in unimmunized controls after oral challenge with virulent SIVmac251 *(74)*. The impact of these vaccines on the oral transmission and evolution of SIV envelope variants was also investigated, and the results showed that there were no consistent differences in the patterns of *env* variants found between vaccinated and unvaccinated infants *(75)*. The reported patterns of viral envelope diversity, immune responses, and course of disease in SIV-infected infant macaques were similar to observations made in HIV-infected children and underscored the relevance of this pediatric animal model.

- *Restoration of Immunity in Late-Stage HIV Infection.* It has been demonstrated that HIV-1–specific CD8$^+$ T-cells proliferate rapidly upon encountering cognate antigens in acute infection but will lose this capacity with ongoing acute viral replication *(76)*. Further data has also shown that a loss of HIV-1–specific CD8$^+$ T-cell function not only correlates with progressive infection but can also be restored in chronic infection by augmenting the HIV-1–specific CD4$^+$ T-helper cells function.

- *Increased Reactogenicity of a Canarypox-Based Vaccine.* In clinical trials, the canarypox ALVAC-HIV vaccines have been shown to elicit human HIV-specific CTL responses in some but not all healthy uninfected adults. A clinical trial was conducted to examine whether the vaccine vCP1452 would elicit a greater HIV-specific CTL response when given at an increased dose. The results of the trial have demonstrated that the high reactogenicity associated with an increased dose of the vCP1452 negated the need to further evaluate this strategy to boost the frequency of the HIV-specific response in seronegative human subjects *(77)*.

- *Identifying How HIV Escapes the Body's Defenses.* The escape from adaptive T-cell immunity through transmutation of viral antigenic structure is a cardinal feature in the pathogenesis of SIV/HIV infection and a major hindrance to antiretroviral vaccine development. However, the molecular determinants of this phenomenon at the T-cell receptor (TCR)-antigen interface are unknown. Recent studies *(78)* have shown that mutational escape has been intimately linked to the structural configuration of constituent TCR clonotypes within virus-specific CD8$^+$ T-cell populations. Thus, fundamental differences in the mode of antigen engagement direct the pattern of adaptive viral evolution.

- *Immunodominance of Virus-Specific CTL Responses.* Although immunodominance is variably used to describe either the most frequently detectable response among tested individuals or the strongest response within a single individual, the factors that determine either interindividual or intraindividual immunodominance are still not well understood. The impact of the HLA-B alleles, epitope binding affinity, functional avidity, and the viral co-infection on the immunodominance of virus-specific CTL responses has been studied in human subjects against HIV- and EBV-derived, previously defined CTL epitopes *(79)*. The data have demonstrated that HLA-B–restricted epitopes were significantly more frequently recognized and also able to induce responses of higher magnitude compared with the HLA-A–restricted or HLA-C–restricted epitopes. Furthermore, the presence or absence of HIV co-infection did not significantly affect the EBV epitope immunodominance patterns.

- *Control of Human HIV Replication by Cytotoxic T-Lymphocyte Targeting Subdominant Epitopes.* Research has been conducted to address the function of subdominant responses in HIV infection by analyzing the CTL responses restricted by HLA-B∗ 1503, a rare allele in a cohort infected with clade B, although common in one infected with clade C. The obtained data suggest that subdominant responses can contribute to *in vivo* viral control and that high HLA allele frequencies may drive the elimination of subdominant yet effective epitopes from circulating viral populations, thereby helping to control the viral load. This last finding should be considered when designing potent antigens for HIV vaccines *(80)*.

- *A Novel Assay for Differential Diagnosis of HIV Infection in the Face of Vaccine-Generated Antibodies.* A study to differentiate vaccine- from virus-induced antibodies has been carried out using a whole-HIV-genome phage display library *(81)*. Conserved sequences in env-gp41 and gag-p6, which are recognized soon after infection, do not contain protective epitopes, and are not part of most of the current vaccines, have been identified. As a result, a new HIV seroselective assay (HIV-SELECTEST) based on these peptides, which showed more than 99% specificity and sensitivity, has been developed *(82)*.

35.3 The Failure of the STEP Trial

The scientific community has recently learned that the STEP HIV vaccine trial, which used an rAd5-based vaccine developed by Merck & Co., failed to protect Ad5-seronegative individuals against infection and may even have enhanced infection in vaccinees with prior immunity to adenoviruses *(83–86)*. The rationale for the Merck candidate vaccine was to generate robust T-cell responses by expressing HIV antigens in replication-defective recombinant adenoviral vaccines *(87, 88)* (see also Section 32.2.5). These vectors elicit protection in some primate models of HIV infection and induce detectable CD8$^+$ T-cell responses in humans, suggesting that this approach could help limit viral load and disease progression *(88–91)*. However, several concerns have been raised about the use of recombinant adenovirus serotype 5 (rAD5) as a vaccine vector, including preexisting vector-specific immunity and uncertainty about whether these vectors can induce long-lasting, broad, and protective immune responses *(92–94)*.

Working with the academic-based HIV Vaccine Trials Network (HVTN) and the NIAID, Merck researchers stopped the multicountry study after an interim analysis revealed that the vaccine did not work *(95)*. In fact, further analysis suggested that the vaccine may have helped HIV infect a subset of participants who at the trial's start had high levels of antibody to adenovirus 5 (Ad5), which causes the common cold and is also a component of the vaccine.

To trigger the T-cell response, the vaccine uses a modified adenovirus, or cold virus, as a vector to shuttle three HIV genes into the body. But many vaccinees have strong immunity to that adenovirus, which theoretically could cripple the vector and render the vaccine ineffective. To assess the magnitude of this problem and increase chances that the vaccine would work, half of the participants enrolled in the study had to have low antibody levels against that adenovirus. The interim analysis focused on only those 1500 participants, most of whom were men who have sex with men *(95)*. In participants who received at least one dose of the vaccine, 24 of the 741 vaccinated people became infected, compared with 21 of the 762 participants who received a placebo. More discouraging still, there was virtually no difference in viral loads between the two groups *(95)*.

In the first full accounting of the trial results, Merck researchers and their partners reported that, as of October 17, 2007, HIV had infected 83 participants in the placebo-controlled trial. Of these, 49 were vaccinated and 34 received saltwater injections. This difference clearly indicated that the vaccine did not protect against HIV, but the increased infections in vaccinees have no statistical import and were likely due to chance *(95)*.

A more recently launched study of the same vaccine in South Africa was also stopped and quickly "unblended" after learning the STEP trial results, notifying everyone of their vaccine status *(96)*.

The STEP trial involved the immunization of almost 3,000 healthy uninfected volunteers with three rAD5 vectors, each expressing an HIV gene: Ad5-gag, Ad5-pol, and Ad5-nef (http://www.hvtn.org/media/pr/step111307.html). This proof-of-concept trial was intended to test the capacity of the vaccine to reduce infection and to reduce the viral load (or "set point") in vaccinated individuals who nevertheless became infected *(87)*. Each individual in the trial received three injections of the three rAD5 vectors, with the last two injections spaced 6 months apart. The same vaccine was being administered in South Africa to 3,000 individuals in

the Phambili trial when the initial results of the STEP trial were made public *(87)*.

The development of the STEP trial included 12 Phase I trials with more than 1,300 volunteers, which showed that the vaccine was safe and immunogenic as measured by a standardized interferon (IFN)-enzyme-linked immunospot (Elispot) assay *(87)*. Furthermore, experiments in non-human primates have also shown some protection. Immunization with the defective rAD5 vector followed by challenge with a hybrid SHIV (SIV with an HIV envelope) resulted in a 1 to 3 log decrease in viral load *(88)*. However, these experiments were performed on only a limited number of macaques. And a more stringent challenge with the SIV mac239 strain resulted in a more modest decrease of viral load ($\sim$1 log, leaving an average of 10^5 copies of RNA/mL plasma in vaccinated animals) *(3, 28)*. In addition, this immunization strategy was effective only in monkeys carrying a specific human histocompatibility leukocyte antigen (HLA) allele known to present a dominant epitope from the gag protein. Thus, the Merck vaccine had limited efficacy in a stringent primate model *(87)*.

The Merck candidate vaccine showed good HIV-specific immunogenicity in Phase I and Phase II studies (see http://www.hvtn.org/science/1107.html for the recently released STEP trial results) as measured mostly by a single parameter: the IFN-γ ELISPOT assay. The rAd vaccine also induced long-lasting, multifunctional responses as monitored by polychromatic flow cytometry (http://www.hvtn.org/fgm/1107slides/McElrath.pdf).

The foremost issue facing any rAd5-based vaccine is the high prevalence of adenovirus-specific antibodies as a result of prior exposure to the virus, particularly in sub-Saharan Africa. Adenovirus vectors, and many other viral vectors currently used in HIV vaccines, will induce a rapid memory immune response against the vector. The resulting elimination of the vector was anticipated to be an impediment to the development of a T-cell response against the inserted antigen *(87)*. *What was completely unexpected, however, was the possibility that previous adenovirus infection might enhance susceptibility to HIV infection in vaccinated subjects.* Although the statistical analysis has not been completed, the initial results showed that vaccinated subjects who had high titers of antibodies against adenovirus tended to have a higher incidence of HIV infection than did those without anti-adenovirus antibodies. One possible explanation for this outcome is that the presence of both antibody and virus could lead to the activation of T cells, thus providing an environment that favors HIV replication *(87)*.

Although some may have predicted disappointing results based on the relatively weak protection in macaques and the lack of a broad T-cell response, no one could have predicted the correlation between preexisting vector-specific immunity and an increase in susceptibility to infection—a result that led to the immediate halting of both the STEP and Phambili trials *(87)*.

To address the consequences of the failure of the STEP trial and discuss future directions of HIV vaccine research, on March 25, 2008, the NIAID convened a *Summit on HIV Vaccine Research and Development* (http://www3. niaid.nih.gov/news/events/summitHIVVaccine.htm).

At the summit, many investigators were concerned that the STEP trial was based on a vaccine that showed minimal protection against SIV infection in macaques and the need for a predictive animal model. Participants agreed that the rhesus macaque system now used to test potential vaccines is not working well. There is a need to create more simian strains of the AIDS virus and develop standard testing protocols, as well as to explore basic biology questions. Such plans will be constrained, however, by the high cost of animal studies and shrinking budgets of primate centers.

It is well known that animal studies offer many distinct advantages *(97–99)*. They can be optimized in terms of the viral strain used, as well as the route and dose of challenge. Animals can also be challenged with heterologous viral isolates, thereby mimicking the situation in humans where it is very unlikely that one will be naturally exposed to the same virus strain used in a vaccine. Hence, proof that viral infection is attenuated in a heterologous infection model should be a minimal requirement for a vaccine to be tested for efficacy in humans *(87)*.

With the input of experts in the field (http://sciencenow. sciencemag.org/cgi/content/full/2008/205/1), NIAID has decided to review its HIV vaccine research portfolio and seek to determine the most appropriate balance between vaccine discovery and development by increasing funding away from product development and toward "discovery research" (http://www3.niaid.nih.gov/news/events/summitHIVVaccine.htm).

References

1. Johnston, M. I. and Fauci, A. S. (2007) An HIV vaccine—evolving concepts, *N. Engl. J. Med.*, **356**(20), 2073–2081.
2. Letvin, N. L. (2005) Progress toward an HIV vaccine, *Annu. Rev. Med.*, **56**, 213–223.
3. Girard, M. P., Osmanov, S. K., and Kieny, M. P. (2006) A review of vaccine research and development: the human immunodeficiency virus (HIV), *Vaccine*, **24**(19), 4062–4081.
4. Weiner, D. B. (2006) Progress in development and testing of novel recombinant vaccine platforms for HIV, *Springer Seminars in Immunopathology*, **28**(3), 195–196.
5. Ensoli, B. (2005) Criteria for selection of HIV vaccine candidates—general principles, *Microbes Infect.*, **7**(14), 1433–1435.
6. Taub, D. D., Turcovski–Corrales, S. M., Key, M. L., Longo, D. L., and Murphy, W. J., (1986) Chemokines and T lymphocyte activation: I. Beta chemokines costimulate human T lymphocyte activation in vitro, *J. Immunol.*, **156**(6), 2095–2103.
7. Walker, C. M., Moody, D. J., Stites, D. P., et al. (1986) CD8+ lymphocytes can control HIV infection in vitro by suppressing virus replication, *Science*, **234**, 1563–1566.
8. Janeway, C. A., Jr., Travers, P., Hunt, S., and Walport, M. (1997) *Immunobiology: The Immune System in Health and Disease*, 3rd ed., Garland, New York.
9. Spearman, P. (2006) Current progress in the development of HIV vaccines, *Curr. Pharm. Des.*, **12**, 1147–1167.
10. McMichael, A. J. (2006) HIV vaccines, *Annu. Rev. Immunol.*, **24**, 227–255.
11. Cocchi, F., DeVico, A. L., Garzino-Demo, A., Arya, S. K., Gallo, R. C., and Lusso, P. (1995) Identification of RANTES, MIP-1 alpha, and MIP-1 beta as the major HIV-suppressive factors produced by CD8$^+$ T cells, *Science*, **270**, 1811–1815.
12. Zhao, A. and Kent, S. (1996) HIV-specific cytotoxic lymphocyte (CTL) responses control initial viremia in HIV infected macaques, *8th Annu. Conf. Australas. Soc. HIV Med., Sydney, Australia*, November 14–17; 8:119 (Poster 139).
13. Pantaleo, G. and Koup, R. A. (2004) Correlates of immune protection in HIV-1 infection: what we know, what we don't know, what we should know, *Nat. Med.*, **10**, 806–810.
14. Ogg, G. S., Jin, X., Bonhoeffer, S., et al. (1998) Quantitation of HIV-1 specific cytotoxic T lymphocytes and plasma load of viral RNA, *Science*, **279**, 2103–2106.
15. Koup, R. A., Safrit, J. T., Cao, Y., et al. (1994) Temporal association of cellular immune responses with the initial control of viremia in primary human immunodeficiency virus type 1 syndrome, *J. Virol.*, **68**, 4650–4655.
16. Schmitz, J. E., Kuroda, M. J., Santra, S., et al. (1999) Control of viremia in simian immunodeficiency virus infection by CD8$^+$ lymphocytes, *Science*, **283**, 857–860.
17. Richman, D. D., Wrin, T., Little, S. J., et al. (2003) Rapid evolution of the neutralizing antibody response to HIV type-1 infection, *Proc. Natl. Acad. Sci. U.S.A.*, **100**, 4144–4149.
18. Wei, X., Decker, J. M., Wang, S., et al. (2003) Antibody neutralization and escape by HIV-1, *Nature*, **422**, 307–312.
19. Allen, T. M., O'Connor, D. H., and Jing P. (2000) Tat-specific cytotoxic T lymphocytes select for SIV escape variants during resolution of primary viremia, *Nature*, **407**, 386–390.
20. Goulder, P. J., Phillips, R. E., and Colbert, R. A. (1997) Late escape from an immunodominant cytotoxic T lymphocyte response associated with progression to AIDS, *Nat. Med.*, **3**, 212–217.
21. Letvin, N. L., Mascola, J. R., Sun, Y., et al. (2006) Preserved CD4(+) central memory T cells and survival in vaccinated SIV-challenged monkeys, *Science*, **312**, 1530–1533.
22. Polacino, P. S., Stallard, V., Klaniecki, J. E., et al. (1999) Role of immune responses against the envelope and the core antigens of simian immunodeficiency virus SIVmne in protection against homologous cloned and uncloned virus challenge in macaques, *J. Virol.*, **73**, 8201–8215.
23. Amara, R. R., Villinger, F., Altman, J. D., et al. (2001) Control of a mucosal challenge and prevention of AIDS by a multiprotein DNA/MVA vaccine, *Science*, **292**, 69–74.
24. Mattapallil, J. J., Douek, D. C., Buckler-White, A., et al. (2006) Vaccination preserves CD4 memory T cells during acute simian immunodeficiency virus challenge, *J. Exp. Med.*, **203**, 1533–1541.
25. Gupta, S. B., Jacobson, L. P., Margolick, J. B., et al. (2207) Estimating the benefit of an HIV-1 vaccine that reduces viral load set point, *J. Infect. Dis.*, **195**, 546–550.
26. Barouch, D. H., Kunstman, J., Kuroda, M. J., et al. (2002) Eventual AIDS vaccine failure in a rhesus monkey by viral escape from cytotoxic T lymphocytes, *Nature*, **415**, 335–339.
27. Cohen, J. (2003) AIDS vaccine trial produces disappointment and confusion, *Science*, **299**, 129–1291.
28. Yewdell, J. W. and Bennink, J. R. (1999) Immunodominance in major histocompatibility complex class I-restricted T lymphocyte

responses, *Annu. Rev. Immunol.*, **17**, 51–88.

29. Ishioka, G. Y., Fikes, J., Hermanson, G., et al. (1999) Utilization of MHC class I transgenic mice for development of minigene DNA vaccines encoding multiple HLA-restricted CTL epitopes, *J. Immunol.*, **162**(7), 3915–3925.

30. McMichael, A. and Hanke, T. (2002) The quest for an AIDS vaccine: is the CD8$^+$ T- cell approach feasible? *Nat. Rev. Immunol.*, **2**(4), 283–291.

31. Hanke, T., Samuel, R. V., Blanchard, T. J., et al. (1999) Effective induction of simian immunodeficiency virus-specific cytotoxic T lymphocytes in macaques by using a multiepitope gene and DNA prime-modified vaccinia virus Ankara boost vaccination regimen, *J. Virol.*, **73**(9), 7524–7532.

32. Allen, T. M., Vogel, T. U., Fuller, D. H., et al. (2000) Induction of AIDS virus- specific CTL activity in fresh, unstimulated peripheral blood lymphocytes from rhesus macaques vaccinated with a DNA prime/modified vaccinia virus Ankara boost regimen, *J. Immunol.*, **164**(9), 4968–4978.

33. Subbramanian, R. A., Kuroda, M. J., Charini, W. A., et al. (2003) Magnitude and diversity of cytotoxic-T-lymphocyte responses elicited by multiepitope DNA vaccination in rhesus monkeys, *J. Virol.*, **77**(18), 10113–10118.

34. McEvers, K., Elrefaei, M., Norris, P., et al. (2005) Modified anthrax fusion proteins deliver HIV antigens through MHC class I and II pathways, *Vaccine*, **23**(32), 4128–4135.

35. Mortara, L., Gras-Masse, H., Rommens, C., Venet, A., Guillet, J. G., and Bourgault- Villada, I. (1999) Type 1 CD4(+) T-cell help is required for induction of antipeptide multispecific cytotoxic T lymphocytes by a lipopeptidic vaccine in rhesus macaques, *J. Virol.*, **73**(5), 4447–4451.

36. Gahery-Segard, H., Pialoux, G., Charmeteau, B., et al. (2000) Multiepitopic B- and T-cell responses induced in humans by a human immunodeficiency virus type 1 lipopeptide vaccine, *J. Virol.*, **74**(4), 1694–1703.

37. Pialoux, G., Gahery-Segard, H., Sermet, S., et al. (2001) Lipopeptides induce cell- mediated anti-HIV immune responses in seronegative volunteers, *AIDS*, **15**(10), 1239–1249.

38. Duerr, A., Wasserheit, J. N., and Corey, L. (2006) HIV vaccines: new frontiers in vaccine development, *Clin. Infect. Dis.*, **43**, 500–511.

39. Elbasha, E. H. and Gumel, A. B. (2006) Theoretical assessment of public health impact of imperfect prophylactic HIV-1 vaccines with therapeutic benefits, *Bull. Math. Biol.*, **68**, 577–614.

40. Shiver, J. W. and Emini, E. A. (2004) Recent advances in the development of HIV-1 vaccines using replication-incompetent adenovirus vectors, *Annu. Rev. Med.*, **55**, 355–372.

41. Roberts, D. M., Nanda, A., Havenga, M. J., et al. (2006) Hexon-chimaeric adenovirus serotype 5 vectors circumvent pre-existing anti-vector immunity, *Nature*, **441**, 239–243.

42. Daniel, M. D., Kirchhoff, F., Czajak, S. C., et al. (1992) Protective effects of a live attenuated SIV vaccine with a deletion of the nef gene, *Science*, **258**, 1938–1941.

43. Baba, T. W., Jeong, Y. S., Penninck, D., et al. (1995) Pathogenicity of live, attenuated SIV after mucosal infection of neonatal macaques, *Science*, **267**, 1820–1825.

44. Learmont, J. C., Geczy, A. F., Mills, J., et al. (1999) Immunologic and virologic status after 14 to 18 years of infection with an attenuated strain of HIV-1, *N. Engl. J. Med.*, **340**, 1715–1722.

45. Donnelly, J. J., Ulmer, J. B., Shiver, J. W., et al. (1997) DNA vaccines, *Annu. Rev. Immunol.*, **15**, 617–648.

46. Egan, M. A., Charini, W. A., Kuroda, M. J., et al. (2000) Simian immunodeficiency virus (SIV) gag-DNA-vaccinated rhesus monkeys develop secondary cytotoxic T lymphocyte responses and control viral replication after pathogenic SIV infection, *J. Virol.*, **74**, 7485–7495.

47. Shen, L., Chen, Z. W., Miller, M. D., et al. (1991) Recombinant virus-vaccine- induced SIV-specific CD8$^+$ cytotoxic T lymphocytes, *Science*, **252**, 440–443.

48. Yasutomi, Y., Koenig, S., Haun, S. S., et al. (1993) Immunization with recombinant BCG-SIV elicits SIV-specific cytotoxic T lymphocytes in rhesus monkeys, *J. Immunol.*, **150**, 3101–3107.

49. Redfield, R. R., Wright, D. C., James, W. D., et al. (1987) Disseminated vaccinia in a military recruit with human immunodeficiency virus (HIV) disease, *N. Engl. J. Med.*, **316**, 673–676.

50. Hirsch, V. M., Fuerst, T. R., Sutter, G., et al. (1996) Patterns of viral replication correlate with outcome in simian immunodeficiency virus (SIV)-infected macaques: effect of prior immunization with a trivalent SIV vaccine in modified vaccinia virus Ankara, *J. Virol.*, **70**, 3741–3752.

51. Santra, S., Schmitz, J. E., Kuroda, M. J., et al. (2002) Recombinant canarypox vaccine-elicited CTL specific for dominant and subdominant simian immunodeficiency virus epitopes in rhesus monkeys, *J. Immunol.*, **168**, 1847–1853.

52. Evans, T. G., Keefer, M. C., Weinhold, K. J., et al. (1999) A canarypox vaccine expressing multiple human immunodeficiency virus type 1 genes given alone or with rgp 120 elicits broad and durable CD8$^+$ cytotoxic T lymphocyte responses in seronegative volunteers, *J. Infect. Dis.*, **280**, 290–298.

53. Shiver, J. W. and Emini, E. A. (2004) Recent advances in the development of HIV-1 vaccines using replication-incompetent adenovirus vectors, *Annu. Rev. Med.*, **55**, 355–372.

54. Shiver, J. W., Fu, T. M., Chen, L., et al. (2002) Replication-incompetent adenoviral vaccine vector elicits effective anti-immunodeficiency-virus immunity, *Nature*, **415**, 331–335.

55. Barouch, D. H., Pau, M. G., Custers, J. H., et al. (2004) Immunogenicity of recombinant adenovirus serotype 35 vaccine in the presence of pre-existing anti-Ad5 immunity, *J. Immunol.*, **172**, 6290–6297.

56. Letvin, N. L., Huang, Y., Chakrabarti, B. K., et al. (2004) Heterologous envelope immunogens contribute to AIDS vaccine protection in rhesus monkeys, *J. Virol.*, **78**, 7490–7497.

57. Reitter, J. N., Means, R. E., and Desrosiers, R. C. (1998) A role for carbohydrates in immune evasion in AIDS, *Nat. Med.*, **4**, 679–684.

58. Ye, Y., Si, Z. H., Moore, J. P., et al. (2000) Association of structural changes in the V2 and V3 loops of the gp120 envelope glycoprotein with acquisition of neutralization resistance in simian-human immunodeficiency virus passaged in vivo, *J. Virol.*, **74**, 955–962.

59. Chan, D. C., Fass, D., Berger, J. M., et al. (1997) Core structure of gp41 from the HIV envelope glycoprotein, *Cell*, **93**, 681–684.

60. D'Souza, M. P., Livnat, D., Bradac, J. A., et al. (1997) Evaluation of monoclonal antibodies to human immunodeficiency virus type-1 primary isolates by neutralization assays: performance criteria for selecting candidate antibodies for clinical trials, *J. Infect. Dis.*, **175**, 1056–1062.

61. Darren, P. W. H. I. and Burton, D. R.. (2001) The antiviral activity of antibodies in vitro and in vivo, *Adv. Immunol.*, **77**, 195–262.

62. Haynes, B. F., Fleming, J., St. Clair, E. W., et al. (2005) Cardiolipin polyspecific autoreactivity in two broadly neutralizing HIV-1 antibodies, *Science*, **308**, 1906–1908.

63. Haynes, B. F., Moody, M. A., Verkoczy, L., Kelsoe, G., and Alam, S. M. (2005) Antibody polyspecificity and neutralization of HIV-1: a hypothesis, *Hum. Antibodies*, **14**, 59–67.

64. Alam, S. M., McAdams, M., Boren, D., et al. (2007) The role of antibody polyspecificity and lipid reactivity in binding of broadly neutralizing anti-HIV-1 envelope human monoclonal antibodies 2F5 and 4E10 to glycoprotein 41 membrane proximal envelope epitopes, *J. Immunol.*, **178**, 4424–4435.

65. Parren, P. W., Marx, P. A., Hessell, A. J., et al. (2001) Antibody protects macaques against vaginal challenge with a pathogenic R5 simian/human immunodeficiency virus at serum levels giving complete neutralization in vitro, *J. Virol.*, **75**, 8340–8347.

66. O'Leary, J. G., Goodarzi, M., Drayton, D. L., and von Andrian, U. H. (2006) T cell- and B cell-independent adaptive immunity mediated by natural killer cells, *Nat. Immunol.*, **7**, 507–516.

67. Kawai, T. and Akira, S. (2006) Innate immune recognition of viral infection, *Nat. Immunol.*, **7**, 131–137.

68. Sugaya, M., Loré, K., Koup, R. A., Douek, D. C., and Blauvelt, A. (2004) HIV- infected Langerhans cells preferentially transmit virus to proliferating autologous CD4$^+$ memory T cells located within Langerhans cell-T cell clusters, *J. Immunol.*, **172**, 2219–2224.

69. Roberts, D. M., Nanda, A., Havenga, M. J. E., Abbink, P., Lynch, D. M., Ewald, B. A., Liu, J., Thorner, A. R., Swanson, P. E., Gorgone, D. A., Lifton, M. A., Lemckert, A. A. C., Holterman, L., Chen, B., Dilraj, A., Carville, A., Mansfield, K. G., Goudsmit, J., and Barouch, D. H. (2006) Hexon-chimaeric adenovirus serotype 5 vectors circumvent pre-existing anti-vector immunity, *Nature*, **441**, 239–243.

70. Liao, H.-X., Sutherland, L. L., Xia, S.-M., Brock, M. E., Scearce, R. M., Vanleeuwen, S., Alam, S. M., McAdams, M., Weaver, E. A., Camacho, Z. T., Ma, B.-J., Li, Y., Decker, J. M., Nabel, G. J., Montefiori, D. C., Hahn, B. H., Korber, B. T., Gao, F., and Haynes, B. F. (2006) A group M consensus envelope lycoprotein induces antibodies that neutralize subsets of subtype B and C HIV-1 primary viruses, *Virology*, **353**(2) 268–282.

71. Zuñiga, R., Lucchetti, Z. R., Galvan, P., Sanchez, S., Sanchez, C., Hernandez, A., Sanchez, H., Frahm, N., Linde, C. H., Hewitt, H. S., Hildebrand, W., Altfeld, M., Allen, T. M., Walker, B. D., Korber, B. T., Leitner, T., Sanchez, J., and Brander, C. (2006) Relative dominance of gag p24-specific cytotoxic T lymphocytes is associated with human immunodeficiency virus control, *J. Virol.* **80**(6), 3122–3125.

72. Moore, P. L., Crooks, E. T., Porter, L., Zhu, P., Cayanan, C. S., Grise, H., Corcoran, P., Zwick, M. B., Franti, M., Morris, L., Roux, K. H., Burton, D. R., and Binley, J. M. (2006) Nature of nonfunctional envelope proteins on the surface of the human immunodeficiency virus, *J. Virol.*, **80**(5), 2515–2528.

73. Song, R. J., Chenine, A.-L., Rasmussen, R. A., Ruprecht, C. R., Mirshahidi, S., Grisson, R. D., Xu, W., Whitney, J. B., Goins, L. M., Ong, H., Li, P.-L., Shai-Kobiler, E., Wang, T., McCann, C. M., Zhang, H., Wood, C., Kankasa, C., Secor, W. E., McClure, H. M., Strobert, E., Else, J. G., and Ruprecht, R. M. (2006) Molecularly cloned SHIV-1157ipd3N4: a highly replication-competent, mucosally transmissible R5 simian-human immunodeficiency virus encoding HIV clade C *env*, *J. Virol.*, **80**(17), 8729–8738.

74. Van Rompay, K. K. A., Greenier, J. L., Cole, K. S., Earl, P., Moss, B., Steckbeck, J. D., Pahar, B., Rourke, T., Montelaro, R. C., Canfield, D. R., Tarara, R. P., Miller, C., McChesney, M. B., and Marthas, M. L. (2003) Immunization of newborn rhesus macaques with simian immunodeficiency virus (SIV) vaccines prolongs survival after oral challenge with virulent SIVmac251, *J. Virol.*, **77**, 179–190.

75. Greenier, J. L., Van Rompay, K. K. A., Montefiori, D., Earl, P., Moss, B., and Marthas, M. L. (2005) Simian immunodeficiency virus (SIV) envelope quasispecies transmission and evolution in infant rhesus macaques after oral challenge with uncloned SIVmac251: increased diversity is associated with neutralizing antibodies and improved survival in previously immunized animals, *Virol. J.*, **2**, 11.

76. Lichterfeld, M., Kauffman, D. E., Yu, X. G., Mui, S. K., Addo, M. M., Johnston, M. N., Cohen, D., Robbins, G. K., Pae, E., Alter, G., Wurcel, A., Stone, D., Rosenberg, E. S., Walker, B. D., and Altfeld, M. (2004) Loss of HIV-1-specific CD8$^+$ T cell proliferation after acute HIV-1 infection and restoration by vaccine-induced HIV- specific CD4$^+$ T cells, *J. Exp. Med.*, **200**(6), 701–712.

77. Goepfert, P. A., Horton, H., McElrath, M. J., Gurunathan, S., Ferrari, G., Tomaras, G. D., Montefiori, D. C., Allen, M., Chiu, Y-L., Spearman, P., Fuchs, J. D., Koblin, B. A., Blattner, W. A., Frey, S., Keefer, M. C., Baden, L. R., Corey, L., and the NIAID HIV Vaccine Trials Network (2005) High-dose recombinant canarypox vaccine expressing HIV-1 protein in seronegative human subjects, *J. Infect. Dis.*, **192**(7), 1249–1259.

78. Price, D. A., West, S. M., Betts, M. R., Ruff, L. E., Brenchley, J. M., Ambrozak, D. R., Edghill-Smith, Y., Kuroda, M. J., Bogdan, D., Kunstman, K., Letvin, N. L., Franchini, G., Wolinsky, S. M., Koup, R. A., and Douek, D. C. (2004) T cell receptor recognition motifs govern immune escape patterns in acute SIV infection, *Immunity*, **21**, 793–803.

79. Bihl, F., Frahm, N., Di Giammarino, L., Sidney, J., John, M., Yusin, K., Woodberry, T., Sango, K., Hewitt, H. S., Henry, L., Linde, C. H., Chisholm III, J. V., Zaman, T. M., Pae, E., Mallal, S., Walker, B. D., Sette, A., Korber, B. T., Heckerman, D., and Brander, C. (2006) The impact of HLA-B alleles, epitope binding affinity, functional avidity, and viral coinfection on the immunodominance of virus-specific CTL responses, *J. Immunol.*, **176**(7), 4094–4101.

80. Frahm, N., Kiepiela, P., Adams, S., Linde, C. H., Hewitt, H. S., Sango, K., Feeney, M. E., Addo, M. M., Lichterfeld, M., Lahaie, M. P., Pae, E., Wurcel, A. G., Roach, T., St. John, M. A., Altfeld, M., Marincola, F. M., Moore, C., Mallal, S., Carrington, M., Heckerman, D., Allen, T. M., Mullins, J. I., Korber, B. T., Goulder, P. J. R., Walker, B. D., and Brander, C. (2006) Control of human immunodeficiency virus replication by cytotoxic T lymphocytes targeting subdominant epitopes, *Nat. Immunol.*, **7**, 173–178.

81. Khurana, S., Needham, J., Mathieson, B., Rodriguez-Chavez, I. R., Catanzaro, A. T., Bailer, R. T., Kim, J., Polonis, V., Cooper, D. A., Guerin, J., Peterson, M. L., Gurwith, M., Nguyen, N., Graham, B. S., Golding, H., and the HIV Vaccine Trial Network (2006) Human immunodeficiency virus (HIV) vaccine trials: a novel assay for differential diagnosis of HIV infections in the face of vaccine-generated antibodies. *J. Virol.*, **80**(5), 2092–2099.

82. Khurana, S., Needham, J., Park, S., et al. (2006) Novel approach for differential diagnosis of HIV infections in the face of vaccine-generated antibodies: utility for detection of diverse HIV-1 subtypes, *J. Acquir. Immune Defic. Syndr.*, **43**(3), 304–312.

83. Pantaleo, G. (2008) HIV-1 T-cell vaccines: evaluating the next step, *Lancet Infect. Dis.*, **8**(2), 82–83.

84. Cohen, J. (2007) AIDS research. Did Merck's failed HIV vaccine cause harm? *Science*, **318**, 1048–1049.

85. Ledford, H. (2007) HIV vaccine may raise risk, *Nature*, **450**, 325.

86. Desrosiers, R. (2008) Scientific obstacles to an effective HIV vaccine, *15th Conference on Retroviruses and Opportunistic Infections, Boston, MA*, February 3–6, abstract 92.

87. Sekaly, R.-P. (2007) The failed HIV Merck vaccine study: a step back or a launching point for future vaccine development? *J. Exp. Med.*, **205**(1), 7–12.

88. Shiver, J. W., Fu, T. M., Chen, L., Casimiro, D. R., Davies, M. E., Evans, R. K., Zhang, Z. Q., Simon, A. J., Trigona, W. L., Dubey, S. A., et al. (2002) Replication- incompetent adenoviral vaccine vector elicits effective anti-immunodeficiency-virus immunity, *Nature*, **415**, 331–335.

89. Casimiro, D. R., Wang, F., Schleif, W. A., Liang, X., Zhang, Z. Q., Tobery, T. W., et al. (2005) Attenuation of simian immunodeficiency virus SIVmac239 infection by prophylactic immunization with DNA and recombinant adenoviral vaccine vectors expressing Gag, *J. Virol.*, **79**, 15547–15555.

90. Gomez-Roman, V. R., Florese, R. H., Peng, B., Montefiori, D. C., Kalyanaraman, V. S., Venzon, D. et al. (2006) An adenovirus-based HIV subtype B prime/boost vaccine regimen elicits antibodies mediating broad antibody-dependent cellular cytotoxic-

ity against non-subtype B HIV strains, *J. Acquir. Immune Defic. Syndr.*, **4**, 270–277.

91. Barouch, D. H., and Nabel. G. J. (2005) Adenovirus vector-based vaccines for human immunodeficiency virus type 1, *Hum. Gene Ther.*, **16**,149–156.

92. Kostense, S., Koudstaal, W., Sprangers, M., Weverling, G. J., Penders, G., et al. (2004) Adenovirus types 5 and 35 seroprevalence in AIDS risk groups supports type 35 as a vaccine vector, *AIDS,* **18**, 1213–1216.

93. Sumida, S. M., Truitt, D. M., Lemckert, A. A., Vogels, R., Custers, J. H., et al. (2005) Neutralizing antibodies to adenovirus serotype 5 vaccine vectors are directed primarily against the adenovirus hexon protein, *J. Immunol.*, **174**, 7179–7185.

94. Roberts, D. M., Nanda, A., Havenga, M. J., Abbink, P., Lynch, D. M., Ewald, B. A., et al. (2006) Hexon-chimaeric

adenovirus serotype 5 vectors circumvent pre-existing anti-vector immunity, *Nature*, **441**, 239–243.

95. Cohen, J. (2007) Did Merck's failed HIV vaccine cause harm? *Science*, **318**(5853), 1048–1049.

96. NIAID Statement (2007) Immunizations are discontiued in two HIV vaccine trials (http://www3.niaid.nih.gov/news/newsreleases/2007/step_statement.htm).

97. Borkow, G. (2005) Mouse models for HIV-1 infection, *IUBMB Lif*, **57**, 819–823.

98. Hu, S.L. (2005) Non-human primate models for AIDS vaccine research, *Curr. Drug Targets Infect. Disord.*, **5**, 193–201.

99. ScienceScope. (2007) New scrutiny on vaccine trial, *Science*, **318**(5851), 529.

Chapter 36

Opportunistic Infections

In contrast with normal hosts, in which many infectious diseases are usually self-limited, in immunocompromised patients such infections have the potential of becoming serious illnesses characterized by high morbidity and mortality rates. There are also the opportunistic infections that occur almost exclusively in immunocompromised hosts such as patients with HIV disease. Usually widely distributed in the environment, opportunistic pathogens rarely cause serious illness in immunocompetent hosts *(1, 2)*. In this context, it is important to note that prompt and correct diagnosis of disseminated opportunistic infections may become crucial as a result of overt differences in the susceptibility to anti-infectious drugs of sometimes closely related opportunistic pathogens. For example, although both *Pseudallescheria boydii* and *Scedosporium prolificans* have been recognized as causes of opportunistic hyalohyphomycoses in immunocompromised patients, diagnosis of disseminated disease caused by *S. prolificans* has been difficult to attain because its signs and symptoms strongly resemble those of pseudallescheriasis and pulmonary aspergillosis. However, early positive identification of *S. prolificans* may prove to be essential because of its extreme drug tolerance and the related poor prognosis of disseminated disease caused by this fungal pathogen *(2)*.

The impaired immunity of patients with HIV disease frequently results in HIV-associated opportunistic infections and co-infections. These life-threatening conditions are caused by a wide range of microorganisms, including protozoa, viruses, fungi, and bacteria, and often are associated with the progression from early to advanced HIV disease (AIDS). Diseases caused by these pathogens are less common nowadays in AIDS patients receiving highly active antiretroviral therapy (HAART); however, the incidence of co-infections with hepatitis C virus (HCV) (see Section 15.3 in Chapter 15) or tuberculosis (see Chapter 14) has increased, especially in countries where the risk of co-infection is high. *Tuberculosis and hepatitis C are fast becoming of increasing concern for the proper management of HIV/AIDS and lead to significant morbidity and mortality among these patients. Moreover, as a result of pro-longed survival, greater numbers of HIV-infected patients may develop long-term complications of HCV infection, such as end-stage liver disease and hepatocellular carcinoma.* In addition, active HCV infection may interfere with HAART and other medications needed to treat HIV infection and its complications (http://www3.niaid.nih.gov/research/topics/HIV/therapeutics/intro/drug_discovery.htm).

36.1 Fungal Infections

During the past two decades or so, the incidence of fungal infections has increased significantly. Deep-seated mycoses are creating serious problems for clinicians working with immunocompromised patients, including those with HIV/AIDS *(2–4)*. Thus, the need for effective antifungal drugs has been felt more and more acutely with the emergence of the HIV/AIDS pandemic and the AIDS-related complex (ARC), both of which are nearly always associated with opportunistic fungal infections.

Another factor facilitating the spread of opportunistic mycoses has been the significant improvement achieved in the management of bacterial infections *(2)*. Several conditions have been identified that favor the predominance of *Candida* spp. over the normal microbial flora, namely, the elimination of bacterial competition after oral or parenteral antibacterial therapy, the use of cimetidine or histamine-2 blockers, as well as the significant elevation of extracellular glucose concentrations in diabetic patients *(5–9)*. The danger posed by the histamine-2 antagonists is because of their ability to elevate the local pH, thereby creating an environment more conducive to fungal growth *(10)*.

Clinicians are particularly concerned that the increasing use of antifungal drugs will lead to drug-resistant fungi, especially in settings such as hospitals where nosocomial (hospital-acquired) infections are a growing problem. Recent studies have documented resistance of *Candida* species to fluconazole and other azole and triazole drugs widely used to treat patients with systemic fungal diseases *(10–12)* (see Section 36.1.3). In addition, primary or inherent resistance limits the activity of currently available antifungal drugs for fungi such as *Aspergillus* and other emerging molds.

Fungi present an especially complex challenge to researchers, in part because pathogenicity is often associated with certain morphologic forms or a certain part of the life cycle of a fungal species. For example, pathogens such as *Histoplasma capsulatum*, *Coccidioides immitis*, or *Sporothrix schenckii* convert from one morphologic form to another in the host tissue before they propagate to cause disease. *Cryptococcus neoformans* causes infection only in the asexual form of its life cycle (yeast cells). The molecular biological progress made in *Cryptococcus neoformans* over the past 5 years attests to the importance of collaborative research between medical and molecular biology researchers. Scientists are identifying a series of antigenic peptides from fungal pathogens that can generate immune responses, which may assist in developing an antifungal vaccine (http://www3.niaid.nih.gov/research/topics/fungal/introduction.htm).

36.1.1 NIAID Plans, Priorities, and Goals

Research on fungal diseases focuses on three goals: providing better means of diagnosis, treatment, and prevention of the most important human fungal infections (http://www3.niaid.nih.gov/research/topics/fungal/introduction.htm). Objectives leading to the achievement of these goals are grouped in the following five research areas:

- *Molecular biology*: transferring the technology developed in model systems to the medically important fungi to address topics of clinical relevance, including vaccine candidates and new drug and diagnostic targets.
- *Immunobiology*: identifying immunologically protective antigens, antibodies, and pathways to plan vaccine approaches and improve therapy.
- *Pathogenesis*: identifying mechanisms of pathogenesis to interrupt or prevent the infectious process.
- *Therapy*: facilitating improvements in available treatment through study, including clinical trials, of new treatments and comparative treatments of the systemic fungal diseases.
- *Genome sequencing and genomics/proteomics*: providing complete genomic sequences for the community and facilitating genomics/proteomics approaches that address the key fungal pathogens of humans.

36.1.2 Mycoses Study Group

The Mycoses Study Group (MSG) is a self-governed organization with its own scientific agenda and its own process to determine what will be evaluated in its clinical trials. Non-MSG investigators wishing to evaluate potential therapies in the MSG must collaborate with MSG investigators.

In general, the MSG is a collaborative network of academic and private research institutions conducting clinical trials for improved antimicrobial therapies for systemic fungal infections in immunocompromised patients, including HIV-infected and uninfected subjects. The MSG is composed of investigators at 66 main and affiliate institutions and a Coordinating Center that provides operational support, data management, statistical consultation, and analysis functions. The Coordinating Center is funded by NIAID. The MSG coordinates its scientific agenda and often collaborates with the Adult AIDS Clinical Trials Group (http://www.niaid.nih.gov/daids/pdatguide/msg.htm).

MSG Research Agenda. The MSG was established by NIAID in 1978 to conduct controlled clinical trials for improved antimicrobial prophylaxis and treatment of systemic mycotic infections. The MSG provides scientific expertise and access to patients with serious fungal diseases to evaluate established and experimental agents as potential therapies. Major studies have been conducted in the treatment or prevention of histoplasmosis, fluconazole-refractory candidiasis, and cryptococcosis in AIDS patients. Subprojects are configured around coccidioidomycosis, endemic mycoses, cryptococcosis, aspergillosis, and candidiasis occurring in HIV-infected and non–HIV-infected populations (http://www.niaid.nih.gov/daids/pdatguide/msg.htm).

Examples of Clinical Studies

- A study to compare the safety and efficacy of AmBisome with conventional amphotericin B for induction therapy of histoplasmosis in patients with AIDS
- A randomized double-blind protocol comparing amphotericin B with flucytosine to amphotericin B alone followed by a comparison of fluconazole and itraconazole in the treatment of acute cryptococcal meningitis
- A Phase IV randomized study of the use of fluconazole as chronic suppressive therapy versus episodic therapy in HIV-positive subjects with recurrent oropharyngeal candidiasis
- A Phase I evaluation of the safety and pharmacodynamic activity of a murine-derived anticryptococcal antibody in patients who have recovered from AIDS-associated cryptococcal meningitis
- A prospective, randomized, double-blind trial comparing liposomal amphotericin B with fluconazole for prophylaxis of invasive fungal infections in liver transplant recipients at high risk for these infections and a prospective

observational cohort study of liver transplant recipients at low risk for invasive fungal infection

- A comparative trial of AmBisome versus amphotericin B in the empiric treatment of febrile neutropenic patients
- A randomized, open-label, comparative multicenter trial of voriconazole versus AmBisome for empirical antifungal therapy in immunocompromised patients with persistent fever and neutropenia

36.1.3 Human Candidiasis

Candidiasis is an acute or chronic, superficial or disseminated mycosis caused by species of the genus *Candida (10)*. This is a genus of nearly 200 yeast-like anamorphic (sexually imperfect) fungi characterized by a polymorphic nature because of their ability to produce budding yeast cells (blastoconidia), mycelia, pseudomycelia, and blastospores. Some *Candida* species have been found capable of mating and producing the teleomorphic (sexually perfect) form.

Based on pathology studies, three distinct forms of human candidiasis have been distinguished: superficial, locally invasive, and systemic (deep) mycoses. Systemic candidiasis is the most serious manifestation of the disease that can affect any organ, but most frequently it involves the heart, kidneys, liver, spleen, lung, and the brain. Usually, dissemination is defined as an invasive infection striking the parenchyma of two or more visceral organs. The most likely organ combinations involved have included the gastrointestinal tract, liver, kidneys, and the lung *(10)*.

Candidal Infections in HIV-Infected Patients. Oral candidiasis is the opportunistic infection that affects HIV-infected patients the most and usually the earliest *(11–13)*. It has been viewed as an initial manifestation of AIDS in all high-risk populations *(14)*, although by some accounts it is considered more prevalent in the homosexual HIV-infected population *(15, 16)*. Risk factors for esophageal candidiasis in HIV-infected patients include initial low CD4$^+$ T-cell count and plasma viremia. The occurrence of oropharyngeal or esophageal candidiasis is recognized as an indicator of immune suppression, and these are most often observed in patients with CD4$^+$ T-lymphocyte counts of <200 cells/μL. In addition, that risk may be influenced by such factors as homosexual/bisexual behavior, prior zidovudine therapy, recent antibacterial therapy, and oral candidiasis *(16)*.

Low levels of serum testosterone may have negative effect on the morbidity of esophageal candidiasis in HIV-infected men *(17)*. In this regard, early detection of low serum testosterone would allow for expedient testosterone supplementation therapy to lessen the morbidity of the disease.

If oral candidiasis is not treated, it may progress to candidal esophagitis *(18, 19)*. In HIV-infected persons, the latter may present with similar manifestations as herpes virus or cytomegalovirus disease, necessitating the use of esophagoscopy and biopsy to establish the diagnosis.

Hairy leukoplakia, which is a more imminent sign of impending AIDS, should be differentiated from candidal infection by its reticulate, smooth plaque that is typically found on the lateral side of the tongue and that will not come off by scraping. Hairy leukoplakia is caused by the Epstein-Barr virus and often will carry herpes virus, papillomavirus, and *Candida* as secondary invaders *(20)*.

Virtually all patients with HIV disease having cutaneous candidiasis will harbor *C. albicans* as the pathogen, with *C. tropicalis* only rarely being diagnosed *(20)*. In patients with ARC, the observed perirectal pain and ulceration has often been associated with *C. albicans*. In female patients with HIV infection, candidal vaginitis is a recurrent problem *(10)*.

As the CD4$^+$ T-helper cell population is progressively depleted, the development of systemic candidiasis in AIDS patients becomes increasingly likely *(10, 20)*.

Treatment. Whereas *C. albicans* is usually susceptible to all major antifungal drugs (fluconazole, itraconazole, flucytosine, and amphotericin B), at present little is known about the optimal duration of treatment *(10)*. Findings from a retrospective study to determine whether there were any correlations between the length of treatment and the development of delayed complications, such as metastatic foci, have indicated that whereas the early failure rate of treatment of candidemia was high, there were few instances of delayed complications due to hematologic dissemination *(21)*. Furthermore, there were no correlations between the duration of treatment and the development of late complications, suggesting that treatment of 2 weeks or less may be sufficient, provided that the initial response to therapy was favorable *(21)*.

Despite continuing efforts *(22, 23)*, to date there are no effective prophylactic and/or therapeutic vaccines developed against *C. albicans (24)*.

A study was conducted to identify prescribing policies likely to potentiate or limit *Candida* resistance to fluconazole in a clinical setting *(25)*. The amount of fluconazole used was determined by the number of fluconazole treatment-days per 100 hospitalization days (penetration index) after prescription of either low-dose fluconazole (50 mg prescribed as intermittent or prolonged treatment) or higher-dose fluconazole regimens (200 mg). The data obtained have suggested that a prolonged or repeated exposure to low-dose fluconazole, rather than total cumulative use, was associated with fluconazole resistance. Moreover, restoration of a normal ecology has been observed when low-dose prolonged or intermittent prescriptions of fluconazole were reduced *(25)*.

HAART and Candidiasis. The initiation of HAART in HIV-infected populations has had a positive impact on the immunologic recovery of such patients, thereby leading to decreased frequency of symptomatic *Candida* infections and an overall decline in some opportunistic infections *(10, 26)*. Thus, in patients receiving HAART, there has been a significant increase in the functional measures of innate immunity, such as fungicidal activity, chemotaxis, and oxidative metabolism of polymorphonuclear leukocytes and monocytes from HIV-positive, naïve patients *(27)*. However, results from a longitudinal study of the relationship between HAART and recurrent oropharyngeal candidiasis in advanced HIV-infected patients have demonstrated that unless HAART is accompanied by a significant decrease in the viral load and increase in the CD4$^+$ T-cell count, HAART alone may not lead to a reduced recurrence rate of oropharyngeal candidiasis *(28)*.

Data from another study have demonstrated that refractory (fluconazole-resistant) AIDS-related mucosal candidiasis has been resolved after initiation of retroviral therapy consisting of didanosine (125 mg, twice daily) and saquinavir (600 mg, thrice daily) *(29)*.

Continuous improvement of oral *Candida* colonization and skin-test reactivity have also been noticed after 1 year of treatment with anti-HIV protease inhibitors (ritonavir) of a cohort of advanced HIV-infected patients *(30, 31)*. Fungal proteinase inhibitors inhibit the *Candida* aspartyl proteinase, resulting in reduced fungal growth, as well as directly inhibiting the virulence of *Candida* *(32, 33)*.

36.1.4 Azole Drug Resistance and Refractory Candidiasis

There have been a number of reports of resistance to azole agents in HIV-infected patients with relapsing oropharyngeal candidiasis, as well as invasive candidiasis *(10, 11)*. For example, daily or every-other-day use of fluconazole has been associated with the development of refractory candidal infection *(12)*. Therefore, susceptibility testing for azole derivatives has become increasingly important in establishing an effective therapy *(34)*. Even though most *Candida* isolates still remain susceptible to amphotericin B *(35)*, the emergence of resistance and cross-resistance to antifungal drugs would necessitate *in vitro* and clinical correlations *(10)*.

The genotypes and susceptibilities to fluconazole of two sets of samples of *C. albicans* (a total of 78 strains), one from HIV-infected patients and one from healthy volunteers, were compared in an attempt to define the clonal and spontaneous origins of fluconazole resistance *(36)*. Although the analysis revealed little evidence for genotypic clustering according to HIV status or body site, a small group of fluconazole-resistant strains from HIV-infected patients formed a distinct cluster. The overall results suggested both clonal and spontaneous origins of fluconazole resistance in *C. albicans (36)*.

The phospholipid and sterol composition of plasma membranes of five fluconazole-resistant clinical *C. albicans* isolates has been compared with that of three fluconazole-sensitive ones *(37)*. Whereas the three azole-sensitive strains tested and four of the five azole-resistant strains did not exhibit any major difference in their phospholipid and sterol composition, the remaining strain showed a decreased amount of ergosterol and a lower phosphatidylcholine:phosphatidylethanolamine ratio in the plasma membrane. It has been postulated that these changes in the plasma membrane lipid and sterol composition may be responsible for an altered uptake of drugs and thus for a reduced intracellular accumulation of fluconazole, thereby providing a possible mechanism of azole resistance *(37)*.

C. albicans resistance to azole antimycotics is thought to be initiated by multiple mechanisms, including alterations in the target enzyme and increased efflux of drugs *(36)*. For example, overexpression of the ABC-transporter genes CDR1 and CDR2 were found in 20 azole-resistant *C. albicans* clinical isolates from seven HIV-infected patients, and overexpression of the *Major Facilitator gene MDR1* was found in nine azole-resistant isolates from six patients *(38)*. The overall results suggested the existence of multiple combinations of mechanisms for the development of azole resistance in *C. albicans*. In another study, the expression of ERG11, MDR1, and CDR2 genes involved in *C. albicans* resistance to fluconazole was monitored using Northern-blot technique *(39)*. The obtained results demonstrated the complexity of the epidemiology of the molecular mechanisms of antifungal resistance and indicated that different subpopulations of yeast may coexist at a given time in the same patient and may develop resistance through different mechanisms.

36.1.5 Human Cryptococcosis

Cryptococcus neoformans is a yeast-like fungus that is pathogenic to both animals and humans *(40)*. This fungus is a saprophytic organism found in soil, in a variety of fruits, and in pigeon nests. It exists in two varieties: *C. neoformans* var. *neoformans*, and *C. neoformans* var. *gattii*. Each of these two varieties, in turn, has two serotypes: A and D for var. *neoformans*, and B and C for var. *gattii*. In addition, there have been reports of human infections caused by two other *Cryptococcus* species: *C. albidus* and *C. laurentii* *(40)*.

Infection with *C. neoformans* is usually acquired by inhalation. Although the fungus is common in pigeon feces, the birds are not clinically infected *(41)*. Furthermore, there is no observation of human-to-human transmission of the disease *(42)*.

Cell-mediated immunity seems to provide the major defense against cryptococcal infections, leaving patients with compromised cell-mediated responses more vulnerable and, therefore, more likely to develop cryptococcal infection *(43–52).*

The alveolar macrophages represent the initial host's defense against the cryptococcal pathogen and may arrest infection before dissemination can occur. Experimental data have shown that the innate fungicidal activity of primary human alveolar macrophages against *C. neoformans* was impaired after HIV-1 infection *in vitro* by a mechanism that might have involved a defect of intracellular antimicrobial processing *(53).*

Human neutrophils are also known to inhibit and kill *C. neoformans in vitro* and are thought to play an important role in the host's defense against cryptococcosis through both oxidative and nonoxidative mechanisms *(54).*

Both interferon-γ (IFN-γ) and the tumor necrosis factor-α (TNF-α) are important factors in mediating acquired resistance to cryptococcal meningoencephalitis *(55).*

Cryptococcosis may develop as an acute, subacute, and chronic pulmonary, systemic, or meningeal mycosis. The pulmonary form is usually transitory, mild, and often asymptomatic. However, the involvement of the central nervous system (CNS) is manifested by subacute or chronic meningitis that in immunocompromised hosts could be life threatening.

During dissemination of the disease, skeletal and visceral lesions may occur. Nearly all immunocompromised patients, including those with HIV disease, are likely to develop disseminated cryptococcosis *(56, 57)* affecting the skin, bone, prostate, kidneys, eyes, liver, spleen, adrenals, lymph nodes, and gastrointestinal tract *(40).*

A persistent cryptococcal infection has been reported of the prostate in AIDS patients even after an adequate therapy with amphotericin B alone or in combination with flucytosine; this observation suggests the possibility of the prostate serving as a sequestered reservoir of infection from which a systemic relapse may occur *(58).*

The coexistence of different diseases within the same lesion is a distinct possibility in HIV-infected patients. For example, there have been several reports of simultaneous Kaposi's sarcoma and cutaneous cryptococcosis occurring at the same site in a patient with AIDS *(59).* Limbal nodules and multifocal choroidal lesions due to *C. neoformans* may also occur in AIDS patients *(60).*

Currently, cryptococcosis is considered to be one of the most life-threatening mycoses in patients with AIDS *(61–67).* It is associated with high relapse rate and poor response to treatment *(68–77).* Disseminated cryptococcosis presenting as molluscum-like lesions has been described as the first manifestation of AIDS *(73, 78).*

Cryptococcal meningitis is by far the most dangerous form of the disease. Because some of the patients with cryptococcal meningitis may be asymptomatic *(43,45,74–76),* it is important that the cerebrospinal fluid be examined whenever *C. neoformans* is isolated from or detected at any site. The onset of cryptococcal meningitis would most likely be insidious, but often it is acute in cases of severely immunocompromised hosts. In the latter case, if untreated, the infection is always fatal *(43,79–81).*

Treatment. The choice of therapy for cryptococcal disease is largely dependent on both the anatomic site of infection and the patient's immune status *(40, 82).* The optimal therapeutic approaches for managing cryptococcal meningitis, especially in HIV/AIDS patients with underlying T-cell dysfunction and those with neoplasia or on corticosteroid therapy, are not completely defined and still subject to discussion *(40,82–85).*

Although fluconazole and itraconazole have been associated with response rates of 50% to 60%, amphotericin B is still the drug of choice for inducing a rapid clearance of the fungus and, therefore, a preferable option for initial therapy *(40).* Results from a large clinical trial (MSG 17/ACTG 159) *(83)* have indicated that initial treatment for 2 weeks with amphotericin B (0.7 mg/kg once daily), followed by triazole (fluconazole at 400 mg daily, or itraconazole at 400 mg daily) therapy for a further 8 weeks resulted in a mortality rate of less than 8%, which is substantially lower than that previously reported *(86).*

Based on the results of a retrospective review of 30 consecutive AIDS patients with cryptococcal infection (median $CD4^+$ T-cell count of 0.042×10^9 cells/L), the use of fluconazole at 400 mg daily was recommended as initial therapy for AIDS-associated cryptococcosis in these patients *(87).* In the largest comparative study *(88),* there was no difference found in the response rates associated with amphotericin B and fluconazole.

Furthermore, high-dose (800 mg daily) of fluconazole was well tolerated by HIV-infected patients and appeared to be an effective primary therapy for cryptococcal disease in AIDS patients *(89).* First-line fluconazole therapy (200 to 400 mg daily) has also been found effective and well tolerated in patients with AIDS-associated nonmeningeal cryptococcosis *(90).*

The preferred therapy for disseminated cryptococcosis, particularly cerebral manifestations, is still amphotericin B–flucytosine combination *(66, 78, 84, 91).* The use of high-dose oral fluconazole for treating disseminated cryptococcosis has also been recommended *(92).*

However, the use of flucytosine (5-FC; 5-fluorocytosine) would be difficult to recommend for AIDS patients because of its adverse bone-marrow-suppressive *(93, 94)* and gastrointestinal *(70)* effects, which often are superimposed on symptoms caused by the human immunodeficiency virus (HIV) *(95, 96)*. Thus, in a multicenter, prospective, randomized trial *(97)* that lasted for either 4 or 6 weeks, the treatment with intravenous amphotericin B (0.3 mg/kg daily) and oral flucytosine (150 mg/kg daily) of 194 patients with cryptococcal meningitis led to the development of one or more adverse side effects in 103 patients. The toxicity included azotemia (*n* = 51), renal tubular necrosis (*n* = 2), leukopenia (*n* = 30), thrombocytopenia (*n* = 22), diarrhea (*n* = 26), hepatitis (*n* = 10), and nausea/vomiting (*n* = 10). Overall, both the 4- and 6-week regimens were complicated by toxicity in 44% and 43% of patients, respectively. In general, the observed side effects appeared during the first 2 weeks of therapy in 56% and during the first 4 weeks in 87% of the patients *(97)*.

Another randomized clinical trial of AIDS patients with cryptococcal meningitis compared the therapeutic efficacies of fluconazole with a combination of amphotericin B and flucytosine *(98)*. The all-male group was randomly assigned to receive either oral fluconazole (400 mg daily) for 10 weeks or amphotericin B (0.7 mg/kg daily) for 1 week, then 3 times weekly for 9 weeks combined with flucytosine (150 mg/kg daily, in 4 divided doses). Eight of 14 patients (57%) assigned to fluconazole failed to respond, compared with none of 6 patients assigned to amphotericin-flucytosine therapy. Although such results show that combined amphotericin B–flucytosine medication may be superior to fluconazole in the treatment of cryptococcal meningitis in AIDS patients, the intravenous administration of amphotericin B has been associated with frequent and often severe side effects compared with oral fluconazole given once daily *(40)*.

After a review of the records of 106 patients with cryptococcal infection and AIDS (criteria included: efficacy of treatment with amphotericin B alone and in combination with flucytosine, efficacy of suppressive therapy, prognostic clinical characteristics, and the course of nonmeningeal cryptococcosis), it was concluded that the addition of flucytosine to amphotericin B neither enhanced survival nor prevented relapse, but long-term suppressive therapy appeared to be beneficial *(99)*. Nevertheless, in a significant number of patients, the flucytosine medication had to be stopped because of cytopenia *(99, 100)*.

Disease relapses are frequent in HIV/AIDS patients (20% to 60%) if a long-term maintenance therapy is not applied promptly. In this regard, fluconazole at 200 mg daily has been shown to be superior to itraconazole at the same dosage level *(83)*.

Fluconazole has also been used prophylactically *(101–103)*. At 200 to 400 mg daily, it reduced significantly the incidence of cryptococcosis (and mucosal candidiasis as well), especially in AIDS patients with CD4$^+$ T-cell counts of less than 50 cells/mm^3.

36.1.6 *Pneumocystis jirovecii Pneumonia*

The genus *Pneumocystis* comprises noncultivable, highly diversified fungal pathogens dwelling in the lungs of mammals. The genus includes numerous host-species–specific species that are able to induce severe pneumonitis, especially in severely immunocompromised hosts. *Pneumocystis* organisms attach specifically to type 1 epithelial alveolar cells, showing a high level of subtle and efficient adaptation to the alveolar microenvironment *(104)*.

Pneumocystis pneumonia (PCP) is a form of pneumonia caused by the yeast-like fungus *Pneumocystis jirovecii*. The causative agent was originally described as a protozoan and spelled *P. jiroveci*, and prior to that was classified as a form of *Pneumocystis carinii*, a name still in common use *(105, 106)*. As a result, *Pneumocystis* pneumonia (PCP) has also been known as *Pneumocystis jiroveci[i]* pneumonia and as *Pneumocystis carinii* pneumonia *(107–109)*.

Pneumocystis pneumonia is relatively rare in people with normal immune systems but common among people with weakened immune systems, such as premature or severely malnourished children, the elderly, and especially AIDS patients, in whom it is most commonly observed today *(110, 111)*. PCP can also develop in patients who are taking immunosuppressant medications (e.g., patients who have undergone solid-organ transplantation) and in patients who have undergone bone marrow transplantation *(111)*.

Taxonomy. The realization that *Pneumocystis* from humans could not infect experimental animals such as rats, and that the rat form of *Pneumocystis* differed physiologically and had different antigenic properties, has led to the recognition *(112)* of the human pathogen as a distinct species. In 1976, it was named *Pneumocystis jirovecii* to honor Otto Jirovec, who first described *Pneumocystis* pneumonia in humans in 1952. Because DNA analysis has shown significant differences between the rat and the human variants, the proposal to change the name to *jirovecii* was made again in 1999 and the new name has come into common use; *P. carinii* still describes the species found in rats *(105)*, and that name is typified by an isolate from rats *(106)*. The International Code of Botanical Nomenclature (ICBN) requires that the name be spelled *jirovecii* rather than *jiroveci*. The latter spelling originated when *Pneumocystis* was believed to be a protozoan, rather than a fungus, and therefore was spelled using the International Code of Zoological Nomenclature. Both spellings are now commonly used.

Initially, it was commonly believed that all *Pneumocystis* were protozoans, but soon afterwards evidence began accumulating that *Pneumocystis* was a fungal genus. Recent studies have demonstrated it to be an unusual, in some ways a primitive, genus of Ascomycota, related to a group of yeasts *(113)*. Every tested primate, including humans, appears to have its own type of *Pneumocystis* that is incapable of cross-infecting other host species and has coevolved with each mammal species *(114)*. Currently only five species have been formally named: *P. jirovecii* from humans, *P. carinii* as originally named from rats, *P. murina* from mice *(115)*, *P. wakefieldiae (116,117)* also from rats, and *P. oryctolagi* from rabbits *(118)*.

The term PCP, which was widely used by practitioners and patients, has been retained for convenience, with the rationale that it now stands for the more general **P**neumo**c**ystis **p**neumonia rather than **P**neumocystis **c**arinii **p**neumonia.

Pneumocystis Pneumonia and AIDS. Before the epidemic of AIDS in the early 1980s, *Pneumocystis* pneumonia (PCP) was a rare infection that occurred in immunosuppressed patients with protein malnutrition or acute lymphocytic leukemia or in patients receiving corticosteroid therapy. This opportunistic infection is now most commonly associated with advanced HIV infection (http://www.aafp.org/afp/991015ap/1699.html).

The appearance of PCP in previously healthy gay men was one of the initial signs of the emergence of AIDS *(111, 119)*. An unusual rise in the number of PCP cases in North America, noticed when physicians began requesting large quantities of the rarely used antibiotic pentamidine, was the first clue to the existence of AIDS in the early 1980s *(120, 121)*.

Before the widespread use of prophylaxis, PCP was the AIDS-defining illness in 60% of cases and eventually affected 80% of patients with AIDS *(122, 123)*. Although PCP remains the most common AIDS-defining illness, earlier diagnosis of HIV, antiretroviral therapy, and effective prophylaxis have all contributed to a 75% decline in cases *(124)*. Intravenous drug users, noncompliant patients, and persons whose HIV serostatus is unknown are at particularly high risk for PCP. Intolerance of anti-*Pneumocystis* agents is common, making management challenging (http://www.aafp.org/afp/991015ap/1699.html).

Controversy exists over whether PCP represents reactivation of infection acquired early in life or whether repeated exposure and reinfection cause the disease. Experiments in immunosuppressed animals and reports of case clusters support the latter theory *(125)*. The organism is acquired by inhalation and adheres to type I alveolar cells. Proliferation produces a foamy, eosinophilic exudate that fills the alveolar spaces, leading to decreased oxygenation, a thickened interstitium, and, eventually, fibrosis *(126)*.

Defective T-cell immunity is the primary risk factor for PCP. Associated clinical signs are well defined in HIV infection and reflect the degree of CD4$^+$ T-cell depletion *(127, 128)*.

Treatment. Prior to the development of more effective treatments, PCP was a common and rapid cause of death in persons living with AIDS. Much of the incidence of PCP has been reduced by instituting a standard practice of using oral co-trimoxazole to prevent the disease in patients with CD4$^+$ T-cell counts of less than 200/mm^3. In populations that do not have access to preventive treatment, PCP continues to be a major cause of death in AIDS *(111)*.

In immunocompromised patients (e.g., cancer patients on chemotherapy or persons living with AIDS with a CD4$^+$ T-cell count below 200/μL), prophylaxis with regular pentamidine inhalations or trimethoprim-sulfamethoxazole (co-trimoxazole, or TMP-SMZ) may be necessary to prevent PCP *(111)*.

The risk of pneumonia due to *Pneumocystis jirovecii* increases when CD4 levels are less than 200 cells/μL. In these immunosuppressed individuals, the manifestations of the infection are highly variable. The disease attacks the interstitial, fibrous tissue of the lungs, with marked thickening of the alveolar septa and alveoli and leading to significant hypoxia that can be fatal if not treated aggressively; hence, lactate dehydrogenase (LDH) levels increase and gas exchange is compromised. Oxygen is less able to diffuse into the blood, leading to hypoxia. Hypoxia, along with high arterial carbon dioxide (CO$_2$) levels, stimulates ventilation, thereby causing dyspnea *(111)*.

Available therapies have many adverse effects, and treatment is more often limited by toxicity than by lack of response. Patients with AIDS require 3 weeks of treatment for PCP compared with 2 weeks in other populations *(129)*. Hospitalized patients should receive intravenous therapy until they improve enough to reliably absorb oral medication; those with mild disease can be treated orally from the outset. All patients should be monitored closely for signs of toxicity and clinical deterioration.

The mainstay of treatment is trimethoprim-sulfamethoxazole (Bactrim, Septra), given intravenously or orally. Trimethoprim-sulfamethoxazole sequentially inhibits two enzymes in the folate metabolism essential for DNA synthesis: dihydrofolate reductase (DHFR) and dihydropteroate synthetase (DHPS) *(130)*. Treatment failure occurs in 9% to 20% of cases, depending on the severity of the disease *(131, 132)*. However, adverse effects have been reported in more than one half of cases, and treatment-limiting toxicities may occur in up to one third *(130)*. Common problems include nausea and vomiting, maculopapular rash, bone marrow suppression, hepatitis, and drug fever *(132)*. Management of adverse effects by means of antiemetics, antihistamines, or antipyretics may enable completion of a course of therapy (http://www.aafp.org/afp/991015ap/1699.html).

Intravenous pentamidine may be somewhat less effective than trimethoprim-sulfamethoxazole to treat moderate-to-severe PCP *(132)*. It is usually reserved for use in patients who do not respond to, or cannot tolerate, trimethoprim-sulfamethoxazole. Serious adverse effects include nephrotoxicity, hyperglycemia and hypoglycemia, pancreatitis, arrhythmias (including torsade de pointes), and the subsequent development of frank diabetes *(130)*. It is important to monitor blood glucose and creatinine levels and to watch for QT (the QT interval is a measure of the total time of ventricular depolarization and repolarization) prolongation, especially during the last 2 weeks of therapy.

Trimetrexate (Neutrexin) is a significantly more potent inhibitor of DHFR than trimethoprim (Proloprim) *(130)*, so potent that hematopoietic cells must be protected through the coadministration of leucovorin. Although trimetrexate is significantly less toxic than trimethoprim-sulfamethoxazole, it is also less effective *(133)*. Because it is administered once daily, trimetrexate can be used in outpatients even though it is given intravenously. To mimic the sequential enzyme blockade provided by trimethoprim-sulfamethoxazole, dapsone (100 mg orally) can be added to the regimen *(131)*.

Besides trimethoprim-sulfamethoxazole, several alternative treatment regimens can be used in patients with mild or moderate PCP. Therapy with dapsone and trimethoprim duplicates the sequential enzyme blockade of trimethoprim-sulfamethoxazole *(131)*. Although dapsone can trigger hemolytic anemia in patients with absolute (homozygous) glucose-6-phosphate dehydrogenase (G6PD) deficiency, black patients typically have relative (heterozygous) G6PD deficiency and tolerate dapsone therapy without significant hemolysis (http://www.aafp.org/afp/991015ap/1699. html).

Clindamycin (Cleocin) plus primaquine is another useful oral combination. Anemia has been a common complication of this therapy, but it is rarely due to hemolysis. Rash, which typically appears in the second week of use, may be severe and is more common than rash related to trimethoprim-sulfamethoxazole *(131)*.

When trimethoprim-sulfamethoxazole, dapsone-trimethoprim, and clindamycin-primaquine were compared in patients with mild-to-moderate PCP, no significant differences were found in terms of either therapeutic failure or treatment-limiting toxicity; 54% of the subjects did not complete a full course of assigned treatment, primarily because of toxicity. Different problems occurred: the trimethoprim-sulfamethoxazole group had a higher incidence of hepatitis; the dapsone-trimethoprim group had more nausea and vomiting; and the clindamycin-primaquine group had more anemia than did the other groups *(131)*. These results suggest that treatment selection may be tailored to the individual patient's preexisting laboratory abnormalities or other medical problems (http://www.aafp.org/ afp/991015ap/1699.html).

Atovaquone (Mepron), an antiprotozoal agent, has shown good activity against PCP but is limited by its modest and unpredictable bioavailability. Although it is less effective than either trimethoprim-sulfamethoxazole or pentamidine, it has been better tolerated *(134, 135)*.

Despite the presence of an effective antimicrobial therapy, mild-to-moderate episodes of PCP can still carry a mortality risk of up to 9% *(134)*. Determination of the alveolar-arterial oxygen gradient [A-a]DO_2 is critical because the degree of impairment is the most important prognostic indicator. Almost all patients experience some deterioration in oxygenation within the first few days of therapy, probably because of the inflammatory response triggered by dying organisms *(136)*. The [A-a]DO_2 gradient represents the difference between the amount of oxygen in the arterial blood and the amount of oxygen actually delivered to the alveoli—the [A-a]DO_2 gradient can be used to assess the ventilation/perfusion imbalances and abnormal gas exchange in the lung. Although the [A-a]DO_2 decrease is not clinically important in mild disease, patients with poor pulmonary reserve may develop respiratory failure (http://www. aafp.org/afp/991015ap/1699.html).

Administration of corticosteroids within the first 72 hours of anti-*Pneumocystis* treatment helps to prevent respiratory failure and death in AIDS patients *(136)*. All patients with an [A-a]DO_2 greater than 35 mm Hg or a PaO_2(oxygen pressure) of less than 70 mm Hg should receive corticosteroids when antimicrobial therapy is initiated *(137)*. The standard approach has been to use prednisone for 21 days. Patients who are severely ill or unable to take oral medication may be given an equivalent dosage of intravenous methylprednisolone. The risk of reactivating tuberculosis or acquiring another infection appeared to be minimal *(136)*.

The prognosis for patients who develop respiratory failure has been poor, although those who required mechanical ventilation early were more likely to recover than were those who developed late respiratory failure *(138)*. In unventilated patients, pneumothorax resulted in prolonged hospitalization but did not increase mortality, whereas pneumothorax in ventilator-dependent patients almost always had a fatal outcome *(139)* (http://www.aafp.org/afp/991015ap/1699. html).

Pneumocystis Pneumonia Prophylaxis. Trimethoprim-sulfamethoxazole is the first choice for prophylaxis. In a meta-analysis of 35 randomized trials *(140)*, patients regularly taking trimethoprim-sulfamethoxazole had only a 5% likelihood of developing PCP. Even though the dosage used for prophylaxis is much lower than that used for treatment, side effects were still common. Lower dosage regimens should be considered, because they may diminish the risk of side effects without compromising protection *(128, 140)*. If a mild reaction to trimethoprim-sulfamethoxazole develops, antihistamines often permit continued use of the agent *(140, 141)*. Desensitization has not been studied rigorously but has been useful in some cases *(142)*. Other benefits of the trimethoprim-sulfamethoxazole regimen include protection against toxoplasmosis and bacterial infections *(143)*.

Dapsone has been reported as a reasonable alternative to trimethoprim-sulfamethoxazole. Dapsone in combination with weekly pyrimethamine (Daraprim) protected against PCP and toxoplasmosis *(128, 144)*. Atovaquone is considerably more expensive than dapsone and is not yet sanctioned for this use by the U.S. Public Health Service.

Aerosolized pentamidine (NebuPent) is another option, although it is the least effective form of prophylaxis, particularly in patients with very low CD4$^+$ T-cell counts *(141)*. Although this agent is well tolerated, it is expensive and does not protect against systemic pneumocystosis, toxoplasmosis, or bacterial infections. Patients should be screened for active tuberculosis before starting aerosolized pentamidine therapy to avoid the unnecessary exposure of others. Pretreatment with inhaled bronchodilators minimizes cough and bronchospasm (http://www.aafp.org/afp/991015ap/1699.html).

36.2 Viral Infections

36.2.1 Cytomegalovirus

Cytomegaloviruses are ubiquitous pathogens that commonly infect animals and humans *(145)*. In humans, the cytomegalovirus (CMV) is commonly known as human herpesvirus 5 (HHV-5) *(146)*. CMV belongs to the Betaherpesvirinae subfamily of Herpesviridae, which also includes Roseolovirus. Other herpesviruses fall into the subfamilies of Alphaherpesvirinae (including HSV-1 and HSV-2 and varicella) or Gammaherpesvirinae (including Epstein-Barr virus) *(146)*. All herpesviruses share a characteristic ability to remain latent within the body over long periods.

The human cytomegaloviruses (HCMVs) are highly species-specific both for replication and pathogenesis. Whereas some host cells are more susceptible to infection, others do not succumb to the virus but may play an important role in harboring the pathogen. Such harboring of the pathogen may persist for longer periods of time, after which it may establish latency *(145)*. It is likely that the thousands of genetically different strains of HCMV currently in existence circulate in the general population throughout the world *(147)*. Humans are believed to be the only reservoir for HCMV. Cytomegalovirus infection is acquired throughout life, with more than 50% of the adult population being infected by age 50. Although neonatal HCMV infections can be severe, in healthy populations the disease is usually asymptomatic *(145)*.

Transmission is carried out by direct or indirect person-to-person contact *(148)*. Among the various sources of infection, oropharyngeal secretions, cervical and vaginal excretions, spermic fluids, urine, feces, breast milk, tears, and

blood are predominant *(149–151)*. Oral and respiratory spread appear to be the primary routes of transmission during childhood and possibly adulthood. Multiple or large quantities of blood transfusion also convey a greater risk of both primary and recurrent HCMV infections *(145)*.

HCMV infection in immunocompetent hosts *(152, 153)* usually is benign and asymptomatic, although occasionally it may be associated with a heterophile-negative mononucleosis syndrome. Whether symptomatic or not, there may be shedding of virus in the urine and oral secretions for several months to several years after the primary infection *(154)*.

After a primary infection, HCMV remains latent in the cells. However, similarly to other herpesviruses, HCMV can reactivate in immunosuppressed hosts. The primary HCMV infection is frequently followed by persistent and/or recurrent infections. Although most often recurrent infections result from latent viral reactivation, reinfection may also occur, possibly because of the antigenic diversity of the cytomegaloviruses *(145, 155)*.

In severe disseminated disease, evidence of HCMV can be observed in virtually all organs *(156–159)*, but ductal epithelial cells are the major site of involvement. In infants and young children, the salivary glands are most frequently affected *(157, 159)*. Viruria resulting from renal infection has been consistently observed in all age groups. The lungs have been another organ affected by HCMV, especially in immunosuppressed older patients and bone marrow and lung transplant recipients *(160)*. Other organs, although less frequently involved in HCMV infections, include the adrenals, ovaries, bones, pancreas, and skin *(145, 156)*.

It is noteworthy to mention that the term "recurrent infection" is generally used to refer to intermittent excretion of virus from single or multiple sites over a prolonged period of time, and should be differentiated from "chronic" or "prolonged excretion of virus" that characterizes certain forms of HCMV infection *(145)*.

HCMV Infection in HIV Disease. Owing to the high rate of seropositivity (90% to 100%) among AIDS patients, HCMV was originally thought by some to be the etiologic agent of HIV disease *(161, 162)*.

Approximately 40% of AIDS patients present with HCMV visceral involvement in the advanced stage of the disease *(163, 164)*. The most common localizations are retinitis and gastrointestinal infection *(165)*, and to a lesser extent CNS disorders. Despite the presence of HCMV in the lungs, no evidence has been found of HCMV-induced pneumonitis in AIDS patients, presumably owing to the inability of the lungs to mount the T-cell response necessary for immunopathology *(166)*.

The profound and progressive immune suppression caused by HIV creates optimal conditions for reactivation of a latent intracellular HCMV infection, which becomes chronic with a high frequency of relapses due to the progression of HIV infection over time. Furthermore, because multiple strains of HCMV have been identified in populations at risk, reinfection remains a distinct possibility *(155)*.

Treatment. HCMV infection is common in both homosexual and heterosexual HIV-infected patients, especially those with low CD4$^+$ T-cell counts *(145, 167)*.

Ganciclovir *(168–172)* and foscarnet *(173–177)* are currently the drugs of choice for the treatment of HCMV retinitis *(1353–1358)*. Their therapeutic efficacy is similar, resulting in a 90% to 95% response rate among patients treated for a first episode of HCMV retinitis during induction therapy *(145, 163, 178)*.

A number of clinical studies have documented the efficacy of ganciclovir in the treatment of HCMV retinitis *(145,168,179–192)*. In spite of the treatment, retinitis recurred in nearly all cases after cessation of therapy, which indicated a virostatic activity for ganciclovir *(184,189–191,193,194)*. Ganciclovir is usually administered intravenously in a 1-hour-long infusion with 5.0 mg/kg daily dose during induction therapy *(163, 165)*. Because of its renal excretion, the dosage of ganciclovir should be adjusted to compensate for renal insufficiency. The mean intravitreal concentration of ganciclovir after intravenous administration to AIDS patients with retinal detachments was 0.93 µg/mL (3.6 µg/mM). This value, which was significantly lower than the concentration of ganciclovir required to achieve 50% of viral plaque formation for many human CMV strains, did suggest that the intravenous administration of ganciclovir resulted in near-steady-state subtherapeutic intravitreal concentrations for many HCMV isolates *(195)*. This may also explain the difficulty of long-term complete suppression of HCMV retinitis *(145)*.

The use of intravenous or intravitreous ganciclovir for the treatment of HCMV retinitis has also been associated with the development of drug-resistant HCMV, which results from mutations in the viral UL97 and polymerase genes *(196)*.

Patients with AIDS who developed clinically resistant HCMV retinitis may show progression of retinitis despite extended intravenous induction of single-drug therapy or alternative therapy with induction of ganciclovir or foscarnet. In several clinical studies *(197–199)*, such patients were treated with a combination of ganciclovir and foscarnet. The recommended dosing regimen for induction combination therapy was ganciclovir (5.0 mg/kg, every 12 hours) and foscarnet at 60 mg/kg, three times daily. Maintenance combination therapy was ganciclovir (5.0 mg/kg, every 12 to 24 hours) and foscarnet (90 to 120 mg/kg, once daily). All patients exhibited a favorable response to the combination therapy, with complete healing of retinitis in 12 of 14 eyes, and partial healing of retinitis with decreased border activity and a cessation of border advancement in 2 of 14 eyes. The combined drug regimen was generally well tolerated with no toxic effects to require cessation of therapy *(197)*.

An intraocular sustained-release ganciclovir implant was reported to be a safe new procedure for the treatment of HCMV retinitis, avoiding the systemic side effects caused by the intravenous medications and improving the quality of life of the patients *(200)*. The intraocular implant was effective in controlling the progression of retinitis for up to 8 months, even in patients for which systemic therapy with either ganciclovir or foscarnet or both had failed. However, a later report *(201)* described a patient who developed oxacillin-resistant *Staphylococcus aureus* endophthalmitis after insertion of a ganciclovir intraocular implant, making bacterial endophthalmitis an infrequent but serious complication of ganciclovir intraocular implants.

An open-pilot, noncomparative, multicenter study was designed to evaluate the efficacy and safety of the ganciclovir-foscarnet combination as induction therapy and maintenance therapy for HCMV-induced central neurologic disorders in 31 HIV-infected patients with acute HCMV encephalitis (*n* = 17) or myelitis (*n* = 14); none of the patients had received HAART *(202)*. All patients received intravenous induction therapy consisting of foscarnet (90 mg/kg) and ganciclovir (5.0 mg/kg) twice daily, followed by maintenance therapy. Clinical efficacy was assessed at the end of the induction phase. Overall, the ganciclovir-foscarnet as induction therapy resulted in a 74% clinical improvement or stabilization *(202)*

Concurrent therapy of ganciclovir and zidovudine has been shown to significantly enhance the risk of granulocytopenia and *in most cases should be avoided (203–205)*. The data from several *in vitro* studies have also demonstrated the presence of synergistic toxicity between ganciclovir and zidovudine *(206–208)*. Nevertheless, a treatment protocol has been proposed that allowed for the coadministration of zidovudine and ganciclovir under certain *controlled conditions* depending on the values of the absolute granulocyte counts *(209)*.

The tolerance of neutropenia caused by ganciclovir has been increased by adjunctive therapy with granulocyte macrophage colony-stimulating factor (GM-CSF) *(210,211)*.

The effectiveness of HAART in suppressing HIV infection and restoring some immune-system functions *(212–218)* led to discontinuing additional maintenance therapy for HCMV-induced retinitis *(219–226)* and encephalitis *(227)*.

Valganciclovir hydrochloride (Valcyte) is an antiviral medication used to treat cytomegalovirus infections. As the *L*-valyl ester of ganciclovir, it is actually a prodrug for ganciclovir. After oral administration, it is rapidly converted to ganciclovir by intestinal and hepatic esterases.

Valganciclovir was approved by the FDA in 2001 for the treatment of CMV retinitis in patients with weakened immune systems, including individuals with HIV and AIDS. It is currently being investigated to determine its efficacy in preventing CMV end-organ disease in HIV-infected patients. It is also being investigated for safety and efficacy in treating congenital CMV disease in neonates. Valganciclovir was approved by the FDA in 2003 for preventing CMV disease in kidney, heart, and kidney-pancreas transplant patients at high risk (donor CMV seropositive/recipient CMV seronegative). It is being investigated for its efficacy in treating and preventing CMV disease in stem cell transplant recipients. Valganciclovir is in the FDA Pregnancy Category C drugs (http://aidsinfo.nih.gov/DrugsNew/ DrugDetailT.aspx?int_id=271).

The absolute bioavailability of ganciclovir after oral administration of valganciclovir is approximately 60%, about 10-fold higher than that after oral administration of ganciclovir. The mean 24-hour area under the plasma concentration-time curve (AUC24) for ganciclovir after once-daily administration of 900 mg of oral valganciclovir is comparable with that for once-daily administration of 5 mg/kg intravenous ganciclovir and exceeds the AUC24 for 1.0 g of oral ganciclovir administered three times daily. Peak plasma concentration of ganciclovir was approximately 5.6 μg/mL, and its time to peak concentration after administration of 450 mg to 2,625 mg valganciclovir tablets was from 1 to 3 hours (http://www.rocheusa.com/products/ valcyte/pi.html).

There have been no adequate or well-controlled studies in pregnant women; however, data obtained using an *ex vivo* human placental model showed that ganciclovir crosses the placenta, likely through simple diffusion. Because valganciclovir is rapidly converted to ganciclovir *in vivo*, it is expected to have reproductive toxicity similar to that of ganciclovir. It is not known whether valganciclovir is excreted in human milk; however, valganciclovir caused granulocytopenia, anemia, and thrombocytopenia in clinical trials, and ganciclovir was mutagenic and carcinogenic in animal studies. Because of the potential for HIV transmission and for serious adverse events from valganciclovir to breast-fed infants, women should be instructed not to breast-feed while taking valganciclovir (http://www.rocheusa.com/products/valcyte/pi.htm).

Because of valganciclovir's rapid conversion to ganciclovir after oral administration, protein binding of valganciclovir has not been established. Plasma protein binding of ganciclovir is 1% to 2% over concentrations of 0.5 and 51 μg/mL. In one study, the steady-state volume of intravenous ganciclovir was reported to be 0.703 ± 0.134 L/kg (http://www.rocheusa.com/products/valcyte/pi.html).

The most frequent and clinically significant adverse effects of valganciclovir are fever; retinal detachment; and hematologic reactions, including anemia, neutropenia, and thrombocytopenia. Other frequently reported but less serious adverse effects include abdominal pain, diarrhea, headache, insomnia, nausea and vomiting, paresthesia, and peripheral neuropathy (http://www.rocheusa.com/products/ valcyte/pi.html).

Oral valganciclovir (900 mg) has provided a daily exposure of ganciclovir comparable with that of intravenous ganciclovir 5 mg/kg. A single, randomized, non-blinded study indicated that oral valganciclovir (900 mg twice daily for 3 weeks then 900 mg once daily) and intravenous ganciclovir (5 mg/kg twice daily for 3 weeks then 5 mg/kg once daily) were equally effective in treating newly diagnosed CMV retinitis in 160 patients with AIDS *(228)*.

Valganciclovir appeared to have a similar tolerability profile to intravenous ganciclovir during induction therapy in patients with AIDS and newly diagnosed CMV retinitis. During maintenance therapy with valganciclovir, the most commonly reported adverse events included neutropenia, anemia, thrombocytopenia, gastrointestinal abnormalities (including diarrhea, nausea, vomiting, and abdominal pain), fever, headache, insomnia, peripheral neuropathy, paraesthesia, and retinal detachment *(228)*.

36.3 Parasitic Infections

36.3.1 Cryptosporidiosis

Over the past 20 years or so, the reported incidence of cryptosporidiosis and isosporiasis, two invasive parasitic opportunistic/nosocomial infections in humans, has risen dramatically *(229)*. Large populations of immunocompromised patients—as a result of underlying diseases such as hematologic malignancies and AIDS, or as a result of cancer chemotherapy or immunosuppressive therapy—are particularly susceptible to the effects of these infections. With the spread of the HIV/AIDS epidemic, the subject of actual and potential therapy for cryptosporidiosis became increasingly important and of considerable interest to clinicians. *Cryptosporidium* spp. represent coccidian protozoans classified in the suborder Eimeriina, order Eucoccidia. Taxonomically, *Cryptosporidium parvum* is related to *Toxoplasma gondii* and *Plasmodium* spp. *(229)*.

Before 1982, cryptosporidiosis was considered to be an infrequent parasitic disease occurring in animals, and with only eight reported cases in humans *(230–234)*. In the past several years, however, because of improved diagnostic techniques and the rising tide of the AIDS epidemic, *Cryptosporidium*-induced infections are considered to be one of the world's most commonly found causes of diarrheal illness in humans, especially infants and children *(235–237)*, the elderly *(238, 239)*, and AIDS patients in particular *(240–251)*.

Cryptosporidial infections are not limited to gastrointestinal illness. Respiratory, conjunctival, gastric, and gall bladder infections caused by *Cryptosporidium* have also been reported *(252–259)*. Acute pancreatitis in HIV-infected patients due to *Cryptosporidium* infection has also been described *(260)*.

Outbreaks of water-borne disease attributed to *Cryptosporidium* linked to drinking water and surface water have also been reported *(261–269)*. Further experiments have demonstrated that oocysts of *C. parvum* in water can retain viability and infectivity after freezing *(270)* and that oocysts may survive longer at freezing temperatures as low as –20°C *(271)*. In this regard, based on environmental occurrence, the risk of *Cryptosporidium* transmission by the water route may be equal to, or greater than, that of *Giardia (229)*. As a result, methods have been developed and optimized for simultaneously detecting *C. parvum* and *Giardia* cysts in water, including cartridge or membrane titration and calcium carbonate flocculation *(272)*. The knowledge of the hydrophobic and cell surface charge properties of *C. parvum* is important for the appropriate choice of various flocculation treatments, membrane filters, and cleaning agents in connection with the recovery of oocysts *(273)*. A rapid procedure for detecting *Cryptosporidium* using *in vitro* cell culture combined with polymerase chain reaction (PCR) has also been developed *(274)*.

The Genome. The analysis of the complete genome sequence of *C. parvum*, type II isolate, identified extremely streamlined metabolic pathways and a reliance on the host for nutrients *(275)*. In contrast with *Plasmodium* and *Toxoplasma*, *C. parvum* lacks an apicoplast in its genome and possesses a degenerate mitochondrion that has lost its genome. Several novel classes of cell-surface and secreted proteins with a potential role in host interactions and pathogenesis were also detected. Elucidation of the core metabolism, including *enzymes with high similarities to bacterial and plant counterparts,* would open new avenues for drug development *(275)*.

36.3.1.1 Treatment of Cryptosporidiosis

Because it invades surface epithelial cells that line the intestinal tract, but not the deeper layers of the intestinal mucosa, *C. parvum* can be regarded as a minimally invasive mucosal pathogen in the immunocompetent host. In patients, cryptosporidial infections result in a self-limited, flu-like gastrointestinal disorder *(276–280)* and mucosal inflammation that resolves spontaneously in 1 to 4 weeks *(279–282)*. Patients will develop immunity and recover completely from the infection. The highest incidence of cryptosporidiosis has

been reported in infant populations of the tropical and subtropical climate zones during the warmer months of the year *(283, 284)*.

In immunocompromised hosts, however, *Cryptosporidium* usually produces a severe and prolonged illness with high morbidity, which in AIDS patients has been clearly associated with lower CD4$^+$ T-cell counts *(242,285–288)*. The mortality rate from cryptosporidiosis in immunocompromised patients has also been high *(289)*: in adults it was associated mainly with AIDS patients *(230, 290, 291)* and children having hypogammaglobulinemia *(292, 293)* or severe combined immunodeficiency (SCID) *(294, 295)*, patients receiving immunosuppressive therapy for malignancies *(296–299)*, or renal-transplant recipients *(300)*.

Currently, there is no clinically effective chemotherapy of cryptosporidial diarrhea in immunocompromised patients *(301–307)*. Moreover, the lack of clinical improvement in such patients after chemotherapy alone may be the result, at least partially, of the presence of multiple concurrent infections and therapies aggravating the already-existing immune deficiency *(308, 309)*. Prophylaxis has been equally ineffective, although in one report *(310)* rifabutin or clarithromycin, when taken for *Mycobacterium avium* complex (MAC) prophylaxis, have been associated with a reduced risk for cryptosporidiosis.

There is also no known treatment for pulmonary cryptosporidiosis, a rare complication of intestinal cryptosporidiosis in AIDS patients *(229)*.

Over the years, a number of therapeutic approaches to cure cryptosporidiosis have been attempted using different agents, including macrolide antibiotics, peptides, and immunotherapy. To date, the results have been rather disappointing *(229)*.

Supportive therapy by fluids and nutrients given orally or intravenously is used to treat severe illness (http://www.aegis.org/news/NIAID/1991/NI910502.html).

Macrolide Antibiotics. Most notably among the macrolide antibiotics, spiramycin has been tested extensively both *in vitro* and *in vivo* for activity against cryptosporidiosis *(229, 311)*. In several anecdotal reports *(312–322)*, spiramycin has been described as useful against cryptosporidial diarrhea and with relatively low toxicity—most often gastrointestinal irritation and hypersensitivity reaction *(321, 323)*. With regard to data reporting anticryptosporidial efficacy of spiramycin *(324–326)*, especially in immunocompromised hosts *(327)*, it is important to emphasize that, to date, all results regarding its clinical efficacy originated mainly from uncontrolled studies involving a limited number of patients. Those results, therefore, should be viewed as premature and treated with skepticism; the accuracy of such reports must be evaluated in and corroborated by multicenter, placebo-controlled trials *(229)*. To lend credence to this skepticism, in a number of reports *(328–331)*, spiramycin has been described as completely lacking in activity against cryptosporidiosis. Some contributing factors to the perceived clinical efficacy of spiramycin may be traced to the observed tendency of the infection to disappear spontaneously *(332)* or to clinical improvement due to concomitant discontinuation of immunosuppressive medication *(318, 319)*, as well as better control of cryptosporidial diarrhea in the early stage of AIDS, as opposed to cryptosporidiosis in the advanced stages of AIDS when the state of immune deficiency is much worse *(333)*. In addition, it has been reported that two of three AIDS patients with cryptosporidiosis receiving high doses of spiramycin have developed acute intestinal injury as the likely result of direct damage to the epithelium by the drug *(334)*.

A multicenter, placebo-controlled clinical trial of chronic cryptosporidiosis was conducted in AIDS patients treated with spiramycin (1.0 g) three times daily for 3 weeks. No difference was noted between the drug and placebo *(335, 336)*. Subsequent pharmacokinetic studies suggested that poor absorption of spiramycin may have affected that finding. Because of concerns that oral spiramycin is poorly absorbed, the AIDS Clinical Trials Group undertook ACTG 113, a placebo-controlled, multicenter safety and efficacy trial of intravenous spiramycin for cryptosporidiosis, testing doses of 3 million units and 4.5 million units. Five of 31 patients met criteria for clinical and parasitologic improvement, and 16 achieved a partial response. Although there was a statistically significant drop in *Cryptosporidium* counts in the stools of those who received drug versus placebo, the intravenous spiramycin had toxicities including paresthesia, nausea, vomiting, and, at high doses, severe colitis *(336)*.

Other macrolide antibiotics tested for activity against cryptosporidiosis included azithromycin *(337–339)* and clarithromycin *(340, 341)*. These studies involved a limited number of patients, and the anticryptosporidial efficacy of these drugs has been questioned *(334)*.

Paromomycin. Paromomycin, a poorly orally absorbed aminoglycoside antibiotic known for its activity against *Giardia* and amebic intestinal infections, has been tested for activity against cryptosporidiosis both in experimental animals and humans *(342–359)*. The clinical results were inconclusive due, to a major degree, to the variable nature of the disease, during which some patients had improved without intervention *(229, 360)*.

Nitazoxanide (NTZ, Cryptaz). Nitazoxanide, an anthelmintic agent, has been available in developing countries for treating infestations of tapeworm and liver fluke *(361, 362)*. Initial trials conducted in Mali and Mexico have shown promising results in controlling cryptosporidial diarrhea and lowering the level of the parasite in the stools of AIDS patients *(362)*. Adverse side effects, although rare, included impaired liver function, discolored urine, and hives *(361)*. However, an NIAID-sponsored study (ACTG 336) failed to provide convincing supportive data because of poor enrollment *(363, 364)*. Ultimately, a FDA Advisory Committee rejected the drug because of insufficient and incomplete evidence (small and not randomized controlled trial) *(364–368)*.

Rifaximin. At doses of 600 mg twice daily for 2 weeks, rifaximin, a nonabsorbable, locally active antibiotic with broad antimicrobial activity, was found effective in resolving the clinical symptoms and clearing cryptosporidial infection in HIV-1–positive patients with CD4$^+$ T-cell counts of ≥ 200 cells/mm^3 *(369)*.

Diclazuril. Diclazuril is a benzene acetonitrile derivative that was first studied for cryptosporidiosis because of its activity against the related protozoan parasite *Eimeria (370)*. In 1989, a dose-escalating Phase I/II placebo-controlled study found that the drug was poorly absorbed and generally ineffective. Only at the highest dose (800 mg daily) were significant diclazuril serum levels achieved. Patients who achieved significant serum levels were the only responders *(370, 371)*.

Letrazuril. Letrazuril, a more bioavailable analogue of diclazuril, was later tested in a randomized, double-blind, placebo-controlled, multicenter trial (ACTG 198) *(370)*. When taken orally, letrazuril was found to be well absorbed and appeared to eradicate the parasite when stool samples were examined by acid-fast staining *(370)*. The lack of significant reduction in diarrhea among patients on active drug, however, led researchers to reexamine the stool smears using ELISA antigen capture methods and the indirect immunofluorescent assay. In fact, stool samples that were negative by the acid-fast method were positive using the other methods, leading investigators to conclude that letrazuril does not kill *Cryptosporidium* but rather affects its acid-fast staining pattern *(370)*.

A recently published open-label study of letrazuril in 35 patients with AIDS-related cryptosporidiosis documented a complete clinical response in only one patient. Twenty-two patients had a partial response defined as a "greater than 50% reduction in bowel movements per day for at least one week." Fifteen (69%) of the responses were short-lived, suggesting that the patients may have experienced a placebo effect *(370, 372)*. This placebo effect, common in cryptosporidiosis, testifies to the power of a patient's own belief that a treatment may be efficacious, whether or not it really is, and is manifested in double-blind trials when patients on placebo experience symptomatic relief. Thus, to determine efficacy of marginally active drugs, the proportion of patients responding symptomatically on placebo must be compared with those responding to the drug *(370)*.

Somatostatin and Analogues. Somatostatin, a tetradecapeptide factor inhibiting the release of somatotropin, has been found useful in the treatment of secretory diarrhea related to various diseases, such as Zollinger-Ellison syndrome, Verner-Morrison syndrome, the carcinoid syndrome, glucagonomas, and ileostomy *(229)*. Somatostatin is known to prolong the intestinal transit time and to induce the net intestinal water and electrolyte reabsorption in patients with diarrhea. Because the native form of somatostatin has a short half-life (3 to 4 minutes), necessitating its intravenous administration *(373)*, analogues with longer half-lives have subsequently been developed *(374)*.

For the past decade or so, attention has been focused on one somatostatin analogue, octreotide (Sandostatin, SMS 201–995). Structurally, octreotide represents a small peptide comprising eight amino acid residues that share homology with a four-amino-acid sequence present in somatostatin *(375)*. The biological activity of octreotide mimicked to a great extent that of the endogenous somatostatin, especially its potent ability to inhibit the release of the vasoactive intestinal peptide and/or its action on the intestinal mucosal target tissue *(376, 377)*.

Octreotide has a longer half-life (90 to 120 minutes) and duration of activity of up to 8 hours *(378, 379)*.

The clinical efficacy of octreotide against cryptosporidial diarrhea in AIDS patients has been the subject of several reports *(380–382)*.

In an open-label, multicenter, controlled clinical trial of 49 AIDS patients with profuse diarrhea, octreotide was administered subcutaneously for 14 days (50 µg every 8 hours for 3 days, then 100, 250, and 500 µg every 8 hours for 3 days each, if no response to the prior dose was observed) *(380)*. Four patients responded completely and 13 partially for an overall rate of 34.7%. After ceasing the therapy, diarrhea recurred in all patients who had initially responded *(380)*. In general, octreotide was well tolerated, and its toxicity was limited to mild adverse reactions such as pain in the injection site, nausea, abdominal pain, and discomfort or bloating *(378, 383)*

36.3.1.2 Cryptosporidial Diarrhea in AIDS

In the broader context of *Cryptosporidium*-induced diarrhea, especially the inability to treat this condition in AIDS patients, the probable mode of action of octreotide deserves special consideration *(229)*. Severe manifestations of watery diarrhea observed in AIDS patients have frequently been associated with infection by cryptosporidia. This, however, has not always been the case, as the human immunodeficiency virus itself may directly cause mucosal hypersecretory response *(379)*, which would result in enteropathy *(384–386)* and diarrhea. Furthermore, an HIV invasion into the enterochromaffin cells of the intestinal mucosa [which is known to occur *(384–386)*] may create a local deficiency of somatostatin. Such a deficiency, if developed, may explain the beneficial effect of octreotide in ameliorating the cryptosporidial diarrhea in some AIDS patients *(387)*.

Alternatively, the protein coat of HIV was found to contain amino acid sequences that are homologous with the vasoactive intestinal peptide (VIP) *(388)*. Based on the fact that VIP is an effective stimulant of intestinal fluid secretion *(389)*, a hypothesis was advanced postulating that HIV may activate the VIP receptors, thereby triggering, at least partially, a diarrheal response *(376)*.

The mechanism of action of octreotide on cryptosporidial diarrhea, although still not fully elucidated, may involve a nonspecific effect on the gastrointestinal fluid and electrolyte secretion *(379)*. The fact that both somatostatin and octreotide inhibited the effect of VIP on the intestinal secretion may explain one aspect of the mechanism of action of octreotide, namely, its ability to act on the membrane receptor that recognizes VIP *(292)*.

Although it is still possible that octreotide may prove to be useful against some cases of AIDS-associate intestinal cryptosporidiosis, this would require not only stringently conducted placebo-controlled trials but also the participation of patient populations that were homogenous in regard to their probable cause of diarrhea and better compliance with stool collections *(390)*.

36.3.1.3 Immunotherapy of Cryptosporidiosis

The lack of effective anticryptosporidial chemotherapy in immunocompromised patients on the one hand, and the importance of the immune system in determining the host's response toward invading pathogens on the other, have prompted the evaluation of some immunotherapeutic approaches for preventing and treating cryptosporidiosis *(229)*.

Some of the novel immunotherapeutic approaches to the treatment of cryptosporidiosis include the use of cow's milk globulin *(391)* and hyperimmune bovine colostrums *(293, 294, 392)*.

Initial reports have indicated that bovine colostrum, obtained from cows that were naturally infected with *Cryptosporidium*, when administered orally to three patients with cryptosporidiosis failed to exert any beneficial effect *(393)*. However, in later experiments *(294, 394)* it was demonstrated that a specially produced hyperimmune bovine colostrum (HBC) was effective in three patients (one of them with AIDS) with intestinal cryptosporidiosis.

This potentially new anticryptosporidial therapy was tested successfully in one AIDS patient with fulminant cryptosporidial diarrhea by passively transferring large amounts of immune elements present in HBC to the affected host; the patient showed remission of diarrhea and elimination of *Cryptosporidium* oocysts from stool specimens *(395)*. A randomized, double-blind, controlled pilot study in five AIDS patients with cryptosporidial diarrhea was conducted, in which HBC was administered by continuous naso-gastric infusion at 20 mL/h (approximately 30 mg total immunoglobulin/mL) for 10 days (396). Although the study was hampered by such factors as the small number of patients, significant differences among patients (oocyst load and severity of diarrhea at the onset of the trial), and the inability to obtain adequate baseline information about daily stool volumes before treatment was started, the overall results have demonstrated that HBC may prove to be effective in treating patients with cryptosporidiosis (396).

The active ingredient(s) of HBC is currently unknown. However, it may be possible that the bovine IgG_1 immunoglobulin, which is very closely related to human IgA, may elicit a protective effect similar to the one already postulated for bovine IgG_1 in enteropathogenic and enterotoxigenic E. coli–related diarrheas and enteric infection caused by rotavirus (397–400). It is also plausible that the active ingredient of HBC is a cytokine (229).

"Colostrum Specific" has been used successfully against cryptosporidiosis in regimens that included four-times-daily administration for 3 weeks (401). Colostrums specific is enteric-coated formulation to protect immunoglobulins from gastric hydrolysis. It contains a minimum of 35% immunoglobulins (IgGs), which is double the strength of typical colostrum products because it is obtained from the first milking after calving (393).

Fourteen AIDS patients with symptomatic cryptosporidiosis were treated with either a specific bovine dialyzable leukocyte extract (immune DLE) prepared from lymph node lymphocytes of calves immunized with cryptosporidia or with a nonspecific (nonimmune) DLE prepared from nonimmunized calves (402, 403). Of the seven patients who received immune DLE, six gained weight and had a decrease in bowel movement frequency; eradication of oocysts from stools was observed in five patients. By comparison, six of seven recipients of nonimmune DLE showed no decrease in bowel movements, and in four of them no clearing of oocysts from stools was observed; five of the patients continued to lose weight. When five of the nonimmune DLE recipients were treated with immune DLE, four experienced a decrease in bowel movement frequency and considerable weight gain, with eradication of oocysts from stools in two patients (402). Even though sustained symptomatic improvement of patients given immune DLE was evident, the lack of an appropriate cryptosporidial antigen would only allow a postulation that the observed microbiologic and clinical improvements were indeed caused by the immune DLE–induced augmentation of cellular immunity toward C. parvum. In this regard, DLE has been found to contain an antigen-binding product of T-helper lymphocytes that enhanced the cell-mediated immune responses in humans (404, 405). In several studies, DLE was found beneficial in the treatment of various bacterial, fungal, and viral infections (406–408), as well as against

parasites such as Eimeria bovis in cattle (409) and Eimeria ferrisi in mice (410).

Because the intestinal cytokine signals involved with eradication of cryptosporidiosis are unknown, a study (411) was initiated to assess the role of cytokines in human cryptosporidiosis in healthy adult volunteers experimentally infected with C. parvum and in AIDS patients with naturally acquired chronic cryptosporidiosis, using endoscopy and jejunal biopsies for human interferon-γ (IFN-γ) and interleukin-15 (IL-15). The overall data suggested key roles for intestinal IFN-γ and IL-15 in controlling human cryptosporidiosis. IL-15 seemed to function in initiating the immune response, and IFN-γ functions in the anamnestic response that limits re-infection (411).

The effects of recombinant interleukin-2 (rIL-2) against cryptosporidiosis have been studied (412) in patients who have AIDS or persistent lymphadenopathy syndrome (LAS). Increasing doses of rIL-2 (from 10^3 U/m^2 to 10^6 U/m^2) were administered as an intravenous bolus injection. The diarrhea of two of the patients with severe intestinal cryptosporidiosis ceased under the treatment with rIL-2 and did not recur during the following 2 months. At the high-dose level, the rIL-2 caused some minor adverse reactions, such as fever, chills, and malaise or vomiting (412). The observed anticryptosporidial effect of rIL-2 was likely due to its ability to enhance immune responses to foreign antigens (413, 414) by acting as a second messenger of T-lymphocyte activation (414,415). After its release from IL-2–producer lymphocytes (mainly within the T4$^+$ subsets), IL-2 facilitates an adequate reaction by the T-responder lymphocytes against infectious pathogens or allogeneic malignant cells (413, 414, 416).

In another study (417), the therapeutic efficacy of recombinant human granulocyte-macrophage colony-stimulating factor (rHuGM-CSF) was evaluated in HIV-positive patients (CD4$^+$ T-cell counts of <50 cells/mm^3) with paromomycin-resistant cryptosporidiosis. rHuGM-CSF was given subcutaneously at 300 mg daily for 14 days, then on every other day for an additional 14 days, together with zidovudine (500 mg) and paromomycin. The patients did show prompt clinical response to rHuGM-CSF (cessation of diarrhea in 2 days), but relapsed when therapy was discontinued (417).

36.3.1.4 Antiretroviral Therapies and Cryptosporidiosis

There have been a number of studies aimed at better understanding whether or not potent antiretroviral therapies can modify the natural history of HIV-associated cryptosporidiosis (418–422). Effective antiretroviral therapy has been associated with restoration of the immune response and accompanying resolution of opportunistic infections including cryptosporidiosis. Thus, retrospective data (418) collected for 50 HIV-positive patients with chronic diarrhea with regard to demographics, clinical and microbiological characteristics of cryptosporidial and microsporidial infections, antiretroviral therapies, and prophylaxis against these parasitic infections have strongly supported the hypothesis that combination antiretroviral therapy significantly modified the course of both cryptosporidiosis and microsporidiosis in HIV-1–infected patients. The resolution of diarrhea seemed to be related to an increased CD4$^+$ T-cell count rather than viral load *(418)*.

Treatment of HIV-1 infections with protease inhibitors has resulted in dramatic decreases in the HIV-1 viral load, with concomitant increases in CD4$^+$ T-cell counts. In a case of progressive cryptosporidiosis, an HIV patient with a CD4$^+$ T-cell count of 33 cells/mm^3 cleared parasite oocysts in stool samples and had the symptoms resolved after treatment with indinavir *(419)*. In another study, there was clearance of *Cryptosporidium* and Microsporidia and clinical improvement in 85% of the cases after treatment with indinavir (nine patients) or ritonavir in combination with two nucleoside analogues (six patients) *(420)*.

36.3.2 *Toxoplasmosis*

Toxoplasma is a genus of coccidian protozoa classified into the suborder Eimeriina and comprising intracellular parasites of many organs and tissues of birds and mammals, including humans. The only known complete hosts of these parasites are cats and other Felidae, in which both asexual and sexual developmental cycles occur in the intestinal epithelium, culminating in the passage of oocysts in the feces. The intestinal stages do not occur in other hosts *(423)*.

Toxoplasma gondii is considered to be the causative agent of toxoplasmosis. It is a widespread intracellular parasite infecting a wide range of birds and mammals, including humans. The sexual cycle of the organism takes place in the intestinal epithelium of the cat, which is the definitive host. *T. gondii* exists in three forms: tachyzoite, tissue cysts (pseudocysts), and oocysts *(423)*.

While persistence of *Toxoplasma* cysts within host tissues may contribute to maintenance of immunity against reinfection, their presence may also represent, under certain conditions, a potential danger for reactivation of infection, especially in immunocompromised patients and infants with congenital toxoplasmosis *(424)*.

Transmission of infection is caused by ingestion of either parenteral cysts (trophozoites) from raw, infected meat, or oocysts from feces of domestic pets (cats), by transplantation of infected organs *(425,426)*, by tainted blood transfusion *(427)*, or even by accidental inoculation in a laboratory setting *(428)*. In immunocompetent hosts, toxoplasmosis is asymptomatic and benign *(429, 430)*. The incidence of the disease is most frequent between ages 16 and 25 *(431)*.

Human toxoplasmosis is expressed either as congenital or acquired. Congenital toxoplasmosis is present in newborn infants and is characterized by encephalitis, rash, jaundice and hepatomegaly, usually associated with chorioretinitis, hydrocephalus, and microcephaly, and with a high mortality rate *(432–434)*. *T. gondii* can be transmitted from mother to fetus during primary maternal infection acquired after, or possibly slightly before, conception *(435)*. The incidence of congenital toxoplasmosis is highest in the third trimester, whereas severity is most pronounced when maternal infection is acquired during the first trimester *(435)*. Studies of congenital toxoplasmosis in twins confirmed the definite role of the placenta in the modalities and mechanisms of fetal contamination by *Toxoplasma (436)*.

By and large, acquired (i.e., noncongenital) toxoplasmosis is manifested by lymphadenopathy, fatigue or malaise, fever, sore throat, headache, myocardial disease, chorioretinitis, and seizures *(429)*. The lymphadenopathy is most likely to be cervical (97%) with lymph nodes being usually enlarged, rubbery, and nontender. Lymphadenopathy may also be febrile, nonfebrile, or subclinical *(431)*.

Chorioretinitis associated with toxoplasmosis is believed to be the most frequent infection of the posterior segment of the eye, which may also lead to blindness *(437–439)*. Encysted *T. gondii* bradyzoites, when persisting in ocular tissues, may cause recurrence of the disease. Chemotherapeutic eradication of encysted bradyzoites from chronically infected tissues is usually hampered by the structure of the cyst walls, as well as by the organism's low metabolism.

Cerebral toxoplasmosis is manifested by fever, encephalitis, convulsions, delirium, lymphadenopathy, and mononuclear pleocytosis, followed by death. In the brain, *T. gondii* multiplies in the neurons and other cells, causing cellular and interstitial necrosis. Occasionally, the infarction necrosis may lead to the formation of extensive lesions *(431, 440)*.

Until recently, toxoplasmic encephalitis (TE) was diagnosed predominately in immunocompromised patients with malignancies of the reticuloendothelial system or organ transplant recipients *(426, 441, 442)*. However, after the advent of the AIDS epidemic, TE has become one of the most common causes of encephalitis in this population *(443–451)*. Toxoplasmosis comprises about 75% of all cases of nonviral infections in AIDS patients *(444)*, and the incidence of CNS toxoplasmosis alone has been estimated to range between 3% and 44% *(442, 443, 452)*. It is believed that the occurrence of TE in AIDS patients has most likely been the result of reactivation of a latent infection rather than an acute acquired infection *(433)*. A study encompassing 31 medical centers and 61 patients with AIDS concluded that currently the overall prognosis of TE is poor—the median survival time after initiation of therapy was 4 months

(453). Clinically, TE is characterized mainly by neurologic disorders such as seizures, change in mental status, coma, confusion, psychosis, and anemia, as well as focal neurologic abnormalities (hemiparesis, hemiplegia, hemisensory loss, cranial nerve palsies, aphasia, ataxia, and alexia), and meningeal symptoms *(445, 446, 454)*. Computed axial tomography (CAT) has been of considerable help in diagnosing TE—mild to severe edema is observed on the CAT scan of almost every patient *(445)*. Lesions were rounded, single or multiple, and isodense or hypodense *(446)*. Furthermore, contrast studies have revealed the presence of ring or nodular enhancement in more than 90% of patients *(455)*. Recently, magnetic resonance imaging (MRI) has been used to detect lesions not shown by CAT *(441)*. It is recommended, therefore, that MRI be performed in seropositive AIDS patients with neurologic signs or symptoms even though the CAT scan did not produce evidence for TE *(441)*. In several reports *(456–459)*, the diagnosis and treatment strategies of CNS toxoplasmosis in AIDS patients have been reviewed.

Pulmonary toxoplasmosis in AIDS patients is the second most frequent localization after the brain *(460–462)*. Its frequency has been estimated to be between 0.2% and 3.7%, and it is seldom identified prior to autopsy. Clinical manifestations include severe interstitial pneumonitis occurring in profoundly immunodeficient patients *(463)*. Disseminated *T. gondii* infection may also present with fulminant pneumonia *(464)*. A retrospective and descriptive study of *T. gondii*–induced pneumonia in AIDS patients *(465)* discussed the clinical presentation, diagnostic procedures, results of therapy, and hypotheses on the pathophysiology of the infection.

Cardiac *(466, 467)* and liver *(468–470)* toxoplasmosis have been described in only a limited number of patients.

A case of toxoplasmosis disseminated in the bladder of an AIDS patient has also been reported *(471)*.

Another rare case of reversible anterior bilateral opercular syndrome (Foix-Chavany-Marie syndrome) secondary to cerebral *Toxoplasma* abscesses has been described in an AIDS patient *(472)*.

36.3.2.1 Treatment of Toxoplasmosis

Current therapeutic strategies and future prospects for the treatment of congenital and acquired toxoplasmosis have been extensively reviewed *(473–478)*. One of the major problems confronting the development of successful anti-*Toxoplasma* agents has been the ability of the parasite to differentiate from the actively growing tachyzoite form, which is susceptible to drug action, into the chronic, almost latent bradyzoite state, which is not susceptible and, therefore, cannot be eradicated by any of the currently known antitoxoplasmic agents. Because the bradyzoites remain as a source

of recrudescing infection, drug therapy must be maintained for the life of the patient *(423)*.

The molecular signals and mechanism(s) involved in the tachyzoite-bradyzoite interconversion are not known *(479)*. Blocking this differentiation process would be a major breakthrough in the cure of toxoplasmosis by preventing reactivation of the latent forms, and thereby attenuating disease. Similarly, stimulating bradyzoites to differentiate back to the drug-sensitive tachyzoites would facilitate chemotherapy that might completely clear the body of the protozoan *(479)*.

Therapy of congenital toxoplasmosis, in general, is based on spiramycin, which is capable of achieving high concentrations in the placenta; if the fetus is uninfected, pyrimethamine and sulfonamides are administered from the fourth month of pregnancy *(435)*. It was found that prenatal therapy of congenital toxoplasmosis is beneficial in reducing the frequency of infant infection *(480)*. The potential of using co-trimoxazole has been considered *(481)* for the prenatal prevention and treatment of toxoplasmic fetal death. Various options for prevention of ocular toxoplasmosis associated with congenital toxoplasmosis have also been suggested *(482)*.

For primary therapy of severe cases of toxoplasmosis in immunocompromised patients and in congenital toxoplasmosis, treatment with synergistic combinations of either trimethoprim or pyrimethamine and sulfonamide (e.g., co-trimoxazole) is widespread *(483)*.

Spiramycin, alone or in combination with pyrimethamine-sulfonamide, is often used in pregnant women with acute infection to prevent congenital toxoplasmosis *(474)*.

Clindamycin is used frequently in managing acute flare-ups of toxoplasmic chorioretinitis and as second-line therapy for toxoplasmic encephalitis in AIDS patients *(448,474)*. The effect of folate supplements in the therapy for cerebral toxoplasmosis has been discussed *(484)*. In another report, the therapy for *T. gondii*–induced myocarditis in AIDS patients has also been surveyed *(485)*.

Immunomodulating drugs such as IFN-γ, alone or in combination with roxithromycin, were found effective in murine models of toxoplasmosis; interleukin-2 was also found to be effective in a murine model *(474)*.

When treating toxoplasmosis in immunocompromised patients, it has been important to take into consideration the tendency of such patients to simultaneously develop other opportunistic diseases, such as cytomegalovirus infection or *Pneumocystis jirovecii* pneumonia *(486)*. If it occurs, the management of such conditions would, undoubtedly, be very difficult. In this regard, gross alterations of the host's microbial flora, as a result of excessive antimicrobial medication and unduly prolonged treatment, must be avoided in order to prevent undesired superinfections *(423)*.

Pyrimethamine-Sulfonamide Combinations

Results from an open, randomized, multicenter trial have shown no difference in the survival rate of HIV-infected patients with toxoplasmic encephalitis following a twice-weekly regimen of pyrimethamine-sulfadiazine combination (consisting of 1.0 g sulfadiazine given twice, 50 mg pyrimethamine, and 15 mg folinic acid) versus the same regimen administered daily (containing 25 mg pyrimethamine instead) (487, 488).

A satisfactory response to sulfonamide-pyrimethamine medication of 20 AIDS patients with toxoplasmosis has been reported, although a high incidence of toxicity has been present (489). Eleven of 13 AIDS patients with CNS toxoplasmosis receiving pyrimethamine-sulfadiazine combination showed clinical and radiologic improvement; toxic side effects included neutropenia, fever, and rash. Autopsies performed in five patients revealed evidence of T. gondii (490).

Pyrimethamine-sulfadiazine (1.0 g four times daily and 25 mg four times daily, respectively) resistant cerebral toxoplasmosis in AIDS patients has been reported (491, 492).

Contrary to a previous report (493), which described successful therapy of cerebral toxoplasmosis using pyrimethamine and clindamycin in place of sulfadiazine, progression of cerebral lesions has been observed in one patient receiving the pyrimethamine-clindamycin combination simultaneously (494). It was this finding that necessitated sulfadiazine desensitization as a useful alternative. The sulfadiazine desensitization was carried out in three AIDS patients with cerebral toxoplasmosis and prior severe sulfonamide reactions (diffused maculopapular rash) (494). The achieved maximum tolerated daily doses were 2.0 g of the drug in one patient and 4.0 g for the remaining two patients. Side effects comprised transient fever, mild pruritus, and hyperglycemia (presumably exacerbated by the steroid given before desensitization) (494).

In this regard, a study was conducted to assess the efficacy of a sulfadiazine desensitization protocol to treat patients with AIDS and cerebral toxoplasmosis and known sulfonamide allergy and to ensure that an adequate dose of sulfadiazine (2.0 to 4.0 g daily) was achieved rapidly (within 4 to 5 days) (495). In addition, the effect of concurrent corticosteroid therapy on the success rate of the sulfadiazine regimen was evaluated. The proposed desensitization protocol employed the oral administration of gradually increasing increments of sulfadiazine every 3 hours over a 5-day period. The overall success rate of desensitization was reported to be 62%; 7 patients achieved a final dose of 4.0 g daily, and for 3 patients the dose was 2.0 g daily. The concurrent corticosteroid administration did not appear to affect the outcome in the patients studied (total of 16) (495).

Results from potential interactions of multiple drug regimens (pyrimethamine-clindamycin, pyrimethamine-

sulfadiazine, and pyrimethamine alone) administered to 35 AIDS patients receiving maintenance therapy for toxoplasmosis have been evaluated (496). Adverse side effects were associated with pyrimethamine in 10 cases, with clindamycin in 7, and with sulfadiazine in 8 patients (496). The application of low-dose alternate-day pyrimethamine medication as a maintenance therapy for cerebral toxoplasmosis in AIDS was also reported (497).

Twelve patients with toxoplasmic chorioretinitis were treated with Fansidar (pyrimethamine and sulfadoxine at 25 and 500 mg/kg, respectively), starting with a loading zone of two tablets of Fansidar, followed by one tablet daily; prednisone (0.5 mg/kg daily) was added and gradually tapered off. The duration of treatment was 21 to 50 days (median, 28 days). In 83% of patients, the scar was considerably smaller than the original lesion (on average 25% of original lesion), with no side effects observed (498).

In utero treatment of congenital toxoplasmosis with pyrimethamine-sulfadiazine has also been reported (498, 499). Mothers in 52 cases of toxoplasmic fetopathy (group 1) were treated in utero with a combination of pyrimethamine and sulfadiazine (or sulfisoxazole) and with spiramycin (499). The results were compared with those obtained from 51 infants with congenital toxoplasmosis whose mothers (group 2) had received spiramycin alone. Patients of both groups received the same medication of pyrimethamine-sulfadiazine and spiramycin after birth. Parasitologic examination of the placenta was positive in 42% of group 1 and 76.6% of group 2, and specific IgM titers in newborns were detected in 17.4% and 69.2% of cases, respectively; these findings indicated that prenatal treatment with pyrimethamine-sulfonamides resulted in less progressing infection at birth (499).

Acute Renal Failure Due to Sulfadiazine Therapy in AIDS Patients. Acute renal failure due to crystal deposition of sulfadiazine in the urinary tract should be of growing concern if appropriate prophylactic measures are not taken promptly (500–512).

There has been evidence that due to the high prevalence of potential risk factors, the incidence of sulfadiazine-associated renal impairment was 1.9% to 7.5% in patients with AIDS compared with 1% to 4% in HIV-seronegative controls. Furthermore, its occurrence appeared to be delayed in HIV-infected individuals with a median of 3 weeks of medication compared with about 10 days in HIV-negative subjects; in conformity, the cumulative sulfadiazine dose at time of manifestation has doubled in AIDS patients (median of 84 g vs. 40 g in controls) (503).

Four cases have been reported of AIDS patients with toxoplasmic encephalitis who developed sulfadiazine-induced crystalluria after receiving a combination of sulfadiazine and pyrimethamine (513). The crystalluria can rapidly reverse by rehydration and urine alkalinization (503, 507, 513, 514).

It was recommended that after high doses of sulfadiazine, patients be adequately hydrated and their urinary pH maintained above 7.5 *(513)*. In one report, an AIDS patient with sulfadiazine-induced urolithiasis acute renal failure (acute lumbar pain, dysuria, urinary frequency, and hematuria) was treated with intravenous fluids and alkalinization of the urine *(501)*.

Adverse Cutaneous Reactions to Pyrimethamine Combinations in AIDS Patients. The value of various clinical and laboratory parameters in predicting the occurrence of skin reactions in AIDS patients with toxoplasmic encephalitis induced by pyrimethamine combinations with either sulfadiazine or clindamycin, and the effects of continued therapy for patients with these reactions, have been studied retrospectively *(515)*. Seventy-five percent of patients (18 of 25) treated with pyrimethamine-sulfadiazine developed cutaneous reactions after a mean of 11 days, whereas 58% (15 of 26) of patients who received pyrimethamine-clindamycin had cutaneous reactions after a mean of 13 days ($p = 0.56$). Nine (50%) of the 18 patients continued to receive pyrimethamine-sulfadiazine throughout the duration of hypersensitivity, compared with all 15 patients who were treated with pyrimethamine-clindamycin ($p = 0.002$). Thus, treatment throughout the duration of hypersensitivity is more likely to succeed for patients receiving the pyrimethamine-clindamycin combination, whereas therapy with pyrimethamine-sulfadiazine has been associated with more pronounced cutaneous side effects and a high risk of developing Lyell's syndrome and Stevens-Johnson syndrome *(515)*.

Trimethoprim-Sulfonamide Combinations

In patients with toxoplasmosis, therapy with trimethoprim (160 mg) and sulfamethoxazole (800 mg), daily for 10 days resulted in a significant remission of symptoms *(516)*.

Treatment of five patients with lymphadenopathy due to toxoplasmosis was reported to yield good therapeutic results using co-trimoxazole for a period of 4 weeks. No adverse effects on the bone marrow were observed during a 3-month trial; however, a transient stomatitis was present, as well as allergic exanthema *(517)*.

In another study, one case of recurrent toxoplasmosis has been described in which the patient required repeated (on three different occasions) treatment with co-trimoxazole *(518)*. This and other reports *(519, 520)* of recurrent toxoplasmosis (which seemed to be independent of the type of drug combination therapy) stressed the need for long-term monitoring of patients, especially in those cases where an immune deficiency is present (or might develop) resulting in increased virulence of the *Toxoplasma* pathogen.

A dramatic recovery of a child with generalized toxoplasmosis after therapy with co-trimoxazole (400 mg sulfamethoxazole and 80 mg trimethoprim, twice daily for 1 month) has been described, leading to the recommendation that co-trimoxazole be used as the treatment of choice for acquired toxoplasmosis, especially in immunocompromised patients and cases of congenital toxoplasmosis *(521)*. Subsequently, however, this recommendation has been seriously questioned *(522)*.

In one study, use of co-trimoxazole in the management of cerebral encephalitis in AIDS patients showing severe hematologic damage caused by pyrimethamine and concurrent zidovudine therapy led to a complete resolution of the lesions after 3 weeks of therapy *(523)*.

A retrospective study on the use of co-trimoxazole as diagnostic support and treatment of suspected cerebral toxoplasmosis in AIDS patients revealed that the drug was effective, as evidenced by improved clinical and radiologic status *(524)*. However, further prospective randomized therapeutic trials seem to be in order to confirm these observations.

Antibiotic Therapy of Toxoplasmosis

Spiramycin

Over the years, spiramycin has been used extensively in the treatment of human congenital toxoplasmosis *(525–530)*. Fetuses infected with *T. gondii* often developed impaired vision or neurologic disorders, even after 5 years postpartum *(531)*. The risk of congenital infections due to acute toxoplasmosis acquired during the first trimester of pregnancy has been estimated at 15% *(526)*. Although such a risk is usually higher during the second (30%) and third (60%) trimesters, only acute toxoplasmosis acquired in the first trimester has been associated with severe congenital infections *(526)*. Alternating 3 weeks of therapy with oral spiramycin with 2 weeks of no treatment resulted in a diminished incidence of congenital toxoplasmosis from 61% to 23% *(525)*.

Results from treating 98 cases of fetal *Toxoplasma* infection with spiramycin during pregnancy have shown that of the 52 pregnancies allowed to proceed, 43 were treated additionally with pyrimethamine and sulfonamides. After a mean follow-up period of 19 months, 41 infants showed evidence of subclinical toxoplasmosis. The therapeutic efficacy of the additional treatment with pyrimethamine and sulfonamides was evidenced by a marked reduction of severe congenital toxoplasmosis and the relative decrease in the ratio of benign to subclinical forms *(532)*.

In a clinical trial involving 67 patients, spiramycin was reported to be effective in treating posterior uveitis caused by *Toxoplasma* *(533)*. However, in another report *(534)*, data have shown that in 87 patients with posterior uveitis, therapy with combination pyrimethamine-sulfadiazine was superior to that of spiramycin (and/or steroids). In two other studies (535, 536), spiramycin was reported to be ineffective in treating toxoplasmic uveitis.

In a study of 54 patients with active toxoplasmic chorioretinitis, the therapy with pyrimethamine-sulfadiazine was found to be statistically more effective than a corresponding treatment with systemic steroids given either alone or in combination with spiramycin (537).

As reported, there has been little serious toxicity associated with spiramycin (538). Contrary to other macrolide antibiotics, spiramycin was not damaging to the liver. It caused mild gastrointestinal disturbance, and allergic reactions were confined to transient skin eruptions (538).

Clindamycin and Clindamycin-Pyrimethamine Combinations

One case of acute toxoplasmic lymphadenitis has been treated with 600 mg daily of oral clindamycin. The therapy was continued for 28 days, after which the patient was apyrexial and clinically well (539).

Clindamycin was used with promising results to treat 15 AIDS patients with toxoplasmic encephalitis (540, 541) as part of either primary or alternative therapy (542). Eleven of the patients responded as shown by clinical or radiologic improvement after receiving the antibiotic either alone or in combination with pyrimethamine. Twelve patients continued to receive oral clindamycin as suppressive therapy on an outpatient basis. The adverse reactions of clindamycin were mainly diarrhea, reversible granulocytopenia, and skin reaction (542).

One side effect often associated with the use of clindamycin (as much as 80% of recorded cases) has been the development of colitis of pseudomembranous type (543). A protocol for clindamycin desensitization in AIDS patients has been recommended (544).

Clinical data have indicated that in the treatment of AIDS patients with cerebral toxoplasmosis, combination regimens consisting of pyrimethamine, clindamycin, and spiramycin, and pyrimethamine-clindamycin proved to be equally effective, and that the addition of spiramycin did not provide additional benefit. Myelosuppressive side effects due to pyrimethamine prevented the addition of folinic acid at the start of the antitoxoplasmic therapy (545).

Interim data from an ongoing large-scale, prospective, randomized study to determine the potential role of clindamycin in the management of toxoplasmic encephalitis has been reported on 33 patients, 15 of whom received oral pyrimethamine and clindamycin (intravenously, then orally), and 18 of whom received pyrimethamine and sulfadiazine (both drugs given orally) (546). The interim evaluation did not reveal any significant differences between the two regimens in the clinical and radiologic response. Both regimens caused similar adverse side effects; however, patients on pyrimethamine-clindamycin medication had more pronounced gastrointestinal side effects and more adverse hematologic reactions than did those receiving pyrimethamine-sulfadiazine (546). In a further study, a randomized unblinded Phase II, multicenter clinical trial was conducted in California to compare the therapeutic efficacy of combination of pyrimethamine and clindamycin to that of pyrimethamine and sulfadiazine (547). The study allowed for crossover in the event of failure or intolerance of the assigned regimen. The patients were treated for 6 weeks with pyrimethamine and folinic acid, plus either sulfadiazine or clindamycin (the latter injected intravenously during the first 3 weeks). The results of several end-points for efficacy, when taken together, indicated that the relative efficacies of clindamycin and sulfadiazine appeared to be approximately the same. Hence, the use of clindamycin should be considered as an acceptable alternative to sulfadiazine in patients unable to tolerate sulfadiazine (547).

A combination of 5-fluorouracil and clindamycin was also used to treat a case of cerebral toxoplasmosis in AIDS (548).

Azithromycin

A prospective study was conducted to evaluate azithromycin in combination with pyrimethamine for treating acute toxoplasmic encephalitis in AIDS patients (549). Fourteen patients were given 75 mg of pyrimethamine and 500 mg azithromycin daily for 4 weeks. Of the eight patients who were evaluable for clinical response, five responded favorably, one had an intermediate response, and two patients did not respond. Based on the adverse effects observed (rash, abnormal liver function, vomiting, and hypoacousia), it seemed that the azithromycin dosage used in the combination was not optimal.

In another study, the use of azithromycin in the treatment of cerebral toxoplasmosis has also been described (550).

Doxycycline

Two reports of treating cerebral toxoplasmosis with a combination of doxycycline and pyrimethamine have appeared (551, 552). Clinical improvement was described in a patient with AIDS and toxoplasmic encephalitis after daily treatment with doxycycline (400 mg) and pyrimethamine (25 mg)—computed tomography scanning of the brain showed complete resolution of two ring-enhanced lesions within 5 weeks of therapy (552).

Clarithromycin

Clarithromycin (1.5 to 2.0 g) combined with pyrimethamine (25 mg) was used successfully (regression of neurologic signs and encephalitic abnormalities) to treat cerebral toxoplasmosis in two AIDS patients *(553)*. The use of clarithromycin-pyrimethamine was suggested as an alternative treatment of toxoplasmosis in AIDS patients who cannot receive or tolerate sulfonamides.

The role of clarithromycin-minocycline combination treatment *(554)* and in maintenance *(555)* therapies of toxoplasmosis in AIDS patients was also examined.

The use of clarithromycin for the treatment of cerebral toxoplasmosis associated with HIV infection has also been discussed *(556)*.

Atovaquone

To date, atovaquone has been studied in a small number of patients (*n* = 5 to 24) with cerebral toxoplasmosis who were mostly unresponsive to conventional chemotherapy *(557–560)*. When given at doses of 750 mg, four times daily, atovaquone produced a complete or partial radiologic response ranging from 37% to 87.5% of patients.

Atovaquone was used to resolve successfully cerebral toxoplasmic lesions in a child and in an adult HIV-positive patient who failed to respond to conventional therapy with high-dose (3.0 mg/kg daily) pyrimethamine, as well as clindamycin and azithromycin *(561)*. A rapid oral desensitization was initiated in the adult patient because of maculopapular rash developed during the attempted treatment with pyrimethamine *(561)*. However, treatment failure of atovaquone in one patient with cerebral toxoplasmosis has also been reported *(562)*.

An uncontrolled open-label study was designed to evaluate the efficacy and tolerance of atovaquone as a long-term maintenance therapy in patients with toxoplasmic encephalitis and intolerant to conventional anti-*Toxoplasma* drugs *(563)*. The patients, who received 750 mg of the drug four times daily, were followed up for a mean period of 1 year. Though 17 (26%) patients experienced a toxoplasmic encephalitis relapse, the survival probability was 70% at 1 year after the episode of TE. The overall results suggested that atovaquone has been a well-tolerated and effective maintenance therapy in patients who were intolerant to conventional anti-*Toxoplasma* drugs *(563)*.

Trimetrexate

The therapeutic efficacy of trimetrexate has been evaluated in nine sulfonamide-intolerant AIDS patients and biopsy-proven cerebral toxoplasmosis *(564)*. Patients received trimetrexate (30 to 280 mg/m^2 daily) plus leucovorin (20 to 90 mg/m^2, every 6 hours) for 28 to 149 days. Radiographic responses were documented in eight patients and clinical responses in five patients. However, despite the improvement, all patients showed both clinical and radiographic dete-

rioration within 12 to 109 days of their initial improvement. The activity of trimetrexate administered alone, although dramatic in sulfonamide-intolerant patients, has been transient in nature, making this drug inappropriate as a single-agent therapy for AIDS-associated toxoplasmosis *(564)*.

36.3.2.2 Management of Ocular Toxoplasmosis

The frequency of ocular toxoplasmosis in AIDS patients has been on the increase *(565)*. It rose from 3.3% in 1983, to 6.1% in 1988, to 5.9% during the first four months of 1989 *(566)*.

Earlier studies conducted in the 1990s have demonstrated the use of systemic corticosteroids as part of the initial treatment regimen in 95% of cases *(567)*. Systemic corticosteroids are usually administered to patients whose vision is threatened *(428)*; however, there is no consensus about their use in ocular toxoplasmosis, as it has been repeatedly demonstrated that fulminant ocular toxoplasmosis may occur after both systemic and periocular administration *(568)*. When patients with unilateral focal chorioretinitis (without associated old scars in the posterior pole) presumably caused by acquired toxoplasmosis have been treated with systemic or periocular corticosteroids not accompanied by antiparasitic medication, they have exhibited rapid increase of inflammation *(569)*.

The most frequently used therapy for ocular toxoplasmosis *(570–573)* consisted of a combination of pyrimethamine, sulfadiazine, and corticosteroids (32% of cases) *(574–576)* or pyrimethamine, sulfadiazine, clindamycin, and corticosteroids (27%) *(577)*; adjunct therapies involving photocoagulation, cryotherapy, or vitrectomy have been used in 33% of the cases *(577)*.

A prospective multicenter study to evaluate the efficacy of therapeutic strategies for treatment of ocular toxoplasmosis was conducted in 106 patients *(578)*. Medication was given for at least 4 weeks and consisted of three combinations, namely, pyrimethamine, sulfadiazine, and corticosteroids (group 1; 29 patients); clindamycin, sulfadiazine, and corticosteroids (group 2; 37 patients); and cotrimoxazole (trimethoprim-sulfamethoxazole) and corticosteroids (group 3; 8 patients). Patients with peripheral retinal lesions remained without systemic therapy (group 4; 32 patients). Patients from group 1 received leucovorin (5.0 mg twice weekly). No difference in the duration of inflammatory activity was noticed between the separate groups of patients. The investigators concluded that independently of the therapy given, the size of the retinal focus was the most important factor in predicting the duration of inflammatory activity ($p < 0.05$). There was a 52% reduction in the size of the retinal inflammatory focus in the pyrimethamine-treated patients compared with only 25% in untreated cases. The most frequently observed side effects of pyrimethamine treatment included hematologic complications (thrombocytopenia and leukopenia, despite the leucovorin medication) *(578)*.

Another prospective, randomized study in 29 patients with presumed toxoplasmic retinochoroiditis was conducted to compare the efficacy of oral pyrimethamine-sulfadiazine with subconjunctival injections of clindamycin *(579)*. Results from both treatments showed no difference in the mean visual acuity after therapy was completed, with similar mean healing times (1.80 months for clindamycin and 1.88 months for pyrimethamine-sulfadiazine). At the 14-month follow-up examination, recurrence of ocular toxoplasmosis had developed in both groups—21% (clindamycin) and 36% (pyrimethamine-sulfadiazine) of patients. In general, other than discomfort, the subconjunctival injection of clindamycin did not produce any significant adverse side effects, thus providing a useful alternative in the choice of anti-*Toxoplasma* ocular therapy *(579)*.

Evaluation of data of 33 patients with active toxoplasmic retinochoroiditis who were followed up for 2 to 9 years has shown no real differences between treatment with argon laser and medication in terms of success rate, time of regression of lesion recurrences, and complications. The regression of the active lesion in the laser-treated group was accomplished in 25 to 50 days, whereas in the medication-treated group it took 50 to 150 days *(580)*.

The intraocular penetration of antitoxoplasmic drugs administered either by subconjunctival, retrobulbar, or intramuscular routes has also been examined *(581)*. Drug measurements were performed in the anterior chamber, the vitreous, and the retina-choroid of a healthy rabbit eye; the best results were obtained for spiramycin, trimethoprim-sulfamethoxazole, and clindamycin. The therapeutic efficacy on *Toxoplasma*-infected rabbit eye was investigated using indirect method; pyrimethamine and especially doxycycline have shown the best results *(581)*.

Neuroretinitis is a distinct clinical entity manifested by moderate to severe visual loss, optic nerve head edema, macular exudate in a stellate pattern, and a variable vitreous inflammation. Several cases of neuroretinitis associated with *T. gondii* infection have been described *(582)*. Treatment with systemic antibiotics and corticosteroids resulted in restoration of visual acuity to 20/25 or better, thereby suggesting that although rare, toxoplasmic neuroretinitis is a potentially treatable ocular disorder *(582)*.

36.3.2.3 Prophylaxis of Cerebral Toxoplasmosis

In a comparative study to evaluate the efficacy and safety of three regimens for primary prophylaxis of toxoplasmic encephalitis (TE), researchers have found co-trimoxazole [160 mg trimethoprim (TMP) and 800 mg sulfamethoxazole

(SMZ) every other day] to significantly reduce the risk of TE *(583)*. The double-strength tablet daily dose of TMP-SMZ, which is recommended as the preferred regimen for *P. jirovecii* pneumonia prophylaxis *(584)*, appeared to be effective against TE and has been recommended for this infection as well *(449)*.

In patients who cannot tolerate TMP-SMZ, the combination dapsone-pyrimethamine (100 mg weekly dapsone and 25 mg biweekly pyrimethamine) was equally effective *(585)*.

Pyrimethamine has been used alone (50 mg daily) as prophylaxis for toxoplasmic encephalitis in 56 patients with advanced HIV infection (38 patients with CD4$^+$ T-cell counts of $\leq$200 cells/mL) and presence of serum IgG antibodies to *T. gondii* *(586)*. All patients received folinic acid (7.5 mg daily) as supplement. During prophylaxis (697 months; mean, 12.5 $\pm$ 12.1), only one patient developed TE, and four patients had their treatment discontinued because of adverse side effects.

However, based on the results of a randomized trial in patients with advanced AIDS (absolute CD4$^+$ T-cell counts of <200 cells/mL) who had been treated with trimethoprim-sulfamethoxazole for toxoplasmic encephalitis, additional prophylaxis for TE with pyrimethamine did not appear necessary *(587)*. Still, it is believed that the continuing occurrence of toxoplasmic encephalitis among AIDS patients is due to the lack of prophylaxis *(588)*—according to data obtained from a Swiss HIV cohort study, at least one half of the cases of TE could have been prevented with a combination of prophylaxis, better motivation of physicians, and increased compliance of patients. High doses of co-trimoxazole prophylaxis appeared to be more effective than were low doses in decreasing the risk of toxoplasmic encephalitis in HIV-infected patients *(589)*.

Meta-analysis of data from 16 trials has suggested that dapsone may be used safely as a primary prophylactic regimen for toxoplasmosis *(590)*. In a randomized trial of HIV-infected patients, the combination of dapsone (50 mg, daily) and pyrimethamine (50 mg, weekly) plus leucovorin (25 mg, weekly) was found superior to co-trimoxazole as primary prophylaxis against toxoplasmosis as well as *P. jirovecii* pneumonia *(591)*.

The use of pyrimethamine in combination with folinic acid was found beneficial as secondary prophylaxis for ocular toxoplasmosis and may be helpful in preventing recurrence of sight-threatening and/or frequent ocular toxoplasmosis *(592)*.

36.3.2.4 Prophylaxis Against Toxoplasmosis and HAART in HIV-Infected Patients

Recent reports have suggested that interruption of primary prophylaxis against toxoplasmosis in HIV patients receiving

HAART may be possible when the CD4$^+$ T-cell counts surpass the 200 cells/μL threshold *(585,593–600)*. However, data on the feasibility of discontinuing secondary prophylaxis are more scarce and involve a limited number of patients *(601)*.

Nonetheless, although reported results have lent credence to the efficiency of immune restoration after HAART and have been beneficial to patients *(602)*, because of the potential for reinfection *(593)* caution must be applied before making a decision based on immunologic and virologic considerations, especially shortly after instituting HAART *(603)*.

36.3.2.5   Immunotherapy of Toxoplasmosis

Ultimately, the control of severe *Toxoplasma* infections will rest with the ability of the host to develop an adequate cell-mediated immune response *(423, 475, 476)*. With the advance of recombinant lymphokines, as well as drugs capable of enhancing the cell-mediated immunity, immunotherapy alone or in conjunction with specific chemotherapy will play an increasing role in the management of toxoplasmosis, especially in immunocompromised patients *(441,604)*.

IFN-γ with its pleiotropic adjuvant effects on host defenses plays an active role in the development of appropriate cell-mediated immune responses by the host *(605)*. It is thought that endogenous interleukin-12 is required for the development and long-term maintenance of IFN-γ–dependent resistance against *T. gondii (606)*. The activation of microglia and astrocytes by IFN-γ or its combination with TNF-α appears to be an important effector mechanism in the host immunity. GM-CSF, IL-1β, and IL-6 may participate in this activation. Alternatively, IL-10 may play a pathogenic role by downregulating IFN-γ production *(607)*.

Administration of IFN-γ can enhance the antibody production and survival time of mice infected with *Toxoplasma (608)*. Furthermore, IFN-γ also augments the activity of natural killer (NK) cells and activates the macrophages, making these cells important factors in the development of viable host resistance against *Toxoplasma (609)*.

Use of levamisole to boost the immune response in five patients with toxoplasmosis has been reported *(610)*. The drug, when given alone (at 150 mg daily for 3 days, every 14 days during a 2-month period) or in combination with trimethoprim-sulfamethoxazole (300 mg daily for 30 days), induced significant increase and normalization of the T-lymphocyte counts and consequently enhanced the cellular immune response while suppressing antitoxoplasmic antibody titers. The lower T-lymphocyte counts in *T. gondii*–infected patients correlated with the depressed thymus activity found in *T. gondii*–infected animals *(610)*. Later, however,

the reported results using levamisole to boost the immune response *(610)* were contradicted by other investigators *(611)* who did not find any activity of levamisole against experimental toxoplasmosis in mice—the drug was administered in the stomach at the same doses and schedule (2.5 mg/kg for 3 consecutive days, every 2 weeks for a 2-month period), as described in Ref. *(610)*.

The effect of levamisole on toxoplasmosis during pregnancy in guinea pigs was also investigated *(612)*.

36.4   Recent NIAID-Supported Clinical Studies on HIV Disease Complications and Co-Infections

Recently, NIAID has supported a number of domestic clinical research studies involving HIV disease complications and co-infections:

- University of California at San Diego (R21AI058765). "Bisphosphonate Therapy for HIV-Associated Osteopenia." This is a study to determine whether zoledronate increases bone density and reduces ongoing bone loss in subjects with HIV-associated osteopenia.
- Case Western Reserve University (R01-AI-60484). "Role of mitochondria in HIV lipoatrophy." This project comprises two studies. An observational study will examine the effect of nucleoside reverse transcriptase inhibitor (NRTI)-containing regimens on content and function of mitochondrial DNA and lipoatrophy over time in HIV-infected patients initiating their first antiretroviral regimen. An interventional study will perform these same detailed evaluations to assess the effect of substituting tenofovir for d4T (stavudine) in HIV-infected patients with established lipoatrophy versus the effect of uridine supplementation in HIV-infected patients on NRTI-containing regimens with established lipoatrophy.
- Columbia University Health Sciences (R01-AI-65200). "Osteoporosis in HIV-infected Postmenopausal Women." This study will examine the impact of traditional risk factors for osteoporosis and characteristics of HIV infection and antiretroviral therapy on the prevalence of osteoporosis and the rate of bone loss in HIV-infected postmenopausal African-American and Hispanic women.
- University of California (ACTG Study 5030). "A Phase III prospective, randomized, double-blind trial of valganciclovir preemptive therapy for cytomegalovirus (CMV) viremia as detected by plasma CMV DNA PCR assay has completed accrual." ACTG 5030 was designed to evaluate the safety and efficacy of valganciclovir for the prevention of CMV end-organ disease in persons with detectable plasma CMV DNA. Given the added pill burden and

toxicity, this study targets a population at greatest risk for CMV end-organ disease. Participants with detectable CMV DNA at entry or during the course of the study were randomized to receive valganciclovir or placebo. All participants have been monitored closely for evidence of CMV disease. Participants developing CMV disease are evaluated for evidence of clinical and virologic resistance.

- University of California at Los Angeles (ACTG Study 5079). "A prospective, multicenter, randomized, placebo-controlled trial of physiologic testosterone supplementation for HIV-positive men with mildly to moderately reduced serum testosterone levels and abdominal obesity." Follow-up studies have been completed, and the final analysis is in progress. A5079 was designed to evaluate the safety and efficacy of testosterone gel to reduce visceral fat as detected by CT scan in males with mild-to-moderate reduced serum testosterone levels. Abdominal obesity is associated with increased risk for cardiovascular disease.

- Duke University (ACTG Study 5084). "Evaluation of metabolic complications associated with antiretroviral medications in HIV-1 infected pregnant women." Follow-up studies have been completed and the final analysis is in progress. A5084 is an observational study designed to determine whether pregnant women receiving protease inhibitors are at a greater risk for glucose intolerance.

- San Francisco General Hospital (ACTG Study 5092s). "Pharmacokinetic evaluation of the effects of ribavirin on zidovudine or stavudine triphosphate formation." Follow-up studies have been completed and the final analysis is in progress. A5092 is a pharmacokinetic study exploring the potential interactions between ribavirin and zidovudine or stavudine. Ribavirin has demonstrated variable effects on NRTIs triphosphate formation *in vitro*. Coexposure with ribavirin has resulted in antagonistic effects upon zidovudine and d4T.

- Indiana University School of Medicine (ACTG Study 5148). "Pilot study of the safety, efficacy, and tolerability of extended-release niacin for the treatment of elevated non-HDL cholesterol and elevated triglycerides in HIV-infected subjects." Follow-up studies have been completed and the final analysis is in progress.

- Case Western Reserve University (ACTG Study 5163). "A Phase II, randomized, placebo-controlled study of once-weekly alendronate in HIV-infected subjects with decreased bone mineral density receiving calcium and vitamin D." A5163 is designed to evaluate the safety and efficacy of alendronate in combination with calcium and vitamin D in men and women with HIV-associated osteopenia. It is not known if alendronate is effective in the treatment of HIV-associated osteopenia.

- University of Cincinnati (ACTG Study 5178). "Suppressive long-term antiviral management of hepatitis C virus (HCV) and HIV-1 co-infected subjects (SLAM-C)." ACTG 5178 will evaluate the safety and efficacy of long-term treatment with pegylated interferon to control liver fibrosis in persons infected with both HIV and HCV who did not have an adequate response to at least 12 weeks of interferon-based treatment.

- New York University (ACTG Study 5206). "A pilot study to determine the impact on dyslipidemia of the addition of tenofovir to stable background antiretroviral therapy in HIV-infected subjects." This study will evaluate the decline in non-HDL levels after the addition of tenofovir to a stable background, highly active antiretroviral regimen for 12 weeks compared with the change after 12 weeks of placebo instead of tenofovir.

- University of Alabama at Birmingham (Pediatric ACTG Study 1045). "Prevalence of morphologic and metabolic abnormalities in vertically HIV-infected and uninfected children and youth." This is an observational study to compare the prevalence of abnormalities in glucose metabolism, serum lipid levels, body composition, fat deposition and distribution, and bone density in vertically acquired HIV children receiving *or* not receiving protease inhibitors–containing antiretroviral therapy (ART) and HIV-negative controls.

- Stanford University (ACTG Study 5164). "A phase IV study of antiretroviral therapy for HIV-infected adults presenting with acute opportunistic infections: immediate vs. deferred initiation of antiretroviral treatment." This study will compare the outcome at 48 weeks of immediate versus deferred antiretroviral therapy in patients presenting with an acute AIDS-defining opportunistic infection or severe bacterial infection.

- Case Western Reserve University (ACTG Study 5229). "A randomized, double-blind, placebo-controlled trial of uridine supplementation in HIV lipoatrophy." This study will examine the effect of NucleomaxX on limb fat in HIV-1–infected subjects receiving stable antiretroviral therapy containing stavudine or zidovudine. It will also assess the safety and tolerability of NucleomaxX in this population.

- Indiana University (ACTG Study 5177). "An observational study of the pharmacokinetics of efavirenz, nevirapine, and lopinavir/ritonavir in HIV-infected subjects requiring hemodialysis." This study will examine the pharmacokinetic parameters of efavirenz, nevirapine, and lopinavir/ritonavir in HIV-infected patients with end-stage renal disease.

- Northwestern University (ACTG Study 5184). "An open label, randomized study to determine the impact of antiretroviral treatment in HCV/HIV-coinfected subjects with high $CD4^+$ T-cell counts on the efficacy of hepatitis C treatment with pegylated interferon alfa-2A and ribavirin." This study will compare virologic response to

ART followed by ART plus IFN plus RBV versus IFN plus RBV alone.

- Ohio State University (ACTG Study 5209). "A pilot study of the safety, efficacy, and tolerability of ezetimibe (Zetia) in combination with statin therapy for the treatment of elevated LDL cholesterol in HIV-infected subjects." This study will measure the change in LDL-C after the addition of ezetimibe to a stable ART regimen compared with the addition of placebo to ART.
- Social and Scientific Systems (ACTG Study 5213). "Safety, tolerability, and pharmacokinetic interactions of atazanavir and rifampin in healthy volunteers." This study will determine whether 300 or 400 mg atazanavir coadministered with rifampin will achieve steady-state levels.
- New York University (ACTG Study 5220). "Improving immune response to HBV vaccine in HIV positive patients with granulocyte-macrophage colony-stimulating factor (GMCSF) as a vaccine adjuvant: a pilot study." This study will evaluate the efficacy and safety of vaccinating HIV-infected subjects with HBV vaccine with or without GMCSF as an adjuvant.
- Case Western Reserve University (ACTG Study 5232). "Optimizing vaccine responsiveness in HIV-1 and HCV infections and identifying determinants of responsiveness: a pilot study." This study will investigate the magnitude of innate and adaptive immune defects present in patients who have hepatitis C, HIV, or have both HIV and hepatitis C. This will be done by giving a tetanus booster shot and hepatitis A and B vaccine to persons who have never had hepatitis A and/or B and seeing how they will respond.

References

1. Georgiev, V. St. (1998) *Infectious Diseases in Immunocompromised Hosts*, CRC Press, Boca Raton, FL.
2. Georgiev, V. St. (2003) *Opportunistic Infections: Treatment and Prophylaxis*, Humana Press, Totowa, NJ.
3. Georgiev, V. St. (ed.) (1988) *Antifungal Drugs*, Ann. N.Y. Acad. Sci., vol. 544. The New York Academy of Sciences, New York.
4. Georgiev, V. St. (1988) Fungal infections and the search for novel antifungal agents, *Ann. N.Y. Acad. Sci.*, **544**, 1–3.
5. Nicholls, P. E. and Henry, K. (1978) Gastritis and cimetidine: a possible explanation, *Lancet*, **1**, 1095.
6. Ruddell, W. S. J., Azon, A. T. R., Findlay, J. M., et al. (1980) Effect of cimetidine on the gastric bacterial flora, *Lancet*, **1**, 672.
7. Seelig, M. S. (1966) The role of antibiotics in the pathogenesis of *Candida* infections, *Am. J. Med.*, **40**, 887.
8. McVay, L. V., Jr. and Sprunt, D. H. (1951) A study of moniliasis in aureomycin therapy, *Proc. Soc. Exp. Biol. Med.*, **78**, 759.
9. Hughes, W. T., Kuhn, S., Chaudhary, S., et al. (1977) Successful chemoprophylaxis for *Pneumocystis carinii* pneumonia, *N. Engl. J. Med.*, **297**, 1419–1426.
10. Georgiev, V. St. (2003) *Candida albicans*. In: *Opportunistic Infections: Treatment and Prophylaxis*, Humana Press, Totowa, NJ, pp. 239–268.

11. Vazquez, J. A., Boikov, D., and Sobel, J. D. (1998) Antifungal cross-resistance among *Candida* spp. recovered from fluconazole-refractory thrush in AIDS patients, *5th Conference on Retroviruses and Opportunistic Infections, Chicago, IL*, February 1–5 [abstract 490].
12. Fichtenbaum, C. J., Koletar, S., Yiannoutsos, C., et al. (2000) Refractory mucosal candidiasis in advanced human immunodeficiency virus infection, *Clin. Infect. Dis.*, **30**, 749–756.
13. Wilcox, C. M. and Karowe, M. W. (1994) Esophageal infections: etiology, diagnosis, and management, *Gastroenterologist*, **2**, 188.
14. Selik, R. M., Starcher, E. T., and Curran, J. W. (1987) Opportunistic diseases reported in AIDS patients: frequencies, associations, and trends, *AIDS*, **1**, 175.
15. Torssander, J., Morfeldt-Manson, L., Biberfeld, G., et al. (1987) Oral *Candida albicans* in HIV infection, *Scand. J. Infect. Dis.*, **19**, 291.
16. Abgrall, S., Charreau, I., Bloch, J., et al. (1998) Risk factors for esophageal candidiasis in HIV infection, *5th Conf. Retroviruses Opportunistic Infections, Chicago, IL*, February 1–5 [abstract 492].
17. Kopicko, J. J., Momodu, I., Adedokun, A., et al. (1999) Characteristics of HIV- infected men with low serum testosterone levels, *Int. J. STD AIDS*, **10**, 817–820.
18. Tavitian, A., Raufman, J. P., and Rosenthal, L. E. (1986) Oral candidiasis as a marker for esophageal candidiasis in the acquired immunodeficiency syndrome, *Ann. Intern. Med.*, **104**, 54.
19. Pedersen, C., Gerstoff, J., Lindhardt, B. O., and Sindrup, J. (1987) *Candida* esophagitis associated with acute human immunodeficiency virus infection, *J. Infect. Dis.*, **156**, 529.
20. Green, B. I. (1990) Treatment of fungal infections in the human immunodeficiency virus-infected individual. In: *Antifungal Drug Therapy: A Complete Guide for the Practitioner* (Jacobs, P. H. and Nall, L., eds.), Marcel Dekker, New York, p. 237.
21. Oude Lashof, A. M., Donnelly, J. P., Meis, J. F., et al. (1998) Duration of antifungal treatment and development of delayed complications in patients with candidemia, *38th Intercience Conference on Antimicrobial Agents and Chemotherapy, San Diego, CA*, September 24–27 [abstract J-97].
22. Palma-Carlos, A. G. and Palma-Carlos, M. L. (2001) Chronic mucocutaneous candidiasis revisited, *Allerg. Immunol. (Paris)*, **33**, 229–232.
23. Mulero-Marchese, R. D., Blank, K. J., and Sieck, T. G. (1998) Genetic basis for protection against experimental vaginal candidiasis by peripheral immunization, *J. Infect. Dis.*, **178**, 227–234.
24. Elahi, S., Clancy, R., and Pang, G. (2001) A therapeutic vaccine for mucosal candidiasis, *Vaccine*, **19**, 2516–2521.
25. Lopez, J., Pernot, C., Aho, S., et al. (2001) Decrease in *Candida albicans* strains with reduced susceptibility to fluconazole following changes in prescribing policies, *J. Hosp. Infect.*, **48**, 122–123.
26. Bini, E. J., Micale, P. L., and Weinshel, E. H. (2000) Natural history of HIV- associated esophageal disease in the era of protease inhibitor therapy, *Dig. Dis. Sci.*, **45**, 1301–1307.
27. Vullo, V., Mastroianni, C. M., Mengoni, F., et al. (1998) Restoration of innate immunity in HIV-infected patients after protease-inhibitr therapy, *38th Interscience Conference on Antimicrobial Agents and Chemotherapy, San Diego, CA*, September 24–27 [I-182].
28. Revankar, S. G., Sanche, S. E., Dib, O. P., Caceres, M., and Patterson, T. F. (1998) Effect of highly active anti-retroviral therapy (HAART) on recurrent oropharyngeal candidiasis in HIV-infected patients: a complex relationship, *5th Conference on Retroviruses and Opportunistic Infections, Chicago, IL*, February 1–5 [abstract 488].
29. Zingman, B. S. (1996) Resolution of refractory AIDS-related mucosal candidiasis after initiation of didanosine plus sequinavir, *N. Engl. J. Med.*, **334**, 1674.

30. Arribas, J. R., Hernandez-Albujar, S., Gonzalez-Garcia, J., et al. (1999) Continuous improvement of oral *Candida* colonization and skin test reactivity after one year of treatment with protease inhibitors, *6th Conference on Retroviruses and Opportunistic Infections, Chicago, IL*, January 31-February 4 [abstract 185].

31. Arribas, J. R., Hernandez-Albujar, S., Gonzalez-Garcia, J., et al. (1998) Prospective study of oral *Candida* colonization in advanced AIDS patients treated with ritonavir, *5th Conference on Retroviruses and Opportunistic Infections, Chicago, IL*, February 1–5 [abstract 485].

32. Tacconelli, E., De Bernardis, F., Tumbarello, M., et al. (1999) A direct effect of HIV protease inhibitors on *Candida albicans*: prevention of oral candidiasis through inhibition of fungal proteinase, *6th Conference on Retroviruses and Opportunistic Infections, Chicago, IL*, January 31–February 4 [abstract 184].

33. Cassone, A., Adriani, D., Tacconelli, E., Cauda, R., and De Bernardis, F. (1998) HIV protease inhibitors have a direct anti-*Candida* effect by inhibition of *Candida* aspartyl proteinase, *12th International Conference on AIDS, Geneva, Switzerland*, June 28–July 3 [abstract 31211].

34. McNeil, M. M., Reiss, E., Elie, C. M., et al. (1999) Molecular analysis of serial *Candida albicans* isolates from HIV-infected patients with oropharyngeal candidiasis (OPC) demonstrating clinical resistance to fluconazole, *99th Gen. Meet. Am. Soc. Microbiol., Chicago, IL*, May 27–June 2 [abstract F-104].

35. Rex, J. H., Walsh, T. J., Sobel, J. D., et al. (2000) Practice guidelines for the treatment of candidiasis. Infectious Diseases Society of America, *Clin. Infect. Dis.*, **30**, 662–678.

36. Xu, J., Ramos, A. R., Vilgalys, R., and Mitchell, T. G. (2000) Clonal and spontaneous origins of fluconazole resistance in *Candida albicans*, *J. Clin. Microbiol.*, **38**, 1214–1220.

37. Loffler, J., Einsele, H., Hebart, H., et al. (2000) Phospholipid and sterol analysis of plasma membranes of azole-resistant *Candida albicans* strains, *FEMS Microbiol. Lett.*, **185**, 59–63.

38. Calabrese, D. C., Bille, J., Barchiesi, F., and Sanglard, D. (1998) Incidence of resistance mechanisms to azole antifungal agents in *Candida* species from HIV+ patients with oropharyngeal candidosis (OPC), *38th Interscience Conference on Antimicrobial Agents and Chemotherapy, San Diego, CA*, September 24–27 [abstract C-152].

39. Vennwald, I., Seebacher, C., and Roitsch, E. (1998) Post-mortem findings in patients with repeatedly mycological demonstration of *Candida glabrata*, *Mycoses*, **41**, 125–132.

40. Georgiev, V. St. (2003) *Cryptococcus neoformans*. In: *Opportunistic Infections: Treatment and Prophylaxis*, Humana Press, Totowa, NJ, pp. 213–237.

41. Littman, M. C. and Walter, J. E. (1968) Cryptococcosis: current status, *Am. J. Med.*, **45**, 922.

42. Sabetta, J. R. and Andriole, V. T. (1985) Cryptococcal infection of the central nervous system, *Med. Clin. North Am.*, **69**, 333.

43. Butler, W. T., Alling, D. W., Spickard, A., and Utz, J. P. (1964) Diagnostic and prognostic value of clinical and laboratory findings in cryptococcal meningitis, *N. Engl. J. Med.*, **270**, 59.

44. De Witt, C. N., Dickson, P. L., and Holt, G. W. (1982) Cryptococcal meningitis: a review of 32 years' experience, *J. Neurol. Sci.*, **53**, 283.

45. Sarosi, G. A., Parker, J. D., Doto, I. L., and Tosh, F. E. (1969) Amphotericin B in cryptococcal meningitis: long-term results of treatment, *Ann. Intern. Med.*, **71**, 1079.

46. Spikard, A., Butler, W. T., Andriole, V., and Utz, J. P. (1963) The improved prognosis of cryptococcal meningitis with amphotericin B therapy, *Ann. Intern. Med.*, **58**, 66.

47. Utz, J. P., Garriques, I. L., Sande, M. A., et al. (1975) Therapy of cryptococcosis with a combination of flucytosine and amphotericin B, *J. Infect. Dis.*, **132**, 368.

48. Zimmerman, L. E. and Rappaport, H. (1954) Occurrence of cryptococcosis in patients with malignant disease of the reticuloendothelial system, *Am. J. Clin. Pathol.*, **24**, 1050.

49. Perfect, J. R., Durack, D. T., and Gallis, H. A. (1983) Cryptococcemia, *Medicine (Baltimore)*, **62**, 98.

50. Graybill, J. R. and Alford, R. H. (1974) Cell-mediated immunity in cryptococcosis, *Cell. Immunol.*, **14**, 12.

51. Schimpff, S. C. and Bennett, J. E. (1975) Abnormalities in cell-mediated immunity in patients with *C. neoformans* infections, *J. Allergy Clin. Immunol.*, **55**, 430.

52. Krick, J. A. (1981) Familial cryptococcal meningitis, *J. Infect. Dis.*, **143**, 133.

53. Ieong, M. H., Reardon, C. C., Levitz, S. M., and Kornfeld, H. (2000) Human immunodeficiency virus type 1 infection of alveolar macrophages impairs their innate fungicidal activity, *Am. J. Respir. Crit. Care Med.*, **162**(3 Part 1), 966–970.

54. Mambula, S. S., Simons, E. R., Hastey, R. P., and Levitz, S. M. (1999) Human neutrophil-mediated nonoxidative antifungal activity against *Cryptococcus neoformans*, *99th Gen. Meet. Am. Soc. Microbiol., Chicago, IL*, May 27–June 2 [abstract F-42].

55. Aguirre, K., Havell, E. A., Gibson, G. W., and Johnson, L. L. (1995) Role of tumor necrosis factor and gamma interferon in acquired resistance to *Cryptococcus neoformans* in the central nervous system of mice, *Infect. Immun.*, **63**, 1725.

56. Kerkering, T. M., Duma, R. J., and Shadomy, S. (1981) The evolution of pulmonary cryptococcosis, *Ann. Intern. Med.*, **94**, 611.

57. Reblin, T., Meyer, A., Albrecht, H., and Greten, H. (1994) Disseminated cryptococcosis in a patient with AIDS, *Mycoses*, **37**, 275.

58. Larsen, R. A., Bozzette, S., McCutchan, J. A., et al. (1989) Persistent *Cryptococcus neoformans* infection of the prostate after successful treatment of meningitis, *Ann. Intern. Med.*, **111**, 125.

59. Glassman, S. J. and Hale, M. J. (1995) Cutaneous cryptococcosis and Kaposi's sarcoma occurring in the same lesions in a patient with the acquired immunodeficiency syndrome, *Clin. Exp. Dermatol.*, **20**, 480.

60. Muccioli, C., Belfort Junior, R., Neves, R., and Rao, N. (1995) Limbal and choroidal *Cryptococcus* infection in the acquired immunodeficiency syndrome, *Am. J. Ophthalmol.*, **120**, 539.

61. Castro Guardiola, A., Ocana Rivera, I., Gasser Laguna, I., et al. (1991) 16 Cases of infectious *Cryptococcus neoformans* in patients with AIDS, *Enferm. Infec. Microbiol. Clin.*, **9**, 90.

62. Sugar, A. M. (1990) Overview: cryptococcosis in the treatment of AIDS, *Mycopathologia*, **114**, 153.

63. Fur, B. (1990) Cryptococcosis in AIDS: therapeutic concepts, *Mycoses*, **33**(Suppl. 1), 55.

64. Kirchner, J. T. (1996) Opportunistic fungal infections in patients with HIV disease: combating cryptococcosis and histoplasmosis, *Postgrad. Med.*, **99**, 209.

65. Mitchell, T. G. and Perfect, J. R. (1995) Cryptococcosis in the era of AIDS: 100 years after the discovery of *Cryptococcus neoformans*, *Clin. Microbiol. Rev.*, **8**, 515.

66. Just-Nübling, G. (1994) Therapy of candidiasis and cryptococcosis in AIDS, *Mycoses*, **37**(Suppl. 2), 56.

67. Emmons, III, W. W., Luchsinger, S., and Miller, L. (1995) Progressive pulmonary cryptococcosis in a patient who is immunocompetent, *South. Med. J.*, **88**, 657.

68. Zuger, A., Louie, E., Holzman, R. S., Simberkoff, M. S., and Rahal, J. J. (1986) Cryptococcal disease in patients with acquired immunodeficiency syndrome: diagnostic features and outcome of treatment, *Ann. Intern. Med.*, **104**, 234.

69. Kovacs, J. A., Kovacs, A. A., Polis, M., et al. (1985) Cryptococcosis in the acquired immunodeficiency syndrome, *Ann. Intern. Med.*, **103**, 533.

70. Dismukes, W. E., Cloud, G., Gallis, H. A., et al. (1987) Treatment of cryptococcal meningitis with combination amphotericin B and flucytosine for four as compared with six weeks, *N. Engl. J. Med.*, **317**, 334.

71. Eng, R. H. K., Bishburg, E., Smith, S. M., and Kapila, R. (1986) Cryptococcal infections in patients with acquired immune deficiency syndrome, *Am. J. Med.*, **81**, 19.

72. Theunissen, A. W. J. and Zanen, H. C. (1987) Dertig petienten net een "verborgen" ziekte: cryptococcen-memnigitis, *Ned. Tijdschr. Geneeskd.*, **131**, 1123.

73. Munoz-Peréz, M. A., Colmenero, M. A., Rodriguez-Pichardo, A., et al. (1996) Disseminated cryptococcosis presenting as moluscum-like lesions as the first manifestation of AIDS, *Int. J. Dermatol.*, **35**, 646.

74. Hellman, R. N., Hinrichs, J., Sicard, G., Hoover, R., Golden, P., and Hoffsten, P. (1984) Cryptococcal pyelonephritis and disseminated cryptococcosis in a renal transplant recipient, *Arch. Intern. Med.*, **141**, 128.

75. Liss, H. P. and Rimland, D. (1981) Asymptomatic cryptococcal meningitis, *Am. Rev. Respir. Dis.*, **124**, 88.

76. Tarala, R. A. and Smith, J. D. (1980) Cryptococcosis treated by rapid infusion of amphotericin B, *Br. Med. J.*, **281**, 28.

77. Mosberg, W. H. and Arnold, J. G. (1950) Torulosis of the central nervous system: review of the literature and report of five cases, *Ann. Intern. Med.*, **32**, 1153.

78. Picon, L., Vaillant, L., Duong, T., et al. (1989) Cutaneous cryptococcosis resembling molluscum contagiosum: a first manifestation of AIDS, *Acta Derm. Venereol. (Stockholm)*, **69**, 365.

79. Beeson, P. B. (1952) Cryptococcal meningitis of nearly sixteen years' duration, *Arch. Intern. Med.*, **89**, 797.

80. Campbell, G. D., Carrier, R. D., and Busey, J. F. (1981) Survival in untreated cryptococcal meningitis, *Neurology*, **31**, 1154.

81. Carton, C. A. and Mount, L. A. (1951) Neurosurgical aspects of cryptococcosis, *J. Neurosurg.*, **8**, 143.

82. Saag, M. S., Graybill, R. J., Larsen, R. A. (2000) Practice guidelines for the management of cryptococcal disease. Infectious Diseases Society of America, *Clin. Infect. Dis.*, **30**, 710–718.

83. Powderly, W. G. (1996) Recent advances in the management of cryptococcal meningitis in patients with AIDS, *Clin. Infect. Dis.*, **22**(Suppl. 2), S119.

84. Dismukes, W. E. (1993) Management of cryptococcosis, *Clin. Infect. Dis.*, **17**(Suppl. 2), S507 [see also: *Clin. Infect. Dis.*, **19**, 975 (1994)].

85. Powderly, W. G. (2000) Current approach to the acute management of cryptococcal infections, *J. Infect.*, **41**, 18–22.

86. Van der Horst, C., Saag, M., Cloud, G., et al. (1995) Randomized double blind comparison of amphotericin B (AMB) plus flucytosine to AMB alone (step 1) followed by a comparison of fluconazole to itraconazole (step 2) in the treatment of acute cryptococcal meningitis in patients with AIDS. Part I, *35th Interscience Conference on Antimicrobial Agents and Chemotherapy, San Francisco, CA*, September 17–20 [I-216].

87. Nightingale, S. D. (1995) Initial therapy for acquired immunodeficiency syndrome- associated cryptococcosis with fluconazole, *Arch. Intern. Med.*, **13**, 538.

88. Saag, M. S., Powderly, W. G., Cloud, G. A., et al. (1992) Comparison of amphotericin B with fluconazole in the treatment of acute AIDS-associated cryptococcal meningitis, *N. Engl. J. Med.*, **326**, 83.

89. Haubrich, R. H., Haghighat, D., Bozzette, S. A., Tilles, J., and McCutchan, J. A. (1994) High-dose fluconazole for treatment of cryptococcal disease in patients with human immunodeficiency virus infection, *J. Infect. Dis.*, **170**, 238.

90. Meyohas, M. C., Meynard, J. L., Bollens, D., et al. (1996) Treatment of non- meningeal cryptococcosis in patients with AIDS, *J. Infect.*, **33**, 7.

91. Carney, M. D., Combs, J. L., and Waschler, W. (1990) Cryptococcal choroiditis, *Retina*, **10**, 27.

92. Sitbon, O., Fourme, T., Bouree, P., Du Pasquier, L., and Salmeron, S. (1993) Successful treatment of disseminated cryptococcosis with high-dose oral fluconazole, *AIDS*, **7**, 1685.

93. Sahai, J. (1988) Management of cryptococcal meningitis in patients with AIDS, *Clin. Pharmacy*, **7**, 528.

94. Kauffman, C. A. and Frame, P. T. (1977) Bone marrow toxicity associated with 5- fluorocytosine therapy, *Antimicrob. Agents Chemother.*, **11**, 244.

95. Donahue, R. E., Johnson, M. M., Zon, L. I., Clark, S. C., and Groopman, J. E. (1987) Suppression of in vitro haematopoiesis following human immunodeficiency virus infection, *Nature*, **326**, 200.

96. Kotler, D. P., Gaetz, H. P., Lange, M., Klein, E. B., and Holt, P. R. (1984) Enteropathy associated with acquired immunodeficiency syndrome, *Ann. Intern. Med.*, **101**, 421.

97. Stamm, A. M., Diasio, R. B., Dismukes, W. E., et al. (1987) Toxicity of amphotericin B plus flucytosine in 194 patients with cryptococcal meningitis, *Am. J. Med.*, **83**, 236.

98. Larsen, R. A., Leal, M. A., and Chan, L. S. (1990) Fluconazole compared with amphotericin B plus flucytosine for cryptococcal meningitis in AIDS: a randomized trial, *Ann. Intern. Med.*, **113**, 183.

99. Chuck, S. L. and Sande, M. A. (1989) Infections with *Cryptococcus neoformans* in the acquired immunodeficiency syndrome, *N. Engl. J. Med.*, **321**, 794.

100. Dismukes, W. E. (1992) Treatment of systemic fungal diseases in patients with AIDS. In: *Recent Progress in Antifungal Chemotherapy* (Yamaguchi, H., Kobayashi, G. S., and Takeuchi, H., eds.), Marcel Dekker, New York, pp. 227–238.

101. Ammassari, A., Linzalone, A., Murri, R., Marasca, G., Morace, G., and Antinori, A. (1995) Fluconazole for primary prophylaxis of AIDS-associated cryptococcosis: a case controlled study, *Scand. J. Infect. Dis.*, **27**, 235.

102. Nelson, M. R., Fisher, M., Cartledge, J., Rogers, T., and Gazzard, B. G. (1994) The role of azoles in the treatment and prophylaxis of cryptococcal diseases in HIV infection, *AIDS*, **8**, 652 [see also: *AIDS*, **9**, 300 (1995)].

103. Manfredi, R., Mastroianni, A., Coronado, O. V., and Chiodo, F. (1997) Fluconazole as prophylaxis against fungal infection in patients with advanced HIV infection, *Arch. Intern. Med.*, **157**, 64.

104. Dei-Cas, E., Chabé, M., Moukhlis, R., et al. (2006) *Pneumocystis oryctolagi* sp. nov., an uncultured fungus causing pneumonia in rabbits at weaning: review of current knowledge, and description of a new taxon on genotypic, phylogenetic and phenotypic bases, *FEMS Micriobiol. Rev.*, **30**(6), 853–871.

105. Stringer, J. R., Beard, C. B., Miller, R. F., and Wakefield, A. E. (2002) A new name (*Pneumocystis jiroveci*) for *Pneumocystis* from humans, *Emerg. Infect. Dis*, **8** (9), 891–896.

106. Redhead, S. A., Cushion, M. T., Frenkel, J. K., and Stringer, J. R. (2006) *Pneumocystis* and *Trypanosoma cruzi*: nomenclature and typifications, *J. Eukaryot. Microbiol.*, **53**(1), 2–11.

107. Cushion, M. T. (1998) *Pneumocystis carinii*. In: *Topley and Wilson's Microbiology and Microbial Infections* (Collier, L., Balows, A., and Sussman, M., eds.), 9th ed., Arnold and Oxford Press, New York, pp. 645–683.

108. Cushion, M. T. (1998) Taxonomy, genetic organization, and life cycle of *Pneumocystis carinii*, *Semin. Respir. Infect.*, **13**(4), 304–312.

109. Cushion, M. T. (2004) *Pneumocystis*: unraveling the cloak of obscurity, *Trends Microbiol.*, **12**(5), 243–249.

110. Ryan, K. J., and Ray, C. G. (eds.) (2004) *Sherris Medical Microbiology*, 4th ed., McGraw-Hill, New York.

111. Georgiev, V. St. (2003) *Pneumocystis carinii*. In: *Opportunistic Infections: Treatment and Prophylaxis*, Humana Press, Totowa, NJ, pp. 507–533.

112. Frenkel, J. K. (1976) *Pneumocystis jiroveci* n. sp. from man: morphology, physiology, and immunology in relation to pathology, *Natl. Cancer Inst. Monogr,* **43**, 13–27.

113. James, T. Y., Kauff, F., Schoch, C. L., et al. (2006) Reconstructing the early evolution of fungi using a six-gene phylogeny, *Nature*, **443**(7113), 818–822.

114. Hugot, J., Demanche, C., Barriel, V., Dei-Cas, E., and Guillot, J. (2003) Phylogenetic systematics and evolution of primate-derived *Pneumocystis* based on mitochondrial or nuclear DNA sequence comparison, *Syst. Biol.*, **52**, 735–744.

115. Keely, S., Fischer, J., Cushion, M., and Stringer, J. (2004) Phylogenetic identification of *Pneumocystis murina* sp. nov., a new species in laboratory mice, *Microbiology*, **150**(Part 5), 1153–1165.

116. Cushion, M. T., Keely, S. P., and Stringer, J. R. (2004) Molecular and phenotypic description of *Pneumocystis wakefieldiae* sp. nov., a new species in rats, *Mycologia*, **96**, 429–438.

117. Cushion, M. T., Keely, S. P., and Stringer, J. R. (2005) Validation of the name *Pneumocystis wakefieldiae*, *Mycologia*, **97**, 268.

118. Dei-Cas, E., Chabé, M., Moukhlis, R., et al (2006) *Pneumocystis oryctolagi* sp. nov., an uncultured fungus causing pneumonia in rabbits at weaning: review of current knowledge, and description of a new taxon on genotypic, phylogenetic and phenotypic bases, *FEMS Micriobiol. Rev.*, **30**(6), 853–871.

119. Centers for Disease Control and Prevention (1981) *Pneumocystis* pneumonia—Los Angeles, *Morb. Mortal. Wkly Rep.*, **30**, 250–252.

120. Fannin, S., Gottlieb, M. S., Weisman, J. D., et al. (1982) A cluster of Kaposi's sarcoma and *Pneumocystis carinii* pneumonia among homosexual male residents of Los Angeles and Range Counties, California, *Morb. Mortal. Wkly Rep.*, **31**(32), 305–307.

121. Masur, H., Michelis, M. A., Greene, J. B., et al. (1981) An outbreak of community- acquired *Pneumocystis carinii* pneumonia, *N. Engl. J. Med.*, **305**, 1431–1438.

122. Centers for Disease Control and Prevention (1986) Update: acquired immunodeficiency syndrome—United States, *Morb. Mortal. Wkly Rep.*, **35**, 757–766.

123. Centers for Disease Control and Prevention (1986) Update: acquired immunodeficiency syndrome—United States, *Morb. Mortal. Wkly Rep.*, **35**, 17–21.

124. Palella, F. J., Jr., Delaney, K. M., Moorman, A. C., Loveless, M. O., et al. (1998) Declining morbidity and mortality among patients with advanced human immunodeficiency virus, *N. Engl. J. Med.*, **338**, 853–860.

125. Cushion, M. T. (1994) Transmission and epidemiology. In: *Pneumocystis carinii Pneumonia,* 2nd ed. (Walzer, P. D., ed.), Marcel Dekker, New York, pp. 251–268.

126. Walzer, P. D. (1994) Pathogenic mechanisms. In: *Pneumocystis carinii Pneumonia,* 2nd ed. (Walzer, P. D., ed.), Marcel Dekker, New York, pp. 123–140.

127. Phair, J., Munoz, A., Detels, R., Kaslow, R., Rinaldo, C., and Saah, A. (1990) The risk of *Pneumocystis carinii* pneumonia among men infected with human immunodeficiency virus type 1, *N. Eng. J. Med.*, **322**, 161–165.

128. USPHS/IDSA (1997) USPHS/IDSA guidelines for the prevention of opportunistic infection in persons infected with human immunodeficiency virus: disease specific recommendations, *Clin. Infect. Dis.*, **25**(Suppl. 3), S313–S335.

129. Kovacs, J. A., Hiemenz, J. W., Macher, A. M., Stover, D., et al. (1984) *Pneumocystis carinii* pneumonia: a comparison between patients with acquired immunodeficiency syndrome and patients with other immunodeficiencies, *Ann. Intern. Med.*, **100**, 663–671.

130. Waler, R. E. and Masur, H. (1994) Current regimens of therapy and prophylaxis. In: *Pneumocystis carinii Pneumonia,* 2nd ed. (Walzer, P. D., ed.), Marcel Dekker, New York, pp. 439–466.

131. Safrin, S., Finkelstein, D. M., Feinberg, J., et al. (1996) Comparison of three regimens for treatment of mild to moderate *Pneumocystis carinii* pneumonia in patients with AIDS, *Ann. Intern. Med.*, **124**, 792–802.

132. Sattler, F. R., Cowan, R., Nielsen, D. M., and Rushkin, J. (1988) Trimethoprim- sulfamethoxazole compared with pentamidine for treatment of *Pneumocystis carinii* pneumonia in the acquired immunodeficiency syndrome, *Ann. Intern. Med.*, **109**, 280–287.

133. Sattler, F. R., Frame, P. T., Davis, R., et al. (1994) Trimetrexate with leucovorin versus trimethoprim-sulfamethoxazole for moderate to severe episodes of *Pneumocystis carinii* pneumonia in patients with AIDS: a prospective, controlled multicenter investigation of the AIDS Clinical Trials Group Protocol 029/031, *J. Infect. Dis.*, **170**, 165–172.

134. Hughes, W., Leoung, G., Kramer, F., et al. (1993) Comparison of atovaquone (566C80) with trimethoprim-sulfamethoxazole to treat *Pneumocystis carinii* pneumonia in patients with AIDS, *N. Engl. J. Med.*, **328**, 1521–1527.

135. Dohn, M. N., Weinberg, W. G., Torres, R. A., et al. (1994) Oral atovaquone compared with intravenous pentamidine for *Pneumocystis carinii* pneumonia in patients with AIDS, *Ann. Intern. Med.*, **121**, 174–180.

136. Bozzette, S. A., Sattler, F. R., Chiu, J., et al. (1990) A controlled trial of early adjunctive treatment with corticosteroids for *Pneumocystis carinii* pneumonia in the acquired immunodeficiency syndrome, *N. Engl. J. Med.*, **323**, 1451–1457.

137. Consensus statement on the use of corticosteroids as adjunctive therapy for *Pneumocystis* pneumonia in the acquired immunodeficiency syndrome (1990) *N. Engl. J. Med.*, **323**, 1500–1504.

138. De Palo, V. A., Millstein, B. H., Mayo, P. H., Salzmann, S. H., and Rosen, M. J. (1995) Outcome of intensive care in patients with HIV infection, *Chest*, **107**, 506–510.

139. Pastores, S. M., Garay, S. M., Naidich, D. P., and Rom, W. N., (1996) Review: pneumothorax in patients with AIDS-related *Pneumocystis carinii* pneumonia, *Am. J. Med. Sci.*, **312**, 329–334.

140. Ioannidis, J. P., Cappelleri, J. C., Skolnik, P. R., Lau, J., and Sacks, H. S. (1996) A meta-analysis of the relative efficacy and toxicity of *Pneumocystis carinii* prophylactic regimens, *Arch. Intern. Med.*, **156**, 177–188.

141. Bozzette, S. A., Finkelstein, D. M., Spector, S. A., et al. (1995) A randomized trial of three antipneumocystis agents in patients with advanced human immunodeficiency virus infection, *N. Engl. J. Med.*, **332**, 693–699.

142. Gluckstein, D. and Rushkin, J. (1995) Rapid oral desensitization to trimethoprim- sulfamethoxazole (TMP-SMZ): use in prophylaxis for *Pneumocystis carinii* pneumonia in patients with AIDS who were previously intolerant to TMP-SMZ, *Clin. Infect. Dis.*, **20**, 849–853.

143. Hardy, W. D., Feinberg, J., Finkelstein, D. M., et al. (1992) A controlled trial of trimethoprim-sulfamethoxazole or aerosolized pentamidine for secondary prophylaxis of *Pneumocystis carinii* pneumonia in patients with the acquired immunodeficiency syndrome. AIDS Clinical Trials Group Protocol 021, *N. Engl. J. Med.*, **327**, 1842–1848.

144. Mallolas, J., Zamora, L., Gatell, J. M., et al. (1993) Primary prophylaxis for *Pneumocystis carinii* pneumonia: a randomized trial comparing cotrimoxazole, aerosolized pentamidine and dapsone plus pyrimethamine, *AIDS*, **7**, 59–64.

145. Georgiev, V. St. (2003) Cytomegalovirus. In: *Opportunistic Infections: Treatment and Prophylaxis*, Humana Press, Totowa, NJ, pp. 3–22.

146. Ryan, K. J. and Ray, C. G. (eds.) (2004) *Sherris Medical Microbiology*, 4th ed., McGraw-Hill, New York, pp. 566–569.

147. Alford, C. A., Stagno, S., Pass, R. F., and Huang, E.-S. (1981) Epidemiology of cytomegalovirus. In: *The Human Herpesviruses: An Interdisciplinary Perspective* (Hahmias, A., Dowdle, W., and Schinazi, R., eds.), Elsevier, New York, p. 159.

148. Lang, D. J. (1975) The epidemiology of cytomegalovirus infections: interpretations of recent observations. In: *Infections of the Fetus and the Newborn Infant*, vol. 3 (Krugman, S. and Gershon, A. A., eds.), Alan R. Liss, New York, p. 35.

149. Lang, D. J. and Krammer, J. F. (1975) Cytomegalovirus in the semen: observations in selected populations, *J. Infect. Dis.*, **132**, 472.

150. Reynolds, D. W., Stagno, S., Hosty, T. S., Tiller, M., and Alford, C. A., Jr. (1981) Maternal cytomegalovirus excretion and perinatal infection, *N. Engl. J. Med.*, **289**, 1.

151. Stagno, S., Reynolds, D. W., Pass, R. F., and Alford, C. A. (1980) Breast milk and the risk of cytomegalovirus infection, *N. Engl. J. Med.*, **302**, 1073.

152. Manian, F. A. and Smith, T. (1993) Ganciclovir for the treatment of cytomegalovirus pneumonia in an immunocompetent host, *Clin. Infect. Dis.*, **17**, 137.

153. Blair, S. D., Forbes, A., and Parkins, R. A. (1992) CMV colitis in an immunocompetent child, *J. R. Soc. Med.*, **85**, 238.

154. Drew, W. L. (1988) Diagnosis of cytomegalovirus infection, *Rev. Infect. Dis.*, **10**(Suppl. 3), 468.

155. Drew, W. L., Sweet, E. S., Miner, R. C., and Mocarski, E. S. (1984) Multiple infections by cytomegalovirus in patients with acquired immunodeficiency syndrome: documentation by Southern blot hybridization, *J. Infect. Dis.*, **150**, 952.

156. Ho, M. (1982) Pathology of cytomegalovirus infection. In: *Cytomegalovirus, Biology and Infection: Current Topics in Infectious Disease* (Greenough III, W. B. and Merigan T. C., eds.), Plenum Press, New York, p. 119.

157. Becroft, D. M. O. (1981) Prenatal cytomegalovirus infection: epidemiology, pathology and pathogenesis. In: *Perspectives in Pediatric Pathology* (Rosenberg, H. S. and Bernstein, J., eds.), Mason Press, New York, p. 203.

158. Weiss, D. J., Greenfield, J. W., Jr., O'Rourke, K. S., and McCune, W. J. (1993) Systemic cytomegalovirus infection mimicking an exacerbation of Wegener's granulomatosis, *J. Rheumatol.*, **20**, 155.

159. Stagno, S., Pass, R. F., Dworsky, M. E., and Alford, C. A. (1983) Congenital and perinatal cytomegalovirus infections, *Semin. Perinatol.*, **7**, 31.

160. Salomon, N. and Perlman, D. C. (1999) Cytomegalovirus pneumonia, *Semin. Respir. Infect.*, **14**, 353–358.

161. Jacobson, M. A. and Mills, J. (1988) Serious cytomegalovirus disease in acquired immune deficiency syndrome (AIDS): clinical findings, diagnosis and treatment, *Ann. Intern. Med.*, **108**, 585.

162. Drew, W. L. and Mintz, L. (1984) Cytomegalovirus infection in healthy and immune-deficient homosexual men. In: *The Acquired ImmuneDeficiency Syndrome and Infections of Homosexual Men* (Ma, P. and Armstrong, D., eds.), Yorke Medical Books, New York, p. 117.

163. Katlama, C. (1993) Cytomegalovirus infection in acquired immune-deficiency syndrome, *J. Med. Virol.*, **1**(Suppl.), 128.

164. Salmon, D., Lacassin, F., Harzic, M., et al. (1990) Predictive value of cytomegalovirus viremia for the occurrence of CMV organ involvement in AIDS, *J. Med. Virol*, **32**, 160.

165. Haas, C., Marteau, P., Roudiere, L., Gisselbrecht, M., Lowenstein, W., and Durand, H. (2000) Severe cytomegalovirus enteritis in AIDS. Favorable outcome of medical treatment, *Presse Med.*, **29**, 596–597.

166. Millar, A. B., Patou, G., Miller, R. F., et al. (1990) Cytomegalovirus in the lungs of patients with AIDS: respiratory pathogen or passenger? *Am. Rev. Respir. Dis.*, **141**, 1474.

167. Jacobson, M. A. (1994) Current management of cytomegalovirus disease in patients with AIDS, *Acquir. Immune Defic. Syndr. Human Retrovir.*, **10**, 917.

168. Markham, A. and Faulds, D. (1994) Ganciclovir: an update of its therapeutic use in cytomegalovirus infection, *Drugs*, **48**, 455.

169. Stevens, C. and Roberts, W. B., Jr. (1994) Ganciclovir: treatment of cytomegalovirus in immunocompromised individuals, *ANNA*, **21**, 204; 209.

170. Bachman, D. M. (1992) Treatment of CMV retinitis, *N. Engl. J. Med.*, **326**, 1702.

171. Deray, G., Katlama, C., and Jacobs, C. (1992) Treatment of CMV retinitis, *N. Engl. J. Med.*, **326**, 1702.

172. Skolnik, P. R. (1992) Treatment of CMV retinitis, *N. Engl. J. Med.*, **326**, 1701.

173. Wagstaff, A. J. and Bryson, H. M. (1994) Foscarnet: a reappraisal of its antiviral activity, pharmacokinetic properties and therapeutic use in immunocompromised patients with viral infections, *Drugs*, **48**, 199.

174. Greening, J. G. (1994) Intravenous foscarnet administration for treatment of cytomegalovirus retinitis, *J. Intraven. Nurs.*, **17**, 74.

175. Wagstaff, A. J., Faulds, D., and Goa, K. L. (1994) Aciclovir: a reappraisal of its antiviral activity, pharmacokinetic properties and therapeutic efficacy, *Drugs*, **47**, 153.

176. Polis, M. A., de Smet, M. D., Baird, B. F., et al. (1993) Increased survival of a cohort of patients with acquired immunodeficiency syndrome and cytomegalovirus retinitis who received sodium phosphonoformate (foscarnet), *Am. J. Med.*, **94**, 175.

177. Smith, D. G., Jr. and Handy, C. M. (1992) A protocol for foscarnet administration, *J. Intraven. Nurs.*, **15**, 274.

178. Yoser, S. L., Forster, D. J., and Rao, N. A. (1993) Systemic viral infections and their retinal and choroid manifestations, *Surv. Ophthalmol.*, **37**, 313.

179. Spector, S. A., Weingeist, T., Pollard, R. B., et al. (1993) A randomized, controlled study of intravenous ganciclovir therapy for cytomegalovirus peripheral retinitis in patients with AIDS, *J. Infect. Dis.*, **168**, 557.

180. Collaborative DHPG Treatment Study Group (1986) Treatment of serious cytomegalovirus infection with 9-(1,3-dihydroxy-2-propoxymethyl)guanine in patients with AIDS and other imunodeficiencies, *N. Engl. J. Med.*, **314**, 801.

181. Hooymans, J. M. M., Sprenger, H. G., and Weits, J. (1987) Treatment of cytomegalovirus retinitis with DHPG in a patient with AIDS, *Doc. Ophthalmol.*, **67**, 5.

182. Orellana, J., Teich, S. A., Friedman, A. H., Lerebours, F., Winterkorn, J., and Mildvan, D. (1987) Combined short- and long-term therapy for the treatment of cytomegalovirus retinitis using ganciclovir (BW B759U), *Ophthalmology*, **94**, 831.

183. Henderly, D. E., Freeman, W. R., Causey, D. M., and Rao, N. A. (1987) Cytomegalovirus retinitis and response to therapy with ganciclovir, *Ophthalmology*, **94**, 425.

184. Cantrill, H. L., Henry, K., Melroe, N. H., et al. (1989) Treatment of cytomegalovirus retinitis with intravitreal ganciclovir: long-term results, *Ophthalmology*, **96**, 367.

185. Felsenstein, D., d'Amico, D. J., Hirsch, M. S., et al. (1983) Treatment of cytomegalovirus retinitis with 9-[2-hydroxy-1- (hydroxymethyl)ethoxymethyl]guanine, *Ann. Intern. Med.*, **103**, 377.

186. Holland, G. N., Sidikaro, Y., Kreiger, A. E., et al. (1987) Treatment of cytomegalovirus retinopathy with ganciclovir, *Ophthalmology*, **94**, 815.

187. Jabs, D. A., Enger, C., and Bartlett, J. G. (1989) Cytomegalovirus retinitis and acquired immunodeficiency syndrome, *Arch. Ophthalmol.*, **107**, 75.

188. Jabs, D. A., Newman, C., de Bustros, S., and Polk, B. F. (1987) Treatment of cytomegalovirus retinitis with ganciclovir, *Ophthalmology*, **94**, 824.

189. Palestine, A. G., Stevens, G., Jr., Lane, H. C., et al. (1986) Treatment of cytomegalovirus retinitis with dihydroxy propoxymethyl guanine, *Am. J. Ophthalmol.*, **101**, 95.

190. Rosecan, L. R., Stahl-Bayliss, C. M., Kalman, C. M., and Laskin, O. L. (1986) Antiviral therapy for cytomegalovirus retinitis in AIDS with dihydroxy propoxymethyl guanine, *Am. J. Ophthal.*, **101**, 405.

191. Holland, G. N. and Shuler, J. D. (1992) Progression rates of cytomegalovirus retinopathy in ganciclovir-treated and untreated patients, *Arch. Ophthalmol.*, **110**, 1435.

192. Blini, M., Chiama, M., Plebani, A., and Bertoni, G. (1991) Use of intravitreal ganciclovir for cytomegalovirus (CMV) retinitis in a child with AIDS, *7th International Conference on AIDS Florence, Italy*, June 16–21, (abstract M.B.2369).

193. Neuwirth, J., Gutman, I., Hofeldt, A. J., et al. (1982) Cytomegalovirus retinitis in a young homosexual male with acquired immunodeficiency, *Ophthalmology*, **89**, 805.

194. Mar, E. C., Cheng, Y. C., and Huang, E.-S. (1983) Effect of 9-(1,3-dihydroxy-2-propoxymethyl)guanine on human cytomegalovirus replication in vitro, *Antimicrob. Agents Chemother.*, **24**, 518.

195. Kuppermann, B. D., Quiceno, J. I., Flores-Aguilar, M., et al. (1993) Intravitreal ganciclovir concentration after intravenous administration in AIDS patients with cytomegalovirus retinitis: application for therapy, *J. Infect. Dis.*, **168**, 1506.

196. Smith, I. L., Hong, C., Pilcher, M. L., Shapiro, A. M., Jiles, R. E., and Spector, S. A. (1998) Development of resistant cytomegalovirus genotypes during oral ganciclovir prophylaxis/preemptive therapy, *38th Interscience Conference on Antimicrobial Agents and Chemotherapy, San Diego, CA*, September 24–27 [abstract H-120].

197. Kupperman, B. D., Flores-Aguilar, M., Quiceno, J. I., Rickman, L. S., and Freeman, W. R. (1993) Combination ganciclovir and foscarnet in the treatment of clinically resistant cytomegalovirus retinitis in patients with acquired immunodeficiency syndrome, *Arch. Ophthalmol.*, **111**, 1359.

198. Flores-Aguilar, M., Kupperman, B. D., and Quiceno, J. I., et al. (1993) Pathophysiology and treatment of clinically resistant cytomegalovirus retinitis, *Ophthalmology*, **100**, 1022.

199. Dieterich, D. T., Poles, M. A., Lew, E. A., et al. (1993) Concurrent use of ganciclovir and foscarnet to treat cytomegalovirus infection in AIDS patients, *J. Infect. Dis.*, **167**, 1184.

200. Miccioli, C. and Belfort, R., Jr. (2000) Treatment of cytomegalovirus retinitis with an intraocular sustained-release ganciclovir implant, *Braz. J. Med. Biol. Res.*, **33**, 779–789.

201. Williamson, J. C., Virata, S. R., Raasch, R. H., and Kylstra, J. A. (2000) Oxacillin-resistant *Staphylococcus aureus* endophthalmitis after ganciclovir intraocular implant, *Am. J. Ophthalmol.*, **129**, 554–555.

202. Anduze-Faris, B. M., Fillet, A. M., Gozlan, J., et al. (2000) Induction and maintenance therapy of cytomegalovirus central nervous system infection in HIV-infected patients, *AIDS*, **14**, 517–524.

203. Hochster, H., Dieterch, D., Bozzette, S., et al. (1990) Toxicity of combined ganciclovir and zidovudine for cytomegalovirus disease associated with AIDS, *Ann. Intern. Med.*, **113**, 111.

204. Jacobson, M. A., de Miranda, P., Gordon, S. M., Blum, M. R., Volberding, P., and Mills, J. (1988) Prolonged pancytopenia due to combined ganciclovir and zidovudine therapy, *J. Infect. Dis.*, **158**, 489.

205. Millar, A. B., Miller, R. F., Patou, G., Mindel, A., Marsh, R., and Semple, S. J. G. (1990) Treatment of cytomegalovirus retinitis with zidovudine and ganciclovir in patients with AIDS: outcome and toxicity, *Genitourin. Med.*, **66**, 156.

206. Prichard, M. N., Prichard, L. E., Baguley, W. A., Nassiri, M. R., and Shipman, C., Jr. (1991) Three-dimensional analysis of the synergisitic cytotoxicity between ganciclovir and zidovudine, *Antimicrob. Agents Chemother.*, **35**, 1060.

207. Tian P. Y., Crouch, J. Y., and Hsiung, G. D. (1991) Combined antiviral effect and cytotoxicity of ganciclovir and azidothymidine against cytomegalovirus infection in cultured cells, *Antivir. Res. Suppl. 1*, **115**, abstract 134.

208. Medina, D. J., Hsiung, G. D., and Mellors, J. W. (1992) Ganciclovir antagonizes the anti-human immunodeficiency virus type 1 activity of zidovudine and didanosine in vitro, *Antimicrob. Agents Chemother.*, **36**, 1127–1130.

209. Causey, D. (1991) Concomitant ganciclovir and zidovudine treatment for cytomegalovirus retinitis in patients with HIV infection: an approach to treatment, *J. Acquir. Immune Defic. Syndr.*, **4**, 515.

210. Patel, J. E., Anderson, J. R., Duncombe, A. S., Carrington, D., and Murday, A. (1994) Granulocyte colony-stimulating factor: a new application for cytomegalovirus-induced neutropenia in cardiac allograft recipients, *Transplantation*, **58**, 863–867.

211. Hardy, D., Spector, S., Polsky, B., et al. (1994) Combination of ganciclovir and granulocyte-macrophage-colony-stimulating factor in the treatment of cytomegalovirus retinitis in AIDS patients, *Eur. J. Clin. Microbiol. Infect. Dis.*, **13**(Suppl. 2), S34.

212. Boivin, G. and LeBlanc, R. P. (2000) Clearance of cytomegalovirus viremia after initiation of highly active antiretroviral therapy, *J. Infect. Dis.*, **181**, 1216–1218.

213. Macdonald, J. C., Torriani, F. J., Morse, L. S., Karavellas, M. P., Reed, J. B., and Freeman, W. R. (1998) Lack of reactivation of cytomegalovirus (CMV) retinitis after stopping CMV maintenance therapy in AIDS patients with sustained elevations in CD4 T cells in response to highly active antiretroviral therapy, *J. Infect. Dis.*, **177**(5), 1182–1187.

214. O'Sullivan, C. E., Drew, W. L., McMullen, D. J., Miner, R., et al. (1999) Decrease of cytomegalovirus replication in human immunodeficiency virus-infected patients after treatment with highly active antiretroviral therapy, *J. Infect. Dis.*, **180**(3), 847–849.

215. Casado, J. L., Arrizabalaga, J., and Gutierrez, C. (1999) Risk of cytomegalovirus viremia and disease in HIV-infected patients with protease inhibitor treatment failure, *6th Conference on Retroviruses and Opportunistic Infections, Chicago, IL*, January 31–February 4, [abstract 458].

216. Arrizabalaga, J., Casado, J. L., Tural, C., et al. (1999) Incidence and risk factors for developing CMV retinitis in HIV-infected patients receiving protease inhibitor therapy, *6th Conference on Retroviruses and Opportunistic Infections, Chicago, IL*, January 31–February 4, [abstract 251].

217. Deayton, J., Mocroft, A., Wilson, P., Emery, V. C., Johnson, M. A., and Griffiths, P. D. (1998) Highly active antiretroviral therapy (HAART) including protease inhibitors can completely suppress asymptomatic CMV viremia in the absence of specific anti-CMV therapy, *38th Interscience Conference on Antimicrobial Agents and Chemotherapy, San Diego, CA*, September 24–27 [abstract I-268].

218. Verbraak, F. D., Boom, R., Wertheim-van Dillen, P. M., van den Horn, G. J., Kijlstra, A., and de Smet, M. D. (1999) Influence of highly active retroviral therapy on the development of CMV disease in HIV positive patients at high risk for CMV disease, *Br. J. Ophthalmol.*, **83**, 1186–1189.

219. Dunn, J. P. (1999) Discontinuation of maintenance CMV therapy in HAART responders, *Hopkins HIV Rep.*, **11**, 5.

220. Soriano, V., Dona, C., Rodriguez-Rosado, R., Barreiro, P., and Gonzalez-Lahoz, J. (2000) Discontinuation of secondary prophylaxis for opportunistic infections in HIV-infected patients receiving highly active antiretroviral therapy, *AIDS*, **14**, 383–386.

221. MacDonald, J. C., Karavellas, M. P., Torriano, F. J., et al. (2000) Highly active antiretroviral therapy-related immune recovery in AIDS patients with cytomegalovirus retinitis, *Ophthalmology*, **107**, 877–882.

222. Margolis, T. P. (2000) Discontinuation of anticytomegalovirus therapy in patients with HIV infection and cytomegalovirus, *Surv. Opthalmol.*, **44**, 455.

223. Labetoulle, M., Goujard, C., Frau, E., et al. (1999) Cytomegalovirus retinitis in advanced HIV-infected patients treated with protease inhibitors: incidence and outcome over 2 years, *J. Acquir. Immune Defic. Syndr.*, **22**, 228–234.

224. Jouan, M., Saves, M., Tubiana, R., et al. (1999) Restimop (ANRS 078): a prospective multicentre study to evaluate the discontinuation of maintenance therapy for CMV retinitis in HIV patients receiving HAART, *6th Conference on Retroviruses and Opportunistic Infections, Chicago, IL*, January 31–February 4, [abstract 256].

225. Chiller, T., Park, A., Chiller, K., Skiest, D., and Keiser, P. (1998) HIV protease inhibitor therapy is associated with increased time to relapse and death in AIDS patients with cytomegalovirus retinitis, *38th Interscience Conference on Antimicrobial Agents and Chemotherapy, San Diego, CA*, September 24–27 [abstract I-267].

226. Whitcup, S. M. (2000) Cytomegalovirus retinitis in the era of highly active retroviral therapy [clinical conference], *J. Am. Med. Assoc.*, **283**, 653–657.

227. Maschke, M., Kastrup, O., Esser, S., Ross, B., Hengge, U., and Hufnagel, A. (2000) Incidence and prevalence of neurological disorders associated with HIV since the introduction of highly active antiretroviral therapy (HAART), *J. Neurol. Neurosurg. Psychiatry*, **69**, 376–380.

228. Curran, M. and Noble, S. (2001) Valganciclovir, *Drugs*, **61**(8), 1145–1150; discussion: 1151–1152.

229. Georgiev, V. St. (2003) *Cryptosporidium* spp. In: *Opportunistic Infections: Treatment and Prophylaxis*, Humana Press, Totowa, NJ, pp. 143–157.

230. Berkowitz, C. D. (1985) AIDS and parasitic infections, including *Pneumocystis carinii* and cryptosporidiosis, *Pediatr. Clin. North Am.*, **32**, 933.

231. Current, W. L. and Blagburn, B. L. (1991) *Cryptosporidium* and microsporidia: some closing comments, *J. Protozool.*, **38**, 244S.

232. Current, W. L. and Garcia, L. S. (1991) Cryptosporidiosis, *Clin. Microbiol. Rev.*, **4**, 325.

233. Garcia, L. S. and Current, W. L. (1989) Cryptosporidiosis: clinical features and diagnosis, *Crit. Rev. Clin. Lab.*, **27**, 439.

234. Current, W. L. and Garcia, L. S. (1991) Cryptosporidiosis, *Clin. Lab. Med.*, **11**, 873.

235. Bhan, M. K., Bhandari, N., Bhatnagar, S., and Bahl, R. (1996) Epidemiology and management of persistent diarrhea in children in developing countries, *Indian J. Med. Res.*, **104**, 103.

236. Assefa, T., Mohammed, H., Abebe, A., Abebe, S., and Tafesse, B. (1996) Cryptosporidiosis in children seen at the children's clinic of Yakatit 12 Hospital, Addis Abeba, *Ethiop. Med. J.*, **34**, 43.

237. Fraser, D., Naggan, L., El-On, J., Deckelbaum, R. J., and Dagan, R. (1996) Risk factors for symptomatic and asymptomatic *Cryptosporidium* (CR) and *Giardia lamblia* (GL) infection in a cohort of Israeli Bedouin children, *36th Interscience Conference on Antimicrobial Agents and Chemotherapy, San Diego, CA*, September 24–27 [abstract K153].

238. Neill, M. A., Rice, S. K., Ahmad, N. V., and Flanigan, T. P. (1996) Cryptosporidiosis: an unrecognized cause of diarrhea in elderly hospitalized patients, *Clin. Infect. Dis.*, **22**, 168.

239. Gerba, C. P., Rose, J. B., and Haas, C. N. (1996) Sensitive populations: who is at the greatest risk? *Int. J. Food Microbiol.*, **30**, 113.

240. Poirot, J. L., Deluol, A. M., Antoine, M., et al. (1996) Bronchopulmonary cryptosporidiosis in four HIV-infected patients, *J. Eukariot. Microbiol.*, **43**, 78S.

241. Farthing, M. J., Kelly, M. P., and Veitch, A. M. (1996) Recently recognized microbial enteropathies and HIV infection, *J. Antimicrob. Chemother.*, **37**(Suppl. B), 61.

242. Greenberg, P. D., Koch, J., and Cello, J. P. (1996) Diagnosis of *Cryptosporidium parvum* in patients with severe diarrhea and AIDS, *Dig. Dis. Sci.*, **41**, 2286.

243. Manatsathit, S., Tansupaswaskul, S., Wanachiwanawin, D., et al. (1996) Causes of chronic diarrhea in patients with AIDS in Thailand: a prospective clinical and microbiological study, *J. Gastroenterol.*, **31**, 533.

244. Tarimo, D. S., Killewo, J. Z., Minjas, J. N., and Msamanga, G. I. (1996) Prevalence of intestinal parasites in adult patients with enteropathic AIDS in north-eastern Tanzania, *East Afr. Med. J.*, **73**, 397.

245. Ghorpade, M. V., Kulkarni, S. A., and Kulkarni, A. G. (1996) *Cryptosporidium*, *Isospora* and *Strongyloides* in AIDS, *Natl. Med. J. India*, **9**, 201.

246. Lanjewar, D. N., Rodrigues, C., Saple, D. G., Hira, S. K., and DuPont, H. L. (1996) *Cryptosporidium*, *Isospora* and *Strongyloides* in AIDS, *Natl. Med. J. India*, **9**, 17.

247. Dieng, T., Ndir, O., Diallo, S., Coll-Seck, A. M., and Dieng, Y. (1994) Prevalence of *Cryptosporidium* sp. and *Isospora belli* in patients with the acquired immunodeficiency syndrome (AIDS) in Dakar (Senegal), *Dakar Med.*, **39**, 121.

248. Gunthard, M., Meister, T., Luthy, R., and Weber, R. (1996) Intestinal cryptosporidiosis in HIV infection: clinical features, course and therapy, *Dtsch. Med. Wochenschr.*, **121**, 686.

249. Moolsart, P., Eampokalap, B., Ratanasrithong, M., Kanthasing, P., Tansupaswaskul, S., and Tanchanpong, C. (1995) Cryptosporidiosis in HIV infected patients in Thailand, *Southeast Asian J. Trop. Med. Public Health*, **26**, 335.

250. Esfandiari, A., Jordan, W. C., and Brown, C. P. (1995) Prevalence of enteric parasitic infection among HIV-infected attendees of an inner city AIDS clinic, *Cell. Mol. Biol. (Noisy-le-Grand)*, **41**(Suppl. 1), S19.

251. Lopez-Velez, R., Tarazona, R., Garcia Camacho, A. et al. (1995) Intestinal and extraintestinal cryptosporidiosis in AIDS patients, *Eur. J. Clin. Microbiol. Infect. Dis.*, **14**, 677.

252. Moon, H. W. and Woodmansee, D. B. (1986) Cryptosporidiosis, *J. Am. Vet. Med. Assoc.*, **189**, 643.

253. Angus, K. W. (1983) Cryptosporidiosis in man, domestic animals and birds: a review, *J. R. Soc. Med.*, **76**, 62.

254. Forgacs, P., Tarshis, A., Ma, P., et al. (1983) Intestinal and bronchial cryptosporidiosis in an immunodeficient homosexual man, *Ann. Intern. Med.*, **99**, 793.

255. Guarda, L. A., Stein, S. A., Cleary, K. A., and Ordonez, N. G. (1983) Human cryptosporidiosis in the acquired immune deficiency syndrome, *Arch. Pathol. Lab. Med.*, **107**, 562.

256. Pitlik, S. D., Fainstein, V., Rios, A., Guarda, L., Mansell, P. W. A., and Hersh, E. M. (1983) Cryptosporidial cholecystitis, *N. Engl. J. Med.*, **308**, 967.

257. Blumberg, R. S., Kelsey, P., Perrone, T., Dickersin, R., Laguaglia, M., and Ferruci, J. (1984) Cytomegalovirus- and *Cryptosporidium*-associated acalculous gangrenous cholesystitis, *Am. J. Med.*, **76**, 1118.

258. French, A. L., Beaudet, L. M., Benator, D. A., Levy, C. S., Kassa, M., and Orenstein, J. M. (1995) Cholecystectomy in patients with AIDS: clinicopathologic correlations in 107 cases, *Clin. Infect. Dis.*, **21**, 852.

259. Mifsud, A. J., Bell, D., and Shafi, M. S. (1994) Respiratory cryptosporidiosis as a presenting feature of AIDS, *J. Infect.*, **28**, 227.

260. Talens, A., Montoya, E., Cubells, M. L., et al. (1996) Acute pancreatitis and acquired immunodeficiency syndrome, *Rev. Esp. Enferm. Dig.*, **88**, 155.

261. Rose, J. B. (1988) Occurrence and significance of *Cryptosporidium* in the water, *J. Am. Water Works Assoc.*, **80**, 53.

262. Dworkin, M. S., Goldman, D. P., Wells, T. G., Kobayashi, J. M., and Herwaldt, B. L. (1996) Cryptosporidiosis in Washington State: an outbreak associated with well water, *J. Infect. Dis.*, **174**, 1372.

263. Kuroki, T., Watanabe, Y., Asai, Y., et al. (1996) An outbreak of waterborne cryptosporidiosis in Kanagawa, Japan, *Kansenshogaku Zasshi*, **70**, 132.

264. Osewe, P., Addiss, D. G., Blair, K. A., Hightower, A., Kamb, M. L., and Davis, J. P. (1996) Cryptosporidiosis in Wisconsin: a case-control study of post-outbreak transmission, *Epidemiol. Infect.*, **117**, 297.

265. Addiss, D. G., Pond, R. S., Remshak, M., Juranek, D. D., Stokes, S., and Davis, J. P. (1996) Reduction of risk of watery diarrhea with point-of-use water filters during a massive outbreak of waterborne *Cryptosporidium* infection in Milwaukee, Wisconsin, 1993, *Am. J. Trop. Med. Hyg.*, **54**, 549.

266. Goldstein, S. T., Juranek, D. D., Ravenholt, O., et al. (1996) Cryptosporidiosis: an outbreak associated with drinking water despite state-of-the-art water treatment, *Ann. Intern. Med.*, **124**, 459.

267. Kramer, M. H., Herwaldt, B. L., Craun, G. F., Calderon, R. L., and Juranek, D. D. (1996) Surveillance for waterborne-disease outbreaks – United States, 1993–1994, *Morb. Mortal. Wkly. Rep. [CDC Surveil. Summ.]*, **45**, 1.

268. Bridgman, S. A., Robertson, R. M., Syed, O., Speed, N., Andrews, N., and Hunter, P. R. (1995) Outbreak of cryptosporidiosis associated with a disinfected groundwater supply, *Epidemiol. Infect.*, **115**, 555.

269. Mackenzie, W. R., Kazmierczak, J. J., and Davis, J. P. (1995) An outbreak of cryptosporidiosis associated with a resort swimming pool, *Epidemiol. Infect.*, **115**, 545.

270. Fayer, R. and Nerad, T. (1996) Effects of low temperature on viability of *Cryptosporidium parvum* oocysts, *Appl. Environ. Microbiol.*, **62**, 1431.

271. Fayer, R., Trout, J., and Nerad, T. (1996) Effects of a wide range of temperatures on the infectivity of *Cryptosporidium parvum* oocysts, *J. Eukaryot. Microbiol.*, **43**, 64S.

272. Shepherd, K. M. and Wyn-Jones, A. P. (1996) An evaluation of methods for the simulateneous detection of *Cryptosporidium* oocysts and *Giardia* cysts from water, *Appl. Environ. Microbiol.*, **62**, 1317–1322.

273. Drozd, C. and Schwartzbrod, J. (1996) Hydrophobic and electrostatic cell surface properties of *Cryptosporidium parvum*, *Appl. Environ. Microbiol.*, **62**, 1227–1232.

274. Rochelle, P. A., Ferguson, D. M., Handojo, T. J., De Leon, R., Stewart, M. H., and Wolfe, R. L. (1996) Development of a rapid detection procedure for *Cryptosporidium*, using in vitro cell culture combined with PCR, *J. Eukaryot. Microbiol.*, **43**, 72S.

275. Abrahamsen, M. S., Templeton, T. J., Enomoto, S., Abrahante, J. A., et al. (2004) Complete genome sequence of the Apicomplexan, *Cryptosporidium parvum*, *Science*, **304**(5669), 441–445.

276. Anderson, B. C., Donndelinger, T., Wilkins, R. M., and Smith, J. (1982) Cryptosporidiosis in a veterinary student, *J. Am. Vet. Med. Assoc.*, **180**, 498.

277. Baxby, D., Hart, C. A., and Blundell, N. (1985) Shedding of oocysts by immunocompetent individuals with cryptosporidiosis, *J. Hyg.*, **95**, 708.

278. Brasseur, P., Lemeteil, D., and Mallet, E. (1987) La cryptosporidiose chez l'enfant immunocompetent, *Presse Med.*, **16**, 177.

279. Current, W. L., Reese, N. C., Ernest, J. V., Bailey, W. S., Heyman, M. B., and Weinstein, W. M. (1983) Cryptosporidiosis in immunocompetent and immunodeficient persons, *N. Engl. J. Med.*, **308**, 1252.

280. Laurent, F., McCole, D., Eckmann, L., and Kagnoff, M. F. (1999) Pathogenesis of *Cryptosporidium parvum* infection, *Microbes Infect.*, **1**, 141–148.

281. Navin, T. R. and Juranek, D. D. (1984) Cryptosporidiosis: clinical, epidemiologic and parasitologic review, *Rev. Infect. Dis.*, **6**, 313.

282. Reese, N. C., Current, W. L., Ernest, J. V., and Bailey, W. S. (1982) Cryptosporidiosis of man and calf: a case report and results of experimental infections in mice and rats, *Am. J. Trop. Med. Hyg.*, **31**, 226.

283. Casemore, D. P. (1988) The epidemiology of human cryptosporidiosis. In: *Cryptosporidiosis, Proc. 1st Int. Workshop, Edinburgh, U.K.* (Angus, K. W. and Blewett, D. A., eds.), Moredun Research Institute Edinburgh, p. 65.

284. Malla, N., Sehgal, R., Ganguly, N. K., and Mahajan, R. C. (1989) Cryptosporidiosis – the Indian scene, *Indian J. Pediatr.*, **56**, 6.

285. Hoepelman, A. I. (1996) Current therapeutic approaches to cryptosporidiosis in immunocompromised patients, *J. Antimicrob. Chemother.*, **37**, 871.

286. Colford, J. M., Jr., Tager, I. B., Hirozawa, A. M., Lemp, G. F., Aragon, T., and Petersen, C. (1996) Cryptosporidiosis among patients infected with human immunodeficiency virus: factors related to symptomatic infection and survival, *Am. J. Epidemiol.*, **144**, 807.

287. Heyworth, M. F. (1996) Parasitic diseases in immunocompromised hosts: cryptosporidiosis, isosporiasis, and strongyloidasis, *Gastroeneterol. Clin. North Am.*, **25**, 691.

288. Ballal, M., Prabhu, T., Chandran, A., and Shivananda, P. G. (1999) *Cryptosporidium* and *Isospora belli* diarrhea in immunocompromised hosts, *Indian J. Cancer.*, **36**, 38–42.

289. Issacs, D. (1985) *Cryptosporidium* and diarrhea, *Arch. Dis. Child.*, **60**, 608.

290. Malenbranche, R., Arnous, E., Guerin, J. M., et al. (1983) Acquired immunodeficiency syndrome with severe gastrointestinal manifestations, *Lancet*, **2**, 873.

291. Vakil, N. B., Schwartz, S. M., Buggy, B. P., et al. (1996) Biliary cryptosporidiosis in HIV-infected people after waterborne outbreak of cryptosporidiosis in Milwaukee, *N. Engl. J. Med.*, **334**, 19.

292. Lasser, K. H., Lewin, K. J., and Ryning, F. W. (1979) Cryptosporidial enteritis in a patient with congenital hypogammaglobulinaemia, *Hum. Pathol.*, **10**, 234.

293. Sloper, K. S., Dourmashkin, R. R., Bird, R. B., Slavin, G., and Webster, A. D. B. (1982) Chronic malabsorption due to cryptosporidiosis in a child with immunoglobulin deficiency, *Gut*, **23**, 80.

294. Tzipori, S., Robertson, D., and Chapman, C. (1986) Remission of diarrhea due to cryptosporidiosis in an immunodeficient child treated with hyperimmune bovine colostrums, *Br. Med. J.*, **293**, 1276.

295. Kocoshis, S. A., Cibull, M. L., Davis, T. E., Hinton, J. T., Seip, M., and Banwell, J. G. (1984) Intestinal and pulmonary cryptosporidiosis in an infant with severe combined immunoglobulin deficiency, *J. Pediatr. Gastroenterol. Nutr.*, **3**, 149.

296. Miller, R. A., Holmberg, R. E., and Clausen, C. R. (1983) Life-threatening diarrhea caused by *Cryptosporidium* in a child undergoing therapy for acute lymphocytic leukaemia, *J. Pediatr.*, **103**, 256.

297. Lewis, I. J., Hart, C. A., and Baxby, D. (1985) Diarrhoea due to *Cryptosporidium* in acute lymphoblastic leukaemia, *Arch. Dis. Child.*, **60**, 60–62.

298. Foot, A. B., Oakhill, A., and Mott, M. G. (1990) Cryptosporidiosis and acute leukaemia, *Arch. Dis. Child.*, **65**, 236.

299. Gentile, G., Venditti, M., Micozzi, A., et al. (1991) Cryptosporidiosis in patients with hematologic malignancies, *Rev. Infect. Dis.*, **13**, 842.

300. Weisburger, W. R., Hutcheon, D. F., Yardley, J. H., Roche, J. C., Hillis, W. D., and Charache, P. (1979) Cryptosporidiosis in an immunosuppressed renal-transplant recipient with IgA deficiency, *Am. J. Clin. Pathol.*, **72**, 473.

301. Griffiths, J. K. (1988) Treatment for AIDS-associated cryptosporidiosis, *J. Infect. Dis.*, **178**, 915–916.

302. Connolly, G. M., Dryden, M. S., Shanson, D. C., and Gizzard, B. G. (1988) Cryptosporidial diarrhea in AIDS and its treatment, *Gut*, **29**, 593.

303. Soave, R. and Johnson, W. D., Jr., (1988) *Cryptosporidium* and *Isospora belli* infections, *J. Infect. Dis.*, **157**, 225.

304. Hudson, R. (1989) No treatment for cryptosporidiosis in AIDS patients, *J. Am. Osteopath.*, **89**, 716.

305. Soave, R. (1990) Treatment strategies for cryptosporidiosis, *Ann. N.Y. Acad. Sci.*, **616**, 442–451.

306. Georgiev, V. St. (1993) Opportunistic infections: treatment and developmental therapeutics of cryptosporidiosis and isosporiasis, *Drug Dev. Res.*, **28**, 445–459.

307. Sterling, C. R. (2000) Cryptosporidiosis: the treatment dilemma, *J. Med. Microbiol.*, **49**, 207–208.

308. Centers for Disease Control and Prevention (1982) Cryptosporidiosis: assessment of chemotherapy of males with acquired immunodeficiency syndrome (AIDS), *Morb. Mortal. Wkly. Rep.*, **31**, 589.

309. U.S. Public Health Service (USPHS) and Infectious Diseases Society of America (IDSA) (2000) 1999 USPHS/IDSA guidelines for the prevention of opportunistic infections in persons infected with human immunodeficiency virus, *Infect. Dis. Obstet. Gynecol.*, **8**, 5–74.

310. Holmberg, S. D., Moorman, A. C., Von Bargen, J. C., et al. (1998) Possible effectiveness of clarithromycin and rifabutin for cryptosporidiosis chemoprophylaxis in HIV disease, *J. Am. Med. Assoc.*, **279**, 384–386.

311. Brasseur, P., Lemeteil, D., and Ballet, J. J.(1991), Anti-cryptosporidial activity screened with an immunosuppressed rat model, *J. Protozool.*, **38**, 230S.

312. Gross, T. L., Wheat, J., Bartlett, M., and O'Connor, K. W. (1986) AIDS and multiple system involvement with *Cryptosporidium*, *Am. J. Gastroenterol.*, **8**, 456.

313. Pilla, A. M., Rybak, M. J., and Chandrasekar, P. H. (1987) Spiramycin in the treatment of cryptosporidiosis, *Pharmacotherapy*, **7**, 188.

314. Centers for Disease Control (1984) Update: treatment of cryptosporidiosis in patients with acquired immunodeficiency syndrome (AIDS), *Morb. Mortal. Wkly Rep.*, **33**, 117.

315. Portnoy, D., Whiteside, M. E., Buckley, E., and MacLeod, C. L. (1984) Treatment of intestinal cryptosporidiosis with spiramycin, *Ann. Intern. Med.*, **101**, 202.

316. Decaux, G. M. and Devroeda, C. (1978) Acute colitis related to spiramycin, *Lancet*, **2**, 993.

317. Moskovitz, B. L., Stanton, T. L., and Kusmierek, J. J. (1988) Spiramycin therapy for cryptosporidial diarrhoea in immunocompromised patients, *J. Antimicrob. Chemother.*, **22** (Suppl. B), 189.

318. Collier, A. C., Miller, P. A., and Meyers, J. D. (1984) Cryptosporidiosis after marrow transplantation: person-to-person transmission and treatment with spiramycin, *Ann. Intern. Med.*, **101**, 205.

319. Mead, G. M., Sweetenham, J. W., Ewins, D. L., Furlong, M., and Lowes, J. A. (1986) Intestinal cryptosporidiosis: a complication of cancer treatment, *Cancer Treat. Rep.*, **70**, 769.

320. Fafard, J. and Lalonde, R. (1990) Long-standing symptomatic cryptosporidiosis in a normal man: clinical response to spiramycin, *J. Clin. Gastroenterol.*, **12**, 190.

321. Galvano, G., Cattaneo, G., and Reverso-Giovantin, E. (1993) Chronic diarrhea due to *Cryptosporidium*: the efficacy of spiramycin treatment, *Pediatr. Med. Chir.*, **15**, 297.

322. Wilmsmeyer, B., Dopfer, R., Hoppe, J. E., and Niethammer, D. (1993) Cryptosporidium enteritis, *Monatsschr. Kinderheilkd.*, **141**, 130.

323. Descotes, J., Vial, T., Delattre, D., and Evreux, J.-C. (1988) Spiramycin: safety in man, *J. Antimicrob. Chemother*, **22**, 207.

324. Kotler, D. P., Gaetz, H. P., Lange, M., Klein, E. B., and Holt, P. R. (1984) Enteropathy associated with the acquired immunodeficiency syndrome, *Ann. Intern. Med.*, **101**, 421.

325. Saez-Llorens, X., Odio, C. M., Umana, M. A., and Morales, M. V. (1989) Spiramycin vs. placebo for treatment of acute diarrhea caused by *Cryptosporidium*, *Pediatr. Infect. Dis. J.*, **8**, 136.

326. Saez-Llorens, X. (1989) Spiramycin for treatment of *Cryptosporidium* enteritis, *J. Infect. Dis.*, **160**, 342.

327. Connolly, G. M., Dryden, M. S., Shanson, D. C., and Gazzard, B. G. (1988) Cryptosporidial diarrhoea in AIDS and its treatment, *Gut*, **29**, 593.

328. Casemore, D.P., Sands, R. L., and Curry, A. (1985) *Cryptosporidium* species: a "new" human pathogen, *J. Clin. Pathol.*, **38**, 1321.

329. Woolf, G. M., Townsend, M., and Guyatt, G. (1987) Treatment of cryptosoridiosis with spiramycin in AIDS: an "N of 1," *J. Clin. Gastroenterol.*, **9**, 632.

330. Wittenberg, D. F., Miller, N. M., and van den Ende, J. (1989) Spiramycin is not effective in treating *Cryptosporidium* diarrhea in infants: results of a double-blind rendomized trial, *J. Infect. Dis.*, **159**, 131.

331. Wittenberg, D. F. (1989), Spiramycin for treatment of *Cryptosporidium* enteritis, *J. Infect. Dis.*, **160**, 342.

332. Berkowitz, C. D. and Seidel, J. S. (1985) Spontaneous resolution of cryptosporidiosis in a child with acquired immunodeficiency syndrome, *Am. J. Dis. Child.*, **139**, 967.

333. Current, W. L. (1986) *Cryptosporidium: Its Biology and Potential for Environmental Transmission [CRC Crit. Rev. Environ. Control, vol. 17]*, p. 21.

334. Weikel, C., Lazenby, A., Belitsos, P., McDewitt, M., Fleming, H. E. Jr., and Barbacci, M. (1991) Intestinal injury associated with spiramycin therapy of *Cryptosporidium* infection in AIDS, *J. Protozool.*, **38**, 147S.

335. Soave, R. (1988) Cryptosporidiosis and isosporiasis in patients with AIDS, *Infect. Dis. Clin. North Am.*, **2**, 485.

336. Chen, X. M., Keithly, J. S., Paya, C. V., and LaRusso, N. F. (2002) Cryptosporidiosis, *N. Engl. J. Med.*, **346**(22), 1723–1731 [comments in *N. Engl. J. Med.*, **347**(16), 1287 (2002)].

337. Dupont, C., Bougnoux, M. E., Turner, L., Rouveix, E., and Dorra, M. (1996) Microbiological findings about pulmonary cryptosporidiosis in two AIDS patients, *J. Clin. Microbiol.*, **34**, 227.

338. Hicks, P., Zwiener, R. J., Squires, J., and Savell, V. (1996) Azithromycin therapy for *Cryptosporidium parvum* infection in four children infected with human immunodeficiency virus, *J. Pediatr.*, **129**, 297.

339. Vargas, S. L., Shenep, J. L., Flynn, P. M., Pui, C. H., Santana, V. M., and Hughes, W. T. (1993) Azithromycin for treatment of severe *Cryptosporidium* diarrhea in two children with cancer, *J. Pediatr.*, **123**, 154.

340. Jordan, W. C. (1996) Clarithromycin prophylaxis against *Cryptosporidium* enteritis in patients with AIDS, *J. Natl. Med. Assoc.*, **88**, 425.

341. Holmberg, S. D., Moorman, A. C., Von Bargen, J. C., Palella, F. J., Loveless, M. O., and Navin, T. R. (1997) Apparent chemoprophylaxis of cryptosporidiosis with clarithromycin and rifabutin, *4th Conference on Retroviruses and Opportunistic Infections,Washington, D.C.*, January 22–26 [191, abstract 685].

342. Tzipori, S., Rand, W., Griffiths, J., Widmer, G., and Crabb, J. (1994) Evaluation of an animal model system for cryptosporidiosis: therapeutic efficacy of paromomycin and hyperimmune bovine colostrum-immunoglobulin, *Clin. Diagn. Lab. Immunol.*, **1**, 450.

343. Cirioni, O., Giacometti A., Balducci, M., Drenaggi, D., Del Prete, M. S., and Scallise, G. (1995) Anticryptosporidial activity of paromomycin, *J. Infect. Dis.*, **172**, 1169.

344. Verdon, R., Polianski, J., Gaudebout, C., and Pocidalo, J. J. (1995) Paromomycin for cryptosporidiosis in AIDS, *J. Infect. Dis.*, **171**, 1070;1071.

345. Tsipori, S., Griffiths, J., and Theodus, C. (1995) Paromomycin treatment against cryptosporidiosis in patients with AIDS, *J. Infect. Dis.*, **171**, 1069;1071.

346. Mancassola, R., Reperant, J. M., Naciri, M., and Chartier, C. (1995) Chemoprophylaxis of *Cryptosporidium parvum* infection with paromomycin in kids and immunological study, *Antimicrob. Agents Chemother.*, **39**, 75.

347. Jimenez-Beatty Navarro, M. D., de la Fuente Aguado, J., Sopena Arguelles, B., and Martinez Vazquez, C. (1995) Paromomycin in the treatment of cryptosporidiosis, *Rev. Clin. Esp.*, **195**, 62.

348. Healey, M. C., Yang, S., Rasmussen, K. R., Jackson, M. K., and Du, C. (1995) Therapeutic efficacy of paromomycin in immunosuppressed adult mice infected with *Cryptosporidium parvum*, *J. Parasitol.*, **81**, 114.

349. Mohri, H., Fujita, H., Asakura, Y., Katoh, K., Okamoto, R., Tanabe, J., Harano, H., Noguchi, T., Inayama, Y., and Amano, T. (1995) Case report: inhalation therapy of paromomycin is effective for respiratory infection and hypoxia by cryptosporidium with AIDS, *Am. J. Med. Sci.*, **309**, 60.

350. Verdon, R., Polianski, J., Gaudebout, C., Marche, C., Garry, L., and Pocidalo, J.-J. (1994) Evaluation of curative anticryptosporidial activity of paromomycin in a dexamethasone-treated rat model, *Antimicrob. Agents Chemother.*, **38**, 1681.

351. Scaglia, M., Atzori, C., Marchetti, G., Orso, M., Maserati, R., Orani, A., Novati, S., and Olliaro, P. (1994) Effectiveness of aminosidine (paromomycin) sulfate in chronic *Cryptosporidium* diarrhea in AIDS patients: an open, uncontrolled, prospective clinical trial, *J. Infect. Dis.*, **170**, 1349.

352. Rehg, J. E. (1994) A comparison of anticryptosporidial activity of paromomycin with that of other aminoglycosides and azithromycin in immunosuppressed rats, *J. Infect. Dis.*, **170**, 934.

353. Youssef, M. M., Hammam, S. M., Abou Samra, L. M., and Khalifa, A. M. (1994) Aminosidine sulphate in experimental cryptosporidiosis, *J. Egypt. Soc. Parasitol.*, **24**, 239.

354. White, A. C. Jr., Chappell, C. L., Hayat, C. S., Kimball, K. T., Flanigan, T. P., and Goodgame, R. W. (1994) Paromomycin for cryptosporidiosis in AIDS: a prospective, double-blind trial, *J. Infect. Dis.*, **170**, 419.

355. Forester, G., Sidhom, O., Nahass, R., and Andavolu, R. (1994) AIDS-associated cryptosporidiosis with gastric structure and a therapeutic response to paromomycin, *Am. J. Gastroenterol.*, **89**, 1096.

356. Wallace, M. R., Nguyen, M. T., and Newton, J. A., Jr. (1993) Use of paromomycin for the treatment of cryptosporidiosis in patients with AIDS, *Clin. Infect. Dis.*, **17**, 1070.

357. Anand, A. (1993) Cryptosporidiosis in patients with AIDS, *Clin. Infect. Dis.*, **17**, 297.

358. Fichtenbaum, C. J., Ritchie, D. J., and Powderly, W. G. (1993) Use of paromomycin for treatment of cryptosporidiosis in patients with AIDS, *Clin. Infect. Dis.*, **16**, 298.

359. Goodgame, R. W., Genta, R. M., White, A. C., and Chappell, C. L. (1993) Intensity of infection in AIDS-associated cryptosporidiosis, *J. Infect. Dis.*, **167**, 704.

360. Hewitt, R. G., Yiannoutsos, C. T., Carey, J., Geiseler, P. J., Soave, R., Rosenberg, R., Vazquez, G. J., Wheta, J., Fass, R. J., Higgs, E. S., Antoninjevic, Z., Walawander, A. L., Flanigan, T., and Bender, J. (1997) A double-blind, placebo-controlled trial of paromomycin for the treatment of cryptosporidiosis in patients with advanced HIV disease and CD4 counts under 150 (ACTG 192),

361. Bowers, M. (1998) Nitazoxanide for cryptosporidial diarrhea, *BETA (April)*, 30–31.

362. Bornhoeft, M. A. (1998) Cryptosporidiosis gets a new treatment, *Body Posit.*, **XI**(3), 13.

363. James, J. S. (1998) NTZ: advisory committee votes against approval, *AIDS Treat. News*, (No. 295), 7.

364. James, J. S. (1998) Prospective case series in clinical trial design – proposal, and NTZ example, *AIDS Treat. News*, (No. 296), 5–6.

365. Baker, R. (1998) FDA panel rejects drug for cryptosporidial diarrhea. Food and Drug Administration, *BETA (July)*, 7.

366. Roehr, B. (1998) Another failed promise? NTZ gets the nix, *J. Int. Assoc. Physicians AIDS Care*, **4**, 26–27; 29.

367. Learned, J. (1998) NTZ—still promising but Unimed walks, *Notes Undergr.* (No. 37), 10.

368. Cadman, J. (1998) Diarrhea drug rejection raises a ruckus, *GMHC Treat Issues*, **12**, 1–3.

369. Amenta, M., Dalle Nogare, E. R., Colomba, C., Prestileo, T. S., Di Lorenzo, F., Fundaro, S., Colomba, A., and Ferrieri, A. (1999) Intestinal protozoa in HIV- infected patients: effect of rifaximin. *Cryptosporidium parvum* and *Blastocystis hominis* infections, *J. Chemother.*, **11**, 391–395.

370. Morrison, L. (1998) Cryptosporidiosis. In: *The OI Report: A Critical Review of the Treatment & Prophylaxis of AIDS-Related Opportunistic Infections (OIs)*, Treatment Action Group (http://aidsinfonyc.org/tag/comp/ois98/index.html).

371. Soave, R., Dieterich, D., Kotler, D., Gassyuk, E., Tierney, A. R., Liebes, L., and Legendre, R. (1990) Oral diclazuril therapy for cryptosporidiosis, *6th International Conference on AIDS, San Francisco, CA*, June 20–24 [6: 252, abstract Th.B 520].

372. Walach , C., Loeb, M., Phillips, J., Salit, I., Rachlis, A., Fong, I., and Walmsley, S. (1993) Use of letrazuril in refractory cryptosporidiosis in AIDS, *9th International Conference on AIDS, Berlin, Germany*, June 6–11 [9: 380 abstract PO-B10-1472].

373. Sheppard, M., Shapiro, B., Pimstone, B., Kronheim, M. B., and Gregory, M. (1979) The metabolic clearance and plasma half disappearance time of exogenous somatostatin in man, *J. Clin. Endocrinol. Metab.*, **49**, 50–53.

374. Bauer, W., Briner, U., Doepfner, W., Haller, R., Huguenin, R., Marbach, P., Petcher, T. J., and Pless, J. (1982) SMS 201–995: a very potent and selective octapeptide analogue of somatostatin with prolonged action, *Life Sci.*, **31**, 1133.

375. Longnecker, S. M. (1988) Somatostatin and octreotide: literature review and description of therapeutic activity in pancreatic neoplasia, *Drug Intell. Clin. Pharm.*, **22**, 99–106.

376. Gaginella, T. S. and O'Dorisio, T. M. (1988) Octreotide: entering the new era of peptodomimetic therapy, *Drug Intell. Clin. Pharm.*, **22**, 154.

377. Santangelo, W. C., O'Dorisio, T. M., Kim, J. G., Severino, G., and Krejs, G. (1986) VIPoma syndrome: effect of a synthetic somatostatin analogue, *Scand. J. Gastroenterol.*, **21**, 187.

378. Gorden, P. (1989) Somatostatin and somatostatin analogue (SMS 201–995) in the treatment of hormone-secreting tumors of the pituitary and gastrointestinal tract and non-neoplastic diseases of the gut, *Ann. Intern. Med.*, **110**, 35.

379. Katz, M. D., Erstad, B. L., and Rose, C. (1988) Treatment of severe *Cryptosporidium*-related diarrhea with octreotide in a patient with AIDS, *Drug Intell. Clin. Pharm.*, **22**, 134.

380. Cello, J. P., Grendell, J. H., Basuk, P., Simon, D., Weiss, L., Rood, R., Wilcox, C., Forsmark, C., Read, A., Satow, J., Weikel, C., and Beaumont, C. (1990) Controlled clinical trial of octreotide (sandostatin) for refractory AIDS-associated diarrhea, *Gastroenterology*, **98**, A163.

381. Fanning, M., Monte, M., Sutherland, L. R., Broadhead, M., Murphy, G. F., and Harris, A. G. (1991) Pilot study of sandostatin

4th Conference on Retroviruses and Opportunistic Infections, Washington, D.C., January 22–26 [65, abstract 4].

(octreotide) therapy of refractory HIV-associated diarrhea, *Dig. Dis. Sci.*, **36**, 476.

382. Moroni, M., Esposito, R., Cernuschi, M., Franzetti, F., Carosi, G. P., and Fiori, G. P. (1993) Treatment of AIDS-related refractory diarrhoea with octreotide, *Digestion*, **54**(Suppl. 1), 30.

383. Crawford, F. G. and Vermund, S. H. (1988) Human cryptosporidiosis, *CRC. Crit. Rev. Microbiol.*, **16**, 113.

384. Nelson, J. A., Wiley, C. A., Reynolds-Kohler, C., Reese, C. E., Margaretten, W., and Levy, J. A. (1988) Human immunodeficiency virus detected in bowel epithelium from patients with gastrointestinal symptoms, *Lancet*, **1**, 259.

385. Levy, J. A., Margaretten, W., and Nelson, J. (1989) Detection of HIV in enterochromaffin cells in the rectal mucosa of an AIDS patient, *Am. J. Gastroenterol.*, **84**, 787.

386. Bigornia, E., Simon, D., Weiss, L., Tanowitz, H., Jones, J., Wittner, M., and Lyman, W. (1990) Detection of HIV-1 viral protein and genomic sequences in enterochromaffin cells of HIV-1-seropositive patients, *Am. J. Gastroenterol.*, **85**, 1264.

387. Kreinik, G., Burstein, O., Landor, M., Bernstein, L., Weiss, L. M., and Wittner, M. (1991) Successful management of intractable cryptosporidial diarrhea with intravenous octreotide, a somatostatin analogue, *AIDS*, **5**, 765–767.

388. Ruff, M. R., Martin, B. M., Guins, E. I., Farrar, W. L., and Pert, C.B. (1987) CD4 receptor-binding peptides that block HIV infectivity cause human monocyte chemotaxis: relationship to vasoactive intestinal polypeptide, *FEBS Lett.*, **211**, 17.

389. Gaginella, T. S., Hubel, K. A., and O'Dorisio, T. M. (1982) Vasoactive intestinal polypeptide and intestinal chloride secretion. In: *Vasoactive Intestinal Peptide* (Said, I., ed.), Raven Press, New York, p. 211.

390. Friedman, L. S. (1991) Somatostatin therapy for AIDS diarrhea: muddy waters, *Gastroenterology*, **101**, 1446.

391. Kotler, D. P. (1987) Preliminary observations of the effect of cow's milk globulin upon intestinal cryptosporidiosis in AIDS, *3rd International Conference on AIDS, Washington D.C.*, January 22–26, abstract.

392. Saxon, A. and Weinstein, W. (1987) Oral administration of bovine colostrum anti- cryptosporidia antibody fails to alter the course of human cryptosporidiosis, *J. Parasitol.*, **73**, 413.

393. Anonymous (1998) Jarrow formulas: "colostrums specific" for cryprosporidiosis, *Posit. Health News*, (17), 22.

394. Tzipori, S., Robertson, D., Chapman, C., and White, L. (1987) Chronic cryptosporidial diarrhoea and hyperimmune cow colostrum, *Lancet*, **2**, 344.

395. Ungar, B. L. P., Ward, D. J., Fayer, R., and Quinn, C. A. (1990) Cessation of *Cryptosporidium*-associated diarrhea in an acquired immunodeficiency syndrome patient after treatment with hyperimmune bovine colostrum, *Gastroenterology*, **98**, 486.

396. Nord, J., Ma, P., DiJohn, D., Tzipori, S., and Tacket, C.O. (1990) Treatment with bovine hyperimmune colostrum of cryptosporidial diarrhea in AIDS patients, *AIDS*, **4**, 581.

397. Mietens, C., Keinhorst, H., Hilpert, H., Gerber, H., Amster, H., and Pahud, J. J. (1979) Treatment of infantile *E. coli* gastroenteritis with specific bovine anti-*E. coli* milk immunoglobulins, *Eur. J. Pediatr.*, **132**, 239.

398. Brussow, H., Hilpert, H., Walther, I., Sidoti, J., Mietens, C., and Bachmann, P. (1987) Bovine milk immunoglobulin for passive immunity to infantile rotavirus gastroenteritis, *J. Clin. Microbiol.*, **25**, 982.

399. Hilpert, H., Brussow, H., Mietens, C., Sidoti, J., Lerner, L., and Werchau, H. (1987) Use of bovine milk concentrate containing antibody to rotavirus to treat rotavirus gastroenteritis in infants, *J. Infect. Dis.*, **156**, 158.

400. Tacket, C. O., Losonsky, G., Link, H., Hoany, Y., Guersy, P., Hilpert, H., and Levine, M. M. (1988) Protection by milk immunoglobulin concentrate against oral challenge with enterotoxigenic *Escherichia coli*, *N. Engl. J. Med.*, **318**, 1240.

401. Perryman, L. E., Riggs, M. W., Mason, P. H., and Fayer, R. (1990) Kinetics of *Cryptosporidium parvum* sporozoite neutralization by monoclonal antibodies, immune bovine serum, and immune bovine colostral antibodies, *Infect. Immun.*, **58**, 257.

402. McMeeking, A., Borkowsky, W., Klesius, P. H., Bonk, S., Holzman, R. S., and Lawrence, H. S. (1990) A controlled trial of bovine dialyzable leukocyte extract for cryptosporidiosis in patients with AIDS, *J. Infect. Dis.*, **161**, 108.

403. Louie, E., Borkowsky, W., Klesius, P. H., Haynes, T. B., Gordon, S., Bonk, S., and Lawrence, H. S. (1987) Treatment of cryptosporidiosis with oral bovine transfer factor, *Clin. Imunol. Immunopathol.*, **44**, 329.

404. Borkowsky, W. and Lawrence, H. S. (1983) Antigen-specific inducer factor in human leukocyte dialysates: a product of T_H cells which binds to anti-V region and anti-Ia region antibodies. In: *Immunology of Transfer Factor* (Kirkpatrick, C. H., Burger, D. R., and Lawrence, H. S., eds.), Academic Press, New York, p. 75.

405. Jeter, W. S., Kibler, R., Soli, T. C., and Stephens, C. A. (1979) Oral administration of bovine and human dyalizable transfer factor to human volunteers. In: *Immune Regulators in Transfer Factor* (Kahn, A., Kirkpatrick, C. H., and Hill, N. O., eds.), Academic Press, New York, p. 451.

406. Lawrence, H. S. (1974) Transfer factor in cellular immunity, *Harvey Lecture Series 68*, Academic Press, New York, p. 239.

407. Schulkind, M. L. and Ayoub, E. M. (1980) Transfer factor and its clinical applications. In: *Advances in Pediatrics* (Barness, L. A., ed.), Year Book Medical Publishers, Chicago, IL, p. 89.

408. Jones, J. F., Jeter, W. S., Fulginiti, V. A., Munnich, L. L., Pritchett, R. F., and Wedgwood, R. J. (1991) Treatment of childhood combined Epstein-Barr virus/cytomegalovirus infection with oral bovine transfer factor, *Lancet*, **2**, 122.

409. Klesius, P. H. and Kristensen, F. (1977) Bovine transfer factor: effect on bovine and rabbit coccidiosis, *Clin. Immunol. Immunopathol.*, **7**, 240.

410. Klesius, P. H., Quals, D. F., Elston, A. L., and Fudenberg, H. H. (1987) Effects of bovine transfer factor (TFd) in mouse coccidiosis (*Eimeria ferrisi*), *Clin. Immunol. Immunopathol.*, **10**, 214.

411. Okhuysen, P., Robinson, P., Watson, V., Actor, J., Lewis, D., Lahoti, S., Cron, S., Shahab, I., Chappell, C., and White, A. C., Jr. (1999) Intestinal IL-15 and interferon-gamma (IFNgamma) in cryptosporidiosis, *6th Conference on Retroviruses and Opportunistic Infections., Chicago, IL*, January 31–February 4 [113, abstract 243].

412. Kern, P., Toy, J., and Dietrich, M. (1985) Preliminary clinical observations with recombinant interleukin-2 in patients with AIDS or LAS, *Blut*, **50**, 1.

413. Donahue, J. H., Resenstein, M., Chang, A. E., Lotze, M. T., Robb, R. J., and Rosenberg, S. A. (1984) The systemic administration of purified interleukin 2 enhances the ability of sensitized murine lymphocytes to cure a disseminated syngeneic lymphoma, *J. Immunol.*, **132**, 2123.

414. Ruscetti, F. W. and Gallo, R. C. (1981) Human T-lymphocyte growth factor: regulation of growth and function of T lymphocytes, *Blood*, **57**, 379.

415. Wagner, H., Kronke, M., Solbach, W., Scheurich, P., Rollinghoff, M., and Pfizenmaier, K. (1982) Murine T cell subsets and interleukins: relationships between cytotoxic T cells, helper T cells and accessory cells, *Clin. Haematol.*, **11**, 607.

416. Pearlstein, K. T., Palladino, M. A., Welte, K., and Vilcek, J. (1983) Purified human interleukin-2 enhances induction of immune interferon, *Cell Immunol.*, **80**, 1.

417. Capetti, A., Bonfanti, P., Rizzardini, G., and Milazzo, F. (1996) Can rHuGM-CSF help treating drug-resistant cryptosporidiosis

in AIDS, *36th Interscience Conference on Antimicrobial Agents and Chemotherapy, New Orleans, LA*, September 15–18 [abstract G33].

418. Maggi, P., Larocca, A. M., Quarto, M., Serio, G., Brandonisio, O., Angarano, G., and Pastore, G. (2000) Effect of antiretroviral therapy on cryptosporidiosis and microsporidiosis in patients infected with human immunodeficiency virus type 1, *Eur. J. Clin. Microbiol. Infect. Dis.*, **19**, 213–217.

419. Mileno, M. D., Tashima, K., Farrar, D., Elliot, B. C., Rich, J. D., and Flanigan, T. P. (1997) Resolution of AIDS-related opportunistic infections with addition of protease inhibitor treatment, *4th Conference on Retroviruses and Opportunistic Infections, Washington, D.C.*, January 22–26 [129, abstract 355].

420. Benhamou, Y., Bochet, M. V., Carriere, J., Tubiana, R., Anduze-Faris, B., Valantin, M. A., Datry, A., Bricaire, F., and Katlama, C. (1997) Effects of triple antiretroviral therapies including a HIV protease inhibitor on chronic intestinal cryptosporidiosis and microsporidiosis in HIV-infected patients, *4th Conference on Retroviruses and Opportunistic Infections, Washington, D.C.*, January 22–26 [130, abstract 357].

421. Landau, A., Aaron, L., Pialoux, G., Eliaszewicz, M., Zylberberg, H., Poncelet, H., and Dupont, B. (1998) Impact of antiretroviral therapy (ART) on cryptosporidiosis outcome and factors of clinical resistance, *5th Conference on Retroviruses and Opportunistic Infections, Chicago, IL*, February 1–5 [169, abstract 480].

422. Moore, R. D., Keruly, J. C., and Chaisson, R. E. (1998) Decline in CMV and other opportunistic disease with combination antiretroviral therapy, *5th Conference on Retroviruses and Opportunistic Infections, Chicago, IL*, February 1–5 [113, abstract 184].

423. Georgiev, V. St. (2003) *Toxoplasma gondii*. In: *Opportunistic Infections: Treatment and Prophylaxis*, Humana Press, Totowa, NJ, pp. 163–182.

424. Nguyen, B. T. and Stadtsbaeder, S. (1983) Comparative effects of cotrimoxazole (trimethoprim-sulfamethoxazole), pyrimethamine-sulfadiazine and spiramycin during avirulent infection with *Toxoplsma gondii* (Beverley strain) in mice, *Br. J. Pharmacol.*, **79**, 923.

425. Renoult, E., Biava, M. F., Hulin, C., Frimat, L., Hestin, D., and Kessler, M. (1996) Transmission of toxoplasmosis by renal transplant: a report of four cases, *Transplant. Proc.*, **28**, 181.

426. Gallino, A., Maggiorini, M., Kiowski, W., Martin, X., Wunderli, W., Schneider, J., Turina, M., and Follath, F. (1996) Toxoplasmosis in heart transplant recipients, *Eur. J. Clin. Microbiol. Infect. Dis.*, **15**, 389.

427. Kimball, A. C., Kean, B. H., and Kellner, A. (1965) The risk of transmitting toxoplasmosis by blood transfusion, *Transfusion*, **5**, 447.

428. Feldman, H. A. (1968) Toxoplasmosis, *N. Engl. J. Med.*, **279**, 1370.

429. Jones, T. C., Kean, B. H., and Kimball, A. C. (1969) Acquired toxoplasmosis, *N. Y. State J. Med.*, **69**, 2237.

430. Bamford, C. R. (1975) Toxoplasmosis mimicking a brain abscess in an adult with treated scleroderma, *Neurology*, **25**, 343.

431. Levine, N. D. (1973) *Protozoan Parasites of Domestic Animals and of Man*, Burgess Publishing Co., Minneapolis, MN, p. 294.

432. Feldman, H. A. (1953) The clinical manifestations and laboratory diagnosis of toxoplasmosis, *J. Trop. Med. Hyg.*, **2**, 420, 1953.

433. Feldman, H. A. and Miller, L. T. (1956) Congenital human toxoplasmosis, *Ann. N.Y. Acad. Sci.*, **64**, 180.

434. Conyn-van Spaendonck, M. A., van Knapen, F., and de Jong, P. T. (1990) Congenital toxoplasmosis, *Tijdschr. Kindergeneeskd.*, **58**, 227.

435. Russo, M. and Calanti, B. (1990) Prevention of congenital toxoplasmosis, *Clin. Ter.*, **134**, 383.

436. Couvreur, J., Thulliez, T., Daffos, F., Aufrant, C., Bompart, Y., Goumy, P., and Tournier, G. (1991) 6 cases of toxoplasmosis in twins, *Ann. Pediatr. (Paris)*, **38**, 63.

437. Woods, A.C. (1960) Modern concepts of the etiology of uveitis, *Am. J. Ophthalmol.*, **50**, 1170.

438. O'Connor, G. R. (1975) Ocular toxoplasmosis, *Jpn. J. Ophthalmol.*, **19**, 1.

439. Pivetti-Pezzi, P., Accorinti, M., Tamburi, S., Ciapparoni, V., and Abdulaziz, M. A. (1994) Clinical features of toxoplasmic retinochoroiditis in patients with acquired immunodeficiency syndrome, *Ann. Ophthalmol.*, **26**, 73.

440. Martin-Duverneuil, N., Cordoliani, Y. S., Sola-Martinez, M. T., Miaux, Y., Weill, A., and Chiras, J. (1995) Cerebral toxoplasmosis: neuroradiologic diagnosis and prognostic monitoring, *J. Neuroradiol.*, **22**, 196.

441. Luft, B. J. and Remington, J. S. (1988) Toxoplasmic encephalitis, *J. Infect. Dis.*, **157**, 1.

442. Rostaing, L., Baron, E., Fillola, O., Roques, C., Durand, D., Massip, P., Lloveras, J. J., and Suc, J. M. (1995) Toxoplasmosis in two renal transplant recipients: diagnosis by bone marrow aspiration, *Transplant. Proc.*, **27**, 1733.

443. Luft, B. J. and Remington, J. S. (1985) Toxoplasmosis of the central nervous system. In: *Current Clinical Topics in Infectious Diseases*, vol. 6 (Remington, J. S. and Swartz, M. N. eds.), McGraw-Hill, New York, p. 315.

444. Levy, R. M., Bredersen, D. E., and Rosenblum, M. L. (1985) Neurobiological manifestations of the acquired immunodeficiency syndrome (AIDS): experience of UCSF and review of the literature, *J. Neurosurg.*, **621**, 475.

445. Tuazon, C. U. (1989) Toxoplasmosis in AIDS patients, *J. Antimicrob. Chemother.*, **23**(Suppl. A), 77–82.

446. Ferrer, S., Fuentes, I., Domingo, P., Munoz, C., et al. (1996) Cerebral toxoplasmosis in patients with human immunodeficiency virus (HIV) infection: clinico-radiological and therapeutic aspects in 63 patients, *An. Med. Interna*, **13**, 4.

447. Winstanley, P. (1995) Drug treatment of toxoplasmic encephalitis in acquired immunodeficiency syndrome, *Postgrad. Med. J.*, **71**, 404.

448. Luft, B. J., Hafner, R., Korzun, A. H., Leport, C., Antoniskis, D., Bosler, E. M., Bourland III, D. D., Uttamchandani, R., Fuhrer, J., Jacobson, J., Morlat, P., Vildé, J.-L., Remington, J. S., and the members of the ACTG 077p/ANRS 009 Study Team (1993) Toxoplasmic encephalitis in patients with the acquired immunodeficiency syndrome, *N. Engl. J. Med.*, **329**, 995.

449. Carr, A., Tindall, B., Brew, B. J., et al. (1992) Low-dose trimethoprim- sulfamethoxazole prophylaxis for toxoplasmic encephalitis in patients with AIDS, *Ann. Intern. Med.*, **117**, 106–111.

450. Alappat, J. P., Mathew, C. F., Jayakumar, K., Suresh, I. C., and Kumar, S. (2000) A case of cerebral toxoplasmosis, *Neurol. India*, **48**, 185–187.

451. Schlager, S. I. (1998) Management of opportunistic infections in acquired immunodeficiency syndrome. I. Treatment, *Am. J. Ther.*, **5**, 45–49.

452. Wilson, C. B., Remington, J. S., Stagno, S., and Reynolds, D. W. (1980) Development of adverse sequelae in children born with subclinical congenital *Toxoplasma* infection, *Pediatrics*, **66**, 767.

453. Haverkos, H. W. (coordinator) (1987) Assessment of therapy for *Toxoplasma* encephalitis. The TE Study Group, *Am. J. Med.*, **82**, 907.

454. Leport, C., Raffi, F., Metherton, S., Katlama, C., Regnier, B., Saimot, A. G., Marche, C., Vedrenne, C., and Vildé J.-L. (1988) Treatment of central nervous system toxoplasmosis with pyrimethamine/sulfadiazine combination in 35 patients with acquired immunodeficiency syndrome: efficacy of long-term continuous therapy, *Am. J. Med.*, **84**, 94.

455. Post, M. J. D., Kusunoglu, S. J., Hensley, C. T., Chan, J. C., Moskowitz, L. B., and Hoffman, T. A. (1985) Cranial CT in acquired immunodeficiency syndrome: spectrum of diseases

and optimal contrast enhancement technique, *Am. J. Radiol.*, **145**, 929.

456. Costa, B., Tacconi, P., Cannas, A., Pinna, L., and Fiaschi, A. (1988) Cerebral toxoplasmosis in AIDS. Case report, *Ital. J. Neurol. Sci.*, **9**(2), 161–163.

457. Altes, J., Salas, A., Ricart, C., Villalonga, C., Riera, M., and Casquero, P. (1989) Cerebral toxoplasmosis in patients with AIDS, *Arch. Neurobiol. (Madr.)*, **52**(Suppl. 1), 121.

458. Carrazana, E. J., Rossitch, E., Jr., and Samuels, M. A. (1994) Cerebral toxoplasmosis in the acquired immune deficiency syndrome, *Clin. Neurol. Neurosurg.*, **91**, 291.

459. Artigas, J., Grosse, G., Niedobitek, F., Kassner, M., Risch, W., and Heise, W. (1994) Severe toxoplasmic ventriculomeningoencephalomyelitis in two AIDS patients following treatment of cerebral toxoplasmic granuloma, *Clin. Neuropathol.*, **13**, 120.

460. Mortier, E., Poirot, J. L., Marteau, M., Febvre, M., Meynard, J. L., Duvivier, C., Maury, E., Picard, O., and Cabane, J. (1996) Pulmonary toxoplasmosis in patients with human immunodeficiency virus infection: 21 cases, *Presse Med.*, **25**, 485.

461. Halme, M., Jokipil, L., Jokipil, A. M., Ristola, M., and Lahdevirta, J. (1995) *Toxoplasma* pneumonia in a patient with AIDS, *J. Infect.*, **31**, 252.

462. Gadea, I., Cuenca, M., Benito, N., Pereda, J. M., and Soriano, F. (1995) Bronchoalveolar lavage for the diagnosis of disseminated toxoplasmosis in AIDS patients, *Diagn. Microbiol. Infect. Dis.*, **22**, 339.

463. Knani, L., Bouslama, K., Varette, C., Gonzalez Canali, G., Cabane, J., Lebas, J., and Imbert, J. C. (1990) Pulmonary toxoplasmosis in AIDS: report of 3 cases, *Ann. Med. Interne (Paris)*, **141**, 469.

464. Miller, R. F., Lucas, S. B., and Bateman, N. T. (1996) Disseminated *Toxoplasma gondii* infection presenting with a fulminant pneumonia, *Genitourin. Med.*, **72**, 139.

465. Oksenhendler, E., Cadranel, J., Sarfati, C., Katlama, C., Datrym, A., Marche, C., Wolf, M., Roux, P., Derouin, F., and Clauvel, J. P. (1990) *Toxoplasma gondii* pneumonia in patients with the acquired immunodeficiency syndrome, *Am. J. Med.*, **88**(5N), 18N.

466. Albrecht, H., Stellbrink, H. J., Fenske, S., Schafer, H., and Greten, H. (1994) Successfull treatment of *Toxoplasma gondii* myocarditis in an AIDS patient, *Eur. J. Clin. Microbiol. Infect. Dis.*, **13**, 500.

467. Duffield, J. S., Jacob, A. J., and Miller, H. C. (1996) Recurrent, life-threatening atrioventricular dissociation associated with toxoplasma myocarditis, *Heart*, **76**, 453.

468. Mastroianni, A., Coronado, O., Scarani, P., Manfredi, R., and Chiodo, F. (1996) Liver toxoplasmosis and acquired immunodeficiency syndrome, *Recenti Prog. Med.*, **87**, 353.

469. Bonacini, M., Kanel, G., and Alamy, M. (1996) Duodenal and hepatic toxoplasmosis in a patient with HIV infection: review of the literature, *Am. J. Gastroenterol.*, **91**, 1838.

470. Kume, H. and Takai, T. (1995) Toxoplasmosis of the liver, *Ryoikibetsu Shokogun Shirizu*, (7), 93.

471. Besnier, J. M., Verdier, M., Cotty, F., Fétissof, F., Besancenez, A., and Choutet, P. (1995) Toxoplasmosis of the bladder in a patient with AIDS, *Clin. Infect. Dis.*, **21**, 452.

472. Grassi, M. P., Borella, M., Clerici, F., Perin, C., Bini, M. T., and Mongoni, A. (1994) Reversible bilateral opercular syndrome secondary to AIDS-associated cerebral toxoplasmosis, *Ital. J. Neurol. Sci.*, **15**, 115.

473. Piens, M. A. and Garir, J. P. (1989) New perspectives in the chemoprophylaxis of toxoplasmosis, *J. Chemother.*, **1**, 46.

474. McCabe, R. E. and Oster, S. (1989) Current recommendations and future prospects in the treatment of toxoplasma, *Drugs*, **38**, 973.

475. Georgiev, V. St. (1993) Opportunistic/nosocomial infections: treatment and developmental therapeutics. Toxoplasmosis, *Med. Res. Rev.*, **13**, 529.

476. Georgiev, V. St. (1994) Management of toxoplasmosis, *Drugs*, 48, 179.

477. Boyer, K. M. (1996) Diagnosis and treatment of congenital toxoplasmosis, *Adv. Pediatr. Infect. Dis.*, **11**, 449.

478. Behbahani, R., Moshfeghi, M., and Baxter, J. D. (1995) Therapeutic approaches for AIDS-related toxoplasmosis, *Ann. Pharmacother.*, **29**, 960 [comment in *Ann. Pharmacother.*, **29**, 1303 (1995)].

479. Tomavo, S. and Boothroyd, J. C. (1995) Interconnection between organellar functions, development and drug resistance in the protozoan parasite, *Toxoplasma gondii*, *Int. J. Parasitol.*, **25**, 1293–1299.

480. Lambotte, R. (1976) Toxoplasmose congenitale: evaluation du benefice therapeutique prenatal, *J. Gynecol. Obstet. Biol. Reprod. (Paris)*, **5**, 265.

481. Derouin, F., Jacqz-Aigrain, E., Thulliez, P., Couvreur, J., and Leport, C. (2000) Cotrimoxazole for prenatal treatment of congenital toxoplasmosis? *Parasitol. Today*, **16**, 254–256.

482. Bloch-Michel, E. (1989) Ocular toxoplasmosis in 1989, *Bull. Soc. BeIge Ophthalmol.*, **230**, 53.

483. Finielz, P., Chuet, C., Ramdane, M., and Guiserix, J. (1995) Treatment of cerebral toxoplasmosis in AIDS with cotrimoxazole, *Presse Med.*, **24**, 917.

484. Holliman, R. E. (1989) Folate supplements and the treatment of cerebral toxoplasmosis, *Scand. J. Infect. Dis.*, **21**, 475.

485. Grange, F., Kinney, E. L., Monsuez, J. J., Rybojad, M., Derouin, F., Khuong, M. A., and Janier, M. (1990) Successful therapy for *Toxoplasma gondii* myocarditis in acquired immunodeficiency syndrome, *Am. Heart J.*, **120**, 443.

486. McNamara, J. J. (1973) Antibiotic therapy in compromised hosts, *Calif. Med.*, **119**, 49.

487. Podamczer, D., Miró, J. M., Ferrer, E., Gatell, J. M., Ramon, J. M., Ribera, E., Sirera, G., Cruceta, A., Knobel, H., Domingo, P., Polo, R., Leyes, M., Cosin, J., Farinas, M. C., Arrizabalaga, J., Martinez-Lacasa, J., and Gudiol, F. (2000) Thrice- weekly sulfadiazine-pyrimethamine for maintenance therapy of toxoplasmic encephalitis in HIV-infected patients. Spanish Toxoplasmosis Study Group, *Eur. J. Clin. Microbiol. Infect. Dis.*, **19**, 89–95.

488. Podzamczer, D., Miró, J. M., Ferrer, E., and Gatell, J. M. (1998) Thrice-weekly vs. daily sulfadiazine-pyrimethamine (SP) for maintenance therapy of toxoplasmic encephalitis (TE), *5th Conference on Retroviruses and Opportunistic Infections, Chicago, IL*, Feb. 1–5 [167, abstract 468].

489. Holliman, R. E. (1991) Clinical and diagnostic findings in 20 patients with toxoplasmosis and acquired immune deficiency syndrome, *J. Med. Microbiol.*, **35**, 1.

490. Wanke, C., Tuazon, C. U., Kovacs, A., Dina, T., Davis, D. O., Barton, N., Katz , D., Lunde, M., Levy, C., Conley, F. K., Lane, H. C., Fauci, A. S., and Mazur, H. (1987) *Toxoplasma* encephalitis in patients with acquired immune deficiency syndrome: diagnosis and response to therapy, *Am. J. Trop. Med. Hyg.*, **36**, 509.

491. Langmann, P., Klinker, H., and Richter, E. (1995) Pyrimethamine-sulphadiazine resistant cerebral toxoplasmosis in AIDS, *Dtsch. Med. Wochenschr.*, **120**, 780.

492. Huber, W., Bautz, W., Classen, M., and Schepp, W. (1995) Pyrimethamine- sulfadiazine resistant cerebral toxoplasmosis in AIDS, *Dtsch. Med. Wochenschr.*, **120**, 60.

493. Luft, B. J., Brooks, R. G., Conley, P. K., McCabe, R. E., and Remington, J. S. (1984) Toxoplasmic encephalitis in patients with acquired immune deficiency syndrome, *J. Am. Med. Assoc.*, **252**, 913.

494. Bell, E. T., Tapper, M. L., and Pollock, A. A. (1985) Sulphadiazine desensitization in AIDS patients, *Lancet*, **1**, 163.

495. Tenant-Flowers, M., Boyle, M. J., Carey, D., Marriott, D. J., Harkness, J. L., Penny, R., and Cooper, D. A. (1991) Sulphadiazine desensitization in patients with AIDS and cerebral toxoplasmosis, *AIDS*, **5**, 311.

496. Leport, C., Tournerie, C., Raguin, G., Fernandez-Martin, J., Niyongabo, T., and Vildé, J.-L. (1991) Long-term follow-up of patients with AIDS on maintenance therapy for toxoplasmosis, *Eur. J. Clin. Microbiol. Infect. Dis.*, **10**, 191.

497. Bhatti, N. and Larson, E. (1990) Low-dose alternate-day pyrimethamine for maintenance therapy in cerebral toxoplasmosis complicating AIDS, *J. Infect.*, **21**, 119.

498. Couvreur, J. (1991) In utero treatment of congenital toxoplasmosis with a pyrimethamine-sulfadiazine combination, *Presse Med.*, **20**, 1136.

499. Couvreur, J., Thulliez, P., Daffos, F., Aufrant, C., Bompard, Y., Gesquiere, A., and Desmonts, G. (1993) Fetal toxoplasmosis: in utero treatment of toxoplasmic fetopathy with the combination pyrimetamine-sulfadiazine, *Fetal Diagn Ther.*, **8**(1), 45–50.

500. Simon, D. I., Brosius III, F. C., and Rothstein, D. M. (1990) Sulfadiazine crystalluria revisited: the treatment of *Toxoplasma* encephalitis in patients with acquired immunodeficiency syndrome, *Arch. Intern. Med.*, **150**, 2379.

501. Diaz, F., Collazos, J., Mayo, J., and Martinez, E. (1996) Sulfadiazine-induced multiple urolithiasis and acute renal failure in a patient with AIDS and Toxoplasma encephalitis, *Ann. Pharmacother.*, **30**, 41, 1996.

502. Rodriguez-Carballeira, M., Casagran, A., More, J., Argilaga, R., and Garcia, M. (1996) Acute renal insufficiency caused by sulfadiazine in a patient with cerebral toxoplasmosis and AIDS, *Enfer. Infecc. Microbiol. Clin.*, **14**, 125.

503. Becker, K., Jablonowski, H., and Haussinger, D. (1996) Sulfadiazine-associated nephrotoxicity in patients with the acquired immunodeficiency syndrome, *Medicine (Baltimore)*, **75**, 185.

504. Peh, C. A., Kimber, T. E., Shaw, D. R., and Clarkson, A. R. (1995) Acute renal failure due to sulphadiazine in a patient with acquired immunodeficiency syndrome (AIDS), *Aust. N. Z. J. Med.*, **25**, 58.

505. Potter, J. L. and Kofron, W. G. (1994) Sulfadiazine/N^4-acetylsulfadiazine crystalluria in a patient with the acquired immune deficiency syndrome (AIDS), *Clin. Chim. Acta*, **230**, 221.

506. Bressolette, L., Carlhant, D., Bellein, V., Morand, C., Mottier, D., and Riche, C. (1994) Crystalluria induced by sulfadiazine in an AIDS patient, *Therapie*, **49**, 154–155.

507. Furrer, H., von Overbeck, J., Jaeger, P., and Hess, B. (1994) Sulfadiazine nephrolithiasis and nephropathy, *Schweiz. Med. Wochenschr.*, **124**, 2100.

508. Marques, L. P., Madeira, E. P., and Santos, O. R. (1994) Renal alterations induced by sulfadiazine therapy in an AIDS patient, *Clin. Nephrol.*, **42**, 68 [comment in *Clin. Nephrol.*, **39**, 254 (1993)].

509. Kronawitter, U., Jacob, K., Zoller, W. G., Rauh, G., and Goebel, F. D. (1993) Acute kidney failure caused by sulfadiazine stones: a complication of the therapy of toxoplasmosis in AIDS, *Dtsch. Med. Wochenschr.*, **118**, 1683.

510. Hein, R., Brunkhorst, R., Thon, W. F., Schedel, I., and Schmidt, R. E. (1993) Symptomatic sulfadiazine crystalluria in AIDS patients: a report of two cases, *Clin. Nephrol.*, **39**, 254 [comment in *Clin. Nephrol.*, **42**, 68 (1994)].

511. Farinas, M. C., Echevarria, S., Sampedro, I., Gonzalez, A., Gonzalez, A., Pérez del Molino, A., and Gonzalez-Macias, J. (1993) Renal failure due to sulphadiazine in AIDS patients with cerebral toxoplasmosis, *J. Intern. Med.*, **233**, 365.

512. Diaz, F., Collazos, J., Mayo, J., and Martinez, E. (1996) Sulfadiazine-induced multiple urolithiasis and acute renal failure in a patient with AIDS and Toxoplasma encephalitis, *Ann. Pharmacother.*, **30**, 41.

513. Molina, J. M., Belefant, X., Doco-Lacompte, T., Idatte, J. M., and Modai, J. (1991) Sulfadiazine induced crystalluria in AIDS patients with toxoplasma encephalitis, *AIDS*, **5**, 587, 1991.

514. Oster, S., Hutchinson, F., and McCabe, R. (1990) Resolution of acute renal failure in toxoplasmic encephalitis despite continuance of sulfadiazine, *Rev. Infect. Dis.*, **12**, 618.

515. Caumes, E., Bocquet, H., Guermonprez, G., Rogeaux, O., Bricaire, F., Katlama, C., and Gentilini, M. (1995) Adverse cutaneous reactions to pyrimethamine/sulfadiazine and pyrimethamine/clindamycin in patients with AIDS and toxoplasmic encephalitis, *Clin. Infect. Dis.*, **21**, 656.

516. Lafrenz, M., Ziegler, K., Saender, R., Budde, E., and Naumann, G. (1973) Treatment of toxoplasmosis, *Muenchen. Med. Wochenschr.*, **115**, 2057.

517. Norrby, R., Eilard, T., Svedhen, A., and Lycke, E. (1975) Treatment of toxoplasmosis with trimethoprim-sulphamethoxazole, *Scand. J. Infect.Dis.*, **7**, 72.

518. Norrby, R. and Eilard, T. (1976) Recurrent toxoplasmosis, *Scand. J. Infect. Dis.*, **8**, 275.

519. Burchall, J. J. (1973) Mechanism of action of trimethoprim-sulfamethoxazole. II., *J. Infect. Dis.*, **128**(Suppl.-Nov), S473.

520. Greenlee, J. E., Johnson, W. D., Jr., Campa, J. F., Adelman, L. S., and Sande, M. A. (1975) Adult cerebellar ataxia, *Ann. Intern. Med.*, **82**, 367.

521. Williams, M. and Savage, D. C.L. (1978) Acquired toxoplasmosis in children, *Arch. Dis. Child.*, **53**, 829.

522. Remington, J. S. (1980) Acquired toxoplasmosis in children, *Arch. Dis. Child.*, **55**, 80.

523. Esposito, R., Lazzarin, A., Orlando, G., Gallo, M., and Foppa, C. U. (1987) ABC of AIDS: treatment of infections and antiviral agents, *Br. Med. J. (Clin. Res.)*, **295**, 668.

524. Solbreux, P., Sonnet, J., and Zech, F. (1990) A retrospective study about the use of cotrimoxazole as diagnostic support and treatment of suspected cerebral toxoplasmosis in AIDS, *Acta Clin. Belg.*, **45**, 85.

525. Desmonts, G. and Couvreur, J. (1979) Congenital toxoplasmosis: a prospective study of the offspring of 542 women who acquired toxoplasmosis during pregnancy. Pathophysiology of congenital disease. In: *Proceedings of the 6th European Congress of Perinatal Medicine, Vienna, Austria* (Thalhammer, O., Baumgarten, K., and Polak, A. eds.), Georg Thieme, Stuttgart, p. 51.

526. Chang, H. R. and Pechère, J. C. (1988) Activity of spiramycin against *Toxoplasma gondii* in vitro, in experimental infections and in human infection, *J. Antimicrob. Chemother.*, **22**(Suppl.), 87.

527. Martin, C. and Mahon, R. (1974) Traitment de la toxoplasmose, *Nouv. Presse Med.*, **2**, 2202.

528. Desmonts, G. and Couvreur, J. (1974) Congenital toxoplasmosis: a prospective study of 378 pregnancies, *N. Engl. J. Med.*, **290**, 1110.

529. Desmonts, G., Couvreur, J., and Thulliez, P. (1988) Prophylaxis of congenital toxoplasmosis: effects of spiramycin on placental injection, *J. Antimicrob. Chemother.*, **22**(Suppl.), 193.

530. Fortier, B., Ajana, F., Pinto de Sousa, M. I., Aissi, E., and Camus, D. (1991) Prevention and treatment of materno-fetal toxoplasmosis, *Presse Med.*, **20**, 1374.

531. Koppe, J. G., Loewer-Siegler, D. H., and De Roever-Bonnet, H. (1986) Results of 20-year follow-up of congenital toxoplasmosis, *Lancet*, **1**, 254.

532. Hohfeld, P., Daffos, F., Thilliez, P., Aufrant, C., Couvreur, J., MacAleese, J., Descombey, D., and Forestier, F. (1989) Fetal toxoplasmosis: outcome of pregnancy and infant follow-up after in utero treatment, *J. Pediatr.*, **115**, 765.

533. Chodos, J. B. and Habegger-Chodos, H. E. (1961) The treatment of ocular toxoplasmosis with spiramycin, *Arch. Ophthalmol.*, **65**, 401.

534. Fajardo, R. V., Furguiele, F. P., and Leopold, J. M. (1962) Treatment of toxoplasmosis uveitis, *Arch. Ophthalmol.*, **67**, 712.

535. Cassidy, J. V., Bahler, J. W., and Minken, M. V. (1964) Spiramycin for toxoplasmosis, *Am. J. Ophthalmol.*, **57**, 227.

536. Canamucio, C. J., Hallet, J. W., and Leopold, J. M. (1963) Recurrence of treated toxoplasmic uveitis, *Am. J. Ophthalmol.*, **55**, 1035.

537. Timsit, J. C. and Bloch-Michel, E. (1987) Efficacite de la chimiotherapie specifique dans la prevention des recidives des chorioretinitis toxoplasmiques dans les quatre annees qui suivent la traitment, *J. Fr. Ophthalmol.*, **10**, 15.

538. Descotes, J., Vial, T., Delattre, D., and Evreux, J. C. (1988) Spiramycin: safety in man, *Antimicrob. Agents Chemother.*, **22**(Suppl. B), 207–210.

539. Burke, G. J. and Mills, A. F. (1979) Toxoplasmosis and clindamycin, *S. Afr. Med. J.*, **55**, 156.

540. Remington, J. S. and Vildé, J.-L. (1991) Clindamycin for toxoplasma encephalitis in AIDS, *Lancet*, **338**, 1142.

541. Santos Gil, I., Noguerado Asensio, A., del Arco Galan, C., and Garcia Polo, I. (1989) Clindamycin in the treatment of cerebral toxoplasmosis in a patient with AIDS, *Rev. Clin. Esp.*, **185**, 47.

542. Dannemann, B. R., Israelski, D. M., and Remington, J. S. (1988) Treatment of toxoplasmic encephalitis with intravenous clindamycin, *Arch. Intern. Med.*, **148**, 2477.

543. Goldsmith, J. M. (1980) Toxoplasmosis and clindamycin, *S. Afr. Med. J.*, **57**, 37.

544. Marcos, C., Sopena, B., Luna, I., Gonzalez, R., de la Fuente, J., and Martinez- Vazquez, C. (1995) Clindamycin desensitization in an AIDS patient, *AIDS*, **9**, 1201.

545. Ruf, B. and Pohle, H. D. (1991) Role of clindamycin in the treatment of acute toxoplasmosis of the central nervous system, *Eur. J. Clin. Microbiol. Infect. Dis.*, **10**, 183.

546. Dannemann, B. R., McCutchan, J. A., Israelski, D. M., Antoniskis, D., Leport, C., Luft, B. J., Chiu, J., Vildé, J.-L., Nussbaum, J. N., Orellana, M., Heseltine, P. N. C., Leedom, J. M., Clumeck, N., Morlat, P., Remington, J. S., and the California Collaborative Treatment Group. (1991) Treatment of acute toxoplasmosis with intravenous clindamycin, *Eur. J. Clin. Microbiol. Infect. Dis.*, **10**, 193.

547. Dannemann, B., MacCutchan, J. A., Israelski, D., Antoniskis, D., Leport, C., Luft, B., Nussbaum, J., Clumeck, N., Morlat, P., Chiu, J., Vildé, J.-L., Orellana, M., M., Feigal, D., Bartok, A., Heseltine, P., Leedom, J., Remington, J. S., and the California Collaborative Treatment Group (1992) Treatment of toxoplasmic encephalitis in patients with AIDS: a randomized trial comparing pyrimethamine plus clindamycin to pyrimethamine plus sulfadiazine, *Ann. Intern. Med.*, **116**, 33.

548. Dhiver, C., Milandre, C., Poizot-Martin, I., Drogoul, M. P., Gastaut, J. L., and Gastaut, J. A. (1993) 5-Fluoro-uracil-clindamycin for treatment of cerebral toxoplasmosis, *AIDS*, **7**, 143.

549. Saba, J., Morlat, P., Raffi, F., Hazebroucq, V., Joly, V., Leport, C., and Vildé, J.-L. (1993) Pyrimethamine plus azithromycin for treatment of acute toxoplasmic encephalitis in patients with AIDS, *Eur. J. Clin. Microbiol. Infect. Dis.*, **12**, 853.

550. Godofsky, E. W. (1994) Treatment of presumed cerebral toxoplasmosis with azithromycin, *N. Engl. J. Med.*, **330**, 575.

551. Valencia, M. E., Laguna, F., Soriano, V., and Gonzalez Lahoz, J. (1993) Favorable course of cerebral toxoplasmosis treated with doxycycline and pyrimetamine, *Rev. Clin. Esp.*, **192**, 197.

552. Hagberg, L., Palmertz, B., and Lindberg, J. (1993) Doxycycline and pyrimethamine for toxoplasmic encephalitis, *Scand. J. Infect. Dis.*, **25**, 157.

553. Dalston, M. O., Tavares, W., Bazin, A. R., Hahn, M. D., et al. (1995) Clarithromycin combined with pyrimethamine in cerebral toxoplasmosis: a report of 2 cases, *Rev. Soc. Bras. Med. Trop.*, **28**, 409.

554. Lacassin, F., Schaffo, D., Perronne, C., Longuet, P., Leport, C., and Vildé, J.-L. (1995) Clarithromycin-minocycline combination as salvage therapy for toxoplasmosis in patients infected with human immunodeficiency virus, *Antimicrob. Agents Chemother.*, **39**, 276.

555. Sellal, A., Rabaud, C., Amiel, C., Hoen, B., May, T., and Canton, Ph. (1996) Maintenance treatment of cerebral toxoplasmosis in AIDS: role of clarithromycin-minocycline combination, *Presse Med.*, **25**, 509.

556. Alba, D., Molina, F., Ripoli, M. M., and del Arco, A. (1993) Clarithromycin in the treatment of cerebral toxoplasmosis associated with HIV infection, *Rev. Clin. Esp.*, **192**, 458.

557. Clumeck, N., Katlama, C., Ferrero, T., et al. (1992) Atovaquone (1,4- hydroxynaphthoquinone, 566C80) in the treatment of acute cerebral toxoplasmosis (CT) in AIDS patients, *32nd Intersci. Conf. Antimicrob. Agents Chemother., Anaheim, CA*, October 11–14 [abstract 1217].

558. Grundman, M., Torres, R. A., Thorn, M., Hriso, and Britton, D. (1992) Neuroradiologic response to 566C80 salvage therapy for CNS toxoplasmosis, *Proc. VIIth International Conference on AIDS, Amsterdam*, July 19–24 [abstract PoB 3185].

559. Kovacs, J. A. (1992) NIAID-Clinical CIAIDSP: efficacy of atovaquone in treatment of toxoplasmosis in patients with AIDS, *Lancet*, **340**, 637.

560. Lafeuillade, A., Pellegrino, P., Poggi, C., Profizi, N., Quilichini, R., Chonette, I., and Navarreté, M. S. (1993) Efficacité de l'atovaquone dans les toxoplasmoses résistantes du SIDA, *Presse Med.*, **22**, 1708.

561. Bouboulis, D. A., Rubinstein, A., Shliozberg, J., Madden, J., and Frieri, M. (1995) Cerebral toxoplasmosis in childhood and adult HIV infection treated with 1,4- hydroxynaphthoquinone and rapid desensitization with pyrimethamine, *Ann. Allergy Asthma Immunol.*, **74**, 491.

562. Durand, J. M., Cretel, E., Bagneres, D., Guillemot, E., Kaplanski, G., and Soubeyrand, J. (1995) Failure of atovaquone in the treatment of cerebral toxoplasmosis, *AIDS*, **9**, 812.

563. Katlama, C., Mouthon, B., Gourdon, D., Lapierre, D., and Rousseau, F. (1996) Atovaquone as long-term suppressive therapy for toxoplasmic encephalitis in patients with AIDS and multiple drug intolerance, *AIDS*, **10**, 1107.

564. Masur, H., Polis, M. A., Tuazon, C. U., Ogata-Arakaki, D., Kovacs, J. A., Katz, D., Hilt, D., Simmons, T., Feuerstein, I., Lundgren, B., Lane, H. C., Chabner, B. A., and Allegra, C. J. (1993) Salvage trial of trimetrexate-leucovorin for the treatment of cerebral toxoplasmosis in patients with AIDS, *J. Infect. Dis.*, **167**, 1422.

565. Tabbara, K. F. (1995) Ocular toxoplasmosis: toxoplasmic retinochoroiditis, *Int. Ophthalmol. Clin.*, **35**, 15.

566. Chakroun, M., Meyohas, M. C., Pelosse, B., Zazoun, L., Vacherot, B., Derouin, F., and Leport, C. (1990) Ocular toxoplasmosis in AIDS, *Ann. Med. Interne (Paris)*, **141**, 472.

567. Engstrom, R. E., Jr., Holland, G. N., Nussenblatt, R. B., and Jabs, D. A. (1991) Current practices in the management of ocular toxoplasmosis, *Am. J. Ophthalmol.*, **111**, 601.

568. Commentary. (1998) Sense and nonsense of corticosteroid administration in the treatment of ocular toxoplasmosis, *Br. J. Ophthalmol.*, **82**, 858–860.

569. Ronday, M. J., Luyendijk, L., Baarsma, G. S., Bollemeijer, J. G., Van der Lelij, A., and Rothova, A. (1995) Presumed acquired ocular toxoplasmosis, *Arch. Ophthalmol.*, **113**, 1524.

570. Mittelviefhaus, H. (1993) Treatment of ocular toxoplasmosis. Part 1: basic principles and diagnosis, *Kinderarztl. Prax.*, **61**, 90.

571. Mittelviefhaus, H. (1993) Treatment of ocular toxoplasmosis. Part 2: therapeutic approaches, *Kinderarztl. Prax.*, **61**, 154.

572. Rothova, A. (1993) Ocular involvement in toxoplasmosis, *Br. J. Ophthalmol.*, **77**, 371 [correction in *Br. J. Ophthalmol.*, **77**, 683 (1993)].

573. Rothova, A., Meenken, C., Buitenhuis, H. J., Brinkman, C. J., Baarsma, G. S., Boen-Tan, T. N., de Jong, P. T. V. M., Klaasen-Broekma, N., Schweitzer, C. M. C., Timerman, Z., de Vries, J., Zaal, M. J. W., and Kijlstra, A. (1993) Therapy of ocular toxoplasmosis, *Am. J. Ophthalmol.*, **115**, 517.

574. Psilas, K., Petroutsos, G., and Aspiotis, M. (1990) Treatment of toxoplasmosis, *J. Fr. Ophthalmol.*, **13**, 551–553.

575. Lebech, A. M., Lebech, M., Borme, K. K., and Mathiesen, L. R. (1996) Toxoplasmosis-chorioretinitis: clinical course and treatment of seven patients, *Ugeskr. Laeger.*, **158**, 3935.

576. Holland, G. N. and Lewis, K. G. (2002) An update on current practices in the management of ocular toxoplasmosis, *Am. J. Ophthalmol.*, **134**, 102–114.

577. Lam, S. and Tessler, H. H. (1993) Quadruple therapy for ocular toxoplasmosis, *Can. J. Ophthalmol.*, **28**, 58.

578. Rothova, A., Buitenhuls, H. J., Meenken, C., Baarsma, G. S., Boen-Tan, T. N., de Jong, P. T., Schweitzer, C. M., Timmerman, Z., de Vries, J., Zaal, M. J., and Kijlstra, A. (1989) Therapy of ocular toxoplasmosis, *Int. Ophthalmol.*, **13**, 415.

579. Colin, J. and Harie, J. C. (1989) Presumed toxoplasmic chorioretinitis: comparative study of treatment with pyrimethamine and sulfadiazine or clindamycin, *J. Fr. Ophthalmol.*, **12**, 161.

580. Theodossiadis, G. P., Koutsandrea C., and Tzonou, A. (1989) A comparative study concerning the treatment of active toxoplasmic retinochoroiditis with argon laser and medication (follow-up 2-9 years), *Ophthalmologica*, **199**, 77.

581. Tassignon, M. J., Brihaye, M., De Meuter, F., Vercruysse, A., Van Hoof, F., and De Wilde, F. (1989) Efficacy of treatments in experimental toxoplasmosis, *Bull. Soc. Belge Ophthalmol.*, **230**, 59.

582. Fish, R. H., Hoskins, J. C., and Kline, L. B. (1993) Toxoplasmosis neuroretinitis, *Ophthalmology*, **100**, 1177.

583. Antinori, A., Murri, R., Ammassari, A., De Luca, A., Linzalone, A., Cingolani, A., Damiano, F., Maiuro, G., Vecchiet, J., Scoppettuolo, G., Tamburrini, E., and Ortona, L. (1995) Aerosolized pentamidine, cotrimoxazole and dapsone-pyrimethamine for primary prophylaxis of *Pneumocystis carinii* pneumonia and toxoplasmic encephalitis, *AIDS*, **9**, 1343.

584. Dworkin, M. S., Williamson, J., Jones, J. L., Kaplan, J. E., and the Adult and Adolescent Spectrum of HIV Disease Project (2001) Prophylaxis with trimethoprim-sulfamethoxazole for human immunodeficiency virus–infected patients: impact on risk for infectious diseases, *Clin. Infect. Dis.*, **33**, 393–398.

585. U.S. Public Health Service and Infectious Diseases Society of America (2000) 1999 USPHS/IDSA guidelines for prevention of opportunistic infections in persons infected with human immunodeficiency virus, *Infect. Dis. Obstet. Gynecol.*, **8**, 5–74.

586. Klinker, H., Langmann, P., and Richter, E. (1996) Pyrimethamine alone as prophylaxis for cerebral toxoplasmosis in patients with advanced HIV infection, *Infection*, **24**, 324.

587. Jacobson, M. A., Besch, C. L., Child, C., Hafner, R., Matts, J. P., Muth, K., Wentworth, D. N., Neaton, J. D., Abrams, D., Rimland, D., Perez, G., Grant, I. H., Sarovalatz, L. D., Brown, L. S., Deyton, L., and the Terry Bairn Community Programs for Clinical Research on AIDS (1994) Primary prophylaxis with pyrimethamine for toxoplasmic encephalitis in patients with advanced human immunodeficiency virus disease: results of a randomized trial, *J. Infect. Dis.*, **169**, 384.

588. Van Delden, C., Gabriel, V., Sudre, P., Flepp, M., von Overbeck, J., Hirschel, B., and the Swiss HIV Cohort Study (1996) Reasons for failure of prevention of *Toxoplasma* encephalitis, *AIDS*, **10**, 509.

589. Ribera, E., Fernandez-Sola, A., Juste, C., Rovira, A., Romero, F. J., Armadans-Gil, L., Ruiz, I., Ocana, I., and Pahissa, A. (1999) Comparison of high and low doses of trimethoprim-sulfamethoxazole for primary prevention of toxoplasmic encephalitis in human immunodeficiency virus-infected patients, *Clin. Infect. Dis.*, **29**, 1461–1466.

590. Saillourglenisson, F., Chene, G., Salmi, L. R., Hafner, R., and Salamon, R. (2000) Effet de la dapsone sur la survie des patients infectes par le VIH: une metanalyse des essais termines, *Rev. Epidemiol. Sante Publique*, **48**, 17–30.

591. Antinori, A., Murri, R., Ammassari, A., Pezzotti, P., Cingolani, A., De Luca, A., Pallavicini, F., and Ortona, L. (1998) Risk of bacterial infections in a cohort of HIV-positive patients receiving anti *P. carinii/T. gondii* prophylaxis, *38th Interscience Conference on Antimicrobial Agents and Chemotherapy, San Diego, CA*, September 24–27 [549, abstract L-9].

592. Gourdon, F., Laurichesse, H., Dalens, H., Cambon, M., Baud, O., Rigal, D., and Beytout, J. (1998) Ocular toxoplasmosis: clinical experience using pyrimethamine as secondary prophylaxis, *38th Interscience Conference on Antimicrobial Agents Chemotherapy, San Diego, CA*, September 24–27 [566, abstract L-66].

593. Jubault, V., Pacanowski, J., Rabian, C., and Viard, J. P. (2000) Interruption of prophylaxis for major opportunistic infections in HIV-infected patients receiving triple combination antiretroviral therapy, *Ann. Med. Interne (Paris)*, **151**, 163–168.

594. Maenza, J. (1999) Discontinuation of prophylaxis in HAART-responders, *Hopkins HIV Rep.*, **11**, 2–3.

595. Furrer, H., Opravil, M., Bernasconi, E., Telenti, A., and Egger, M. (2000) Stopping primary prophylaxis in HIV-1-infected patients at high risk of toxoplasma encephalitis. Swiss HIV Cohort Study, *Lancet*, **355**(9222), 2217–2218.

596. Mussini, C., Pezzotti, P., Govoni, A., Borghi, V., Antinori, A., d'Arminio Monforte, A., De Luca A., Mongiardo, N., Cerri, M. C., Chiodo, F., Concia, E., Bonazzi, L., Moroni, M., Ortona, L., Esposito, R., Cossarizza, A., and De Rienzo, B. (2000) Discontinuation of primary prophylaxis for *Pneumocistis carinii* pneumonia and toxoplasmic encephalitis in human immunodeficiency virus type I-infected patients: the changes in opportunistic prophylaxis study, *J. Infect. Dis.*, **181**, 1635–1642.

597. Guex, A. C., Radziwill, A. J., and Bucher, H. C. (2000) Discontinuation of secondary prophylaxis for toxoplasmic encephalitis in human immunodeficiency virus infection after immune restoration with highly active antiretroviral therapy, *Clin. Infect. Dis.*, **30**, 602–603.

598. Antinori, A., Cingolani, A., Ammassari, A., Pezzotti, P., Murri, R., de Luca, A., Larocca, L. M., and Ortona, L. (1999) AIDS-related focal brain lesions in the era of HAART, *6th Conference on Retrovirures and Opportunistic Infections, Chicago, IL*, January 31–February 4 [145, abstract 413].

599. Ravaux, I., Quinson, A. M., Chadapaud, S., and Gallais, H. (1998) Discontinue primary and secondary prophylaxis regimens in selected HIV-infected patients treated with HAART, *38th Interscience Conference on Antimicrobial Agents and Chemotherapy, San Diego, CA*, September 24–27 [429, abstract I-203].

600. Moore, R. D., Keruly, J. C., and Chaisson, R. E. (1998) Decline in CMV and other opportunistic diseases with combination antiretroviral therapy, *5th Conference on Retroviruses and Opportunistic Infections, Chicago, IL*, February 1–5 [113, abstract 184].

601. Soriano, V., Dona, C., Rodriguez-Rosado, R., Barreiro, P., and Gonzalez-Lahoz, J. (2000) Discontinuation of secondary prophylaxis for opportunistic infections in HIV-infected patients receiving highly active antiretroviral therapy, *AIDS*, **14**, 383–386.

602. Michaels, S., Clark, R., and Kissinger, P. (1998) Differences in the incidence rates of opportunistic processes before and after the

availability of protease inhibitors, *5th Conference on Retroviruses and Opportunistic Infections, Chicago, IL*, February 1–5 [112, abstract 180].

603. Rodriguez-Rosado, R., Soriano, V., Dona, C., and Gonzalez-Lahoz, J. (1998) Opportunistic infections shortly after beginning highly active antiretroviral therapy, *Antiviral Ther.*, **3**, 229–231.

604. Krahenbuhl, J. L. and Remington, J. S. (1982) The immunology of toxoplasma and toxoplasmosis. In: *Immunology of Parasitic Infections* (Cohen, S. and Warren, K. S. eds.), Blackwell, Oxford, p. 356.

605. Gallin, J. I., Farber, J. M., Holland, S. M., and Nitman, T. B. (1995) Interferon- gamma in the management of infectious diseases [clinical conference], *Ann. Intern. Med.*, **123**, 216 [comment in *Ann. Intern. Med.*, 124, 1095, (1996)].

606. Yap, G., Pesin, M., and Sher, A. (2000) Cutting edge: IL-12 is required for the maintenance of IFN-gamma production in T cells mediating chronic resistance to the intracellular pathogen, *Toxoplasma gondii, J. Immunol.*, **165**, 628–631.

607. Suzuki, Y. (1999) Genes, cells and cytokines in resistance against development of toxoplasmic encephalitis, *Immunobiology*, **201**, 255–271.

608. McCabe, R. E., Luft, B. J., and Remington, J. S. (1984) Effect of murine interferon gamma on murine toxoplasmosis, *J. Infect. Dis.*, **150**, 961.

609. Luft, B. J. and Remington, J. S. (1988) AIDS Commentary. Toxoplasmic encephalitis, *J. Infect. Dis.*, **157**, 1–6.

610. Fegies, M. and Guerrero, J. (1977) Treatment of toxoplassmic encephalitis with levamisole, *Trans. R. Soc. Trop. Med. Hyg.*, **71**, 178.

611. Zastera, M., Fruehbauer, Z., and Pokorny, J. (1982) Levamisole therapy of experimental toxoplasmosis in white mice, *Cesk. Epidemiol. Mikrobiol. Immunol.*, **31**, 94.

612. Youssef, M. Y., el-Ridi, A. M., Arafa, M. S., el-Sawy, M. T., and el-Sayed, W. M. (1985) Effect of levamisole on toxoplasmosis during pregnancy in guinea pigs, *J. Egypt. Soc. Parasitol.*, **15**, 41.

Part III
Immunology Research

Chapter 37

Introduction

Many of the world's major diseases—infection, cancer, autoimmunity, and allergy—critically involve the immune system. Continued progress in understanding basic immune mechanisms is essential for developing new abilities to treat and prevent diseases that affect millions of people worldwide *(1)*.

There have been enormous advances in the field of immunology over the past three decades, and those advances have had a positive effect on many subspecialties of medicine. In this regard, the NIAID plays an increasingly important role in supporting immunology research through a host of programs, investigator-initiated research, as well as by the efforts of the institute's intramural research scientists *(1,2)* (http://www.niaid.nih.gov/publications/). At present, the NIAID appropriation falls into three approximately equal categories aligned with the institute's main mission areas: human immunodeficiency virus (HIV) and AIDS; biodefense; and immunology and infectious diseases, a category that includes research on basic immunology, immune-mediated diseases, microbiology, and infectious diseases not in the HIV/AIDS or biodefense categories. Although most immunology research has traditionally been supported by the appropriation for immunology and infectious diseases, the discipline of immunology has also received support from HIV/AIDS and biodefense appropriations *(1)*.

Major Areas of NIAID-Supported Immunology Research. The genetic control of immune responses demonstrates both complexity and flexibility. Of the 20,000 to 25,000 genes estimated to compose the human genome *(3)*, more than 4,000 are broadly associated with immune system functions *(1)*. For example, frontline recognition of pathogens falls mainly to 10 Toll-like receptors (TLRs) and several nucleotide-binding oligomerization domain proteins *(4,5)*, whereas just two genetic loci, the immunoglobulin variable-diversity-joining-constant regions and the corresponding T-cell receptor genes, rearrange to provide millions of distinct T-cell and B-cell specificities, enabling responses to almost any biological molecule *(6)*.

New discoveries about the way the immune system functions has led the way to ever-increasing capabilities in preventing and treating immune-mediated and infectious diseases. However, even the considerable capacity of the immune system can be overwhelmed by organisms naturally adapted for virulence and immune evasion. Thus, orthopoxviruses, which include the smallpox agent variola major, are capable of allowing as many as one half of their genes to be involved in virus-host interactions *(7)*. Understanding of the complexities of the scope of interactions between microorganisms and the immune system will remain one of the most important goals of immunology research *(1)*.

Research on HIV/AIDS, emerging infectious diseases, including influenza, and biodefense is a public health priority with substantial funding support by the U.S. federal government. Notably, basic immunology research is central to future progress in those areas, including the development of effective therapeutics, diagnostics, and vaccines *(1)*. For example, at present the ability to induce broadly protective immune responses to HIV or to elicit heterotypic immunity to the ever-evolving influenza virus is lacking. Similarly, protective strategies cannot yet be defined that would thwart many potential agents of bioterrorism, especially those that could be genetically engineered to lack immunodominant epitopes or to incorporate immune-evasion molecules. In this regard, immunology research can play a crucial role by addressing the challenging questions posed in those priority areas *(1)*.

References

1. Hackett, C. J., Rotrosen, D., Auchincloss, H., and Fauci, A. S. (2007) Immunology research: challenges and opportunities in a time of budgetary constraint, *Nat. Immunol., 8, 114–117.*
2. Bishop, J. M. and Varmus, H. (2006) Re-aim blame for NIH's hard times, *Science,* **312**(5773), 499.
3. Ezekowitz, R. A. B. and Hoffmann, J. A. (eds.) (2003) *Innate Immunity,* Humana Press, Totowa, NJ.

4. Gordon, S. (2003) Mammalian host defenses. In: *Innate Immunity* (Ezekowitz, R. A. B. and Hoffmann, J. A. eds.), Humana Press, Totowa, NJ, pp. 175–265.

5. Kaisho, T. and Akira, S. (2003) Toll-like receptors. In: *Innate Immunity* (Ezekowitz, R. A. B. and Hoffmann, J. A. eds.), Humana Press, Totowa, NJ, pp. 177–189.

6. Aderem, A. and Ulevitch, R. J. (2000) Toll-like receptors in the induction of the innate immune response, *Nature*, **406**, 782–787.

7. Akira, S., Takeda, K., and Kaisho, T. (2001) Toll-like receptors: critical proteins linking innate and acquired immunity, *Nat. Immunol.*, **2**, 675–680.

Chapter 38

Mammalian Host Defenses: Innate and Adaptive Immunity

The mammalian host defense is categorized into *innate* and *adaptive* immunity *(1–3)*. Host defense relies on a concerted action of both antigen (Ag)-nonspecific innate immunity and Ag-specific adaptive immunity *(4–6)*.

It is unquestionably clear that the human immune system is the culmination of a defense system directed at eliminating foreign antigens or pathogens by using a sophisticated network of interactive processes ranging from the nonspecific preprogrammed reaction to pattern recognition molecules of the innate immunity to the exquisitely specific cell-mediated response to a single antigen carried out by the adaptive immune system *(7)*.

Adaptive immunity is mediated by B- and T-lymphocytes, which carry antigen-specific receptors that can bind antigen with high affinity owing to somatic gene recognition *(3)*. The clonally selected lymphocytes can mount a specific response against virtually any pathogen via nearly infinite repertoire of antibodies with random specificity *(8)*. In case of infection, adaptive immunity benefits the host by its high-affinity recognition of the pathogen and memory responses but has the disadvantage because of its gradual response, resulting from the selection and propagation of specific lymphocyte populations, before an effective systematic response can be initiated *(8)*. Hence, the necessity for a rapidly triggered response that will act as the first line of defense, a function that is best served by the innate immune response.

Although innate immunity is the most ancient form of host defense, it is a key area of discovery in contemporary immunology *(1)*. In contrast with the adaptive response, the innate immune response, which is activated by the recognition of pathogenic ligands by germ-line–encoded receptors, provides a rapid response to an invading pathogen, thereby playing a major role especially during the early phase of infection. Innate immunity receptors have been selected through evolution to recognize highly conserved and widely distributed features of common pathogens *(9)*. Furthermore, accumulating evidence has suggested that innate immunity can discriminate pathogens as nonself from self through a group of transmembrane proteins known as the Toll-like receptor family *(3, 10, 11)*.

Recent research, however, has suggested that the distinction between innate and adaptive immunity is not as distinct as previously thought as both arms of the immune system have been shown to share several common features including an extensive degree of specificity for pathogens and foreign antigens *(12, 13)*. For example, there is increasing evidence that the induction of different types of effector adaptive responses has been directed by the innate immune system after its highly selective recognition of particular groups of pathogens through pattern recognition molecules, such as the Toll-like receptors and the elaboration of soluble protein signals that activate the relevant lymphoid cell population *(12)*. Furthermore, before terminating its activity, the innate response can induce key costimulatory molecules on antigen-presenting cells largely due to the generation of potent adjuvants. The antigen-presenting cells then direct the antigen-driven clonal expansion of T- and B-cells and other antigen-specific cells of the acquired (adaptive) immune response *(14)*. In addition, the concerted innate and acquired immune responses would ensure that self-antigens are clearly discriminated from nonself-antigens thereby not only avoiding inappropriate autoimmune events but also allowing for both rapid responses and dynamic regulation of inflammation *(15, 16)*.

The invariant features on microbial pathogens are referred to as *pathogen-associated molecular patterns (PAMPs)*, and the molecules that recognize them are termed *pattern recognition receptors (PRR)*. The PRRs, which have a broad ligand specificity that can recognize pathogens, are expressed by particular subsets of cells that include macrophages, dendritic cells, and natural killer cells, generally known as *antigen-presenting cells (APCs)*. Upon binding to a ligand expressed on the surface of an invading pathogen, the PRRs can mediate their phagocytic uptake and/or generate intracellular signals leading to host cell activation *(8)*.

38.1 Toll-like Receptors

The innate immune system in *Drosophila* and mammals senses the invasion of microorganisms by using the family of Toll receptors, the stimulation of which initiates a range of host defense mechanisms *(17)*. In *Drosophila*, antimicrobial responses rely on two signaling pathways: the Toll pathway and the immune deficiency (IMD) pathway, which can synergistically activate an innate immune response *(18)*. In mammals, there are at least 10 members of the Toll-like receptor (TLR) family (designated as TLR1-10) that recognize specific components conserved among microorganisms. Activation of the TLRs leads not only to the induction of inflammatory responses but also to the development of antigen-specific adaptive immunity. The TLR-induced inflammatory response is dependent on a common signaling pathway that is mediated by the adaptor molecule MyD88. However, there is evidence for additional pathways that mediate TLR ligand-specific biological responses *(17, 19–23)*.

The TLRs function mainly as sensors for pathogens. So far, a number of TLR ligands have been identified, and most of them can be classified as PAMPs *(24)*. Some ligands are non-PAMPs; nevertheless, they play a critical role through TLRs in host immune and inflammatory responses *(3)*.

TLR4. The *lipopolysaccharide (LPS)* is the most well known PAMP. It is a major component of the outer membrane of *Gram-negative bacteria* and contains a hydrophilic polysaccharide and a hydrophobic lipid A, which is the biologically active component *(3)*. LPS can stimulate APCs to produce proinflammatory cytokines and can upregulate surface expression of costimulatory molecules such as CD40. Excess amount of LPS can also cause endotoxin shock with high mortality *(3)*. Genetic studies have revealed that TLR4 is responsible for LPS signaling and acts as a critical signal transducer for LPS *(3)*.

TLR2. Similar to Gram-negative bacteria, the *Gram-positive bacteria* can provoke not only immune responses but also shock status. However they do not contain LPS in their cell wall. Instead, the Gram-positive bacteria carry a thick layer of *peptidoglycan (PGN)*, which represents an alternating β- *(1, 4)*-linked *N*-acetylmuramyl and *N*-acetylglucosaminyl glucans cross-linked with tetrapeptides that can induce macrophages to produce inflammatory cytokines *(3)*. Data from analysis of TLR2-deficient mice has demonstrated that PGN acts as a PAMP through TLR2 *(25)*. Furthermore, TLR2 can recognize a variety of lipopeptides, lipoproteins, mycobacterial lipoarabinomanns, yeast extracts, and glycosyl-phosphatidylinositol (GPI)-anchoring proteins from *Treponema pallidum (11)*.

TLR5. Most bacilli, including *Salmonella*, contain flagella – common protein structures involved in motility and projecting from the bacterial cell surface. *Flagellin*, a monomeric subunit of flagella, can induce proinflammatory activity such as induction of IL-8 or inducible nitric oxide (NO) synthase in intestinal epithelial cells *(26, 27)*. Data have indicated that TLR5 can sense flagellin *(28)*. Furthermore, flagellin expression rendered nonflagellated *E. coli* capable of activating TLR5 *(3)*. *Salmonella* translocates flagellin

across intestinal epithelia, possibly through a type III secretion apparatus, and can elicit inflammatory responses with flagellin *(29)*.

TLR9. Bacillus Calmette-Guérin (BCG), a *Mycobacterium bovis* strain, is known as an effective adjuvant of cell-mediated immunity. Experimental findings have indicated that BCG-derived DNA has contributed to the immunostimulatory activity of BCG *(30)*. It was found that the unmethylated cytidine-phosphate-guanosine (CpG) motif has been responsible for this and other activities [inhibition of tumor growth, enhanced natural killer cell activity, and increased interferon production by lymphocytes *(30)*] of the BCG-derived DNA. Because CpG motif could also activate the B cells *(31)*, it can be regarded as PAMP *(3)*. Because all effects of CpG DNA have been abolished in TLR9-deficient mice, TLR9 is considered to be a critical signal transducer for CpG DNA *(22)*.

38.2 The Macrophage Mannose Receptor and Innate Immunity

The macrophage mannose receptor (MR) is one of four multilectin receptors belonging to a class of molecules having *multiple lectin domains* present within a single peptide backbone *(8, 32–34)*.

The mannose receptor is the prototype of a new family of receptors currently consisting of four members: (i) the mannose receptor; (ii) the receptor for secretory phospholipase A2 (PLA$_2$R); (iii) DEC-205, which functions in the internalization of the antigens for processing and presentation in dendritic cells; and (iv) Endo 180/uPARAP, the newest member, which is associated with the urokinase-type plasminogen activator receptor and recognized *N*-acetylglucosamine moieties *(8)*.

Lectins. The multiple lectin domains, known as *carbohydrate recognition domains (CRDs)*, are structurally homologous in all lectins *(8)*. Potential carbohydrate targets that can be recognized by the CDRs include mannans, glucans, lipophosphoglycans, and glycoinositol-phospholipids with mannose, glucose, fucose or *N*-acetylglucosamine as terminal hexoses *(8)*.

Pathogenic organisms display an array of carbohydrate structures on their surfaces that can be recognized by the lectins *(8, 35)*. Because the interaction between a unique CRD and its corresponding oligosaccharide ligand is generally weak, it would require the recognition of multiple oligosaccharides or multiple sites on an oligosaccharide to provide a high-affinity interaction *(36)*. Another mechanism to circumvent weak affinity is the formation of lectin multimers. Furthermore, lectins are also capable of recognizing sugars with different spatial arrangements (i.e., sugars coupled with different glycosidic linkages), which is common in branched oligosaccharides.

In contrast with other lectins, the macrophage mannose receptor, however, appears to recognize only terminal sugars *(37)*. Analysis of spent media taken from macrophage cultures led to the identification of a soluble form of MR, which happened to be fully active with respect to mannose binding. It is produced by a proteolytic clip and is present in normal sera *(38)*. Experimental results have indicated that the soluble MR could transport an antigen to a specific subset of cells as part of the immune response against specific targets *(39)*.

Mannose Receptor Structure and Function. Structurally, the mannose receptor has a transmembrane domain followed by a relatively short 45-amino-acid C-terminal cytoplasmic tail, which has no homology to the tails of any other known receptor *(8)*. A tyrosine residue similar to that present in the low-density lipoprotein (LDL) receptor and known to be critical for the localization and internalization of some endocytic receptors in clathrin-coated pits is also seen in MR *(40)*. Deletion of the cytoplasmic tail abolished the ability of MR to internalize ligands and to phagocytose yeast particles *(41)*. Although there are a few potential phosphorylation sites in MR, none has yet been shown to be a target site for a cellular kinase *(8)*.

The mannose receptor, being an integral membrane protein, is synthesized in the rough endoplasmic reticulum (ER) and is shuttled via the Golgi body to the plasma membrane *(8)*. Pulse chase experiments with newly synthesized MR provided evidence for *N*- and *O*-linked oligosaccharide chain additions during maturations. An initial signal peptide cleavage step is also observed before the ER docking. The initially synthesized form of MR is inactive and unable to bind to ligands. An activation event, which may involve the formation of disulfide bonds, will be required for the mannose receptor to achieve competency for ligand binding *(8, 42)*.

At 37°C, complete receptor/ligand internalization was found to occur within 5 minutes. The internalized MRs will rapidly recycle back to the plasma membrane. The reversibility of the receptor binding to its ligand is pH-dependent, and dissociation occurred at pH <6 *(43)*. In macrophages, internalized ligands reached the lysosomes within 20 minutes *(44)*. The mannose receptor has been localized to clathrin-coated vesicles, and internalization through this mechanism appeared to rely on the internalization motif in the cytoplasmic tail of the receptor. Furthermore, there have also been experiments to suggest that other motifs in the cytoplasmic tail of the MR may also play a role in the receptor recycling during endocytosis *(40)*.

The mannose receptor has also mediated phagocytosis by what appears to be a zipper mechanism *(8)*. Experiments using CV-1 (**S**imian cell lime in **O**rigin containing Simian SV40 virus mutants) cells have shown that these cells expressing full-length MR efficiently internalized particles and that the cytoplasmic tail of the MR was required for internalization *(41)*.

Based on its cell biollogy, it is clear that the mannose receptor can act both as an endocytic and a phagocytic receptor. Because the phagocytosis and receptor-mediated endocytosis are essentially different processes, they would require different cellular proteins and would exhibit sensitivity to different inhibitors. Thus, treatment of macrophages with interleukin-4 (IL-4) did elevate the MR expression and enhanced the mannose glyco-conjugate uptake. Concomitant with the elevated MR expression, the endocytic apparatus of the macrophages is selectively expanded, reflecting elevated membrane traffic. Alternatively, treatment of macrophages with interferon-γ (IFN-γ) did result in a reduction of MR expression; also, the receptor-mediated endocytosis via the mannose receptor was likewise reduced. However, the efficiency of the endocytosis through the MR (the phagocytic index) is enhanced. IFN-γ treatment unlike IL-4 resulted in elevated particle sorting to the lysosomal compartment *(45)*.

38.3 Lung Collectins in Pulmonary Innate Immunity

The lung is being constantly challenged by a wide array of infectious pathogens as well as other organic antigens and toxic substances. Consistent with the diversity of these potential challenges, the airways and airspaces of the lung represent a complex and multilayered pulmonary host defense comprising various anatomic and cellular components coupled with secreted molecules of the natural and acquired immune system *(39)*. Two of the most important components of the mammalian innate and natural defense are the lung collectins A (SP-A) and D (SP-D) *(46–50)*.

The lung collectins are surface proteins (SP) that belong to a growing family of collagenous C-type lectins that also includes the serum mannose-binding lectin (MBL, mannose-binding protein), two serum collectins (conglutinin and CL-43) *(46, 49, 51)*, and the intracellular collectin, CL-L1 *(52)*.

The lung collectins are synthesized and secreted into the pulmonary airspaces and airways by alveolar type II cells and subsets of bronchial epithelial cells *(46)*. In contrast with SP-A, which is expressed in the submucosal glands of the trachea, the eustachian tube, and possibly a few other tissues *(53, 54)*, the SP-D is widely expressed at many epithelial sites including the upper airways, tracheal-bronchial glands, and the oropharynx *(55)*.

The minimal functional unit of each collectin is a trimer *(56)* that confers high-affinity saccharide binding.

Structurally, each trimeric subunit consists of a short amino-terminal cross-linking domain; a triple helical collagenous domain; a triple coiled-coil linking or neck domain; and a mannose-subtype, C-type lectine carbohydrate recognition domain (CRD) *(51, 57)*. In the case of the primate SP-A family of collectins, an additional complexity relates to the capacity of the molecules to assemble as heterotrimers of the two, genetically different, chain types *(58)* that are subject to differential regulation *(59, 60)*. The functional significance of these heteropolymers is not known. By contrast, all known members of the SP-D family are assembled as homotrimers *(57)*. Furthermore, although the lung collectins show comparable domain structures, there is significant divergence in the primary sequence within all domains of the molecule.

There are also conspicuous differences in the distribution of the attached carbohydrates that could influence the function or interactions with microbial lectins. In particular, the collectins vary with respect to asparagine-linked glucosylation—although there are species variations in the number and sites of Asn-linked glycosylation, all known SP-As and SP-Ds contain at least one conserved complex oligosaccharide *(61)*.

Role of Lung Collectins in Microbial Clearance and Neutralization. SP-A and SP-D interact with or modify the phagocytic response to a wide array of both Gram-negative and Gram-positive microbial pathogens, fungi, respiratory viruses, and mycobacteria *(50, 57, 62)*. The mechanisms involved in the pathogen clearance and neutralization may be carried out by either direct effects of the lung collectin on the phagocytes or by prior recognition or opsonization of the organism by the collectin *(57)*.

One extensively studied example is the collectin-associated clearance of *Aspergillus fumigatus*, in which human SP-A and SP-D acted via CRD-dependent binding to the *N*-linked oligosaccharides of the cell wall glycoproteins of *A. fumigatus (63, 64)*. Circumstantial evidence has suggested that SP-D may also interact with β(1-6)-glucans associated with the *Aspergillus* cell wall. Pustulan, a β(1-6) glucose homopolymer, but not a β(1-3) homopolymer, was found to be a potent inhibitor of the SP-D binding to *A. fumigatis* and *Saccharomyces cerevisiae (57)*. *In vivo* experiments have shown that in murine model of fatal, invasive aspergillosis, intranasal administration of human lung collectins, or recombinant trimeric human SP-D neck+CRDs significantly enhanced the survival (80%) of SP-D–treated mice (versus 0% in untreated mice) *(65)*.

In the case of *Pneumocystis jirovecii*, where infection is characterized by massive accumulation of organisms within the airspace (often in association with characteristic foamy exudates containing surfactant lipids and proteins), SP-A and SP-D collectins acted by CRD-dependent binding to the trophozoites and the cyst forms of the pathogen *(66–68)*. This, in part, involved CRD-dependent interactions with a heavily mannosylated, cell wall glycoprotein, gpA (gp 140) *(68, 69)*, as well as SP-D binding to cell wall–associated β-glucans *(70)*. Furthermore, the lung collectins have increased the attachment of *P. jirovecii* to rat alveolar macrophages *(66, 71)*.

There has been considerable evidence showing that both SP-A and SP-D modulate the host response by binding to the lipopolysaccharide (LPS), particularly the rough forms lacking extended O-antigens *(72–74)*. The interactions of collectins with LPS could result in altered or decreased presentation of LPS to host cell receptors, alteration in the cellular metabolism of LPS, or effects on the interactions of LPS binding proteins or receptors to LPS *(57)*. *In vivo*, SP-A– and SP-D–deficient mice were highly susceptible to LPS-induced pulmonary inflammation *(75, 76)*.

Another study has suggested that SP-A and SP-D had direct inhibitory effects on the lipid peroxidation, protecting lipoproteins, surfactant phospholipids, and macrophages from oxidation *(77)*. Currently, however, there is relatively little information relating to the effects of the lung collectins on oxidant metabolism *in vivo (57)*.

38.4 Complement Control Proteins

The complement system is an element of the innate immunity comprising approximately 30 interacting plasma proteins and surface receptors normally circulating in the blood as inactive zymogens *(78)*. This group of glycoproteins can be stimulated in a cascading fashion to produce biologically active fragments that either directly attack foreign substances or enhance the functions of certain types of inflammatory leukocytes.

When stimulated by one of several triggers, proteases in the system cleave specific proteins to release cytokines and initiate an amplifying cascade of further cleavages. The end result of this activation cascade is massive amplification of the response and activation of the cell-killing membrane attack complex. The complement proteins are synthesized mainly in the liver and account for about 5% of the globulin fraction of blood serum *(79, 80)*.

As part of the innate immunity, the complement system is not adaptable and does not change over the course of an individual's lifetime. However, it can be recruited and brought into action by the adaptive immune system. Three biochemical pathways activate the complement system: the classical complement pathway, the alternative complement pathway, and the mannose-binding lectin pathway, either of which may lead to the formation of a cell membrane attack complex *(78–80)*.

The Classical Pathway. The classical pathway of the complement system may be activated by antigen-antibody complexes of the IgG, IgG3, or IgM isotypes by their binding to the C1q subunit of the first component of complement *(80)*. Consequently, the C1qrs subunits of C1 component will form an esterase that will cleave the next component, C4, into two fragments, the larger of which, C4b, binds covalently to hydroxyl or amino groups on cellular membranes. The next component, C2, after binding to C4b is partially digested by C1s esterase to form C2b. The resultant membrane-bound complex, C4b2a, is an enzyme (C3 convertase) that cleaves C3 into two biologically active fragments, C3a and C3b *(80)*.

The Alternative Pathway. The alternative pathway of the complement system is activated independently of the antigen-antibody complexes *(80)*. The major exogenous activators of the pathway are microbial agents and their products. The major components of the pathway are the serum protein factors B, D, and P (properdin). A small amount of C3 in the fluid phase, which normally is spontaneously activated, will interact with factor B to form C3Bb, which cleaves other C3 molecules to form C3b. C3b in turn attaches to surfaces and binds factor B. The resultant protein C3bB is then cleaved by factor D to form C3bBb, the C3 convertase of the alternative pathway. That enzyme is distinct from the one generated from the classical pathway but serves the same purpose. This complex then is stabilized by factor P *(80)*.

The binding of C3 to factor B is prevented, particularly in the fluid phase, by a regulatory molecule, factor H. The more vigorous activation of this pathway occurs when the host is exposed to microorganisms that are poor in sialic acid. In those circumstances, the binding of factor B to C3 is favored, and the activation of the alternative pathway is not readily inhibited by factor H. Therefore, more C3b is generated, and a positive amplification loop that generates more C3bBb (C3 convertase) is created. In contrast, sialic acid–rich encapsulated microorganisms such as *Streptococcus pneumoniae*, *Haemophilus influenzae*, and *Neisseria meningitides* are incapable of activating the alternative pathway and require binding to specific IgG or IgM antibodies to activate the classical pathway and generate the C3b for phagocytosis and the formation of the membrane attack complex. The receptors for activated complement fragments are (i) CR1, principally on phagocytic cells for C3b; (ii) CR2, principally on B cells for a fragment called C3d (receptor for EBV); and (iii) CR3 (Mac-1), on phagocytic and NK cells for inactivated C3b (C3bi) and C3d-g fragments *(80)*.

The Membrane Attack Complex. The activation of the complement system eventually leads to the formation of the membrane attack complex (MAC) that consequently lyses cells. The membrane attack complex is formed in the following manner. As a result of the formation of C3b, C5 is cleaved into two fragments, C5b and C5a. The larger fragment, C5b, combines with C6 and the complex attaches to the cell surface, where it forms the foundation for the sequential binding of C7, 8, and 9 (e.g., the membrane attack complex). C3b and its degradation product, C3bi, are opsonins. C3a and C5a are chemotaxins and anaphylotoxins; C5a is the more potent of the two factors *(80)*.

Once the membrane attack complex is formed, discrete holes are created in the surface membranes of the target cells. Consequently, extracellular fluid accumulates in the target cell, eventually leading to its lysis *(80)*.

38.4.1 Regulators of Complement Activation

A family of proteins, known as the regulators of complement activation (RCA), is playing a key role in this process by interacting with fragments of complement proteins C3 and/or C4 *(81–86)*. The RCA proteins are defined by (i) the presence of *short consensus repeat (SCR) domains*; (ii) the ability to bind the complement molecules C3b and C4b; and (iii) their clustering on chromosome 1 at the q3.2 locus *(81, 82)*. The RCA family includes the *soluble plasma proteins C4 binding protein (C4bp)* and *factor H*, as well as the *integral membrane proteins CD46 (membrane cofactor protein)*, *CD55 (decay accelerating factor)*, *CD35 (complement receptor type 1)*, and *CD21 (complement receptor type 2) (78)*. A C9 binding protein as the membrane attack complex inhibition factor is also able to inhibit complement activation but is not formally considered an RCA protein *(78)*.

In addition to their function in complement regulation, many RCA family members are used as receptors by a surprisingly large and diverse number of pathogens *(78)*. Thus, CD46 is a receptor for the measles virus *(87, 88)*, group A *Streptococcus pyogenes (89)*, *Neisseria gonorrhoeae* and *Neisseria meningitides (90)*, and human herpesvirus 6 *(91)*. CD55 has been identified as a receptor for enterovirus 70 *(92)*, some echoviruses *(93–95)*, and some coxsackieviruses *(96,97)*. Another protein, CD21, is a receptor for the Epstein-Barr virus *(98–100)*. The plasma proteins factor H and C4bp were found to bind to *Streptococcus pyogenes (101, 102)*, and factor H also binds to the surface protein OspE of *Borrelia burgdorferi (103)*.

Structurally, the RCA proteins contain short consensus repeats (SCRs), which represent modules of about 60 amino acids with four invariant cysteines linked in a Cys1–Cys3, Cys2–Cys4 pattern *(82)*. One striking feature of these molecules is that they each have several SCR domains concatenated in an uninterrupted series *(78)*.

Results from NMR studies *(104–109)* and x-ray crystallography *(110–115)* have demonstrated that the SCR domain adopts a β-barrel fold that consists of a central four-stranded antiparallel β-sheet. The SCR fold efficiently exposes most of the side chains to the solvent, giving domains a high surface-to-volume ratio. At structural level, the large difference in sequence has translated into a profound heterogeneity of the SCR domains (107–115).

38.4.2 Complement Activation

One strength of the complement response is its capacity to target its accumulative activation toward foreign substances while, under normal circumstances, it is being tightly controlled on self-surfaces (116). The stages of complement activation can be divided into early and late events.

The early events, which are initiated by one of the three distinct pathways (classical, alternative, or the mannose-binding lectin pathway), consist of a series of proteolytic steps leading to the formation of C3 convertase. Split-products resulting from the activation of the complement cascade then mediate inflammation by recruiting and activating the host's phagocytes. Furthermore, the assembly of the terminal complement components in the membrane of the pathogens would proceed to cell lysis.

In this regard, the complement component C3 is playing a key role at the point where the initiating pathways converge (116). One critical event that follows the complement activation is the covalent attachment of C3 to the pathogen surface. Both complement proteins, C3 and C4, possess an internal thioester moiety that would enable these molecules to form either ester or amide covalent bonds with acceptor sites on the pathogen surface (117, 118). Once it is covalently bound onto the nonself surfaces, the C3 protein would become a part of its own convertase creating an amplification loop that activates and then deposits increasing amounts of C3. The deposition of C3 on the surface of foreign substances will then target them for destruction by either the lytic pathway or by uptake by phagocytes through various specific complement receptors (116).

The activation of the complement is tightly controlled by several mechanisms, namely (i) by being covalently attached to foreign surfaces - the convertases ensure that the complement activation takes place only in close proximity to the nonself substance; (ii) the fast hydrolysis of the activated thioester bond of C3 (or C4) would prevent attachment to occur beyond its site of activation, thereby keeping deposition localized; and (iii) regulatory proteins found on cell surfaces and in circulation would protect the host cells from opsonization and lysis (116).

IgM is the most efficient initiator of classical complement activation. It is constitutively produced by a long-lived, self-renewing population of B1 lymphocytes and is nearly 1,000 times more effective than IgG (119) by showing a broad range of avidities for both foreign and self-antigens (120). It has been demonstrated that B-cell responses to IgM-antigen-

C3 complexes were significantly increased compared with the that for antigen alone (121).

38.4.3 Complement Receptors

Complement receptors play an important role in the uptake and clearance of opsonized antigens, as well as in the enhancement of both the innate and adaptive immunity (116). Based on their cell distribution and binding specificities, several types of complement receptors have been described. For example, the chemokine-like receptors C3aR and C5aR are known to specifically recognize the anaphylotoxins of C3 and C5, respectively, and to be important in the activation of the leukocytes.

Among the receptors that bind opsonizing complement fragments, the complement receptors 1, 2, 3, and 4 have been the subject of particular attention.

Complement Receptor 1 (CR1). CR1 (CD35) (122, 123) has been described as a receptor for opsonizing activation products C3 (C3b), C4 (C4b) (124), human C1q (125), and the mannose-binding lectin (MBL) (126). In human erythrocytes, CR1 fulfill an important role in the clearance of immune complexes and microorganisms by targeting them to the liver and spleen. Once in the spleen, the complexed antigen can be removed and degraded. In monocytes, CR1 promotes phagocytosis, and in dendritic and B cells, it serves to internalize antigens for processing and presentation. In addition, the CR1 regulates C3 convertase deposited on the host cells (116).

Complement Receptor 2 (CR2). CR2 (CD21) plays a key function in directly linking adaptive and innate immunity (116). It possesses binding specificity for C3d, C3dg, and iC3b. In the B cell, CR2 forms in conjunction with CD19 and CD81, a coreceptor for the antigen-specific B-cell receptor (BCR).

Complement Receptors 3 (CR3) and 4 (CR4). CR3 (CD11b/CD18, Mac-1) and CD4 (CD11c/CD18) share a number of characteristics (116). Both receptors, which have considerable structural homology, consist of two noncovalently associated type I membrane glycoproteins known as subunits α (CD11b or c, respectively) and β (CD18). As adhesion molecules in phagocytes, CR3 and CR4 facilitate the migration through the vascular endothelium into the sites of inflammation. Expression of CR3 and CR4 is detected mainly on cells of the myeloid lineage. However, nonmyeloid cells expressing CR3 include natural killer (NK) cells and CD5$^+$ B-lymphocytes. High levels of CR4 were found on tissue macrophages and dendritic cells (109).

Both CR3 and CR4 bind iC3b, a proteolytic breakdown product of antigen-bound C3b (127).

38.5 Lipopolysaccharide-Binding Protein and CD14

Human lipopolysaccharide (LPS)-binding protein (LBP) *(128)* is a serum glycoprotein belonging to a family of lipid-binding proteins that includes the bactericidal/permeability-increasing protein (BPI), the phospholipid ester transfer protein, and the cholesterol ester transfer protein *(129–131)*. It consists of 456 amino acid residues preceded by a hydrophobic signal sequence of 25 residues *(132)*. LBP is synthesized by hepatocytes *(133)* and intestinal epithelial cells *(134)* and is present in normal serum at concentrations of 5 to 10 μg/mL, rising up to 200 μg/mL 24 hours after induction of an acute-phase response *(135)*. This rise in LBP levels is caused by transcriptional activation of the LBP gene mediated by interleukin-1 (IL-1) and IL-6 *(136)*. LBP has a concentration-dependent dual role: low concentrations of LBP enhance the LPS-induced activation of mononuclear cells (MNCs), whereas the acute-phase rise in LBP concentrations inhibits LPS-induced cellular stimulation *(137)*. LBP binds a variety of LPS (endotoxin) chemotypes from rough and smooth strains of Gram-negative bacteria and even lipid A, the lipid moiety of LPS *(138, 139)*. The LPS molecules, components of the outer membrane of Gram-negative bacteria, are important mediators in the pathogenesis of Gram-negative sepsis and septic shock *(140)*. Because the lipid A moiety has been shown to be responsible for the biological activity of LPS in most *in vivo* and *in vitro* test systems, it has been termed the *endotoxic principle of LPS (141)*.

The LPS or endotoxin elicits a broad, nonspecific cascade of events *in vivo*, resulting in secretion of a variety of potent mediators and cytokines produced primarily by activated macrophages and monocytes through an intracellular signal amplification pathway *(141, 142)*. The overproduction of these effector molecules, such as interleukin-1 and tumor necrosis factor-α (TNF-α), in turn, contributes to the pathophysiology of cardiovascular shock, multisystem organ failure, and septic shock *(143, 144)*, one of the major causes of death in intensive care units. Specific cellular responses in organisms are generally mediated by receptors. For endotoxin recognition, a binding protein/receptor system has been postulated that involves LBP, the membrane-bound and soluble CD14 molecules, members of the family of TLRs *(145)*, and a K^+ channel *(146, 147)*.

Cellular recognition of LPS involves several different molecules, including the *"cluster of differentiation antigen 14" (CD14) (141)*. CD14 is a 55-kDa glycoprotein expressed on the surfaces of monocytes, macrophages, and neutrophils *(148–150)*. Although its expression on B cells has been reported *(151–153)*, it is generally accepted that normal B cells are CD14-negative *(142)*. CD14 has been initially characterized as a myeloid differential antigen, present in mature

cells but absent in myeloid precursors. In subsequent studies, CD14 has been assigned a functional role serving as a receptor of LPS in association with LBP in which heparinized human blood cultured for 16 hours with LPS resulted in the production of TNF-α, whose synthesis and release could be nearly eliminated by pretreatment with CD14-blocking mAb *(154)*. Thus, the LBP-mediated complexation of LPS with CD14, followed by the interaction of LPS-CD14 complexes with a receptor capable of initiating signaling that leads to inflammatory mediator production is a major functional role of CD14 *(155)*.

Structurally, CD14 has 10 leucine-rich repeats. It is both a membrane-bound receptor (via a glycosylphosphatidyl inositol tail) and a soluble plasma glycoprotein. It functions similarly in both environments to enhance activation of cells by LPS *(154, 156, 157)*.

The relevance of CD14 to acute disease mediated by Gram-negative bacteria has been well established from studies with CD14-deficient mice and models wherein the CD14 function was blocked by antibodies *(154, 155)*. The blockade of inflammation is essentially universally observed *(158, 159)*, although some cytokine responses were still found to persist *(160)*.

CD14 Polymorphisms and Asthma and Heart Disease. The relationship between CD14 polymorphisms and the chronic conditions of asthma and heart disease has emerged as an important subject of research *(155)*. The CD14 promoter has a polymorphism at an Sp1 site resulting in allelic variation in the levels of soluble CD14 produced *(161, 162)*. Because inflammation will alter the cytokine levels and Th2 responses, the altered CD14 levels may be related to a potential for allergic sensitization *(163)*. Hence, the possibility has been suggested for CD14 to be involved in the so-called *hygiene hypothesis* whereby exposure to environmental LPS or higher CD14 levels would lead to a diminished tendency for allergic responses *(164, 165)*. Thus, soluble CD14 was found to interact with B cells to lower IgE production *(166)*. Results from other studies have suggested that the same CD14 allele protecting against allergy may predispose to myocardial infarction *(167)* and to atherosclerosis *(168, 169)*, but not to ischemic cerebral disease *(170)*.

38.6 Chemokines in Innate and Adaptive Immunity

The chemokines belong to a supergene family of soluble 8- to 10-kDa protein mediators capable of attracting and activating specific leukocyte populations in the context of inflammatory and immune events *(12, 171, 172)*. In addition, they have also been implicated in playing an important role in the development and homeostasis of the inflammatory and immune responses *(173, 174)*. Because of their differing effects on the recruitment of specific leukocytes, the chemokines will ultimately determine which cells will regulate and participate in localized innate and adaptive immune responses *(12)*.

Nearly every mammalian cell appears to possess the ability to respond to pathogen invasion through the production of chemokines, which is carefully regulated to ensure that the kinetics and phenotype of the localized inflammatory response is tailored to the specific pathogen threat by directing only appropriate inflammatory cells to the target tissue *(12)*. Given the direct association between the chemokine expression and the severity of the inflammatory and immune responses in several tissues, blocking the actions of chemokines is now considered to be a novel therapeutic strategy for the treatment of diseases resulting from excessive immune activation *(175)*.

Chemokines Nomenclature. Bioinformatics-based analysis of nucleotide databases has defined at least 50 chemokines in four distinct structural families distinguished by the positioning of the cysteine moieties at the amino terminus in these proteins *(176)*.

The chemokine nomenclature has been standartized to mirror the sequential classification scheme currently used for chemokine receptors. Thus, chemokines are numbered consecutively as C–C ligand (CCL), C–X–C ligand (CXCL), C ligand (XCL), and C–X_3–C ligand (CX3CL). The two largest families are the C–C and C–X–C chemokines *(12, 176)*.

Chemokine Receptor Nomenclature. The chemokine superfamily of leukocyte chemoattractants coordinates the development and deployment of the immune system by signaling through a family of distinct rhodopsin-like GTP-binding protein-coupled receptors *(177)*. It should be noted, however, that most of the chemokine receptors are not selective for a single chemokine. For example, the C–C chemokines interact with at least 11 distinct receptors designated as CCR1 to CCR11. The C–X–C chemokines interact with at least six distinct CXCRs, of which CXCR1 and CXCR2 bind the prototypical human C–X–C chemokine, IL-8/CXCL8 *(12)*.

Nevertheless, the selectivity of the chemokine effects in the immune responses appeared to be tightly regulated at the level of chemokine receptor expression and the cell distribution of these receptors *(12)*.

38.6.1 Chemokines in Linking the Innate and Acquired Immune Systems in Cell-Specific Fashion

There has been clear evidence that chemokines play a major role in linking the innate and acquired immune systems *(12)*.

One way by which chemokines coordinate both arms of the immune response is through cell-specific activation and migration.

Neutrophils. Owing to their ability to perform a series of aggressive effector functions, the neutrophils represent key cellular innate immunity elements (phagocytes) in the inflammatory responses to injuries and infections *(12)*. In particular, neutrophils can be induced to express a variety of chemokines such as IL-8/CXCL8, GRO/CXCL1-3, MIP-1α/CCL3, MIP-1β/CCL4, IP-10/CXCL10, and MIG/CXCL9 *(178)*. Through its ability to elaborate these chemokines, it is conceivable to assume that chemokines can further initiate the chemotaxis of other leukocyte subsets including monocytes, immature dendritic cells (DCs), and T-lymphocyte subsets. However, the manner in which neutrophils regulate mononuclear cell recruitment to the sites of infection or inflammation is currently unknown *(12)*.

Dendritic Cells. The dendritic cells represent a heterogenous family that functions as sentinels of the immune system and are critical for moving antigens from peripheral sites to regional lymph nodes to allow appropriate transmission of antigenic specificity to T cells *(12, 179, 180)*.

Dendritic cells (DCs) are APCs with a unique ability to induce primary immune responses *(4)*. DCs capture and transfer information from the outside world to the cells of the adaptive immune system. DCs are not only critical for the induction of primary immune responses but may also be important for the induction of immunologic tolerance, as well as for the regulation of the type of T-cell–mediated immune response. Although current understanding of the biology of dendritic cells is still in its infancy, the use of DC-based immunotherapy protocols to elicit immunity against cancer and infectious diseases is the subject of a number of studies *(4)*.

In the lymphoid organs, DCs undergo maturation process during which they are capable of priming naïve T cells. Immature DCs respond to a number of C–C and C–X–C chemokines, including MIP-1α/CCL3, MIP-1β/CCL4, MIP-3α/CCL20, MCP-3/CCL7, MCP-4/CCL13, RANTES/CCL5, TECK/CCL25, and SDF-1/CXCL12; however, each immature DC population appeared to respond to a particular subset of chemokines *(12)*.

Conversely, the mature dendritic cells in the lymphoid tissue will lose their responsiveness to most of the inflammatory chemokines through receptor downregulation or desensitization *(12)*. Instead, these cells would subsequently acquire responsiveness to MIP-3β/CCL19 and SLC/CCL21 via CCR67 upregulation *(181–183)*. This change in DCs responsiveness would ensure the migration of mature DCs (also referred as *interdigitating DCs*) to the T-cell–rich areas in lymphoid tissues where MIP-3β/CCL19 and SLC/CCL21 chemokines are specifically expressed *(184)*. Furthermore, because dendritic cells serve as the major APCs in the induction of cellular responses to intracellular pathogens (e.g., mycobacteria), they control directly the development of the Th1-type protective immunity *(185)*.

On the whole, through their actions the chemokines trigger the rapid movement of dendritic cells during the first wave of cells into the inflamed tissues *(186)*, which in turn would participate in the further elaboration of chemokines necessary for the recruitment and activation of other inflammatory cells *(187)*. These events taken together clearly demonstrate the major role of chemokines and dendritic cells in the link between the innate and acquired immune response *(12)*.

CD1 Molecules. Recent studies have identified the CD1 family as nonclassical, Ag-presenting molecules involved in regulation of T-cell responses to microbial lipids and glycolipids-containing Ag *(4, 188, 189)*. Both endogenous and exogenous lipids can be presented, and this pathway may contribute not only to microbial immunity but also to autoimmunity and antitumor responses *(4)*.

CD1 molecules, a hallmark of the DC phenotype, constitute a family of β2-microglobulin–associated nonpolymorphic glycoproteins that assemble with a nonprocessed antigen (Ag) in the endosomal/lysosomal compartments and present Ag in a TAP-independent manner. In humans, four CD1 proteins (CD1a to CD1d) are expressed by myeloid DCs, whereas in mice only CD1d has been identified. CD1 proteins are functionally heterogeneous, and two subgroups can be identified. Subgroup I, including human CD1b-c, can present glycolipids to a large repertoire of T cells. Indeed, mycobacteria-specific, CD1b-restricted CD8$^+\alpha/\beta$ TCR T-cells have been demonstrated. Binding of the lipids to these CD1 molecules requires endosomal acidification. Subgroup II includes mouse and human CD1d and binds a limited set of antigens (α-galactosyl ceramide) and activates a restricted set of T cells as well as NK T-cells *(190)*. CD1-restricted presentation appears to also regulate γ/δ T-cells and intestinal intraepithelial lymphocytes. Much remains to be learned about this presentation pathway and the possibilities of its use in vaccine protocols *(4)*.

Natural Killer Cells. The natural killer (NK) cells comprise the major lymphocyte population *(191–194)* and can be distinguish from other lymphocytes by the absence of B- and T-cell antigen receptors, that is, surface immunoglobulin (sIg) and T-cell receptor (TCR), respectively *(191, 192)*. Although freshly isolated NK cells express the ξ-chain of the TCR/CD3 complex *(195, 196)*, they do not display other component of the complex; do not express mRNA for mature TCR chains; and do not rearrange TCR genes *(197)*.

The natural killer cells represent a population of unique lymphocytes that exhibit cytotoxic activity and produce high levels of certain cytokines and chemokines making them an important part of the innate and adaptive immune responses

to a number of infectious pathogens, such as in antiviral defense (e.g., herpesvirus) *(198–200)*.

The regulation of NK cells migration to inflammatory sites and subsequent activation have been the subject of intense research that have shown specificity in their response to different chemokines *(12, 191, 192)*. For example, while MIP-3α/CCL20, SLC/CCL21, and MIP-3β/CCL19 failed to induce detectable chemotaxis of resting peripheral blood NK cells, the latter two chemokines stimulated the migration of various types of activated peripheral blood NK cells *(201)*. Because of their ability to respond to these chemokines (normally expressed in defined lymphoid tissues), the NK cell may be able to interact directly with T cells in such defined lymphoid organs *(12)*.

In patients with HIV disease, the NK cell activity has been markedly diminished *(202, 203)* by infection with herpesvirus 6, inducing cytopathic changes and *de novo* expression of CD4 (a cellular receptor for HIV-1 not normally expressed by NK cells) *(204)*. This effect will render the NK cells susceptible to infection by HIV-1 resulting in an NK deficiency and possibly accounting, at least in part, for the increased susceptibility of HIV-positive patients to other infections such as cytomegalovirus *(191)*.

In general, the NK cell responses in innate immunity to infections involved two major effector mechanisms: *cytokine production and target killing (191)*. Thus, NK cells can respond to several different cytokines resulting in the production of other cytokines; for example, the induction of NK cell production of IFN-γ by IL-12 and the type I interferons. Studies in mice have shown that NK cells did not appear to respond directly to *Listeria* infection, but rather macrophage production of IL-12 was required for the production of IFN-γ by NK cells as well as infection control *(205, 206)*. Furthermore, TNF-α can synergize with IL-12 to induce NK cell production by IFN-γ, whereas IL-10 was an antagonist *(205)*. Additional studies have demonstrated that during viral infections, including lymphocytic choriomeningitis virus (LCMV), the cytotoxicity of NK cells was enhanced and proliferation ensued. These events constituted some of the systemic effects directly or indirectly mediated by the type I interferons *(207)*.

An emerging area of investigation has been the role of IL-15 in NK cell responses *in vivo (208)* because mice deficient in IL-15 or IL-15Rα were found to lack NK cells *(209, 210)*. Nevertheless, a number of studies have indicated that NK cells were stimulated during the course of infection by IL-15 and have increased activity against virus-infected cells *(208, 211–214)*.

Normally, the NK cells will kill their targets by triggering the release of preformed cytoplasmic granules containing perforin and granzymes, a process termed *granule exocytosis (215)*. The conventional thinking has been that during the exocytosis, perforin will polymerize in the target cell plasma membrane, producing a pore through which the granzymes would enter and after being activated will trigger the target cell apoptosis *(191)*. However, subsequent studies have suggested that granzymes may also enter the cell via the mannose-6-phosphate receptor rather than through the perforin-formed pore *(216)*. Further studies have also indicated that NK cells can kill certain targets by other means, including Fas and TNF-α–related apoptosis-inducing ligand (TRAIL), although these pathway are still not well understood *(217)*. In addition, resting NK cells apparently did not express Fas ligand on their cell surface and therefore must be triggered to mediate Fas-induced death *(218)*.

Early studies on the molecular basis for NK cell recognition of cellular targets have described an inverse correlation between target cell expression of MHC class I and the susceptibility to NK cells *(219)*. For example, target cells that have not expressed MHC class I proteins were killed by NK cells, whereas MHC class I–bearing targets were generally resistant *(220)*. These findings have provided the major insights into NK cell recognition, termed the *missing-self hypothesis (191)*. Accordingly, it has been postulated *(221)* that NK cells would survey tissues for normal expression of MHC class I proteins that are ubiquitously expressed. Then, if a cell is lacking expression of MHC I class proteins (such as in tumorigenesis or viral infection) thereby evading MHC class I–restricted T-cells, the chronic inhibitory influence of MHC class I is lost, permitting NK cell to lyse the target *(191)*.

It is now clearly recognized that NK cells express *MHC class I–specific inhibitory receptors*, which fall into two general structural types *(222, 223)*. The human killer Ig-like receptors (KIRs) represent type I integral membrane proteins with Ig-like domains encoded in the leukocyte receptor complex. By contrast, human and rodent CD94/NKG2A and rodent Ly49 receptors have type II orientation and are disulfide-linked dimers with domains that are distantly related to the C-type lectins and encoded in the NK gene complex (NKC) *(191)*. The two structural types share common features such as immunoreceptor tyrosine-based inhibitory motifs (ITIMs) in their cytoplasmic domains *(224)*. Contrary to T cells, the NK cell receptors for MHC class I have different requirements for MHC-associated peptides. For example, while some receptors appeared to have no peptide selectivity *(225, 226)*, other NK receptors displayed an apparent peptide selectivity *(227, 228)*.

In addition to inhibitory receptors, the NK cell recognition also appeared to involve *activation receptors* compatible with a two-receptor model for the mechanism of NK cell activation *(229)*. That is, the fate of a target cell will be determined by the engagement (or not) of both activation and inhibitory receptors on the NK cell by their target cell ligands and the integration of signals transduced by such receptors *(191)*. During such an event, inhibitory receptors appeared

to regulate activation receptors (or vice versa) that may have their own specificity for ligands on targets *(230–233)*. In general, however, the simultaneous engagement of activation and inhibitory receptors has been associated with inhibition, indicating that inhibition is dominant over activation *(234, 235)*. Nevertheless, the outcome of activation or inhibition would likely result from a balance between the kinases and phosphatases activated by respective ligand interactions *(236)*.

There has been recent evidence to suggest the important role that NK cell activation receptors may play in viral evasion strategies through viral-encoded proteins that interfere with natural killing *(191, 237–243)*. In many cases, this interference is caused by enhanced function of inhibitory MHC class I–specific NK cell receptors as documented with human cytomegalovirus (HCMV) *(191)*. Another example of viral evasion is the selective downregulation of MHC class I molecules by HIV-1 *(237)*. In that case, the virus down-regulated HLA-A and HLA-B but not HLA-C or HLA-E. In both cases, HCMV and HIV have evolved mechanisms that resulted in inhibition due to selective engagement of both structural types of inhibitory receptors *(191)*.

The Kaposi's sarcoma–associated herpesvirus (KSHV) has also been shown to possess mechanism to avoid NK cells *(243)*. In this case, the KSHV protein K5 downregulated the expression of the intracellular adhesion molecule (ICAM)-1 and B7-2, which are ligands for NK cell receptors involved in cytotoxicity. In this regard, the interaction of leukocyte function-associated antigen-1 (LFA-1) on the NK cell with ICAM-1 on the target was one of the first receptor-ligand interactions important in NK cell killing of targets to be recognized *(244)*. In contrast with the limited distribution of most NK cell activation and inhibitory receptors, LFA-1 in particular, is broadly expressed and its function has been required for target cytoxicity *(191)*.

Ly49H is another NK cell activation receptor found to play a key role in the resistance of murine cytomegalovirus (MCMV). Thus, a genome-wide scan identified autosomal dominant *Cmv1* resistance gene as being responsible for the genetically determined resistance of ceratin strains of mice to MCMV *(245)*. The identification of Ly49H as a resistance factor for MCMV infections also suggested that it may be involved in defense against other pathogens, such as the mousepox (ecromelia) virus and herpes simplex virus (HSV), for which resistant loci have also been genetically mapped to the NK cells *(246, 247)*.

T Cells. The adaptive immune response is initiated by the interaction of T-cell antigen receptors with MHC molecule-peptide complexes *(248)*. Although the interaction between chemokines and their receptors is an important step in the control of T-cell migration into the sites of inflammation, it has become apparent that chemokines also play a major role in determining the T-cell cytokine generation *(12)*.

Activated T cells differentiate into two major effector subtypes, Th1 and Th2, which secrete cytokines that enhance the cell-mediated (IFN-γ) and humoral immunity (Il-4 and IL-13), respectively. These cytokines, which define either a type 1 or type 2 inflammatory phenotype, have the ability to induce a set of either IFN-γ–inducible chemokines or a set of IL-4/IL-13–inducible chemokines *(12)*.

Chemokines have also been involved in the mediation of multiple effects independent of chemotaxis, including the induction and enhancement of Th1- and Th-2–associated cytokine responses *(249)*. When activated under polarizing conditions with polyclonal stimuli *in vitro*, human Th1 and Th2 clones displayed distinct patterns of chemokine receptor expression: Th1 clones preferentially expressed CCR5 and CXCR3 *(250)*, whereas many Th2 clones expressed CCR4, CCR8 *(251, 252)*, and, to a lesser extent, CCR3. Such differential patterns of chemokine receptor expression did suggest a mechanism for selective induction of migration and activation of Th1- and Th2-type cells during the inflammation and (perhaps) normal immune homeostasis *(253)*.

Epithelial Cells. Although not normally associated with either the innate or acquired immune systems by being ideally situated between the host and its environment, the epithelial cells from various tissues have been established to respond to innate immune signals and consequently to secrete an array of chemokines that participate in both arms of the immune response when penetrated by invasive microbial pathogens *(254)*. For example, MIP-3α/CCL20 was constitutively expressed by human intestinal epithelium, and the levels of this CCR6 ligand, which is expressed on dendritic cells, T cells, and NK cells, could be markedly upregulated by inflammatory cytokines such as TNF-α and IL-1β *(12)*. RANTES/CCL5 is another chemokine (chemotactic for T cells) that is produced by lymphoid and epithelial cells at several mucosal sites in response to various external stimuli. Evidence that RANTES/CCL5 can serve as a link between the initial innate signals of the host and the adaptive immune system has been derived by the fact that this C-C chemokine enhanced the mucosal and systemic humoral antibody responses through help provided by the Th1- and select Th2-type cytokines *(255)*. In addition, RANTES/CCL5 has also been shown to induce the expression of costimulatory molecules and cytokine receptors on T cells *(255)*.

Fibroblasts. As in the case of epithelial cells, fibroblasts are normally not considered in the context of innate or adaptive immune responses, but these cells have been clearly associated with the production of chemokines during inflammatory reactions in several tissues *(12)*. Fibroblasts are a major source of constitutive and cytokine-induced MCP-1/CCL2, MIP-1α/CCL3, RANTES/CCL5, IP-10/CXCL10, and eotaxin/CCL11 *(256)*, but in their capacity as sentinel cells *(257)*, fibroblasts have also been able to produce different patterns of chemokines in response to different

alarm stimuli *(12)*. In this regard, an important regulator of chemokine production by fibroblasts appeared to be ReIB, a transcription factor that increases rapidly after the activation of fibroblasts with inflammatory stimuli such as IL-1β, TNF-α, and LPS *(258)*.

38.6.2 Chemokines in Linking the Innate and Acquired Immune Systems During Disease

A series of studies have provided convincing evidence of the role of chemokines in linking the innate and acquired immune responses during disease, especially in HIV infection and in models of pulmonary disease and septic shock syndrome *(12)*.

Chemokines, HIV, and Other Viruses. Since the discovery that MIP-1α/CCL3, RANTES/CCL5, and MIP-1β/CCL4 inhibited the binding of the M-tropic HIV to macrophages *(256)*, and that an array of herpesviruses and poxviruses have encoded chemokine mimics capable of blocking chemokine action *(259)*, the relationship between viruses and chemokines has been the subject of extensive investigation *(12)*.

During their evolution, viruses have developed effective means to elude the normal host defense. Thus, infection with HIV has affected both the innate and acquired immune responses by the ability of the virus during its dissemination to target macrophages and T cells via the CCR5 and CXCR4 coreceptors, respectively *(260, 261)*. In addition, the HIV infection also changes the phagocytic function of the macrophages *(262)*. The latter effect has been manifested by the patients' reduced capacity to deal with subsequent pathogen exposure, such as chronic pulmonary infections caused by mycobacteria *(263)*.

However, recent findings have also suggested a therapeutic potential in using the various evasive molecular "piracy" and mimicry tactics developed by the viral pathogens. For example, the Kaposi's sarcoma–associated herpesvirus (KSHV) or the human herpesvirus 8 have been able to encode C–C chemokine-like molecules, such as KSHV vMIP-I *(264, 265)* and vMIP-II *(265)*, which exerted potent agonist effects on CCR8, a C–C chemokine receptor that regulates the chemotaxis of Th2-type lymphocytes *(265)*. However, vMIP-II and vMMC-I have also been found to exhibit potent *in vitro* antagonistic activities against CCRs, CXCRs, and CX3CR1 *(266)*. The anti-inflammatory activity of recombinant vMIP-II was documented in a rat model of experimental glomerulonephritis demonstrating that this viral chemokine potently inhibited the leukocyte infiltraton to the glomeruli and markedly attenuated proteinuria *(267)*. Hence, although viruses presumably use chemokines and chemokine receptors to ensure their survival or to create a tissue environment that facilitates their dissemination *(268)*, it is conceivable that these viral chemokines could also be modified to benefit humans undergoing an inflammatory or immune event *(12)*.

Chemokine Regulation of Pulmonary Inflammatory and Immune Responses. In order to facilitate an adequate gas exchange, the lung contains the largest epithelial surface area of the body. Because of its contact with the external environment, the upper and lower airways of the lung are constantly exposed to a bevy of potentially harmful airborne particles and microorganisms, necessitating an elaborate system of defense mechanisms to prevent the harmful effects of invading pathogens *(12)*.

The initial clearance of microorganisms from the lung is carried out by a dual phagocytic system involving both alveolar macrophages and polymorphonuclear leukocytes. When the host is challenged by a pathogen, a number of systems are set in motion for the production of chemokines *(12)*. For example, tissue macrophages, such as the alveolar macrophages in the lung, can generate early response cytokines, IL-1 and TNF-α. These early response cytokines will further involve surrounding cells in the lung tissue to produce a set of chemokines facilitating the moving of leukocytes from the lumen of the vasculature to the site of inflammation *(269)*. The manner in which the chemokine actions in the lung affect not only the acute inflammatory response but also the much later acquired response has been investigated in mice by examining the role of MIP-2 and SLC/CCL21 in the development of acute pulmonary inflammation induced by an intrathracheal injection of *Propionibacterium acnes (270)*. Immunoneutralization of MIP-2 and CXCR2 (neutrophil-specific chemokine and chemokine receptor) was shown to alleviate the *P. acnes*–induced pulmonary inflammation, as has been shown for a number of acute infectious-type insults in the lung *(271)* including pneumonia *(272)*. However, in the same study *(271)*, the immunoneutralization of SLC/CCL21 did exacerbate the pulmonary inflammation due to a significant increase in the number of mature dendritic cells, macrophages, and neutrophils but decreased CD4$^+$ T-cell counts in the *P. acnes*–challenged lungs. This finding was attributed to the fact that dendritic cells that were detained in the lungs of *P. acnes*–challenged mice prevented the development of an antigen-specific T-cell response in the regional lymph nodes *(271)*.

Systemic overexpression of MCP-1/CCL2 via an adenoviral vector during the sensitization phase of Th1 (PPD-induced)- and Th2 [*Schistosoma* egg antigen (SEA)-induced]-type pulmonary granulomatous responses had a major impact on the overall phenotype associated with these lesions *(249)*. Systematic overexpression of MCP-1 during the sensitization phase of the Th1 model markedly reduced the granulomatous response, whereas increased MCP-1 dur-

ing the sensitization phase of the Th2 model enhanced the granulomatous reaction *(249)*. Furthermore, restimulation of splenocytes *ex vivo* from both models revealed an altered cytokine profile in which IFN-γ and IL-12 levels were significantly reduced in the Th1 model, and IL-10 and IL-13 were increased in the Th2 model *(249)*.

38.6.3 Chemokines and Sepsis

In spite of significant advances in antibiotic research and in intensive care unit technology, the sepsis-associated morbidity and mortality continue to be a major health care problem worldwide *(12, 273)*. The clinicopathologic manifestations and ultimate mortality of sepsis to a very large degree have been the result of intense cellular and molecular interactions that contribute to the systemic inflammatory state, the so-called *systemic inflammatory response syndrome (SIRS) (274)*. A number of immune and anti-inflammatory modulating therapies have been used in an attempt to limit the progression of SIRS. However, the results of these interventions have not led to significant improvement in survival; in some cases even the results proved to be deleterious *(275)*. In addition, patients with sepsis often develop nosocomial infections due to a global anergic state of their immune systems *(276)*.

In a murine model of septic peritonitis, MCP-1/CCL2 appeared to have a distinct role in the recruitment of leukocytes, including neutrophils, necessary for the containment of bacteria that have leaked in the peritoneal cavity *(277)*. The mechanism of action of MCP-1/CCL2 is thought to involve shifting the immune balance in favor of anti-inflammatory cytokine expression and away from the production of proinflammatory cytokines *(278, 279)*.

Further studies have shown that two other chemokines, MDC/CCL22 and C10, shared some key characteristics with MCP-1/CCL2 during septic responses. However, some notable differences have also been observed. For example, contrary to MCP-1/CCL2, either exogenous MDC/CCL22 or the C10 chemokines could be administered to mice after the induction of septic peritonitis to achieve a clear survival benefit *(280, 281)*. Furthermore, both MDC/CCL22 and C10 have a distinct effect on the phagocytic activities of resident peritoneal macrophages (through upregulation of TNF-α), but these macrophage-activating effects have appeared to be limited to the peritoneal cavity *(12)*.

38.6.4 Antimicrobial Peptides

A number of endogenous antimicrobial polypeptides, typically containing fewer than 100 amino acids, have increasingly been recognized as integral components of the human innate immunity *(282)*. Structurally, they represent, in general, cationic (positively charged) and amphipathic molecules. Such configuration would facilitate their binding and integration into the anionic cell walls and phospholipid membranes of the microorganisms. The structures of the antimicrobial peptides are diverse, but amphipathic peptides that assume α-helical conformations in membrane-mimetic environments and disulfide-stabilized β-sheet–rich peptides are particularly common *(282)*. Also presented are peptides with repetitive motifs (often containing prolines) and peptides with a high percentage of tryptophan.

In mammals, two major antimicrobial peptides have been defined: *defensins*, characterized by a β-sheet–rich structure stabilized by three disulfides, and *cathelicidins*, characterized by a conserved precursor motif (the "cathelin" domain) joined by a highly variable *C*-terminal mature peptide. In addition, there are histidine-rich peptides (*histatins*) produced by the salivary glands, and several peptides (e.g., lactoferricin, buforin, etc.) generated by partial hydrolysis of macromolecular precursors (lactoferrin and histone H2A) *(282)*.

Antimicrobial peptides exist in the innate immunity of all living organisms (vertebrates, invertebrates, plants, and protozoa). Antimicrobial peptides are also produced by some prokaryotes *(283)* and even Archaea *(284)*.

Mechanism of Action. In general, the antimicrobial peptides would bind initially to the microbial membranes resulting in the increased membrane's permeability. It is generally accepted that the antimicrobial peptides will act through different mechanisms to facilitate traverse through the microbial cell wall barriers, often involving multiple phases as the peptide concentration increases *(285–289)*.

Nearly all of the antimicrobial peptides can exert their activity by disrupting the microbial membrane causing interference with the bacterial metabolism, homeostasis, and the proton-motive force. If severe, these will cause leakage of the cellular contents and allow noxious substances and/or the peptides themselves to enter the bacterial cytoplasm *(282)*.

The microbial damage can be exacerbated by osmotic stresses resulting from the excessive entry of water or by displacing the bacterium's autolytic enzymes from their cell wall docking sites, thereby inducing inappropriate cell wall remodeling. Moreover, other host defense molecules, including oxidants, lytic enzymes, pore-forming proteins, and binders of essential nutrients, may also act concomitantly to potentiate further damage to the target *(282)*. In addition to acting on cell wall structures (outer membrane, peptidoglycan, plasma membrane), the antimicrobial peptides may also enter the microbial cytoplasm through pores or by flip-flop movements through the phospholipid membranes *(290)*.

Defensins. Human defensins are members of a widely distributed family of microbicidal peptides having a three-dimensional fold and a six-cystein/three-disulfide pattern *(291, 292)*. Depending on the spacing and connectivity of the cysteines, these peptides have been classified as α- and β-defensins. In addition, cyclic demidefensins (θ-defensins), isolated from rhesus leukocytes, are generated by posttranslational circularization of two demidefensin segments; there are no human counterparts of θ-defensins *(293)*.

The crystal structures of human α-defensin HNP-3 *(294)* and human β-defensin HBD-2 *(295)* have been determined, as well as the solution structures of the human β-defensin HNP-1, rabbit α-defensins NP-1 and NP-5, human β-defensin HBD-2, and the bovine β-defensin BNBD-12 *(295–298)*. Common features indicate similarities of the three-dimensional structures of the α- and β-defensins including the presence of an antiparallel β-sheet. The difference in the activities of the α- and β-defensins may be largely due to variations in charge and its distribution, as well as the length and composition of the *N*-terminal segment *(282)*.

Three closely related α-defensins, HNP-1, -2, and -3, are major components of the myeloperoxidase-containing azurophil granules of the neutrophils. A fourth α-defensin, HNP-4, has been found in the same location but is much less abundant *(299–301)*. When neutrophils that have ingested *Salmonella typhimurium* were assayed by radioiodination and subcellular fractionation, defensins appeared to be the most abundant neutrophil-derived polypeptides within the phagocytic vacuoles *(302)*. It has also been reported that α-defensins were also expressed by certain populations of human T-lymphocytes and natural killer cells *(303)*.

The three best characterized β-defensins, HBD-1, -2, and -3, differ slightly from the classical α-defensins in the placement and connectivity of their cysteines *(304–307)*. Their mRNAa were expressed in epithelial cells and some glands. Although HBD-2 is not expressed constitutively by the skin keratinocytes, its synthesis is induced by inflammation, most likely by a transcriptional control mechanism analogous to that described for bovine epithelial defensins in the trachea and the tongue *(308–310)*.

The microbicidal and cytotoxic activities of the defensins are thought to involve several steps *(311–315)*. Initially, the defensins will bind to the target cell membranes and make them permeable to small molecules such as trypan blue (MW = 960.8), various β-lactams, or β-galactosides. Both electrostatic interaction and transmembrane electromotive force play a role in defensin-mediated permeabilization of biologic membranes *(311, 313, 314, 316–329)*.

In anionic phospholipid liposomes (but not zwitterionic or mixed liposomes), the human defensin HNP-2 induced leakage of vesicle contents through stable pores large enough to pass dextran molecules of several kilodaltons in mass, yielding an estimated pore size of 25 Å *(282)*.

In a rare human genetic disease, *specific granule deficiency*, neutrophil defensins were found present at 10% of the normal amount *(320)*. The affected patients suffer from frequent bacterial infections, and their neutrophils have been defective in killing bacteria *(321)*. However, because multiple other components of neutrophil granules are also found deficient, including the human cationic antimicrobial peptide of 18 kDa (hCAP-18) and the bactericidal/permeability-increasing protein (BPI) *(327)*, the phenotype (frequent infections) cannot be attributed solely to the lack of defensins *(282)*.

Cathelicidins. The cathelicidins comprise a large family of microbicidal pro-peptides with a conserved *N*-terminal precursor cathelin domain of about 100 amino acid residues and an antimicrobial *C*-terminal that is typically 10 to 40 amino acid residues long. Many cathelicidin pro-peptides, including hCAP-18, have antimicrobial domains that comprise α-helical peptides, typically containing 23 to 37 residues *(282)*. Unlike defensins, the α-helical cathelicidin peptides retain a strong, broad-spectrum antimicrobial activity in the presence of physiologic concentrations of NaCl and divalent cations *(323)*.

Most mammalian cathelicidins will undergo an extracellular proteolytic cleavage freeing the active *C*-terminal antimicrobial peptide from the cathelin domain of the precursor *(324–327)*. However, some cathelicidins appeared to be active in the uncleaved form *(328, 329)*.

In contrast with defensins, which are confined within the neutrophil's primary (azurophil) granules in a fully processed form, the human cathelicidin, hCAP-18/LL-37, is found in specific (secretory) granules of the neutrophils in its 17-kDa (140 amino acid), cathelin-containing hCAP-18 proform *(282)*. During or after its secretion, the hCAP-18 proform can undergo processing into mature 5-kDa (37 amino acid) peptide, LL37 *(330, 331)*.

Biophysical measurements in model systems revealed that LL-37 has predominately assumed α-helical conformation oriented nearly parallel with the surface of zwitterionic-lipid membranes. This finding could be interpreted to be consistent with a detergent-like (rather than a pore-forming) mechanism *(332)*. LL-37 was found to be chemotactic for human neutrophils, monocytes, and T lymphocytes, apparently acting through the formyl peptide receptor-like-1 (FPRL1) receptor. Consequently, LL-37 may also contribute to adaptive immunity by recruiting monocytes and T cells *(333)*.

Although hCAP-18/LL37 has been initially recognized as a constitutive component of the human neutrophil, it is also expressed in other cells and by nonmyeloid tissues such as the squamous epithelia of the mouth, tongue, esophagus, cervix, and the vagina *(334)*, as well as in service epithelial cells and submucosal glands of the conducting airway *(335)*. The hCAP-18 is also produced in the epididymis and could play a prominent role in host defense of the genitourinary tract *(336)*.

In a recent observation *(337)*, during early *Shigella* spp. infections and other dysenteries, the rectal expression of the antibacterial peptides LL-37 and β-defensin-1 has been reduced or turned off for up to several weeks. When this phenomenon was studies in *Shigella*-infected epithelial and monocyte cultures, it appeared that the *Shigella* plasmid DNA could mediate the effect. It has been suggested that downregulation of these endogenous antimicrobial peptides may have promoted both the bacterial adherence and their subsequent invasion into host epithelium *(337)*.

Respiratory epithelia of cystic fibrosis (CF) patients are abnormally susceptible to bacterial infections. In this regard, overexpression of hCAP-18/LL-37 by recombinant adenovirus in CF respiratory epithelial cell cultures was shown to increase the epithelial resistance to infection with *Pseudomonas aeruginosa* and *Staphylococcus aureus (338)*. Moreover, the adenovirus construct also augmented the resistance of mice against airway challenge with *P. aeruginosa (339)*. The observed effect of CAP-18/LL-37 may be partly mediated by its ability to bind LPS, as systemic administration of the adenovirus construct had also protected against systemic challenge with LPS *(339)*.

38.7 Innate Immune Signaling During Phagocytosis

Phagocytosis of pathogens is a general and effective innate mechanism of mammalian host defense that also initiates the highly specific adaptive immune response *(340, 341)*. It is a process by which foreign particles larger than about 0.5 μm in diameter are engulfed by the plasma membrane of a cell and internalized into an intracellular membrane-bound phagosome *(341–343)*.

The mechanism of phagocytosis is a succession of events that involve several steps, namely (i) receptors on the host cell surface (most likely, Fc or the mannose receptors) recognize and bind to a foreign particle; (ii) a signal is generated that induces actin polymerization under the membrane at the site of contact; (iii) actin-rich membrane extensions reach out around the particle; (iv) the membranes fuse behind the particle, pulling it in toward the center of the cell; and (v) the newly formed phagosome matures into an acidic, hydrolytic compartment *(340)*. The precise mechanism of internalization, however, exhibits surprising heterogeneity and will depend largely on the type of receptor(s) that participate in the particle recognition *(341)*. In addition, the immunologic consequences of the particle internalization will vary. For example, particles internalized by receptors, such as the Fc receptor and the mannose receptor, evoke potent proinflammatory responses, whereas particles internalized by the complement receptor appear largely silent, and the phagocytosis of apoptotic cells induces anti-inflammatory responses *(341)*.

As a host immune response, phagocytosis lies in the interface of the innate and adaptive immune responses. Thus, the inflammatory responses associated with pathogen internalization by immune recognition receptors facilitate the elaboration of the adaptive immune response. Similarly, the adaptive immune response would use the phagocytes as effector cells; antibody-opsonized particles are recognized by the Fc receptors on the phagocytes, leading to particle internalization and sterilization *(341, 344, 345)*.

38.7.1 Recognition Receptors

Currently, an extremely high number of proteins have been implicated in direct recognition of pathogens. Nevertheless, only relatively few types of innate immune recognition receptors, such as the Fc receptors, appear to be individually competent to generate the signals that are required for both particle ingestion and inflammatory responses *(341, 343, 345)*. Therefore, the processes associated with pathogen recognition are likely to be caused by the simultaneous engagement of different receptors that taken together will influence the phagocytic responses *(340)*.

Integrin Receptors. Foreign particles entering the host may be opsonized by a variety of serum proteins, such as complement iC3b, fibronectin, and vitronectin, all of which are defined as members of the integrin family of receptors. Thus, particles coated with iC3b are recognized by the $\alpha_M\beta_2$-integrin (also known as complement receptor 3, CD11b/CD18, or Mac 1) found on monocytes, macrophages, neutrophils, granulocytes, dendritic cells, and natural killer cells *(346)*. An additional integrin, $\alpha_X\beta_2$ (also called complement receptor 4, CD11c/CD18, or gp150/95), also binds iC3b-opsonized particles; this receptor, however, is expressed highly only on tissue macrophages and dendritic cells and has not been as well characterized as $\alpha_M\beta_2$ *(346)*.

The extracellular binding domain structure of the leukocyte integrins has been extensively studied, and most of the properties of the protein domains were well documented. Thus, similarly to other α-integrins, the extracellular domains of α_M and α_X were found to consist of seven tandem repeats that mediate divalent cation binding. In addition, their extracellular domains also contain a 200-amino-acid inserted domain (I-domain) that is required by leukocyte β_2-integrins for ligand recognition *(346, 347)*.

Leukocyte α- and β-integrins possess short 45- and 23-amino-acid cytoplasmic tails, respectively, that together mediate the intracellular signaling *(348)*. Furthermore, internalization signaled by $\alpha_M\beta_2$ integrin would require a second activation step *(inside-out signaling)* that would increase the number of receptors at the cell surface *(347, 349, 350)* and the infinity of the receptors *(351)*, and would allow the receptors to trigger phagocytosis *(352–354)*.

Overall, the integrin engagement activates multiple downstream signaling pathways that can not only mediate particle internalization but are also likely to be involved in mediating the inflammatory responses *(340)*.

Mannose Receptor. The macrophage mannose receptor is a type I transmembrane protein with a short, 45-amino-acid cytoplasmic tail. The extracellular domain of the receptor consists of eight C-type lectin carbohydrate recognition domains (CRDs) together with a short amino-terminal cystein-rich region and a fibronectin type II repeat *(340)*. The expression of the mannose receptor in normally non-phagocytic COS cells was found to be sufficient in mediating the internalization of zymosan, a yeast wall particle made primarily of α-mannan/mannoproteins and β-glucans *(355, 356)*. However, the molecular mechanisms by which mannose receptors activate downstreams signals for particle internalization have not yet been defined *(340)*.

β-Glucan Receptor. Soluble forms of both α-mannan and β-glucan were found to inhibit the phagocytosis of zymosan by macrophages, indicating that receptors for both of these sugars participate in the particle recognition and uptake *(357–360)*.

Scavenger Receptors. The scavenger receptors are a family defined initially for their ability to bind and internalize modified lipoproteins such as acetylated low-density lipoprotein *(340)*. However, the spectrum of targets recognized by these receptors has expanded to include polyribonucleotides, lipopolysaccharides, and silica particles *(361)*.

Currently, there is significant evidence that several scavenger receptors participate in phagocytosis *(340)*. Thus, macrophages from mice lacking scavenger receptor A have been significantly less effective at phagocytosing heat-killed *E. coli (362, 363)*. One additional member of the class A scavenger receptors, macrophage structure with collagenous structure (MARCO), has been shown to be expressed constitutively on certain subpopulations of macrophages such as those in the marginal zone of the spleen *(364)* and could be induced in other macrophage populations by exposure to inflammatory stimuli such as LPS *(365)*. MARCO was observed to bind to a variety of Gram-positive and Gram-negative bacteria, as well as artificial particles such as latex, and antibodies to MARCO markedly blocked the internalization of each of these targets *(365, 366)*.

CD36 (a class B scavenger receptor) is required for the phagocytosis of apoptotic cells by macrophages and dendritic cells *(367, 368)*. A CD36-related protein, croquemort, was also found necessary for phagocytosis of apoptotic cells in *Drosophila (369)*.

Whereas scavenger receptors clearly mediate clearance of soluble ligands such as acetylated low-density polyprotein by trigering receptor-mediated endocytosis, there has been no evidence to suggest that the scavenger receptors were capable of generating phagocytic signal directly. That is to say that while expression of the mannose receptor or the complement receptor 3 in nonphagocytic cells can make these cells competent to internalize a target, the expression of scavenger receptors would mediate binding without notable internalization *(362, 364, 365)*.

38.7.2 Signaling Mechanisms for Particle Internalization

Particle internalization necessitates the activation of an array of signaling pathways that taken together would elicit the rearrangement of the actin cytoskeleton, extension of the plasma membrane, and the fusion to form a phagosome *(340)*. To this end, whereas some signaling molecules such as the PI-3-kinase appear to be required for internalization mediated by any phagocytic receptor, other proteins such as the tyrosine kinases are required for some types of internalization but not for others. In addition, many of the same molecules that coordinate events associated with the particle ingestion also participate in signaling events leading to gene transcription and protein secretion, alterations in cell morphology, and the activation of antimicrobial mechanisms. This extensive overlap of processes involving signaling molecules when coupled with the recruitment of these molecules together to phagosomes would make it likely that different signaling pathways will interact functionally *(340)*.

Tyrosine Kinases. Tyrosine phosphorylation of phagosome-associated and cytosolic proteins accompanies all types of phagocytosis, suggesting that many types of phagocytic receptors stimulate tyrosine kinase activation *(341, 345, 347, 348)*. However, an absolute requirement for tyrosine kinase activation has been demonstrated only for the internalization of igG-opsonized particles by Fc receptors *(370, 371)*.

Upon ligation, the immunoreceptor tyrosine-based activation motifs (ITAMs) of Fc receptors are phosphorylated by src family tyrosine kinases, and this would probably account for the blockade imposed by tyrosine kinase inhibitors *(372)*.

The requirement for tyrosine kinase activation during internalization through innate immune recognition, however, is less clear. Macrophages from syk-deficient mice did internalize complement-opsonized particles, bacteria, and zymosan normally *(372)*. Even though general tyrosine kinase inhibitors did not block internalization of particles such as complement-opsonized particles or bacteria, these inhibitors did reduce the efficiency of the uptake, indicating that other tyrosine kinases might be eventually involved *(370, 373)*. Furthermore, proinflammatory responses initiated

during phagocytosis via innate immune recognition receptors would require tyrosine kinase activation, and some of this requirement can be attributed to activation of the mitogen-activated protein (MAP) kinases *(374, 375)*.

Protein Kinase C. The protein kinase C (PKC) is known to exist in 12 isoforms, and at least five of them (PKC-α, -β, -ε, -δ, and -ζ) are expressed in macrophages and recruited to membranes during phagocytosis where their activities are necessary for particle internalization *(376–378)*. General inhibitors of protein kinase C activity would inhibit internalization of IgG-opsonized and complement-opsonized particles as well as unopsonized zymosan particles *(376, 379)*.

It is important to note that PKC is required at the earliest stages of particle internalization because inhibition of PKC would block the formation of actin filaments beneath the site of the particle binding *(376)*. Hence, activation of PKC is a general requirement for phagocytosis through a broad variety of receptors. Downstream effects of PKC activation include phosphorylation of myristoylated alanine-rich protein kinase C substrate (MARCKS) family of proteins and activation of integrin receptors *(341)*. The MARCKS proteins regulate actin cytoskeletal interactions with the plasma membrane and have been associated with phagocytosis and membrane trafficking *(380)*. PKC-mediated activation of integrin receptors like the $\alpha_M\beta_2$ complement receptor is required for phagocytosis through these receptors *(340)*.

Moreover, PKCs have also been required for cytokine production and antimicrobial activation induced by a variety of stimuli; LPS-induced production of cyclooxygenase-2 (COX-2), TNF-α, and IL-1β, and activation of the respiratory burst have been blocked by pharmacologic inhibitors of PKC *(381–384)*. Similarly, expression of a dominant-negative PKC-α in macrophages inhibited the LPS- and Fc receptor–induced cytokine production *(384–386)*. Other protein kinase C isoforms probably mediate particle ingestion, as DN-PKC-α expression and depletion of Ca^{2+} (required for activation of classic PKCs such as PKC-α and PKC-β) did not effect the internalization of IgG-opsonized particles *(387)*. The same separation of functions is likely to apply to internalization via the innate immune receptors, as DN-PKC-α expression did not alter internalization of a number of pathogens including *Leishmania donovani*, *Legionella pneumophila*, and *Pseudomonas aeruginosa (386)*.

Phosphoinositide Signaling. One classic mechanism for activation of PKCs is via phospholipase C (PLC)-mediated cleavage of phosphatidyl inositol-4,5-biphosphate [$PI(4,5)P_2$] to release inositol triphosphate (IP_3) and diacylglycerol (DAG), second messengers that mobilize intracellular Ca^{2+} stores and activated PKC family members, respectively *(340)*.

Protein kinase C is recruited to phagosomes containing IgG-opsonized particles, and inhibition of its activity would prevent the particle internalization by completely blocking the formation of actin filaments beneath the site of particle contact *(388)*.

PI-3-kinase catalyzes the phosphorylation of PI(4,5)P$_2$ to PI(3,4,5)P$_3$, a phospholipid important in recruiting signaling molecules such as the kinase analogous tumor killing (AKT) protein kinase B (PKB) to specific regions of the membranes *(389)*. Inhibitors of PI-3-kinase would impede the phagocytosis of a broad array of particles including IgG- and complement-opsonized particles, unopsonized zymosan, and bacteria, clearly demonstrating a universal role for PI-3-kinase in particle internalization *(390–393)*. However, blockage of the PI-3-kinase will not inhibit the binding of particles or initial actin polymerization beneath the particle, indicating that the initial phagocytic signaling would stay intact. Instead, PI-3-kinase is required for membrane extension and fusion behind the particle, perhaps because of the failure to insert new membrane at the site of the particle internalization *(392, 393)*.

In addition to their roles in particle internalization, PI-3-kinase and protein kinase C have also been implicated in the proinflammatory signaling induced by particulate stimuli *(340)*. For example, PI-3-kinase was recruited to Toll-like receptors when cells have been stimulated with heat-killed *Staphylococcus aureus*, and activation of PI-3-kinase has been implicated in inducing translocation of NF-κB to the nucleus and the induction of cytokine production in macrophages by pathogens *(394)*.

Rho Family of GTPases. Members of the Rho family of small-molecular-weight GTPases act as key regulators of the actin cytoskeleton, as well as play a central role for these proteins in phagocytosis *(395)*. Thus, the Rho family members Cdc42, Rac, and Rho have been involved in coordinating the actin dynamics during cell adhesion and motility, as well as participating in a number of signaling cascades, including activation of MAP kinases and transporting factors such as the activator protein (AP)-1 *(395, 396)*.

Expression of inhibitory mutants of the Cdc42 and Rac 1 proteins prevented the internalization of IgG-opsonized particles by macrophages and mast cells *(397–400)*, signifying a role of these proteins in the Fc-mediated phagocytosis. Rho seemed not to be required for Fc receptor–mediated phagocytosis, as expression of C3 transferase (a Rho-specific inhibitor) did not impede internalization of IgG-opsonized particles, whereas C3 transferase did block the internalization of complement-opsonized particles *(397)*.

Overall, there has been ample demonstration that the Rho family proteins played an important role in the internalization of unopsonized bacteria, as a number of pathogenic bacteria have evolved mechanisms to regulate the Rho family GTPases as a means of avoiding immune clearance *(342)*. Thus, *Yersinia* species did avoid phagocytosis by host immune cells in part by secreting (via a type III secretion system) the YopE protein into the cytoplasm of host cells. The YopE cytotoxin serves as a GAP (GTPase activating protein) for Cdc42, Rac, and Rho and thus rapidly deactivating these proteins resulting in inhibition of the actin rearrangements necessary for phagocytosis *(342, 401)*. Similarly, *P. aeruginosa* secretes the ExoT cytotoxin (a protein with Rho family GAP activity) into the host cell cytoplasm to avoid uptake and clearance *(342, 402)*.

38.7.3 Particle Internalization and Inflammatory Responses

The internalization of particles during phagocytosis is often accompanied by the production of inflammatory mediators and the activation of antimicrobial mechanisms, and coordination of these responses represents an integral part of an effective and controlled innate immune response *(340)*. The molecular mechanisms that mediate particle internalization share much in common with the mechanisms that mediate many inflammatory responses. For example, the tyrosine kinases, protein kinase C, and the Rho family of GTPase proteins all play roles in both phagocytosis and proinflammatory signaling. On the other hand, relatively few phagocytic receptors are capable themselves of eliciting both phagocytic and inflammatory responses *(340)*. To this end, there is clear evidence that ligation of Fc receptors has been sufficient to induce both the morphologic rearrangements necessary for particle internalization and the production and release of inflammatory mediators *(344, 345)*.

Furthermore, although different phagocytic receptors often would function cooperatively in eliciting inflammatory responses, it is less clear whether such cooperation between receptors involved in phagocytosis will occur both at the level of direct interaction between their downstream signaling components and by their co-association with phagosomes *(340)*.

Superoxide Production. During phagocytosis, different host cells including monocytes, macrophages, and especially neutrophils kill the newly internalized pathogens in part by producing caustic reactive superoxide ions *(340)*.

The secretion of superoxide ions can be induced by soluble stimuli such as PMA (phorbol-12-myristate-14-acetate), FMLP (*N*-formyl-methionyl-leucyl-phenylamine), or calcium ionophores, which induce the assembly of the reduced nicotineamide adenine dinucleotide phosphate (NADPH) oxidase on the plasma membranes, whereas during phagocytosis, the assembly of NADPH oxidase on phagosomal membranes stimulates the localized production of superoxide *(403–405)*. Such localized secretion of superoxide during phagocytosis is thought to be beneficial, as an immune cell would not initiate the killing mechanism until the pathogen is confined to the phagosome, where locally high superoxide concentrations can be generated with as little collateral damage to the surrounding tissue as possible (340).

Whereas the signaling components required to activate the oxidase vary depending on the receptor system activated, there has been a remarkable overlap between these components and the signaling molecules required for particle internalization (405).

Despite several shared signaling pathways and a mutual requirement for regulation of actin cytoskeleton, the superoxide production was not inevitably linked to phagocytosis (340). For instance, it has been long known that internalization through the complement receptor 3 in macrophages was not accompanied by the production of superoxide (406, 407). In addition, downregulation of the receptor systems required for internalization of non-opsonized zymosan did not block internalization of serum-opsonized zymosan or IgG-opsonized particles, but it did prevent NADPH oxidase activation by these particles (408). Hence, phagocytosis can clearly take place without inducing superoxide production, and conversely, several soluble stimuli including PMA and FMLP could induce NADPH oxidase activation without concurrent phagocytosis (403, 405).

Although cross-linking of Fc receptors was found sufficient to induce superoxide production and phagocytosis (341, 405), and phagocytosis through complement receptor 3 was not accompanied by NADPH oxidase activation (406, 407), it has been less clear whether NADPH oxidase activation has been stimulated directly by other innate immune phagocytic receptors (340).

Even though integrin ligation can be linked to NADPH oxidase stimulation, it was highly dependent on the type of integrin, the cell type examined, and whether the cell has been exposed to a priming stimulus (340). Thus, resting neutrophils challenged with immobilized antibodies to leukocyte function-associated antigen-1 (LFA-1, $\alpha_L\beta_2$) or to CR4 (gp150/95, $\alpha_X\beta_2$) produced superoxide, whereas stimulation through CR3 ($\alpha_M\beta_2$) did not (409). In macrophages, CR3 stimulation did not activate the oxidase (406, 407), whereas in eosinophils, ligation of LFA-1 and CR3 both did (410). Such variability of responses to receptor ligation indicated that in different cell types, integrins would signal differently, or that oxidase activation has been regulated by the presence or absence of another coreceptor (340).

Cytokine and Chemokine Production. Activation of gene transcription during phagocytosis has been a critical event for the development of an effective immune response, and in order to detect pathogen-derived products, the innate immune recognition receptors must have access to their ligands. However, because many pathogen-derived products recognized by the innate immune system (such as peptidoglycan or bacterial DNA) are presumably not displayed on the surface of the pathogens, they become accessible only after killing and lysis of the cell, thereby making phagocy-

tosis and killing an integral part of the recognition mechanism (340). Thus, the TLR family of proteins has been actively recruited to phagosomes during pathogen internalization, where they have been able to sample the contents of the phagosome to determine the nature of the pathogen being ingested. Hence, the recruitment of TLRs to phagosomes provided a mechanism by which phagocytosis and the associated inflammatory responses could be linked, even though recruitment itself did not require TLR activation (411, 412). TLRs are also recruited to phagosomes during the internalization of IgG-opsonized particles by Fc receptors, a process that did not require TLP activation, thereby indicating that *TLR recruitment is a general feature of phagocytosis* and that TLRs are simply in position to recognize ligands should they become present in the phagosome (411). This mechanism suggests that particle internalization and inflammatory responses can be disassociated.

However, despite the ability to disassociate these two processes, there remains a significant overlap in the signaling molecules whose activation is required for particle internalization and those activated during proinflammatory signaling. This overlap implies that at some level it is likely that signaling by phagocytic receptors could influence or modify proinflammatory signaling through other receptors (340).

38.8 Mast Cells and Innate Immunity

Mast cells (MCs) are bone marrow–derived, tissue-dwelling immune effector cells characterized by their distinctive metachromatically staining secretory granules (413). Abundantly present in tissues and organs that are in contact with the environment (414), the mast cell responds to both immunologic and nonimmunologic stimulation by secreting an array of preformed granule-associated inflammatory mediators such as histamine and protease/proteoglycan complexes, as well as newly formed eicosanoid products of the arachidonic acid metabolism (cysteinyl leukotrienes, prostaglandin D_2), and by inducing the expression of several proinflammatory cytokines and chemokines (413). Hence, their ability to respond to a variety of nonimmune stimuli coupled with their anatomic distribution would allow the MCs to act as initiators of innate immunity responses.

In both rodents and humans, MCs develop from c-*kit*–bearing committed progenitor cells (PrMCs) that transit through the systemic circulation from the bone marrow to the tissues. As with all circulating leukocytes, the movement of the prMCs from blood to tissues will require the service of both chemoattractants and adhesion receptors. Because the MCs populate tissues under baseline conditions, the receptors and ligands responsible for PrMC homing would likely be constitutively expressed (413). Results from experiments in mice have demonstrated that the number of PrMCs in the small intestine was exceedingly large when compared with that in the bone marrow *(415, 416)* and the lung *(416)*, clearly suggesting a difference between the small intestine and the lung in expressing the necessary ligands and receptors for PrMCs homing under basal conditions. Further experiments have shown that blockade of the α_4- and β_7-integrin subunits of the $\alpha_4\beta_7$ heterodimer with specific antibodies each resulted in a diminished reconstitution of intestinal PrMCs after sublethal irradiation and reconstitution with normal congenic bone marrow. These observations have indicated a critical requirement for the $\alpha_4\beta_7$/ MadCAM-1 adhesion pathway in the maintenance of the normal constitutive small intestinal pool of PrMCs *(413)*. However, even though the $\alpha_4\beta_7$ has been critical for PrMC homing to the small intestine, the assumption is likely that other adhesion pathways would dictate constitutive PrMC homing and localization of mature MCs in other tissues. Thus, the targeted deletion of the α_M (CD11b) integrin subunit, which pairs with the β_2 to form a heterodimeric counterligand for intracellular adhesion molecule (ICAM)-1, was associated with a baseline deficit in MCs in the peritoneal cavity and dorsal skin *(413)*. In contrast, the numbers of mature MCs appearing in response to helminth infection were unaffected *(417)* in this mouse model, and small intestine PrMCs were not enumerated.

Human PrMCs derived *in vitro* from cord blood–associated CD34$^+$ hematopoietic progenitor cells expressed another member of the β_2-integrin family, $\alpha_L\beta_2$, which did decrease in its level of expression with increasing maturation of the cultured MC *(418)*.

In addition to adhesin receptors, chemoattractants are also required for the transendothelial movement of leukocytes including PrMCs to facilitate direct migration and ensure activation of the integrins *(413)*. In this regard, recombinant stem cell factor (SCF) has served as chemoattractant for both mouse MCs and a transformed human MC line *in vitro (419, 420)*. Thus, the absence of constitutive populations of PrMCs in the lungs and intestines in mice in the c-*kit*–deficient *W/Wv* strain – even though PrMCs can be identified in their bone marrow *(416)* – could reflect the *in situ* function of stem cell factor (SCF) as a chemoattractant for PrMCs *in vivo*, in addition to its function in maintaining normal PrMC viability and differentiation *(413)*.

38.8.1 Mast Cells–Associated Mediators and Effector Mechanisms

38.8.1.1 Preformed Mediators

Histamine. Histamine, a biogenic amine–containing molecule [2-(3*H*-imidazol-4-yl)ethanamine], is derived from the decarboxylation of the amino acid histidine, a reaction catalyzed by the enzyme *L*-histidine decarboxylase. It is a hydrophilic vasoactive amine stored in the secretory granules of both human and rodent mast cells *(421, 422)*. After exocytosis, histamine dissociates from the carboxyl groups of proteoglycans in MC granules at neutral pH and acts through at least three classes of receptors *(423, 424)*. Functionally, histamine is associated with both proinflammatory and immunomodulatory activities potentially relevant to both innate and adaptive immunity. Thus, histamine elicits bronchial and gastrointestinal smooth muscle contraction, vasodilation and vasopermeability, secretion of gastric acid, and induction of cutaneous pruritus. Furthermore, histamine exerts both stimulatory and inhibitory effects on immune cells *in vitro*, including (i) enhancement of natural killer cell activation; (ii) stimulation of IL-6 synthesis by B cells; (iii) inhibition of mitogen- and antigen-mediated T-cell proliferation; (iv) inhibition of neutrophil activation; and (v) inhibition of TNF-α, IL-1, IFN-γ, and IL-2 production by monocytes and T cells *(424)*.

Mast Cell Proteases. Mast cells are abundantly and uniquely endowed with proteolytic enzymes with both trypsin-like (tryptases) *(425)* and chymotrypsin-like *(426)* substrate specificity. Human tryptase genes reside in chromosome 16 *(427)*, and at least four of these [(tryptases-α, -βII, and -γ, and the murine mast cell protease 7 (mMCP-7)-like tryptase)] are transcribed by mast cells *(413)*. In addition, human MCs also express a cathepsin G–like chymase that is nearly identical to the neutrophil cathepsin G *(428)*. Further, both the human and mouse MCs express an exopeptidase, carboxypeptidase (CP)A *(429, 430)*. Contrary to mice where the repertoire of chymase genes would allow a wide diversity of expression patterns in different tissues, the human MCs have shown only two distinct patterns of protease composition: the skin and submucosa of the small intestine are immunoreactive for tryptase, chymase, cathepsin G, and carboxypeptidase A (CPA), whereas those in the intestinal and bronchial mucosa and the alveoli of the lung express tryptase but lack immunoreactivity for other proteases *(431)*. MCs expressing tryptase but not chymase are depleted at the gastrointestinal tract mucosal surface in humans with acquired T-cell immunodeficiencies, whereas the numbers of submucosal MCs expressing both tryptase and chymase were normal in the same specimens *(432)*.

All chymases have been found to cleave angiotensin I to form angiotensin *(433, 434)*, which may permit MCs to participate in the homeostasis of local vascular tone and perfusion *(413)*. MCs have also been able to cleave and activate various angiogenic factors *(435)* and initiate collagen fibril formation by cleaving type 1 procollagen *(436)*. Human MC chymase would cleave stem cell factor (SCF) *(437)* resulting in a product that retains activating and mitogenic functions *(438)*. Further studies have also revealed that human MC chymase stimulated the secretion by bronchial mucous glands *(439)*.

Mast Cell Proteoglycans. Mast cells contain proteoglycans in their secretory granules with a peptide core common to cells of hematopoietic lineage *(440–442)*, known as *serglycin* for its repetitive serine and glycidine residues that would allow negatively charged glycosaminoglycans to polymerize at every second and/or third serine residue *(413)*.

An intracellular proteoglycan, serglycin is found particularly in the storage granules of the connective tissue MCs. The core protein consists of 153 amino acids with 24 serine glycine repeats between amino acids 89 and 137, hence the name. This structure probably is responsible for the resistance of the proteoglycans to degradation by bound proteases that have been freed from their activating peptide. Furthermore, the MC granules contain biochemically distinct species of proteoglycans that differ in sulfation of their respective glycosaminoglycan side chains. Both heparin-rich and chondroitin sulfate E–rich proteoglycan species have been identified in MCs obtained from various dispersed human tissues *(443–446)*.

An intracellular function of the proteoglycans has been the storage and packaging of MC granule contitiuents *(413)*. The negatively charged proteoglycans form the basic structural components of large macromolecular complexes that are stored by and released from the MC granules during exocytosis *(447–449)*. These acidic proteoglycans associate with basically charged proteases, as well as histamine and β-hexosaminidase. With the exocytosis and release into the extracellular environment at neutral pH, both the histamine and β-hexosaminidase dissociate from the complex along with mMCP-7, ionically linked by histidine rather than lysine or arginine, which serves to retain many of the proteases *(413)*.

In human MCs, chymase and carbopeptidase A (CPA) (which are expressed in the same subset of mast cells) are complexed with proteoglycan subspecies (probably heparin-containing) that is different from the subspecies complexed with tryptase (probably chondroitin sulfate E) *(450)*.

38.8.1.2 Eicosanoids

After activation by either cross-linking with FcεRI or engagement of the *c-kit* receptor, MCs start rapidly producing the eicosanoid inflammatory mediators leukotriene (LT)C_4 and LTB_4 and prostaglandin (PG)D_2 from the endogenous membrane arachidonic acid (AA) stores *(413, 451–454)*. The eicosanoid synthesis is initiated by a calcium-dependent cytosolic phospholipase (PL)A_2 (cPLA$_2$) that liberates AA from the perinuclear membrane phospholipids *(455)*. The arachidonic acid is then converted sequentially to 5-hydroperoxyeicosatetranoic acid (5-HPETE) and then to LTA_4 by the actions of 5-lipoxygenase (5-LO) after its reversible translocation from the cytosol to the perinuclear

envelope *(456)* where it requires the cooperation of an integral membrane protein, 5-lipoxygenase–activating protein (FLAP) *(457)*, for its metabolic function *(413)*. Next, LTA_4 is either converted by a cytosolic LTA_4 hydrolase to LTB_4 *(458)* or is conjugated to reduced gluthatione by LTC_4 synthase (LTC$_4$S) *(459)*, an integral perinuclear membrane protein with homology to FLAP, to generate LTC_4. Both LTB_4 *(460)* and LTC_4 *(461)* are exported to the extracellular space by distinct, energy-dependent steps *(413)*.

LTB_4 is a potent neutrophil chemotactic factor *(462)* acting through at least two 7-transmembrane–spanning G-protein–coupled receptors (GPCRs), a high-affinity receptor (BLT1 receptor) *(463)* and a low-affinity receptor (BLT2 receptor) *(464)*. LTB_4 is then sequentially converted extracellularly to the receptor-active cysteinyl leukotrienes (cys-LTs) LTD_4 and LTE_4 *(465)*. The cys-LTs caused bronchoconstriction *(466, 467)* and eosinophil recruitment when experimentally instilled into the airways of human subjects *(468)*.

The activity of the cys-LTs is mediated through at least two 7-transmembrane receptors, CysLT1 and CysLT2, respectively *(469, 470)*. The CysLT1 receptor is expressed on the bronchial smooth muscle, alveolar macrophages, CD34-bearing progenitor cells, peripheral blood eosinophils, and B cells as well as on human cultured MCs *(471)*, whereas the CysLT2 receptor is expressed by brain and hematopoietic tissues, the bronchial smooth muscle, and the peripheral blood leukocytes *(413)*.

The secretion of both cys-LTs and LTB_4 by MCs could facilitate the innate immune responses through induction of the venular permeability and transudation of plasma proteins and recruitment of neutrophils, respectively *(472)*.

Prostaglandin D_2 (PGD_2) is generated by the conversion of arachidonic acid through the sequential actions of prostaglandin endoperoxide synthase (PGHS)-1 and -2 and the hemopoietic form of PGD_2 synthase *(473)*. Similarly to the cysteinyl leukotrienes, PGD_2 is a bronchoconstrictor *(474)*, and its active metabolite 9α,11β-PGF_2 is a potent constrictor of the coronary arteries *(475)*. Two receptors of PGD_2 (DP and CRTH2 receptors) have been identified and cloned *(476, 477)*. The findings that the CRTH2 receptor was selectively expressed on human eosinophils, basophils, and Th2 lymphocytes, coupled with its selective chemotactic actions on these cell types *(476)*, have clearly supported a role for PGD_2 in inflammatory responses, especially in circumstances such as helminth infection, in which the Th2-dominated inflammation is typical *(413)*.

38.8.1.3 Mast Cell–Produced Cytokines

Early-Acting Cytokines. When stimulated through FcεRI, both human and mouse MCs secreted a number of cytokines [TNF-α *(478)*, IL-1 *(479)*, and IL-6 *(480, 481)*] that have been associated with the early phases of an inflammatory response *(413)*. The early stage acting cytokines trigger hepatic acute-phase protein production, endothelial cell adhesion molecule expression, and leukocyte recruitment *(413)*.

The immunolocalization of TNF-α to the MCs of the human skin *(482)*, nasal mucosa *(483)*, and the bronchial submucosa *(484)* implies that some TNF-α has been constitutively synthesized and stored by human MCs *in vivo (413)*. However, although the IgE-dependent TNF-α release by the MCs may favor recruitment of cell populations that sustain the allergic response, the capacity of the MCs to secrete TNF-α rapidly through non-IgE–dependent mechanisms would normally facilitate a protective role against bacteria *(485)*.

Th2-Type Cytokines/Co-mitogens. The helminth-induced expansion of intestinal mucosal MC populations has depended on both the cytoprotective functions of stem cell factor (SCF) and the co-mitogenic effects of cytokines such as IL-3, IL-4, IL-5, and others *(413)*. Even though the Th2 lymphocytes have been considered to be the major source of these co-mitogens, the capacity for the mast cells to generate these same cytokines did indicate a possible autocrine priming function that may have arisen before the evolution of the adaptive lymphocyte response *(413)*. Using immunohistochemistry techniques has allowed for the IL-4 and IL-5 each to be localized in MCs in the lung tissue of patients with asthma *(484)* and to MCs in the nasal mucosa of patients with allergic rhinitis *(483)*. Both immunodetectable IL-4 and IL-5 and their corresponding mRNA species have been localized to human skin MCs after cutaneous allergen challenge *(486)* and were detectable, along IL-6, in nasal mucosal MCs in biopsy specimens from patients with allergic rhinitis *(487)*.

IL-3, another cytokine with co-mitogenic activity on MCs, is transcribed *de novo* along with IL-5 when human lung MCs are stimulated with anti-IgE *(488, 489)*.

Chemokines. The MCs of both humans and mice produce several members of the C-C and C-X-C families of chemokines *(413)*. For example, the human MCs generate IL-8, a potent neutrophil-active chemokine *(490, 491)*, and those derived from cord blood *in vitro* generated the C-C chemokine macrophage inflammatory protein-1α (MIP-1α) in response to IgE-dependent activation *(492)*. Another C-C chemokine, monocyte chemoattractant protein-1 (MCP-1), is generated by human lung MCs when stimulated *in vitro* by stem cell factor (SCF) and anti-IgE *(493)*. Contact between mouse MCs and fibroblasts induced the production of the C-C chemokine eotaxin *(494)*. These induced mediators selectively targeted neutrophils (IL-8, ENA-78), lymphocytes (MIP-α, MIP-1β, MCP-1), and eosinophils (eotaxin), respectively, and may act in sequence with preformed exocytosed mediators and newly formed eicosanoids to recruit different leukocyte subsets selectively *(413)*.

Fibrogenic and Angiogenic Growth Factors. Mast cells generate factors that are involved in fibroblast proliferation,

extracellular matrix deposition, and angiogenesis, including the vascular permeability/vascular endothelial cell growth factor *(495)*, transforming growth factor-β (TGF-β) *(496)*, and basic fibroblast growth factor *(497)*. The latter finding supported the role of MCs as modulators of tissue repairs, fibrosis, and remodeling *(413)*. Moreover, the fact that the MCs store and secrete stem cell factor (SCF) *(498, 499)* has indicated another potential autocrine capability of their survival.

38.8.2 Mast Cells Involvement in Innate Microbial Immunity

The presence of MCs at the interface with the external environment has long implicated their involvement in the innate immune responses. Such a role would require that invading pathogens initiate MC activation leading to direct or indirect involvement of MCs in microbial clearance *(413)*. The involvement of MCs in innate microbial immunity was initially supported by the observation that MCs phagocytized Gram-negative bacteria *in vitro* at least partly through their complement receptors *(500)*.

The role for MCs in the recruitment of neutrophils to a tissue site has been confirmed in a mouse model of immune complex–mediated peritonitis, which elicits biphasic peaks of peritoneal fluid TNF-α and subsequent neutrophil recruitment in WBB6/F1 MC-sufficient mice, but not in MC-deficient *W/Wv* mice *(501)*. The experimental results did indicate that MCs *in vivo* would respond to immune complexes by providing both preformed and newly synthesized TNF-α, leading to neutrophil influx. These findings were later extended to experimental models of acute septic peritonitis. Two original studies that *W/Wv* mice when subjected to cecal ligation and puncture (CLP) *(485)* or directly inoculated with a virulent strain of *Klebsiella pneumoniae* intraperitonealy *(502)* each had shown substantially greater rates of mortality compared with their congenic, MC-sufficient WBB6/F1 controls *(485, 502)*. In both cases, the increased mortality correlated with impaired neutrophil recruitment to the peritoneum. Moreover, in a separate study *(503)*, the repeated instillation of recombinant SCF into the peritoneum of normal C57B1/6 mice has augmented the MC number and survival rate after cecal ligation and puncture. Taken together, the results of these studies provide a strong case that resident constitutive MCs played an essential role in the initiation of neutrophil recruitment in response to bacterial infection *(413)*. In this regard, it is likely that several effector mechanisms have been involved in the observed protection in the cecal ligation and puncture (CLP) model, notably, that MCs store some preformed TNF-α in their secretory granules *(478)*, as well as that they can also generate TNF-α rapidly through *de novo* transcription and translation *(504, 505)*. As in the immune complex-mediated model of peritonitis, a sharp transient increase in peritoneal fluid-associated TNF-α has been observed in MC-sufficient but not MC-deficient mice in the CLP model, presumably reflecting the preformed and rapidly released MC-associated product. Thus, the provision of TNF-α by resident constitutive MCs seemed to be an important component of their role in neutrophil recruitment in innate immune responses to Gram-negative pathogens *(413)*.

In addition to TNF-α, other MC-derived factors were found also to support neutrophil recruitment to the peritoneum and other tissue sites. For example, the augmentative effects of SCF injection on CLP-induced mortality have been observed even in TNF-α–deficient mice, thus supporting the involvement of these additional factors in neutrophil recruitment *(503)*. Also, the mouse tryptase mMCP-6 generated a marked and sustained local neutrophilia when administered into the peritoneal cavity *(506)*, and more recently, the instillation of purified recombinant human MC-specific human tryptase-β1 has been shown to induce significant neutrophilia in the lungs of mice *(507)* and to protect *W/Wv* mice from mortality in response to experimentally induced *Klebsiella* pneumonitis. These findings suggested that the MC tryptases are involved as mediators in the MC-dependent aspects of innate immunity, and that *the diversity of the tryptase genes may permit selective, tissue-specific responses (413)*.

The CD48-mediated secretion of TNF-α by MCs has been linked to the phosphorylation of Janus kinase 3 (JAK3). Thus, mice lacking JAK3 exhibited significantly lower levels of TNF-α in their peritoneal fluids sampled 1 hour after CLP, and both peritoneal recruitment and bacterial clearance have been similarly impaired *(508)*.

Taken together, all these studies have demonstrated at least two receptors through which Gram-negative organisms can directly initiate MC-dependent neutrophil recruitment and TNF-α generation. CD48 and TLR4 are known to signal through distinct pathways. Thus, the FimH1/CD48-mediated stimulation involved JAK3-initiated signal transduction pathway, which is probably necessary for exocytosis and release of preformed TNF-α, but not for CD48 expression or endocytosis *(413)*. LPS/TLR4-mediated stimulation of MCs elicited NF-κB–dependent generation of newly formed TNF-α, which was released over several hours independently of exocytosis. Hence, the original observation that MC-dependent peritonitis elicited both early and late peaks of TNF-α production has been consistent with the involvement of both of these direct receptor-mediated mechanisms of MC activation *in vivo (413)*.

In vivo studies have also shown a key role for the complement cascade and complement MC-mediated defense against Gram-negative pathogens *(413)*. For example, mice that were deficient by targeted disruption of the gene in the complement components C3 and C4 were much more susceptible to mortality from cecal ligation and puncture than were the congenic controls *(509)*. These complement-null mice also exhibited impaired TNF-α generation and MC degranulation *in vivo* after CLP, defects that were restored by the exogenous administration of C3 to the C3-deficient mice *(509)*. Similarly to complement-null mice, mice deficient in complement receptor (CR)1 (CD35) and CR2 (CD21), which arise from a single gene in mice, or deficient in CD19, which forms a functional heterodimer with CD21, have also been shown to be more susceptible to CLP-induced mortality than were the wild-type control mice *(510)*.

Finally, the large pool of prMCs constitutively residing in the mouse small intestine represents an important feature of the innate host defense against helminths *(413)*. Thus, mice lacking this normal PrMC pool, such as those with a deletion of the β7-integrin *(416, 511)* or with natural occuring disruptions in either the *c-kit* or SCF genes *(485, 502)*, were profondly impaired in their ability to clear helminthic parasites *in vivo*. Furthermore, although T cells have been required to provide the cytokines that amplify the development of mucosal MCs from the constitutive PrMC pool, the elimination of helminthic parasites by mast cells did not depend on either IgE or B-cells *(413)*.

38.9 CD1-Restricted T Cells as Effectors of Innate Immunity

In general, the primary signals for T-cell activation are not mediated by soluble antigens. Rather, T-cell receptors (TCRs) interact with antigens complexed to proteins on the surface of antigen-presenting cells (APCs) *(512)*. Until recently, it was thought that peptides bound to MHC-encoded antigen-presenting molecules were the only natural targets of T-cell responses *in vivo (513)*. However, subsequent studies have demonstrated that T cells respond to a variety of nonpeptide antigens including lipids bound to CD1 proteins *(514–520)*. This finding has clearly expanded the traditional paradigms of T-cell function in innate and acquired immunity, especially *the fundamentally new function of T cells involving the recognition of alterations in the lipid content of cellular membranes that result from infection, transformation, or cellular stress (512)*.

To explain the newly discovered function of the lipid-specific T cells in the integrated immune responses, a comparison was drawn with cells that have established roles in either innate or acquired immunity *(512)*. For example, contrary to MHC-restricted T cells that expressed myriads of unique receptors (TCRs) and *function in acquired immunity*, certain CD1d-restricted natural killer (NK) T cells displayed a strickingly limited TCR repertoire and responded to a very limited number of antigens *(519, 521–523)*. Hence, these NK T-cells have been linked *as effectors of innate immunity*, which use germ-line–encoded, pattern recognition receptors to interact with foreign antigens *(524, 525)*.

Alternatively, other CD1-restricted T cells expressed clonally varied receptors and recognized a moderately varied spectrum of antigens *(526–529)*. Hence, it is at least posssible that infection could shape the CD1-restricted T-cell repertoire over time *(512)*.

On the whole, the biologic functions of CD1-restricted T-cell function emphasize criteria that would differentiate effectors of innate and acquired immunity, namely (i) receptor diversity; (ii) ligand diversity; (iii) precursor frequency; and (iv) the generation of antigen-specific memory. Overall, CD1-restricted T cells appear to mediate immunologic functions that are intermediate between classic notions of acquired or innate immunity, leading to a more nuanced understanding of these concepts *(512)*.

38.9.1 The CD1 Family of Antigen-Presenting Molecules

CD1 genes are present in all mammalian species studied to date *(530–538)*. In humans, five CD1 genes have been defined: CD1A, CD1B, CD1C, CD1D, and CD1E, which all are encoded outside the MHC on chromosome 1 *(515)*. All of the five CD1 genes are known to be translated into proteins, and four of these, CD1a, CD1b, CD1c, and CD1d, have been shown in antigen presentation to T cells *(519, 520, 539–543)*.

Because the CD1 genes do not possess the high level of allelic polymorphism [which is characteristic of MHC class I and II antigen presentation molecules *(514, 544)*], they are often described as being nonpolymorphic *(512)*.

Based on their sequence similarities, the five human CD1 genes have been separated into two groups *(539)*. CD1A, CD1B, and CD1C genes have the highest levels of sequence homology to one another and were designated as group 1, whereas CD1D was designated group 2; CD1E has shown features of both groups. This classification, originally based on gene structure, was subsequently supported by studies on CD1 protein expression and T-cell function: the group 2 CD1d protein mediates presentation of α-galactosyl ceramides and phosphatidylinositols to T cells with a *conserved* T-cell receptor (TCR) repertoir, whereas the group 1 CD1 proteins presented a variety of microbial glycolipids to a population of T cells with *diverse* TCRs *(512)*.

Structurally, the CD1 proteins are transmembrane glycoproteins that contain short cytoplasmic domains and three extracellular domains (α_1, α_2, and α_3), which noncovalently associate with β_2-microglobulin (β_2-M) *(545)*. Owing to their similar domain organization and β_2-M–dependent expression, the CD1 proteins are occasionally referred to as *MHC class I–like proteins*. However, in terms of amino acid sequence homology, the CD1 proteins are *similarly related to both MHC class I and MHC class II proteins*. Consequently, it is thought that these three families of antigen-presenting molecules had diverged at a similar time point of evolution, and CD1 proteins should be more appropriately viewed as a *distinct family* of antigen-presenting proteins *(512)*.

38.9.2 CD1-Glycolipid Antigen Complexes

The detailed structures of the murine CD1d and CD1b have been elucidated by x-ray studies *(546, 547)*. The CD1 α_3-domain has an immunoglobulin-like fold, and the α_1- and α_2- domains form a hollow groove in the distal surface of the protein, which functions as an antigen binding site. The overall configuration of the CD1 grooves was similar to that of the MHC-encoded antigen-presenting molecules insofar as the CD1 grooves have been composed of a β-sheet floor that supported antiparallel α-helices that form the lateral margins of the grooves. However, the CD1d has two large pockets, A′ and F′, rather than the seven pockets of a typical MHC class I groove *(547)*. The groove of the human CD1b is much larger and comprises four pockets: A′, C′, F′, and T′. Importantly, the amino acids that line the inner surface of the CD1 grooves possessed predominately nonpolar side chains, providing hydrophobic surfaces for interaction with antigens *(546)*. Although it has become common to refer to the CD1 antigen binding site as a groove, its depth and enclosed nature can be be more readily likened to a pocket or a shallow cave.

Furthermore, interdomain interactions between the amino acids in the α_1- and α_2-helices of mCD1d would close the groove at both ends thereby rectricting the access to the top of the groove, so that the route for the entry into the hollow interior of the protein will be through a relatively narrow portal above the F′ pocket. Such configuration would allow the CD1d groove to more fully sequester antigens within the globular head of the protein formed by the α_1- and α_2- domains, in contrast with the MHC class I and class II grooves, which are open to solvent over their entire length *(547)*. Thus, the enclosed and hydrophobic architecture of the CD1 groove will make it well suited to bind the antigens (small amphipathic lipids and glycolipids) that it presents *(412)*.

The antigen-presenting function of the CD1 proteins was first demonstrated using human T-cell lines that have been specifically activated by components of the mycobacterial cell wall *(420)*. Structural characterizations of the antigens presented by the CD1b proteins have shown that they represent lipids or glycolipids including mycolic acid, lipoarabinomannan, or glucose monomycolate *(517–519)*. These CD1b-presented microbial lipids, along with the CD1c-presented mannosyl phosphoisoprenoids, differed in structure from the glycolipids that compose mammalian cells and were therefore foreign antigens *(548)*. However, self glycolipids of normal structure such as phosphatidylethanolamine, phosphatidylinositol, and gangliosides can also be presented by APCs to CD1-resticted T cells *(549–551)*. Synthetic α-galactosyl ceramides and hydrophobic peptides can also bind to CD1d and mediate CD1d-restricted responses *(519, 552)*.

The molecular mechanism of antigen presentation involved an initial insertion of the lipid molecules into the CD1 groove, thereby allowing the aliphatic hydrocarbon chains of the antigen to interact with the hydrophobic interior of the CD1 groove. Such binding mechanism would make it possible for the carbohydrate portions and other hydrophilic components of the antigen to protrude from the groove into the aqueous solvent, allowing them to establish direct contact with antigen-specific TCRs *(518, 526, 529, 547, 553)*.

These studies coupled with other studies that have shown CD1d-restricted T-cell binding to CD1d-glycolipid tetramers have clearly demonstrated that CD1-glycolipid antigen complexes have been the molecular targets of the CD1-restricted T-cell responses *(554–556)*.

Taken as a whole, the T-cell activation by glycolipids occurs by a molecular mechanism that is analogous to the recognition of peptide-MHC complexes, a trimolecular interaction of the variable regions of the antigen-specific TCRα- and β-chains with lipid-CD1 complexes *(512, 529)*.

38.9.3 Cellular Pathways of Lipid Antigen Presentation

The CD1 antigen-presenting molecules are predominately expressed on hematopoietic cells with specialized immunologic functions, including myeloid dendritic cells, Langerhans cells, B cells, and thymocytes *(557)*. Whereas the thymocytes and dendritic cells express all four of the known CD1 isoforms with an established function in antigen presentation, other APCs selectively express only certain CD1 isoforms *(535, 557)*. In addition, each of the human CD1 proteins differred from one another in their patterns of expression within the intracellular compartments of APCs, reflecting their different patterns of trafficking through secretory, cell surface, and endosomal compartments *(558–562)*.

After translation and folding in the endoplasmic reticulum, the CD1 proteins are thought to exit to the cell surface through the secretory pathway *(512)*. The CD1b, CD1c, and CD1d proteins reached the endosomal network by one of two known mechanisms. The first mechanism involves the CD1d proteins associating with the invariant chain, which would promote their delivery to late endosomes *(563)*. In the second mechanism, the cytoplasmic tails of CD1b, CD1c, and CD1d proteins contain a sequence that conforms to a tyrosine-based

amino acid motif that will interact with clathrin adaptor protein complexes that will promote the trafficking of these CD1 proteins from the cell surface into the endosomal network *(559–565)*.

Although CD1b, CD1c, and CD1d have all been found in the endosomes, CD1b proteins did appear to traffic more deeply into the endosomal network, as evidenced by their more extensive co-localizations with markers of late endosomes and lysosomes such as LAMP-1 *(561)*. In contrast, CD1a has been found nearly exclusively at the cell surface, presumably owing to its particularly short cytoplasmic tail, which is lacking an endosomal localization motif *(558)*.

The different trafficking patterns of the human CD1 isoforms has indicated that each one of them will function to survey the glycolipid content of different subcellular locations *(566, 567)*. For example, there is substantial evidence to suggest that the trafficking of the CD1b and CD1d proteins through the late endosomal compartments had influenced the development and activation of the antigen-specific T cells *(520, 562, 563, 568–570)*. In addition, the antigen structure can also influence which glycolipids were loaded onto the CD1 proteins for T-cell recognition, as CD1b-presented antigens with longer alkyl chains have been preferentially presented by myeloid dendritic cells *(571)*.

Because of the fact that the CD1-restricted T cells have been highly specific for lipid antigen structure, the cellular mechanisms that control which particular families of lipids are loaded onto the CD1 proteins could exert a profound effect on the outcome of the immune responses *in vivo (12)*. These observations have led to a growing research on the cellular pathways of processing glycolipid antigens for recognition by T cells. However, the precise molecular mechanism of loading glycolipid antigens into the hydrophobic groove of the CD1 proteins is yet to be determined *(512)*.

38.9.4 CD1d-Restricted T Cells

The natural killer (NK) T cells have been defined as a specialized CD4$^+$ or CD4$^-$/CD8$^-$ T cells (see Section 38.6.1) that were MHC-unrestricted and expressed receptors encoded in the NK locus, including MK1.1 in the mouse and NKRP-1 in humans *(374, 512, 572, 573)*. However, even though NK receptors can modulate the activation state of NK T-cells, there has been evidence to clearly substantiate the notion that their activation is controlled primarily by TCR interactions with lipid-loaded CD1d proteins *(512, 513, 554–556, 574, 575)*.

One stricking feature of a major population of NK T-cells *in vivo* is the marked limitation of the TCR gene usage *(512)*. Thus, a large population of NK T-cells was observed to express an invariant TCR α-chain that paired with a limited number of Vβ-chains. In humans, the invariant Vα24JαQ chain usually paired with Vβ11 *(521, 523)*. This limited TCR variability did not result from elements that control the rearrangements of the TCR α-chains but instead resulted from the positive selection of T cells bearing these TCRs by CD1d proteins *(576–581)*. This relative lack of complexity of receptor expression has distinguished the NK T-cells from the much more complex repertoire of the MHC-restricted T cells, which has been shaped by antigen exposure over time *(512)*.

The identities of the natural antigenic targets of the T cells are not precisely known, although some observations have described them as autoreactive to CD1d proteins, based on experiments in which the T-cell activation had required that APCs expressed the CD1d heavy chain and β$_2$-M, but did not required the addition of an exogenous glycolipid antigen *(575)*. However, this finding did not imply that these T cells would recognize unliganded CD1d proteins *(512)*. Instead, it is likely that CD1d would bind and present self or altered self lipids for recognition by the T cells, as this was demonstrated with phosphatidylinositol-containing compounds and other lipids with similar structure, which have activated the T cells under certain circumstances *in vitro (550, 551, 582–584)*. Hence, the current notion is that nonantigenic phosphatidylinositols or other self compounds would occupy the CD1d groove, functioning as chaperones prior to insertion of more strongly antigenic lipids into the groove *(512)*.

Currently, the most potent antigens for NK T-cells activation are a family of structurally related synthetic compounds known as α-galactosyl ceramides *(519)*. These molecules have been shown to bind CD1d proteins, forming complexes that interacted with invariant TCRs *(554–556, 585)*.

Experiments studying the functions of CD1d-restricted T cells *in vivo* included injecting mice with α-galactosyl ceramides, using germ-line deletion of CD1s, or deletion of the Jα281 gene, which has been necessary for the expression of the invariant TCR α-chain in mice *(513, 576, 581, 585)*. These studies led to strong immunologic effects and systemically detectable levels of interferon-γ, interleukin-4 (IL-4), and other cytokines.

In a number of other studies, it has been shown that treatment of mice with α-galactosyl ceramides did also protect against the development of autoimmune diabetes and allergic encephalomyelitis (EAE) *(586–589)*. These apparently immunosuppressive effects of α-galactosyl ceramide antigens have been confirmed in studies demonstrating that CD1d deletion has exacerbated autoimmune diabetes *(590)*.

These and other studies have clearly indicated that by and large, the selective activation of CD1d-restricted T cells can influence significantly the integrated immune response to antigens, self tissues, and tumors *in vivo*. In this regard, there has been evidence that antigen-mediated signals through the TCR can lead to activation, apopotic cell death, or Th1/Th2 polarized responses, depending on the stimulation conditions *(586, 591, 592)*.

The NK T-cells did differ from the peptide-specific MHC-restricted T cells in their precursor frequency as well as in their requirements for priming and maturation prior to development of effector functions *(512)*. The high precursor frequency, limited receptor variability, limited antigen variability, and strong activation by a primary immune response have suggested that the NK T-cells and the peptide-specific MHC-restricted T cells may have fundamentally different functions in the immune response. In this regard, the NK T-cells have more in common with the effector cells of the innate immune system, which use pattern recognition receptors to respond to a limited number of nonself-antigens of conserved structure. Hence, the NK T-cells like other effectors of innate immunity would play a role early in the immune response, either to combat infection directly or to regulate the other cells, including the peptide-specific T cells *(512)*.

38.9.5 T Cells Restricted by Group 1 CD1 Proteins

T cells that recognized glycolipid antigens presented by group 1 CD1 proteins (CD1a, CD1b, CD1c) appeared to be somewhat more diverse in their TCR repertoire and range of antigenic targets than were the NK T-cells *(512)*.

In contrast with NK T-cells, analysis of the TCR expression in CD1a-, CD1b-, and CD1c-restricted T cells has failed to find evidence for a conserved TCR structure *(512)*. TCRs that have mediated recognition of antigens presented by CD1a, CD1b, and CD1c proteins have been found to incorporate varied Vα and Vβ gene segments and apparently random N-region additions *(526)*. These varied TCRs mediate recognition of structurally distinct antigens, and those T cells that did recognize a given antigen did not generally cross-react with structurally related glycolipids or with other known CD1-presented glycolipids *(519, 548)*.

Most of the known antigens for group 1 CD1-restricted T cells, such as mycolic acids, lipoarabinomannans, glucose monomycolates, and mannosyl phosphoisoprenoids, have been produced by mycobacteria and related species *(516–518, 520, 593)*. Because these glycolipids do not possess readily identifiable homologues in mammalian cells, these molecules are intrinsically foreign to the mammalian immune system and therefore would allow the group1 CD1 proteins to play a role in the host defense against infections *(512)*. Moreover, the CD1b isoform can bind and present antigens comprising at least three different classes of antigens: mycolates, diacylglycerols, and sphingolipids *(516, 517, 549)*. Because each of these larger classes contains many different naturally occuring glycosylated molecules, it is possible that the number of glycolipid antigens recognized by CD1-restricted T cells may be substantially greater than is currently recognized.

In addition, the regulated expression of group 1 CD1 proteins on myeloid dendritic cells provided further evidence for their role in host defense. Thus, dendritic cells undergo a program of differentiation as they migrate from the bone marrow to the peripheral blood, through inflamed tissues and subsequently to secondary lymphoid tissues. Owing to the ability of dendritic cells to control the activation of peptide-specific T cells by acquiring antigen-presenting functions at discrete stages of development, the development regulation of group 1 CD1 proteins now provides evidence that this is also the case for glycolipid-specific T cells *(594)*.

Because group 1 CD1 proteins are abundantly expressed on myeloid cells in skin biopsies of patients infected with *Mycobacterium leprae*, this finding provided direct evidence for the upregulation of group 1 CD1 proteins on dendritic cells during natural infections *(595)*. All together, these observations did suggest that myeloid cells when migrating to the sites of infection would selectively upregulate group 1 CD1 proteins (CD1a, CD1b, CD1c) for antigen presentation during the host response to infection *(512)*.

Mycobacterium Infections and Group 1 CD1 Proteins. The CD1a-, CD1b-, and CD1c-restricted T cells possess effector mechanisms that have promoted host defense against mycobacteria and other pathogens *(512)*. *In vitro* experiments of human group 1 CD1-restricted T cells have shown that these proteins have secreted interferon-γ, synthesized granulysin, and displayed cytolytic properties *(596, 597)*, which led to the killing of target cells infected with mycobacteria *(562, 596)*. There has also been evidence suggesting the generation of glycolipid-specific T-cell responses during the natural human immune response to *Mycobacterium tuberculosis*, as CD1c-resticted T cells isolated from patients with tuberculosis showed greater stimulation by mannosyl phosphoisoprenoid antigens than did those from uninfected patients *(548)*. However, there has not been a conclusive evidence for a protective function in animal models other than mice (which do not express homologues of group 1 CD1 proteins) *(531)*.

38.10 Interleukin-17 Family of Cytokines

Cytokines are secreted proteins that regulate many biological activities, including hemopoiesis and the immune response *(598, 599)*. One recently discovered related group of cytokines is the interleukin-17 (IL-17) family *(599, 600)*. The IL-17 family has no sequence similarity to any other known cytokines. However, a viral homologue of IL-17 was found in the open reading frame 13 of herpesvirus saimiri (HVS13) *(601)*. IL-17 binds to a type I transmembrane receptor termed IL-17R *(602)*. IL-17R is a large ubiquitously expressed protein that also shows no sequence similarity to any other known cytokine receptors, suggesting a new ligand-receptor family *(598, 603)*.

IL-17 Family Relationships, Origins, and Nomenclature. The IL-17 family now includes six members, at least three of which are produced by T cells and have potent proinflammatory properties *(604)*. A cDNA encoding IL-17 was isolated from a murine cytotoxic T lymphocyte (CTL) hybridoma cDNA library in a screen to identify inducible CTL-associated transcripts and was originally called CTLA-8 (cytotoxic T lymphocyte-associated-8) *(600)*. Subsequently, the homologous T-lymphotrophic herpesvirus saimiri gene 13 was cloned and used to isolate a cDNA encoding a receptor that bound CTLA-8 *(602)*. The mammalian and viral homologue were renamed IL-17 and vIL-17, respectively, and the receptor was named IL-17R. Five homologous cytokines were later identified through database searches and degenerative PCR strategies *(605)*.

Note: IL-17 has also been designated as IL-17A to indicate that it is the founding member of this extended, six-member cytokine family, which now includes IL-17A–F. IL-17E was independently identified and named IL-25 (606), a nomenclature that is being used here.

IL-17F has the highest homology with IL-17A, as they are 50% identical at the protein level. IL-17B to D have lower homology, and IL-25 (IL-17E) is the least related, sharing only 16% identity at the primary amino acid sequence in humans. IL-17A and IL-17F are syntenic, tightly linked in all species examined to date; the remaining family members each map to different chromosomes. IL-17 shares no sequence homology with other known mammalian proteins and therefore constitutes a distinct cytokine family *(604)*.

IL-17 Family Structures and Functions. The crystal structure of a single IL-17 family member, IL-17F, has been solved *(607)*. It reveals that IL-17F is a structural homologue of the *cysteine knot* family of proteins, so named for their unusual pattern of intrachain disulfide bonds. A similar structural motif is found in growth factors such as TGF-β, nerve growth factor (NGF), bone morphogenetic proteins, and platelet-derived growth factor-BB, except that in these other growth factors the cysteine knot is formed with six cysteines rather than four. The four cysteines that form the cysteine knot structure in IL-17F are conserved in all IL-17 family members and across species.

Other IL-17 family members, including IL-17B *(608, 609)*, IL-17C *(608)*, IL-17D *(598)*, IL-17E *(610)*, and IL-17F *(607, 611, 612)*, were cloned by several laboratories *(598)*. Each of these IL-17 family members shares four highly conserved cysteine residues that are involved in the formation of intrachain disulfide linkages. All of the IL-17 family members also have two or more cysteine residues that may be involved in interchain disulfide linkages as suggested by the homodimeric cysteine knot fold crystal structure of IL-17F *(607)*.

Multiple functions have been reported for the IL-17 family of cytokines that mainly involve regulating the immune response *(598)*. IL-17 has been shown to induce the production of IL-6, IL-8, G-CSF, GM-CSF, growth-related oncogene-α, IL-1β, TGF-β, TNF-α, PGE$_2$, and MCP-1 from multiple different cell types including fibroblasts, endothelial cells, epithelial cells, keratinocytes, and macrophages *(613–615)*. IL-17 can induce fibroblasts to secrete IL-6 and G-CSF, which can induce proliferation and differentiation of CD34$^+$ hemopoietic progenitors *(616, 617)*. IL-17 can stimulate granulopoiesis *in vivo (618)* and induce murine stem cells to rescue lethally irradiated mice *(619)*, suggesting its importance in hemopoiesis *(598)*. For example, IL-17D was found to regulate cytokine production in endothelial cells and showed an inhibitory effect on hemopoiesis *in vitro (598)*. Furthermore, whereas recombinant human IL-17F did not stimulate the proliferation of hematopoietic progenitors or the migration of mature leukocytes, it markedly inhibited the angiogenesis of human endothelial cells and induced endothelial cells to produce IL-2, TGF-β, and MCP-1 *(611)*.

IL-17 Involvement in Disease Pathogenesis. IL-17 is a T-cell–derived cytokine produced by activated T cells, predominately activated CD4$^+$ CD45RO$^+$ memory T-cells *(601, 616, 617)*. This cytokine may play a role in T-cell–triggered inflammation by stimulating stromal cells to secrete various cytokines and growth factors associated with inflammation *(601, 602, 616)*. A pathogenic role for IL-17 was found in organ allograft rejection *(618, 619)*, and increased IL-17 expression was detected in several diseases, such as systemic sclerosis *(620)*, nephrotic syndrome *(621)*, systemic lupus erythematosus *(622)*, rheumatoid arthritis *(623, 624)*, as well as in tumorigenicity *(625)* and antitumor immunity *(611, 626)*. In contrast with the restricted expression of IL-17, the IL-17 receptor is ubiquitously expressed in virtually all cells and tissues. It is a type I transmembrane protein that has no sequence similarity with any other known cytokine receptor *(602)*. Binding of IL-17 to its unique receptor results in activation of the adaptor molecule, TNF receptor–associated factor 6, which is required for IL-17 signaling *(627)*.

Furthermore, IL-17 cytokines are also key mediators in a diverse range of autoinflammatory disorders. The identification of Th17 cells as the principal pathogenic effectors in several types of autoimmunity previously thought to be Th1-mediated promises new approaches for therapies of these disorders, as does identification of IL-25 (IL-17E) as a potentially important mediator of dysregulated Th2 responses that cause asthma and other allergic disorders *(604)*.

38.10.1 IL-17 Family Receptors

Like the IL-17 cytokine family, the IL-17 receptors form a unique family *(528, 604)*. There are five family members, including the founding member, IL-17R (or IL-17RA), and four additional members have been identified through sequence homology searches. Individual family members share only limited sequence similarity with each other and do not contain domains found in other proteins. They, therefore, constitute a novel family of cytokine receptors. All are predicted to be single-pass transmembrane proteins with an extracellular amino terminus and large intracellular tails. Four of the IL-17 receptor family members map to human chromosome 3 in two tightly linked clusters: IL-17RB (also called IL-17RH1 or IL-25R) with IL-17RD (also called SEF or IL-17RLM), and IL-17RC (also IL-17RL) with IL-17RE. There is similar clustering of these pairs in the mouse. Evidence suggests that, with the notable exception of IL-17RA, each of these receptors has an alternative splice variant. Alternative splicing of IL-17RB and IL-17RC creates frameshifts and introduces stop codons that result in secreted soluble proteins *(628, 629)*.

Presumably these soluble receptors retain their ligand-binding properties and act as decoys, although this has not been demonstrated *(604)*.

Detailed functional studies of the IL-17 receptor family have not yet been reported. The best-studied member to date, IL-17RA, binds both IL-17A and IL-17F, although IL-17A binds with more than 10-fold higher affinity *(607)*. Expression of IL-17RA appears to be ubiquitous, hence the broad tissue responsiveness to IL-17A. Mice with targeted deletion of *Il17ra* have profound defects in host protection *(630)*, consistent with a critical role for IL-17A and IL-17F in host defense. Of the four remaining family members, only IL-17RH1 has been shown to bind IL-17 cytokines, namely IL-17B and IL-25 *(609, 610)*; IL-17RL, IL-17RD, and IL-17RE have only been identified by sequence similarities to IL-17R, and their ligand specificities are not yet reported *(604)*.

Similarly to all other known cytokine receptors, IL-17RA appears to be expressed as a multimer, existing as a preformed complex prior to ligand binding *(631)*. Interestingly, the IL-17RA complex undergoes a conformational change upon binding of IL-17A or IL-17F, which leads to dissociation of the intracellular domains *(604)*. Whether IL-17R family members can interact with other, nonfamily member components for signal transduction is unknown, although the cytoplasmic domains do not appear to contain identifiable catalytic motifs *(602, 603)*. In this regard, it is notable that the neurotrophins, with which the IL-17R ligands have structural homology, not only bind specific Trk receptors but also bind simultaneously to p75^{NTR}, a common second receptor component. Although not yet proven, the IL-17 receptors may be multicomponent signal transducers analogous to neurotrophin receptors *(607)*. A single report has identified the participation of a second IL-17R family member, IL-17RC, as a component of a heteromeric IL-17R that includes IL-17RA *(632)*, suggesting greater complexity in the IL-17R family than previously appreciated.

38.10.2 Th1-Th2 Paradigm

CD4 T-cells play a central role in orchestrating immune responses through their capacity to provide help to other cells of the adaptive or innate immune systems *(604)*. In early studies of CD4 T-cell biology, it became apparent that two classes of CD4 T-cells could be defined: those that helped B cells for class switching, or promoted humoral immunity, and those that enhanced macrophage activation, or promoted cell-mediated immunity. With the advent of techniques for cloning T cells *(633)*, investigators found that these activities typically resided in distinct cloned populations *(634)* and correlated with differential production of factors that promoted or inhibited B-cell class switching to IgE *(635)*, indicating interclonal functional heterogeneity of CD4 T-cells. The activities responsible for these disparate functions were identified as T-cell–derived cytokines, initially defined using specific bioassays, and subsequently using cloned cytokines and specific neutralizing antibodies *(604)*. On the basis of these findings, the T-helper type 1 (Th1)-Th2 hypothesis *(636)* was proposed, which postulated that subsets of CD4 T-cells produce reciprocal patterns of immunity through their production of distinct profiles of cytokine secretion—either delayed-type hypersensitivity/cell-mediated immunity (Th1) or allergic/humoral immunity (Th2). Furthermore, each subset promotes its own development and inhibits the development of the other subset, also via their secreted cytokines *(637, 638)*, such that the induction of one type of response suppresses the induction of the other *(639)*. This hypothesis established a new paradigm for understanding immune regulation by CD4 T-cells and led to the appreciation that effector CD4 T-cells, like class-switched B cells, are functionally heterogeneous *(604)*.

Th1 cells were defined on the basis of their production of IFN-γ, a potent macrophage-activating cytokine important in the clearance of certain intracellular pathogens and a switch factor for induction of IgG2a production by B cells. Th2 cells became defined as producers of IL-4 and IL-5, which promote IgG1 and IgE class switching and eosinophil recruitment. Th2 cells were later shown also to produce IL-13, which participates in IgE class switching and is important for mucosal activation (mucus hypersecretion and increased contractility) *(604)*. Accordingly, the cytokines produced by Th2 cells also became identified as factors involved in the clearance of helminths *(640)*. The importance

of an appropriate Th1 or Th2 response was demonstrated in early studies that examined host protection to challenge by the obligate intracellular protozoal parasite, *Leishmania major*, by genetically resistant and susceptible strains *(641)*. Protection of a resistant mouse strain, C57Bl/6, correlated with an appropriate Th1-mediated IFN-γ response, whereas susceptibility of BALB/c mice correlated with an inappropriate Th2-mediated IL-4 response *(642)*. Susceptible BALB/c mice could be protected by transfer of a Th1 cell line specific to an immunodominant *L. major* antigen, whereas transfer of a Th2 cell line exacerbated disease *(643)*. Thus, the Th1-Th2 hypothesis explained the divergence of distinct types of immunity—types 1 and 2, induction of which could determine success or failure of host protection, depending on the type of pathogen *(604)*.

Discovery of the factors that induce Th1 development followed from studies that directly examined the effects of a Th1-associated pathogen, *Listeria monocytogenes*, on the differentiation of naïve CD4 T-cells. It was found that macrophages activated by heat-killed *L. monocytogenes* induced strongly polarized Th1 responses and that this effect could be blocked by neutralization of IFN-γ, although IFN-γ alone could not induce as robust a Th1 response as that of macrophage-derived factors elicited by heat-killed *L. monocytogenes (644)*. This implicated an additional factor acting in concert with IFN-γ to induce Th1 differentiation. IL-12, a heterodimeric cytokine that had been defined as a potent inducer of IFN-γ production by NK cells *(645)*, was soon identified as the Th1-inducing cofactor responsible for Th1 development *(646, 647)*. This provided a mechanism linking pathogen-driven innate immune activation to a directed adaptive T-cell response and introduced a new cytokine pathway involved in coordination of innate and adaptive immune responses. Thus, cytokine signals induced by first-line innate responses could guide the adaptive response to enhance pathogen clearance *(648)*.

After establishment of the cytokines that polarize Th1 or Th2 differentiation, delineation of key signaling pathways followed *(649)*. Notably, each of the Th1- or Th2-polarizing cytokines are members of the type I cytokine superfamily, receptors for which are heterodimers that signal via JAK/STAT complexes *(650)*.

The cellular sources of the polarizing cytokines responsible for Th1 and Th2 development *in vivo* have been the subject of considerable debate. Although Th1 and Th2 cells can themselves provide IFN-γ or IL-4 for the recruitment of Th1 or Th2 differentiation, respectively, it was not yet definitively determined which cells initiate effector T-cell differentiation in primary versus secondary responses *(604)*. Plasmacytoid DCs, NK cells, or NK T-cells appear to be involved in early production of type I and II IFNs for induction of Th1 cells, but which cells initiate Th2 development is less clear. Basophils, eosinophils, mast cells, and NK T-cells are sources of IL-4 that may be important for Th2 differentiation *(651–655)*, and each of these cell populations may be important for initiating Th2 responses to distinct pathogens or in distinct settings.

38.10.3 IL-17A Cytokine in Innate and Adaptive Immunity

Members of the IL-17 family play a central role in various arms of the adaptive immune response and have become important to an expanded understanding of cytokine networks that coordinate innate and adaptive immunity to certain pathogens. Although current understanding of the links between members of the IL-17 cytokine family and adaptive immunity is relatively new, many features of the landscape and logic of its contribution to innate and adaptive immunity, whether protective or pathogenic, are well documented *(656)*.

IL-17A is a proinflammatory cytokine that is primarily secreted from T lymphocytes, mediators of adaptive immunity. *Recently, IL-17A was shown to be the defining cytokine of a new T-helper subset termed Th17. Discovery of the Th17 population was a groundbreaking discovery that has triggered major revisions of the prevailing paradigms in T-cell biology (656).*

Innate immune cells in mammals, represented primarily by monocytes/macrophages, dendritic cells, and granulocytes, are activated by pathogen-associated molecular patterns (PAMPs) and act to remove foreign bodies from the host as well as process and transport antigens to lymphocytes. The adaptive immune system represented by B- and T-lymphocytes is characterized by clonal expansion of cells that bind to a highly specific antigen. Although often described separately, cross-talk between the adaptive and innate immune systems is frequent and IL-17A represents an intriguing new bridge between adaptive and innate immunity *(656)*.

Since its discovery in 1993 *(600)*, many studies have demonstrated that IL-17A plays a nonredundant role in directing innate immune responses. Its receptor, IL-17RA, is nearly ubiquitous and is expressed on hematopoietic cells as well as many nonimmune cell types such as osteoblasts, fibroblasts, endothelial cells, and epithelial cells *(602, 603)*. Gene expression studies have demonstrated that signaling through IL-17RA promotes the expression of numerous genes relevant to the recruitment of innate immune cells to sites of infection or tissue damage *(630, 657–661)*. Inflammatory proteins such as matrix metalloproteinases (MMPs), acute phase proteins, IL-6 and chemokine ligands, particularly C-X-C chemokines that function to recruit neutrophils,

are among the gene products that are most strongly regulated by IL-17 *(630, 659, 662, 663)*.

Although IL-17A clearly has functional and structural similarities to innate immune molecules, the vast majority of IL-17A is T-cell derived *(660)*. Indeed, IL-17A was discovered in a cDNA library of a murine cytotoxic T-lymphocyte hybridoma and originally termed *cytotoxic T lymphocyte antigen 8 (CTLA-8) (600)*. Soon after its discovery, IL-17A was found to be secreted from CD4$^+$ T-cells with an effector memory phenotype *(664)*, and was correlated with T-cell–mediated autoimmune diseases such as rheumatoid arthritis *(665,666)*. Early attempts in humans to classify IL-17A into a particular T-helper subset (i.e., Th1 or Th2) were inconsistent and unconvincing *(656)*. For example, human T-cell clones isolated from arthritic synovial fluid have been characterized as Th1 (secrete IFN-γ but not IL-4), Th2 (secrete IL-4 but not IFN-γ), or Th0 (secrete both IFN-γ and IL-4). Among these subsets, IL-17A was found to be secreted from Th1 and Th0 cells but not Th2 cells *(667)*. Thus, for some time, IL-17A was considered a Th1 or pre-Th1 cytokine *(656)*.

However, recent studies examining requirements for IL-17A production in T cells in mice have resulted in an upheaval in the Th1-Th2 paradigm *(668, 669)*. Whereas CD4$^+$ T-cells have been classically divided as either Th1 or Th2, which secrete IFN-γ or IL-4, respectively, there is now ample evidence for the existence of a new T-helper effector subset, Th17, which is distinguishable in lineage and function from Th1 and Th2 cells. Th17 cells arise from T-helper progenitor (Thp) cells in a cytokine environment consisting of TGF-β and IL-6 *(604, 668, 670–672)*. This differentiation is under the control of the transcription factor retinoic acid orphan receptor gamma t (RORgammat) *(673)* and is inhibited by IFN-γ and IL-4 *(661)* and, by extension, inhibited by *signal transducer and activator of transcription 1* (STAT1)/T-bet and STAT6/GATA-3 *(674)*. Th17 cells secrete IL-17A and a related family member IL-17F, as well as TNF-α, IL-6 *(675)* and IL-22 *(676,677)*. Similar to IL-17A, Th17 cells function to promote inflammation for host defense or, in other contexts, to promote pathology through excess inflammation *(678)*.

Another source of IL-17A that is likely to be highly significant is the γ/δ T-cell population. Unlike conventional CD4$^+$ or CD8$^+$ T-cells with highly diverse α/β TCR, γ/δ T-cells are enriched at mucosal and epithelial surfaces, such as the gut, lung, and skin, and express a limited TCR antigen-binding repertoire. The role of γ/δ T-cells at these sites is uncertain, but studies have shown that IL-17A production from γ/δ T-cells is important in controlling mouse *Mycobacterium tuberculosis* lung infections *(679)* as well as mouse intraperitoneal *Escherichia coli* infections *(680)*. These discoveries help explain the observation that pathology in IL-17RA^{KO} mice occurs within a few days of infection, before mature effector T-cell responses are likely to be involved *(630)*. Therefore, IL-17A from γ/δ T-cells may be important for initiating an immediate and early neutrophil response to mucosal infections. Furthermore, IL-17A may be a mechanism by which gamma-delta T-cells provide defense responses until adaptive immune cells are recruited to combat remaining pathogens *(656)*.

38.10.4 IL-17 in Rheumatoid Arthritis

Rheumatoid arthritis (RA) is considered a systemic Th1-associated inflammatory joint disease that is characterized by chronic synovitis and destruction of cartilage and bone *(681)*. T cells represent a large proportion of the inflammatory cells invading the synovial tissue. Because the etiology of RA is still unknown, regulating the cytokine imbalance might represent an effective way to control this disease. The proinflammatory cytokines TNF-α and IL-1β play a crucial role in the pathology of arthritis, causing enhanced production of cytokines, chemokines, and degradative enzymes *(682)*. *In vivo* studies have shown that neutralizing TNF-α or IL-1β control chronic inflammation and cartilage degradation, respectively *(683–685)*. Consistent with these findings, clinical studies revealed efficacy after blocking of TNF-α or IL-1β. However, a subset of patients did not respond to these inhibitors, and none of the treatments cured the disease. Therefore, it is tempting to speculate that cytokines or factors other than TNF-α or IL-1β would also participate in the proinflammatory cytokine cascade *(681)*.

T-cell cytokine IL-17, which is spontaneously produced by RA synovial membrane cultures *(686)*, and high levels have been detected in the synovial fluid of patients with rheumatoid arthritis *(687, 688)* and triggers human synoviocytes to produce IL-6, IL-8, granulocyte macrophage colony-stimulating factor, and prostaglandin E_2 *(689, 690)*, thereby suggesting that IL-17 could be an upstream mediator in the pathogenesis of arthritis. Early neutralization of endogenous IL-17 prior to the development of arthritis in the experimental arthritis model suppresses the onset of disease *(691, 692)*. Furthermore, IL-17 may be involved in tissue destruction. IL-17 has biologic activities similar to those of IL-1β, and additive/synergistic effects with TNF-α and IL-1β have been reported *(693)*. *In vitro*, IL-17 suppresses matrix synthesis by articular chondrocytes through enhancement of nitric oxide (NO) production *(694, 695)*. In addition, *in vitro* studies suggested a role for IL-17 in bone erosion by induction of receptor activator of NF-κB ligand (RANKL) expression *(696)*. Recently, it was shown that IL-17 promoted bone erosion in murine collagen-induced arthritis (CIA) through loss of the RANKL/osteoprotegerin (OPG) balance *(697)*. These observations indicate that IL-17 may promote joint inflammation as well as tissue destruction during the initial phase of arthri-

tis. However, the role of T-cell IL-17 during the effector phase of arthritis has still not been identified *(681)*.

Recently, the therapeutic effect of anti-IL-17 antibody treatment in CIA was demonstrated, implying that the T-cell cytokine IL-17 not only plays a role in the early stage of arthritis but also has a function in propagating and prolonging the arthritis *(681)*. Furthermore, fewer synovial IL-1β–positive and RANKL-positive cells were found after treatment with neutralizing endogenous IL-17. This suggests that IL-17 might be a novel target for the treatment of destructive arthritis and implies that neutralization of this T-cell factor during the effector phase of arthritis has therapeutic potential, and that the anti-IL-17 cytokine therapy could be an interesting new approach that may contribute to the prevention of joint destruction and could provide an important additional strategy to the current anti-TNF-α and anti-IL-1β therapy for rheumatoid arthritis *(681)*.

38.10.5 Th17 Cells in Inflammatory Conditions

CD4$^+$ T-cells have been subdivided into a range of different subsets on the basis of the cytokines they produce and the functions they perform *(698)*. Th1, Th2, and regulatory T-cells (Tregs) have been well characterized with respect to factors influencing their development, the cytokines they produce, and their respective roles in response to pathogens, tumors, and self-antigens *(639, 699–704)*. Another population of Th cells, Th17, characterized by their production of the cytokine IL-17, has also been described *(674)*, and it is only recently that factors determining their generation have been identified *(671, 672)*.

It is well known that IL-12 regulates Th1, while IL-4 regulates Th2 differentiation. Studies have shown that TGF-β and IL-6 are required for naïve CD4$^+$ T-cells to differentiate into Th17 cells *(671, 672)*. This differentiation is facilitated by the absence of IFN-γ and IL-4. As TGF-β has usually been associated with the development of Treg cells *(705)* and the inhibition of Th1 and Th2 cell differentiation *(706)*, it is interesting to note that in the presence of an inflammatory cytokine, such as IL-6, the inhibition of Treg cell development and differentiation of naïve CD4$^+$ T-cells into Th17 could be observed *(672)*. This data confirms the view that Th17 cells are a completely separate lineage of CD4$^+$ T-cells *(698)*.

It is known that the signal transducer and activator of transcription (STAT)-4 and the transcription factor T-bet are essential for development of Th1 whereas STAT-6 and GATA-3 are needed for Th2 development. However, only recently was it shown that STAT-3 is also involved in Th17 development together with the suppression of cytokine signaling 3 (Socs3), which acts as a regulator of

IL-23–induced STAT-3 phosphorylation and Th17 development *(698)*.

IL-23 has also been shown to regulate IL-17 production and to promote the expansion of Th17 cells *(707, 708)*. It is a heterodimeric cytokine composed of p40 and p19 subunits. The p40 subunit is also found in IL-12. The receptors for IL-23 and IL-12 share a subunit, IL-12 Rβ1. The IL-12Rβ1 subunit combines with IL-23R to give the functional IL-23 receptor and, together with IL-12Rβ2, to give a functional IL-12R. It can be seen that this subunit sharing by these cytokines and their receptors could have been a source of confusion in assigning a role for IL-12 and Th1 cells in certain pathologic conditions *(698)*. Early studies suggested that effects on inflammatory responses can be observed after the blockade of p40 with antibody or its targeted mutation. These results were interpreted as demonstrating an involvement of IL-12 and correspondingly Th1 cells in the pathogenesis of inflammatory conditions. However, subsequent studies showed that the specific targeting of IL-23 resulted in the alleviation of several inflammatory conditions *(709–711)*, and the lack of IL-12 in some situations actually exacerbated inflammation *(709)*. In summary, these studies emphasized the potential importance of Th17 cells in inflammatory responses *(698)*.

38.10.5.1 Th17 Cells and Autoimmune Disease

The role of Th17 cells in mediating autoimmune pathology is also now becoming recognized, interestingly in events that were previously thought to be Th1-mediated. As type 1 diabetes is thought to be a Th1-mediated disease, it would be appropriate to examine the involvement of Th17 in beta cell destruction *(698)*. The role of these cells, however, in type 1 diabetes remains to be clarified.

There is little information, as yet, regarding the role of IL-17 and Th17 cells in type 1 diabetes. The ability of IL-17 to induce inducible nitric oxide synthase (iNOS) in chondrocytes *(712)* could be observed to occur in mouse islets exposed to this cytokine *(713)*. A potential role for Th17 cells in the exacerbation of diabetes is suggested by the observation that IL-23 induces diabetes in mice if coadministered with sub-diabetogenic multiple low doses of streptozotocin *(714)*. Whether Th17 cells and cytokines IL-23 and IL-17 play a role in the spontaneous onset of diabetes remains to be clarified *(698)*.

IL-17 levels are elevated in a range of inflammatory conditions including systemic sclerosis, psoriasis, and rheumatoid arthritis synovium *(623, 686, 715–717)*. Collagen-induced arthritis (CIA) and experimental-induced encephalomyelitis (EAE) were thought to be Th1-mediated autoimmune diseases. As discussed above, this assumption arose in part from experiments that did not distinguish between effects on IL-12 or IL-23. More recently, it has been shown that these two experimentally induced autoimmune conditions as well as some others are mediated by Th17 cells. The absence of IL-6, which is needed for Th17 development, protected mice against both EAE and CIA *(718–721)*. Neutralization of IL-17 by specific antibody treatments *in vivo* has been shown to prevent the induction of EAE, and the deficiency in IL-23 has been demonstrated to protect mice against both EAE and CIA. The involvement of Th17 cells in mediating pathology in EAE has recently been demonstrated *(672)*.

References

1. Ezekowitz, R. A. B. and Hoffmann, J. A. (eds.) (2003) *Innate Immunity*, Humana Press, Totowa, NJ.
2. Gordon, S. (2003) Mammalian host defenses. In: *Innate Immunity* (Ezekowitz, R. A. B. and Hoffmann, J. A. eds.), Humana Press, Totowa, NJ, pp. 175–176.
3. Kaisho, T. and Akira, S. (2003) Toll-like receptors. In: *Innate Immunity* (Ezekowitz, R. A. B. and Hoffmann, J. A. eds.), Humana Press, Totowa, NJ, pp. 177–189.
4. Banchereau, J., Briere, F., Caux, C., Davoust, J., Lebecque, S., Liu, Y.-J., Pulendran, B., and Palucka, K. (2000) Immunobiology of dendritic cells, *Annu. Rev. Immunol.*, **18**, 767–811.
5. Fearon, D.T. and Locksley, R. M. (1996) The instructive role of innate immunity in the acquired immune response, *Science*, **272**, 50–53.
6. Hoffmann, J.A., Kafatos, F. C., Janeway, C. A., and Ezekowitz, R. A. (1999) Phylogenetic perspectives in innate immunity, *Science*, **284**, 1313–1318.
7. Kunkel, S. L. (2003) Mamalian host defenses: links between innate and adaptive immunity. In: *Innate Immunity* (Ezekowitz, R. A. B. and Hoffmann, J. A. eds.), Humana Press, Totowa, NJ, pp. 267–268.
8. Ramkumar, T. P., Hammache, D., and Stahl, P. D. (2003) The macrophage mannose receptor and innate immunity. In: *Innate Immunity* (Ezekowitz, R. A. B. and Hoffmann, J. A. eds.), Humana Press, Totowa, NJ, pp. 191–204.
9. Janeway, C. A., Jr. (1992) The immune system evolved to discriminate infectious nonself from noninfectious self, *Immunol. Today*, **13**, 11–16.
10. Aderem, A. and Ulevitch, R. J. (2000) Toll-like receptors in the induction of the innate immune response, *Nature*, **406**, 782–787.
11. Akira, S., Takeda, K., and Kaisho, T. (2001) Toll-like receptors: critical proteins linking innate and acquired immunity, *Nat. Immunol.*, **2**, 675–680.
12. Hogaboam, C. M. and Kunkel, S. L. (2003) The role of chemokines in linking innate and adaptive immunity. In: *Innate Immunity* (Ezekowitz, R. A. B. and Hoffmann, J. A. eds.), Humana Press, Totowa, NJ, pp. 269–286.
13. Palucka, K. and Banchereau, J. (1999) Linking innate and adaptive immunity, *Nat. Med.*, **5**, 868–870.
14. Bromley, S. K., Burack, W. R., Johnson, K. G., et al. (2001) The immunological synapse, *Annu. Rev. Immunol.*, **19**, 375–369.
15. Parish, C. R. and O'Neill, E. R. (1997) Dependence of the adaptive immune response on innate immunity: some questions answered but new paradoxes emerge, *Immunol. Cell Biol.*, **75**, 523–527.
16. Lo, D., Feng, L., Li, L., et al. (1999) Integrating innate and adaptive immunity in the whole animal, *Immunol. Rev.*, **169**, 225–239.

17. Takeda, K., Kaisho, T., and Akira, S. (2003) Toll-like receptors, *Annu. Rev. Immunol.*, **21**, 335–376.

18. Tanji, T., Hu, X., Weber, A. N. R., and Ip, Y. Y. (2007) Toll and IMD pathways synergistically activate an innate immune response in *Drosophila melanogaster*, *Mol. Cell Biol.*, **27**(12), 4578–4588.

19. Rock, F. L., Hardiman, G., Timans, J. C., Kastelein, R. A., and Bazan, J. F. (1998) A family of human receptors structurally related to *Drosophila* Toll, *Proc. Natl. Acad. Sci. U.S.A.*, **95**, 588–593.

20. Takeuchi, O., Kawai, T., Sanjo, H., et al. (1999) TLR6: a novel member of an expanding Toll-like receptor family, *Gene*, **231**, 59–65.

21. Du, X., Poltorak, A., Wei, Y., and Beutler, B. (2000) Three novel mammalian Toll-like receptors: gene structure, expression, and evolution, *Eur. Cytokine Netw.*, **11**, 362–371.

22. Hemmi, H., Takeuchi, O., Kawai, T., et al. (2000) Toll-like receptor recognizes bacterial DNA, *Nature*, **408**, 740–745.

23. Chuang, T. and Ulevitch, R. J. (2001) Identification of hTLR10: a novel human Toll-like receptor preferentially expressed in immune cells, *Biochim. Biophys. Acta*, **1518**(1–2), 157–161.

24. Takeda, K. and Akira, S. (2004) TLR signaling pathways, *Semin. Immunol.*, **16**(1), 3–9.

25. Underhill, D. M., Ozinsky, A., Smith, K. D., and Aderem, A. (1999) Toll-like receptor-2 mediates mycobacteria-induced proinflammatory signaling in macrophages, *Proc. Natl. Acad. Sci. U.S.A.*, **96**, 14459–14463.

26. Steiner, T. S., Nataro, J. P., Poteet-Smith, C. E., Smith, J. A., and Guerrant, R. L. (2000) Enteroaggregative Escheria coli express a novel flagellin that caused IL-8 release from intestinal epithelial cells, *J. Clin. Invest.*, **105**, 1769–1777.

27. Eaves-Pyles, T., Murthy, K., Liaudet, L., et al. (2001) Flagellin, a novel mediator of *Salmonella*-induced epithelial activation and systemic inflammation: IκBα degradation, induction of nitric oxide synthase, induction of proinflammatory mediators, and cardiovascular dysfunction, *J. Immunol.*, **166**, 1248–1260.

28. Hayashi, F., Smith, K. D., Ozinsky, A., et al. (2001) The innate immune response to bacterial flagellin is mediated by Toll-like receptor-5, *Nature*, **410**, 1099–1103.

29. Gewirtz, A. T., Simon, J., Schmitt, C. K., et al. (2001) *Salmonella typhimurium* translocates flagellin across intestinal epithelia, inducing a proinflammatory response, *J. Clin. Invest.*, **107**, 99–109.

30. Tokunaga, T., Yamamoto, H., Shimada, S., et al. (1984) Antitumor activity of deoxyribonucleic acid fraction from *Mycobacterium bovis* BCG. I. Isolation, physicochemical characterization, and antitumor activity, *J. Natl. Cancer Inst.*, **72**, 955–962.

31. Krieg, A. M., Yi, A. K., Matson, S., et al. (1995) CpG motifs in bacterial DNA trigger direct B cell activation, *Nature*, **374**, 546–549.

32. Stahl, P. D. and Ezekowitz, R. A. (1998) The mannose receptor is a pattern recognition receptor involved in host defense, *Curr. Opin. Immunol.*, **10**, 50–55.

33. Linehan, S. A., Martinez-Pomares, L., and Gordon, S. (2000) Macrophage lectins in host defence, *Microbes Infect.*, **2**, 279–288.

34. Taylor, M. E. (2001) Structure and function of the macrophage mannose receptor, *Results Probl. Cell Differ.*, **33**, 105–121.

35. Medzhitov, R. and Janeway, C. A., Jr. (1997) Innate immunity: impact on the adaptive immune response, *Curr. Opin. Immunol.*, **9**, 4–9.

36. Hille-Rehfeld, A. (1995) Mannose 6-phosphate receptors in sorting and transport of lysosomal enzymes, *Biochim. Biophys. Acta*, **1241**, 177–194.

37. Stahl, P. D., Wileman, T. E., Diment, S., and Shepherd, V. L. (1984) Mannose- specific oligosaccharide recognition by monomeric phagocytes, *Biol. Cell*, **51**, 215–218.

38. Martinez-Pomares, L., Mahoney, J. A., Kaposzta, R., et al. (1998) A functional soluble form of the murine mannose receptor is produced by macrophages in vitro and is present in mouse serum, *J. Biol. Chem.*, **273**, 23376–23380.

39. Martinez-Pomares, L. and Gordon, S. (1999) Potential role of the mannose receptor in antigen transport, *Immunol. Lett.*, **65**, 9–13.

40. Schweizer, A., Stahl, P. D., and Rohrer, J. (2000) A di-aromatic motif in the cytosolic tail of the mannose receptor mediates endosomal sorting, *J. Biol. Chem.*, **275**, 29694–29700.

41. Kruskal, B. A., Sastry, K., Warner, A. B., Mathieu, C. E., and Ezekowitz, R. A. (1992) Phagocytic chimeric receptors require both transmembrane and cytoplasmic domains from the mannose receptor, *J. Exp. Med.*, **176**, 1673–1680.

42. Pontow, S. E., Blum, J. S., and Stahl, P. D. (1996) Delayed activation of the mannose receptor following synthesis. Requirement for exit from the endoplasmic reticulum, *J. Biol. Chem.*, **271**, 30736–30740.

43. Tietze, C., Schlesinger, P., and Stahl, P. (1982) Mannose-specific endocytosis receptor of alveolar macrophages: demonstration of two functionally distinct intracellular pools of receptor and their roles in receptor recycling, *J. Cell. Biol.*, **92**, 417–424.

44. Wileman, T., Boshans, R. L., Schlesinger, P., and Stahl, P. (1984) Monesin inhibits recycling of macrophage mannose-glycoprotein receptors and ligand delivery to lysosomes, *Biochem. J.*, **220**, 665–675.

45. Montaner, L. J., da Silva, R. P., Sun, J., et al. (1999) Type 1 and type 2 cytokine regulation of macrophage endocytosis: differential activation by IL-4/IL-13 as opposed to IFN-gamma or IL-10, *J. Immunol.*, **162**, 4606–4613.

46. Crouch, E. C. (1998) Collectins and pulmonary host defense, *Am. J. Respir. Cell. Mol. Biol.*, **19**, 177–201.

47. Wright, J. R. (1997) Immunomodulatory functions of surfactant, *Physiol. Rev.*, **77**, 931–962.

48. Haagsman, H. P. (1998) Interactions of surfactant protein A with pathogens, *Biochim. Biophys. Acta*, **1408**, 264–277.

49. Holmskov, U. L. (2000) Collectins and collectin receptors in innate immunity, *APMIS Suppl.*, **100**, 1–59.

50. Lawson, P. R. and Reid, K. B. (2000) The roles of surfactant proteins A and D in innate immunity, *Immunol. Rev.*, **173**, 66–78.

51. Hakansson, K. and Reid, K. B. (2000) Collectin structure: a review, *Protein Sci.*, **9**, 1607–1617.

52. Ohtani, K., Suzuki, Y., Eda, S., et al. (1999) Molecular cloning of a novel human collectin from liver (CL-L1), *J. Biol. Chem.*, **274**, 13681–13689.

53. Khoor, A., Gray, M. E., Hull, W. M., Whisett, J. A., and Stahlman, M. T. (1993) Developmental expression of SP-A and SP-A mRNA in the proximal and distal respiratory epithelium in the human fetus and newborn, *J. Histochem. Cytochem.*, **41**, 1311–1119.

54. Khubchandani, K. R. and Snyder, J. M. (2001) Surfactant protein A (SP-A): the alveolus and beyond, *FASEB J.*, **15**, 59–69.

55. Madsen, J., Kliem, A., Tornoe, I., et al. (2000) Localization of lung surfactant protein D (SP-D) on mucosal surfaces in human tissues, *J. Immunol.*, **164**, 5866–5870.

56. Hakansson, K., Lim, N. K., Hoppe, H. J., and Reid, K. B. (1999) Crystal structure of the trimeric alpha-helical coiled-coil and the three lectin domains of human lung surfactant protein D, *Structure Fold. Des.*, **7**, 255–264.

57. Crouch, E. C. and Whitsett, J. A. (2003) Diverse roles of lung collectins in pulmonary innate immunity. In: *Innate Immunity* (Ezekowitz, R. A. B. and Hoffmann, J. A. (eds.), Humana Press, Totowa, NJ, pp. 205–229.

58. Voss, T., Melchers, K., Scheirle, G., and Schafer, K. P. (1991) Structural comparison of recombinant pulmonary composition of natural protein SP-A derived from two human coding sequences:

implication for the chain composition of natural human SP-A, *Am. J. Respir. Cell. Mol. Biol.*, **4**, 88–94.

59. Karinch, A. M., Deiter, G., Ballard, P. L., and Floros, J. (1998) Regulation of expression of human SP-A1 and SP-A2 genes in fetal lung explant culture, *Biochim. Biophys. Acta*, **1398**, 192–202.

60. McCormick, S. M. and Mendelson, C. R. (1994) Human SP-A1 and SP-A2 genes are differentially regulated during development and by cAMP and glucocorticoids, *Am. J. Physiol.*, **266**, L367–L374.

61. Van Eijk, M., Haagsman, H. P., Skinner, T., et al. (2000) Porcine lung surfactant protein D: complementary DNA cloning, chromosomal localization, and tissue distribution, *J. Immunol.*, **164**, 1442–1450.

62. Crouch, E. and Wright, J. R. (2001) Surfactant proteins A and D and pulmonary host defense, *Annu. Rev. Physiol.*, **63**, 521–554.

63. Madan, T., Kishore, U., Shah, A., et al. (1997) Lung surfactant proteins A and D can inhibit specific IgE binding to the allergens of *Aspergillus fumigatus* and block allergen-induced histamine release from human basophils, *Clin. Exp. Immunol.*, **110**, 241–249.

64. Allen, M. J., Harbeck, R., Smith, B., Voelker, D. R., and Mason, R. J. (1999) Binding of rat and human surfactant proteins A and D to *Aspergillus fumigatus* conidia, *Infect. Immun.*, **67**, 4563–4569.

65. Madan, T., Kishore, U., Singh, M., et al. (2001) Protective role of lung surfactant protein D in a murine model of invasive pulmonary aspergillosis, *Infect. Immun.*, **69**, 2728–2731.

66. Williams, M. D., Wright, J. R., March, K. L., and Martin, W. J. (1996) Human surfactant protein A enhances attachment of *Pneumocystis carinii* to rat alveolar macrophages, *Am. J. Respir. Cell. Mol. Biol.*, **14**, 232–238.

67. Zimmerman, P. E., Voelker, D. R., McCormack, F. X., Paulsrud, J. R., and Martin, W. J. (1992) 120-kD surface glucoprotein of *Pneumocystis carinii* is a ligand for surfactant protein A, *J. Clin. Invest.*, **89**, 143–149.

68. O'Riordan, D. M., Standing, J. E., Kwon, K. Y., et al. (1995) Surfactant protein D interacts with *Pneumocystis carinii* and mediates organism adherence to alveolar macrophages, *J. Clin. Invest.*, **95**, 2699–2710.

69. McCormack, F. X., Festa, A. L., Andrews, R. P., Linke, M., and Walzer, P. D. (1997) The carbohydrate recognition domain of surfactant protein A mediates binding to the major surface glycoprotein of *Pneumocystis carinii*, *Biochemistry*, **36**, 8092–8099.

70. Vuk-Pavlovic, Z., Diaz-Montes, T., Standing, J. E., and Limper, A. H. (1998) Surfactant protein D binds to cell wall β-glucans, *Am. J. Respir. Cell. Mol. Biol.*, **157**, A236.

71. Limper, A. H., Crouch, E. C., O'Riordan, D. M., et al. (1995) Surfactant protein D modulates interaction of *Pneumocystis carinii* with alveolar macrophages, *J. Lab. Clin. Med.*, **126**, 416–422.

72. Kuan, S. F., Rust, K., and Crouch, E. (1992) Interactions of surfactant protein D with bacterial lipopolysaccharides. Surfactant protein D is an *Escherichia coli*-binding protein in bronchoalveolar lavage, *J. Clin. Invest.*, **90**, 97–106.

73. Kalina, M., Blau, H., Riklis, S., and Kravtsov, V. (1995) Interaction of surfactant protein A with bacterial lipopolysaccharide may affect some biological functions, *Am. J. Physiol.*, **268**, L144–L151.

74. Van Iwaarden, J. F., Pikaar, J. C., Storm, J., et al. (1994) Binding of surfactant protein A to the lipid A moiety of bacterial lipopolysaccharides, *Biochem. J.*, **303**, 407–411.

75. Borron, P., McIntosh, J. C., Korfhagen, T. R., et al. (2000) Surfactant-associated protein A inhibits LPS-induced cytokine and nitric oxide production in vivo, *Am. J. Physiol. (Lung Cell Mol. Physiol.)*, **278**, L840–L847.

76. Greene, K. E., Whitsett, J. A., Korfhagen, T. R., and Fisher, J. H. (2000) SP-D expression regulates endotoxin mediated lung inflammation in vivo, *Am. J. Respir. Crit. Care*, **161**, A515.

77. Bridges, J. P., Davis, H. W., Damodarasamy, M., et al. (2000) Pulmonary surfactant proteins A and D are potent endogenous inhibitors of lipid peroxidation and oxidative cellular injury, *J. Biol. Chem.*, **275**, 38848–38855.

78. Stehle, T. and Larvie, M. (2003) Structures of complement control proteins. In: *Innate Immunity* (Ezekowitz, R. A. B. and Hoffmann, J. A., eds.), Humana Press, Totowa, NJ, pp. 231–253.

79. Janaway, C. A., Jr., Travers, P., Walport, M., and Shlomchik, M. J. (eds.) (2001) *Immunobiology: The Immune System in Health and Disease*, 5th ed., Garland Publishing, New York.

80. Baron, S. (ed.) (1996) *Medical Microbiology*, 4th ed., The University of Texas Branch at Galveston, Galveston, TX.

81. Hourcade, D., Holers, V. M., and Atkinson, J. P. (1989) The regulators of complement activation (RCA) gene cluster, *Adv. Immunol.*, **45**, 381–416.

82. Liszewski, M. K., Post, T. W., and Atkinson, J. P. (1991) Membrane cofactor protein (MCP or CD46): newest member of the regulators of complement activation gene cluster, *Annu. Rev. Biochem.*, **9**, 431–455.

83. Hourcade, D., Liszewski, M. K., Krych-Goldberg, M., and Atkinson, J. P. (2000) Functional domains, structural variation and pathogen interactions of MCP, DAF and CRI, *Immunopharmacology*, **49**, 103–116.

84. Pangburn, M. K. (2000) Host recognition and target differentiation by factor H, a regulator of the alternative pathway of complement, *Immunopharmacology*, **49**, 149–157.

85. Kirkitadze, M. D. and Barlow, P. N. (2001) Structure and flexibility of the multiple domain proteins that regulate complement activation, *Immunol. Rev.*, **180**, 146–157.

86. Kirschfink, M. (2001) Targeting complement in therapy, *Immunol. Rev.*, **180**, 177–189.

87. Dörig, R. E., Marcil, A., Chopra, A., and Richardson, C. D. (1993) The human CD46 molecule is a receptor for measles virus (Edmonston strain), *Cell*, **75**, 295–305.

88. Naniche, D., Varior-Krishnan, G., Cervoni, F., et al. (1993) Human membrane cofactor protein (CD46) acts as a cellular receptor for measles virus, *J. Virol.*, **67**, 6025–6032.

89. Okada, N., Liszewski, M. K., Atkinson, J. P., and Caparon, M. (1995) Membrane cofactor protein (CD46) is a keratinocyte receptor for the M protein of the group A *Streptococcus*, *Proc. Natl. Acad. Sci. U.S.A.*, **92**, 2489–2493.

90. Kallstrom, H., Liszewski, M. K., Atkinson, J. P., and Jonsson, A. B. (1997) Membrane cofactor protein (MCP or CD46) is a cellular pilus receptor for pathogenic *Neisseria*, *Mol. Microbiol.*, **25**, 639–647.

91. Santoro, F., Kennedy, P. E., Locatelli, G., et al. (1999) CD46 is a cellular receptor for human herpesvirus 6, *Cell*, **99**, 817–827.

92. Karnauchow, T. M., Dawe, S., Lublin, D. M., and Dimock, K. (1998) Short consensus repeat domain 1 of decay-accelerating factor is required for enterovirus 70 binding, *J. Virol.*, **72**, 9380–9383.

93. Bergelson, J. M., Chan, M., Solomon, K. R., et al. (1994) Decay-accelerating factor (CD55), a glycosylphosphatidyl-inositol-anchored complement regulatory protein, is a receptor for several echoviruses, *Proc. Natl. Acad. Sci. U.S.A.*, **91**, 6245–6249.

94. Ward, T., Pipkin, P. A., Clarkson, N. A., et al. (1994) Decay-accelerating factor CD55 is identified as a receptor for echovirus-7 using CELICS, a rapid immuno-focal cloning method, *EMBO J.*, **13**, 5070–5074.

95. Clarkson, N. A., Kaufman, R., Lublin, D. M., et al. (1995) Characterization of the echovirus 7 receptor: domains of CD55 critical for virus binding, *J. Virol.*, **69**, 5497–5501.

96. Bergelson, J. M., Modlin, J. F., Wieland-Alter, W., et al. (1997) Clinical coxsackievirus B isolates differ from laboratory strains in their interaction with two cell-surface receptors, *J. Infect. Dis.*, **175**, 697–700.

97. Bergelson, J. M., Cunningham, J. A., Droguett, G., et al. (1997) Isolation of a common receptor for coxsackie B viruses and adenoviruses 2 and 5, *Science*, **275**, 1320–1323.

98. Fingeroth, J. D., Weis, J. J., Tedder, T. F., et al. (1984) Epstein-Barr virus receptor of human B lymphocytes is the C3d receptor CR2, *Proc. Natl. Acad. Sci. U.S.A.*, **81**, 4510–4514.

99. Weis, J. J., Tedder, T. F., and Fearon, D. T. (1984) Identification of a 145,000 Mr membrane protein as the C3d receptor (CR2) of human B lymphocytes, *Proc. Natl. Acad. Sci. U.S.A.*, **81**, 884–885.

100. Nemerow, G. R., Wolfert, R., McNaughton, M. E., and Cooper, N. R. (1985) Identification and characterization of the Epstein-Barr virus receptor on human B lymphocytes and its relationship to the C3d complement receptor (CR2), *J. Virol.*, **55**, 347–351.

101. Sharma, A. K. and Pangburn, M. K. (1997) Localization by site-directed mutagenesis of the site in human complement factor H that binds to Streptomyces pyogenes M protein, *Infect. Immun.*, **65**, 484–487.

102. Thern, A., Stenberg, L., Dahlback, B., and Lindahl, G. (1995) Ig-binding surface proteins of *Streptococcus pyogenes* also bind human C4b-binding protein (C4BP), a regulatory component of the complement system, *J. Immunol.*, **154**, 375–386.

103. Hellwage, J., Meri, T., Heikkila, T., et al. (2001) The complement regulator factor H binds to the surface protein OspE of *Borrelia burgdorferi*, *J. Biol. Chem.*, **276**, 8427–8435.

104. Norman, D. G., Barlow, P. N., Baron, M., et al. (1991) Three-dimensional structure of a complement control protein module in solution, *J. Mol. Biol.*, **219**, 717–725.

105. Barlow, P. N., Baron, M., Norman, D. G., et al. (1991) Secondary structure of a complement control protein module by two-dimensional ^{1}H NMR, *Biochemistry*, **30**, 997–1004.

106. Barlow, P. N., Norman, D. G., Steinkasserer, A., et al. (1992) Solution structure of the fifth repeat of factor H: a second example of the complement control protein module, *Biochemistry*, **31**, 3626–3634.

107. Barlow, P. N., Steinkasserer, A., Norman, D. G., et al. (1993) Solution structure of a pair of complement modules by nuclear magnetic resonance, *J. Mol. Biol.*, **232**, 268–284.

108. Wiles, A. P., Shaw, G., Bright, J., et al. (1997) NMR studies of a viral protein that mimicks the regulators of complement activation, *J. Mol. Biol.*, **272**, 253–265.

109. Henderson, C. E., Bromek, K., Mullin, N., et al. (2001) Solution structure and dynamics of the central CCP module pair of a poxvirus complement control protein, *J. Mol. Biol.*, **307**, 323–339.

110. Casasnovas, J. M., Larvie, M., and Stehle, T. (1999) Crystal structure of two CD46 domains reveals an extended measles virus-binding surface, *EMBO J.*, **18**, 2911–2922.

111. Szakonyi, G., Guthridge, J. M., Li, D., et al. (2001) Structure of complement receptor 2 in complex with its C3d ligand, *Science*, **292**, 1725–1728.

112. Murthy, K. H. M., Smith, S. A., Ganesh, V. K., et al. (2001) Crystal structure of a complement control protein that regulates both pathways of complement activation and binds heparin sulfate proteoglycans, *Cell*, **104**, 301–311.

113. Schwarzenbacher, R., Zeth, K., Diederichs, K., et al. (1999) Structure of human beta2-glycoprotein I: implications for phospholipid binding and the antiphospholipid syndrome, *EMBO J.*, **18**, 6228–6239.

114. Bouma, B., de Groot, P. G., van den Elsen, J. M., et al. (1999) Adhesion mechanism of human beta(2)-glycoprotein I to phospholipids based on its crystal structure, *EMBO J.*, **18**, 5166–5174.

115. Gaboriaud, C. G., Rossi, V., Bally, I., Arlaud, G. J., and Fontecilla-Camps, J. C. (2000) Crystal structure of the catalytic domain of human complement C1s: a serine protease with a handle, *EMBO J.*, **19**, 1755–1765.

116. Gadjeva, M., Verschoor, A., and Carroll, M. C. (2003) The role of complement in innate and adaptive immunity. In: *Innate Immunity* (Ezekowitz, R. A. B. and Hoffmann, J. A., eds.), Humana Press, Totowa, NJ, pp. 305–319.

117. Law, S. K. and Dodds, A. W. (1997) The internal thioester and the covalent binding properties of the complement proteins C3 and C4, *Protein Sci.*, **6**, 263–274.

118. Law, S. K., Lichtenberg, N. A., and Levine, R. P. (1980) Covalent binding and hemolytic activity of complement proteins, *Proc. Natl. Acad. Sci. U.S.A.*, **77**, 7194–7198.

119. Cooper, N. R. (1985) The classical complement pathway: activation and regulation of the first complement component, *Adv. Immunol.*, **37**, 151–216.

120. Boes, M. (2000) Role of natural and immune IgM antibodies in immune responses, *Mol. Immunol.*, **37**, 1141–1149.

121. Heyman, B. (2000) Regulation of antibody responses via antibodies, complement, and Fc receptors, *Annu. Rev. Immunol.*, **18**, 709–737.

122. Fearon, D. T. (1980) Identification of the membrane glycoprotein that is the C3b receptor of the human erythrocyte, polymorphonuclear leukocyte, B lymphocyte, and monocyte, *J. Exp. Med.*, **152**, 20–30.

123. Carroll, M. C., Alicot, E. M., Katzman, P. J., et al. (1988) Organization of the genes encoding complement receptors type 1 and 2, decay-accelerating factor, and C4- binding protein in the RCA locus on human chromosome 1, *J. Exp. Med.*, **167**, 1271–1280.

124. Tas, S. W., Klickstein, L. B., Barbashov, S. F., and Nicholson-Weller, A. (1999) C1q and C4b bind simultaneously to CR1 and additively support erythrocyte adhesion, *J. Immunol.*, **163**, 5056–5063.

125. Klickstein, L. B., Barbashov, S. F., Liu, T., Jack, R. M., and Nicholson-Weller, A. (1997) Complement receptor type 1 (CR1, CD35) is a receptor for C1q, *Immunity*, **7**, 345–355.

126. Ghiran, I., Barbashov, S. F., Klickstein, L. B., et al. (2000) Complement receptor 1/CD35 is a receptor for mannan-binding lectin, *J. Exp. Med.*, **192**, 1797–1808.

127. Law, S. K. (1988) C3 receptors on macrophages, *J. Cell Sci. Suppl.*, **9**, 67–97.

128. Gutsmann, T., Müller, M., Carroll, S. F., MacKenzie, R. C., Wiese, A., and Seydel, U. (2001) Dual role of lipopolysaccharide (LPS)-binding protein in neutralization of LPS and enhancement of LPS-induced activation of mononuclear cells, *Infect. Immun.*, **69**(11), 6942–6950.

129. Agellon, L. B., Quinet, E. M., Gillette, T. G., Drayna, D. T., Brown, M. L., and Tall, A. R. (1990) Organization of the human cholesteryl ester transfer protein gene, *Biochemistry*, **29**, 1372–1376.

130. Kirschning, C. J., Au-Young , J., Lamping, N., Reuter, D., Pfeil, D., Seilhamer, J. J., and Schumann, R. R. (1997) Similar organization of the lipopolysaccharide-binding protein (LBP) and phospholipid transfer protein (PLTP) genes suggests a common gene family of lipid-binding proteins, *Genomics*, **46**, 416–425.

131. Tobias, P. S., Mathison, J. C., and Ulevitch, R. J. (1988) A family of lipopolysaccharide binding proteins involved in responses to gram-negative sepsis, *J. Biol. Chem.*, **263**, 13479–13481.

132. Schumann, R. R., Leong, S. R., Flaggs, G. W., Gray, P. W., Wright, S. D., Mathison, J. C., Tobias, P. S., and Ulevitch R J. (1990) Structure and function of lipopolysaccharide binding protein, *Science*, **249**, 1429–1431.

133. Ramadori, G., Meyer zum Buschenfelde, K. H., Tobias, P. S., Mathison, J. C., and Ulevitch R. J. (1990) Biosynthesis of

lipopolysaccharide-binding protein in rabbit hepatocytes, *Pathobiology*, **58**, 89–94.

134. Vreugdenhil, A. C., Dentener, M. A., Snoek, A. M., Greve, J. W., and Buurman, W. A. (1999) Lipopolysaccharide binding protein and serum amyloid A secretion by human intestinal epithelial cells during the acute phase response, *J. Immunol.*, **163**, 2792–2798.

135. Tobias, P. S., Mathison, J., Mintz, D., Lee, J. D., Kravchenko, V., Kato, K., Pugin, J., and Ulevitch, R. J. (1992) Participation of lipopolysaccharide-binding protein in lipopolysaccharide-dependent macrophage activation, *Am. J. Respir. Cell Mol. Biol.*, **7**, 239–245.

136. Kirschning, C., Unbehaun, A., Lamping, N., Pfeil, D., Herrmann, F., and Schumann, R. R. (1997) Control of transcriptional activation of the lipopolysaccharide binding protein (LBP) gene by proinflammatory cytokines, *Cytokines Cell. Mol. Ther.*, **3**, 59–62 [Erratum: *Cytokines Cell. Mol. Ther.*, **3**:137 (1998)].

137. Lamping, N., Dettmer, R., Schroeder, N. W. J., Pfeil, D., Hallatschek, W., Burger, R., and Schumann, R. R. (1998) LPS-binding protein protects mice from septic shock caused by LPS or gram-negative bacteria, *J. Clin. Invest.*, **101**, 2065–2071.

138. Tobias, P. S., Soldau, K., and Ulevitch, R. J. (1986) Isolation of a lipopolysaccharide-binding acute phase reactant from rabbit serum, *J. Exp. Med.*, **164**, 777–793.

139. Tobias, P. S., Soldau, K., and Ulevitch, R. J. (1989) Identification of a lipid A binding site in the acute phase reactant lipopolysaccharide binding protein, *J. Biol. Chem.*, **264**, 10867–10871.

140. Morrison, D. C. and Ryan, J. L. (1987) Endotoxins and disease mechanisms, *Annu. Rev. Med.*, **38**, 417–432.

141. Rietschel, E. T., Brade, H., Brade, L., Brandenburg, K., Schade, U., Seydel, U., Zahringer, U., Galanos, C., Luderitz, O., and Westphal, O. (1987) Lipid A, the endotoxic center of bacterial lipopolysaccharides: relation of chemical structure to biological activity, *Prog. Clin. Biol. Res.*, **231**, 25–53.

142. Kielian, T. L. and Blecha, F. (1995) CD14 and other recognition molecules for lipopolysaccharide: a review, *Immunopharmacology*, **29**(3), 187–205.

143. Bone, R. C. (1991) The pathogenesis of sepsis, *Ann. Intern. Med.*, **115**, 457–469.

144. Glauser, M. P., Zanetti, G., Baumgartner, J. D., and Cohen, J. (1991) Septic shock: pathogenesis, *Lancet*, **338**, 732–736.

145. Ulevitch, R. J. and Tobias, P. S. (1999) Recognition of gram-negative bacteria and endotoxin by the innate immune system, *Curr. Opin. Immunol.*, **11**, 19–22.

146. Blunck, R., Scheel, O., Müller, M., Brandenburg, K., Seitzer, U., and Seydel, U. (2001) New insights into endotoxin-induced activation of macrophages: involvement of a K^+ channel in transmembrane signaling, *J. Immunol.*, **166**, 1009–1015.

147. Maruyama, N., Yasunori, K., Yamauchi, K., Aizawa, T., Ohrui, T., Nara, M., Oshiro, T., Ohno, L., Tanura, G., Shimura, S., Saschi, H., Tahishima, T., and Shirato, K. (1994) Quinine inhibits production of tumor necrosis factor-α from human alveolar macrophages, *Am. J. Respir. Cell. Mol. Biol.*, **10**, 514–520.

148. Todd, R. F., Bhan, A. K., Kabawat, S. E., and Schlossman, S. F. (1984) Human myelomonocytic differentiation antigens defined by monoclonal antibodies. In: *Leucocyte Typing, Human Leucocyte Differentiation Antigens Detected by Monoclonal Antibodies* (Bernard, A., Boumsell, L., Dausset, J., Milstein, C., and Schlossman, S. F., eds.), Springer-Verlag, Oxford, pp. 424–433.

149. Griffin, J. D. and Schlossman, S. F. (1984) Expression of myeloid differentiation antigens in acute myeloblastic leukemia. In: *Leucocyte Typing, Human Leucocyte Differentiation Antigens Detected by Monoclonal Antibodies* (Bernard, A., Boumsell, L., Dausset, J., Milstein, C., and Schlossman, S. F., eds.), Springer-Verlag, Oxford, pp. 404–410.

150. Hogg, N. and Horton, M. A. (1986) Myeloid antigens: new and previously defined clusters. In: *Leucocyte Typing III, White Cell Differentiation Antigens* (McMichael, A. J., ed.), Oxford University Press, New York, pp. 576–602.

151. Labeta, M. O., Landmann, R., Obrecht, J. P., and Obrist, R. (1991) Human B cells express membrane-bound and soluble forms of the CD 14 myeloid antigen, *Mol. Immunol.*, **28**, 115–122.

152. Morabito, F., Prasthofer, E. F., Dunlap, N. E., Grossi, C. E., and Tilden, A. B. (1987) Expression of myelomonocytic antigens on chronic lymphocytic leukemia B cells correlates with their ability to produce interleukin 1, *Blood*, **70**, 1750–1757.

153. Zeigler-Heitbrock, H. W. L., Pechumer, H., Petersmann, I., Durieux, J. J., Vita, N., Labeta, M. O., and Strobel, M. (1994) CD14 is expressed and functional in human B cells, *Eur. J. Immunol.*, **24**, 1937–1940.

154. Wright, S. D., Ramos, R. A., Tobias, P. S., Ulevitch, R. J., and Mathison, J. C. (1990) CD14, a receptor for complexes of lipopolysaccharide (LPS) and LPS binding protein, *Science*, **249**, 1431–1433.

155. Tobias, P. S. (2003) Lipopolysaccharide-binding protein and CD14. In: *Innate Immunity* (Ezekowitz, R. A. B. and Hoffmann, J. A., eds.), Humana Press, Totowa, NJ, pp. 255–265.

156. Pugin, J., Schurer-Maly, C.-C., Leturcq, D., et al. (1993) Lipopolysaccharide activation of human endothelial and epithelial cells is mediated by lipopolysaccharide-binding protein and soluble CD14, *Proc. Natl. Acad. Sci. U.S.A.*, **90**, 2744–2748.

157. Simmons, D. L., Tan, S., Tenen, D. G., Nicholson Weller, A., and Seed, B. (1989) Monocyte antigen CD14 is a phospholipid anchored membrane protein, *Blood*, **73**, 284–289.

158. Haziot, A., Ferrero, E., Xing, Y. L., Stewart, C. L., and Goyert, M. (1994) CD14- deficient mice are exquisitely insensitive to the effects of LPS. In: *Bacterial Endotoxins* (Levin, J., Alving, C. R., Munford, R. S., and Redl, H., eds.), Wiley-Liss, New York, pp. 349–351.

159. Moore, K. J., Andersson, L. P., Ingalls, R. R., et al. (2000) Divergent response to LPS and bacteria in CD14-deficient murine macrophages, *J. Immunol.*, **165**, 4272–4280.

160. Haziot, A., Lin, X. Y., Zhang, F., and Goyert, S. M. (1998) The induction of acute phase proteins by lipopolysaccharide uses a novel pathway that is CD14- independent, *J. Immunol.*, **160**, 2570–2572.

161. Le Van, T. D., Bloom, J. W., Bailey, T. J., et al. (2001) A common single nucleotide polymorphism in the CD14 promoter decreases the affinity of Sp protein binding and enhances transcriptional activity, *J. Immunol.*, **167**, 5838–5844.

162. Zhang, D. E., Hetherington, C. J., Tan, S., et al. (1994) Sp1 is a critical factor for the monocytic specific expression of human CD14, *J. Biol. Chem.*, **269**, 11425–11434.

163. Vercelli, D., Baldini, M., Stern, D., et al. (2001) CD14: a bridge between innate immunity and adaptive IgE responses, *J. Endotoxin Res.*, **7**, 45–48.

164. Williams, H., Robertson, C., Stewart, A., et al. (1999) Worldwide variations in the prevalence of symptoms of atopic eczema in the International Study of Asthma and Allergies in Childhood, *J. Allergy Clin. Immunol.*, **103**, 125–138.

165. Strachan, D., Sibbald, B., Weiland, S., et al. (1997) Worldwide variations in prevalence of symptoms of allergic rhinoconjunctivitis in children: the Internaltional Study of Asthma and Allergies in Childhood (ISAAC), *Pediatr. Allergy Immunol.*, **8**, 161–176.

166. Arias, M. A., Rey Nores, J. E., Vita, N., et al. (2000) Cutting edge: human B cell function is regulated by interaction with soluble CD14: opposite effects on IgG1 and IgE production, *J. Immunol.*, **164**, 3480–3486.

167. Shimada, K., Watanabe, Y., Mokuno, H., et al. (2000) Common polymorphism in the promoter of the CD14 monocyte receptor gene is associated with acute myocardial infarction in Japanese men, *Am. J. Cardiol.*, **86**, 682–684.

168. Unkelbach, K., Gardemann, A., Kostrzewa, M., et al. (1999) A new promoter polymorphism in the gene of lipopolysaccharide receptor CD14 is associated with expired myocardial infarction in patients with low atherosclerotic risk profile, *Arterioscler. Thromb. Vasc. Biol.*, **19**, 932–938.

169. Hubacek, J. A., Rothe, G., Pit'ha, J., et al. (1999) C(–260)→T polymorphism in the promoter of the CD14 monocyte receptor gene as a risk factor for myocardial infarction, *Circulation*, **99**, 3218–3220.

170. Ito, D., Murata, M., Tanahashi, N., et al. (2000) Polymorphism in the promoter of lipopolysaccharide receptor CD14 and ischemic cerebrovascular disease, *Stroke*, **31**, 2661–2664.

171. Moser, B. and Loetscher, P. (2001) Lymphocyte traffic control by chemokines, *Nat. Immunol.*, **2**, 123–128.

172. Thelen, M. (2001) Dancing to the tune of chemokines, *Nat. Immunol.*, **2**, 129–134.

173. Yoshie, O. (2000) Immune chemokines and their receptors: the key elements in the genesis, homeostasis and function of the immune system, *Springer Semin. Immunopathol.*, **22**, 371–391.

174. Gerard, C. and Rollins, B. J. (2001) Chemokines and disease, *Nat. Immunol.*, **2**, 108–115.

175. Matsukawa, A., Hogaboam, C. M., Lukacs, N. W., and Kunkel, S. L. (2000) Chemokines and innate immunity, *Rev. Immunogenet.*, **2**, 339–358.

176. Kunkel, S. L. (1999) Through the looking glass: the diverse in vivo activities of chemokines, *J. Clin. Invest.*, **104**, 1333–1334.

177. Rossi, D. and Zlotnik, A. (2000) The biology of chemokines and their receptors, *Annu. Rev. Immunol.*, **18**, 217–242.

178. Scapini, P., Lapinet-Vera, J. A., Gasperini, S., et al. (2000) The neutrophil as a cellular source of chemokines, *Immunol. Rev.*, **177**, 195–203.

179. Clark, G. J., Angel, N., Kato, M., et al. (2000) The role of dendritic cells in the innate immune system, *Microbes Infect.*, **2**, 257–272.

180. Stockwin, L. H., McGonagle, D., Martin, I. G., and Blair, G. E. (2000) Dendritic cells: immunological sentinels with a central role in health and disease, *Immunol. Cell Biol.*, **78**, 91–102.

181. Caux, C., Ait-Yahia, S., Chemin, K., et al. (2000) Dendritic cell biology and regulation of dendritic cell trafficking by chemokines, *Springer Semin. Immunopathol.*, **22**, 345–369.

182. Gunn, M. D., Kyuwa, S., Tam, C., et al. (1999) Mice lacking expression of secondary lymphoid organ chemokine have defects in lymphocyte homing and dendritic cell localization, *J. Exp. Med.*, **189**, 451–460.

183. Chan, V. W., Kothakota, S., Rohan, M. C., et al. (1999) Secondary lymphoid-tissue chemokine (SLC) is chemotactic for mature dendritic cells, *Blood*, **93**, 3610–3616.

184. Willimann, K., Legler, D. F., Loetscher, M., et al. (1998) The chemokine SLC is expressed in T cell areas of lymph nodes and mucosal lymphoid tissues and attracts activated T cells via CCR7, *Eur. J. Immunol.*, **28**, 2025–2034.

185. Demangel, C. and Britton, W. J. (2000) Interaction of dendritic cells with mycobacteria: where the action starts, *Immunol. Cell Biol.*, **78**, 318–324.

186. McWilliam, A. S., Napoli, S., Marsh, A. M., et al. (1996) Dendritic cells are recruited into airway epithelium during the inflammatory response to a broad spectrum of stimuli, *J. Exp. Med.*, **184**, 2429–2432.

187. Rescigno, M., Granucci, F., and Ricciardi-Castagnoli, P. (2000) Molecular events of bacterial-induced maturation of dendritic cells, *J. Clin. Immunol.*, **20**, 161–166.

188. Burdin, N. and Kronenberg, M. (1999) CD1mediated immune responses to glycolipids, *Curr. Opin. Immunol.*, **11**, 326–331.

189. Porcelli, S.A. and Modlin, R. L. (1999) The CD1 system: antigen-presenting molecules for T cell recognition of lipids and glycolipids, *Annu. Rev. Immunol.*, **17**, 297–329.

190. Kitamura, H., Iwakabe, K., Yahata, T., Nishimura, S., Ohta, A., Ohmi, Y., Sato, M., Takeda, K., Okumura, K., Van Kaer, L., Kawano, T., Taniguchi, M., and Nishimura, T. (1999) The natural killer T (NKT) cell ligand α-galactosylceramide demonstrates its immunopotentiating effect by inducing interleukin (IL)-12 production by dendritic cells and IL-12 receptor expression on NKT cells, *J. Exp. Med.*, **189**, 1121–1128.

191. Yokoyama, W. M. (2003) The role of natural killer cells in innate immunity to infection. In: *Innate Immunity* (Ezekowitz, R. A. B. and Hoffmann, J. A., eds.), Humana Press, Totowa, NJ, pp. 321–339.

192. Yokoyama, W. M., Kim, S., and French, A. R. (2004) The dynamic life of natural killer cells, *Annu. Rev. Immunol.*, **22**, 405–429.

193. Trinchieri, G. (1989) Biology of natural killer cells, *Adv. Immunol.*, **47**, 187–376.

194. Yokoyama, W. M. (1999) Natural killer cells. In: *Fundamental Immunology* (Paul, W. E., ed.), Lippincott-Raven, New York, pp. 575–603.

195. Anderson, P., Caligiuri, M., Ritz, J., and Schlossman, S. F. (1989) CD3-negative natural killer cells express zeta TCR as part of a novel molecular complex, *Nature*, **341**, 159–162.

196. Lanier, L. L., Yu, G., and Phillips, J. H. (1989) C-association of CD3 zeta with receptor (CD16) for IgG on human natural killer cells, *Nature*, **342**, 803–805.

197. Lanier, L. L., Phillips, J. H., Hackett, J., Jr., Tutt, M., and Kumar, V. (1986) Natural killer cells: definition of a cell type rather than a function, *J. Immunol.*, **137**, 2735–2739.

198. Biron, C. A., Nguyen, K. B., Pien, G. C., Cousens, L. P., and Salazar-Mather, T. P. (1999) Natural killer cells in antiviral defense: function and regulation by innate cytokines, *Annu. Rev. Immunol.*, **17**, 189–220.

199. Biron, C. A., Byron, K. S., and Sullivan, J. L. (1989) Severe herpesvirus infections in an adolescent without natural killer cells, *N. Engl. J. Med.*, **320**, 1731–1735.

200. Jawahar, S., Moody, C., Chan, M., et al. (1996) Natural killer (NK) cell deficiency associated with an epitope-deficient Fc receptor type IIIA (CD16-II), *Clin. Exp. Immunol.*, **103**, 408–413.

201. Robertson, M. J., Williams, B. T., Christopherson, K., Brahmi, Z., and Hromas, R. (2000) Regulation of human natural killer cell migration and proliferation by the exodus subfamily of CC chemokines, *Cell. Immunol.*, **199**, 8–14.

202. Rook, A. H., Masur, H., Lane, H. C., et al. (1983) Interleukin-2 enhances the depressed natural killer and cytomegalovirus-specific cytotoxic activities of lymphocytes from patients with the acquired immune deficiency syndrome, *J. Clin. Invest.*, **72**, 398–403.

203. Bonavida, B., Katz, J., and Gottlieb, M. (1986) Mechanism of defective NK cell activity in patients with acquired immunodeficiency syndrome (AIDS) and AIDS- related complex. I. Defective trigger on NK cells for NKCF production by target cells, and partial restoration by IL-2, *J. Immunol.*, **137**, 1157–1163.

204. Lusso, P., Malnati, M. S., Garzino-Demo, A., et al. (1993) Infection of natural killer cells by human herpesvirus 6, *Nature*, **362**, 458–462.

205. Tripp, C. S., Wolf, S. F., and Unanue, E. R. (1993) Interleukin 12 and tumor necrosis factor alpha are costimulators of interferon gamma production by natural killer cells in severe combined immunodeficiency mice with listeriosis, and interleukin 10 is a

physiologic antagonist, *Proc. Natl. Acad. Sci. U.S.A.*, **90**, 3725–3729.

206. Tripp, C. S., Gately, M. K., Hakimi, J., Ling, P., and Unanue, E. R. (1994) Neutralization of IL-12 decreases resistance to *Listeria* in SCID and S.B-17 mice, reversal by IFN-gamma, *J. Immunol.*, **152**, 1883–1887.

207. Guidotti, L. G. and Chisari, F. V. (2001) Noncytolytic control of viral infections by the innate and adaptive immune response, *Annu. Rev. Immunol.*, **19**, 65–91.

208. Waldmann, T. A. and Tagaya, Y. (1999) The multifaceted regulation of interleukin-15 expression and the role of this cytokine in NK cell differentiation and host response to intracellular pathogens, *Annu. Rev. Immunol.*, **17**, 19–49.

209. Kennedy, M. K., Glaccum, M., Brown, S. N., et al. (2000) Reversible defects in natural killer and memory CD8 T cell lineages in interleukin 15-deficient mice, *J. Exp. Med.*, **191**, 771–780.

210. Lodolce, J. P., Boone, D. L., Chai, S., et al. (1998) IL-15 receptor maintains lymphoid homeostasis by supporting lymphocyte homing and proliferation, *Immunity*, **9**, 669–676.

211. Gosselin, J., Tomoiu, A., Gallo, R. C., and Flamand, L. (1999) Interleukin-15 as an activator of natural killer cell-mediated antiviral response, *Blood*, **94**, 4210–4219.

212. Fawaz, L. M., Sharif-Askari, E., and Menezes, J. (1999) Up-regulation of NK cytotoxic activity via IL-15 induction by different viruses: a comparative study, *J. Immunol.*, **163**, 4473–4480.

213. Ahmad, A., Sharif-Askari, E., Fawaz, L., and Menezes, J. (2000) Innate immunity response of the human host to exposure with herpes simplex virus type 1: in vitro control of the virus infection by enhanced natural killer activity via interleukin-15 induction, *J. Virol.*, **74**, 7196–7203.

214. Tsunobuchi, H., Nishimura, H., Goshima, F., et al. (2000) A protective role of interleukine-15 in a mouse model for systemic infection with herpes simplex virus, *Virology*, **275**, 57–66.

215. Henkart, P. A. (1994) Lymphocyte-mediated cytotoxicity: two pathways and multiple effector molecules, *Immunity*, **1**, 343–346.

216. Motyka, B., Korbutt, G., Pinkoski, M. J., et al. (2000) Mannose 6-phosphate/insulin-like growth factor II receptor is a death receptor for granzyme B during cytotoxic T cell-induced apoptosis, *Cell*, **103**, 491–500.

217. Zamai, L., Ahmad, M., Bennett, I. M., et al. (1998) Natural killer (NK) cell-mediated cytotoxicity: differential use of TRAIL and Fas ligand by immature and mature primary human NK cells, *J. Exp. Med.*, **188**, 2375–2380.

218. Bradley, M., Zeytun, A., Rafi-Janajreh, A., Nagarkatti, P. S., and Nagarkatti, M. (1998) Role of spontaneous and interleukin-2-induced natural killer cell activity in the cytotoxicity and rejection of Fas+ and Fas- tumor cells, *Blood*, **92**, 4248–4255.

219. Kärre, K., Ljunggren, H. G., Piontek, G., and Kiessling, R. (1986) Selective rejection of H-2-deficient lymphoma variants suggests alternative immune defence strategy, *Nature*, **319**, 675–678.

220. Ljunggren, H. G. and Kärre, K. (1990) In search of the "missing self": MHC molecules and NK cell recognition, *Immunol. Today*, **11**, 237–244.

221. Kärre, K. (1985) Role of target histocompatibility antigens in regulation of natural killer activity: a reevaluation and a hypothesis. In: *Mechanisms of Cytotoxicity by NK Cells* (Herberman, R. B. and Callewaert, D. M., eds.), Academic Press, Orlando, FL, pp. 81–92.

222. Karlhofer, F. M., Ribaudo, R. K., and Yokoyama, W. M. (1992) MHC class I alloantigen specificity of Ly-49+ IL-2-activated natural killer cells, *Nature*, **358**, 66–70.

223. Yokoyama, W. M. (1997) What goes up must come down: the emerging spectrum of inhibitory receptors, *J. Exp. Med.*, **186**, 1803–1808.

224. Long, E. O. (1999) Regulation of immune responses through inhibitory receptors, *Annu. Rev. Immunol.*, **17**, 875–904.

225. Correa, I. and Raulet, D. H. (1995) Binding of diverse peptides to MHC class I molecules inhibits target cell lysis by activated natural killer cells, *Immunity*, **2**, 61–71.

226. Orihuela, M., Margulies, D. H., and Yokoyama, W. M. (1996) The natural killer cell receptor Ly-49A recognizes a peptide-induced conformational determinant on its major histocompatibility complex class I ligand, *Proc. Natl. Acad. Sci. U.S.A.*, **93**, 11792–11797.

227. Michaelsson, J., Achour, A., Salcedo, M., et al. (2000) Visualization of inhibitory Ly49 receptor specificity with soluble major histocompatibility complex class I tetramers, *Eur. J. Immunol.*, **30**, 300–307.

228. Mandelboim, O., Wilson, S. B., Vales-Gomez, M., Reyburn, H. T., and Strominger, J. L. (1997) Self and viral peptides can initiate lysis by autologous natural killer cells, *Proc. Natl. Acad. Sci. U.S.A.*, **94**, 4604–4609.

229. Yokoyama, W. M. (1995) Natural killer cell receptors, *Curr. Opin. Immunol.*, **7**, 110–120.

230. Biassoni, R., Cantoni, C., Falco, M., et al. (1996) The human leucocyte antigen (HLA)-C-specific "activatory" or "inhibitory" natural killer cell receptors display highly homologous extracellular domains but differ in their transmembrane and intracytoplasmic portions, *J. Exp. Med.*, **183**, 645–650.

231. Idriss, A. H., Smith, H. R. C., Mason, L. H., et al. (1999) The natural killer cell complex genetic locus, Chok, encodes Ly49D, a target recognition receptor that activates natural killing, *Proc. Natl. Acad. Sci. U.S.A.*, **96**, 6330–6335.

232. Nakamura, M. C., Linnemeyer, P. A., Niemi, E. C., et al. (1999) Mouse Ly-49D recognizes H-2Dd and activates natural killer cell cytotoxicity, *J. Exp. Med.*, **189**, 493–500.

233. George, T. C., Mason, L. H., Ortaldo, J. R., Kumar, V., and Bennett, M. (1999) Positive recognition of MHC class I molecules by the Ly49D receptor of murine NK cells, *J. Immunol.*, **162**, 2035–2043.

234. Karlhofer, F. M., Ribaudo, R. K., and Yokoyama, W. M. (1992) The interaction of Ly-49 with H-2Dd globally inactivates natural killer cell cytolytic activity, *Trans. Assoc. Am. Physicians*, **105**, 72–85.

235. Correa, I., Corral, L., and Raulet, D. H. (1994) Multiple natural killer cell-activating signals are inhibited by major histocompatibility complex class I expression in target cells, *Eur. J. Immunol.*, **24**, 1323–1331.

236. Storkus, W. J., Alexander, J., Payne, J. A., Dawson, J. R., and Cresswell, P. (1989) Reversal of natural killing susceptibility in target cells expressing transfected class I HLA genes, *Proc. Natl. Acad. Sci. U.S.A.*, **86**, 2361–2364.

237. Cohen, G. B., Gandhi, R. T., Davis, D. M., et al. (1999) The selective downregulation of class I major histopatibility complex proteins by HIV-1 protects HIV-infected cells from NK cells, *Immunity*, **10**, 661–671.

238. Reyburn, H. T., Mandelboim, O., Vales-Gomez, M., et al. (1997) The class I MHC homologue of human cytomegalovirus inhibits attack by natural killer cells, *Nature*, **386**, 514–517.

239. Farrell, H. E., Vally, H., Lynch, D. M., et al. (1997) Inhibition of natural killer cells by a cytomegalovirus MHC class I homologue in vivo, *Nature*, **386**, 510–514.

240. Cosman, D., Fanger, N., Borges, L., et al. (1997) A novel immunoglobulin superfamily receptor for cellular and viral MHC class I molecules, *Immunity*, **7**, 273–282.

241. Tomasec, P., Braud, V. M., Rickards, C., et al. (2000) Surface expression of HLA-E, an inhibitor of natural killer cells, enhanced by human cytomegalovirus gpUL40, *Science*, **287**, 1031.

242. Ulbrecht, M., Martinozzi, S., Grzeschik, M., et al. (2000) Cutting edge: the human cytomegalovirus UL40 gene product contains a ligand for HLA-E and prevents NK cell-mediated lysis, *J. Immunol.*, **164**, 5019–5022.

243. Ishido, S., Choi, J. K., Lee, B. S., et al. (2000) Inhibition of natural killer cell- mediated cytotoxicity by Kaposi's sarcoma-associated herpesvirus K5 protein, *Immunity*, **13**, 365–374.

244. Schmidt, R. E., Bartley, G., Levine, H., Schlossman, S. F., and Ritz, J. (1985) Functional characterization of LFA-1 antigens in the interaction of human NK clones and target cells, *J. Immunol.*, **135**, 1020–1025.

245. Scalzo, A. A., Fitzgerald, N. A., Simmons, A., La Vista, A. B., and Shellam, G. R. (1990) Cmv-1, a genetic locus that controls murine cytomegalovirus replication in the spleen, *J. Exp. Med.*, **171**, 1469–1483.

246. Delano, M. L. and Brownstein, D. G. (1995) Innate resistance to lethal mousepox is genetically linked to the NK gene complex on chromosome 6 and correlates with early restriction of virus replication by cells with an NK phenotype, *J. Virol.*, **69**, 5875–5877.

247. Pereira, R. A., Scalzo, A., and Simmons, A. (2001) Cutting edge: a NK complex- linked locus governs acute versus latent herpes simplex virus infection of neurons, *J. Immunol.*, **166**, 5869–5873.

248. Bromley, S. K., Burack, W. R., Johnson, K. G., et al. (2001) The immunological synapse, *Annu. Rev. Immunol.*, **19**, 375–396.

249. Matsukawa, A., Lukacs, N. W., Standiford, T. J., Chensue, S. W., and Kunkel, S. L. (2000) Adenoviral-mediated overexpression of monocyte chemoattractant protein-1 differentially alters the development of Th1 and Th2 type responses in vivo, *J. Immunol.*, **164**, 1699–1704.

250. Odum, N., Bregenholt, S., Eriksen, K. W., et al. (1999) The CC-chemokine receptor 5 (CCR5) is a marker of, but not essential for the development of human Th1 cells, *Tissue Antigens*, **54**, 572–577.

251. D'Ambrosio, D., Iellem, A., Bonecchi, R., et al. (1998) Selective up-regulation of chemokine receptors CCR4 and CCR8 upon activation of polarized human type 2 Th cells, *J. Immunol.*, **161**, 5111–5115.

252. Zingoni, A., Soto, H., Hedrick, J. A., et al. (1998) The chemokine receptor CCR8 is preferentially expressed in Th2 but not Th1 cells, *J. Immunol.*, **161**, 547–551.

253. Campbell, J. D. and HayGlass, K. T. (2000) T cell chemokine receptor expression in human Th1- and Th2-associated diseases, *Arch. Immunol. Ther. Exp. (Warsz.)*, **48**, 451–456.

254. Naumann, M. (2000) Nuclear factor-kappa B activation and innate immune response in microbial pathogen infection, *Biochem. Pharmacol.*, **60**, 1109–1114.

255. Lillard, J. W., Boyaka, P. N., Taub, D. D., and McGhee, J. R. (2001) RANTES potentiates antigen-specific mucosal immune responses, *J. Immunol.*, **166**, 162–169.

256. Hogaboam, C. M., Smith, R. E., and Kunkel, S. L. (1998) Dynamic interactions between lung fibroblasts and leukocytes: implications for fibrotic lung disease, *Proc. Assoc. Am. Physicians*, **110**, 313–320.

257. Smith, R. S., Smith, T. J., Blieden, T. M., and Phipps, R. P. (1997) Fibroblasts as sentinel cells. Synthesis of chemokines and regulation of inflammation, *Am. J. Pathol.*, **151**, 317–322.

258. Xia, Y., Pauza, M. E., Feng, L., and Lo, D. (1997) RelB regulation of chemokine expression modulates local inflammation, *Am. J. Pathol.*, **151**, 375–387.

259. Murphy, P. M. (2001) Viral exploitation and subversion of the immune system through chemokine mimicry, *Nat. Immunol.*, **2**, 116–122.

260. Scarlatti, G., Tresoldi, E., Bjorndal, A., et al. (1997) In vivo evolution of HIV-1 co- receptor usage and sensitivity to chemokine-mediated suppression, *Nat. Med.*, **3**, 1259–1265.

261. Simmons, G., Reeves, J. D., Hibbits, S., et al. (2000) Co-receptor use by HIV and inhibition of HIV infection by chemokine receptor ligands, *Immunol. Rev.*, **177**, 112–126.

262. Howie, S., Ramage, R., and Hewson, T. (2000) Innate immune system damage in human immunodeficiency virus type 1 infection. Implications for acquired immunity and vaccine design, *Am. J. Respir. Crit. Care Med.*, **162**, S141–S145.

263. Holland, S. M. (1996) Host defense against nontuberculous mycobacterial infections, *Semin. Respir. Infect.*, **11**, 217–230.

264. Endres, M. J., Garlisi, C. G., Xiao, H., Shan, L., and Hedrick, J. A. (1999) The Kaposi's sarcoma-related herpesvirus (KSHV)-encoded chemokine vMIP-I is a specific agonist for the CC chemokine receptor (CCR)8, *J. Exp. Med.*, **189**, 1993–1998.

265. Sozzani, S., Luini, W., Bianchi, G., et al. (1998) The viral chemokine macrophage inflammatory protein-II is a selective Th2 chemoattractant, *Blood*, **92**, 4036–4039.

266. Kledal, T. N., Rosenkilde, M. M., Coulin, F., et al. (1997) A broad-spectrum chemokine antagonist encoded by Kaposi's sarcoma-associated herpesvirus, *Science*, **277**, 1656–1659.

267. Chen, S., Bacon, K. B., Li, L., et al. (1998) In vivo inhibition of CC and CX3C chemokine-induced leukocyte infiltration and attenuation of glomerulonephritis in Wistar-Kyoto (WKY) rats by vMIP-II, *J. Exp. Med.*, **188**, 193–198.

268. Penfold, M. E., Dairaghi, D. J., Duke, G. M. (1999) Cytomegalovirus encodes a potent alpha chemokine, *Proc. Natl. Acad. Sci. U.S.A.*, **96**, 9839–9844.

269. Zhang, P., Summer, W. R., Bagby, G. J., and Nelson, S. (2000) Innate immunity and pulmonary host defense, *Immunol. Rev.*, **173**, 39–51.

270. Itakura, M., Tokuda, A., Kimura, H., et al. (2001) Blockade of secondary lymphoid tissue chemokine exacerbates *Propionibacterium acnes*-induced acute lung inflammation, *J. Immunol.*, **166**, 2071–2079.

271. Standiford, T. J. (1997) Cytokines and pulmonary host defenses, *Curr. Opin. Pulm. Med.*, **3**, 81–88.

272. Standiford, T. J. and Huffnagle, G. B. (1997) Cytokines in host defense against pneumonia, *J. Invest. Med.*, **45**, 335–345.

273. Brun-Bruisson, C. (2000) The epidemiology of the systemic inflammatory response, *Intensive Care Med.*, **26**, S64–S74.

274. Fry, D. E. (2000) Sepsis syndrome, *Am. Surg.*, **66**, 126–132.

275. Glauser, M. P. (2000) Pathophysiologic basis of sepsis: considerations for future strategies of intervention, *Crit. Care Med.*, **28**, S4–S8.

276. Deitch, E. A. and Goodman, E. R. (1999) Prevention of multiple organ failure, *Surg. Clin. North Am.*, **79**, 1471–1488.

277. Matsukawa, A., Hogaboam, C. M., Lukacs, N. W., et al. (1999) Endogenous monocyte chemoattractant protein-1 (MCP-1) protects mice in a model of acute septic peritonitis: cross-link between MCP-1 and leukotrine B4, *J. Immunol.*, **163**, 6148–6154.

278. Matsukawa, A., Hogaboam, C. M., Lukacs, N. W., et al. (2000) Endogenous MCP-1 influences systemic cytokine balance in a murine model of acute septic peritonitis, *Exp. Mol. Pathol.*, **68**, 77–84.

279. Zisman, D. A., Kunkel, S. L., Strieter, R. M., et al. (1997) MCP-1 protects mice in lethal endotoxemia, *J. Clin. Invest.*, **99**, 2832–2836.

280. Matsukawa, A., Hogaboam, C. M., Lukacs, N. W., et al. (2000) Pivotal role of the CC chemokine, macrophage-derived chemokine, in the innate immune response, *J. Immunol.*, **164**, 5362–5368.

281. Steinhauser, M. L., Hogaboam, C. M., Matsukawa, A., et al. (2000) Chemokine C10 promotes disease resolution and survival in an experimental model of bacterial sepsis, *Infect. Immun.*, **68**, 6108–6114.

282. Ganz, T. and Lehrer, R. I. (2003) Antimicrobial peptides. In: *Innate Immunity* (Ezekowitz, R. A. B. and Hoffmann, J. A., eds.), Humana Press, Totowa, NJ, pp. 287–303.

283. Sablon, E., Contreras, B., and Vandamme, E. (2000) Antimicrobial peptides of lactic acid bacteria: mode of action, genetics and biosynthesis, *Adv. Biochem. Eng. Biotechnol.*, **68**, 21–60.

284. Haseltine, C., Hill, T., Montalvo-Rodriguez, R., et al. (2001) Secreted euryarchaeal microhalocins kill hyperthermophillic crenarchaea, *J. Bacteriol.*, **183**, 287–291.

285. Hancock, R. E. and Bell, A. (1988) Antibiotic uptake into gram-negative bacteria, *Eur. J. Clin. Microbiol. Infect. Dis.*, **7**, 713–720.

286. Shai, Y. (1999) Mechanism of the binding, insertion and destabilization of phospholipid bilayer membranes by alpha-helical antimicrobial and cell non-selective membrane-lytic membranes, *Biochim. Biophys. Acta*, **1462**, 55–70.

287. Ludtke, S. J., He, K., Heller, W. T., et al. (1996) Membrane pores induced by magainin, *Biochemistry*, **35**, 13723–13728.

288. Higashimoto, Y., Kodama, H., Jelokhani-Niaraki, M., Kato, F., and Kondo, M. (1999) Structure-function relationship of model Aib-containing peptides as ion transfer intermembrane templates, *J. Biochem. (Tokyo)*, **125**, 705–712.

289. Hara, T., Kodama, H., Kondo, M., et al. (2001) Effects of peptide dimerization on pore formation: antiparallel disulfide-dimerized magainin 2 analogue, *Biopolymers*, **58**, 437–446.

290. Kobayashi, S., Takeshima, K., Park, C. B., Kim, S. C., and Matsuzaki, K. (2000) Interactions of the novel antimicrobial peptide buforin 2 with lipid bilayers: praline as a translocation promoting factor, *Biochemistry*, **39**, 8648–8654.

291. Ganz, T. and Lehrer, R. I. (1995) Defensins, *Pharmacol. Ther.*, **66**, 191–205.

292. Lehrer, R. I., Lichtenstein, A. K., and Ganz, T. (1993) Defensins: antimicrobial and cytotoxic peptides of mammalian cells, *Annu. Rev. Immunol.*, **11**, 105–128.

293. Tang, Y. Q., Yuan, J., Osapay, G., et al. (1999) A cyclic antimicrobial peptide produced in primate leukocytes by the ligation of two truncated alpha-defensins, *Science*, **286**, 498–502.

294. Hoover, D. M., Rajashankar, K. R., Blumenthal, R., et al. (2000) The structure of human beta-defensin-2 shows evidence of higher-order oligomerization, *J. Biol. Chem.*, **275**, 32911–32918.

295. Pardi, A., Zhang, X. L., Selsted, M. E., Skalicky, J. J., and Yip, P. F. (1992) NMR studies of defensin antimicrobial peptides. 2. Three-dimmensional structures of rabbit NP-2 and human HNP-1, *Biochemistry*, **31**, 11357–11364.

296. Skalicky, J. J., Selsted, M. E., and Pardi, A. (1994) Structure and dynamics of neutrophil defensins NP-2, NP-5, and HNP-1: NMR studies of amide hydrogen exchange kinetics, *Proteins*, **20**, 52–67.

297. Zimmermann, G. R., Legault, P., Selsted, M. E., and Pardi, A. (1995) Solution structure of bovine neutrophil beta-defensin-12: the peptide fold of the beta-defensins is identical to that of the classical defensins, *Biochemistry*, **34**, 13663–13671.

298. Sawai, M. V., Jia, H. P., Liu, L., et al. (2001) The NMR structure of human beta-defensin-2 reveals a novel alpha-helical segment, *Biochemistry*, **40**, 3810–3816.

299. Ganz, T., Selsted, M. E., Szklarek, D., et al. (1985) Defensins. Natural peptide antibiotics of human neutrophils, *J. Clin. Invest.*, **76**, 1427–1435.

300. Selsted, M. E., Harwig, S. S., Ganz, T., Schilling, J. W., and Lehrer, R. I. (1985) Primary structures of three human neutrophil defensins, *J. Clin. Invest.*, **76**, 1436–1439.

301. Gabay, J. E., Scott, R. W., Campanelli, D., et al. (1989) Antibiotic proteins of human polymorphonuclear leukocytes, *Proc. Natl. Acad. Sci. U.S.A.*, **86**, 5610–5614.

302. Joiner, K. A., Ganz, T., Albert, J., and Rotrosen, D. (1989) The opsonizing ligand on *Salmonella typhimurium* influences incorporation of specific, but not azurophil, granule constituents into neutrophil phagosomes, *J. Cell. Biol.*, **109**, 2771–2782.

303. Porter, E. M., Liu, L., Oren, A., Anton, P. A., and Ganz, T. (1997) Localization of human intestinal defensin 5 in Paneth cell granules, *Infect. Immun.*, **65**, 2389–2395.

304. Bensch, K. W., Raida, M., Magert, H. J., Schulz-Knappe, P., and Forssmann, W. G. (1995) hBD-1: a novel beta-defensin from human plasma, *FEBS Lett.*, **368**, 331–335.

305. Zhao, C. Q., Wang, I., and Lehrer, R. I. (1996) Widespread expression of beta- defensin HBD-1 in human secretory glands and epithelial cells, *FEBS Lett.*, **396**, 319–322.

306. Harder, J., Bartels, J., Christophers, E., and Schröder, J. M. (1997) A peptide antibiotic from human skin, *Nature*, **387**, 861–862.

307. Harder, J., Bartels, J., Christophers, E., and Schröder, J. M. (2001) Isolation and characterization of human beta-defensin-3, a novel human inducible peptide antibiotic, *J. Biol. Chem.*, **276**, 5707–5713.

308. Diamond, G., Russell, J. P., and Bevins, C. L. (1996) Inducible expression of an antibiotic peptide gene in lipopolysaccharide-challenged tracheal epithelia cells, *Proc. Natl. Acad. Sci., U.S.A.*, **93**, 5156–5160.

309. Schonwetter, B. S., Stolzenberg, E. D., and Zasloff, M. A. (1995) Epithelial antibiotics induced at sites of inflammation, *Science*, **267**, 1645–1648.

310. Diamond, G., Zasloff, M., Eck, H., et al. (1991) Tracheal antimicrobial peptide: a cystein-rich peptide from mammalian tracheal mucosa: peptide isolation and cloning of a cDNA, *Proc. Natl. Acad. Sci. U.S.A.*, **88**, 3852–3956.

311. Lehrer, R. I., Barton, A., Daher, K. A., Harwig, S. S., Ganz, T., and Selsted, M. E. (1989) Interaction of human defensins with *Escherichia coli.* Mechanism of bacterial activity, *J. Clin. Invest.*, **84**, 553–561.

312. Lehrer, R. I., Szklarek, D., Ganz, T., and Selsted, M. E. (1985) Correlation of binding of rabbit granulocyte peptides to *Candida albicans* with candidacidal activity, *Infect. Immun.*, **49**, 207–211.

313. Lehrer, R. I., Barton, A., and Ganz, T. (1988) Concurrent assessment of inner and outer membrane permeability and bacteriolysis in *E. coli* by multiple-wavelength spectrophotometry, *J. Immunol. Methods*, **108**, 153–158.

314. Lichtenstein, A. K., Ganz, T., Nguyen, T. M., Selsted, M. E., and Lehrer, R. I. (1988) Mechanism of target cytolysis by peptide defensins. Target cell metabolic activities, possibly involving endocytosis, are crucial for expression of cytotoxicity, *J. Immunol.*, **140**, 2686–2694.

315. Lichtenstein, A., Ganz, T., Selsted, M. E., and Lehrer, R. I. (1986) In vitro tumor cell cytolysis mediated by peptide defensins of human and rabbit granulocytes, *Blood*, **68**, 1407–1410.

316. Wimley, W. C., Selsted, M. E., and White, S. H. (1994) Interactions between human defensins and lipid bilayers: evidence for formation of multimeric pores, *Protein Sci.*, **3**, 1362–1373.

317. White, S. H., Wimley, W. C., and Selsted, M. E. (1995) Structure, function, and membrane integration of defensins, *Curr. Opin. Struct. Biol.*, **5**, 521–527.

318. Fujii, G., Selsted, M. E., and Eisenberg, D. (1993) Defensins promote fusion and lysis of negatively charged membranes, *Protein Sci.*, **2**, 1301–1312.

319. Kagan, B. L., Selsted, M. E., Ganz, T., and Lehrer, R. I. (1990) Antimicrobial defensin peptides form voltage-dependent ion-permeable channels in planar lipid bilayer membranes, *Proc. Natl. Acad. Sci. U.S.A.*, **87**, 210–214.

320. Ganz, T., Metcalf, J. A., Gallin, J. I., Boxer, L. A., and Lehrer, R. I. (1988) Microbicidal/cytotoxic proteins of neutrophils are deficient in two disorders: Chediak-Higashi syndrome and "specific" granule deficiency, *J. Clin. Invest.*, **82**, 552–556.

321. Gallin, J. I., Fletcher, M. P., Seligmann, B. E., et al. (1982) Human neutrophil- specific granule deficiency: a model to assess the role of neutrophil-specific granules in the evolution of the inflammatory response, *Blood*, **59**, 1317–1329.

322. Gombart, A. F., Shiohara, M., Kwok, S. H., et al. (2001) Neutrophil-specific granule deficiency: homozygous recessive inheritance of a frameshift mutation in the gene encoding transcription factor CCAAT/enhancer binding protein-epsilon, *Blood*, **97**, 2561–2567.

323. Turner, J., Cho, Y., Dinh, N. N., Waring, A. J., and Lehrer, R. I. (1998) Activities of LL-37, a cathelin-associated antimicrobial peptide of human neutrophils, *Antimicrob. Agents Chemother.*, **42**, 2206–2214.

324. Zanetti, M., Gennaro, R., and Romeo, D. (1995) Cathelicidins: a novel protein family with a common proregion and a variable C-terminal antimicrobial domain, *FEBS Lett.*, **374**, 1–5.

325. Panyutich, A., Shi, J., Boutz, P. L., Zhao, C., and Ganz, T. (1997) Porcine polymorphonuclear leukocytes generate extra-cellular microbicidal activity by elastase-mediated activation of secreted proprotegrins, *Infect. Immun.*, **65**, 978–985.

326. Scocchi, M., Skerlavaj, B., Romeo, D., and Gennaro, R. (1992) Proteolytic cleavage by neutrophil elastase converts inactive storage proforms to antibacterial bactenecins, *Eur. J. Biochem.*, **209**, 589–595.

327. Zanetti, M., Litteri, L., Griffiths, G., Gennaro, R., and Romeo, D. (1991) Stimulus- induced maturation of probactenecins, precursors of neutrophil antimicrobial polypeptides, *J. Immunol.*, **146**, 4295–4300.

328. Levy, O., Weiss, J., Zarember, K., Ooi, C. E., and Elsbach, P. (1993) Antibacterial 15-kDa protein isoforms (p15s) are members of a novel family of leukocyte proteins, *J. Biol. Chem.*, **268**, 6058–6063.

329. Zarember, K., Elsbach, P., Shin-Kim, K., and Weiss, J. (1997) p15s (15-kD antimicrobial proteins) are stored in the secondary granules of rabbit granulocytes: implications for antibacterial synergy with the bactericidal/permeability-increasing protein in inflammatory fluids, *Blood*, **89**, 672–679.

330. Gudmundsson, G. H., Agerberth, B., Odeberg, J., et al. (1996) The human gene FALL39 and processing of the cathelin precursor to the antibacterial peptide LL-37 in granulocytes, *Eur. J. Biochem.*, **238**, 325–332.

331. Sorenson, O. E., Follin, P., Johnsen, A. H., et al. (2001) Human cathelicidin, hCAP-18, is processed to the antimicrobial peptide LL-37 by extracellular cleavage with proteinase 3, *Blood*, **97**, 3951–3959.

332. Oren, Z., Lerman, J. C., Gudmunsson, G. H., Agerberth, B., and Shai, Y. (1999) Structure and organization of the human antibacterial peptide LL-37 in phospholipid membranes: relevance to the molecular basis for its non-cell-selective activity, *Biochem. J.*, **341**, 501–513.

333. De, Y., Chen, Q., Schmidt, A. P., et al. (2000) LL-37, the neutrophil granule- and epithelial cell-derived cathelicidin, utilizes formyl peptide receptor-like 1 (FPRL 1) as a receptor to chemoattract human peripheral blood neutrophils, monocytes, and T-cells, *J. Exp. Med.*, **192**, 1069–1074.

334. Frohm, N. M., Sandstedt, B., Sorensen, O., et al. (1999) The human cationic antimicrobial protein (hCAP18), a peptide antibiotic, is widely expressed in human squamous epthelia and colocalizes with interleukin-6, *Infect. Immun.*, **67**, 2561–2566.

335. Bals, R., Wang, X., Zasloff, M., and Wilson, J. M. (1998) The peptide antibiotic LL-37/hCAP-18 is express in epithelia of the human lung where it has broad antimicrobial activity at the airway surface, *Proc. Natl. Acad. Sci. U.S.A.*, **95**, 9541–9546.

336. Malm, J., Sorensen, O., Persson, T., et al. (2000) The human cationic antimicrobial protein (hCAP-18) is expressed in the epithelium of human epididymis, is present in seminal plasma at high concentrations, and is attached to spermatozoa, *Infect. Immun.*, **68**, 4297–4302.

337. Islam, D., Bandholtz, L., Nilsson, J., et al. (2001) Downregulation of bacterial peptides in enteric infections: a novel immune escape mechanism with bacterial DNA as a potential regulator, *Nat. Med.*, **7**, 180–185.

338. Bals, R., Weiner, D. J., Meegalla, R. L., and Wilson, J. M. (1999) Transfer of cathelicidin peptide antibiotic gene restores bacterial killing in a cystic fibrosis xenograft model, *J. Clin. Invest.*, **103**, 1113–1117.

339. Bals, R., Weiner, D. J., Moscioni, A. D., Meegalla, R. L., and Wilson, J. M. (1999) Augmentation of innate host defense by expression of a cathelicidin antimicrobial peptide, *Infect. Immun.*, **67**, 6084–6089.

340. Underhill, D. M. (2003) Innate immune signaling during phagocytosis. In: *Innate Immunity* (Ezekowitz, R. A. B. and Hoffmann, J. A., eds.), Humana Press, Totowa, NJ, pp. 341–359.

341. Aderem, A. and Underhill, D. M. (1999) Mechanisms of phagocytosis in macrophages, *Annu. Rev. Immunol.*, **17**, 593–623.

342. Ernest, J. D. (2000) Bacterial inhibition of phagocytosis, *Cell. Microbiol.*, **2**, 279–386.

343. Greenberg, S. (1999) Modular components of phagocytosis, *J. Leukoc. Biol.*, **66**, 712–717.

344. Revetch, J. V. and Clynes, R. A. (1998) Divergent roles for Fc receptors and complement in vivo, *Annu. Rev. Immunol.*, **16**, 421–432.

345. Daeron, M. (1997) Fc receptor biology, *Annu. Rev. Immunol.*, **15**, 203–234.

346. Ross, G. D. (2000) Regulation of adhesion versus cytotoxic functions of the Mac- 1/CR3/alphaM-beta-2-integrin glycoprotein, *Crit. Rev. Immunol.*, **20**, 197–222.

347. Blystone, S. D. and Brown, E. J. (1999) Integrin receptors of phagocytes. In *Phagocytosis: The Host* (Gordon, S., ed.), JAI Press, Stamford, CT, pp. 102–147.

348. Dib, K. (2000) BETA 2 integrin signaling in leukocyes, *Front. Biosci.*, **5**, D438–D451.

349. Berger, M., O'Shea, J., Cross, A. S., et al. (1984) Human neutrophils increase expression of C3bi as well as C3b receptors upon activation, *J. Clin. Invest.*, **74**, 1566–1571.

350. Sengelov, H., Kjeldsen, L., Diamond, M. S., Springer, T. A., and Borregaard, N. (1993) Subcellular localization and dynamics of Mac-1 (alpha m beta 2) in human neutrophils, *J. Clin. Invest.*, **92**, 1467–1476.

351. Jones, S. L., Knaus, U. G., Bokoch, G. M., and Brown, E. J. (1998) Two signaling mechanisms for activation of alphaM beta2 avidity in polymorphonuclear neutrophils, *J. Biol. Chem.*, **273**, 10556–10566.

352. Wroght, S. D. and Griffin, F. M., Jr. (1985) Activation of phagocytic cells' C3 receptors for phagocytosis, *J. Leukoc. Biol.*, **38**, 327–339.

353. Wright, S. D., Craigmyle, L. S., and Silverstein, S. C. (1983) Fibronectin and serum amyloid P component stimulate C3b- and C3bi-mediated phagocytosis in cultured human monocytes, *J. Exp. Biol.*, **158**, 1338–1343.

354. Pommier, C. G., Inada, S., Fries, L. F., et al. (1983) Plasma fibronectin enhances phagocytosis of opsonized particles by human peripheral blood monocytes, *J. Exp. Med.*, **157**, 1844–1854.

355. Di Carlo, F. J. and Fiore, J. V. (1958) On the composition of zymosan, *Science*, **127**, 756–757.

356. Lipke, P. N. and Ovalle, R. (1998) Cell wall architecture in yeast: new structure and new challenges, *J. Bacteriol.*, **180**, 3735–3740.

357. Sung, S. S., Nelson, R. S., and Silverstein, S. C. (1983) Yeast mannans inhibit binding and phagocytosis of zymosan by mouse peritoneal macrophages, *J. Cell. Biol.*, **96**, 160–166.

358. Goldman, R. (1988) Characteristics of the beta-glucan receptor of murine macrophages, *Exp. Cell. Res.*, **174**, 481–490.

359. Janusz, M. J., Austen, K. F., and Czop, J. K. (1986) Isolation of soluble yeast beta-glucans that inhibit human monocyte phagocytosis mediated by beta-glucan receptors, *J. Immunol.*, **137**, 3270–3276.

360. Giaimis, J., Lombard, Y., Fonteneau, P., et al. (1993) Both mannose and beta- glucan receptors are involved in the phagocytosis of unopsonized, heat-killed *Saccharomyces cerevisiae* by murine macrophages, *J. Leukoc. Biol.*, **54**, 564–571.

361. Platt, N., Haworth, R., da Silva, R. P., and Goedon, S. (1999) Scavenger receptors and phagocytosis of bacteria and apoptotic cells. In: *Phagocytosis: The Host* (Gordon, S., ed.), JAI Press, Stamford, CT, pp. 71–85.

362. Peiser, L., Gough, P. J., Kodama, T., and Goedon, S. (2000) Macrophage class A scavenger receptor-mediated phagocytosis of Escherichia coli: role of the cell heterogeneity, microbial strain, and culture conditions in vitro, *Infect. Immun.*, **68**, 1953–1963.

363. Thomas, C. A., Li, Y., Kodama, T., et al. (2000) Protection from lethal gram- positive infection by macrophage scavenger receptor-dependent phagocytosis, *J. Exp. Med.*, **191**, 147–156.

364. Elomaa, O., Kangas, M., Sahlberg, C., et al. (1995) Cloning of a novel bacteria- binding receptor structurally related to scavenger receptors and expressed in a subset of macrophages, *Cell*, **80**, 603–609.

365. van der Laan, L. J., Dopp, E. A., and Haworth, R., et al. (1999) Regulation and functional involvement of macrophage scavenger receptor MARCO in clearance of bacteria in vivo, *J. Immunol.*, **162**, 939–947.

366. Placecanda, A., Paulauskis, J., Al-Mutairi, E., et al. (1999) Role of the scavenger receptor MARCO in alveolar macrophage binding of unopsonized environmental particles, *J. Exp. Med.*, **189**, 1497–1506.

367. Albert, M. L., Pearce, S. F., Francisco, L. M., et al. (1998) Immature dendritic cells phagocytose apoptotic cells via $\alpha_v\beta_5$ and CD36, and cross-present antigens to cytotoxic T lymphocytes, *J. Exp. Med.*, **188**, 1359–1368.

368. Fadok, V. A., Warner, M. L., Bratton, D. L., and Henson, P. M. (1998) CD36 is required for phagocytosis of apoptotic cells by human macrophages that use either a phosphatidylserine receptor or the vitronectin receptor $\alpha_v\beta_5$, *J. Immunol.*, **161**, 6250–6257.

369. Franc, N. C., Heitzler, P., Ezekowitz, R. A., and White, K. (1999) Requirement for croquemort in phagocytosis of apoptotic cells in *Drosophila*, *Science*, **284**, 1991–1994.

370. Allen, L. A. and Aderem, A. (1996) Molecular definition of distinct cytoskeletal structures involved in complement- and Fc receptor-mediated phagocytosis in macrophages, *J. Exp. Med.*, **184**, 627–637.

371. Allen, L. A. and Aderem, A. (1996) Mechanisms of phagocytosis, *Curr. Opin. Immunol.*, **8**, 36–40.

372. Crowley, M. T., Costello, P. S., Fitzer-Attas, C. J., et al. (1997) A critical role for Syk in signal transduction and phagocytosis mediated by Fcgamma receptors on macrophages, *J. Exp. Med.*, **186**, 1027–1039.

373. Kusner, D. J., Hall, C. F., and Schlesinger, L. S. (1996) Activation of phospholipase D is tightly coupled to the phagocytosis of *Mycobacterium tuberculosis* or opsonized zymosan by human macrophages, *J. Exp. Med.*, **184**, 585–595.

374. Lin, T. H., Aplin, A. E., Shen, Y., Chen, Q., et al. (1997) Integrin-mediated activation of MAP kinase is independent of FAK: evidence for dual integrin signaling pathways in fibroblasts, *J. Cell Biol.*, **136**(6), 1385–1995.

375. Ip, Y. T. and Davis, R. J. (1998) Signal transduction by the c-Jun N-terminal kinase (JNK) – from inflammation to development, *Curr. Opin. Cell. Biol.*, **10**, 205–219.

376. Allen, L. H. and Aderem, A. (1995) A role for MARCKS, the alpha isozyme of protein kinase C and myosin I in zymosan phagocytosis by macrophages, *J. Exp. Med.*, **182**, 829–840.

377. Melendez, A. J., Harnett, M. M., and Allen, J. M. (1999) Differentiation-dependent switch in protein kinase C isoenzyme activation by FcgammaRI, the human high- affinity receptor for immunoglobulin G, *Immunology*, **96**, 457–464.

378. Zheng, L., Zomerdijk, T. P., Aarnoudse, C., van Furth, R., and Nibbering, P. H. (1995) Role of protein kinase C isozymes in Fc gamma receptor-mediated intracellular killing of *Staphylococcus aureus* by human monocytes, *J. Immunol.*, **155**, 776–784.

379. Zheleznyak, A. and Brown, E. J. (1992) Immunoglobulin-mediated phagocytosis by human monocytes requires protein kinase C activation. Evidence for protein kinase C translocation to phagosomes, *J. Biol. Chem.*, **267**, 12042–12048.

380. Aderem, A. (1992) The MARCKS brothers: a family of protein kinase C substrates, *Cell*, **71**, 713–716.

381. Shapira, L., Takashiba, S., Champagne, C., Amar, S., and van Dyke, T. E. (1992) Involvement of protein kinase C and protein tyrosine kinase in lipopolysaccharide-induced TNF-alpha and IL-1 beta production by human monocytes, *J. Immunol.*, **153**, 1818–1824.

382. Kovacs, E. J., Radzioch, D., Young, H. A., and Varesio, L. (1988) Differential inhibition of IL-1 and TNF-alpha mRNA expression by agents which block second messenger pathways in murine macrophages, *J. Immunol.*, **141**, 3101–3105.

383. Huwiler, A. and Pfeilschifter, J. (1993) A role for protein kinase X-alpha in zymosan-stimulated eicosanoid synthesis in mouse peritoneal macrophages, *Eur. J. Biochem.*, **217**, 69–75.

384. Giroux, M. and Descoteaux, A. (2000) Cyclooxygenase-2 expression in macrophages: modulation by protein kinase C-alpha, *J. Immunol.*, **165**, 3985–3991.

385. St-Denis, A., Chano, F., Tremblay, P., St-Pierre, Y., and Descoteaux, A. (1998) Protein kinase C-alpha modulates lipopolysaccharide-induced functions in a murine macrophage cell line, *J. Biol. Chem.*, **273**, 32787–32792.

386. St-Denis, A., Caouras, V., Gervais, F., and Descoteaux, A. (1999) Role of protein kinase C-alpha in the control of infection by intracellular pathogens in macrophages, *J. Immunol.*, **163**, 5505–5511.

387. Larsen, E. C., DiGennaro, J. A., Saito, N., et al. (2000) Differential requirement for classic and novel PKC isoforms in respiratory burst and phagocytosis in RAW 264.7 cells, *J. Immunol.*, **165**, 2809–2817.

388. Botelho, R. J., Teruel, M., Dierckman, R., et al. (2000) Localized biphasic changes in phosphatidylinositol-4,5-biphosphate at sites of phagocytosis, *J. Cell. Biol.*, **151**, 1353–1368.

389. Chan, T. O., Rittenhouse, S. E., and Tsichlis, P. N. (1999) AKT/PKB and other D3 phosphoinositide-regulated kinases: kinase activation by phosphoinositide-dependent phosphorylation, *Annu. Rev. Biochem.*, **68**, 965–1014.

390. Lennartz, M. R. (1999) Phospholipases and phagocytosis: the role of phospholipid- derived second messengers in phagocytosis, *Int. J. Biochem. Cell. Biol.*, **31**, 415–430.

391. Celli, J., Oliver, M., and Finlay, B. B. (2001) Enteropathogenic Escherichia coli mediates antiphagocytosis through the inhibition of PI 3-kinase-dependent pathways, *EMBO J.*, **20**, 1245–1258.

392. Araki, N., Johnson, M. T., and Swanson, J. A. (1996) A role for phosphoinositide 3- kinase in the completion of macropinocytosis and phagocytosis by macrophages, *J. Cell. Biol.*, **135**, 1249–1260.

393. Gold, E. S., Underhill, D. M., Morrissette, N. S., et al. (1999) Dynamin 2 is required for phagocytosis in macrophages, *J. Exp. Med.*, **190**, 1849–1856.

394. Arbibe, L., Mira, J. P., Teusch, N., et al. (2000) Toll-like receptor 2-mediated NF- kappa B activation requires a Rac 1-dependent pathway, *Nat. Immun.*, **1**, 533–540.

395. Chimini, G. and Chavrier, P. (2000) Function of Rho family proteins in actin dynamics during phagocytosis and engulfment, *Nat. Cell. Biol.*, **2**, E191–E196.

396. Schmitz, A. A., Govek, E. E., Bottner, B., and van Aelst, L. (2000) Rho GTPases: signaling, migration, and invasion, *Exp. Cell. Res.*, **261**, 1–12.

397. Caron, E. and Hall, A. (1998) Identification of two distinct mechanisms of phagocytosis controlled by different Rho GTPases, *Science*, **282**, 1717–1721.

398. Massol, P., Montcourrier, P., Guillemot, J. C., and Chavrier, P. (1998) Fc receptor- mediated phagocytosis requires CDC42 and Rac1, *EMBO J.*, **17**, 6219–6229.

399. Guillen, N., Boquet, P., and Sansonetti, P. (1998) The small GTP-binding protein RacG regulates uroid formation in the protozoan parasite *Entamoeba histolytica*, *J. Cell. Biol.*, **111**, 1729–1739.

400. Cox, D., Chang, P., Zhang, Q., et al. (1997) Requirements for both Rac1 and Cdc42 in membrane ruffing and phagocytosis in leukocytes, *J. Exp. Med.*, **186**, 1487–1494.

401. Von Pawel-Rammingen, U., Telepnev, M.V., Schmidt, G., et al. (2000) GAP activity of the *Yersinia* YopE cytotoxin specifically targets the Rho pathway: a mechanism for disruption of actin microfilament structure, *Mol. Microbiol.*, **36**, 737–748.

402. Goehring, U. M., Schmidt, G., Pederson, K. J., Aktories, K., and Barbieri, J. T. (1999) The N-terminal domain of *Pseudomonas aeruginosa* exoenzyme S is a GTPase-activating protein for Rho GTPases, *J. Biol. Chem.*, **274**, 36369–36372.

403. Leusen, J. H. W., Verhoeven, A. J., and Roos, D. (1996) Interactions between the components of the human NADPH oxidase: a review about the intrigues in the phox family, *Front. Biosci.*, **1**, 72–90.

404. DeLeo, F. R., Allen, L. A., Apicella, M., and Nauseef, W. M. (1999) NADPH oxidase activation and assembly during phagocytosis, *J. Immunol.*, **163**, 6732–6740.

405. Segal, A. W., Wientjes, F., Stockely, R. W., and Dekker, L. V. (1999) Components and organization of the NADPH oxidase of phagocytic cells. In: *Phagocytosis: The Host* (Gordon, S., ed.), JAI Press, Stamford, CT, pp. 441–483.

406. Wright, S. D. and Silverstein, S. C. (1983) Receptors for C3b and C3bi promote phagocytosis but not the release of toxic oxygen from human phagocytes, *J. Exp. Med.*, **158**, 2016–2023.

407. Yamamoto, K. and Johnston, R. B., Jr. (1984) Dissociation of phagocytosis from stimulation of the oxidative metabolic burst in macrophages, *J. Exp. Med.*, **159**, 405–416.

408. Berton, G. and Gordon, S. (1983) Modulation of macrophage mannosyl-specific receptors by cultivation on immobilized zymosan. Effects on superoxide-anion release and phagocytosis, *Immunology*, **49**, 705–715.

409. Berton, G., Laudanna, C., Sorio, C., and Rossi, F. (1992) Generation of signals activating neutrophil functions by leukocyte integrins: LFA-1 and gp150/95, but not CR3, are able to stimulate the respiratory burst of human neutrophils, *J. Cell. Biol.*, **116**, 1007–1017.

410. Laudanna, C., Melotti, P., Bonizatto, C., et al. (1993) Ligation of members of the beta 1 or the beta 2 subfamilies of integrins by antibodies triggers eosinophil respiratory burst and spreading, *Immunology*, **80**, 273–280.

411. Ozinsky, A., Underhill, D. M., Fontenot, J. D., et al. (2000) The repertoire for pattern recognition of pathogens by the innate immune system is defined by cooperation between Toll-like receptors, *Proc. Natl. Acad. Sci. U.S.A.*, **97**, 13766–13771.

412. Underhill, D. M., Ozinsky, A., Hajjar, A. M., et al. (1999) The Toll-like receptor 2 is recruited to macrophage phagosomes and discriminates between pathogens, *Nature*, **401**, 811–815.

413. Boyce, J. A. and Austen, K. F. (2003) The role of mast cells in innate immunity. In: *Innate Immunity* (Ezekowitz, R. A. B. and Hoffmann, J. A., eds.), Humana Press, Totowa, NJ, pp. 361–385.

414. McNeil, H. P. and Austen, K. F. (1995) Biology of the mast cell. In: *Sampter's Immunologic Diseases*, 5th ed. (Frank, M. M., Austen, K. F., Claman, H. N., et al., eds.), Williams & Wilkins, Baltimore, MD, pp. 185–204.

415. Guy-Grant, D., Dy, M., Luffau, G., et al. (1984) Gut mucosal mast cells: origin, traffic and differentiaton, *J. Exp. Med.*, **160**, 12–28.

416. Gurish, M. F., Tao, H., Abonia, J. P., et al. 2001) Intestinal mast cell progenitor require CD49dβ7 (α4β7) for tissue-specific homing, *J. Exp. Med.*, **194**, 1243–1252.

417. Rosenkranz, A. R., Coxon, A., Maurer, M., et al. (1998) Impaired mast cell development and innate immunity in Mac-1 (CD11b/CD18, CR3)-deficient mice, *J. Immunol.*, **168**, 6463–6467.

418. Tachimoto, H., Hudson, S. A., and Bochner, B. S. (2001) Acquisition and alteration of adhesion molecules during cultured human mast cell differentiation, *J. Allergy Clin. Immunol.*, **107**, 10–16.

419. Nilsson, G., Butterfield, J. H., Nilsson, K., and Siegbahn, A. (1994) Stem cell factor is a chemotactic factor for human mast cells, *J. Immunol.*, **153**, 3717–3723.

420. Meininger, C. J., Yano, H., Rottapel, R., et al. (1992) The c-kit receptor ligand functions as a mast cell chemoattractant, *Blood*, **79**, 958–963.

421. Schwartz, L. B., Irani, A. M., Roller, K., et al. (1987) Quantitation of histamine, tryptase, and chymase in human T and TC mast cells, *J. Immunol.*, **138**, 2611–2615.

422. Benditt, E. P., Arase, M., and Roeper, M. E. (1956) Histamine and heparine in isolated rat mast cells, *J. Histochem. Cytochem.*, **4**, 419.

423. Leino, L. and Lilius, E.-M. (1990) Histamine receptors on leukocytes are expressed differently in vitro and ex vivo, *Int. Arch. Allergy Appl. Immunol.*, **91**, 30–35.

424. Falus, A. and Meretey, K. (1992) Histamine: an early messenger in inflammatory and immune reactions, *Immunol. Today*, **13**, 154–156.

425. Schwartz, L. B., Lewis, R. A., and Austen, K. F. (1981) Tryptase from human pulmonary mast cells. Purification and characterization, *J. Biol. Chem.*, **256**, 11939–11943.

426. Schechter, N. M., Choi, J. K., Slavin, D. A., et al. (1986) Identification of a chymotrypsin-like proteinase in human mast cells, *J. Immunol.*, **137**, 962–970.

427. Pallaoro, M., Fejzo, M. S., Shayesteh, L., et al. (1999) Characterization of genes encoding known and novel human mast cell tryptases on chromosome 16p13.3, *J. Biol. Chem.*, **274**(6), 3355–3362.

428. Schchter, N. M., Irani, A. M., Sprows, J. L., et al. (1990) Identification of cathepsin G-like proteinase in the MCTC type of human mast cell, *J. Immunol.*, **145**, 2652–2661.

429. Reynolds, D. S., Stevens, R. L., Gurley, D. S., et al. (1989) Isolation and molecular cloning of mast cell carboxypeptidase A: a novel member of the carboxypeptidase gene family, *J. Biol. Chem.*, **264**, 20094–20099.

430. Irani, A. M., Goldstein, S. M., Wintroub, B. U., et al. (1991) Human mast cell carboxypeptidase. Selective localization to MCTC cells, *J. Immunol.*, **147**, 247–253.

431. Irani, A. A., Schechter, N. M., Craig, S. S., et al. (1986) Two types of human mast cells that have distinct neutral protease compositions, *Proc. Natl. Acad. Sci. U.S.A.*, **83**, 4464–4468.

432. Irani, A. M., Craig, S., DeBlois, G., et al. (1987) Deficiency of the tryptase-positive, chymase-negative mast cell type in gastroin-

testinal mucosa of patients with defective T lymphocyte function, *J. Immunol.*, **138**, 4381–4386.

433. Chandrasekharan, U. M., Sanker, S., Glynias, M. J., et al. (1996) Angiotensin II- forming activity in a reconstructed ancestral chymase, *Science*, **271**, 502–505.

434. Sanker, S., Chandrasekharan, U. M., Wilk, D., et al. (1997) Distinct multisite synergistic interactions determine substrate specificities of human chymase and rat chymase-1 for angiotensin II formation and degradation, *J. Biol. Chem.*, **272**, 2963–2968.

435. Coussens, L. M., Raymond, W. W., Bergers, G., et al. (1999) Inflammatory mast cells up-regulate angiogenesis during squamous epithelial carcinogenesis, *Genes Dev.*, **13**, 1382–1397.

436. Kofford, M. W., Schwartz, L. B., Schechter, N. M., et al. (1997) Cleavage of type I procollagen by human mast cell chymase initiates collagen fibril formation and generates a unique carboxyl-terminal propeptide, *J. Biol. Chem.*, **272**, 7127–7131.

437. Longley, B. J., Tyrrell, L., Ma, Y., et al. (1997) Chymase cleavage of stem cell factor yields a bioactive, soluble product, *Proc. Natl. Acad. Sci. U.S.A.*, **94**, 9017–9021.

438. Reynolds, D. S., Gurley, D. S., Stevens, R. L., et al. (1989) Cloning of cDNAs that encode human mast cell carboxypeptidase A, and comparison of the protein with mouse mast cell carboxypeptidase A and rat pancreatic carboxypeptidases, *Proc. Natl. Acad. Sci. U.S.A.*, **86**(23), 9480–9484.

439. Caughey, G. H. (1989) Roles of mast cell tryptase and chymase in airway function, *Am. J. Physiol.*, **257**, L39.

440. Humphries, D. E., Nicodemus, C. F., Schiller, V., et al. (1992) The human serglycin gene. Nucleotide sequence and methylation pattern in human promyelitic leukemia HL-60 cells and T-lymphoblast Molt-4 cells, *J. Biol. Chem.*, **267**, 13558–13563.

441. Avraham, S., Stevens, R. L., Gartner, M. C., et al. (1988) Isolation of a cDNA that encodes the peptide core of the secretory proteoglycan of rat basophilic leukemia-1 cells and assessment of its homology to the human analogue, *J. Biol. Chem.*, **263**, 7292–7296.

442. Avraham, S., Stevens, R. L., Nicodemus, C. F., et al. (1989) Molecular cloning of a cDNA that encodes the peptide core of a mouse mast cell secretory granule proteoglycan and comparison with the analogous rat and human cDNA, *Proc. Natl. Acad. Sci. U.S.A.*, **86**, 3763–3767.

443. Metcalfe, D. D., Soter, N. A., Wasserman, S. I., et al. (1980) Identification of sulfated mucopolysaccharides including heparin in the lesional skin of a patient with systemic mastocytosis, *J. Invest. Dermatol.*, **74**, 210–215.

444. Metcalfe, D. D., Lewis, R. A., Silbert, J. E., et al. (1979) Isolation and characterization of heparin from human lung, *J. Clin. Invest.*, **64**, 1537–1543.

445. Stevens, R. L., Fox, C. C., Lichtenstein, L. M., et al. (1988) Identification of chondroitin sulfate E proteoglycans in the secretory granules of human lung mast cells, *Proc. Natl. Acad. Sci. U.S.A.*, **85**, 2284–2287.

446. Eliakim, R., Gilead, L., Ligumsky, M., et al. (1986) Possible presence of E-mast cells in the human colon, *Proc. Natl. Acad. Sci. U.S.A.*, **83**, 461–464.

447. Schwartz, L. B., Riedel, C., Caufield, J. P., et al. (1981) Cell association of complexes of chymase, heparin proteoglycan, and protein after degranulation by rat mast cells, *J. Immunol.*, **126**, 2071–2078.

448. Schwartz, L. B., Riedel, C., Schratz, J. J., et al. (1982) Localization of carboxypeptidase A to the macromolecular heparin proteoglycan-protein complex in secretory granules of rat serosal mast cells, *J. Immunol.*, **128**, 1128–1133.

449. Serafin, W. E., Katz, H. R., Austen, K. F., et al. (1986) Complexes of heparin proteoglycans, chondroitin sulfate E proteoglycans, and [^{3}H] diisopropyl fluorophosphates-binding proteins are exocytosed from activated mouse bone marrow-mast cells, *J. Biol. Chem.*, **261**, 15017–15021.

450. Goldstein, S. M., Leong, J., Schwartz, L. B., et al. (1992) Protease composition of exocytosed human skin mast cell protease-proteoglycan complexes, *J. Immunol.*, **148**, 2475–2482.

451. Paterson, N. A. M., Wasserman, S. I., Said, J. W., et al. (1976) Release of chemical mediators from partially purified human lung mast cells, *J. Immunol.*, **117**, 1356–1362.

452. Heavey, D. J., Ernst, P. B., Stevens, R. L., et al. (1988) Generation of leukotriene C4, leukotriene B4 and prostaglandin D2 by immunologically activated rat intestinal mucosal mast cells, *J. Immunol.*, **140**, 1953–1957.

453. Murakami, M., Austen, K. F., and Arm, J. P. (1995) The immediate phase of c-*kit* ligand stimulation of mouse bone marrow-derived mast cells elicits rapid leukotriene C_4 generation through posttranslational activation of cytosolic phospholipase A_2 and 5-lipoxygenase, *J. Exp. Med.*, **182**, 197–206.

454. Columbo, M., Horowitz, E. M., Botana, L. M., et al. (1992) The human recombinant c-kit receptor ligand, rhSCF, induces mediator release from human cutaneous mast cells and peripheral blood basophils, *J. Immunol.*, **149**, 599–608.

455. Clark, J. D., Lin, L.-L., Kriz, R. W., et al. (1991) A novel arachidonic acid-selective cytosolic PLA$_2$ contains a Ca_{2+}-dependent translocation domain with homology to PKC and GAP, *Cell*, **65**, 1043–1051.

456. Malavia, R., Malavia, R., and Jakschik, B. A. (1993) Reversible translocation of 5- lipoxygenase in mast cells upon IgE/antigen stimulation, *J. Biol. Chem.*, **268**, 4939–4944.

457. Dixon, R. A. F., Diehl, R. E., Opas, E., et al. (1990) Requirement of a 5- lipoxygenase-activating protein for leukotriene biosynthesis, *Nature*, **343**, 282–284.

458. Evans, J. F., Dupuis, P., and Ford-Hutchinson, A. W. (1985) Purification and characterization of leukotriene A$_4$ hydrolase from rat neutrophils, *Biochem. Biophys. Acta*, **840**, 43–50.

459. Lam, B. K., Penrose, J. F., Freeman, G. J., et al. (1994) Expression cloning of a cDNA for human leukotriene C$_4$ synthase, an integral membrane protein conjugating reduced glutathione to leukotriene A$_4$, *Proc. Natl. Acad. Sci. U.S.A.*, **91**, 7663–7667.

460. Lam, B. K., Gagnon, L., Austen, K. F. et al. (1990) The mechanism of leukotriene B$_4$ export from human polymorphonuclear leukocytes, *J. Biol. Chem.*, **265**, 13438–13441.

461. Lam, B. K., Xu, K., Atkins, M. B., et al. (1992) Leukotriene C$_4$ uses a probenicid-sensitive export carrier that does not recognize leukotriene B$_4$, *Proc. Natl. Acad. Sci. U.S.A.*, **89**, 11598–11602.

462. Lindbom, L., Hedqvist, P., Dahlen, S. E., et al. (1982) Leukotriene B$_4$ induces extravasation and migration of polymorphonuclear leukocytes in vivo, *Acta Physiol. Scand.*, **116**, 105–108.

463. Yokomizo, T., Izumi, T., Chang, K., Takuwa, Y., and Shimizu, T. (1997) A G- protein-coupled receptor for leukotriene B$_4$ that mediates chemotaxis, *Nature*, **387**, 620–624.

464. Yokomizu, T., Kato, K., Terawaki, K., Izumi, T., and Shimizu, T. (2000) A second leukotriene B(4) receptor, BLT2. A new therapeutic target in inflammation and immunological disorders, *J. Exp. Med.*, **192**, 421–432.

465. Raulf, M., Stuning, M., and Konig, W. (1985) Metabolism of leukotrienes by L- gamma-glutamyl-transpeptidase and dipeptidase from human polymorphonuclear granulocytes, *Immunology*, **55**, 135–147.

466. Davidson, A. B., Lee, T. H., Scanlon, P. D., et al. (1987) Bronchoconstrictor effects of leukotriene E$_4$ in normal and asthmatic subjects, *Am. Rev. Respir. Dis.*, **135**, 333–337.

467. Griffin, M., Weiss, J. W., Leitch, A. G., et al. (1983) Effect of leukotriene D$_4$ on the airways in asthma, *N. Engl. J. Med.*, **308**, 436–439.

468. Laitinen, L. A., Laitinen, A., Haahtela, T., et al. (1993) Leukotriene E$_4$ and granulocytic infiltration into asthmatic airways, *Lancet*, **341**, 989–990.

469. Lynch, K. R., O'Neill, G. P., Liu, Q., et al. (1999) Characterization of the human cysteinyl leukotriene CysLT1 receptor, *Nature*, **399**, 789–793.

470. Heise, C. E., O'Dowd, B. F., Figueroa, D. J., et al. (2000) Characterization of the human cysteinyl leukotriene 2 receptor, *J. Biol. Chem.*, **275**, 30531–30536.

471. Mellor, E. A., Maekawa, A., Austen, K. F., and Boyce, J. A. (2001) Cysteinyl leukotriene receptor 1 is also a pyrimidinergic receptor and is expressed by human mast cells, *Proc. Natl. Acad. Sci. U.S.A.*, **98**, 7964–7969.

472. Kanaoka, Y., Maekawa, A., Penrose, J. F., Austen, K. F., and Lam, B. K. (2001) Attenuated zymosan-induced peritoneal vascular permeability and IgE-dependent passive cutaneous anaphylaxis in mice lacking leukotriene C$_4$ synthase, *J. Biol. Chem.*, **276**, 22608–22613.

473. Murakami, M., Matsumoto, R., Urade, Y., et al. (1995) c-*kit* ligand mediates increased expression of cytosolic phospholipase A$_2$, prostaglandin endoperoxide synthase 1, and hematopoietic prostaglandin D$_2$ synthase and increased IgE- dependent PGD$_2$ generation in immature mouse mast cells, *J. Biol. Chem.*, **270**, 3239–3246.

474. Liu, M. C., Bleecker, E. R., Lichtenstein, L. M., et al. (1990) Evidence for elevated levels of histamine, prostaglandin D$_2$ and other bronchoconstricting prostaglandins in the airways of subjects with mild asthma, *Am. Rev. Respir. Dis.*, **142**, 126–132.

475. Roberts, L. J., II, Seibert, K., Liston, T. E., et al. (1987) PGD$_2$ is transformed by human coronary arteries to 9 alpha, 11 beta-PGF$_2$, which contracts human coronary artery rings, *Adv. Prostaglandin Thromboxane Leukotr. Res.*, **17A**, 427–429.

476. Hirai, H., Tanaka, K., Yoshie, O., et al. (2001) Prostaglandin D$_2$ selectively induces chemotaxis in T helper type 2 cells, eosinophils, and basophils via seven- transmembrane receptor CRTH2, *J. Exp. Med.*, **193**, 255–261.

477. Boie, Y., Sawyer, N., Slipetz, D. M., Metters, K. M., and Abramovitz, M. (1995) Molecular cloning and characterization of the human prostanoid DP receptor, *J. Biol. Chem.*, **270**, 18910–18916.

478. Gordon, J. R. and Galli, S. J. (1990) Mast cells as a source of both preformed and immunologically inducible TNF-α/cachectin, *Nature*, **346**, 274–276.

479. Subramanian, N. and Bray, M. A. (1987) Interleukin 1 releases histamine from human basophils and mast cells in vitro, *J. Immunol.*, **138**, 271–274.

480. Lu-Kuo, J. M., Austen, K. F., and Katz, H. R. (1996) Posttranscriptional stabilization by interleukin-1β of interleukin-6 mRNA induced by c-*kit* ligand and interleukin-10 in mouse bone marrow-derived mast cells, *J. Biol. Chem.*, **271**, 22169–22174.

481. Gagari, E., Tsai, M., Lantz, C. S., et al. (1997) Differential release of mast cell interleukin-6 via c-kit, *Blood*, **89**, 2654–2663.

482. Walsh, L. J., Trinchieri, G., Waldorf, H. A., et al. (1991) Human dermal mast cells contain and release tumor nectosis factor α, which induces endothelial leukocyte adhesion molecule 1, *Proc. Natl. Acad. Sci., U.S.A.*, **88**, 4220–4224.

483. Bradding, P., Mediwake, R., Feather, I. H., et al. (1995) TNF-α is localized to nasal mucosal mast cells and is released in acute allergic rhinitis, *Clin. Exp. Allergy*, **25**, 406–415.

484. Bradding, P., Roberts, J. A., Britten, K. M., et al. (1994) Interleukin-4, -5, and -6 and tumor necrosis factor-α in normal and asthmatic airways: evidence for the human mast cell as a source of these cytokines, *Am. J. Respir. Cell. Mol. Biol.*, **10**, 471–480.

485. Echtenacher, B., Mannel, D. N., and Hultner, L. (1996) Critical protective role of mast cells in a model of acute septic peritonitis, *Nature*, **381**, 75–79.

486. Barata, L. T., Ying, S., Meng, Q., et al. (1998) IL-4 and IL-5-positive T lymphocytes, eosinophils, and mast cells in allergen-induced late-phase cutaneous reactions in atopic subjects, *J. Allergy Clin. Immunol.*, **101**, 222–230.

487. Bradding, P., Feather, I. H., Wilson, S., et al. (1993) Immunolocalization of cytokines in the nasal mucosa of normal and perennial rhinitis subjects. The mast cell as a source of IL-4, IL-5, and IL-6 in human allergic mucosal inflammation, *J. Immunol.*, **151**, 3853–3865.

488. Ochi, H., Hirani, W. M., Yuan, Q., et al. (1999) T helper type-2 cytokine-mediated comitogenic responses and CCR3 expression during differentiation of human mast cells in vitro, *J. Exp. Med.*, **190**, 267–280.

489. Okayama, Y., Semper, A., Holgate, S. T., and Church, M. K. (1995) Multiple cytokine mRNA expression in human mast cells stimulated via Fc epsilon RI, *Int. Arch. Allergy Immunol.*, **107**, 158–159.

490. Grutzkau, A., Kruger-Krasagakes, S., Kogel, H., et al. (1997) Detection of intracellular interleukin-β in human mast cells: flow cytometry as a guide for immunoelectron microscopy, *J. Histochem. Cytochem.*, **45**, 935–945.

491. Moller, A., Lippert, U., Lessmann, D., et al. (1993) Human mast cells produce IL-8, *J. Immunol.*, **151**, 3261–3266.

492. Yano, K., Yamaguchi, M., de Mora, F., et al. (1977) Production of macrophage inflammatory protein-1 alpha by human mast cells: increased anti-IgE-dependent secretion after IgE-dependent enhancement of mast cell IgE-binding ability, *Lab. Invest.*, **77**, 185–193.

493. Baghestanian, M., Hofbauer, R., Kiener, H. P., et al. (1997) The c-*kit* ligand stem cell factor and anti-IgE promote expression of monocyte chemoattractant protein-1 in human lung mast cells, *Blood*, **90**, 4438–4449.

494. Hogaboam, C., Kunkel, S. L., Strieter, R. M., et al. (1998) Novel role of transmembrane SCF for mast cell activation and eotaxin production in mast cell-fibroblast interactions, *J. Immunol.*, **160**, 6166–6171.

495. Boesiger, J., Tsai, M., Maurer, M., et al. (1998) Mast cells can secrete vascular permeability factor/vascular endothelial cell growth factor and exhibit enhanced release after immunoglobulin E-dependent upregulation of FcεRI expression, *J. Exp. Med.*, **188**, 1135–1145.

496. Kanbe, N., Kurosawa, M., Nagata, H., et al. (1999) Cord blood-derived human cultured mast cells produce transforming growth factor β1, *Clin. Exp. Allergy*, **29**, 105–113.

497. Reed, J. A., Albino, A. P., and McNutt, N. S. (1995) Human cutaneous mast cells express basic fibroblast growth factor, *Lab. Invest.*, **72**, 215–222.

498. Zhang, S., Anderson, D. F., Bradding, P., et al. (1998) Human mast cells express stem cell factor, *J. Pathol.*, **186**, 59–66.

499. de Paulis, A., Minopoli, G., Arbustini, E., et al. (1999) Stem cell factor is localized in, released from, and cleaved by human mast cells, *J. Immunol.*, **163**, 2799–2808.

500. Sher, A., Hein, A., Moser, G., and Caulfield, J. P. (1979) Complement receptors promote the phagocytosis of bacteria by rat peritoneal mast cells, *Lab. Invest.*, **41**, 490–499.

501. Zhang, Y., Ramos, B. F., and Jaschik, B. A. (1992) Neutrophil recruitment by tumor necrosis factor from mast cells in immune complex peritonitis, *Science*, **258**, 1957–1959.

502. Malaviya, R., Ikeda, T., Ross, E., et al. (1996) Mast cell modulation of neutrophil influx and bacterial clearance at sites of infection through TNF-alpha, *Nature*, **381**, 77–80.

503. Maurer, M., Echtenacher, B., Hulktner, L., et al. (2001) the c-*kit* ligand, stem cell factor, can enhance innate

immunity through effects on mast cells, *J. Exp. Med.*, **188**, 2343–2348.

504. Lorentz, A., Schwengberg, S., Sellge, G., et al. (2000) Human intestinal mast cells are capable of producing different cytokine profiles: role of IgE receptor cross-linking and IL-4, *J. Immunol.*, **164**, 43–48.

505. Ochi, H., De Jesus, N. H., Hsieh, F., Austen, K. F., and Boyce, J. A. (2000) Interleukins 4 and 5 prime human mast cells for different profiles of IgE-dependent cytokine production, *Proc. Natl. Acad. Sci. U.S.A.*, **97**, 10509–10513.

506. Huang, C., Friend, D. S., Qui, W. T., et al. (1998) Induction of a selective and persistent extravasation of neutrophils into the peritoneal cavity by tryptase mouse mast cell protease 6, *J. Immunol.*, **160**, 1910–1919.

507. Huang, C., De Sanctis, G. T., O'Brien, P. J., et al. (2001) Evaluation of the substrate specificity of human mast cell tryptase beta 1 and demonstration of its importance in bacterial infections of the lung, *J. Biol. Chem.*, **276**, 26276–26284.

508. Malaviya, R., Navara, C., and Uckun, F. M. (2001) Role of Janus kinase 3 in mast cell-mediated innate immunity against gram-negative bacteria, *Immunity*, **18**, 313–321.

509. Prodeus, A. P., Zhou, X., Maurer, M., Galli, S. J., and Carroll, M. C. (1997) Impaired mast cell-dependent natural immunity in complement C3-deficient mice, *Nature*, **390**, 172–175.

510. Gommerman, J. L., Oh, D. Y., Zhou, X., et al. (2000) A role for CD21/CD35 and CD19 in responses to acute septic peritonitis: a potential mechanism for mast cell activation, *J. Immunol.*, **165**, 6915–6921.

511. Artis, D., Humphreys, N. E., Potten, C. S., et al. (2000) β_7 Integrin-deficient mice: delayed leukocyte recruitment and attenuated protective imminity in the small intestine during enteric helminth infection, *Eur. J. Immunol.*, **30**, 1656–1664.

512. Moody, D. B. (2003) CD1-restricted T-cells. In: *Innate Immunity* (Ezekowitz, R. A. B. and Hoffmann, J. A., eds.), Humana Press, Totowa, NJ, pp. 387–402.

513. Garcia, K. C., Degano, M., Stanfield, R. L., et al. (1996) An alpha beta T cell receptor structure at 2.5 Å and its orientation in the TCR-MHC complex, *Science*, **274**, 209–219.

514. Porcelli, S. A. (1995) The CD1 family: a third lineage of antigen-presenting molecules, *Adv. Immunol.*, **59**, 1–98.

515. Calabi, F. and Milstein, C. (1986) A novel family of human major histocompatibility complex-related genes not mapping to chromosome 6, *Nature*, **323**, 540–543.

516. Beckman, E. M., Porcelli, S. A., Morita, C. T., et al. (1994) Recognition of a lipid antigen by CD1-restricted alpha beta+ T cells, *Nature*, **372**, 691–694.

517. Sieling, P. A., Chatterjee, D., Porcelli, S. A., et al. (1995) CD1-restricted T cell recognition of microbial lipoglycan antigens, *Science*, **269**, 227–230.

518. Moody, D. B., Reinhold, B. B., Guy, M. R., et al. (1997) Structural requirements for glycolipid antigen recognition by CD1b-restricted T cells, *Science*, **278**, 283–286.

519. Kawano, T., Cui, J., Koezuka, Y., et al. (1997) CD1d-restricted and TCR-mediated activation of Vα 14 NKT cells by glycosylceramides, *Science*, **278**, 1626–1629.

520. Porcelli, S., Morita, C. T., and Brenner, M. B. (1992) CD1b restricts the response of human CD4⁻8⁻ T lymphocytes to a microbial antigen, *Nature*, **360**, 593–597.

521. Koseki, H., Imai, K., Nakayama, F., et al. (1990) Homogenous junctional sequence of the V 14+ T-cell antigen receptor alpha chain expanded in unprimed mice, *Proc. Natl. Acad. Sci. U.S.A.*, **180**, 5248–5252.

522. Lantz, O. and Bendelac, A. (1994) An invariant T cell receptor alpha chain is used by a unique subset of major histocompatibility complex class I-specific CD4+ and CD4⁻8⁻ T cells in mice and humans, *J. Exp. Med.*, **180**, 1097–1106.

523. Porcelli, S., Gerdes, D., Fertig, A. M., and Balk, S. P. (1996) Human T cells expressing an invariant V alpha 24-J alpha Q TCR alpha are CD4- and heterogeneous with respect to TCR beta expression, *Hum. Immunol.*, **48**, 63–67.

524. Medzhitov, R. and Janeway, C. A., Jr. (1997) Innate immunity: the virtues of a nonclonal system of recognition, *Cell*, **91**, 295–298.

525. Park, S. H., Chiu, Y. H., Jayawardena, J., et al. (1998) Innate and adaptive functions of the CD1 pathway of antigen presentation, *Semin. Immunol.*, **10**, 391–398.

526. Grant, E. P., Degano, M., Rosat, J. P., et al. (1999) Molecular recognition of lipid antigens by T cell receptors, *J. Exp. Med.*, **189**, 195–205.

527. Cardell, S., Tangri, S., Chan, S., et al. (1995) CD1-restricted CD4⁺ T cells in major histocompatibility complex class II-deficient mice, *J. Exp. Med.*, **182**, 993–1004.

528. Behar, S. M., Podrebarac, T. A., Roy, C. J., Wang, C. R., and Brenner, M. B. (1999) Diverse TCRs recognize murine CD1, *J. Immunol.*, **162**, 161–167.

529. Moody, D. B., Besra, G. S., Wilson, I. A., and Porcelli, S. A. (1999) The molecular basis of CD1-mediated presentation of lipid antigens, *Immunol. Rev.*, **172**, 285–296.

530. Moore, P. F., Schrenzel, M. D., Affolter, V. K., Olivry, T., and Naydan, D. (1996) Canine cutaneous histiocytoma is an epidermotrophic Langerhans cell histiocytosis that expresses CD1 and specific beta 2-integrin molecules, *Am. J. Pathol.*, **148**, 1699–1708.

531. Dascher, C. C., Hiromatsu, K., Naylor, J. W., et al. (1999) Conservation of a CD1 multigene family in the guinea pig, *J. Immunol.*, **163**, 5478–5488.

532. Woo, J. C. and Moore, P. F. (1997) A feline homologue of CD1 is defined using a feline-specific monoclonal antibody, *Tissue Antigens*, **49**, 244–251.

533. Ichimiya, S., Kikuchi, K., and Matsuura, A. (1994) Structural analysis of the rat homologue of CD1. Evidence for evolutionary conservation of the CD1D class and widespread transcription by rat cells, *J. Immunol.*, **153**, 1112–1123.

534. Calabi, F., Belt, K. T., Yu, C. Y., et al. (1989) The rabbit CD1 and the evolutionary conservation of the CD1 gene family, *Immunogenetics*, **30**, 370–377.

535. Sugita, M., Moody, D. B., Jackman, R. M., et al. (1998) CD1-a new paradigm for antigen presentation and T cell activation, *Clin. Immunol. Immunopathol.*, **87**(1), 8–14.

536. Bradbury, A., Belt, K. T., Neri, T. M., Milstein, C., and Calabi, F. (1988) Mouse CD1 is distinct from and co-exists with TL in the same thymus, *EMBO J.*, **7**, 3081–3086.

537. MacHugh, N. D., Bensaid, A., Davis, W. C., et al. (1988) Characterization of a bovine thymic differentiation antigen analogous to CD1 in the human, *Scand. J. Immunol.*, **27**, 541–547.

538. Dutia, B. M. and Hopkins, J. (1991) Analysis of the CD1 cluster in sheep, *Vet. Immunol. Immunopathol.*, **27**, 189–194.

539. Calabi, F., Jarvis, J. M., Martin, L., and Milstein, C. (1989) Two classes of CD1 genes, *Eur. J. Immunol.*, **19**, 285–292.

540. Angenieux, C., Salamero, J., Fricker, D., et al. (2000) Characterization of CD1e, a third type of CD1 molecule expressed in dendritic cells, *J. Biol. Chem.*, **275**, 37757–37764.

541. Mirones, I., Oteo, M., Parra-Cuadrado, J. F., and Martinez-Naves, E. (2000) Identification of two novel human CD1E alleles, *Tissue Antigens*, **56**, 159–161.

542. Rosat, J. P., Grant, E. P., Beckman, E. M., et al. (1999) CD1-restricted microbial lipid antigen-specific recognition found in the CD8⁺ alpha beta T cell pool, *J. Immunol.*, **162**, 366–371.

543. Beckman, E. M., Melian, A., Behar, S. M., et al. (1996) CD1c restricts responses of mycobacteria-specific T cells. Evidence for antigen presentation by a second member of the human CD1 family, *J. Immunol.*, **157**, 2795–2803.

544. Han, M., Hannick, L. I., DiBrino, M., and Robinson, M. A. (1999) Polymorphism of human CD1 genes, *Tissue Antigens*, **54**, 122–127.

545. Bauer, A., Huttinger, R., Staffler, G., et al. (1997) Analysis of the requirement for beta 2-microglobulin for expression and formation of human CD1 antigens, *Eur. J. Immunol.*, **27**, 1366–1373.

546. Gadola, S. D., Zaccai, N. R., Harlos, K., et al. (2002) Structure of human CD1b with bound ligands at 2.3 Å, a maze for alkyl chains, *Nat. Immunol.*, **3**, 721–726.

547. Zeng, Z., Castaño, A. R., Segelke, B. W., et al., (1997) Crystal structure of mouse CD1: an MHC-like fold with a large hydrophobic binding groove, *Science*, **277**, 339–345.

548. Moody, D. B., Ulrich, T., Muhlecker, W., et al. (2000) CD1c-mediated T cell recognition of mycobacterial glycolipids in *M. tuberculosis* infection, *Nature*, **404**, 884–888.

549. Shamshiev, A., Donda, A., Carena, I., et al. (1999) Self glycolipids as T-cell autoantigens, *Eur. J. Immunol.*, **29**, 1667–1675.

550. Gumperz, J., Roy, Makowska, A., et al. (2000) Murine CD1d-restricted T cell recognition of cellular lipids, *Immunity*, **12**, 211–221.

551. Schofield, L., McConville, M. J., Hansen, D., et al. (1999) CD1d-restricted immunoglobulin G formation to GPI-anchored antigens mediated by NKT cells, *Science*, **283**, 225–229.

552. Castaño, A. R., Tangri, S., Miller, J. E., et al. (1995) Peptide binding and presentation by mouse CD1, *Science*, **269**, 223–226.

553. Brossay, L., Naidenko, O., Burdin, N., et al. (1998) Structural requirements for galactosylceramide recognition by CD1-restricted NK T cells, *J. Immunol.*, **161**, 5124–5128.

554. Park, S. H., Weiss, A., Benlagha, K., et al. (2001) The mouse CD1d-restricted repertoire is dominated by a few autoreactive T cell receptor families, *J. Exp. Med.*, **193**, 893–904.

555. Benlagha, K., Weiss, A., Beavis, A., Teyton, L., and Bendelac, A. (2000) In vivo identification of glycolipid antigen-specific T cells using fluorescent CD1d tetramers, *J. Exp. Med.*, **191**, 1895–1903.

556. Matsuda, J. L., Naidenko, O. V., Gapin, L., et al. (2000) Tracking the response of natural killer T cells to a glycolipid antigen using CD1d tetramers, *J. Exp. Med.*, **192**, 741–754.

557. Porcelli, S. A. (1995) The CD1 family: a third lineage of antigen-presenting molecules, *Adv. Immunol.*, **59**, 1–98.

558. Sugita, M., Grant, E. P., van Donselaar, E., et al. (1999) Separate pathways for antigen presentation by CD1 molecules, *Immunity*, **11**, 743–752.

559. Sugita, M., Jackman, R. M., van Donselaar, E., et al. (1996) Cytoplasmic tail- dependent localization of CD1b antigen-presenting molecules to MIICs, *Science*, **273**, 349–352.

560. Sugita, M., van der Wel, N., Rogers, R. A., Petters, P. J., and Brenner, M. B. (2000) CD1c molecules broadly survey the endocytic system, *Proc. Natl. Acad. Sci. U.S.A.*, **97**, 8445–8450.

561. Briken, V., Jackman, R. M., Watts, G. F., Rogers, R. A., and Porcelli, S. A. (2000) Human CD1b and CD1c isoforms survey different intracellular compartments for the presentation of microbial lipid antigens, *J. Exp. Med.*, **192**, 281–288.

562. Jackman, R. M., Stenger, S., Lee, A., et al. (1998) The tyrosine-containing cytoplasmic tail of CD1b is essential for its efficient presentation of bacterial lipid antigens, *Immunity*, **8**, 341–351.

563. Jayawardena-Wolf, J., Benlagha, K., Chiu, Y. H., Mehr, R., and Bendelac, A. (2001) CD1d endosomal trafficking is independently regulated by an intrinsic CD1d-encoded tyrosine motif and by the invariant chain, *Immunity*, **15**, 897–908.

564. Bonifacino, J. S. and Dell'Angelica, E. C. (1999) Molecular bases for the recognition of tyrosine-based sorting signals, *J. Cell. Biol.*, **145**, 923–926.

565. Briken, V., Moody, D. B., and Porcelli, S. A. (2000) Diversification of CD1 proteins: sampling the lipid content of different cellular compartments, *Semin. Immunol.*, **12**, 517–525.

566. Moody, D. B. and Porcelli, S. A. (2001) CD1 trafficking invariant chain gives a new twist to the tale, *Immunity*, **15**(6), 861–865.

567. Sugita, M., Peters, P. J., and Brenner, M. B. (2000) Pathways for lipid antigen presentation by CD1 molecules: nowhere for intracellular pathogens to hide, *Traffic*, **1**, 295–300.

568. Moody, D. B., Reinhold, B. B., Reinhold, V. N., Besra, G. S., and Porcelli, S. A. (1999) Uptake and processing of glycosylated mycolates for presentation to CD1b-restricted T cells, *Immunol. Lett.*, **65**, 85–91.

569. Chiu, Y. H., Jayawardena, J., Weiss, A., et al. (1999) Distinct subsets of DC1d- restricted T cells recognize self-antigens loaded in different cellular compartments, *J. Exp. Med.*, **189**, 103–110.

570. Spada, F. M., Koezuka, Y., and Porcelli, S. A. (1998) CD1d-restricted recognition of synthetic glycolipid antigens by human natural killer T cells, *J. Exp. Med.*, **188**, 1529–1534.

571. Moody, D. B., Briken, V., Cheng, T. Y., et al. (2002) Lipid length controls antigen entry into endosomal and nonendosomal pathways for CD1b presentation, *Nat. Immunol.*, **3**, 435–442.

572. Bendelac, A., Killeen, N., Littman, D. R., and Schwartz, R. H. (1994) A subset of CD4$^+$ thymocytes selected by MHC class I molecules, *Science*, **263**, 1774–1778.

573. Beutner, U., Launois, P., Ohteki, T., Louis, J. A., and MacDonald, H. R. (1997) Natural killer-like T cells develop in SJL mice despite genetically distinct defects in NK1.1 expression and in inducible interleukin-4 production, *Eur. J. Immunol.*, **27**, 928–934.

574. Asea, A. and Stein-Streilein, J. (1998) Signaling through NK1.1 triggers NK cells to die but induces NK T cells to produce interleukin-4, *Immunology*, **93**, 296–305.

575. Bendelac, A., Lantz, O., Quimby, M. E., et al. (1995) CD1 recognition by mouse NK1+ T lymphocytes, *Science*, **268**, 863–865.

576. Smiley, S. T., Kaplan, M. H., and Grusby, M. J. (1997) Immunoglobulin E production in the absence of interleukin-4-secreting CD1-dependent cells, *Science*, **275**, 977–979.

577. Gapin, L., Matsuda, J. L., Surh, C. D., and Kronenberg, M. (2001) NKT cells derive from double-positive thymocytes that are positively selected by CD1d, *Nat. Immunol.*, **2**, 971–978.

578. Coles, M. C. and Raulet, D. H. (2000) NK1.1+ T cells in the liver arise in the thymus and are selected by interactions with class I molecules on CD4$^+$CD8$^+$ cells, *J. Immunol.*, **164**, 2412–2418.

579. Shimamura, M., Ohteki, T., Beutner, U., and MacDonald, H. R. (1997) Lack of directed V alpha 14-J alpha 281 rearrangement in NK1+ T cells, *Eur. J. Immunol.*, **27**, 1576–1579.

580. Mendiratta, S. K., Martin, W. D., Hong, S., et al. (1997) CD1d1 mutant mice are deficient in natural T cells that promptly produce IL-4, *Immunity*, **6**, 469–477.

581. Chen, Y. H., Chiu, N. M., Mandal, M., Wang, N., and Wang, C. R. (1997) Impaired NK1+ T cell development and early IL-4 production in CD1-deficient mice, *Immunity*, **6**, 459–467.

582. Joyce, S., Woods, A. S., Yewdell, J. W. (1998) Natural ligand of mouse CD1d1: cellular glycosylphosphatidylinositol, *Science*, **279**, 1541–1544.

583. Molano, A., Park, S. H., Chiu, Y. H., et al. (2000) Cutting edge: the IgG response to the circumsporozoite protein is MHC class II-dependent and CD1d-independent: exploring the role of GPI in NK T cell activation and antimalarial responses, *J. Immunol.*, **164**, 5005–5009.

584. Romero, J. F., Eberl, G., MacDonald, H. R., and Corradin, G. (2001) CD1d- restricted NK T cells are dispensable for specific antibody responses and protective immunity against liver stage malaria infection in mice, *Parasite Immunol.*, **23**, 267–269.

585. Kawano, T., Nakayama, T., Kamada, N., et al. (1999) Antitumor toxicity mediated by ligand-activated human V alpha24 NKT cells, *Cancer Res.*, **59**, 5102–5105.

586. Miyamoto, K., Miyake, S., Yamamura, T. (2001) A synthetic glycolipid prevents autoimmune encephalomyelitis by inducing TH2 bias of natural killer cells, *Nature*, **413**, 531–534.

587. Hong, S., Wilson, M. T., Serizawa, I., et al. (2001) The natural killer T-cell ligand alpha-galactosylceramide prevents autoimmune diabetes in non-obese diabetic mice, *Nat. Med.*, **7**, 1052–1056.

588. Sharif, S., Arreaza, G. A., Zucker, P., et al. (2001) Activation of natural killer T cells by alpha-galactosylceramide treatment prevents the onset and recurrence of autoimmune type 1 diabetes, *Nat. Med.*, **7**, 1057–1062.

589. Shi, F. D., Flodstrom, M., Balasa, B., et al. (2001) Germ line deletion of the CD1 locus exacerbates diabetes in the NOD mouse, *Proc. Natl. Acad. Sci. U.S.A.*, **98**, 6777–6782.

590. Wang, B., Geng, Y. B., and Wang, C. R. (2001) CD1-restricted NK T cells protect nonobese diabetic mice from developing diabetes, *J. Exp. Med.*, **194**, 313–320.

591. Behar, S. M., Porcelli, S. A., Beckman, E. M., and Brenner, M. B. (1995) A pathway of costimulation that prevents anergy in CD28-T cells: B7-independent costimulation of CD1-restricted T cells, *J. Exp. Med.*, **182**, 2007–2018.

592. Pal, E., Tabira, T., Kawano, T., et al. (2001) Costimulation-dependent modulation of experimental autoimmune encephalomyelitis by ligand stimulation of V alpha 14 NK T cells, *J. Immunol.*, **166**, 662–668.

593. Barry, C. E., Lee, R. E., Mdluli, K., et al. (1998) Mycolic acids: structure, biosynthesis and physiological functions, *Prog. Lipid Res.*, **37**, 143–179.

594. Bhardwaj, N., Friedman, S. M., Cole, B. C., and Nisanian, A. J. (1992) Dendritic cells are potent antigen-presenting cells for microbial superantigens, *J. Exp. Med.*, **175**, 267–273.

595. Sieling, P. A., Jullien, D., Dahlem, M., et al. (1999) CD1 expression by dendritic cells in human leprosy lesions: correlation with effective host immunity, *J. Immunol.*, **162**, 1851–1858.

596. Stenger, S., Hanson, D. A., Teitelbaum, R., et al. (1998) An antimicrobial activity of cytolytic T cells mediated by granulysin, *Science*, **282**, 121–125.

597. Stenger, S., Mazzaccaro, R. J., Uyemura, K., et al. (1997) Differential effects of cytolytic T cell subsets on intracellular infection, *Science*, **276**, 1684–1687.

598. Starnes, T., Broxmeyer, H. E., Robertson, M. J., and Hromas, R. (2002) Cutting edge: IL-17D, a novel member of the IL-17 family, stimulates cytokine production and inhibits hemopoiesis, *J. Immunol.*, **169**, 642–646.

599. Thomson, A. W. (1998) *The Cytokine Handbook*, 3rd ed., Academic Press, San Diego, CA, p. xxii; 1017.

600. Rouvier, E., Luciani, M. F., Mattei, M. G., Denizot, F., and Golstein, P. (1993) CTLA-8, cloned from an activated T cell, bearing AU-rich messenger RNA instability sequences, and homologous to a herpesvirus saimiri gene, *J. Immunol.*, **150**, 5445–5456.

601. Yao, Z., Painter, S. L., Fanslow, W. C., Ulrich, D., Macduff, B. M., Spriggs, M. K., and Armitage, R. J. (1995) Human IL-17: a novel cytokine derived from T cells, *J. Immunol.*, **155**, 5483–5486.

602. Yao, Z., Fanslow, W. C., Seldin, M. F., Rousseau, A. M., Painter, S. L., Comeau, M. R., Cohen, J. I., and Spriggs, M. K. (1995) Herpesvirus saimiri encodes a new cytokine, IL-17, which binds to a novel cytokine receptor, *Immunity*, **3**(6), 811–821.

603. Yao, Z., Spriggs, M. K., Derry, J. M., Strockbine, L., Park, L. S., VandenBos, T., Zappone, J. D., Painter, S. L., and Armitage, R. J. (1997) Molecular characterization of the human interleukin (IL)-17 receptor, *Cytokine*, **9**, 794–800.

604. Weaver, C. T., Hatton, R. D., Mangan, P. R., and Harrington, L. E. (2007) IL-17 family cytokines and the expanding diversity of effector T cell lineages, *Annu. Rev. Immunol.*, **25**, 821–852.

605. Kolls, J. K. and Linden, A. (2004) Interleukin-17 family members and inflammation, *Immunity*, **21**, 467–476.

606. Fort, M. M., Cheung, J., Yen, D., Li, J., Zurawski, S. M., et al. (2001) IL-25 induces IL-4, IL-5, and IL-13 and Th2-associated pathologies in vivo, *Immunity*, **15**, 985–995.

607. Hymowitz, S. G., Filvaroff, E. H., Yin, J. P., Lee, J., Cai, L., et al. (2001) IL-17s adopt a cystine knot fold: structure and activity of a novel cytokine, IL-17F, and implications for receptor binding, *EMBO J.*, **20**(19), 5332–5341.

608. Li, H., Chen, J., Huang, A., Stinson, J., Heldens, S., Foster, J., et al. (2000) Cloning and characterization of IL-17B and IL-17C, two new members of the IL-17 cytokine family, *Proc. Natl. Acad. Sci. U.S.A.*, **97**(2), 773–778.

609. Shi, Y., Ullrich, S. J., Zhang, J., Connolly, K., et al. (2000) A novel cytokine receptor-ligand pair: identification, molecular characterization, and in vivo immunomodulatory activity, *J. Biol. Chem.*, **275**(25), 19167–19176.

610. Lee, J., Ho, W. H., Maruoka, M., Corpuz, R. T., Baldwin, D. T., et al. (2001) IL- 17E, a novel proinflammatory ligand for the IL-17 receptor homolog IL-17Rh1, *J. Biol. Chem.*, **276**(2), 1660–1664.

611. Starnes, T., Robertson, M. J., Sledge, G., Kelich, S., Nakshatri, H., et al. (2001) Cutting edge: IL-17F, a novel cytokine selectively expressed in activated T cells and monocytes, regulates angiogenesis and endothelial cell cytokine production, *J. Immunol.*, **167**, 4137–4140.

612. Kawaguchi, M., Onuchic, L. F., Li, X. D., Essayan, D. M., Schroeder, J., et al. (2001) Identification of a novel cytokine, ML-1, and its expression in subjects with asthma, *J. Immunol.*, **167**, 4430–4435.

613. Aggarwal, S. and Gurney, A. L. (2002) IL-17: prototype member of an emerging cytokine family, *J. Leukocyte Biol.*, **71**, 1–8.

614. Fossiez, F., Banchereau, J., Murray, R., Van Kooten, C., Garrone, P., and Lebecque, S. (1998) Interleukin-17, *Int. Rev. Immunol.*, **16**(5–6), 541–551.

615. Jovanovic, D. V., Di Battista, J. A., Martel-Pelletier, J., Jolicoeur, F. C., He, Y., Zhang, M., Mineau, F., and Pelletier, J. P. (1998) IL-17 stimulates the production and expression of proinflammatory cytokines, IL-β and TNF-α, by human macrophages, *J. Immunol.*, **160**, 3513–3521.

616. Fossiez, F., Djossou, O., Chomarat, P., Flores-Romo, L., Ait-Yahia, S., et al. (1996) T cell interleukin-17 induces stromal cells to produce proinflammatory and hematopoietic cytokines, *J. Exp. Med.*, **183**, 2593–2603.

617. Lubberts, E., Koenders, M. I., Oppers-Walgreen, B., van den Bersselaar, L., Coenen-de Roo, C. J. J., Joosten, L. A. B., and van den Berg, W. B. (2004) Treatment with a neutralizing anti-murine interleukin-17 antibody after the onset of colageninduced arthritis reduces joint inflammation, cartilage destruction, and bone erosion, *Arthritis Rheum.*, **50**(2), 650–659.

618. Antonysamy, M. A., Fanslow, W. C., Fu, F., Li, W., Qian, S., Troutt, A. B., and Thomson, A. W. (1999) Evidence for a role of IL-17 in organ allograft rejection: IL-17 promotes the functional differentiation of dendritic cell progenitors, *J. Immunol.*, **162**, 577–584.

619. Van Kooten, C., Boonstra, J. G., Paape, M. E., Fossiez, F., Banchereau, J., et al. (1998) Interleukin-17 activates human renal epithelial cells in vitro and is expressed during renal allograft rejection, *J. Am. Soc. Nephrol.*, **9**, 1526–1534.

620. Kurusawa, K., Hirose, K., Sano, H., Endo, H., Shinkai, H., Nawata, Y., et al. (2000) Increased interleukin-17 production in patients with systemic sclerosis, *Arthritis Rheum.*, **43**, 2455–2463.

621. Matsumoto K. and Kanmatsuse, K. (2002) Increased urinary excretion of interleukin-17 in nephrotic patients, *Nephron*, **91**, 243–249.

622. Wong, C. K., Ho, C. Y., Li, E. K., and Lam, C. W. (2000) Elevation of proinflammatory cytokine (IL-18, IL-17, IL-12) and Th2 cytokine (IL-4) concentrations in patients with systemic lupus erythematosus, *Lupus*, **9**(8), 589–593.

623. Kotake, S., Udagawa, N., Takahashi, N., Matsuzaki, K., Itoh, K., et al. (1999) IL-17 in synovial fluids from patients with rheumatoid arthritis is a potent stimulator of osteoclastogenesis, *J. Clin. Invest.*, **103**, 1345–1352.

624. Chabaud, M., Garnero, P., Dayer, J. M., Guerne, P. A., Fossiez, F., and Miossec, P. (2000) Contribution of interleukin 17 to synovium matrix destruction in rheumatoid arthritis, *Cytokine*, **12**(7), 1092–1099.

625. Tartour, E., Fossiez, F., Joyeux, I., Galinha, A., Gey, A., Claret, E., et al. (1999) Interleukin 17, a T-cell-derived cytokine, promotes tumorigenicity of human cervical tumors in nude mice, *Cancer Res.*, **59**, 3698–3704.

626. Hirahara, N., Nio, Y., Sasaki, S., Minari, Y., Takamura, M., et al. (2001) Inoculation of human interleukin-17 gene-transfected Meth-A fibrosarcoma cells induces T cell-dependent tumor-specific immunity in mice, *Oncology*, **61**(1), 79–89.

627. Schwandner, R., Yamaguchi, K., and Cao, Z. (2000) Requirement of tumor necrosis factor receptor-associated factor (TRAF) 6 in interleukin 17 signal transduction, *J. Exp. Med.*, **191**, 1233–1240.

628. Tian, E., Sawyer, J. R., Largaespada, D. A., Jenkins, N. A., Copeland, N.G., and Shaughnessy, J. D., Jr. (2000) Evi27 encodes a novel membrane protein with homology to the IL17 receptor, *Oncogene*, **19**, 2098–2109.

629. Haudenschild, D., Moseley, T., Rose, L., and Reddi, A. H. (2002) Soluble and transmembrane isoforms of novel interleukin-17 receptor-like protein by RNA splicing and expression in prostate cancer, *J. Biol. Chem.*, **277**, 4309–4316.

630. Ye, P., Rodriguez, F. H., Kanaly, S., Stocking, K. L., Schurr, J., et al. (2001) Requirement of interleukin 17 receptor signaling for lung CXC chemokine and granulocyte colony-stimulating factor expression, neutrophil recruitment, and host defense, *J. Exp. Med.*, **194**, 519–527.

631. Kramer, J. M., Yi, L., Shen, F., Maitra, A., Jiao, X., et al. (2006) Evidence for ligand-independent multimerization of the IL-17 receptor, *J. Immunol.*, **176**, 711–715.

632. Toy, D., Kugler, D., Wolfson, M., Bos, T. V., Gurgel, J., Derry, J., Tocker, J., and Peschon, J. (2006) Cutting edge: interleukin 17 signals through a heteromeric receptor complex, *J. Immunol.*, **177**, 36–39.

633. Sredni, B., Tse, H. Y., and Schwartz, R. H. (1980) Direct cloning and extended culture of antigen-specific MHC-restricted, proliferating T lymphocytes, *Nature*, **283**, 581–583.

634. Mosmann, T. R., Cherwinski, H., Bond, M. W., Giedlin, M. A., and Coffman, R. L. (1986) Two types of murine helper T cell clone. I. Definition according to profiles of lymphokine activities and secreted proteins, *J. Immunol.*, **136**, 2348–2357.

635. Coffman, R. L. and Carty, J. (1986) A T cell activity that enhances polyclonal IgE production and its inhibition by interferon-γ, *J. Immunol.*, **136**, 949–954.

636. Mosmann, T. R. and Coffman, R. L. (1987) Two types of mouse helper T-cell clone, *Immunol. Today*, **8**, 223–227.

637. Fernandez-Botran, R., Sanders, V. M., Mosmann, T. R., and Vitetta, E. S. (1988) Lymphokine-mediated regulation of the proliferative response of clones of T helper 1 and T helper 2 cells, *J. Exp. Med.*, **168**, 543–558.

638. Gajewski, T. F. and Fitch, F. W. (1988) Anti-proliferative effect of IFN-γ in immune regulation. I. IFN-γ inhibits the proliferation of Th2 but not Th1 murine helper T lymphocyte clones, *J. Immunol.*, **140**, 4245–4252.

639. Mosmann, T. R. and Coffman, R. (1989) Th1 and Th2 cells: different patterns of lymphokine secretion lead to different functional properties, *Annu. Rev. Immunol.* **7**, 145–173.

640. Finkelman, F. D., Shea-Donohue, T., Goldhill, J., Sullivan, C. A., Morris, S. C., et al. (1997) Cytokine regulation of host defense against parasitic gastrointestinal nematodes: lessons from studies with rodent models, *Annu. Rev. Immunol.*, **15**, 505–533.

641. Sadick, M. D., Heinzel, F. P., Shigekane, V. M., Fisher, W. L., and Locksley, R. M. (1987) Cellular and humoral immunity to *Leishmania major* in genetically susceptible mice after in vivo depletion of L3T4+ T cells, *J. Immunol.*, **139**, 1303–1309.

642. Heinzel, F. P., Sadick, M. D., Holaday, B.J., Coffman, R. L., and Locksley, R.M. (1989). Reciprocal expression of interferon γ or interleukin 4 during the resolution or progression of murine leishmaniasis. Evidence for expansion of distinct helper T cell subsets, *J. Exp. Med.*, **169**, 59–72.

643. Scott, P., Natovitz, P., Coffman, R.L., Pearce, E., and Sher, A. (1988) Immunoregulation of cutaneous leishmaniasis. T cell lines that transfer protective immunity or exacerbation belong to different T helper subsets and respond to distinct parasite antigens, *J. Exp. Med.*, **168**, 1675–1684.

644. Hsieh, C. S., Macatonia, S. E., O'Garra, A., and Murphy, K. M. (1993) Pathogen- induced Th1 phenotype development in CD4+αβ-TCR transgenic T cells is macrophage dependent, *Int. Immunol.*, **5**, 371–382.

645. Kobayashi, M., Fitz, L., Ryan, M., Hewick, R. M., Clark, S. C., et al. (1989) Identification and purification of natural killer cell stimulatory factor (NKSF), a cytokine with multiple biologic effects on human lymphocytes, *J. Exp. Med.*, **170**, 827–845.

646. Hsieh, C. S., Macatonia, S. E., Tripp, C. S., Wolf, S. F., O'Garra, A., and Murphy, K. M. (1993) Development of TH1 CD4+ T cells through IL-12 produced by *Listeria*-induced macrophages, *Science*, **260**, 547–549.

647. Seder, R. A., Gazzinelli, R., Sher, A., and Paul, W. E. (1993) Interleukin 12 acts directly on CD4+ T cells to enhance priming for interferon-γ production and diminishes interleukin 4 inhibition of such priming, *Proc. Natl. Acad. Sci. U.S.A.*, **90**, 10188–10192.

648. Seder, R. A. and Paul, W. E. (1994) Acquisition of lymphokine-producing phenotype by CD4+ T cells, *Annu. Rev. Immunol.*, **12**, 635–673.

649. Murphy, K. M. and Reiner, S. L. (2002) The lineage decisions of helper T cells, *Nat. Rev. Immunol.*, **2**, 933–944.

650. Boulay, J. L., O'Shea, J. J., and Paul, W. E. (2003) Molecular phylogeny within type I cytokines and their cognate receptors, *Immunity*, **19**, 159–163.

651. Min, B., Prout, M., Hu-Li, J., Zhu, J. F., Jankovic, D., et al. (2004) Basophils produce IL-4 and accumulate in tissues after infection with a Th2-inducing parasite, *J. Exp. Med.*, **200**, 507–517.

652. Shinkai, K., Mohrs, M., and Locksley, R. M. (2002) Helper T cells regulate type-2 innate immunity in vivo, *Nature*, **420**, 825–829.

653. Seder, R. A., Plaut, M., Barbieri, S., Urban, J. J., Finkelman, F. D., and Paul, W. E. (1991) Purified Fc εR+ bone marrow and splenic non-B, non-T cells are highly enriched in the capacity to produce IL-4 in response to immobilized IgE, IgG2a, or ionomycin, *J. Immunol.*, **147**, 903–909.

654. Yoshimoto, T., Bendelac, A., Watson, C., Hu-Li, J., and Paul, W. E. (1995) Role of NK1.1+ T cells in a TH2 response and in immunoglobulin E production, *Science*, **270**, 1845-1847.

655. Voehringer, D., Reese, T., Huang, X., Shinkai, K., and Locksley, R. M. (2006) Type 2 immunity is controlled by IL-4/IL-13 expression in hematopoietic non- eosinophil cells of the innate immune system, *J. Exp. Med.*, **203**, 1435–1446.

656. Yi, J. J. and Gaffen, S. L. (2008) Interleukin-17: a novel inflammatory cytokine that bridges innate and adaptive immunity, *Front. Biosci.*, **13**, 170–177.

657. Ruddy, M. J., Shen, F., Smith, J., Sharma, A., and Gaffen, S. L. (2004) Interleukin-17 regulates expression of the CXC

chemokine LIX/CXCL5 in osteoblasts: implications for inflammation and neutrophil recruitment, *J. Leukoc. Biol.*, **76**, 135–144.

658. Ruddy, M. J., Wong, G. C., Liu, X. K., Yamamoto, H., et al. (2004) Functional cooperation between interleukin-17 and tumor necrosis factor-alpha is mediated by CCAAT/enhancer binding protein family members, *J. Biol. Chem.*, **279**, 2559–2567.

659. Shen, F., Ruddy, M. J., Plamondon, P., and Gaffen, S. L. (2005) Cytokines link osteoblasts and inflammation: microarray analysis of interleukin-17- and TNF-alpha-induced genes in bone cells, *J. Leukoc. Biol.*, **77**, 388–399.

660. Fossiez, F., Djossou, O., Chomarat, P., Flores-Romo, L., Ait-Yahia, S., et al. (1996) T cell interleukin-17 induces stromal cells to produce proinflammatory and hematopoietic cytokines, *J. Exp. Med.*, **183**, 2593–2603.

661. Park, H., Li, Z., Yang, X. O., Chang, S. H., Nurieva, R., et al. (2005) A distinct lineage of CD4 T cells regulates tissue inflammation by producing interleukin 17, *Nat. Immunol.*, **6**, 1133–1141.

662. Moseley, T. A., Haudenschild, D. R., Rose, L., and Reddi, A. H. (2003) Interleukin- 17 family and IL-17 receptors, *Cytokine Growth Factor Rev.*, **14**, 155–174.

663. Gaffen, S. L., Kramer, J. M., Yu, J. J., and Shen, F. (2006) The IL-17 cytokine family. In: *Vitamins and Hormones* (Litwack, G., ed.), Academic Press, London.

664. Shin, H. C., Benbernou, N., Esnault, S., and Guenounou, M. (1999) Expression of IL-17 in human memory CD45RO+ T lymphocytes and its regulation by protein kinase A pathway, *Cytokine*, **11**, 257–266.

665. Chabaud, M., Fossiez, F., Taupin, J. L., and Miossec, P. (1998) Enhancing effect of IL-17 on IL-1-induced IL-6 and leukemia inhibitory factor production by rheumatoid arthritis synoviocytes and its regulation by Th2 cytokines, *J. Immunol.*, **161**, 409–414.

666. Gaffen, S. L. (2005) Biology of recently discovered cytokines: interleukin-17A unique inflammatory cytokine with roles in bone biology and arthritis, *Arthritis Res. Ther.*, **6**(6), 240–247.

667. Aarvak, T., Chabaud, M., Miossec, P., and Natvig, J. B. (1999) IL-17 is produced by some proinflammatory Th1/Th0 cells but not by Th2 cells, *J. Immunol.*, **162**, 1246–1251.

668. McGeachy, M. J., Bak-Jensen, K. S., Chen, Y., Tato, C. M., et al. (2007) TGF-β and IL-6 drive the production of IL-17 and IL-10 by T cells and restrain Th-17 cell–mediated pathology, *Nat. Immunol.*, **8**, *1390–1397*.

669. Steinman, L. (2007) A brief history of T (H)17, the first major revision in the T (H)1/T (H)2 hypothesis of T cell-mediated tissue damage, *Nat. Med.*, **13**, 139–145.

670. Mangan, P. R., Harrington, L. E., O'Quinn, B., Helms, W. S., et al. (2006) Transforming growth factor-beta induces development of the T (H)17 lineage, *Nature*, **441**, 231–234.

671. Veldhoen, M., Hocking, R. J., Atkins, C. J., Locksley, R. M., and Stockinger, B. (2006) TGFbeta in the context of an inflammatory cytokine milieu supports de novo differentiation of IL-17-producing T cells, *Immunity*, **24**, 179–189.

672. Bettelli, E., Carrier, Y., Gao, W., Korn, T., et. al. (2006) Reciprocal developmental pathways for the generation of pathogenic effector T (H)17 and regulatory T cells, *Nature*, **441**, 235–238.

673. Ivanov, I. I., McKenzie, B. S., Zhou, L., Tadokoro, C. E., Lepelley, A., et al. (2006) The orphan nuclear receptor RORgammat directs the differentiation program of proinflammatory IL-17+ T helper cells, *Cell*, **126**, 1121–1133.

674. Harrington, L. E., Hatton, R. D., Mangan, P. R., Turner, H., et al. (2005) Interleukin 17-producing CD4+ effector T cells develop via a lineage distinct from the T helper type 1 and 2 lineages, *Nat. Immunol.*, **6**, 1123–1132.

675. Langrish, C. L., Chen, Y., Blumenschein, W. M., Mattson, J., et al. (2005) IL-23 drives a pathogenic T cell population that induces autoimmune inflammation, *J. Exp. Med.*, **201**, 233–240.

676. Liang, S. C., Tan, X. Y., Luxenberg, D. P., Karim, R., Dunussi-Joannopoulos, K., Collins, M., and Fouser, L. A. (2006) Interleukin (IL)-22 and IL-17 are coexpressed by Th17 cells and cooperatively enhance expression of antimicrobial peptides, *J. Exp. Med.*, **203**, 2271–2279.

677. Chung, Y., Yang, X., Chang, S. H., Ma, L., Tian, Q., and Dong, C. (2006) Expression and regulation of IL-22 in the IL-17-producing CD4+ T lymphocytes, *Cell Res.*, **16**, 902–907.

678. Cua, D. J. and Kastelein, R. A. (2006) TGF-beta, a "double agent" in the immune pathology war, *Nat. Immunol.*, **7**, 557–559.

679. Lockhart, E., Green, A. M., and Flynn, J. L. (2006) IL-17 production is dominated by gamma-delta T cells rather than CD4 T cells during *Mycobacterium tuberculosis* infection, *J. Immunol.*, **177**, 4662–4669.

680. Shibata, K., Yamada, H., Hara, H., Kishihara, K., and Yoshikai, Y. (2007) Resident V{delta}1+ {gamma} {delta} T cells control early infiltration of neutrophils after *Escherichia coli* Infection via IL-17 production, *J. Immunol.*, **178**, 4466–4472.

681. Shulze-Koops, H. (2003) The balance of Th1/Th2 cytokines in rheumatoid arthritis, *Best Practice & Research Clin. Rheumatol.*, **15**(5), 677–691.

682. Arend, W. P. and Dayer, J. M. (1995) Inhibition of the production and effects of interleukin-1 and tumor necrosis factor α in rheumatoid arthritis, *Arthritis Rheum.*, **38**, 151–160.

683. Thorbecke, G. J., Shah, R., Leu, C. H., Kuruvilla, A. P., Hardison, A. M., and Palladino, M. A. (1992) Involvement of endogenous tumor necrosis factor α and transforming growth factor β during induction of collagen type II arthritis in mice, *Proc. Natl. Acad. Sci. U.S.A.*, **89**, 7375–7379.

684. van den Berg, W. B., Joosten, L. A., Helsen, M., and van de Loo, F. A. (1004) Amelioration of established murine collagen-induced arthritis with anti-IL-1 treatment, *Clin. Exp. Immunol.*, **95**, 237–243.

685. Joosten, L. A. B., Helsen, M. M. A., van de Loo, F. A. J., and van den Berg, W. B. (1996) Anticytokine treatment of established type II collagen-induced arthritis in DBA/1 mice: a comparative study using anti-TNF-α, anti-IL-1α/β, and IL-1Ra, *Arthritis Rheum.*, **39**, 797–809.

686. Chabaud, M., Durand, J. M., Buchs, N., Fossiez, F., Page, G., Frappart, L., et al. (1999) Human interleukin-17: a T cell-derived proinflammatory cytokine produced by the rheumatoid synovium, *Arthritis Rheum.*, **42**, 963–970.

687. Ziolkowska, M., Koc, A., Luszczykiewicz, G., Ksiezopolska-Pietrzak, K., Klimczak, E., Chwalinska-Sadowska, H., et al. (2000) High levels of IL-17 in rheumatoid arthritis patients: IL-15 triggers in vitro IL-17 production via cyclosporin A-sensitive mechanism, *J. Immunol.*, **164**, 2832–2838.

688. Koenders, M., Lubberts, E., Joosten, L., Oppers, B., van den Bersselaar, L., Kolls, J., and van den Berg, W. B. (2003) TNF-α dependency of IL-17-induced joint pathology differs under naive and arthritis conditions *in vivo*, *Arthritis Res. Ther.*, **5**(Suppl. 1), 46.

689. Kehlen, A., Thiele, K., Riemann, D., and Langner, J. (2002) Expression, modulation and signalling of IL-17 receptor in fibroblast-like synoviocytes of patients with rheumatoid arthritis, *Clin. Exp. Immunol.*, **127**(3), 539–546.

690. Chabaud, M., Fossiez, F., Taupin, J. L., and Miossec, P. (1998) Enhancing effect of IL-17 on IL-1-induced IL-6 and leukemia inhibitory factor production by rheumatoid arthritis synoviocytes and its regulation by Th2 cytokines, *J. Immunol.*, **161**, 409–414.

691. Lubberts, E., Joosten, L. A.B., Oppers, B., van den Bersselaar, L., Coenen-de Roo, C. J. J., Kolls, J. K., et al. (2001) IL-1-independent role of IL-17 in synovial inflammation and joint destruction during collagen-induced arthritis, *J. Immunol.*, **167**, 1004–1013.

692. Bush, K. A., Farmer, K. M., Walker, J. S., and Kirkham, B.W. (2002) Reduction of joint inflammation and bone erosion in rat adjuvant arthritis by treatment with interleukin-17 receptor IgG1 Fc fusion protein, *Arthritis Rheum.*, **46**, 802–805.

693. Chabaud, M., Lubberts, E., Joosten, L., van den Berg, W., and Miossec, P. (2001) IL-17 derived from juxta-articular bone and synovium contributes to joint degradation in rheumatoid arthritis, *Arthritis Res.*, **3**, 168–177.

694. Lubberts, E., Joosten, L. A. B., van de Loo, F. A. J., van den Bersselaar, L. A., and van den Berg, W. B. (2000) Reduction of interleukin-17-induced inhibition of chondrocyte proteoglycan synthesis in intact murine articular cartilage by interleukin-4, *Arthritis Rheum.*, **43**, 1300–1306.

695. Martel-Pelletier, J., Mineau, F., Jovanovic, D., Di Battista, J. A., and Pelletier, J. P. (1999) Mitogen-activated protein kinase and nuclear factor κB together regulate interleukin-17-induced nitric oxide production in human osteoarthritic chondrocytes: possible role of transactivating factor mitogen-activated protein kinase-activated protein kinase (MAPKAPK), *Arthritis Rheum.*, **42**, 2399–2409.

696. Kotake, S., Udagawa, N., Takahashi, N., Matsuzaki, K., Itoh, K., Ishiyama, S., et al. (1999) IL-17 in synovial fluids from patients with rheumatoid arthritis is a potent stimulator of osteoclastogenesis, *J. Clin. Invest.*, **103**, 1345–1352.

697. Lubberts, E., van den Bersselaar, L., Oppers-Walgreen, B., Schwarzenberger, P., Coenen-de Roo, C. J. J., Kolls, J. K., et al. (2003) IL-17 promotes bone erosion in murine collagen-induced arthritis through loss of the receptor activator of NF-κB ligand/osteoprotegerin balance, *J. Immunol.*, **170**, 2655–2662.

698. Cooke, A. (2006) Th17 cells in inflammatory conditions, *Rev. Diabet. Stud.*, **3**(2), 72–75.

699. Bottomly, K. (1988) A functional dichotomy in CD4+ T lymphocytes, *Immunol. Today*, **9**(9), 268–274.

700. Fehervari, Z. and Sakaguchi, S. (2004) Development and function of CD25+CD4+ regulatory T cells, *Curr. Opin. Immunol.*, **16**(2), 203–208.

701. Fitch, F. W., McKisic, M. D., Lancki, D. W., and Gajewski, T. F. (1993) Differential regulation of murine T lymphocyte subsets, *Annu. Rev. Immunol.*, **11**, 29–48.

702. Fontenot, J. D. and Rudensky, A. Y. (2005) A well adapted regulatory contrivance: regulatory T cell development and the forkhead family transcription factor Foxp3, *Nat. Immunol.*, **6**(4), 331–337.

703. Szabo, S. J., Jacobson, N. G., Dighe, A. S., Gubler, U., and Murphy, K. M. (1995) Developmental commitment to the Th2 lineage by extinction of IL-12 signaling, *Immunity*, **2**(6), 665–675.

704. O'Garra, A. (1998) Cytokines induce the development of functionally heterogeneous T helper cell subsets, *Immunity*, **8**(3), 275–283.

705. Chen, W., Jin, W., Hardegen, N., Lei, K. J., Li, L., Marinos, N., McGrady, G., and Wahl, S. M. (2003) Conversion of peripheral CD4$^+$CD25- naive T cells to CD4$^+$CD25$^+$ regulatory T cells by TGF-beta induction of transcription factor Foxp3, *J. Exp. Med.*, **198**(12), 1875–1886.

706. Gorelik, L. and Flavell, R. A. (2002) Transforming growth factor-beta in T-cell biology, *Nat. Rev. Immunol.*, **2**(1), 46–53.

707. Aggarwal, S., Ghilardi, N., Xie, M. H., de Sauvage, F. J., and Gurney, A. L. (2003) Interleukin-23 promotes a distinct CD4 T cell activation state characterized by the production of interleukin-17, *J. Biol. Chem.*, **278**(3), 1910–1914.

708. Langrish, C. L., Chen, Y., Blumenschein, W. M., Mattson, J., Basham, B., et al. (2005) IL-23 drives a pathogenic T cell population that induces autoimmune inflammation, *J. Exp. Med.*, **201**(2), 233–240.

709. Murphy, C. A., Langrish, C. L., Chen, Y., Blumenschein, W., McClanahan, T., Kastelein, R. A., Sedgwick, J. D., and Cua, D. J. (2003) Divergent pro- and antiinflammatory roles for IL-23 and IL-12 in joint autoimmune inflammation, *J. Exp. Med.*, **198**(12), 1951–1957.

710. Cua, D. J., Sherlock, J., Chen, Y., Murphy, C. A., Joyce, B., Seymour, B., et al. (2003) Interleukin-23 rather than interleukin-12 is the critical cytokine for autoimmune inflammation of the brain, *Nature*, **421**(6924), 744–748.

711. Yen, D., Cheung, J., Scheerens, H., Poulet, F., McClanahan, T., McKenzie, B., et al. (2006) IL-23 is essential for T cell-mediated colitis and promotes inflammation via IL-17 and IL-6, *J. Clin. Invest.*, **116**(5), 1310–1316.

712. Shalom-Barak, T., Quach, J., and Lotz, M. (1998) Interleukin-17-induced gene expression in articular chondrocytes is associated with activation of mitogen-activated protein kinases and NF-κB, *J. Biol. Chem.*, **273**(42), 27467–27473.

713. Miljkovic, D., Cvetkovic, I., Momcilovic, M., Maksimovic-Ivanic, D., Stosic- Grujicic, S., and Trajkovic, V. (2005) Interleukin-17 stimulates inducible nitric oxide synthase-dependent toxicity in mouse beta cells, *Cell Mol. Life Sci.*, **62**(22), 2658–2668.

714. Mensah-Brown, E. P., Shahin, A., Al-Shamisi, M., Wei, X., and Lukic, M. L. (2006) IL-23 leads to diabetes induction after subdiabetogenic treatment with multiple low doses of streptozotocin, *Eur. J. Immunol.*, **36**(1), 216–223.

715. Kurusawa, K., Hirose, K., Sano, H., Endo, H., Shinkai, H., Nawata, Y., et al. (2000) Increased interleukin-17 production in patients with systemic sclerosis, *Arthritis Rheum.*, **43**, 2455–2463.

716. Teunissen, M. B., Koomen, C. W., de Waal Malefyt, R., Wierenga, E. A., and Bos, J. D. (1998) Interleukin-17 and interferon-gamma synergize in the enhancement of proinflammatory cytokine production by human keratinocytes, *J. Invest. Dermatol.*, **111**(4), 645–649.

717. Albanesi, C., Scarponi, C., Cavani, A., Federici, M., Nasorri, F., and Girolomoni, G. (2000) Interleukin-17 is produced by both Th1 and Th2 lymphocytes, and modulates interferon-gamma- and interleukin-4-induced activation of human keratinocytes, *J. Invest. Dermatol.*, **115**(1), 81–87.

718. Eugster, H. P., Frei, K., Kopf, M., Lassmann, H., and Fontana, A. (1998) IL-6- deficient mice resist myelin oligodendrocyte glycoprotein-induced autoimmune encephalomyelitis, *Eur. J. Immunol.*, **28**(7), 2178–2187.

719. Alonzi, T., Fattori, E., Lazzaro, D., Costa, P., Probert, L., et al. (1998) Interleukin 6 is required for the development of collagen-induced arthritis, *J. Exp. Med.*, **187**(4), 461–468.

720. Ohshima, S., Saeki, Y., Mima, T., Sasai, M., Nishioka, K., et al. (1998) Interleukin 6 plays a key role in the development of antigen-induced arthritis, *Proc. Natl. Acad. Sci. U.S.A.*, **95**(14), 8222–8226.

721. Okuda, Y., Sakoda, S., Bernard, C. C., Fujimura, H., Saeki, Y., Kishimoto, T., and Yanagihara, T. (1998) IL-6-deficient mice are resistant to the induction of experimental autoimmune encephalomyelitis provoked by myelin oligodendrocyte glycoprotein, *Int. Immunol.*, **10**(5), 703–708.

Chapter 39

Immune Adjuvants

Research on innate immunity has provided understanding and practical direction for the observation first made more than 70 years ago that most immunogens would require adjuvants to induce robust adaptive immune responses *(1–4)*. With the knowledge that adjuvants target antigen-presenting cells, especially dendritic cells, by triggering activation through Toll-like receptors and other pattern-recognition receptors, molecular libraries are being screened for their ability to upregulate costimulatory molecules and antigen presentation mediated by major histocompatibility complex class II molecules. Based on those principles, a growing list of adjuvant candidates now promises to provide improved vaccine immunogenicity and reduced nonspecific reactivity while taking advantage of the ability of the innate immune system to channel adaptive immunity toward the type of antibody or cellular responses most appropriate for the control of a particular pathogen *(5)*.

39.1 Adjuvants and the Initiation of T-Cell Responses

The rapidly increasing understanding of the mechanistic basis by which adjuvants initiate and promote the T-cell responses has stemmed from the better understanding and appreciation of the requirements for T-cell activation, the importance of innate immunity in T-cell activation, and the central role that dendritic cells play as antigen-presenting cells (APCs) to activate the T cells *(6)*. In this regard, the ability to activate the dendritic cells and induce the production of inflammatory cytokines is emerging as a critical feature shared by most, if not all, adjuvants.

The use of the *adoptive transfer* approach has been an important step in helping to directly assess the effects of adjuvants on the T-cell responses. Thus, challenging mice with a soluble antigen resulted in tolerance induction although injection of the same antigen along with a bacterial cell wall adjuvant caused a productive response *(7, 8)*. Furthermore, tracking the adoptively transferred CD4 T-cells

revealed that soluble antigens activated the T cells in the lymph node and spleen resulting in substantial clonal expansion at these sites that peaked on day 3 *(9, 10)*. Within a few days, however, the number of antigen-specific cells declined precipitously so that by days 10 to 15, there were fewer cells than were present before the challenge. Moreover, these cells were hyporesponsive after reexposure to antigen. Thus, whereas activation did occur in the absence of adjuvant, the outcome was tolerance because of failure of most of the cells to survive, and because of the induction of nonresponsiveness in the small number of cells that did suvive *(6)*.

By contrast, when mice were challenged with the same peptide antigen with lipopolysaccharide (LPS) as an adjuvant, the outcome was a comparable initial clonal expansion of the antigen-specific T cells, peaking at day 3 at levels only about twofold higher than in the absence of adjuvant. However, after the peak of clonal expansion, the decline in the numbers of antigen-specific cells was much less when adjuvant was used, and an expanded population persisted for a prolonged period of time. Moreover, the remaining cells responded rapidly on rechallenge with the antigen. This result clearly indicated that the adjuvant converted a tolerizing response to one that yielded an expanded and responsive memory population of T cells *(6)*.

Similar results—the presence of an expanded and responsive memory population of T cells—have been observed in experiments examining the responses of adoptively transferred CD8 T-cells after a challenge with an adjuvant; in this case, however, the presence of adjuvant appeared to have a greater effect on the initial clonal expansion *(11, 12)*.

39.1.1 Requirements for Clonal Expansion of Naïve T Cells

As initially proposed *(13)*, the T-lymphocyte activation did require two signals, with signal 1 being provided by the antigen-specific receptor and signal 2 by a second receptor-ligand interaction *(14–19)*. More recent evidence has suggested that, at least for CD8 T-cells, a third signal was required—its presence or absence would have determined whether effective activation or tolerance indiction occurs in response to antigen and costimulation *(11,20–23)*.

To become activated, naïve T cells must first recognize a peptide antigen bound to class I or class II MHC protein on an APC. However, this event has not been sufficient for full activation and can instead lead to the induction of anergy *(18)*, a nonresponsive state characterized by an inability of the T cells to produce interleukin-2 restimulation. For full activation to occur, the T cells must receive a second signal through a costimulatory receptor *(6)*. Even though there have been reports of costimulation-dependent activation of T cells using anti-TCR mAb or high densities of MHC class I/peptide antigen complexes, in most circumstances naïve T cells appeared to require both signal 1 and signal 2 to respond to normal physiologic levels of antigen. Whether or not naïve T cells would encounter sufficient antigen in the lymphoid organs to receive an effective signal 1 can be influenced by adjuvants *(6)*.

A number of studies have demonstrated that binding of the CD28 receptor on the T cell to its ligands, B7-1 or B7-2, on the APC could provide the second signal necessary to activate the cells *(14, 16, 24)*. Several additional receptor-ligand systems have also been shown to exert costimulatory activity for T cells including leukocyte function-associated antigen (LFA)-1/intercellular adhesion molecule (ICAM) and several members of the tumor necrosis factor superfamily *(25)*.

When a panel of cytokines was examined for effects in the artificial APC system, it was found that the addition of IL-12 resulted in vigorous proliferation and development of effector functions by the naïve CD8 T-cells *(21)* thereby confirming that the response of the naïve T cells depended on all three signals (antigen, costimulation, and IL-12). Although known for some time *(26)*, the ability of IL-12 to augment the cytotoxic T-lymphocyte (CTL) responses and provide a requisite third signal to naïve cells (especially, the CD8 T-lymphocytes) had not been previously appreciated *(6)*.

There is also some evidence to suggest that CD4 T-cells may also require a third signal for productive activation, and that IL-1 may provide this signal. Thus, stimulation of naïve CD4 T-cells with antigen and B7 on microspheres has been substantially increased when IL-1 (but not IL-12) was added to the cultures *(21)*. Furthermore, IL-1 was as effective as LPS in enhancing the clonal expansion and persistence of adoptively transferred CD4 T-cells in response to peptide or protein antigen *(10)*. The TNF-α exerted *in vivo* similar effects possibly as the result of its ability to potentiate the IL-1 production *(27)*. However, it still remains to be determined whether or not the observed adjuvant effects of IL-1 and TNF-α were the result of a direct delivery of a third signal to the CD4 T-cells *in vivo (6)*.

39.1.2 Effects of Dendritic Cells Activation on Stimulation of Naïve T Cells

The major function of the Toll-like receptors (TLRs), which are expressed on macrophages and dendritic cells, is to recognize conserved molecular patterns on products of microbial origins, termed *pathogen-associated molecular patterns (6)*. Even though the different TLRs are specific for different ligands, most, if not all of them, can recognize multiple ligands, including most of the conventional adjuvants such as lipids and glycolipids, including LPS, lipoteichoic acid, polynucleotides, including bacterial deoxyribonucleic acid (DNA) and double-stranded ribonucleic acid (RNA) (produced in viral infection), lipoproteins, and zymosan *(6)*.

Signaling through the TLRs would activate the NF-κB pathway resulting in the induction of variety of genes that function in host defense, including the effector molecules of the innate immunity such as microbial peptides and nitric oxide synthase, and molecules with roles in adaptive responses, including chemokines, MHC proteins, costimulatory and inflammatory cytokines *(6)*

Whereas the signaling pathways activated by TLRs are usually shared (activated by all receptors), there have been pathways activated by a specific TLR. Furthermore, whereas the TLR engagement by most adjuvants will result in some common activation event, some adjuvants may differ with respect to other activation events depending on which TLR has been involved *(28–30)*.

Adding to this complexity is the fact that there are several different subsets of dendritic cells *(31, 32)*, and they can express different sets of TLRs. Hence, adjuvants may have different effects depending on the dendritic cells subset that had expressed the TLR for a given adjuvant *(6)*. Moreover, the same TLR can induce different cytokines depending on the dendritic cells subset that has been expressed on; for example, TLR7 ligation would lead to IFN-α by plasmacytoid dendritic cells but IL-12 production by myeloid dendritic cells *(33)*. Consequently, even though the engagement of TLR by different adjuvants would result in many common events associated with the maturation of dendritic cells, *the full spectrum of changes that will occur may differ from one adjuvant to another in ways that will influence the T-cell activation and differentiation (6)*.

The effects of dendritic cells (DCs) activation on the stimulation of naïve T cells can be summarized as follows:

(i) *Migration of DCs to Lymph Nodes and Processing and Presentation of Antigens*. In most nonlymphoid tissues, DCs are located in the T-cell areas of the secondary lymphoid organs and consist of several subpopulations that can be separated broadly into subsets that arrived recently from the blood or nonlymphoid tissues *(34–36)*; for example, the lymph nodes contain blood-derived DCs that have entered via blood vessels and Langerhans cells that have migrated from the skin through afferent lymphatic vessels. While the rate of DC migration from nonlymphoid organs is believed to be relatively low under normal uninflammed conditions, during inflammation most DCs in the inflamed tissue will migrate to the lymph nodes—because of changes in the expression of chemokine receptors—and undergo functional changes known collectively as *dendritic cells maturation (37,38)*. When immature DCs have been stimulated by TLR ligands or by inflammatory cytokines produced in response to adjuvants, further antigen uptake has been inhibited, and the already internalized antigen is processed to produce peptide-class II MHC complexes that were then shuttled to the surface *(39)*. Furthermore, inflammation will also reduce the turnover of peptide-class II MHC complexes on the surface of the DCs *(40)* and will induce the components of the MHC class I peptide processing machinery *(41)*. Hence, inflammation caused by the presence of adjuvants would lead to a much greater antigen presentation because many immature DCs would migrate from the tissue of antigen deposition into the lymphoid organs in which naïve T cells reside and in the process mature to display more stable surface and abundant peptide-MHC complexes *(6)*.

(ii) *Costimulation*. In addition to increasing expression of MHC protein-peptide complexes in response to maturation agents like adjuvants, DCs will also upregulate the expression of adhesion molecules and costimulatory ligands including LFA-3 (CD58), ICAM-1 (CD54), B7-1 (CD80), and B7-2 (CD86) *(6)*. Furthermore, the increased expression of CD28 ligands could enhance the ability of DCs to provide costimulation (signal 2) to T cells. Support for this came from the observation that the ability of LPS to enhance IL-2 production and proliferation by antigen-stimulated CD4 T-cells did require that these T cells expressed CD28 *(42)*. However, this experiment did not rule out the possibility that basal CD28 signaling is necessary for certain T cells (e.g., CD8 cells) to respond to some other signal stimulated by the adjuvant, for example, a cytokine *(23)*. Nevertheless, CD28-dependent costimulation has induced IL-2 production by naïve T cells, thus providing an important growth factor to support proliferation, at least *in vitro*. However, the importance of IL-2 as growth factor in the initial proliferation of naïve T cells *in vivo* has been less clear *(6)*.

(iii) *Multiple Roles of Cytokine Production*. The DCs are capable of secreting a wide array of cytokines including IL-1, IL-2, IL-6, IL-7, IL-12, IL-15, IL-18, and type I interferons. Which cytokines a DC is producing is a function of its lineage and the way in which the cell is activated. In addition, in many instances the engagement of different TLRs and other surface receptors would result in the production of different cytokines. These cytokines can exert a profound influence on the adaptive T-cell responses by providing a third signal for the initial activation of the T cells and by directing the differentiation of the responding cells *(6)*. For example, for the naïve CD8 T-cells to be activated and to undergo clonal expansion and develop effector function, they must, in addition to signals 1 and 2, also require a third signal that can be provided by IL-12 or INF-α *(11, 21, 23, 43)*.

T- Cell Survival and Memory. In order for the T cells to initiate an effector response and develop a responsive memory population, they not only have to undergo clonal expansion but also have to survive in sufficient numbers to be effective. There has been evidence suggesting that the cytokines produced by DCs in response to adjuvants had also influenced this aspect of the T-cell responses *(6)*. Thus, whereas antiapoptotic proteins of the Bcl-2 family, including Bcl-2 and Bcl-X_L, were induced on TCR and CD28 ligation and helped to promote survival, this event was not sufficient and an adjuvant was needed to contribute for a long-term survival in a manner that did not depend on the effects of members of the Bcl-2 family *(44, 45)*. Further experiments using gene array analysis have shown that adjuvants promoted *in vivo* the survival of T cells by inducing the expression of Bcl-3 (a member of the IκB gene family) and suggested that this might be mediated by inflammatory cytokines induced by the adjuvant *(46, 47)*. To this end, it was also found that IL-1, a putative third signal for CD4 T-cells *(10, 21)*, stimulated the upregulation of Bcl-3 in these cells *(47)*

IL-15, another cytokine produced by the DCs in response to adjuvants such as LPS and double-stranded RNA *(48)*, was shown to be necessary for supporting the continuing survival of memory CD8 T-cells by driving a low level of proliferative self-renewal of these cells *(49–51)*. Thus, IL-15 can act early in a virus-specific CD8 response to extend the primary proliferative phase of the response and yield a large memory pool *(52)*.

Similarly to CD8 T-cells, the immune memory of the CD4 T-cell subset has been dependent on the survival of antigen-specific cells at the end of the primary response *(53, 54)*. An initial exposure to antigen during the primary response must take place in the presence of an adjuvant for maximal numbers of memory CD4 T-cells to survive in the secondary lymphoid organs as well as for these cells to retain their capacity to produce rapidly sufficient quantity of IL-2 *(9, 10, 55)*. In addition, an adjuvant must also be present at the time of initial exposure to antigen for the antigen-specific CD4 T-cells to survive as memory cells in nonlymphoid organs *(56)*.

Shaping the T-Cell Response. In addition to providing a third signal to initiate T-cell responses, cytokines produced in response to adjuvants have also played important roles in shaping the resulting T-cell responses by influencing the effector functions that cells develop and the migration patterns of the effector cells *(6)*. One such example involved IL-12, which was unable to provide the third signal for the initial activation of CD4 T-cells, but once they were activated, IL-12 directed their development down the Th1 pathway *(10)*.

39.1.3 Bypassing the Use of Conventional Adjuvants

Conventional adjuvants rapidly induce an innate response by a variety of effector mechanisms, as well as support the induction of adaptive T-cell responses. Although beneficial when the challenge is with live infectious agents, it may be preferable to avoid some of the inflammatory sequelae caused by conventional adjuvants when the goal is to induce T-cell immunity using defined protein or peptide antigens. In fact, such unwanted inflammatory effects may well preclude the use of some of the most potent adjuvants currently available for human immunization *(6)*.

One approach to bypass conventional adjuvants has been use of isolated DCs that had been activated and loaded with antigen *in vitro*, and then administered *(57)*. One serious drawback of this approach is the time and labor intensity, which may well preclude its application for protective immunization on any large scale *(6)*.

Another approach to bypass conventional adjuvants is use of antibody (Ab) or reagents that bind receptors on DCs and directly activates them to mature and effectively present the antigen. To this end, anti-CD40 mAb seemed very promising *(58)*. Ligating CD40 on DCs stimulated their maturation and upregulated the expression of costimulatory ligands *(59)* and the production of cytokines, including IL-12 *(60)*. Subsequent *in vivo* administration of anti-CD40 antibody along with antigen can induce strong T-cell responses.

In a third approach, the use of peptide antigen and the appropriate cytokine(s) would make it possible to bypass the need for DCs activation altogether *(6)*. Thus, the systemic administration of peptide would likely result in the presentation of the antigen on the APCs by binding directly to the MHC proteins on the cell surface, thereby avoiding the need to activate the intracellular antigen-processing pathways *(6)*. Because this will include APCs residing in the spleen and lymph nodes, migration of the antigen-bearing DCs to these sites will not be necessary. Finally, if the appropriate cytokine is administered together with peptide to provide the third signal, a potent T-cell activation would ensue. This has been demonstrated in a murine adoptive transfer system using IL-1

and peptide to induce CD4 T-cell responses *(10)* and IL-12 and peptide to induce CD8 cytolytic responses *(11, 23)*. It remains to be determined, however, whether such strategies will provide protective or therapeutic immunity *(6)*.

39.2 Bacterial Deoxyribonucleic Acid: Cytosine Phosphate Guanine

The bacterial deoxyribonucleic acid (DNA) containing cytosine phosphate guanine (CpG) motifs, but not vertebrate DNA, were shown to activate the innate immune cells *(61)*.

The CpG motifs of vertebrate DNA are suppressed and usually methylated. In contrast, the CpG motifs of bacterial DNA (CpG DNA) are unmethylated and with adequate frequency to cause immune cell activation. Moreover, the CpG DNA activation of immune cells was reproduced with synthetic oligodeoxynucleotides (ODNs) containing CpG motifs (CpG ODN) *(62)*.

In animal models, treatment with CpG DNA was found to induce a potent immune response dominated by Th1 cell–mediated cellular immunity leading to prevention and cure of several infectious and immune diseases *(61)*.

The reason as to why the mammalian immune system is not activated by vertebrate DNA lies in its structural difference from bacterial DNA. Thus, CpG motifs were observed at the expected frequency of 1:16 in the bacterial genomic DNA. By contrast, the frequency of CpG motifs in vertebrate genomic DNA was less than one-fourth that predicted *(CpG suppression)* *(62)*. In addition to CpG frequency, the cytosines of CpG motifs in the vertebrate genomic DNA were highly methylated *(CpG methylation)*. For example, methylation at the C-5 position of the cytosine of the CpG motif has been shown to eliminate the immunostimulatory activity *(63)*. *The mammalian immune system appeared to recognize these distinct CpG frequency and methylation differences and respond only to bacterial DNA (61).*

The molecular mechanism of CpG DNA–induced cellular activation has been extensively investigated and a signaling pathway has been defined *(61)*.

Cells of the innate immune system are lacking highly specific antigen receptors. Rather they rely on a set of pattern recognition receptors (PRRs) that have the general ability to recognize specific patterns of microbial structures [termed *pattern-associated molecular patterns (PAMPs)*] *(3, 62, 64, 65)*. PAMPs are specific molecular structures found in pathogens, but not in self tissues. Many of the PRRs have been found in the family of TLRs. Examples of PAMPs that PRRs are able to detect include endotoxins, flagellin, high mannose proteins, single- and double-stranded viral ribonucleic acids (RNAs), and the unmethylated CpG dinucleotides in particular base context CpG motifs that are prevalent in bacterial and many viral DNAs that are heavily suppressed and methylated in vertebrate genomes *(62)*.

The features of PAMPs can be attributed to their ability to stimulate the innate immune cells and the commonly observed structures (cell wall components) in several microbial organisms. Although not a microbial cell wall component, the bacterial DNA has also been demonstrated to have the ability to activate the innate immune cells *(66–70)*.

Studies on oligonucleotide (OND) sequences that have activated immune cells revealed that a simple sequence motif based on an unmethylated CpG dinucleotide (5′-Pu–Pu–CpG–Pyr–Pyr-3′) accounted for the immunostimulatory activity of oligodeoxyribonucleotide (ODN) in the mouse *(63)*.

DNA Vaccine. Whereas vaccination with a peptide antigen elicits antibody-mediated antigen-specific humoral immune responses, which have been most effective for protection against viral and bacterial infections, cellular immunity characterized by a T-helper 1 (Th1)-biased immune response is required to combat infections caused by intracellular organisms (tuberculosis, malaria, leishmaniasis) *(61)*. To this end, injection of plasmid DNA encoding a bacterial or viral protein has been shown to be protective in several animal models of infection with enhancement of both humoral and Th1-biased cellular immunity *(71–76)*. Subsequently, plasmid DNA is being studied in clinical trials for prevention against several infectious diseases as "DNA vaccine" *(77–79)*.

The effect of the plasmid DNA as a potent DNA vaccine has now been attributed to the CpG motifs present in the bacteria-derived plasmid backbone DNA, and the induction of preferential Th1 response by CpG DNA treatment of intracellular infections (e.g., *Listeria monocytogenes, Leishmania major*) *(61)*.

The introduction of CpG motifs into the backbone of the plasmid DNA has been shown to improve the resultant antigen-specific humoral response and cellular immune responses *(80–82)*. In their role acting as intrinsic adjuvants, CpG motifs enhanced the protective immune response against pathogens *(80, 83)*.

Furthermore, the importance for CpG DNA as an adjuvant for vaccines has been supported by reports that coadministration of CpG DNA and soluble peptide antigen induced Th1-skewed immune responses when compared with administration of peptide antigen alone *(84–87)*.

39.2.1 Mechanism for Recognition of CpG DNA

The mechanism by which CpG DNA did induce a strong Th1 response has been clarified in several models *(67, 68, 88)*. DCs are the main cells linking innate immunity (recognition

of PAMPs and induction of inflammatory responses) with acquired immunity (antigen-specific immune responses; e.g., Th1 responses). Reports from several studies have shown that CpG DNA induced maturation of DCs as demonstrated by the production of IL-12 and expression of costimulatory molecules *(88–90)*. The following model of CpG DNA–induced maturation of DCs has been summarized as follows: CpG DNA is recognized by and induces maturation of DCs leading to production of IL-12. IL-12, in turn, induces the development of Th1 cells from naïve T cells to employ an effective immune response *(61)*.

The major events of CpG DNA–mediated signaling pathways included (i) cellular uptake of CpG DNA; (ii) translocation into the endosome; and (iii) activation of signaling molecules leading to activation of transcriptional factors *(61)*.

Cellular Uptake of CpG DNA. After its binding to the cell surface receptor, the CpG DNA is internalized into the cells *(63)*. The recognition of CpG DNA by the cell surface receptor (still to be defined) and its uptake appeared to have no sequence specificity *(63, 91)*. However, internalization is essential for cellular activation *(91)*.

Localization of CpG DNA in the Endosome. After internalization, CpG DNA is rapidly localized to acidic vesicles of the endosomal-lysosomal compartment in mouse macrophages, which is similar to the endosomal localization of the antisense phosphorothioate oligodeoxyribonucleotide (ODN) in the premyelocytic leukemic cell line HL60 *(92, 93)*.

The CpG DNA–induced activation of immune cells required endosomal activation. There are several hypotheses linking the CpG DNA–induced cellular activation and the endosomal acidification. In the first one, the endosomal acidification is thought to enable the uptaken CpG DNA to dissociate from nonspecific cell surface receptors and bind to a specific receptor in the endosome. In a second hypothesis, the endosomal acidification is essential for the release of the CpG DNA from the endosome to the cytoplasm in which a specific receptor exists. Alternatively, there may be an unknown mechanism for the activation of the CpG DNA signaling pathway *(61)*.

Several inflammatory stimuli, including PAMPs (e.g., LPS), have been shown to activate the mitogen-activated protein kinases (MARKs) such as p38 MARK, the c-JUN NH2-terminal kinase (JNK), and the extracellular receptor kinases (ERKs) *(61, 92, 94)*.

As in the LPS signaling pathway, the CpG DNA–induced activation of JNK was found to lead to phosphorylation of the Ap-1 family of transcription factors, and the activation of p38 led to the activation of transcription factor ATF2 *(61, 92, 94)*.

In addition to these transcription factors, CpG DNA has been demonstrated to activate the NF-κB family of transcription factors responsible for several aspects of inflammatory and immune responses *(95–97)*. In this regard, acidification of the endosome was shown to lead to rapid generation of intracellular reactive oxygen species, followed by NF-κB activation *(96)*.

These and other experiments have clearly indicated that endosomal maturation has been indispensible for activation of nearly all of the CpG DNA–mediated signaling cascades *(61)*.

39.2.2 Recognition of Microbial Components by Innate Immune Cells

Studies on TLR-mediated recognition of microbial pathogens have revealed that both TLR1 and TLR6, which are highly homogeneous *(98)*, did cooperate with TLR2 and have discriminated between the patterns of pathogens *(99–101)*.

39.2.3 Recognition of CpG DNA by Innate Immune Cells

Subsequent to the indication of a role for the TLR family in CpG DNA recognition, experiments on gene deletion led to the elucidation of the CpG receptor, the newly recognized TLR9 *(102)*. The localization of TLR9 is still unknown. Its structural features, however, indicated that TLR9 possess a transmembrane portion as well as signal peptides that are required for extracellular transport of proteins, suggesting that TLR9 is not a cytoplasmic protein *(103)*.

Currently, there has been no evidence to indicate a direct binding of PAMPs (such as CpG DNA) with TLRs *(61)*.

In addition to the role of TLR9 as CpG DNA receptor, data have emerged to demonstrate the involvement of the *catalytic subunit of DNA-dependent protein kinase (DNA-PKcs)* in the CpG DNA–induced immune cell activation *(104)*. DNA-PKcs is a member of the phosphatidyl-inositol-3 kinase (PI-3K) family, localized in the nucleus and cytoplasm. Furthermore, it has been shown that in the nucleus, DNA-PKcs is activated in the process of repair of DNA double-stranded breaks caused by stress-induced damage from ionizing radiation and by programmed DNA rearrangement (the so-called *VDJ recombination*) during the development of T- and B-cells *(105–107)*. However, the role of DNA-PKcs localized in the cytoplasm still remains unclear *(61)*.

39.2.4 CpG ODN as an Th1 Immune Enhancer

Recently, there has been broad interest in the testing and development of oligodeoxynucleotides containing CpG motifs (CpG ODN), which are ligands of TLR9, as enhancers of adaptive immunity and adjuvants for prophylactic and therapeutic vaccines *(62)*.

The ability of CpG DNA to exert direct stimulatory and mitogenic effects on murine and human B-cells and trigger cytokine production, immunoglobulin secretion, and resistance to apoptosis have been well documented *(63,108–112)*. However, not just any unmethylated CpG will be immunostimulatory. Rather, the base context of the CpG dinucleotides is extremely important in establishing whether or not they will be a CpG motif and cause immunostimulatory effects, and what type of immunostimulatory effects they will have *(62)*. For example, if the CpG is preceded by an A, G, or T, and if it is followed by an A, C, or T, then it is likely to trigger immunostimulatory effects *(109)*. In contrast, in vertebrate genomes, CpG dinucleotides are most frequently preceded by a C and/or followed by a G, which will severely reduce their immunostimulatory effects, and the cytosine is almost always methylated, which would abolish any potential stimulatory effect *(113)*. To this end, the immunostimulatory effects of bacterial DNA can be mimicked by synthetic CpG ODN *(62)*.

Based on specific imunostimulatory properties, three main families of CpG ODN with distinct structural and biological characteristics have been identified. Thus, the A class was found to be a potent activator of natural killer (NK) cells and interferon (IFN)-α secretion from DCs, but was a poor stimulator of B cells. In contrast, the B class was a strong B-cell stimulator, but weaker for induction of NK activity or IFN-α. However, both classes had induced Th1-type cytokines *(114)*. The most recently discovered C class has shown properties of both the A and B classes *(115)*.

Because nearly all published studies had been conducted using the *B class CpG ODN* as vaccine adjuvant, it has been commonly accepted to be referred to as the "CpG ODN" *(62)*. However, there has been some experimental evidence that the A and C classes CpG OND may be superior to the B class for induction of CTL responses *(62)*.

Although optimal B class CpG motifs for driving B-cell proliferation have the general formula: purine–purine-C–G-pyrimidine–pyrimidine, there have been some species-specific differences regarding what was the optimal hexamer *(112)*. Thus, the immunostimulatory activity of an ODN is determined not only by the activity of a given hexamer CpG motif but also by several other factors including (i) the number of CpG motifs in an ODN, in which two or three are optimal; (ii) the spacing of the CpG motifs, which are best separated by at least two intervening bases, preferably threonines; (iii) the presence of poly G sequences or other flanking sequences in the ODN; and (iv) the ODN backbone, in which a nuclease-resistant phosphorothioate backbone is best for *in vivo* use *(63, 109, 111, 112, 116, 117)*. In addition, the immunostimulatory effects of the ODN have been enhanced if it has a TpC dinucleotide on the 5' end and is pyrimidine rich on the 3' side *(109, 111, 112)*.

Briefly, the immunostimulatory mechanism of action of CpG ODN effect could be summarized as follows *(114)*: it appears that the CpG ODN would enter the lymphocyte after binding to the cell surface DNA-binding proteins that are not CpG sequence-specific, to end up within the endosomal compartments *(118, 119)*. It appeared that the endosome may be the site of CpG-induced signal initiation *(120–125)*, and this is associated through the TLR9, which would specifically recognize CpG motifs *(62)*.

Other examples in which natural ligands have been identified included TLR2 and TLR6, which have detected proteoglycans, TLR3, which detected double-stranded DNA of RNA viruses, TLR4, which detected endotoxin of Gram-negative bacteria, and TLR5, which detected flagellin *(62)*.

Among human cell types, TLR9 expression was found to be most abundant in B cells and plasmacytoid dendritic cells, which have been the only cell types to be directly activated by CpG ODN *(120, 126)*. The current view is that TLR9 is an essential component of the postulated CpG DNA receptor that is acting upstream of the adaptor protein MyD88 and linking the CpG motif recognition to the TLR/IL-1R signaling pathway *(127)*.

As vaccine adjuvant, the activity of CpG ODN has been identified *(114)*. First, purified B cells have been synergistically activated when stimulated with CpG ODN in the presence of antigen, indicating cross-talk between the B-cell receptor and the CpG signaling pathways *(63)*.

CpG ODN has been shown to exert very potent activity augmenting the humoral and cellular responses to infectious disease antigens including HbsAg *(128–130)*, hepatitis C virus envelope protein *(131)*, herpes simplex virus-2 gD *(132)*, influenza *(133)*, rotavirus *(134)*, HIV gp160 *(135)*, gp120-depleted HIV particles *(136)*, whole killed mycobacterium *(137)*, and the leishmanial protein *(138)*.

Because most pathogens enter the body through one of the vast mucosal surfaces, a number of potentially effective adjuvants have been tested for mucosal immunization. Some effective mucosal adjuvants such as the cholera vaccine and the heat-labile enterotoxin have been studied, and their effects were found to be too toxic for human use and required mutagenesis to reduce the severe adverse effects *(62)*.

In this regard, CpG ODN has been found extremely effective in mice when used as mucosal adjuvant either by intranasal, intraperitoneal, or oral routes *(133,139–145)*. The CpG ODN induced the Th1 immune responses both at systemic and mucosal immune surfaces, as well as mucosal IgA responses at local and distal mucosal sites *(146)*.

The role of CpG ODN as an adjuvant to DNA vaccines is still not clearly identified. By and large, a simple addition of CpG ODN to DNA vaccines has been generally unsuccessful because of the dose-dependent interference of the phospho-

rothioate ODN backbone with the uptake and expression of the plasmid *(147–149)*.

Another factor affecting the CpG optimization of DNA vaccines has been the discovery of neutralizing CpG motifs (CpG-N) *(62)*. To block and/or evade the host defense, some intracellular pathogens have evolved with a reduced number of CpG motifs in their genomes to decrease the immunostimulatory effects. In principle, this evasive mechanism should be much easier for pathogens with small genome than for those with large genomes. Indeed, analyses of the genomes of small DNA viruses and retroviruses have revealed that these pathogens all have very low CpG content *(150–152)*. Nevertheless, large genome viruses, although much less consistent in exhibiting CpG suppression, have evolved CpG-N that can actually block the effects of a stimulatory CpG motif. Thus, serotypes 2 and 5 adenovirus showed a marked skewing in their CpG motifs with a dramatic overrepresentation of immune-neutralizing CpG-N motifs *(62)*.

39.3 Modified Bacterial Toxins

Bacteria produce an array of virulence factors that allow them to invade, colonize, and cause disease in humans and other hosts. Toxins released by bacteria can kill and/or damage host cells and in the process exert powerful immunomodulating activity that can subvert host immune responses. The bacterial toxins target the surface receptors on the host cell causing tissue damage and modulating its signaling pathways involved in multiple physiologic functions such as immune responses *(153)*.

However, because of their immunomodulating properties, bacterial toxins can also enhance immune responses to unrelated antigens, especially when administered via mucosal routes; that is, they can also serve as mucosal adjuvants against a number of infectious diseases.

Bacterial toxins include exotoxins of most Gram-positive and many Gram-negative bacteria that are released extracellularly during multiplication of the organism, as well as endotoxin or LPS, which forms part of the outer layer of the Gram-negative bacterial cell wall and is only released in large amounts following lysis of the cell *(153)*. To counter the effects of bacterial toxins, the host has also evolved a range of strategies including the production of toxin-neutralizing antibodies. Because this adaptive immune response is very effective in a primed host, it has been exploited in the development of antibacterial vaccines based on *detoxified bacterial toxins (153)*.

The local and systemic inflammation is probably the best-characterized immunologic response to bacterial toxins, and although a cause for safety concern, if properly managed, it could provide a powerful means for augmenting the immune responses to coadministered antigens, especially when delivered by mucosal routes. In this regard, the immunogenicity of killed and attenuated bacterial vaccines can be attributed, at least in part, to the adjuvant activity of toxins, together with other cell wall components of the bacteria, as best examplified by killed *Bordetella pertussis,* which as a powerful adjuvant has been used for decades to boost the immune responses to unrelated antigens *(153).*

Furthermore, chemically modified toxoids of diphtheria toxin and tetanus toxin can prevent diseases caused by *Corynebacterium diphtheria* or *Clostridium tetani,* respectively, and genetically or chemically inactivated pertussis toxin (PT) in combination with other virulence factors of *B. pertussis* can protect against whooping cough *(120, 154, 155).* All *pertussis acellar vaccines (Pa)* licenced to date include PT as a component. A monocomponent Pa, based on hydrogen peroxide–treated PT, protected 71% of children in a placebo-controlled trial carried out in Göthenburg, Sweden *(156).* Two-, three-, or five-component Pa, comprising aldehyde or genetically detoxified PT and filamentous hemagglutinin, with or without pertactin and fimbrae, had efficacies of 84% to 85% *(115, 154, 155).*

A genetically detoxified pertussis toxin was created using direct mutagenesis of amino acids in the A subunit involved in ADP-ribosylating activity *(112).* Substitution of Arg_9 to Lys and Glu_{129} to Gly created the mutant PT-9K/129G, which was nontoxic but fully immunogenic. The PT mutant was highly effective at inducing functionally relevant antibody responses at lower doses than those required for the chemically treated PT *(118)* and has induced T-cell responses *(119, 120).*

The diphtheria toxin consists of two disulfide-linked fragments, an enzymatically active A fragment, and a B fragment that is responsible for binding and entry of the toxin into sensitive eukaryotic cells. Protein synthesis in these cells is inhibited by inactivation of the ribosomal elongation factor 2 (caused by the specific ADP-ribosylating activity of fragment A) resulting in cell death *(123).*

Several nontoxic or partially toxic mutants of diphtheria toxin that cross-react immunologically with it [known as *cross-reacting materials (CRMs)*] have been produced and exerted strong immune responses against diphtheria toxin *(153).* One mutant of diphtheria toxin, CRM_{197} (containing a glycine to glutamic acid mutation at position 52 in the A subunit), has been rendered enzymatically inactive and therefore nontoxic *(124).* After stabilization with formaldehyde, the immunogenicity of CRM_{197} has been increased *(125, 157, 158).* In animal models, intranasal immunization with CRM_{197} formulated with chitosan (a cationic polysaccharide derived from chitin with potential for vaccine delivery and as an adjuvant) did induce high levels of antigen-specific IgG, secretory IgA, and toxin-neutralizing

antibodies, as well as predominately Th2 subtype T-cell responses *(158).*

39.4 Cholera Toxin and *Escherichia coli Enterotoxin*

The enterotoxins CT from *Vibrio cholerae* and LT from enterotoxigenic strains of *Escherichia coli* are members of the AB class of bacterial toxins *(153).* Both toxins comprise an enzymatically active A subunit with adenosine-diphosphate (ADP)-ribosyltransferase activity (responsible for toxicity) and a pentameric B oligomer that binds to receptors on the eukaryotic cell surface. The B-subunits of LT (LTB) and CT (CTB) are formed by five monomers that are arranged in a cylinder-like structure with a central cavity *(127, 159–162).* Interaction of LTB and CTB with their cell surface receptors is necessary for internalization of the globular A subunit *(163).*

The basal ADP-ribosyltransferase activity of CT and LT was enhanced by interaction with GTP-binding proteins, known as *ADP-ribosylation factors (ARFs) (164).* The ARFs have played a crucial role in the vesicular membrane trafficking as well as contributing to the maintenance of the organelle integrity and the assembly of coat proteins in eukaryotic cells *(153).*

Both CT and LT have shown powerful mucosal immunogenicity, and low doses induced strong antitoxin secretory and systemic antibody responses, even against bystander molecules that have been present simultaneously at the mucosal surfaces *(160–162, 165, 166).* Consequently, CT and LT have been used extensively as mucosal adjuvants with a wide variety of antigens in animal models and later in clinical trials *(153).*

Coadministration of CT and LT with antigens by nasal, oral, or other mucosal routes has resulted in substantial enhancement of antigen-specific mucosal IgA and serum IgG responses *(153).* In addition, the adjuvant effects of CT and LT have also been demonstrated in studies involving immunization by subcutaneous, intraperitoneal, intravenous, intradermal, and transcutaneous routes *(160–162).*

Besides their ability to enhance humoral immunity, CT and LT have also been shown to augment the cellular immune responses to coadministered antigens. Thus, most studies indicated that CT induced a Th2-biased response to itself and to bystander molecules *(129, 167–177).* However, mixed Th1/Th2 responses have also been reported after oral immunization with CT and keyhole limpet hemocyanin (KLH) *(132),* HIV reverse transcriptase *(133), Helicobacter pylori (134),* or hen egg lysozyme *(135),* and intranasal immunization with fimbrial protein from *Porphyromonas gingivalis (136).*

The B-subunits of LT and CT *(178–184)* have immunomodulatory activities independent of the A subunit *(153)*. Thus, recombinant CTB and LTB have shown activity as mucosal adjuvants, although weaker when compared with holotoxins *(136,169,171,185–187)*. Furthermore, CTB and LTB can also suppress immune responses and induce tolerance to orally or nasally delivered antigens and can prevent experimental autoimmune diseases *(140,141,162,188–192)*.

39.4.1 CT and LT Mutants

During the past few years, site-directed mutagenesis has permitted the generation of LT and CT mutants fully nontoxic or with dramatically reduced toxicity, which still retain their strong adjuvanticity at the mucosal level.

A number of studies have described success in reducing the toxicity of LT and CT without removing the adjuvanticity, mostly by eliminating or attenuating the enzyme activity of the A subunit *(144,145,167,174,193–199)*. Using site-directed mutagenesis to target amino acids in the active site of the toxins that are critical for enzymatic activity has allowed for the preparation of CT and LT mutants with greatly reduced or undetectable toxicity and stability on storage *(153)*.

Initially, it was thought that ADP-ribosylation and accumulation of cAMP were essential for adjuvanticity of CT and LT. However, subsequent efforts have demonstrated that mutants lacking ADP-ribosyltransferase activity have retained their ability to act as mucosal adjuvants *(144,145,167,170,174,193,196–199)*. Thus, two CTA subunit mutants, CTS61F and CTE112K, constructed by site-directed mutagenesis, had no ADP-ribosylation activity and did not promote cAMP production or fluid accumulation in ligated mouse ileal loops; nevertheless, both molecules retained adjuvant activity *(169)*.

CT and LP mutations have also been constructed in the protease sensitive loop of the toxins, rendering the loop insensitive to proteases and therefore eliminating the susceptibility of the toxins to the cleavage required for activation of the enzymatic activity and toxicity *(196–198)*. Like the parent toxins, the mutants enhanced the antibody and T-cell responses to coadministered antigens. For example, the CT mutants CTS61F, CTE112K, and CTE29H have selectively augmented the Th2 responses and IgG1 and IgE *(167, 168, 199)*. Furthermore, the completely nontoxic mutant, LTK63, enhanced the Th2 responses to a protein from serogroup B *Neisseria meningitides* and at high doses the Th1 and Th2 responses, whereas LTR72, which retained 1% of the ADP-ribosyltransferase activity, had a more potent enhancing effect on the Th2 responses; both mutants augmented

the IgG1 and IgG2 antibody responses *(200)*. By contrast, IgG2 was the dominant subclass of antibody induced after intranasal immunization with killed *Candida albicans* and LTR192G *(197)* or influenza virus hemagglutinin and LTR72 *(201)*.

In addition to using site-directed mutagenesis of the A1 subunit, a fusion of the intact CT A1 subunit with a dimer of an Ig-binding fragment D of *Staphylococcus aureus* protein A (CTA1-DD) has also been described. The CTA1-DD was found to be an effective parenteral and mucosal adjuvant able to enhance IgG1 and IgG2 antibodies to coadministered antigens *(202, 203)*.

39.4.2 Mechanism of Adjuvant Action

The mechanism of action of CT and LT has long been controversial, and a number of hypotheses have been put forward to explain the potent immunogenicity and adjuvanticity of these toxins. Thus, the enhanced uptake of antigen at mucosal surfaces has been considered as one mechanism whereby CT and LT may have enhanced the immunogenicity of coupled or coadministered antigens *(153)*.

The activation of cells of the innate immune system leading to potentiation of antigen-presenting cell function and T-cell responses would likely be a key feature in the adjuvant action of CT and LT.

39.5 Pertussis Toxin

The pertussis toxin (PT) is an AB exotoxin and one of the main virulence factors of *Bordetella pertussis (153)*. The B-oligomer, which consists of four noncovalently linked subunits (S2 to S5), in a ratio of 1:1:2:1 *(204,205)*, mediated binding of the toxin to surface glycoproteins (such as lactosylceramide, gangliosides) expressed on a variety of mammalian cells (cilia, macrophages, and lymphocytes) *(206, 207)*. In addition, a 43-kDa plasma-membrane protein *(208)* and CD14 *(209)* have also been proposed as receptors for the pertussis toxin.

Binding of the B-oligomer to host cells will allow the PT's A subunit to enter the host cell where it ADP-ribosylates the G_i proteins. The latter would transmit inhibitory signals to the adenylate cyclase complex (L3) thereby affecting the signaling pathways in many cell types, including cells of the immune system *(210)*, and contributing to the immune dysfunction in infected patients *(153)*. In this regard, it has been shown that the pertussis toxin impaired the delivery of signals promoting the survival of B cells *in vitro (211)*, inhibited macrophage chemotaxis *in vivo (212)*, and neutrophil and lymphocyte chemotaxis *in vitro* by altering the intracellular calcium levels *(213)*. Other abnormalities such as lymphocytosis, histamine sensitization, and hypoglycemia and neurologic responses have also been attributed to the active toxin *(210, 214)*.

Similarly to LT and CT, the pertussis toxin has been shown in mice to possess adjuvant properties by boosting the immune responses to unrelated bystander antigen coadministered by systemic or nasal routes *(215–218)*. There is also indirect evidence for adjuvant effect of PT in humans [e.g., antibody responses to other components of combination vaccines were diminished in the absence of whole cell pertussis vaccines *(219, 220)*]. Furthermore, it has been demonstrated that the adjuvant effect of PT for IgE responses has been associated with augmented production of IL-4 *(217)*.

39.5.1 Pertussis Toxin Mutants

Because of its toxicity and adverse effects on the immune system, the pertussis toxin cannot be used in clinical applications. Although chemical treatment can eliminate the undesirable toxicity of PT, it also affected its antigenicity and immunogenicity and abrogated its adjuvant activity *(122, 123)*. By contrast, recombinant PT molecules with mutations in the S-1 subunit that abrogated the ADP-ribosyltransferase activity were nontoxic and highly immunogenic *(117, 207, 210)*. Moreover, these mutants may also retain their immunopotentiating activities of the native toxin that had been lost through chemical toxoiding *(153)*.

Several genetically engineered mutants of pertussis toxin have been developed and compared with the native toxin for enzymatic activity and immunomodulatory characteristics *(112, 207, 210, 221)*. Replacing the one or two key amino acids within the enzymatically active S-1 subunit yielded PT mutants with indistinguishable subunit binding pattern from the native toxin and the ability to modulate immune responses to unrelated antigens *(153)*.

In contrast with the S-1 mutant, a toxin with mutations in both the enzyme and binding domain did not display adjuvant activity, suggesting that binding of pertussis toxin to its receptor although essential was not necessarily the only feature of adjuvanticity *(215)*.

39.5.2 Mechanisms of Adjuvant Activity

Although the precise mechanism of action is not well understood, it appears that the pertussis toxin functions as an adjuvant by activating both the innate and adaptive immune responses and targeting both the antigen-presenting cells and

T cells *(153)*. Binding of PT to the surface receptors of cells of the innate and acquired immune system will activate the signaling pathways involved in the cytokine secretion as well as the accessory molecule expression.

The pertussis toxin and its nontoxic mutants activated the macrophages to secrete IL-1β and to upregulate surface expression of the costimulatory molecules CD80 and CD86 on macrophages *(215)* and DCs *(222, 223)*. In addition, the pertussis toxin also induced proliferation, IL-2 and INF-γ secretion by T cells, and augmented their surface expression of the costimulatory molecule CD28 *(215)*.

Recent studies have demonstrated the presence of synergy between the pertussis toxin and LPS in enhancing DC maturation, specifically IL-12 *(223)*, and promoting the generation of DCs that direct the differentiation of Th1 cells *(224)*.

39.5.3 Adenylate Cyclase Toxin

The adenylate cyclase toxin (CyaA) from *B. pertussis* is a major virulence factor and plays a central role in the pathogenicity of *B. pertussis (225)*. CyaA is released by the pathogen and can be taken up by many cell types in which it catalyzes the conversion of cellular ATP to cAMP *(226)*.

CyaA represents a bifunctional protein having a hemolysin enzyme domain that is critical for its entry into host cells and an adenylate cyclase domain that elevates the intracellular cAMP *(227)*. When elevated, the intracellular cAMP will interfere with the intracellular signaling in cells of the immune system and will modulate an array of immune effector functions, such as the oxidative responses and the TNF-α production by monocytes or macrophages and will also induce apoptosis of macrophages *(227, 228)* and DCs *(229)*. Similarly to cholera toxin *(230)*, CyaA enhanced the cell surface expression of CD40 and ICAM-1 *(231)*.

Recombinant CyaA mutants with disruptions in the adenylate cyclase catalytic domain (but with cell invasive activity) have been used to deliver unrelated foreign peptides and proteins to the cytosol and for the induction of class I–restricted CTLs *(232)*.

Recent results have shown that CyaA was an effective parenteral adjuvant by being able to induce Th2 and Tr1 (a population of T cells with regulatory or suppressive activity) cells and an IgG1-dominated serum IgG response *(232)*.

39.6 Monophosphoryl Lipid A and Synthetic Lipid A Mimetics

The monophosphoryl lipid A (MPL, a vaccine adjuvant from Corixa Corp., Seattle, US), a derivative of lipopolysaccharide

(LPS), is primarily obtain from *Salmonella minnesota* R595. It retains much of the immunomodulatory properties of LPS but without the inherent toxicity and has been used as an adjuvant for parenteral administration of antigens *(152, 233)*.

RC-529 is a synthetic lipid A mimetic of MPL with promising adjuvant activity *(233)*.

The LPS, a constituent of the outer surface of all Gram-negative bacteria, possesses powerful immunomodulating properties by stimulating the inflammatory responses. Thus, at submicromolar concentrations, LPS was able to dramatically elevate the levels of a number of proinflammatory cytokines (IL-1, IL-6, TNF-α, and IL-12) *(234, 235)*. However, LPS-induced disruption in the balance of proinflammatory and anti-inflammatory mediators can result in endotoxic shock (sometimes fatal) that makes LPS too toxic to be used in humans *(153)*.

A note of historical interest: More than a century ago, a New York physician, William B. Coley, noted that some cancer patients experienced spontaneous tumor regression after episodes of acute bacterial illness *(236)*. Hypothesizing a correlation between the bacterial infection and tumor regression, Dr. Coley started to treat cancer patients successfully with heat-killed bacterial cultures known as the *Coley's Toxins*. It is now realized that the Coley's Toxins contained a number of TLR agonists, including LPS, which undoubtedly stimulated the innate immunity of Dr. Coley's cancer patients leading to nonspecific tumor regression *(233, 236)*.

Because it was the lipid A portion of LPS that was found responsible for its adjuvanticity and toxicity, its chemical modifications resulted in the production of less toxic compounds. Thus, mild acid hydrolysis of lipid A and removal of a base-labile fatty acyl residue attached to carbon 3 of the diglucosamine backbone led to the synthesis of the monophosphoryl lipid A. Subsequent experiments have shown MPL displaying dramatically reduced toxicity compared with LPS coupled with potent adjuvant activity *(237, 238)*.

Drawing from the experience with MPL, a number of novel synthetic lipid A mimetics, known as *aminoalkyl glucosaminide 4-phosphates (AGPs)*, have been synthesized containing chemically unique acylated monosaccharides *(239)*. The rationale for the synthesis of AGPs was that a conformationally flexible aglycon unit would permit energetically favored close packing of the six fatty acyl chains; tight packing of six fatty acids in a hexagonal array is believed to play an essential role in the bioactivity of lipid A–like molecules *(240)*. Moreover, recent evidence has suggested that the interaction of lipid A and its analogues with the pattern recognition receptor TLR4 is determined in part by the conformational shape and supramolecular assembly of the compounds in solution, which in turn is dependent on the fatty acid chain length and their three-dimensional arrangement in space *(241–243)*.

In preclinical studies, one of the AGPs, RC-529, has demonstrated adjuvant activity very similar to to that induced by MPL. Clinical experience with RC-529 (the clinical Good Manufacturing Practice (GMP) product is called *Ribi.529*) did indicate that this synthetic lipid A analogue is a safe and effective vaccine adjuvant *(244)*.

The mechanism of action of MPL has not been defined clearly. Nevertheless, it is believed to be similar to LPS by involving interaction with TLR4 and CD14 that resulted in the activation of NF-κB and the production of proinflammatory cytokines *(245)*. The adjuvant activity of MPL has been primarily attributed to its ability to activate the cell-presenting cells and to elicit cytokine production, in particular IL-12 by DCs and macrophages, resulting in the induction of antigen-specific cellular immunity and enhancement of complement fixing antibodies *(246, 247)*.

39.7 Clinical Experience with Modified Bacterial Toxins

Chemically detoxified diphtheria toxin, tetanus toxin, and chemically or genetically detoxified pertussis toxin have been used in routine pediatric diphtheria, tetanus, and pertussis (DTP) vaccines for several decades *(246, 247)*. Moreover, tetanus toxoid and diphtheria toxoids, because of their acceptance for human use and availability, have been used as carriers for polysaccharide vaccines in humans *(248)*. Recently, CRM[197], a nontoxic analogue of diphtheria toxin, has been used as a carrier for the *Haemophilus influenzae* type b capsular polysaccharide vaccine in humans *(248)*.

The MPL adjuvant has been extensively evaluated in clinical trials with infectious disease, cancer, and allergy vaccines containing the MPL adjuvant alone or in combination with other adjuvants, including alum, cell wall skeleton of *Mycobacterium phlei*, or QS-21 *(233)*.

An adjuvant formulation consisting of MPL and QS-21 in combination with an emulsion system has also been evaluated in clinical trials with malaria *(249)* and HIV *(250)* vaccines. Furthermore, several clinical trials have demonstrated that the inclusion of MPL adjuvant in a hepatitis B vaccine enhanced the rate of seroprotection *(251, 252)*.

A herpes vaccine formulated with MPL adjuvant has been shown to yield significant protection against genital herpes in women who were seronegative for both herpes simplex virus (HSV)-1 and HSV-2 before vaccination *(241)*. The vaccine elicited both binding and neutralizing antibodies against HSV and cellular responses as indicated by the lymphoproliferation and IFN-γ secretion. The results of the trial are deemed to be potentially important because no other vaccine has been shown to prevent genital HSV infection. It is thought that the MPL adjuvant exerted Th1-biasing activity [233].

The safety and efficacy of an investigational nine-valent pneumococcal-CRM[197] protein conjugate vaccine (PCV9) combined with 10, 25, or 50 μg MPL adjuvant in the presence or absence of alum was recently evaluated in 129 healthy children [253]. A dose-dependent effect of the MPL adjuvant on the antigen-specific cellular immune responses has been reported. Addition of 10 μg MPL adjuvant to the antigen in the absence of alum significantly enhanced CRM[197]-specific T-cell proliferation and IFN-γ production compared with that of the antigen plus alum.

To explore the possibility that MPL, a Th1-inducing adjuvant, might have potential utility in vaccines designed to treat human allergies, a placebo-controlled, randomized, double-blind clinical study has been conducted with a standardized allergy vaccine consisting of a tyrosine-absorbed glutaraldehyde-modified grass pollen extract containing MPL adjuvant [254]. The MPL adjuvant–containing vaccine was significantly better than placebo at reducing the nasal and ocular symptoms as well as in eliciting a marked reduction in the sensitivity to skin-prick testing. The vaccine is now available in a number of countries as Pollinex Quattro [233].

39.7.1 Safety Implications for Use of Bacterial Toxins in Vaccines

Parenteral administration of bacterial toxins can result in various adverse reactions ranging from mild local inflammation to severe systemic and neurologic disorders [153]. Nevertheless, bacterial toxins could act as important protective antigens, and antitoxin antibodies can prevent the bacterial disease caused by the parent bacteria. In this regard, modification of toxins by treatment with aldehydes would make them nontoxic without abrogating their capacity to generate toxin-neutralizing antibodies. However, the use of glutaraldehyde or formaldehyde prior to purification may result in relatively impure preparations with other bacterial components including other bacterial components such as cell wall components cross-linked to the toxoids. Such impurities may contribute to the reactogenicity of the DTP (diphtheria, tetanus, pertusis) combination vaccines. For example, DTP was highly reactogenic when the pertussis component was whole cell, and although it has been significantly reduced with the introduction of the acellular pertussis vaccine, DT alone or DTPs vaccines still induce a significant number of local and systemic reactions [153]. In fact, the whole-cell pertussis vaccine is considered one of the most reactogenic vaccines in clinical use today causing systemic centrally controlled responses, including fevers and seizures [214, 255, 256].

Nasal immunization with vaccine formulations that include native or modified bacterial toxins as antigens or adjuvants may also pose a risk of neurologic side effects linked with the direct transport from the nose to the brain through the olfactory bulb [153, 257].

In contrast with the proinflammatory effects associated with the induction of IL-1, TNF-α, and IFN-γ, enhancement of IL-4, IL-5, and IgE responses by vaccines and adjuvants may also carry certain risks in relation to possible induction or enhancement of anaphylactic or allergic reactions. For example, CT (but not LT) has been known to augment the IgE responses [258–261]. To this end, the currently used adjuvant for most subunit vaccines in humans, alum, is also enhancing the IgE production to the antigenic components of the vaccines. Significant local adverse reactions, including swelling, have also been reported with increasing booster doses of DTPs administered parenterally with alum as an adjuvant [262]. Therefore, the substitution of alum (which is known to enhance Th2 and IgE responses) with adjuvants that promote the induction of Th1 cells may not only reduce the incidence of these local reactions but also improve the efficacy of the vaccines [153].

39.8 Glycosylphosphatidylinositol Anchors from Protozoan Parasites

Parasitic invasion of a human host will evolve into an intimate association between two different organisms in which one, the human host, will provide food and shelter for the parasite, which in return may or may not injure the host. In the case of the intracellular protozoan parasites, the host immune system plays a critical role in controlling the parasite replication and maintaining a balanced interaction between the parasite and the host, until the parasite encounters the transmitting factor or is shed to the environment to propagate its life cycle [263].

Taken together, it seems plausible that a successful cohabitation between human hosts and parasites would emerge from parasites being able to manage balancing their mechanisms of *evasion and activation* of the host immune system, so that they can establish parasitism but at the same time limit their replication to avoid excessive tissue damage contributing to host lethality [263].

Cell-mediated immunity is the main compartment of the immune system involved in the resistance of vertebrate hosts against the intracellular protozoan parasites [264]. The activation of the immune system observed during the early stages of infection depends on the ability of the protozoan parasites to elicit the synthesis of the proinflammatory cytokine IL-12 by the monocytic lineage cells of the innate immune system

(265–267), which in turn will initiate the synthesis of high levels of IFN-γ by the natural killer cells *(263)*.

Although the release of IL-12 and IFN-γ appears to be an important stage in host resistance to infection with different protozoan parasites such as *Leishmania* spp., *Plasmodium* spp., *Toxoplasma gondii*, and *Trypanozoma cruzi (268–271)*, the balance between evasion and activation of host immunity would depend on the nature of the protozoan species. Thus, for *Leishmania* spp., which are slow-growing parasites and obligatory macrophage residents, *evasion must prevail* over activation of innate immunity so that they can establish parasitism. In contrast, for more virulent protozoan parasites (*T. gondii* and *T. cruzi*), which infect and replicate inside any nucleated cell from the vertebrate host, *strong stimulation* of the host innate immunity and high levels of proinflammatory cytokines (IL-12, IFN-γ, TNF-α) would be essential *(272–274)*.

Several studies have clearly documented the immunostimulating and regulatory activities of the glycosylphosphatidylinositol (GPI) anchors derived from the membrane of protozoan parasites such as *P. falciparum*, *T. brucei*, and *T. cruzi (275–280)*.

The most fundamental function of the GPI anchors is to allow a stable association of proteins to the cell surface plasma membrane *(281)*. The GPI anchors, which are also found on the surface of protozoan parasites in its free form (i.e., not attached to any surface protein), are known as glycoinositolphospholipids (GIPLs) *(263)*.

Structure of GPI Anchors. The basic GPI structure comprises a hydrophilic core with a conserved domain of Manα1-2Manα1-6Manα1-4GlcNα1-6*myo*-inositol-1-HPO₄. Variant-related structures have been associated with this conserved domain as a result of phosphorylated substituents such as ethanolamine phosphate or 2-aminoethylphosphonate and extra carbohydrate residues. The ethanolamine phosphate or the 2-aminoethylphosphonate will serve as the point of attachment to the GPI for the parasite surface proteins. The other extremity of the conserved hydrophilic domain comprises a *myo*-inositol ring followed by a phosphate that is covalently linked to the hydrophobic moiety of the GPI anchor. In the case of *T. cruzi*, the hydrophobic moiety of the GPI anchors consists, in most cases, of alkylacylglycerol or ceramide lipid *(272, 281)*.

Studies using gas chromatography–mass spectrometry and electrospray ionization–mass spectrometry to define the structures of various GPI anchors and GIPLs from *T. cruzi* have demonstrated that GPI anchors derived from the trypomastigote developmental stage of *T. cruzi* were highly active in inducing TNF-α, IL-12, and nitric oxide by IFN-γ–primed murine macrophages *(276, 277)*.

To exert maximal biological activity, an intact GPI anchor was necessary to contain in its phosphatidylinositol (PI) moiety mainly unsaturated (C18:1 or C18:2) fatty acids in the *sn*-2 position of the glycerol residue of the alkylacylglycerolipid as well as extra galactose residues in the glycan *(263)*. The absence of these components in the less active GPI anchors may be indicative for such structural elements to be responsible for the extreme potency of GPI anchors derived from the *T. cruzi* tripomastigotes in eliciting the synthesis of proinflammatory cytokines by the macrophages *(263)*.

T. cruzi–Derived GPI Anchors as Potential Immunologic Adjuvants. Recent studies have shown that the GPI anchors derived from *T. cruzi* trypomastigotes represent one of the most powerful stimulants of Toll-like receptor 4 (TLR4) *(277, 282)* and have induced macrophages to produce high levels of proinflammatory cytokines leading to IFN-γ production by natural killer cells. Moreover, because DCs express TLR2 *(283, 284)*, *T. cruzi*–derived CPI anchors may potentially stimulate the maturation of DCs. Results from these and other studies may indicate the possibility that using *T. cruzi*–derived GPI anchors as adjuvants would lead to a less polarized Th1 response compared with LPS *(263)*. However, the ability to induce a polarized Th1 response could be circumvented if *T. cruzi*–derived anchors are used in association with other adjuvant molecules such as α-galactosyl ceramide *(285)*, which induces the production of INF-γ response by natural killer cells in an IL-12–independent manner *(263)*.

To date, the main obstacle to use *T. cruzi*–derived GPI anchors as immunologic adjuvants lies in the difficulties of producing large quantities of synthetic glycolipids such as complex oligosaccharides containing defined carbohydrate sequences, which would be a labor-intensive and time-consuming process *(263)*.

39.9 Helminth Glycan LNFPIII/Lewis X

The immune response to most bacterial and viral pathogens is generally associated with the production of proinflammatory cytokines such as IL-12, IFN-γ, TNF-α, and IL-18, leading to maturation of CD4⁺ Th1-type effector cells *(286, 287)*. In contrast, results from numerous studies both in humans and animal experiments have demonstrated that infections with helminth parasites or injecting extracts from helminths have promoted polarized Th2-type CD4⁺ T-cell immune responses characterized by production of IL-4, IL-5, IL-10, IL-13, and often large amounts of IgE antibodies *(288–293)*. Moreover, by producing the immunoregulatory cytokine IL-10, which downregulates IFN-γ, a helminth infection can induce immune anergy by reducing expression of the MHC and costimulatory molecules on the APCs *(294–297)*.

These helminth-induced Th2-type immune responses have been largely directed at helminth-expressed carbohydrates. A number of glycan structures from helminths have been identified with the Lewis X and other fucosylated sugars being prominent *(288)*.

The Lewis X was originally identified from *Schistosoma mansoni*, but now has been found common among many helminths. The human milk sugar lacto-*N*-fucopentaose III (LNFPIII) contains the Lewis X trisaccharide *(288)*. Experiments using synthetically produced LNFPIII, polyvalently linked to a backbone/carrier molecule, have demonstrated that this carbohydrate can produce some of the immunologic effects associated with the Th2 response in schistosome-infected mice, including B-cell proliferation and IL-10 and prostaglandin E$_2$ production *(298)*.

The Lewis X glucan has also been studied in chronically schistosome-infected patients *(297)*. These patients displayed a profound IL-10–induced anergy and showed decreased proliferation of their peripheral blood mononuclear cells to stimulation with the schistosome antigen. However, proliferation has been restored and the IL-10 levels reduced when the peripheral blood mononuclear cells had been pretreated with free monovalent LNFPIII. Hence, it has been hypothesized that although polyvalent LNFPIII activates cells to produce IL-10, the monovalent LNFPIII might actually work to block the same activity by interfering with the interaction between polyvalent LNFPIII and a receptor complex *(288)*.

Studies on LNFPIII/Lewis X conjugate activation on murine DCs to determine whether this is a potential mechanism behind the adjuvant activity of LNFPIII/Lewis X have demonstrated that LNFPIII when used as a multivalent conjugate has been capable of activating immature bone marrow–derived DCs and inducing their maturation to DCs type 2 (DC2) *(299)*. It has been hypothesized that LNFPIII/Lewis X did activate the cells through TLR4 by inducing a MyD88-independent signaling pathway that gave rise to a DC2 maturational pathway.

When the LNFPIII/Lewis X conjugate was mixed with alum, a significant synergistic effect yielded increases in the IgG end-points from 9- to 10-fold higher than the levels seen in mice immunized with human serum albumin (HSA) -LNFPIII of HSA-alum alone *(288)*. The synergy in antibody responses suggested that this combination of adjuvants could safely be employed for antigens that are poorly immunogenic; however, caution should be applied when testing such combination because of the small increase in IgE antibodies *(288)*.

39.10 Muramyl Peptides: Murabutide

Since 1974, when the parent molecule, *N*-acetylmuramyl-*L*-alanyl-*D*-isoglutamine (muramyl dipeptide; MDP) was synthesized *(300)*, several hundred derivatives have been prepared by chemical modifications and substitutions in their sugar and/or amino acid moieties. Currently, the muramyl peptides have been divided into two major classes: hydrophilic and hydrophobic analogues *(301)*.

The hydrophilic derivatives have been synthesized with the aim of reducing the frequently observed MDP toxicities, including pyrogenicity, transient leukopenia, sensitization to endotoxin, and induction of arthritis *(302, 303)*. The lipophilic (hydrophobic) analogues have been prepared to reproduce the antitumor activity of bacterial cell walls, which have a high lipid content, and are able to inhance the limited adjuvant activity of MDP when administered as an aqueous solution *in vivo (301)*.

The biological activities of the different muramyl peptides, which have been well documented *(304–307)*, have been significantly increased by polymerization, conjugation with an appropriate carrier, or incorporation into liposomes *(308, 309)*. These approaches are believed to enhance the uptake by the reticuloendothelial system and the bioavailability of immunostimulants. As a whole, the studies led to the selection of several analogues from both classes. Among the hydrophilic derivatives that eventually have reached the clinical stage of development were murabutide (*N*-acetyl-muramyl-*L*-glutaminyl-*N*-butyl ester), temurtide (threonyl-MDP), nor-MDP (*N*-acetyl-glucosamin-3-yl-acetyl-*L*-alanyl-*D*-isoglutamine), and GMDP [*N*-acetyl-*D*-glucosaminyl-β (1, 4)-*N*-acetyl-muramyl-*L*-alanyl-*D*-isoglutamine]. From the lipophilic class, the three major analogues for clinical development included romurtide [MDP-Lys[L18]; N^2-[(*N*-acetylmuramyl)-*L*-alanyl-*D*-isoglutaminyl]-N^6-stearoyl-*L*-lysine], MTP-PE (muramyl-tripeptide phosphatidylethanolamine), and ImmTher (*N*-acetyl-glucosaminyl-*N*-acetylmuramyl-*L*-alanyl-glyceryl dipalmitate) *(302,305–307)*. In addition, the biological activities of the muramyl dipeptides extended far beyond the initially described adjuvant activity to target cells of the immune, hematopoietic, and central nervous system that have been described extensively *(301, 302, 306, 307, 310)*.

39.10.1 Murabutide: Safety and Adjuvant Activity

Murabutide was selected for clinical development based on its water solubility, apyrogenicity, and adjuvant activity *(301, 311)*. Murabutide did not show the toxicities (CNS and inflammatory responses, including distress syndrome in guinea pigs, autoimmune thyroiditis in the mouse, adjuvant polyarthritis in mice and rats, and toxic synergism with lipopolysaccharide) usually attributed to MDP *(311–314)*.

With regard to the adjuvant activity of murabutide, it has been clearly demonstrated that when given intraperitoneally (but not orally), murabutide exerted adjuvant effects identical to those of MDP *(311)*. Thus, when administered with an antigen, murabutide enhanced the antibody responses *in vivo*, and the titers of total antibodies produced in the presence of murabutide were equivalent to those detected using alum hydroxide as adjuvant *(311, 315)*. To this end, the combination of alum-containing vaccine with murabutide was found to induce higher titers of antibodies than did the vaccine alone. Moreover, cell-mediated immunity against the antigenic component could be detected more efficiently in the murabutide-supplemented vaccine *(301)*.

Using synthetic hepatitis B antigen conjugated to a toxoid carrier and comparing the adjuvanticity of murabutide, alum hydroxide, and Freund's complete adjuvant (FCA), it was shown that high-titered antibodies against the synthetic hepatitis B antigen could be generated with any of the three adjuvants. However, the use of murabutide resulted in modulating the antibody specificity allowing a better recognition of the natural hepatitis antigen *(316)*.

Subsequently, even though the optimal murabutide dosage to include in the vaccine preparations is yet to be determined, murabutide has been evaluated and has shown adjuvant activity to a natural streptococcal M protein vaccine in adults *(317)* and to a weakly immunogenic fluid-phase tetanus vaccine in children *(318)*.

Because murabutide alone or in combination with antigens did not elicit detectable antibodies against its own structure, this nonimmunogenicity would allow its use in the same subject on repeated occasions *(301)*.

39.10.2 Murabutide-Mediated Suppression of HIV-1 Replication

Even with the successful advent of the highly active antiretroviral therapy (HAART) for the management of HIV/AIDS, as the only strategy HAART is insufficient to eliminate the pool of latently infected cells and to bring about normalization of the immune functions. Therefore, immune-based strategies are being investigated to correct the considerable immune dysfunction caused by the HIV infection in cells implicated in the innate and acquired immunity. One such strategy would be to involve the use of nonspecific immunomodulators to restore the capacity of the APCs in mounting an efficient and protective response against HIV *(301)*.

Based on its ability to regulate the function of cells of the innate immune system, murabutide has been evaluated for its effects on HIV-infected macrophages and DCs. Surprisingly, stimulation of acutely infected cells with murabutide led to a marked inhibition of HIV replication and to release of HIV-suppressive β-chemokines *(301)*. However, the two phenomena were not directly linked because neutralization

of the released chemokines by polyclonal antibodies had no measurable effect on the observed viral inhibition *(319)*. On the other hand, experiments aimed at defining the steps in the virus cycle that were blocked or inhibited by murabutide revealed that it significantly interferred with the nuclear transport of the HIV preintegration complexes and with the virus transcription. Whereas these effects did not target the virus directly, they appeared to correlate with the regulation of different cellular factors needed at critical steps of the HIV replication process *(301)*.

Two recent Phase I/IIa clinical studies have been carried out employing single and repeated administrations of murabutide in 30 HIV-1–infected patients under HAART *(320)*. The results have clearly indicated the excellent clinical tolerance of murabutide in HIV-infected patients and provided further evidence on the capacity of murabutide to induce the release of HIV-suppressive β-chemokines without any detrimental effect on viral loads and CD4 counts *(301)*.

Another study, which was conducted in 18 HIV-1–infected, antiretroviral (ARV)-naïve patients, has addressed the safety and biological effects after a 6-week cycle of immunotherapy with murabutide, given for 5 consecutive days per week for a period of 6 weeks, at a daily dose of 7 mg (generally corresponding to 0.1 mg/kg) *(321)*. The results of this clinical trial provided unambiguous evidence for the safety of long-term administration of murabutide in patients who were not receiving any antiretroviral therapy and more importantly for the efficacy of nonspecific immunotherapy to potentiate the immune responses, including those directed against HIV *(321)*.

39.11 Quillaja Saponins: QS-21

The triterpene saponin, QS-21, is a purified natural product isolated from the bark of *Quillaja saponaria* Molina, a tree native to Chile and Argentina *(322)*. Structurally, the plant saponins represent glycosides in which an oligosaccharide or oligosaccharides are linked to an aglycone consisting of a triterpene or steroid *(323)*. Most saponins have the same triterpene base, quillaic acid, and are acylated 3,28-bisdesmonosides in which the oligosaccharide is linked to the 3- and 28-carbons of the quillaic acid.

The structural differences between the unique saponins are primarily found in their glycosylation or acylation patterns. Compared with other non-*Quillaja* saponins, QS-21 has two distinct structural features: the presence of an aldehyde group on the triterpene moiety and a glycosylated acyl domain. The latter can be easily removed by mild alkaline hydrolysis. The predominant site of acylation is the C4-hydroxyl of the fucose moiety, although an intramolecular acyl migration between the hydroxyl groups at C3 and C4 of the fucose did occur in aqueous solution; this acyl migration did not appear to affect the adjuvant activity of QS-21 *(324)*.

Saponin Structure and Adjuvant Activity. The *Quillaja* saponins have long been known for their adjuvant activity *(325–327)*. The differences in their structures have affected their biological activities, such as the adjuvant function, effects on cell membranes, and the toxicity. In this regard, QS-21 has shown strong adjuvant activity coupled with minimal toxicity *(328)*.

The triterpene aldehyde group of QS-21 has been found critical for its adjuvant activity on the antibody and CTL responses *(329)*. Any modification of the aldehyde group would severely diminish the adjuvant effect of QS-21. One possible mechanism involving the aldehyde might be the formation of a Schiff base, with a free amino group on the cellular target to stabilize a cellular interaction such as the one involving free amino groups on APCs and aldehyde on the T cells *(330)*. However, it should be noted that QS-21 was a highly effective adjuvant to hydrophilic polysaccharides that do not possess amino groups, suggesting that formation of a saponin-antigen complex may not be essential for strong immune responses *(322)*.

A broad dose range study (0 to 240 μg) in mice demonstrated that the acyl domain has been critical to Th1-type responses (IgG2a and CTL) but less critical to the Th2 type responses (IgG1) *(331)*. Furthermore, reacylation of DS-1 (the deacylated QS-21) at a *different* site (the glucuronic acid carboxyl group) with dodecilamine of the QS-21 molecule yielded a product (RDS-1) with diminished adjuvant activity *(331)*. RDS-1 did not produce CTL responses to ovalbune (OVA) even at doses above 200 μg.

QS-21 congeners in which the glucuronic acid carboxyl group was modified with ethylamine, ethylenediamine, or glycine through an amide bond (creating neutral, cationic, and anionic analogues at physiologic pH, respectively) retained their adjuvant activity for antibody and CTL responses to OVA albeit at higher (two- to sixfold) threshold doses compared with that of native QS-21 *(329)*.

39.11.1 QS-21 Effects on Adaptive Immune Responses

Humoral Immune Responses. In a number of preclinical and clinical studies, QS-21 has been shown to have strong adjuvant effect for antibody responses with a number of different antigens *(332–337)*. For example, addition of 100 μg QS-21 to HIV-1 gp120 *(338)*, a malaria simplified by removing the "NANP" peptide *(339)*, and to GM2-KLH (a vaccine consisting of GM2 ganglioside conjugated with the immunostimulant keyhole limpet hemocyanin (KLH)) *(340, 341)* resulted in improved antibody responses in clinical studies. In a human clinical vaccine study of an experimental HIV-1 vac-

cine in healthy uninfected volunteers, QS-21 enabled the use of a 100-fold reduced gp120 antigen dose to yield comparable neutralizing antibody titers to an alum hydroxide–adjuvanted vaccine *(338)*.

The use of QS-21 in experimental vaccines in mice typically resulted in both strong IgG1 and IgG2a responses *(328, 332, 333, 342, 343)*. The stimulation of the IgG2a responses suggested that QS-21 stimulated the Th1 cytokines, in contrast with the response induced by standard adjuvants such as aluminum hydroxide, which is primarily limited to IgG1 response (associated with a Th2 cytokine pattern).

In addition to standard parenteral routes of administration, QS-21 has also been used successfully in intranasal immunization with HIV envelope DNA *(335)* and oral administration with tetanus toxoid in mice *(342)*. In the oral administration of QS-21 and tetanus toxoid, it appeared that IL-4 was critical for secretory IgA responses in fecal and vaginal washes *(342)*.

Cellular Immune Responses. The generation of cytotoxic T-lymphocytes (CD8$^+$) generally will require the expression of endogenous antigen that can enter the cytosol and associate with the class I MHC. Subunit antigens, in the absence of adjuvant, will typically act as "exogenous" antigens that will not enter the class I MHC antigen processing/presentation pathway *(344)*. However, certain strategies (the use of liposomal formulations or particulate antigens) can be employed to alter the pathway for exogenous antigens. To this end, QS-21 was also found to facilitate an exogenous antigen to be presented by the class I MHC pathway. It stimulated the CTL responses to subunit vaccines in mice; examples included ovalbumin *(345)*, HIV gp120 *(346)*, respiratory syncytial virus (RSV) fusion protein *(334)*, and the soluble mutant RAS protein *(347)*.

39.11.2 QS-21 Effects on Innate Immune Responses

QS-21 has been shown to stimulate the secretion of cytokines (TNF-α, IL-6) from murine macrophages in *in vitro* culture, as well as natural killer cell activity *(348)*. Administration of a single dose of QS-21 in the absence of adjuvant appeared to protect mice from a subsequent challenge with *Listeria monocytogenes* 3 days later *(322)*.

References

1. Hackett, C. J., Rotrosen, D., Auchincloss, H., and Fauci, A. S. (2007) Immunology research: challenges and opportunities in a time of budgetary constraint, *Nat. Immunol.,* **8**, 114–117.
2. Hackett, C. J. and Harn, D. A. (eds.) (2006) *Vaccine Adjuvants: Immunological and Clinical Principles*, Humana Press, Totowa, NJ, pp. *v–vi*.

3. Janaway, C. A., Jr. (1989) Approaching the asymptote? Evolution and revolution in immunology, *Cold Spring Harb Symp Quant Biol.*, **54**(Part 1), 1–13.

4. Lindblad, E. B. (2004) Aluminum adjuvants – in retrospect and prospects, *Vaccine*, **22**(27–28), 3658–3668.

5. Pulendran, B. and Ahmed, R. (2006) Translating innate immunity into immunological memory: implications for vaccine development, *Cell*, **124**(4), 849–863.

6. Mescher, M. F., Curtsinger, J. M., and Jenkins, M. (2006) Adjuvants and the initiation of T-cell response. In: *Vaccine Adjuvants: Immunological and Clinical Principles* (Hackett, C. J. and Harn, D. A., Jr., eds.), Humana Press, Totowa, NJ, pp. 49–67.

7. Dresser, D. W. (1961) Effectiveness of lipid and lipidophilic substances as adjuvants, *Nature*, **191**, 1169–1171.

8. Dresser, D. W. (1962) Specific inhibition of antibody production. II. Paralysis induced in adult mice by small quantities of protein antigen, *Immunology*, **5**, 378–388.

9. Kearney, E., Pape, K., Loh, D., and Jenkins, M. (1994) Visualization of peptide-specific T cell immunity and peripheral tolerance induction in vivo, *Immunity*, **1**, 327–339.

10. Pape, K. A., Khoruts, A., Mondino, A., and Jenkins, M. K. (1997) Inflammatory cytokines enhance the in vivo clonal expansion and differentiation of antigen-activated CD4$^+$ T cells, *J. Immunol.*, **159**, 591–598.

11. Schmidt, C. S. and Mescher, M. F. (1999) Adjuvant effect of IL-12: conversion of peptide antigen administration from tolerizing to immunizing for CD8$^+$ T cells in vivo, *J. Immunol.*, **163**, 2561–2567.

12. Kiburtz, D., Aichele, P., Speiser, D., Hengartner, H., Zinkernagel, R., and Pircher, H. (1993) T cell immunity after a viral infection versus T cell tolerance induced by soluble viral peptides, *Eur. J. Immunol.*, **23**, 1956–1962.

13. Lafferty, K. J. and Cunningham, A. J. (1975) A new analysis of allogeneic interactions, *Aust. J. Exp. Biol. Med. Sci.*, **53**, 27–42.

14. Allison, J. P. (1994) CD28-B7 interactions in T cell activation, *Curr. Opin. Immunol.*, **6**, 414–419.

15. Janeway, C. A. and Bottomly, K. (1994) Signals and signs for lymphocyte responses, *Cell*, **76**, 275–285.

16. Jenkins, M. K. and Johnson, J. G. (1993) Molecules invoved in T-cell costimulation, *Curr. Opin. Immunol.*, **5**, 361–367.

17. Lafferty, K. J., Prowse, S. J., Simeonovic, C. J., and Warren, H. S. (1983) Immunobiology of tissue transplantation: a return to the passenger leukocyte concept, *Annu. Rev. Immunol.*, **1**, 143–173.

18. Mueller, D., Jenkins, M., and Schwatrz, R. (1989) Clonal expansion vs. functional clonal inactivation, *Annu. Rev. Immunol.*, **7**, 445–480.

19. Jenkins, M. and Schwartz, R. (1987) Antigen presentation by chemically modified splenocytes induces antigen-specific T cell unresponsiveness in vitro and in vivo, *J. Exp. Med.*, **165**, 302–319.

20. Albert, M. L., Jegathesan, M., and Darnell, R. B. (2001) Dendritic cell maturation is required for the cross-tolerization of CD8$^+$ T cells, *Nat. Immunol.*, **2**, 1010–1017.

21. Curtsinger, J. M., Schmidt, C. S., Mondino, A., et al. (1999) Inflammatory cytokines provide third signal for activation of naïve CD4$^+$ and CD8$^+$ T cells, *J. Immunol.*, **162**, 3256–3262.

22. Hernandez, J., Aung, S., Marquardt, K., and Sherman, L. A. (2002) Uncoupling of proliferative potential and gain of effector function by CD8(+) T cells responding to self-antigens, *J. Exp. Med.*, **196**, 323–333.

23. Schmidt, C. S. and Mescher, M. F. (2002) Peptide Ag priming of naïve, but not memory, CD8 T cells requires a third signal that can be provided by IL-2, *J. Immunol.*, **168**, 5521–5529.

24. Sharpe, A. H. and Freeman, G. J. (2002) The B7-CD28 superfamily, *Nat. Rev. Immunol.*, **2**, 116–126.

25. Watts, T. H. and DeBenedette, M. A. (1999) T cell co-stimulatory molecules other than CD28, *Curr. Opin. Immunol.*, **11**, 286–293.

26. Trinchieri, G. (1995) Interleukin-12: a proinflammatory cytokine with immunoregulatory functions that bridge innate resistance and antigen-specific adaptive immunity, *Annu. Rev. Immunol.*, **13**, 251–276.

27. Brouckaert, P., Libert, C., Evereardt, B., Takahashi, N., Cauwels, A., and Fiers, W. (1993) Tumor necrosis factor, its receptors and the connection with interleukin 1 and interleukin 6, *Immunobiology*, **187**, 317.

28. Medzhitov, R. (2001) Toll-like receptors and innate immunity, *Nat. Rev. Immunol.*, **1**, 135–145.

29. Aderem, A. and Ulevitch, R. J. (2000) Toll-like receptors in the induction of the innate immune response, *Nature*, **406**, 782–787.

30. Kaisho, T. and Akira, S. (2002) Toll-like receptors as adjuvant receptors, *Biochim. Biophys. Acta*, **1589**, 1–13.

31. Liu, Y. J. (2001) Dendritic cell subsets and lineages, and their functions in innate and adaptive immunity, *Cell*, **106**, 259–262.

32. Shortman, K. and Liu, Y. I. (2002) Mouse and human dendritic cell subtypes, *Nat. Rev. Immunol.*, **2**, 151–161.

33. Ito, T., Amakawa, R., Kaisho, T., et al. (2002) Interferon-alpha and interleukin-12 are induced differentially by Toll-like receptor 7 ligands in human blood dendritic cell subsets, *J. Exp. Med.*, **195**, 1507–1512.

34. Henri, S., Vremec, D., Kamath, A., et al. (2001) The dendritic cell populations of mouse lymph nodes, *J. Immunol.*, **167**, 741–748.

35. Nakano, H., Yanagita, M., and Gunn, M. D. (2001) CD11c(+)B220(+)Gr-1(+) cells in mouse lymph nodes and spleen display characteristics of plasmacytoid dendritic cells, *J. Exp. Med.*, **194**, 1171–1178.

36. Ruedl, C., Koebel, P., Bachmann, M., Hess, M., and Karjalainen, K. (2000) Anatomical origin of dendritic cells determines their life span in peripheral lymph nodes, *J. Immunol.*, **165**, 4910–4916.

37. Banchereau, J. and Steinman, R. M. (1998) Dendritic cells and the control of immunity, *Nature*, **392**, 245–252.

38. Sallusto, F. and Lanzavecchia, A. (2000) Understanding dendritic cell and T- lymphocyte traffic through the analysis of chemokine receptor expression, *Immunol. Rev.*, **177**, 134–140.

39. Mellman, I. and Steinman, R. M. (2001) Dendritic cells: specialized and regulated antigen processing machines, *Cell*, **106**, 255–258.

40. Cella, M., Engering, A., Pinet, V., Pieters, J., and Lanzavecchia, A. (1997) Inflammatory stimuli induce accumulation of MHC class II complexes on dendritic cells, *Nature*, **388**, 782–787.

41. Epperson, D. E., Arnold, D., Spies, T., Cresswell, P., Pober, J. S., and Johnson, D. R. (1992) Cytokines increase transporter in antigen processing-1 expression more rapidly that HLA class I expression in endothelial cells, *J. Immunol.*, **149**, 3297–3301.

42. Khoruts, A., Mondino, A., Pape, K. A., Reiner, S. L., and Jenkins, M. (1998) A natural immunological adjuvant enhances T cell clonal expansion through a CD28- dependent, IL-2-independent mechanism, *J. Exp. Med.*, **187**, 225–236.

43. Curtsinger, J. M., Valenzuela, J. O., Agarwal, P., Lins, D., and Mescher, M. F. (2005) Cutting edge: type I interferons provide a third signal to CD8 T cells to stimulate clonal expansion and differentiation, *J. Immunol.*, **174**, 4465–4469.

44. Mitchel, T., Kappler, J., and Marrack, P. (1999) Bystander virus infection prolongs activated T cell survival, *J. Immunol.*, **162**, 4527–4535.

45. Vella, A. T., Mitchell, T., Groth, B., et al. (1997) CD28 engagement and proinflammatory cytokines contribute to T cell expansion and long-term survival in vivo, *J. Immunol.*, **158**, 4714–4720.

46. Mitchell, T. C., Hildeman, D., Krdl, R. M., et al. (2001) Immunological adjuvants promote activated T cell survival via induction of Bcl-3, *Nat. Immunol.*, **2**, 397–402.

47. Valenzuela, J. O., Hammerbeck, C., and Mescher, M. F. (2005) Cutting edge: Bcl-3 upregulation by signal 3 cytokine (IL-12) prolongs survival of Ag-activated CD8 T cells, *J. Immunol.*, **174**, 600–604.

48. Mattei, F., Schiavoni, G., Belardelli, F., and Tough, D. F. (2001) IL-15 is expressed by dendritic cells in response to type I IFN, double-stranded RNA, or lipopolysaccharide and promotes dendritic cell activation, *J. Immunol.*, **167**, 1179–1187.

49. Ku, C. C., Murakami, M., Sakamoto, A., Kappler, J., and Marrack, P. (2000) Control of homeostasis of CD8$^+$ memory T cells by opposing cytokines, *Science*, **288**, 675–678.

50. Sprent, J. and Surh, C. D. (2001) Generation and maintenance of memory T cells, *Curr. Opin. Immunol.*, **13**, 248–254.

51. Zhang, X., Sun, S., Hwang, I., Tough, D. F., and Sprent, J. (1998) Potent and selective stimulation of memory-phenotype CD8$^+$ T cell in vivo by IL-15, *Immunity*, **8**, 591–599.

52. Schluns, K. S., Williams, K., Ma, A., Zheng, X. X., and Lefrancois, L. (2002) Cutting edge: requirement for IL-15 in the generation of primary and memory antigen-specific CD8 T cells, *J. Immunol.*, **168**, 4827–4831.

53. Antia, R., Pilyugin, S. S., and Ahmed, R. (1998) Models of immune memory: on the role of cross-reactive stimulation, competition, and homeostasis in maintaining immune memory, *Proc. Natl. Acad. Sci. U.S.A.*, **95**, 14926–14931.

54. Homann, D., Teyton, L., and Oldstone, M. B. (2001) Differential regulation of antiviral T-cell immunity results in stable CD8$^+$ but declining CD4$^+$ T-cell memory, *Nat. Med.*, **7**, 913–919.

55. Pape, K. A., Merica, R., Mondino, A., Khoruts, A., and Jenkins, M. K. (1998) Direct evidence that functionally impaired CD4$^+$ T cells persist in vivo following induction of peripheral tolerance, *J. Immunol.*, **160**, 4719–4729.

56. Reinhardt, R. L., Khoruts, A., Merica, R., Zell, T., and Jenkins, M. K. (2001) Visualizing the generation of memory CD4 T cells in the whole body, *Nature*, **410**, 101–105.

57. Bancherau, J., Schuler-Thurner, B., Palucka, A. K., and Schuler, G. (2001) Dendritic cells as vectors for therapy, *Cell*, **106**, 271–274.

58. Grewal, I. and Flavell, R. (1998) CD40 and CD154 in cell-mediated immunity, *Annu. Rev. Immunol.*, **16**, 111–135.

59. Ranheim, E. A. and Kipps, T. J. (1993) Activated T cells induce expression of B7/BB1 on normal or leukemic B cells through a CD40-dependent signal, *J. Exp. Med.*, **177**, 925–935.

60. Cella, M., Scheidegger, D., Palmer-Lehmann, K., Lane, P., Lanzavecchia, A., and Alber, G. (1996) Ligation of CD40 on dendritic cells triggers production of high levels of interleukin-12 and enhances T cell stimulatory capacity: T–T help via APC activation, *J. Exp. Med.*, **184**, 747–752.

61. Takeda, K., Hemmi, H., and Akira, S. (2006) Mechanism for recognition of CpG DNA. In: *Vaccine Adjuvants: Immunological and Clinical Principles* (Hackett, C. and Harn, D. A., Jr., eds.), Humana Press, Totowa, NJ, pp. 69–86.

62. Krieg, A. M. and Davis, H. L. (2006) CpG ODN as a Th1 immune enhancer for prophylactic and therapeutic vaccines. In: *Vaccine Adjuvants: Immunological and Clinical Principles* (Hackett, C. and Harn, D. A., Jr., eds.), Humana Press, Totowa, NJ, pp. 87–110.

63. Krieg, A. M., Yi, A.-K., Matson, S., et al. (1995) CpG motifs in bacterial DNA trigger direct B cell activation, *Nature*, **374**, 546–549.

64. Medzhitov, R. and Janeway, C. A., Jr. (1997) Innate immunity: the virtues of a nonclonal system of recognition, *Cell*, **91**, 295–298.

65. Medzhitov, R. and Janeway, C. A., Jr. (1997) Innate immunity: impact on the adaptive immune response, *Curr. Opin. Immunol.*, **9**, 4–9.

66. Wagner, H. (1999) Bacterial CpG DNA activates immune cells to signal infectious danger, *Adv. Immunol.*, **73**, 329–367.

67. Krieg, A. M., Hartmann, G. H., and Yi, A.-K. (2000) Mechanism of action of CpG DNA, *Curr. Top. Microbiol. Immunol.*, **247**, 1–21.

68. Stacey, K. J., Sester, D. P., Sweet, M. J., and Hume, D. A. (2000) Macrophage activation by immunostimulatory DNA, *Curr. Top. Microbiol. Immunol.*, **247**, 41–58.

69. Tokunaga, T., Yamamoto, H., Shimada, S., et al. (1984) Antitumor activity of deoxyribonucleic acid fraction from mycobacterium bovis BCG. I. Isolation, physicochemical characterization, and antitumor activity, *J. Natl. Cancer Inst.*, **72**, 955–962.

70. Yamamoto, S., Kuramoto, E., Shimada, S., and Tokunaga, T. (1988) In vitro augmentation of natural killer cell activity and production of interferon-α/β and $-\gamma$ with deoxyribonucleic acid fraction from mycobacterium bovis BCG, *Jpn. J. Cancer Res.*, **79**, 866–873.

71. Ulmer, J. B., Donnelly, J. J., Parker, S. E., et al. (1993) Heterologous protection against influenza by injection of DNA encoding a viral protein, *Science*, **259**, 1745–1749.

72. Sedegah, M., Hedstrom, R., Hobart, P., and Hoffman, S. L. (1994) Protection against malaria by immunization with plasmid DNA encoding circumsporozoite protein, *Proc. Natl. Acad. Sci. U.S.A.*, **91**, 9866–9870.

73. Boyer, J. D., Ugen, K. E., Wang, B., et al. (1997) Protection of chimpanzees from high-dose heterologous HIV-1 challenge by DNA vaccination, *Nat. Med.*, **3**, 526–532.

74. Xu, L., Sanchez, A., Yang, Z., et al. (1998) Immunization for Ebola virus infection, *Nat. Med.*, **4**, 37–42.

75. Lowrie, D. B., Silva, C. L., Colston, M. J., Ragno, S., and Tascon, R. E. (1997) Protection against tuberculosis by a plasmid DNA vaccine, *Vaccine*, **15**, 834–838.

76. Gurunathan, S., Sacks, D. L., Brown, D. R., et al. (1997) Vaccination with DNA encoding the immunodominant LACK parasite antigen confers protective immunity to mice infected with *Leishmania major*, *J. Exp. Med.*, **186**, 1137–1147.

77. Wang, R., Doolan, D. L., Le, T. P., et al. (1998) Induction of antigen specific cytotoxic T lymphocytes in humans by a malaria vaccine DNA, *Science*, **282**, 476–480.

78. Calarota, S., Bratt, G., Nordlund, S., et al. (1998) Cellular cytotoxic response induced by DNA vaccination in HIV-1 infected patients, *Lancet*, **351**, 1320–1325.

79. Gurunathan, S., Wu, C.-Y., Freidag, B. L., and Sedar, R. A. (2000) Vaccine DNA, a key for inducing long term cellular immunity, *Curr. Opin. Immunol.*, **12**, 442–447.

80. Sato, Y., Roman, M., Tighe, H., et al. (1996) Immunostimulatory DNA sequences necessary for effective intradermal gene immunization, *Science*, **273**, 352–354.

81. Klinman, D. M., Yamshchikov, G., and Ishigatsubo, Y. (1997) Contribution of CpG motifs to the immunogenicity of vaccines DNA, *J. Immunol.*, **158**, 3635–3642.

82. Klinman, D. M., Barnhart, K. M., and Conover, J. (1999) CpG motifs as immune adjuvants, *Vaccine*, **17**, 19–25.

83. Klinman, D. M., Verthlyi, D., Takeshita, F., and Ishii, K. J. (1999) Immune recognition of foreign DNA: a cure for bioterrorism? *Immunity*, **11**, 123–129.

84. Roman, M., Martin-Orozco, E., Goodman, J. S., et al. (1997) Immunostimulatory DNA sequences function as T helper-1-promoting adjuvants, *Nat. Med.*, **3**, 849–854.

85. Lipford, G. B., Bauer, M., Blank, C., Reiter, R., Wagner, H., and Heeg, K. (1997) CpG-containing synthetic ologonucleotides promote B and cytotoxic T cell responses to protein antigen: a new class of vaccine adjuvants, *Eur. J. Immunol.*, **27**, 2340–2344.

86. McCluskie, M. J. and Davis, H. L. (1998) CpG DNA is a potent enhancer of systemic and mucosal immune responses against hepatitis B surface antigen with intranasal administration to mice, *J. Immunol.*, **161**, 4463–4466.

87. Manders, P. and Thomas, R. (2000) Immunology of vaccines DNA, CpG motifs and antigen presentation, *Inflamm. Res.*, **49**, 199–205.

88. Hartmann, G., Weiner, G. J., and Krieg, A. M. (1999) CpDNA G, a potent signal for growth, activation, and maturation of human dendritic cells, *Proc. Natl. Acad. Sci. U.S.A.*, **96**, 9305–9310.

89. Sparwasser, T., Koch, E. S., Vabulas, R. M., et al. (1998) Bacterial DNA and immunostimulatory CpG oligonucleotides trigger maturation and activation of murine dendritic cells, *Eur. J. Immunol.*, **28**, 2045–2054.

90. Jacob, T., Walker, P. S., Krieg, A. M., Udey, M. C., and Vogel, J. C. (1998) Activation of cutaneous dendritic cells by CpG-containing oligonucleotides: a role for dendritic cells in the augmentation of Th1 responses by immunostimulatory DNA, *J. Immunol.*, **161**, 3042–3049.

91. Kimua, Y., Sonehara, K., Kuramoto, E., et al. (1994) Binding of oligoguanylate to scavenger receptors is required for oligonucleotides to augment NK cell activity and induce IFN, *J. Biochem.*, **116**, 991–994.

92. Hacker, H., Mischak, H., Miethke, T., et al. (1998) CpG-DNA-specific activation of antigen-presenting cells requires stress kinase activity and is preceded by non-specific endocytosis and endosomal maturation, *EMBO J.*, **17**, 6230–6240.

93. Tonkinson, J. L. and Stein, C. A. (1994) Patterns of intracellular compartmentalization, trafficking and acidification of 5′-fluorescein labeled phosphodiester and phosphorothioate oligodeoxynucleotides in HL60 cells, *Nucleic Acids Res.*, **22**, 4288–4275.

94. Yi, A.-K. and Krieg, A. M. (1998) Rapid induction of mitogen-activated protein kinases by immune stimulatory CpG DNA, *J. Immunol.*, **161**, 4493–4497.

95. Sparwasser, T., Miethke, T., Lipford, G., et al. (1997) Macrophages sense pathogens via DNA motifs: induction of tumor necrosis-α-mediated shock, *Eur. J. Immunol.*, **27**, 1671–1679.

96. Yi, A.-K., Tuetken, R., Redford, T., Waldschmidt, M., Kirsch, J., and Krieg, A. M. (1998) CpG motifs in bacterial DNA activates leukocytes through the pH-dependent generation of reactive oxygen species, *J. Immunol.*, **160**, 4755–4761.

97. Stacey, K. J., Sweet, M., and Hume, D. A. (1996) Macrophages ingest and are activated by bacterial DNA, *J. Immunol.*, **157**, 2116–2122.

98. Zimmerman, P. E., Voelker, D. R., McCormack, F. X., Paulsrud, J. R., and Martin, W. J. (1992) 120-kD surface glycoprotein of *Pneumocystis carinii* is a ligand for surfactant protein A, *J. Clin. Invest.*, **89**, 143–149.

99. Ozinsky, A., Underhill, D. M., Fontenot, J. D., et al. (2000) The repertoire for pattern recognition of pathogens by the innate immune system is defined by cooperation between Toll-like receptors, *Proc. Natl. Acad. Sci. U.S.A.*, **97**, 13766–13771.

100. Wyllie, D. H., Kiss-Toth, E., Visintin, A., et al. (2000) Evidence for an accessory protein function for Toll-like receptor 1, in antibacterial responses, *J. Immunol.*, **165**, 7125–7132.

101. Hajjar, A. M., O'Mahony, D. S., Ozinsky, A., et al. (2001) Cutting edge: functional interactions between Toll-like receptor (TLR) 2, and TLR1, or TLR6, in response to phenol-soluble modulin, *J. Immunol.*, **166**, 15–19.

102. Hemmi, H., Takeuchi, O., Kawai, T., et al. (2000) A Toll-like receptor recognized bacterial DNA, *Nature*, **408**, 740–745.

103. Stehle, T. and Larvie, M. (2003) Structures of complement control proteins. In: *Innate Immunity* (Ezekowitz, R. A. B. and Hoffmann, J. A., eds.), Humana Press, Totowa, NJ, pp. 231–253.

104. Chu, W.-M., Gong, X., Li, Z.-W., et al. (2000) DNA-PKcs is required for activation of innate immunity by immunostimulatory DNA, *Cell*, **103**, 909–918.

105. Gottlieb, T. M. and Jackson, S. P. (1993) The DNA-dependent protein kinase: requirement for DNA ends and association with Ku antigen, *Cell*, **72**, 131–142.

106. Hartley, K. O., Gell, D., Smith, G. C., et al. (1995) DNA-dependent protein kinase catalytic subunit: a relative of phosphatidylinositol 3-kinase and ataxia telangiectasia gene product, *Cell*, **82**, 849–856.

107. Kirchgessner, C. U., Patil, C. K., Evans, J. W., et al. (1995) DNA-dependent protein kinase (p350) as a candidate gene for the murine defect CID, *Science*, **267**, 1178–1183.

108. Liang, H., Nishioka, Y., Reich, C. F., Pisetsky, D. S., and Lipsky, P. E. (1996) Activation of human B cells by phosphorothioate oligodeoxynucleotides, *J. Clin. Invest.*, **98**, 1119–1129.

109. Yi, A.-K., Chang, M., Peckham, D. W., Krieg, A. M., and Ashman, R. F., (1998) CpG oligodeoxyribonucleotides rescue mature spleen B cells from spontaneous apoptosis and promote cell cycle entry, *J. Immunol.*, **160**, 5898–5906.

110. Yi, A.-K., Hornbeck, P., Lafrenz, D. E., and Krieg, A. M. (1996) CpG DNA rescue of murine B lymphoma cells from anti-IgM-induced growth arrest and programmed cell death is associated with increased expression of c-myc and bcl- xL, *J. Immunol.*, **157**, 4918–4925.

111. Hartmann, G., Weeratna, R. D., Ballas, Z. K., et al. (2000) Delineation of a CpG phosphorodithioate oligodeoxynucleotide for activating primate immune responses in vitro and in vivo, *J. Immunol.*, **164**, 1617–1624.

112. Hartmann, G. and Krieg, A. M. (2000) Mechanism and function of a newly identified CpG DNA motif in human primary B cells, *J. Immunol.*, **164**, 944–953.

113. Simmons, C. P., Hussell, T., Sparer, T., Walzl, G., Openshaw, P., and Dougan, G. (2001) Mucosal delivery of a respiratory syncytial virus CTL peptide with entrotoxin-based adjuvants elicits protective immunopathogenic, and immunoregulatory antiviral CD8+ T cell responses, *J. Immunol.*, **166**, 1106–1113.

114. Czerkinsky, C., Anjyere, F., McGhee, J. R., et al. (1999) Mucosal immunity and tolerance: relevance to vaccine development, *Immunol Rev.*, **170**, 197–222.

115. Greco, D., Salmaso, S., Mastrantonio, P., et al. (1996) A controlled trial of two acellular vaccines and one whole-cell vaccine against pertussis, Progetto Pertosse Working Group, *N. Engl. J. Med.*, **334**, 341–348.

116. van Ginkel, F. W., Nguyen, H. H., and McGhee, J. R. (2000) Vaccines for mucosal immunity to combat emerging infectious diseases, *Emerg. Infect. Dis.*, **6**, 123–132.

117. Pizza, M., Covacci, A., Bartoloni, A., et al. (1989) Mutants of pertussis toxin suitable for vaccine development, *Science*, **246**, 497–499.

118. Rappuoli, R. (1997) Rational design of vaccines, *Nat. Med.*, **3**, 374–376.

119. Mills, K. H. G., Ryan, M., Ryan, E., and Mahon, B. P. (1998) A murine model in which protection correlates with pertussis vaccine efficacy in children reveals complementary roles for humoral and cell-mediated immunity in protection against *Bordetella pertussis*, *Infect. Immun.*, **66**, 594–602.

120. Ryan, M. and Mills, K. H. G. (1997) The role of the S-1, and B-oligomer components of pertussis toxin in its adjuvant properties for Th1 and Th2 cells, *Biochem. Soc. Trans.*, **25**, 126S.

121. Mills, K. H. G., Barnard, A., Watkins, S., and Redhead, K. (1990) Specificity of the T cell response to *Bordetella pertussis* in aerosol infected mice. In: *Proc. 6th Int. Symp. Pertussis* (Manclarck, C. R., ed.), Department of Health and Human Services, United States Public Health Service, Bethesda, MD, pp. 166–174.

122. Nencioni, L., Volpini, G., Peppoloni, S., Bugnoli, M., De Magistris, T., Marcili, I., and Pappuoli, R. (1991) Properties of pertussis toxin mutant PT-9k/129G after formaldehyde treatment,
Infect. Immun., **59**, 625–630.

123. Ratti, G., Rappuoli, R., and Giannini, G. (1983) The complete
nucleotide sequence of the gene coding for diphtheria toxin in
the corynephage omega (tox$^+$) genome, *Nucleic Acids Res.*, **11**,
6589–6595.

124. Rappuoli, R. (1997) New and improved vaccines against diphtheria and tetanus. In: *New Generation Vaccines*, 2nd ed. (Levine, M.
M., Woodrow, G. C., Kaper, J. B., and Cobon, G. S., eds.), Marcel
Dekker, New York, pp. 417–436.

125. Gupta, R. K., Collier, R. J., Rappuoli, R., and Siber, G. R. (1997)
Differences in the immunogenicity of native and formalinized
cross reacting material (CRM$_{197}$) of diphtheria toxin in mice and
guinea pigs and their implications on the development and control
of diphtheria vaccine based on CRMs, *Vaccine*, **15**, 1341–1343.

126. Mills, K. H., Cosgrove, C., McNeela, E. A., et al. (2003) Protective levels of diphtheria-neutralizing antibody induced in healthy
volunteers by unilateral priming-boosting intranasal immunization associated with restricted ipsilateral mucosal secretory
immunoglobulin A, *Infect. Immun.*, **71**, 726–732.

127. Spangler, B. D. (1992) Structure and function of cholera toxin
and the related *Escherichia coli* heat-labile enterotoxin, *Microbiol. Rev.*, **56**, 622–647.

128. McGuirk, P., McCann, C., and Mills, K. H. (2002) Pathogen-
specific T regulatory 1 cells induced in the respiratory tract by
a bacterial molecule that stimulates interleukin 10 production by
dendritic cells: a novel strategy for evasion of protective T helper
type 1 responses by *Bordetella pertussis*, *J. Exp. Med.*, **195**, 221–
231.

129. Clarke, C. J., Wilson, A. D., Williams, N. A., and Stokes, C. R.
(1991) Mucosal priming of T-lymphocyte responses to fed protein antigens using cholera toxin as adjuvant, *Immunology*, **72**,
323–328.

130. Richards, C. M., Shimeld, C., Williams, N. A., and Hill, T. J.
(1998) Induction of mucosal immunity against herpes simplex
virus type 1 in the mouse protects against ocular infection and
establishment of latency, *J. Infect. Dis.*, **177**, 1451–1457.

131. Martin, M., Metzger, D. J., Michalek, S. M., Connell, T. D., and
Russell, M. W. (2000) Comparative analysis of the mucosal adjuvanticity of the type II heat-labile enterotoxins LT-IIa and LTIIb,
Infect. Immun., **68**, 281–287.

132. Hornquist, E. and Lycke, N. (1993) Cholera toxin adjuvant
greatly promotes antigen priming of T cells, *Eur. J. Immunol.*,
23, 2136–2143.

133. Pacheco, S. E., Gibbs, R. A., Ansari-Lari, A., and Rogers, P.
(2000) Intranasal immunization with HIV reverse transcriptase:
effect of dose in the induction of helper type 1 and 2 immunity,
AIDS Res. Hum. Retroviruses, **16**, 2009–2017.

134. Akhiani, A. A., Schon, K., and Lycke, N. (2004) Vaccine-induced
immunity against *Helicobacter pylori* infection is impaired in IL-
18-deficient mice, *J. Immunol.*, **173**, 3348–3356.

135. Schaffeler, M. P., Brokenshire, J. S., and Snider, D. P. (1997)
Detection of precursor Th cells in mesenteric lymph nodes after
oral immunization with protein antigen and cholera toxin, *Int.
Immunol.*, **9**, 1555–1562.

136. Yanagita, M., Hiroi, T., Kitagaki, N., et al. (1999)
Nasopharyngeal-associated lymphoreticular tissue (NATL)
immunity: fimbriae-specific Th1 and Th 2 cell-regulated IgA
responses for the inhibition of bacterial attachment to epithelial
cells and subsequent inflammatory cytokine production,
J. Immunol., **162**, 3559–3565.

137. Lavelle, E. C., Jarnicki, A., McNeela, E., et al. (2004) Effects of
cholera toxin on innate and adaptive immunity and its application
as an immunomodulatory agent, *J. Leukoc. Biol.*, **75**, 756–763.

138. Douce, G., Fontana, M., Pizza, M., Rappuoli, R., and Dougan,
G. (1997) Intranasal immunogenicity and adjuvanticity of site-
directed mutant derivatives of cholera toxin, *Infect. Immun.*, **65**,
2821–2828.

139. Weeratna, R., Comanita, L., and Davis, H. L. (2003) CPG ODN
allows lower dose of antigen against hepatitis B surface antigen
in BALB/c mice, *Immunol. Cell Biol.*, **81**, 59–62.

140. Sun, J.-B., Rask, C., Olsson, T., Holmgren, J., and Czerkinsky, C.
(1996) Treatment of experimental autoimmune encephalomyelitis by feeding myelin basic protein conjugated to cholera toxin
subunit B., *Proc. Natl. Acad. Sci. U.S.A.*, **93**, 7196–7201.

141. Williams, N. A., Stasiuk, L. M., Nashar, T. O., et al. (1997) Prevention of autommune disease due to lymphocyte modulation by
the B-subunit of *Escherichia coli* heat-labile enterotoxin, *Proc.
Natl. Acad. Sci. U.S.A.*, **94**, 5290–5295.

142. Ploix, C., Bergerot, I., Durand, A., Czerkinsky, C., Holmgren, J.,
and Thivolet, C. (1999) Oral administration of cholera toxin B-
insulin conjugates protects NOD mice from autoimmune diabetes
by inducing CD4$^+$ regulatory T-cells, *Diabetes*, **48**, 2150–2156.

143. Widermann, U., Jahn-Schmid, B., Repa, A., Kraft, D., and
Ebner, C. (1999) Modulation of an allergic immune response via
the mucosal route in a murine model of inhalative type-1 allergy,
Int. Arch. Allergy Immunol., **118**, 129–132.

144. Ryan, E. J., McNeela, E., Pizza, M., Rappuoli, R., O'Neill, L.,
and Mills, K. H. G. (2000) Modulation of innate and acquired
immune responses by *Escherichia coli* heat-labile toxin: distinct
pro- and anti-inflammatory effects of the nontoxic AB complex
and the enzyme activity, *J. Immunol.*, **165**, 5750–5759.

145. Douce, G., Turcotte, C., Cropley, I., et al. (1995) Mutants of
Escherichia coli heat-labile toxin lacking ADP-ribosyltransferase
activity act as nontoxic mucosal adjuvants, *Proc. Natl. Acad. Sci.
U.S.A.*, **92**, 1644–1648.

146. Haynes, J. R., Arrington, J., Dong, L., Braun, R. P., and Payne, L.
J. (2006) Potent protective cellular immune responses generated
by a DNA vaccine encoding HSV-2 ICP27 and the *E. coli* heat
labile enterotoxin, *Vaccine*, **24**(23), 5016–5026.

147. Li, T. K. and Fox, B. S. (1996) Cholera toxin B subunit binding to an antigen- presenting cell directly co-stimulates cytokine
production from a T cell clone, *Int. Immunol.*, **8**, 1849–1856.

148. Cong, Y., Weaver, C. T., and Elson, C. O. (1997) The mucosal
adjuvanticity of cholera toxin involves enhancement of costimulatory activity by selective up-regulation of B72 expression,
J. Immunol., **159**, 5201–5208.

149. Yamamoto, M., Kiyono, H., Yamamoto, S., et al. (1999) Direct
effects on antigen- presenting cells and T lymphocytes explain
the adjuvanticity of a nontoxic cholera toxin mutant, *J. Immunol.*,
162, 7015–7021.

150. Braun, M. C., He, J., Wu, C. Y., and Kelsall, B. L. (1999) Cholera
toxin suppresses interleukin (IL)-12 production and IL-12 and
receptor β_1 and β_2 chain expression, *J. Exp. Med.*, **189**, 541–552.

151. Panina-Bordignon, P., Mazzeo, D., Lucia, P. D., et al. (1997)
Beta2 agonists prevent Th1 development by selective inhibition
of interleukin 12, *J. Clin. Invest.*, **100**, 1513–1519.

152. Munoz, E., Zubiaga, A. M., Merrow, M., Sauter, N. P., and Huber,
B. T. (1990) Cholera toxin discriminates between T helper 1 and
2 cell in T cell receptor-mediated activation: role of cAMP in T
cell proliferation, *J. Exp. Med.*, **172**, 95–103.

153. Lavelle, E. C., Leavy, O., and Mills, K. H. G. (2006) Modified
bacterial toxins. In: *Vaccine Adjuvants: Immunological and Clinical Principles* (Hackett, C. and Harn, D. A., Jr., eds.), Humana
Press, Totowa, NJ, pp. 111–153.

154. Tozzi, A., Pastore Calentano, L., Ciofi degli Atti, M. L., and
Salmaso, S. (2005) Diagnosis and management of pertussis, *Can.
Med. Assoc. J.*, **172**(4), 509–515.

155. Gustafsson, L., Hallander, H. O., Olin, P., Reizenstein, E., and
Storsaeter, J. (1996) A controlled trial of a two-component

acellular, a five-component acellular, and a whole-cell pertussis vaccine, *N. Engl. J. Med.*, **334**, 349–355.

156. Trollofors, B., Taranger, J., Lagergard, T., et al. (1995) A placebo-controlled trial of a pertussis-toxoid vaccine, *N. Engl. J. Med.*, **333**, 1045–1050.

157. Porro, M., Saletti, M., Nencioni, L., Tagliaferri, L., and Marsili, I. (1980) Immunogenic correlation between cross-reacting material (CRM197) produced by a mutant of *Corynebacterium diphtheriae* and diphtheria toxoid, *J. Infect. Dis.*, **142**, 716–724.

158. McNeela, E. A., O'Connor, D., Jabbal-Gill, I., et al. (2000) A mucosal vaccine against diphtheria: formulation of cross reacting material (CRM$_{197}$) of diphtheria toxin with chitosan enhances local and systemic antibody and Th2 responses following nasal delivery, *Vaccine*, **19**, 1188–1198.

159. Zhang, R. G., Scott, D. L., Westbrock, M. L. (1995) The three-dimensional structure of cholera toxin, *J. Mol. Biol.*, **251**, 563–573.

160. Rappuoli, R., Pizza, M., Douce, G., and Dougan, G. (1999) Structure and mucosal adjuvanticity of cholera and *Escherichia coli* heat-labile enterotoxins, *Immunol. Today*, **20**, 493–500.

161. Pizza, M., Giuliani, M. M., Fontana, M. R., et al. (2001) Mucosal vaccines: non toxic derivatives of LT and CT as mucosal adjuvants, *Vaccine*, **19**(17–19), 2634–2541.

162. Williams, N. A., Hirst, T. R., and Nashar, T. O. (1999) Immune modulation by the cholera-like enterotoxins: from adjuvant to immunotherapeutic, *Immunol. Today*, **20**, 95–101.

163. Holmgren, J., Lonroth, I., and Svennerholm, L. (1973) Tissue receptor for cholera exotoxin: postulated structure from studies with GM1, ganglioside and related glycolipids, *Infect. Immun.*, **8**, 208–214.

164. Tsai, S. C., Noda, M., Adamik, R., Moss, J., and Vaughan, M. (1988) Stimulation of choleragen enzymatic activities by GTP and two soluble proteins purified from bovine brain, *J. Biol. Chem.*, **263**, 1768–1772.

165. Lycke, N., Lindholm, L., and Holmgren, J. (1983) IgA isotype restriction in the mucosal but not in the extramucosal immune response after oral immunizations with cholera toxin or cholera subunit B, *Int. Arch. Allergy Appl. Immunol.*, **72**, 119–127.

166. Lycke, N. and Holmgren, J. (1988) Long-term mucosal memory to cholera toxin in mice after oral immunizations: antitoxin production from isolated lamina propria cells after in vivo or in vitro boosting. In: *Mucosal Immunity and Infections at Mucosal Surfaces* (Strober, W., Lamm, M. E., McGhee, J. R., and James, S. P., eds.), Oxford University Press, New York, pp. 401–404.

167. Xu-Amano, J., Kiyono, H., Jackson, R. L., et al. (1993) Helper T cell subsets for immunoglobulin A responses: oral immunization with tetanus toxoid and cholera toxin as adjuvant selectively induces Th2 cells in mucosa-associated tissues, *J. Exp. Med.*, **178**, 1309–1320.

168. Marinaro, M., Staats, H. F., Hiroi, T., et al. (1995) Mucosal adjuvant effect of cholera toxin in mice results from induction of T helper 2 (Th2) cells and IL-4, *J. Immunol.*, **155**, 4621–4629.

169. Yamamoto, S., Kiyono, H., Yamamoto, M., et al. (1997) A nontoxic mutant of cholera toxin elicits Th2-type responses for enhanced mucosal immunity, *Proc. Natl. Acad. Sci. U.S.A.*, **94**, 5267–5272.

170. Yamamoto, S., Yoshifumi, K., Yamamoto, M., et al. (1997) Mutants in the ADP-ribosyltransferase cleft of cholera toxin lack diarrheagenicity but retained adjuvanticity, *J. Exp. Med.*, **185**, 1203–1210.

171. Yamamoto, M., Rennert, P., McGhee, R. J., et al. (2000) Alternate mucosal immune system: organized Peyer's patches are not required for IgA responses in the gastrointestinal tract, *J. Immunol.*, **164**, 5184–5191.

172. Simecka, J. W., Jackson, R. J., Kiyono, H., and McGhee, J. R. (2000) Mucosally induced immunoglobulin E-associated inflammation in the respiratory tract, *Infect. Immun.*, **68**, 672–679.

173. Haynes, J. R., Arrington, J., Dong, L., Braun, R. P., and Payne, L. J. (2006) Potent protective cellular immune responses generated by a DNA vaccine encoding HSV-2 ICP27 and the *E. coli* heat-labile enterotoxin, *Vaccine*, **24**(23), 5016–5026.

174. Douce, G., Fontana, M., Pizza, M., Parruoli, R., and Dougan, G. (1997) Intranasal immunogenicity and adjuvanticity of site-directed mutant derivatives of cholera toxin, *Infect. Immun.*, **65**, 2821–2828.

175. Pierre, P., Denis, O., Bazin, H., Mbella, E. M., and Vaerman, J.-P. (1992) Modulation of oral tolerance to ovalbumin by cholera toxin and its subunit B, *Eur. J. Immunol.*, **22**, 3127–3128.

176. Glenn, G., Scharton-Kersten, T., Vassell, R., Mallet, C. P., Hale, T. L., and Alving, C. R. (1998) Cutting edge: transcutaneous immunization with cholera toxin protects mice against lethal mucosal toxin challenge, *J. Immunol.*, **161**, 3211–3214.

177. Reudel, C., Rieser, C., Kofler, N., Wick, G., and Wolf, H. (1996) Humoral and cellular immune responses in the murine respiratory tract following oral immunization with cholera toxin or *Escherichia coli* heat-labile enterotoxin, *Vaccine*, **14**, 792–798.

178. Burnett, W. N. (1994) AB$_5$ ADP-ribosylating toxins: comparative anatomy and physiology, *Structure*, **2**, 151–158.

179. Brunton, J. L. (1990) The shiga toxin family: molecular nature and possible role in disease. In: *The Bacteria*, vol. 11 (Iglewski, B. and Clark, U., eds.), Academic Press, New York, pp. 377–397.

180. Moss, J. and Vaughan, M. (1988) ADP-ribosylation of guanyl nucleotide-binding regulatory proteins by bacterial toxins, *Advan. Enzymol.*, **61**, 303–379.

181. Leong, J., Vinal, A. C., and Dallas, W. S. (1985) Nucleotide sequence comparison between heat-labile toxin B subunit citrons from *Escherichia coli* of human and porcine origin, *Infect. Immun.*, **48**, 73–77.

182. Zhang, R.-G., Westbrook, M. L., Westbrook, E. M., et al. (1995) The 2.4 Å crystal structure of cholera toxin B subunit pentamer: choleragenoid, *J. Mol. Biol.*, **251**(4), 550–562.

183. Sixma, T. K., Kalk, K. H., van Zanten, B. A. M., et al. (1993) Refined crystal structure of *Escherichia coli* heat-labile enterotoxin, a close relative of cholera toxin, *J. Mol. Biol.*, **230**, 890–918.

184. Stein, P.E., Boodhoo, A., Armstrong, G. D., et al. (1994) The crystal structure of pertussis toxin, *Structure*, **2**, 45–47.

185. Douce, G., Giuliani, M. M., Giannelli, V., Pizza, M. G., Rappuoli, R., and Dougan, G. (1998) Mucosal immunogenicity of genetically detoxified derivatives of heat labile toxin from *Escherichia coli*, *Vaccine*, **16**, 1065–1073.

186. Tamura, S., Yamanaka, A., Shimohara, M., et al. (1994) Synergistic action of cholera toxin B subunit (and *Escherichia coli* heat-labile toxin B subunit) and a trace amount of cholera whole toxin as an adjuvant for nasal influenza vaccine, *Vaccine*, **12**, 419–426.

187. Richards, C. M., Aman, A. T., Hirst, T. R., Hill, T. J., and Williams, N. A. (2001) Protective mucosal immunity to ocular herpes simplex virus type 1 infection in mice by using *Escherichia coli* heat-labile enterotoxin B subunit as an adjuvant, *J. Virol.*, **75**, 1664–1671.

188. Sun, J.-B., Mielcarek, N., Lakew, M., et al. (1999) Intranasal administration of a *Schistosoma mansoni* glutathione S-transferase-cholera toxoid conjugate vaccine evokes antiparasitic and antipathological immunity in mice, *J. Immunol.*, **15**, 1045–1052.

189. Luross, J. A., Heaton, T., Hirst, T. R., Day, M. J., and Williams, N. A. (2002) *Escherichia coli* heat-labile enterotoxin B subunit prevents autoimmune arthritis through induction of regulatory CD4$^+$ T cells, *Arthritis Rheum.*, **62**(6), 1671–1682.

190. Williams, N. A. (2000) Immune modulation by the cholera-like enterotoxin B-subunits: from adjuvant to immunotherapeutic,

ETOX, *European Workshop on Bacterial Protein Toxins No 9, Ste Maxime, France* (27/06/1999), vol. 290, no. 4–5 (300 p.) (1 p.3/4) [Notes: extended abstracts], pp. 447–453.

191. Nashar, T. O., Webb, H. M., Eagletone, S., Williams, N. A., and Hirst, T. R. (1996) Potent immunogenicity of the B subunits of *Escherichia coli* heat-labile enterotoxin: receptor binding is essential and induces differential modulation of lymphocyte subsets, *Proc. Natl. Acad. Sci. U.S.A.*, **93**(1), 226–230.

192. Raveney, B. J. E., Richards, C. M., Aknin, M.-L., Copland, D. A., et al. (2008) The B subunit of Escherichia coli heat-labile enterotoxin inhibits Th1 but not Th17 cell responses in established autoimmune uveoretinitis, *Investig. Ophthalmol. Visual Sci.* **49**, 4008–4017.

193. Giuliani, M. M., Del Giudice, G., Gianelli, V., Dougan, G., Douce, G., Rappuoli, R., and Pizza, M. (1998) Mucosal adjuvanticity and immunogenicity of LTR72, a novel mutant of *Escherichia coli* heat-labile enterotoxin with partial knockout of ADP-ribosyltransferase activity, *J. Exp. Med.*, **187**, 1123–1132.

194. Martin, M., Metzger, D. J., Michalek, S. M., Connell, T. D., and Russell, M. W. (2000) Comparative analysis of the mucosal adjuvanticity of the type II heat-labile enterotoxins LT-IIa and LT-IIb, *Infect. Immun.*, **68**(1), 281–287.

195. Nawar, H., Arce, S., Russell, M. W., and Connell, T. D. (2005) Mucosal adjuvant properties of mutant LT-IIa and LT-IIb enterotoxins that exhibit altered ganglioside-binding activities, *Infect. Immun.*, **73**(3), 1330–1342.

196. Cárdenes-Freytag, L., Cheng, E., Mayeux, P., Domer, J. E., and Clements, J. D. (1999) Effectiveness of heat-killed *Candida albicans* and novel mucosal adjuvant, LT(R192G) against systemic candidiasis, *Infect. Immun.*, **67**, 826–833.

197. O'Neal, C. M., Clements, J. D., Estes, M. K., and Conner, M. E. (1998) Rotavirus 2/6 virus-like particles administered intranasally with cholera vaccine, *Escherichia coli* heat-labile toxin (LT) and LT-R192G induce protection from rotavirus challenge, *J. Virol.*, **72**, 3390–3393.

198. Chong, C., Friberg, M., and Clements, J. D. (1998) LT(R192G), a non-toxic mutant of the heat-labile enterotoxin of *Escherichia coli*, elicits enhanced humoral and cellular immune responses associated with protection against lethal oral challenge with *Salmonella* ssp., *Vaccine*, **16**, 732–740.

199. Tebbey, P. W., Scheuer, C. A., Peek, J. A., et al. (2000) Effective mucosal immunization against respiratory syncytial virus using purified F protein and a genetically detoxified cholera holotoxin, CT-E29H, *Vaccine*, **18**, 2723–2734.

200. Bowe, F., Lavelle, E. C., McNeela, E. A., et al. (2004) Mucosal vaccination against serogroup B meningococcus: induction of bactericidal antibodies and cellular immunity following intranasal immunization with NadA of *Neisseria meningitides* and mutants of *Escherichia coli* heat-labile enterotoxin, *Infect. Immun.*, **72**, 4052–4060.

201. Barakman, J. D., Ott, G., and O'Hagan, D. T. (1999) Intranasal immunization of mice with influenza virus vaccine in combination with the adjuvant LT-R72 induces potent mucosal and serum immunity which is stronger than that with traditional intramuscular immunization, *Infect. Immun.*, **67**, 4276–4279.

202. Agren, L. C., Ekman, L., Lowenadler, B., and Lycke, N. (1997) Genetically engineered nontoxic vaccine adjuvant that combines B cell targeting with immunomodulation by cholera toxin A1 subunit, *J. Immunol.*, **158**, 3936–3946.

203. Lycke, N. and Schon, K. (2001) The B cell targeted adjuvant, CTA1-DD exhibits potent mucosal immunoenhancing activity despite pre-existing anti-toxin immunity, *Vaccine*, **19**, 2542–2548.

204. Tamura, M., Nogimori, A., Murai, A., et al. (1982) Subunit structure of islet-activation protein, pertussis toxin, in conformity with the A-model B, *Biochemistry*, **21**, 5516–5522.

205. Kaslow, H. R. and Burns, D. L. (1992) Pertussis toxin and target eukaryotic cells: binding, entry and activation, *FASEB J.*, **6**, 2684–2690.

206. Saukkonen, K., Burnette, W. N., Mar, V. L., Masure, H. R., and Tuomanen, E. I. (1992) Pertussis toxin has eukaryotic-like carbohydrate recognition domains, *Proc. Natl. Acad. Sci. U.S.A.*, **89**, 118–122.

207. Lobet, Y., Feron, C., Dequesne, G., Simoen, E., Hauser, P., and Locht, C. (1993) Site-specific alterations in the B oligomer that affect receptor-binding activities and mitogenicity of pertussis toxin, *J. Exp. Med.*, **177**, 79–87.

208. Zhang, X. M., Berland, R., and Rosoff, P. M. (1995) Differential regulation of accessory mitogenic signaling receptors by the T cell antigen receptor, *Mol. Immunol.*, **32**, 323–332.

209. Li, H. and Wong, W. S. (2000) Mechanisms of pertussis toxin-induced myelomonocytic cell adhesion: role of CD14 and urokinase receptor, *Immunology*, **100**, 502–509.

210. Burnette, W. N. (1992) Perspectives in recombinant pertussis toxoid development. In: *Vaccine Research and Development* (Koff, W. and Six, H. R., eds.), Marcel Dekker, New York, pp. 143–193.

211. Lyons, A. B. (1997) Pertussis toxin pretreatment alters the in vivo cell division behaviour and survival of B lymphocytes after intravenous transfer, *Immunol. Cell. Biol.*, **75**, 7–12.

212. Meade, B. D., Kind, P. D., and Manclark, C. R. (1985) Altered mononuclear phagocyte function in mice treated with the lymphocytosis promoting factor of *Bordetella pertussis*, *Dev. Biol. Stand.*, **61**, 63–74.

213. Spangrude, G. J., Sacchi, F., Hill, H. R., Van Epps, D. E., and Daynes, R. A. (1985) Inhibition of lymphocyte and neutrophil chemotaxis by pertussis toxin, *J. Immunol.*, **135**, 4135–4143.

214. Cherry, J. D., Brunel, P. A., Golden, G. S., and Karzon, D. T. (1988) Report of the task force on pertussis immunization – 1988, *Pediatrics*, **88**, 939–984.

215. Ryan, M., McCarthy, L., Mahon, B., Rappuoli, R., and Mills, K. H. G. (1998) Pertussis toxin potentiates Th1 and Th2 responses to co-injected antigen: adjuvant action is associated with enhanced regulatory cytokine production and expression of the co-stimulatory molecules B7-1, B7-2 and CD28, *Int. Immunol.*, **10**, 651–662.

216. Roberts, M., Bacon, A., Rappuoli, R., et al. (1995) A mutant toxin molecule that lacks ADP-ribosyltransferase activity, PT-9K/129G, is an effective mucosal adjuvant for intranasally delivered proteins, *Infect. Immun.*, **63**, 2100–2108.

217. Mu, H.-H. and Sewell, W. A. (1994) Regulation of DTH and IgE responses by IL-4 and IFN-γ in immunized mice given pertussis toxin, *Immunology*, **83**, 639–645.

218. Munoz, J. J. and Peacock, M. G. (1990) Action of Pertussigen (pertussis toxin) on serum IgE and on Fcε receptors on lymphocytes, *Cell Immunol.*, **127**, 327–336.

219. Bell, F., Heath, P., MacLennan, J., et al. (1999) Adverse effects and sero-responses to an acellular pertussis/diphtheria/tetanus vaccine when combined with *Haemophilus influenzae* type b vaccine in an accelerated schedule, *Eur. J. Pediatr.*, **158**, 329–336.

220. Richie, E., Punjabi, N. H., Harjanto, S. J., et al. (1999) Safety and immunogenicity of combined diphtheria-tetanus-pertussis (whole cell and acellular)-*Haemophilus influenzae*-b conjugate vaccines administered to Indonesian children, *Vaccine*, **17**, 1384–1393.

221. Loosmore, S., Zealey, G., Cockle, S., Boux, H., et al. (1993) Characterization of pertussis toxin analogs containing mutations in B-oligomer subunits, *Infect. Immun.*, **61**, 3216–3224.

222. Leavy, O. (2005) Mechanisms of immunomodulatory activity of cholera toxin, *PhD Thesis*, Trinity College, Dublin, Ireland.

223. Ausiello, C. M., Fedele, G., Urbani, F., et al. (2002) Native and genetically inactivated pertussis toxins induce human dendritic cell maturation and synergize with lipopolysaccharide

in promoting T helper type 1 responses, *J. Infect. Dis.*, **186**, 351–360.

224. de Jong, E. C., Vieira, P. L., Kalinski, P., et al. (2002) Microbial compounds selectively induce Th1 cell-promoting or Th2 cell-promoting dendritic cells in vitro with diverse Th cell-polarizing signals, *J. Immunol.*, **168**, 1704–1709.

225. Gross, M. K., Au, D. C., Smith, A. L., and Storm, D. R. (1992) Targeted mutations that ablate either the adenylate cyclase or hemolysine function of the bifunctional CyaA toxin of *Bordetella pertussis* abolish virulence, *Proc. Natl. Acad. Sci., U.S.A.*, **89**, 4898–4902.

226. Mouallem, M., Farfel, Z., and Hanski, E. (1990) *Bordetella pertussis* adenylate cyclase toxin: intoxication of host cells by bacterial invasion, *Infect. Immun.*, **58**, 3759–3764.

227. Pearson, R. D., Symes, P., Conboy, M., Weiss, A. A., and Hewlett, E. L. (1987) Inhibition of monocyte oxidative responses by *Bordetella pertussis* adenylate cyclase toxin, *J. Immunol.*, **139**, 2749–2754.

228. Njamkepo, E., Pinot, F., Francois, D., et al. (2000) Adaptive responses of human monocytes infected with *Bordetella pertussis*: the role of adenylate cyclase hemolysin, *J. Cell. Physiol.*, **183**, 91–99.

229. Gueirard, P., Druilhe, A., Pretolani, M., and Guiso, N. (1998) Role of adenylate cyclase-hemolysin in alveolar macrophage apoptosis during *Bordetella pertussis* infection in vivo, *Infect. Immunol.*, **66**, 1718–1725.

230. Lavelle, E. C., McNeela, E., Armstrong, M. E., et al. (2003) Cholera toxin promotes the induction of regulatory T cells specific for bystander antigens by modulating dendritic cell activation, *J. Immunol.*, **171**, 2384–2392.

231. Ross, P. J., Lavelle, E. C., Mills, K. H., and Boyd, A. P. (2004) Adenylate cyclase toxin from *Bordetella pertussis* synergized with lipopolysaccharide to promote innate interleukin-10 production and enhance the induction of Th2 and regulatory T cells, *Infect. Immun.*, **72**, 1568–1579.

232. Osicka, R., Osickova, A., Basar, T., et al. (2000) Delivery of CD8$^+$ T-cell epitopes into major histocompatibility complex class I antigen presentation pathway by *Bordetella pertussis* adenylate cyclase: delineation of cell invasive structures and permissive insertion sites, *Infect. Immun.*, **68**, 247–256.

233. Baldridge, J., Myers, K., Johnson, D., Persing, D., Cluff, C., and Herschberg, R. (2006) Monophosphoryl lipid A and synthetic lipid A mimetics as TLR4-based adjuvants and immunomodulators. In: *Vaccine Adjuvants: Immunological and Clinical Principles* (Hackett, C. and Harn, D. A., Jr., eds.), Humana Press, Totowa, NJ, pp. 235–255.

234. Dinarello, C. A. (1991) The proinflammatory cytokines interleukin-1 and tumor necrosis factor and treatment of the septic shock syndrome, *J. Infect. Dis.*, **163**, 1177–1184.

235. Higgins, S. C., Lavelle, E. C., McCann, C., et al. (2003) Toll-like receptor 4- mediated innate IL-10 activates antigen-specific regulatory T cell and confers resistance to *Bordetella pertussis* by inhibiting inflammatory pathology, *J. Immunol.*, **171**, 3119–3127.

236. Nauts, H. C., Swift, W. E., and Corley, B. L. (1946) Treatment of malignant tumors by bacterial toxins as developed by the late William B. Coley, M.D., reviewed in light of modern research, *Cancer Res.*, **6**, 205–216.

237. Ribi, E. (1984) Beneficial modification of endotoxin molecule, *J. Biol. Response Mod.*, **3**, 1–9.

238. Ulrich, J. T. and Myers, K. B. (1995) Monophosphoryl lipid A as an adjuvant past experiences and new directions. In: *Vaccine Design: The Subunit and Adjuvant Approach* (Powell, M. F. and Newman, J. M., eds.), Plenum Press, New York, pp. 495–524.

239. Johnson, D. A., Sowell, C. G., and Johnson, C. L., et al. (1999) Synthesis and biological evaluation of a new class of vaccine adjuvants: aminoalkyl glucosaminide 4-phosphates (AGPs), *Biorg. Med. Chem. Lett.*, **9**, 2273–2278.

240. Seydel, U., Labischinski, H., Kastowsky, M., and Brandenburg, K. (1993) Phase behavior, supramolecular structure, and molecular conformation of lipopolysaccharide, *Immunobiology*, **187**, 191–211.

241. Fukuoka, S., Brandenburg, K., Muller, M., et al. (2001) Physicochemical analysis of lipid A fractions of lipopolysaccharide from *Erwinia carotovora* in relation to bioactivity, *Biochim. Biophys. Acta*, **1510**, 185–197.

242. Fukase, K., Oikawa, M., Suda, Y., et al. (1999) New synthesis and conformational analysis of lipid A: biological activity and supramolecular assembly, *J. Endotoxin Res.*, **5**, 46–51.

243. Brandenburg, K., Matsuura, M., Heine, H., et al. (2002) Biophysical characterization of triacyl monosaccharide lipid A partial structures in relation to bioactivity, *Biophys. J.*, **83**, 322–333.

244. Dupont, J.-C., Altclas, J., Sigelchifer, M., Von Eschen, E. B., Timmermans, I., and Wegener, A. (2002) Efficacy and safety of AgB/RC529: a novel two dose adjuvant vaccine against hepatitis B, *42nd Interscience Conference on Antimicrobial Agents and Chemotherapy, San Diego, CA*, September 27–30 [abstract].

245. Martin, M., Michalek, S., and Katz, J. (2003) Role of innate immune factors in the adjuvant activity of monophosphoryl lipid A, *Infect. Immun.*, **71**(5), 2498–2507.

246. Moore, A., McCarthy, L., and Mills, K. H. G. (1999) The adjuvant combination monophosphoryl lipid A and QS21 switches T cell responses induced with a soluble recombinant HIV protein from Th2 to Th1, *Vaccine*, **17**, 2517–2527.

247. Salkowski, C. A. (1997) Lipopolysaccharide and monophosphoryl lipid A differentially regulate interleukin-12, gamma interferon and interleukine-10 mRNA production in murine macrophages, *Infect. Immun.*, **65**, 3239–3247.

248. Peteers, C. C. A. M., Legerman, P. R., De Weers, O., et al. (1996) Polysaccharide- conjugate vaccines. In: *Vaccine Protocols* (Robinson, A., Farrar, G. H., and Wiblin, C. H., eds.), Humana Press, Totowa, NJ, pp.111–134.

249. Stoute, J. A., Kester, K. E., Krzych, U., et al. (1998) Long-term efficacy and immune responses following immunization with the RTSS malaria vaccine, *J. Infect. Dis.*, **178**, 1139–1144.

250. McCormack, S., Tilzey, A., Carmichael, A., et al. (2000) A phase I trial in HIV negative healthy volunteers evaluating the effect of potent adjuvant on immunogenicity of a recombinant gp120W61D derived from dual tropic R5X4, HIV-1ACH320, *Vaccine*, **18**, 1166–1177.

251. Thoelen, S., Van Damme, P., Mathei, C., et al. (1998) Safety and immunogenicity of a hepatitis B vaccine formulated with a novel adjuvant system, *Vaccine*, **16**, 708–714.

252. Thoelen, S., de Clercq, N., and Tornieporth, N. (2001) A prophylactic hepatitis B vaccine with a novel adjuvant system, *Vaccine*, **19**, 2400–2403.

253. Vernacchio, L., Bernstein, H., Pelton, S., et al. (2002) Effect of monophosphoryl lipid A (MPL(R)) on T-helper cells when administered as an adjuvant with pneumococcal-CRM(197) conjugate vaccine in healthy toddlers, *Vaccine*, **20**, 3658–3667.

254. Drachenberg, K. J., Wheeler, A. W., Stuebner, P., and Horak, F. (2001) A well- tolerated grass pollen-specific allergy vaccine containing a novel adjuvant, monophosphoryl lipid A, reduces allergic symptoms after only four preseasonal injections, *Allergy*, **56**, 498–505.

255. Miller, D. L., Ross, E. M., Alderslade, R., Bellman, M. H., and Rawson, N. S. (1981) Pertussis immunisation and serious acute neurological illness in children, *Br. Med. J.*, **282**, 1595–1599.

256. Donnelly, S., Loscher, C., Lynch, M. A., and Mills, K. H. G. (2001) Whole cell but not acellular pertussis vaccines induce convulsive activity in mice: evidence of a role for toxin-induced

IL-1β in a new murine model for analysis of neuronal side effects of vaccination, *Infect. Immun.*, **69**, 4217–4223.

257. van Ginkel, F. W., Jackson, R. J., Yuki, Y., and McGhee, J. R. (2000) Cutting edge: the mucosal adjuvant cholera toxin redirects vaccine proteins into olfactory tissues, *J. Immunol.*, **165**, 4778–4782.

258. Marinaro, M., Staats, H. F., Hiroi, T., et al. (1995) Mucosal adjuvant effect of cholera toxin in mice results from induction of T helper 2 (Th2) cells and IL-4, *J. Immunol.*, **155**, 4621–4629.

259. Yamamoto, S., Kiyono, H., Yamamoto, M., et al. (1997) A nontoxic mutant of cholera toxin elicits Th2-type responses for enhanced mucosal immunity, *Proc. Natl. Acad. Sci. U.S.A.*, **94**, 5267–5272.

260. Simecka, J. W., Jackson, R. J., Kiyono, H., and McGhee, J. R. (2000) Mucosally induced immunoglobulin E-associated inflammation in the respiratory tract, *Infect. Immun.*, **68**, 672–679.

261. Takahashi, I., Kiyono, H., Marinaro, M., et al. (1996) Mechanisms for mucosal immunogenicity and adjuvanticity of *Escherichia coli* labile toxin, *J. Infect. Dis.*, **173**, 627–635.

262. Rennels, M. B., Deloria, M. A., Pichichero, M. E., et al. (2000) Extensive swelling after booster doses of acellular pertussis-tetanus-diphtheria vaccines, *Pediatrics*, **105**: e12.

263. Gazzinelli, R. T., Ropert, C., Almeida, I. C., Silva, J. S., and Campos, M. A. (2006) Glycosylphosphatidylinositol anchors as natural immunological adjuvants derived from protozoan parasites. In: *Vaccine Adjuvants: Immunological and Clinical Principles* (Hackett, C. and Harn, D. A., Jr., eds.), Humana Press, Totowa, NJ, pp. 155–175.

264. Pearce, E., Scott, P. A., and Sher, A. (1999) Immune regulation in parasitic diseases. In: *Fundamentals in Immunology*, 4th ed. (Paul, W., ed.), Lippincott-Raven, Philadelphia, pp. 1271–1295.

265. Aliberti, J. C. S., Cardoso, M. A. G., Martins, G. A., Gazzinelli, R. T., et al. (1996) IL-12 mediates resistance to *Trypanozoma cruzi* infection in mice and is produced by normal murine macrophages in response to live trypomastigote, *Infect. Immun.*, **64**, 1961–1967.

266. Cardillo, F., Voltarelli, J. C., Reed, S. G., and Silva, J. S. (1996) Regulation of *Trypanozoma cruzi* infection in mice by gamma interferon and interleukin 10: role of NK cells, *Infect. Immun.*, **64**, 128–134.

267. Gazzinelli, R. T., Ropert, C., and Campos, M. A. (2004) Role of Toll/interleukin-1 receptor signaling pathway in host resistance and pathogenesis during infection with protozoan parazites, *Immunol. Rev.*, **201**(1), 9–25.

268. Biron, C. and Gazzinelli, R. T. (1995) IL-12 effects on immune responses to microbial infections: a key mediator in regulating disease outcome, *Curr. Opin. Immunol.*, **7**, 485–496.

269. Gazzinelli, R. T., Wysocka, M., Hayashi, S., et al. (1994) Parasite-induced IL-12 stimulates early IFN-g synthesis and resistance during acute infection with *Toxoplasma gondii*, *J. Immunol.*, **153**, 2533–2543.

270. Mattner, F., Magram, J., Ferrante, J., et al. (1996) Genetically resistant mice lacking interleukin-12 are susceptible to infection with *Leishmania major* and mount a polarized Th2 cell response, *Eur. J. Immunol.*, **26**, 1553–1559.

271. Su, Z. and Stevenson, M. M. (2002) IL-12 is required for antibody-mediated protective immunity against blood-stage *Plasmodium chabaudi* AS malaria infection in mice, *J. Immunol.*, **168**, 1348–1355.

272. Roggero, E., Perez, A., Tamae-Kakasu, M., et al. (2002) Differential susceptibility to acute *Trypanozoma cruzi* infection in BALB/c and C57BL/6 mice is not associated with a distinct parasite load but cytokine abnormalities, *Clin. Exp. Immunol.*, **128**, 421–428.

273. Gazzinelli, R. T., Hieny, S., Wysocka, M., et al. (1996) In the absence of endogenous IL-10 mice acutely infected with *Toxoplasma gondii* succumb to a lethal CD41 T cell response associated with type 1 cytokine synthesis, *J. Immunol.*, **157**, 798–805.

274. Hunter, C. A., Ellis-Neyes, L. A., Slifer, T., et al. (1997) IL-10 is required to prevent immune hyperactivity during infection with *Trypanozoma cruzi*, *J. Immunol.*, **158**, 3311–3316.

275. Camargo, M. M., Almeida, I. C., Pereira, M. E. S., et al. (1997) Glycosylphosphatidylinositol anchored mucin-like glycoproteins isolated from *Trypanozoma cruzi* trypomastigotes initiate the synthesis of proinflammatory cytokines by macrophages, *J. Immunol.*, **158**, 5980–5991.

276. Almeida, I. C., Camargo, M. M., Procopio, D. O., et al. (2000) Highly-purified glycosylphosphatidylinositols from *Trypanozoma cruzi* are potent proinflammatory agents, *EMBO J.*, **19**, 1476–1485.

277. Almeida, I. C. and Gazzinelli, R. T. (2001) Proinflammatory activity of glycosylphosphatidylinositol anchors derived from *Trypanozoma cruzi*: structural and functional analyses, *J. Leuk. Biol.*, **70**, 467–477.

278. Schofield, L. and Hackett, F. (1993) Signal transduction in host cells by a glycosylphosphatidylinositol toxin of malaria parasites, *J. Exp. Med.*, **177**, 145–153.

279. Naik, R. S., Branch, O. L. H., and Wood, A. S. (2000) Glycosylphosphatidylinositol anchors of *Plasmodium falciparum*: molecular characterization and naturally elicited antibody response that may provide immunity to malaria pathogenesis, *J. Exp. Med.*, **192**, 1563–1575.

280. Magez, S., Stijlemans, B., Radwanska, M., et al. (1998) The glycosyl-inositol-phosphate and dimyristoylglycerol moieties of the glycosylphosphatidylinositol anchor of the *Trypanozoma* variant-specific surface glycoprotein are distinct macrophage activating factors, *J. Immunol.*, **160**, 1949–1956.

281. Ferguson, M. A. J. (1999) The structure, biosynthesis and functions of glycosylphosphatidylinositol anchors and the contributions of *Trypanozoma* research, *J. Cell Sci.*, **112**, 2799–1809.

282. Campos, M. A. S., Almeida, I. C., Takeuchi, O., et al. (2001) Activation of Toll-like receptor-2 by glycosylphosphatidylinositol anchors from a protozoan parasite, *J. Immunol.*, **167**, 416–423.

283. Janeway, C. A., Jr. and Medzhitov, R. (2002) Innate immune recognition, *Annu. Rev. Immunol.*, **20**, 197–216.

284. Akira, S., Takeda, K., and Kaisho, T. (2001) Toll-like receptors: critical proteins linking innate and acquired immunity, *Nat. Immunol.*, **2**, 675–680.

285. Bendelac, A. and Medzhitov, R. (2002) Adjuvants of immunity: harnessing innate immunity to promote adaptive immunity, *J. Exp. Med.*, **195**, F19-F23.

286. Jankovic, D., Sher, A., and Yap, G. (2001) Th1/Th2 effector choice in parasitic infection: decision making by committee, *Curr. Opin. Immunol.*, **13**, 403–409.

287. O'Garra, A. (1998) Cytokines induce the development of functionally heterogeneous T helper cell subsets, *Immunity*, **8**, 275–283.

288. Okano, M., Nishizaki, K., Da'dara, A., Thomas, P., Carter, M., and Harn, D. A., Jr. (2006) The immunomodulatory glycan LNF-PIII/Lewis X functions as a potent adjuvant for protein antigens. In: *Vaccine Adjuvants: Immunological and Clinical Principles* (Hacket, C. J. and Harn, D. A., Jr., eds.), Humana Press, Totowa, NJ, 177–191.

289. Finkelman, F. D. and Urban, J. F., Jr. (2001) The other side of the coin: the protective role of the TH2 cytokines, *J. Allergy Clin. Immunol.*, **107**, 772–780.

290. Remou, F., Rogerie, F., Gallissot, M. C., et al. (2000) Sex-dependent neutralizing humoral response to *Schistosoma mansoni* 28GST antigen in infected human populations, *J. Infect. Dis.*, **181**, 1855–1859.

291. Urban, J. F., Jr., Fayer, R., Sullivan, C., et al. (1996) Local TH1 and TH2 responses to parasitic infection in the intestine: regulation by IFN-gamma and IL-4, *Vet. Immunol. Immunopathol.*, **54**, 337–344.

292. Urban, J. F., Jr., Schopf, L., Morris, S. C., et al. (2000) Stat6 signaling promotes protective immunity against *Trichinella spiralis* through a mast cell- and T-cell-dependent mechanism, *J. Immunol.*, **164**, 2046–2052.

293. Fallon, P. G., Fookes, R. E., and Wharton, G. A. (1996) Temporal differences in praziquantel- and oxamniquine-induced tegumental damage to adult *Schistosoma mansoni*: implications for drug-antibody synergy, *Parasitology*, **112**(Part 1), 47–58.

294. Vella, A. T. and Pearce, E. J. (1992) CD4$^+$ and Th2 response induced by *Schistosoma mansoni* eggs develops rapidly, through an early, transient Th0-like stage, *J. Immunol.*, **148**, 2283–2290.

295. Cook, G. A., Metwali, A., Blum, A., Mathew, R., and Weinstock, J. V. (1993) Lymphokine expression in granulomas of *Schistosoma mansoni*-infected mice, *Cell Immunol.*, **152**, 13–58.

296. van der Kleij, D., Latz, E., Brouwers, J. F., et al. (2002) A novel host-parasite lipid cross-talk. Schistosomal lysophosphatidylserine activates Toll-like receptor 2 and affects immune polarization, *J. Biol. Chem.*, **227**, 48122–48129.

297. Velupillai, P., dos Reis, E. A., dos Reis, M. G., and Harn, D. A. (2000) Lewis^x- containing oligosaccharide attenuates schistosome egg antigen-induced immune depression in human schistosomias, *Hum. Immunol.*, **61**, 225–232.

298. Velupillai, P. and Harn, D. A. (1994) Oligosaccharide-specific induction of interleukin 10 production by B220+ cells from schistosome-infected mice: a mechanism for regulation of CD+ T-cell subsets, *Proc. Natl. Acad. Sci. U.S.A.*, **91**(1), 18–22.

299. Thomas, P. G., Carter, M. R., Atochina, O., et al. (2003) Maturation of dendritic cell 2 phenotype by a helminth glycan uses a Toll-like receptor 4-dependent mechanism, *J. Immunol.*, **171**, 5837–5841.

300. Ellouz, F., Adam, A., Ciobaru, R., and Lederer, E. (1974) Minimal structural requirements for adjuvant activity of bacterial peptidoglycan derivatives, *Biochem. Biophys. Res. Commun.*, **59**, 1317–1325.

301. Bahr, G. M. (2006) Immune and antiviral effects of the synthetic immunomodulator murabutide. In: *Vaccine Adjuvants: Immunological and Clinical Principles* (Hackett, C. and Harn, D. A., Jr., eds.), Humana Press, Totowa, NJ, pp. 193–219.

302. Bahr, G. M., Darcissac, E., Bevec, D., Dukor, P., and Chedid, L. (1995) Immunopharmacological activities and clinical development of muramyl peptides with particular emphasis on murabutide, *Int. J. Immunopharmacol.*, **17**, 117–131.

303. Waters, R. V., Terrell, T. G., and Jones, G. H. (1986) Uveitis induction in the rabbit by muramyl dipeptides, *Infect. Immun.*, **51**, 816–825.

304. Chedid, L., Audibert, F., Lefrancier, P., Choay, J., and Lederer, E. (1976) Modification of the immune response by a synthetic adjuvant and analogs, *Proc. Natl. Acad. Sci. U.S.A.*, **73**, 2472–2475.

305. Lefrancier, P., Derrien, M. Jamet, X., et al. (1982) Apyrogenic, adjuvant-active *N*- acetyl-muramyl-dipeptides, *J. Med. Chem.*, **25**, 87–90.

306. Werner, G. H. and Jolles, P. (1996) Immunostimulating agents: what next? A review of their present and potential medical applications, *Eur. J. Biochem.*, **242**, 1–19.

307. Azuma, I. and Otani, T. (1994) Potentiation of host defense mechanism against infection by a cytokine inducer, an acyl-MDP derivative, MDP-Lys(L18) (romurtide) in mice and humans, *Med. Res. Rev.*, **14**, 401–414.

308. Phillips, N. C. and Chedid, L. (1988) Muramyl peptides and liposomes. In: *Liposomes as Drug Carriers* (Gregoriadis, G. E., ed.), John Wiley & Sons, Ltd, Chichester, pp. 243–259.

309. Parant, M. (1987) Muramyl peptides as enhancers of host resistance to bacterial infections. In: *Immunopharmacology of Infectious Diseases: Vaccine Adjuvants and Modulators of Non-Specific Resistance* (Majde, J. A. ed.), Alan R. Liss, Inc., New York, pp. 235–244.

310. Parant, M. and Chedid, L. (1988) Muramyl dipeptides. In: *Handbook of Experimental Pharmacology*, vol. 85 (Bray, M. A. and Morley, J., eds.), Springer-Verlag, Berlin, pp. 503–516.

311. Chedid, L. A., Parant, M. A., Audibert, F. M., et al. (1982) Biological activity of a new synthetic muramyl peptide adjuvant devoid of pyrogenicity, *Infect. Immun.*, **35**, 417–424.

312. Byars, N. E. (1984) Two adjuvant-active muramyl dipeptide analogs induce differential production of lymphocyte-activating factor and a factor causing distress in guinea pigs, *Infect. Immun.*, **44**, 344–350.

313. Kong, Y. C., Audibert, F., Giraldo, A. A., Rose, N. R., and Chedid, L. (1985) Effects of natural or synthetic microbial adjuvants on induction of autoimmune thyroiditis, *Infect. Immun.*, **49**, 40–45.

314. Chang, Y. H., Pearson, C. M., and Chedid, L. (1981) Adjuvant polyarthritis. V. Induction by N-acetylmuramyl-L-alanyl-D-isoglutamine, the smallest peptide subunit of bacterial peptidoglycan, *J. Exp. Med.*, **153**, 1021–1026.

315. Audibert, F. M., Przewlocki, G., Leclerc, C. D., et al. (1984) Enhancement by murabutide of the immune response to natural and synthetic hepatitis B surface antigens, *Infect. Immun.*, **45**, 261–266.

316. Przewlocki, G., Audibert, F., Jolivet, M., et al. (1986) Production of antibodies recognizing a hepatitis B virus (HBV) surface antigen by administration of murabutide associated to a synthetic pre-S HBV peptide conjugated to a toxoid carrier, *Biochem. Biophys. Res. Commun.*, **140**, 557–564.

317. Olberling, F., Morin, A., Duclos, B., Lang, J. M., Berchley, E. H., and Chedid, L. (1983) Enhancement of antibody response to a natural fragment of streptococcal M protein by murabutide administered to healthy volunteers, *Int. J. Immunol.*, **7**, 398.

318. Telzak, E., Wolff, S. M., Dinarello, C. A., et al. (1986) Clinical evaluation of the immunoadjuvant murabutide, a derivative of MDP, administered with tetanus toxoid vaccine, *J. Infect. Dis.*, **153**, 628–633.

319. Darcissac, E. C., Truong, M. J., Dewulf, J., Mouton, Y., et al. (2000) The synthetic immunomodulator murabutide controls human immunodeficiency virus type 1 replication at multiple levels in macrophages and dendritic cells, *J. Virol.*, **74**, 7794–7802.

320. Amiel, C., de la Tribonniere, X., Vidal, V., et al. (2002) Clinical tolerance and immunological effects after single or repeated administrations of the synthetic immunomodulator murabutide in HIV-1-infected patients, *J. AIDS*, **30**, 294–305.

321. de la Tribonniere, X., Mouton, Y., Vidal, V., et al. (2003) A phase I study of a six- week cycle of immunotherapy with murabutide in HIV-1 patients naïve to antiretrovirals, *Med. Sci. Monit.*, **9**, 143–150.

322. Kensil, C. R., Liu, G., Anderson, C., and Storey, J. (2006) Effects of QS-21 on innate and adaptive immune responses. In: *Vaccine Adjuvants: Immunological and Clinical Principles* (Hackett, C. and Harn, D. A., Jr., eds.), Humana Press, Totowa, NJ, pp. 221–234.

323. Hostettman, K. and Marston, A. (1995) *Saponins*, Cambridge University Press, Cambridge.

324. Jacobsen, N. E., Fairbrother, W. J., Kensil, C. R., et al. (1996) Structure of the saponin adjuvant QS-21 and its base-catalyzed isomerization product by 1H and natural abundance 13C NMR spectrometry, *Carbohydr. Res.*, **280**, 1–14.

325. Espinet, R. G. (1951) Nouveau vaccine antiaphteux a complexe glucoviral, *Gac. Vet.*, **13**, 268–273.

326. Dalsgaard. K. (1974) Isolation of a substance from *Quillaja saponaria* Molina with adjuvant activity in foot-and-mouth disease vaccines, *Arch. Gesamte Virusforsch.*, **44**, 243–254.

327. van Setten, D. C., van de Werken, G., Zomer, G., and Kersten, G. F. A. (1995) Glycosyl compositions and structural characteristics of the potential immunoadjuvant active saponins in the *Quillaja saponaria* Molina extract Quil A, *Rapid Commun. Mass Spectrom.*, **9**, 660–666.

328. Kensil, C. R., Patel, U., Lennick, M., and Marcianni, D. (1991) Separation and characterization of saponins with adjuvant activity from *Quillaja saponaria* Molina cortex, *J. Immunol.*, **146**, 431–437.

329. Soltysik, S., Wu, J. Y., Recchia, J., et al. (1995) Structure/function studies of QS-21 adjuvant: assessment of triterpene aldehyde and glucuronic acid roles in adjuvant function, *Vaccine*, **13**, 1403–1410.

330. Rhodes, J. (1989) Evidence for an intercellular covalent reaction essential in antigen-specific T cell activation, *J. Immunol.*, **143**, 1482–1489.

331. Liu, G., Anderdon, C., Scaltreto, H., Barbon, J., and Kensil, C. R. (1994) QS-21 structure/function studies: effect of acylation on adjuvant activity, *Vaccine*, **20**, 2808–2815.

332. Kensil, C. R., Newman, M. J., Coughlin, R. T., et al. (1993) The use of Stimulon adjuvant to boost vaccine response, *Vaccine Res.*, **2**, 273–281.

333. Coughlin, R. T., Fattom, A., Chu, C., White, A. C., and Winston, S. (1995) Adjuvant activity of QS-21 for experimental *E. coli* 018 polysaccharide vaccines, *Vaccine*, **13**, 17–21.

334. Hancock, G. E., Speelman, D. J., Frenchick, P. J., et al. (1995) Formulation of the purified fusion protein of respiratory syncytial virus with the saponin QS-21 induces protective immune responses in Balb/c mice that are similar to those generated by experimental infection, *Vaccine*, **13**, 391–400.

335. Sasaki, S., Sumino, K., Hamajima, K., et al. (1998) Induction of systemic and mucosal immune responses to human immunodeficiency virus type 1 by a DNA vaccine formulated with QS-21 saponin adjuvant via intramuscular and intranasal routes, *J. Virol.*, **72**, 4931–4939.

336. Kim, S. K., Ragupathi, G., Musselli, C., et al. (1999) Comparison of the effect of different immunological adjuvants on the antibody and T-cell response to immunization with MUC1-KLH and GD3-KLH conjugate cancer vaccines, *Vaccine*, **18**, 597–603.

337. Chen, D., Endres, R., Maa, Y. F., et al. (2003) Epidermal powder immunization of mice and monkeys with an influenza vaccine, *Vaccine*, **21**, 2830–2836.

338. Evans, T. G., McElrath, M. J., Matthews, T., et al. (2001) QS-21 promotes an adjuvant effect allowing for reduced antigen dose during HIV-1 envelope subunit immunization in humans, *Vaccine*, **19**, 2080–2091.

339. Nardin, E. H., Oliveira, G. A., Calvo-Calle, J. M., et al. (2000) Synthetic malaria peptide vaccine elicits high levels of antibodies in vaccines of defined HLA genotypes, *J. Infect. Dis.*, **182**, 1486–1496.

340. Livingston, P. O., Adluri, S., Helling, F., et al. (1994) Phase I trial of immunological adjuvant QS-21 with GM2 ganglioside-keyhole limpet haemocyanin conjugate vaccine in patients with malignant melanoma, *Vaccine*, **12**, 1275–1280.

341. Helling, F., Zhang, S., Shang, A., et al. (1995) GM2-KLH conjugate vaccine: increased immunogenicity in melanoma patients after administration with immunological adjuvant QS-21, *Cancer Res.*, **55**, 2783–2788.

342. Boyaka, P. N., Marinaro, M., Jackson, P. J., et al. (2001) Oral QS-21 requires early IL-4 help for induction of mucosal and systemic immunity, *J. Immunol.*, **166**, 2283–2290.

343. Chen, D., McMichael, J. C., van der Meid, K. R., et al. (1996) Evaluation of purified UspA from *Moraxella catarrhalis* as a vaccine in a murine model after active immunization, *Infect. Immun.*, **64**, 1900–1905.

344. Yewdell, J. W. and Bennink, J. R. (1990) The binary logic of antigen processing and presentation to T cells, *Cell*, **62**, 203–206.

345. Newman, M. J., Wu, J. Y., Gardner, B. H., et al. (1992) Saponin adjuvant induction of ovalbumin-specific CD8$^+$ cytotoxic T lymphocyte responses, *J. Immunol.*, **148**, 2357–2362.

346. Wu, J. Y., Gardner, B. H., Murphy, C. I., et al. (1992) Saponin adjuvant enhancement of antigen-specific immune responses to an experimental HIV-1 vaccine, *J. Immunol.*, **148**, 1519–1525.

347. Fenton, R. G., Keller, C. J., Hanna, N., and Taub, D. D. (1995) Induction of T cell immunity against Ras oncoproteins by soluble protein or Ras-expressing *Escherichia coli*, *J. Natl. Cancer Inst.*, **87**, 1853–1861.

348. Kensil, C., Mo, A., and Truneh, A. (2004) Current vaccine adjuvants: an overview of a diverse class, *Front. Biosci.*, **9**, 2972–2988.

Chapter 40

Immune Tolerance

Immune tolerance holds the key to controlling unwanted immunologic attacks on self and transplanted tissues. Alloreactive responses to transplanted tissues and organs have long been recognized as among the most powerful known in immunology, being at least 100-fold greater than those elicited by conventional antigens; such responses require potent, nonspecific immunosuppression to maintain organ allografts in clinical practice. In contrast, autoimmune diseases involve the loss of tolerance to self-antigens *(1)*.

The identification of genes involved in the establishment and maintenance of central and peripheral tolerance provides a new level of understanding and, potentially, control of deleterious immune responses. For example, induction of central T-cell tolerance is promoted by thymic expression of peripheral antigens related to the function of the gene encoding the transcription factor AIRE *(2)*. In the peripheral tissues, active antigen-specific suppression mediated by a variety of T cells has been repeatedly and reliably observed over decades. The association of the gene encoding the transcription factor Foxp3 with immune disorders and the linking of that gene to regulatory T cells represent a substantial milestone, allowing new approaches to determine the origin and mode of action of a potentially important regulatory T-cell population *(3)*. An emerging understanding of the genetic and cellular processes involved in central and peripheral tolerance should enable more robust and antigen-specific approaches to prevent organ transplant rejection and provide treatment strategies for autoimmunity *(1)*.

40.1 Concepts of Immune Tolerance

The primary responsibility of the immune system is to protect the host from foreign materials. Immune tolerance is selective in that the immune system disregards molecules native to the host and responds aggressively to remove foreign molecules. Autoimmune diseases are the result of breakdowns in immune tolerance. The development lineages of B cells and T cells contain several checkpoints at which autoreactive cells are blocked from maturation. The immune system maintains control over self/nonself reactivity with functional regulation of mature lymphocytes (http://www.rndsystems.com/mini_review_detail_objectname_MR03_ImmuneTolerance.aspx).

Exposure of B Cells to Antigen. Immature B cells are the earliest cell type in the lineage to express antigen-specific B-cell receptors (BCRs) *(4–7)*. Selection against autoreactive B cells begins at this stage of development and takes place in the bone marrow *(8,9)*. A functional BCR binds extracellular molecules and initiates antigen-specific cytoplasmic signaling *(10–13)*. If the B cell does not bind antigen, BCR signaling remains at a basal level, and the cell enters the transitional stage for release into the peripheral circulation. If the immature B cell encounters extracellular antigen capable of cross-linking its BCR, it will experience an increase in BCR-mediated signaling accompanied by developmental arrest *(14,15)*. This indicates that the B cell has responded to an autoantigen and will be blocked from further development. In addition, the B cell will initiate the receptor editing process to produce BCR with new antigen-binding specificities. If it cannot alter its BCR effectively, the immature B cells will be deleted by apoptosis to prevent development into autoreactive mature B cells. Some autoreactive B-cell clones escape deletion and enter the peripheral circulation in an anergic state *(16)*. These cells are not responsive to antigen stimulation but potentially can be activated with pathogen-derived ligands that mimic the autoantigen *(17)* (http://www.rndsystems.com/mini_review_detail_objectname_MR03_ImmuneTolerance.aspx).

Genetic Recombination and Receptor Editing. Genetic recombination within the immunoglobulin locus is the major source of BCR diversity, as different immunoglobulin variable domain sequences confer different antigen-binding specificities to the receptor. The Rag 1 and Rag 2 proteins, which mediate recombination, are upregulated under conditions when rearrangement of the heavy- and light-chain sequences is required and downregulated at other times *(18,19)*. Once a B cell produces an antigen receptor, it is normally prevented from further rearrangement of the heavy- and light-chain sequences (allelic exclusion) *(20)*. In the process of receptor editing, however, a B-cell re-expresses the Rag proteins and then can produce alternate light-chain sequences *(21–25)*. Replacement light chains are paired with the existing heavy chain and the modified BCR is once again subjected to antigen selection. If receptor editing results in a BCR unresponsive to self-antigen, the B cells continue along the development pathway *(26,27)*. If receptor editing results in a different BCR that is still autoreactive, rearrangement of the light chain locus will continue. Autoreactive B cells that cannot re-express their Rag proteins will be deleted by apoptosis (http://www.rndsystems.com/mini_review_detail_objectname_MR03_ImmuneTolerance.aspx).

B-Cell Receptor Signaling. In resting mature B cells, the BCR associates with the Igα and Igβ accessory proteins *(28–30)* and is separated from them following antigen-induced receptor desensitization *(31)*. Adaptor and accessory proteins are associated with distinct regions of the plasma membrane termed *lipid rafts (32)*. The BCR is able to enter lipid rafts and begin signaling only after it has been cross-linked by antigen binding *(33)*. Positive and negative regulating coreceptors also affect the access of the BCR to the raft *(34,35)*. Cross-linking of the BCR with the positive regulators CD19 and CD21 leads to a longer retention time of the BCR in the raft and, consequently, prolonged signaling *(36,37)*. Involvement of negative regulators, such as Fc gamma RII, CD22, and PIR-B, opposes BCR-mediated signaling *(38)*. The BCR adaptor and accessory proteins as well as the positive and negative regulators directly influence B-cell maturation and are involved in the development of tolerance *(39)*. Deletion of any of these proteins affects the production of normal B lymphocytes (http://www.rndsystems.com/mini_review_detail_objectname_MR03_ImmuneTolerance.aspx).

Central T-Cell Development. During their double-positive stage (expressing CD4 and CD8 coreceptors), thymic T cells complete the assembly of their antigen-specific T-cell receptor (TCR) *(40–42)*. This genetic recombination is similar to that undergone by the B-cell receptor and is also mediated by Rag 1 and Rag 2 *(43,44)*. Like the B cells, the T cells can alter the antigen specificity of their TCR *(45,46)*, although the mechanism and implications for immune tolerance are not as well understood as for BCR editing (http://www.rndsystems.com/mini_review_detail_ objectname_MR03_ImmuneTolerance.aspx).

Antigen-Dependent Selection of T Cells. The T cells are exposed to antigens presented by class I and class II MHC proteins on the surface of thymic epithelial cells and bone marrow–derived dendritic cells *(47,48)*. There are three possible outcomes of these interactions:

- Death by neglect will occur if the TCR-MHC-peptide interaction is absent or too weak. This can be caused by

aberrant T-cell or target cell proteins or by an inability of the two cell types to make contact for physiologic reasons.

- Active deletion of T cells take place if the TCR-MHC-peptide interaction generates a strong signal. This removes T-cell clones that react too strongly with host molecules and would pose a risk of autoimmunity.

- Those T cells that receive intermediate-strength signals continue development into more specialized T-cell subsets *(49–52)*.

Mature single-positive T cells are released from the thymus and enter the peripheral circulation. A certain leakiness in the selection of T cells leads to the presence of some autoreactive cells in the periphery *(53–55)*. The activity of these cells must be regulated to avoid autoimmune reactions (http://www.rndsystems.com/mini_review_detail_objectname_MR03_ImmuneTolerance.aspx).

Peripheral T-Cell Tolerance. The control of T cells is continuing after lymphocytes have exited the thymus and entered the peripheral circulation *(56)*. The activation of the peripheral T cells can be blocked through their negative costimulatory molecules *(57,58)*. The regulatory T cells can effect the functional inactivation of otherwise competent T cells. Access to cognate peptide antigens can be regulated by antigen-presenting cells. In addition, altered T-cell migration can prevent the activation of fully competent autoreactive clones *(59–63)*.

Signaling in T-Cell Activation. The activity of the peripheral mature T cells can be modified by positive and negative regulatory receptors *(64)*. The CD28 and CTLA-4 proteins that are expressed on the T cells bind to B7 family members expressed on antigen-presenting cells *(65,66)*. Ligation of CD28 by either B7-1 or B7-2 would lower the threshold of TCR signaling needed to induce the T-cell activation and will also increase the effect of that signal *(67,68)*. Costimulation via CD28 will intensify the T-cell cytokine responses and will promote T-cell expansion and differentiation *(69,70)*. The stimulatory effects of CD28 ligation are counteracted by the inhibitory signaling of CTLA-4 *(71)*. In addition, the CTLA-4 ligation by B7-1 or B7-2 would result in inhibition of the TCR- and CD28-mediated signals *(72–74)*. The balance of CD28-derived and CTLA-4–derived signals is critical to the T-cell activation and tolerance (http://www.rndsystems.com/mini_review_detail_objectname_MR03_ImmuneTolerance.aspx).

Several more members of the B7-CD28 superfamily have been recently identified and may be potentially involved in the development or maintenance of immune tolerance. For example, inducible co-stimulator (ICOS) is expressed by activated T cells *(75)* but will not bind to B7-1 or B7-2 *(76,77)*. Ligation of ICOS by inducible T-cell co-stimulator ligand (ICOSL) helps to prolong the T-cell proliferation and IL-2 secretion but will not facilitate the initial activation *(78,79)*. The tissue distribution of ICOS is more widespread than that of CD28 to include several nonlymphoid tissues *(80)*.

Another protein, PD-1, which is expressed by activated T cells, B cells, and myeloid cells *(81)*, has a wider distribution than that of the predominately T-cell–expressed CD28 and CTLA-4. The PD-1 engagement by its ligands, PD-L1 or PD-L2 *(82)*, would inhibit the T-cell proliferation and reduce cytokine production *(83)*. Yet another B7 homolog, B7-H3, can be induced on dendritic cells *(84)*. B7-H3 binds to an unidentified protein on activated T cells other than CD28 and CTLA-4 *(84)*.

Regulatory T Cells. Regulatory, or suppressor, T cells (T_{reg}) do not proliferate in response to antigen binding but prevent the activation of helper and cytotoxic T cells *(85–87)*. The T_{reg} can suppress $CD4^+$ and $CD8^+$ T-cell proliferation and the production of effector cytokines regardless of TCR specificity *(86,88)*. This is mediated, at least in part, by inhibition of IL-2 transcription within the target cell *(89)*. Furthermore, the Treg constitutively express CTLA-4 *(90)* and secrete inhibitory TGF-β and IL-10 *(91,92)*.

Treg activity requires direct contact with the target T cells *(89)*, although the molecular mechanism for suppression is not clear. They may constitute a specialized T-cells subset optimized to reduce the activity of autoreactive T cells *(93,94)*.

The regulatory T cells are released from the thymus as $CD4^+CD25^+$ cells *(95)*. The demonstration of T_{reg} generation by a variety of stimuli *(96,97)* leaves open the possibility that there may be additional *in vivo* mechanisms for their generation as well (http://www.rndsystems.com/mini_review_detail_objectname_MR03_ImmuneTolerance.aspx).

Dendritic Cell–Mediated Tolerance. Immature dendritic cells continuously sample and present autoantigens to the T cells *(98,99)*. Because of the low expression levels of class I and class II MHC and costimulatory B7 proteins on immature dendritic cells, these interactions did not lead to productive immune responses. Instead, the cognate T cells become tolerant to the self-antigen *(100–103)*. Mature dendritic cells express high levels of MHC and costimulatory proteins and are much more potent at activating T cells. Activation of dendritic cells can be accomplished by ligation of their Toll-like receptors by microbial molecules *(104–106)* or by binding certain self-proteins released from necrotic cells *(107,108)* (http://www.rndsystems.com/mini_review_detail_objectname_MR03_ImmuneTolerance.aspx).

40.2 Disruption of Immune Tolerance

Immune tolerance is defined as the absence of activation of pathogenic autoreactivity. Autoimmune diseases are syndromes caused by the activation of T- or B-cells or both, with no evidence of other causes, such as infections or malignancies. Once thought to be mutually exclusive, immune tolerance and autoimmunity are now both recognized to be present normally in health and, when abnormal, they represent extremes from the normal state (http://www.accessmedicine.com/content.aspx?aID=93538) *(109)*.

Immune tolerance and autoimmunity are important clinically *(110)*. There are at least 40 known or suspected autoimmune diseases, and many are common illnesses. Overall, 1 in every 31 persons is affected *(111)*. Moreover, autoimmune type 1 diabetes mellitus is the most common of all chronic diseases of children. In addition, autoimmune diseases are poorly diagnosed because the onset can be stealthy and initial symptoms are often nonspecific: tiredness, fatigue, or fever.

Prevalence of autoimmune diseases *(110)*:

- *Thyroid diseases (*includes *Hashimoto's thyroiditis* and *Graves' disease)*: more than 3% of adult women
- *Rheumatoid arthritis*: 1% of general population, but female excess
- *Primary Sjögren's syndrome*: 0.6% to 3% of adult women
- *Systemic lupus erythematosus*: 0.12% of general population, but female excess
- *Multiple sclerosis*: 0.1% of general population, but female excess
- *Type 1 diabetes mellitus*: 0.1% of children
- *Primary biliary cirrhosis*: 0.05% to 0.1% of middle-aged and elderly women
- *Myasthenia gravis*: 0.01% of general population, but female excess

However, new insights are set to revolutionize management of autoimmune diseases by replacing blanket immunosuppression with new selective immunotherapies *(112)*.

40.2.1 Immune Tolerance and the Immune Response

The immune system does not normally respond to self-antigens. This immunologic tolerance was postulated more than 50 years ago, but its multifactorial basis is still controversial *(113–115)*. Tolerance is generated at two levels. The "upper level" of central tolerance develops primarily in fetal life, and the "lower level" of peripheral tolerance develops postnatally as a back-up process. A faulty central tolerance sows the seeds for autoimmune disease, and faulty peripheral tolerance leads to its eruption *(110)*.

Central Tolerance. Lymphocytes learn to react with antigens during lymphopoiesis in the central lymphoid organs, thymus, and the bone marrow *(110)*. During the random rearrangements of genes that encode antigen receptors of nascent lymphocytes, the lymphocytes are exposed to antigenic signals from self-molecules. Weak interactions with low-affinity signals are stimulatory and select lymphocytes suitable for immune repertoires-positive selection. Strong interactions with high-affinity signals are lethal, and self-reactive lymphocytes are eliminated by apoptosis-negative selection (115).

In the bone marrow, developing B lymphocytes receive stimulatory or deletional signals from self-antigens, but the selection processes continue in the germinal centers of peripheral lymphoid tissues as well (116). Exactly how these selection processes operate is uncertain, but among the important influences, the extent of representation and level of exposure to tolerogenic self-molecules, and, in the thymus, the HLA constitution of the individual (117) would certainly play a role. In any event, not all self-antigens are available for efficient negative selection, so that central tolerance is "leaky" and results in export to the periphery of self-reactive lymphocytes that require control throughout life (110).

Peripheral Tolerance. Peripheral tolerance encompasses various safeguards that prevent the activation of self-reactive lymphocytes. These include ignorance, anergy, homeostatic control, and regulation (110):

- *Ignorance.* Autoimmune lymphocytes are kept in ignorance by sequestration of autoantigens behind cellular or vascular barriers; by the occurrence of cell death by apoptosis, which normally precludes spillage of autoantigenic intracellular constituents, and by the presence on the surface of potentially autoimmune (but nonactivated) T lymphocytes of signaling molecules that preclude entry of the cell into tissue parenchyma (118).

- *Anergy* describes a state of unstable metabolic arrest affecting lymphocytes that can lead to apoptosis (119). It occurs when a lymphocyte receives an antigenic signal without the normally necessary costimulatory second signal (120). Anergy is a protective (tolerogenic) outcome after interaction between an autoimmune T cell and a self-peptide on a parenchymal cell that is not competent to deliver a costimulatory signal (121).

- *Homeostatic control* occurs by expression of cytotoxic T-lymphocyte antigen 4 (CTLA-4, CD152) on activated T lymphocytes as an alternative to the CD28 ligand. When CD80/86 on the antigen-presenting cell interacts with CTLA-4, the T cell is switched off (110).

- *Regulation* by dedicated T cells inhibits the induction or effector functions of other classes of lymphocytes, either by the production of downregulatory cytokines or interference with receptor signaling pathways. More information is needed on markers that identify regulatory T cells (122) and their role in the development of autoimmunity (110).

Apoptosis. Apoptosis represents physiologic as opposed to pathologic (necrotic) cell death (123). It is of pivotal importance for tolerance and autoimmunity. Deficiency or dysregulation of apoptosis will result in lymphocytes becoming unresponsive to death signals essential for deletional tolerance. Alternatively, when apoptosis is overwhelming or apoptotic fragments are not effectively removed, as can occur with deficiency of serum complement, a risk of autoimmunity exists (124).

Two families of proteins mediate apoptosis (110). The cysteine aspartate proteases (caspases) are activated by the binding of the cell-surface molecule fas (CD95) to its ligand, fas L. The Bcl2 family contains some 20 proteins, among which Bcl2 itself protects against apoptosis whereas others promote apoptosis. Because apoptosis normally eliminates self-reactive lymphocytes, gene mutations that disrupt apoptosis are conducive to autoimmunity. Thus, mutations affecting fas or fas L cause autoimmune lymphoproliferative syndromes of childhood and analogous diseases in inbred mouse models (125).

40.2.2 Role of AIRE Gene in Autoimmunity

The genesis of autoimmunity involves environmental and genetic mechanisms, both contributing to the disruption or deregulation of central or peripheral tolerance, allowing autoreactive pathogenetic T- and B-cell clones to arise (126).

Among genetic factors, the *autoimmune regulator (AIRE) gene (127,128)*, correlated with the development of organ-specific autoimmune disease with monogenic autosomal recessive inheritance, has recently been identified. The AIRE gene, located on chromosome 21q22.3, coding for a protein of 552 amino acids, *functions as a transcription factor*. It has recently been shown that the PHD1 domain of AIRE gene acts as an E3 ubiquitin ligase, mediating transfer of ubiquitin to specific proteins, which resulted in several effects such as proteasome degradation, downregulation of cell surface receptors, and proteolysis independent activities (129). In autoimmunity, AIRE plays an important role due to its limited tissue expression in medullary thymic epithelial cells and cells of the monocytes' dendritic cell lineage of the thymus (130). Both cell types are considered to play a major role in the establishment of self-tolerance by eliminating autoreactive T cells (negative selection) and/or by producing immunoregulatory T cells, which prevent CD4 T-cell–mediated organ-specific autoimmune diseases (131). It has been demonstrated that AIRE regulates expression in the thymus of several mRNA genes of ectopic peripheral proteins (132) in a dosage-dependent manner (133); a slight decrease in AIRE gene function can lead to a consequent decrease in thymic protein expression, allowing delivery of autoreactive T-cell clones in the periphery (126).

Forty mutations of AIRE gene, responsible for a rare autosomal recessive disease, *autoimmune polyendocrinopathy candidiasis ectodermal dystrophy (APECED)*, also known as *autoimmune polyglandular syndrome type 1 (APS1)*, have been identified. APECED is characterized by at least two of the following conditions: chronic mucocutaneous candidiasis, hypoparathyroidism and/or Addison's disease; however APECED patients show a high incidence of many other organ-specific autoimmune diseases, such as thyroid autoimmune disease, diabetes mellitus type 1, gonadal failure, as well as extraendocrine autoimmune diseases, such as hepatitis, vitiligo, alopecia, pernicious anemia, intestinal malabsorption, keratinopathy, and dystrophy of dental enamel and nails. AIRE gene mutations have also been identified in several patients with atypical or incomplete manifestations (126).

Studies in patients with type 1 diabetes, Graves' disease, and Addison disease (134), as well as inflammatory bowel disease (135), have failed to show an association with AIRE gene polymorphisms. On the other side, variants of AIRE gene have been correlated with autoimmune manifestations in the immune deficiency Omenn syndrome (136), with alopecia areata (137), and with lupus-like panniculitis in patients with APECED (138). Furthermore, knockout mice for AIRE gene develop Sjögren's syndrome–like pathologic changes in the exocrine organs, correlated with the presence of T-cell autoreactive clones against α-fodrin (131).

Although AIRE gene is the disease locus for APECED, with a strictly recessive inheritance pattern, in other autoimmune manifestations, which range from isolated organ target belonging to APECED criteria to other autoimmune diseases, AIRE variants act in a semidominant manner. Heterozygosity for AIRE mutations, which leads to a reduction in AIRE protein amount per cell, causes a marked decrease in ectopic proteins expression in the thymus. The consequence in the periphery of this semidominant effect in thymic deletion is an increase in susceptibility to autoimmunity attack (126).

40.3 NIAID-Supported Research in Immune Tolerance

NIAID is supporting a wide range of programs to turn the promise of immune tolerance therapies into reality (http://www3.niaid.nih.gov/research/topics/immune/research_activities.htm). Many of these programs are carried out by NIAID's Division of Allergy, Immunology, and Transplantation (DAIT), which supports basic research into the mechanisms responsible for immune tolerance, translational research to facilitate the application of immune-tolerance approaches to human diseases, and clinical research to evaluate new therapies that can induce and maintain immune tolerance. New approaches are being investigated to:

- Improve understanding of the molecular mechanisms responsible for the induction and maintenance of immune tolerance
- Replace or improve suboptimal treatment protocols for immune-mediated diseases
- Discover methods to prevent or reverse immune-mediated disorders for which no effective therapies are currently available
- Create an efficient research infrastructure for the development and rapid testing of tolerogenic agents in human immune-mediated diseases
- Clarify mechanisms by which tolerogenic agents suppress disease

In collaboration with the National Institute of Diabetes and Digestive and Kidney Diseases, DAIT supports the Nonhuman Primate Transplant Tolerance Cooperative Study Group (NHPCSG). The goal of this program is to evaluate the safety and efficacy of novel tolerogenic regimens in preclinical models of kidney and islet transplantation. Scientists in this study group have demonstrated long-term graft acceptance using tolerogenic regimens in both kidney and islet allograft recipients. In 2002, this program was expanded from 3 to 10 research grants. This expansion has allowed a larger number of tolerance-induction strategies to be rigorously evaluated, allowed the sharing of valuable resources, and facilitated the development of new collaborations. The NHPCSG will be further expanded to include heart and lung transplantation. To accelerate research conducted through this program, DAIT maintains breeding colonies of specific pathogen-free rhesus and cynomolgus macaques.

Other DAIT-supported research programs that include studies on immune tolerance are the Autoimmunity Centers of Excellence; Innovative Grants on Immune Tolerance; and program projects in basic biology, basic immunology, and transplantation tolerance (http://www3.niaid.nih.gov/research/topics/immune/research_activities.htm).

40.4 Immune Tolerance Network

NIAID, along with the National Institute of Diabetes and Digestive and Kidney Diseases (NIDDK) and the Juvenile Diabetes Research Foundation International, cosponsors the Immune Tolerance Network (ITN), an international consortium of more than 80 investigators in the United States, Canada, Europe, and Australia.

The ITN is a collaborative effort that is soliciting, developing, implementing, and assessing clinical strategies and biological assays for the purposes of inducing, maintaining, and monitoring tolerance in humans for kidney, liver, and islet transplantations, autoimmune diseases, and allergy and asthma. (http://www.immunetolerance.org/overview/).

To achieve its goals, the ITN is providing subcontracted research funds as well a number of key tools to help investigators in their research, whether it is academic or industry initiated. Key services of ITN include (i) conducting clinical trials or research on assays for tolerance; (ii) assistance identifying potential collaborators and clinical sites; (iii) an in-house "CRO-style" Clinical Trials Group for trial planning, development, monitoring, and analysis; (iv) access to cutting-edge biological assays and equipment; (v) scientific and administrative support; and (vi) assistance in procuring vital agents and equipment *(112)*. In addition, ITN investigators have access to the expertise of some of the field's most prominent figures.

Every clinical trial supported by the ITN is augmented by a series of mechanistic studies designed to uncover the basic biological features of clinical tolerance. The ITN works with investigators to choose an ideal set of assays that will provide direct feedback for subsequent trial development. The ITN operates a number of Core Facilities providing investigators with cutting-edge technologies designed to increase our understanding of tolerance (http://www.immunetolerance.org/overview/).

Research supported by the ITN comes from a year-round, open call for proposals from tolerance researchers around the world. The highly interactive peer-review process ensures that all applicants are given thorough and fair consideration. Once funded, the ITN provides an interactive platform for developing ideas into high-impact clinical and tolerance assay research. The ITN's Clinical Trials Group offers a wealth of scientific, technical, and administrative support, including trial development and regulatory assistance, as well as monitoring staff and experts, and tools for data analysis. The ITN's Tolerance Assay Group assists investigators with the development, data acquisition, and analysis for mechanistic and marker studies associated with every trial.

40.4.1 Specific Research Areas

Islet Transplantation. The ITN investigates novel strategies aimed at creating and maintaining long-term tolerance to transplanted islet cells. The goal of the program is the restoration of normal insulin production in type 1 diabetes patients, without the need for long-term immunosuppressive therapy. A key issue in this regard is finding ways to alleviate both the alloimmune response and the ongoing autoimmune response in these affected individuals (http://www.immunetolerance.org/overview/).

Solid-Organ Transplantation. Clinical trials in liver and renal transplantation are closely related to those performed in islet transplant recipients. In addition, the network aims to test potential tolerance induction strategies against the backdrop of maintenance immunosuppression that does not include calcineurin inhibitors. Combination drug therapies, including use of hematopoietic stem cell chimerization, are a key focus of the ITN (http://www.immunetolerance.org/overview/).

Autoimmune Diseases. The ITN conducts clinical trials and mechanistic studies aimed at alleviating the autoimmune responses that characterize these diseases. The main disease entities studied include systemic lupus erythematosus, rheumatoid arthritis, multiple sclerosis, and type 1 diabetes. Nevertheless, the ITN is also keenly interested in clinical studies of other diseases (http://www.immunetolerance.org/overview/).

Allergy and Asthma. Studies in allergy and asthma supported by ITN are focused at ameliorating the allergen-specific Th2-driven processes and replacing these processes with allergen-specific, protective immune responses. Among the diseases supported by the Asthma and Allergic Diseases Subgroup are allergic rhinitis (seasonal and perennial) and allergic asthma (http://www.immunetolerance.org/overview/).

Tolerance Assays and Core Facilities. In each of the disease areas, the ITN Tolerance Assay Group (TAG) is supporting clinical trials by (i) examining the mechanism(s) that create and maintain the tolerant state and (ii) developing a set of assays that will function as a road map to guide clinicians in their attempt to create and monitor immune tolerance in individual patients. The TAG oversees several core assay facilities and the standardization of assay protocols performed at local clinical centers (http://www.immunetolerance.org/overview/).

40.4.2 Immune Tolerance Therapies

All tolerance-induction strategies share a common goal: to selectively prevent or diminish specific harmful immune responses without disabling the immune system as a whole. In autoimmune diseases, the goal is to make the immune system tolerant to the specific, normally occurring antigens that cause it to attack the body's own organs, tissues, or cells. In asthma and allergic diseases, the goal is to prevent responses to allergens such as cockroaches and house dust mites, which cause or exacerbate these diseases. For transplant rejection, the goal is to selectively block immune responses directed against the foreign antigens on the graft and thereby allow long-term graft survival without the heightened risks of infection, malignancy, and atherosclerosis associated with current immunosuppressive therapies (http://www3.niaid. nih.gov/research/topics/immune/introduction.htm).

Immune tolerance therapies are designed to reprogram immune cells in a highly specific fashion to eliminate pathogenic responses while preserving protective immunity *(112)*.

A concept that has been researched for decades, the development of tolerance-inducing therapies, would revolutionize the management of a wide range of chronic and often debilitating diseases by obviating the need for lifelong immunosuppressive regimens. The advances of the past decade have provided a more detailed understanding of the molecular events associated with T-cell recognition and activation. Building on these advances, recent research has demonstrated the feasibility of various tolerance-inducing approaches in small- and large-animal models of autoimmunity, allergy, and transplant graft rejection. Unprecedented opportunities to test these approaches in a variety of human diseases have now emerged. To capitalize on these advances, the ITN is using a unique interactive approach to accelerate the development of clinical tolerance therapies by partnering with the biotechnology and pharmaceutical industries to examine innovative tolerogenic approaches in a range of allergic and autoimmune diseases and to prevent graft rejection after transplantation *(112)*.

40.4.3 Clinical Trials in Immune Tolerance

The ITN is conducting integrated studies on the mechanisms that underlie immune tolerance and developing markers and assays to measure the induction, maintenance, and loss of tolerance in humans. The network has established several state-of-the-art core facilities and has supported 18 approved clinical protocols as well as several additional studies of the immune mechanisms involved in tolerance (http://www3.niaid.nih.gov/research/topics/immune/clinical.htm). The ITN is currently involved in the following areas of clinical research:

Allergy	Islet cell, kidney, and liver
Asthma	transplantation
Diabetes	Bone marrow transplantation
Multiple sclerosis (MS)	Systemic lupus
Psoriatic arthritis	erythematosus

Examples of active ITN clinical research studies include:

- A Phase I trial to analyze and monitor the safety of immunization with a fragment of the human insulin B chain in subjects newly diagnosed with type 1 diabetes; the hope is that this "autoimmunization" therapy will increase the immune tolerance of insulin-producing cells.

- A pilot study to evaluate the safety and efficacy of a treatment regimen to induce tolerance in kidney transplant recipients. In this study, patients will receive low-dose steroid-free immunosuppression, two donor stem cell infusions, and an antibody called Campath-1H, which selectively eliminates immune system T cells involved in organ rejection. Treatment will be withdrawn after 1 year and the patients will be followed to see if long-term tolerance has been achieved.

- A Phase I study in 16 patients with relapsing-remitting MS to assess the safety of one dose of CTLA4-IgG4m, an antibody that may block a pathway that allows the immune system to attack nervous system tissue.

- A Phase II multicenter trial to evaluate the lipid-lowering drug atorvastatin in patients at high risk of developing MS.

Tolerance assays. Tests and procedures to monitor patient responses to tolerance therapies are critically needed to better evaluate tolerance-inducing therapies during and after clinical trials. ITN has, therefore, established a set of core laboratories to develop assays for the induction, maintenance, or loss of immune tolerance. These core facilities carry out microarray analyses of gene expression, develop analytic tools for clinical and scientific data sets from ITN-sponsored trials, and conduct enzyme-linked immunospot (Elispot) assay analyses of protein expression and cellular assays for T-cell reactivity.

Examples of current ITN efforts to develop mechanistic assays include:

- Development of antigen-specific assays for donor-specific tolerance in renal transplant recipients
- Cytokine production in children with preclinical and clinical type 1 diabetes
- Identification and mechanistic investigations of tolerant kidney transplant patients

40.5 Recent Scientific Advances

HLA-Mismatched Renal Transplantation Without Maintenance Immunosuppression. Five patients with end-stage renal disease received combined bone marrow and kidney transplants from HLA single-haplotype mismatched living related donors, with the use of a nonmyeloablative preparative regimen. Transient chimerism and reversible capillary leak syndrome developed in all recipients. Irreversible humoral rejection occurred in one patient. In the other four recipients, it was possible to discontinue all immunosuppressive therapy 9 to 14 months after the transplantation, and renal function has remained stable for 2.0 to 5.3 years since transplantation. The T cells from these four recipients, tested *in vitro*, showed donor-specific unresponsiveness, and in specimens from allograft biopsies, obtained after withdrawal of immunosuppressive therapy, there were high levels of P3 (FOXP3) messenger RNA (mRNA) but not granzyme B mRNA *(139)*.

Chimerism and Tolerance in a Recipient of a Deceased-Donor Liver Transplant. Complete hematopoietic chimerism and tolerance of a liver allograft from a deceased male donor have developed in a 9-year-old girl, with no evidence of graft-versus-host disease 17 months after transplantation. The tolerance was preceded by a period of severe hemolysis, reflecting partial chimerism that was refractory to standard therapies. The hemolysis resolved after the gradual withdrawal of all immunosuppressive therapy *(140)*.

Tolerance and Chimerism After Renal and Hematopoietic Cell Transplantation. A combined kidney and hematopoietic cell transplant from an HLA-matched donor has been described. A posttransplantation conditioning regimen of total lymphoid irradiation and antithymocyte globulin allowed engraftment of the donor's hematopoietic cells. The patient had persistent mixed chimerism, and the function of the kidney allograft has been normal for more than 28 months since discontinuation of all immunosuppressive drugs. Adverse events requiring hospitalization were limited to a 2-day episode of fever with neutropenia. The patient has had neither rejection episodes nor clinical manifestations of graft-versus-host disease *(141)*.

A Novel Subset of Memory B Cells Is Enriched in Autoreactivity and Correlates with Adverse Outcomes in Systemic Lupus Erythematosus. It has previously been reported that some systemic lupus erythematosus (SLE) patients have a population of circulating memory B-cells with greater than twofold higher levels of CD19. In this study, the presence of CD19^{hi} B-cells correlated with long-term adverse outcomes. These B cells did not appear anergic, as they exhibited high basal levels of phosphorylated Syk and ERK1/2, signal transduced in response to BCR cross-linking and can become plasma cells (PCs) *in vitro*. Autoreactive anti-Smith (Sm) B-cells were enriched in this population, and the degree of enrichment correlated with the log of the serum anti-Sm titer, arguing that they had undergone clonal expansion before PC differentiation. PC differentiation may occur at sites of inflammation, as CD19^{hi} B-cells have elevated CXCR3 levels and chemotax in response to its ligand CXCL9. Thus, CD19^{hi} B-cells acted as precursors to anti-self PCs and will identify an SLE patient subset likely to experience poor clinical outcomes *(142)*.

Decrease of CD4+CD25highFoxp3$^+$ Regulatory T Cells and Elevation of CD19$^+$BAFF-R$^+$ B Cells and Soluble ICAM-1 in Myasthenia Gravis. Myasthenia gravis (MG) is caused by T-cell–dependent autoantibodies against muscle acetylcholine receptors (AChR) at the neuromuscular

junction. Recently, ELISA and flow cytometry techniques have been used to measure the levels of Th1, Th2, Th3 cytokines, inflammatory cytokine, and chemokine soluble ICAM-1 (sICAM-1), and to analyze the phenotypes of CD4$^+$ and CD8$^+$ regulatory cells, as well as the expression of the newly identified receptor BAFF-R on CD19$^+$ B-cells in peripheral blood from 75 MG patients and 50 healthy controls *(143)*. There were no differences in the levels of IL-2, IL-4, IL-10, IL-13, IFN-γ, TNF-α, TGF-β, and sCTLA-4 in both sera and culture supernatants between MG patients and healthy controls. The level of IL-12 was decreased in culture supernatants from MG patients, and the level of sICAM-1 was increased in both sera and culture supernatants from MG patients. Although the populations of CD8$^+$CD28$^-$ and CD8$^+$CD122$^+$ regulatory T cells were not different between MG patients and healthy controls, MG patients exhibited the decrease of CD4$^+$CD25^{high}Foxp3$^+$ regulatory T cells and the increase of CD19$^+$BAFF-R$^+$ B cells, revealing that MG patients should display the dysfunction of T-cell balance and the activation of B-cell maturation *(143)*.

Effect of Immunosuppressants on the Expansion and Function of Naturally Occurring Regulatory T Cells. The induction of immune tolerance is one of the final therapeutic goals in clinical transplantation. Regulatory T lymphocytes are important for the induction and maintenance of immune tolerance to grafts. If immunosuppressive drugs used clinically to prevent immune rejection also inhibit regulatory T lymphocytes, tolerance would not be achieved. The effect of several immunosuppressants with different mechanisms of action has been tested on the proliferation and suppressive activity of CD4$^+$CD25$^+$ regulatory T cells. Highly purified CD4$^+$CD25h$^+$ T-cells from C57BL/6 (H-2^b) mice were stimulated with allogeneic T-depleted splenocytes (BALB/c; H-2^d) in the presence of various immunosuppressants. After 1 week in culture, viable T cells were recovered, their regulatory capacity was assessed by their ability to inhibit responder T-cell proliferation in mixed lymphocyte reaction (MLR), and their cytokine production profile was measured by ELISA. The immunosuppressive drugs rapamycin, cyclosporin A, and methylprednisolone significantly inhibited the expansion of regulatory T cells upon stimulation with alloantigen, whereas mycophenolic acid and the costimulatory blockers, anti-CD40L and CTLA4Ig, did not. None of these immunosuppressants, however, reduced the suppressive capacity of regulatory T cells. Pretreatment with immunosuppressive drugs did not induce significant changes in the cytokine production profile of regulatory T cells. These results suggested that costimulatory blockers and mycophenolate mofetil can be used therapeutically in the induction of immune tolerance. In contrast, use of rapamycin, cyclosporin A, and methylprednisolone should be reconsidered, due to their deleterious effects on the expansion of naturally occurring regulatory T cells *(144)*.

References

1. Hackett, C. J., Rotrosen, D., Auchincloss, H., and Fauci, A. S. (2007) Immunology research: challenges in a time of budgetary constraints, *Nat. Immunol.* **8**, 114–117.

2. Anderson, M. S., Venanzi, E., Chen, Z., Berzins, S., Benoist, C., and Mathis, D. (2005) The cellular mechanism of Aire control of T cell tolerance, *Immunity,* **23**(2), 227–239.

3. Fontenot, J. D. and Rudensky, A. Y. (2005) A well-adapted regulatory contrivance: regulatory T cell development and the forkhead family transcription factor Foxp3, *Nat. Immunol.*, **6**, 331–337.

4. Liu, Y.-J. and Banchereau, J. (1996) The paths and molecular controls of peripheral B cell development, *Immunologist*, **4**, 55–66.

5. Kee, B. L. and Murre, C. (2001) Transcription factor regulation of B lineage commitment, *Curr. Opin. Immunol.*, **13**(2), 180–185.

6. Hardy, R. R. and Hayakawa, K. (2001) B cell development pathways, *Annu. Rev. Immunol.*, **19**, 595–621.

7. Banchereau, J. and Rousset, F. (1992) Human B lymphocytes: phenotype, proliferation and differentiation, *Adv. Immunol.*, **52**, 125–262.

8. Hardin, J.A., Yamaguchi, K., and Sherr, D. H. (1995) The role of peritoneal stromal cells in the survival of sIgM$^+$ peritoneal B lymphocyte populations, *Cell. Immunol.*, **161**(1), 50–60.

9. Pillai, S. (1999) The chosen few? Positive selection and the generation of naive B lymphocytes, *Immunity*, **10**(5), 493–502.

10. Agenès, F., Rosado, M. M., and Freitas, A. A. (1997) Independent homeostatic regulation of B cell compartments, *Eur. J. Immunol.*, **27**(7), 1801–1807.

11. Benschop, R. J. and Cambier, J. C. (1999) B cell development: signal transduction by antigen receptors and their surrogates, *Curr. Opin. Immunol.*, **11**, 143–151.

12. Nemazee, D. (2000) Receptor selection in B and T lymphocytes, *Annu. Rev. Immunol.*, **18**, 19–51.

13. Rolink, A. G., Schaniel, C., Andersson, J., and Melchers. F. (2001) Selection events operating at various stages in B cell development, *Curr. Opin. Immunol.*, **13**, 202–207.

14. Rolink, A. G., Brocker, T., Bluethmann, H., Kosco–Vilbois, M.H., Andersson, J., and Melchers, F. (1999) Mutations affecting either generation or survival of cells influence the pool size of mature B cells, *Immunity*, **10**, 619–628.

15. Ceredig, R., Rolink, A. G., Melchers, F., and Andersson, J. (2000) The B cell receptor, but not the pre-B cell receptor, mediates arrest of B cell differentiation, *Eur. J. Immunol.*, **30**(3), 759–767.

16. Hayakawa, K., Asano, M., Shinton, S. A., et al. (1999) Positive selection of natural autoreactive B cells, *Science*, **285**(5424), 113–116.

17. Kouskoff, V., Lacaud, G., and Nemazee, D. (2000) T cell-independent rescue of B lymphocytes from peripheral immune tolerance, *Science*, **287**, 2501–2503.

18. Grawunder, U., Leu, T. M., Schatz, D. G., et al. (1995) Downregulation of RAG 1 and RAG2 gene expression in preB cells after functional immunoglobulin heavy chain rearrangement, *Immunity*, **3**, 601–608.

19. Tarlinton, D. M. and Smith, G. C. (2000) Targeting plasma cells in autoimmune diseases, *Immunol. Today*, **21**, 436–441.

20. Papavasiliou, F., Jankovic, M., Suh, H., and Nussenzweig, M. C. (1995) The cytoplasmic domains of immunoglobulin (Ig) α and Igβ can independently induce the precursor B cell transition and allelic exclusion, *J. Exp. Med.*. **182**, 1389–1394.

21. Tiegs, S. L., Russell, D. M., and Nemazee, D. (1993) Receptor editing in self-reacting bone marrow B cells, *J. Exp. Med.*, **177**, 1009–1020.

22. Gay, D., Saunders, T., Camper, S., and Weigert, M. (1993) Receptor editing: an approach by autoreactive B cells to escape tolerance, *J. Exp. Med.*, **177**, 999–1008.

23. Retter, M. W. and Nemazee, D. (1998) Receptor editing occurs frequently during normal B cell development, *J. Exp. Med.*, **188**, 1231–1238.

24. Casellas, R., Sish, T. A., Kleinewietfeld, M., et al. (2001) Contribution of receptor editing to the antibody repertoire, *Science*, **291**, 1541–1544.

25. Kouskoff, V. and Nemazee, D. (2001) Role of receptor and revision in shaping the B and T lymphocyte repertoire, *Life Sci.*, **69**, 1105–1113.

26. Meffre, E., Davis, E., Schiff, C., et al. (2000) Circulating human B cells that express surrogate light chains and edited receptors, *Nat. Immunol.*, **1**(3), 207–208.

27. Calame, K. L. (2001) Plasma cells: finding new light at the end of B cell development, *Nat. Immunol.*, **2**, 1103–1108.

28. Sanchez, M., Misulovin, Z., Burkhardt, A. L., et al. (1993) Signal transduction by immunoglobulin is mediated through Ig alpha and Ig beta, *J. Exp. Med.*, **178**, 1049–1055.

29. Tsubata, T. (1999) Co-receptors on B lymphocytes, *Curr. Opin. Immunol.*, **11**, 249–255.

30. Martensson, I.-L. and Ceredig, R. (2000) The pre-B cell receptor in mouse B cell development, *Immunology*, **101**, 435–441.

31. Vilen, B., Nakamura, T., and Cambier, J. C. (1999) Antigen-stimulated dissociation of BCR mIg from Ig-α/Ig-β: implications for receptor desensitization, *Immunity*, **10**, 239–248.

32. Pierce, S. K. (2002) Lipid rafts and B-cell activation, *Nat. Rev. Immunol.*, **2**, 96–105.

33. Cheng, P. C., Dykstra, M. L., Mitchell, R. N., and Pierce, S. K. (1999) A role for lipid rafts in B cell antigen receptor signaling and antigen targeting, *J. Exp. Med.*, **190**, 1549–1560.

34. Malapati, S. and Pierce, S. K. (2001) The influence of CD40 on the association of the B cell antigen receptor with lipid rafts in mature and immature cells, *Eur. J. Immunol.*, **31**(12), 3789–3797.

35. Kurosaki, T. (2002) Regulation of B-cell signal transduction by adaptor proteins, *Nat. Rev. Immunol.*, **2**, 354–363.

36. Fearon, D. T. and Carroll, M. C. (2000) Regulation of B lymphocyte responses to foreign and self-antigens by the CD19/CD21 complex, *Annu. Rev. Immunol.*, **18**, 393–422.

37. Cherukuri, A., Cheng, P. C., Sohn, H. W., and Pierce, S. K. (2001) The CD19/CD21 complex functions to prolong B cell antigen receptor signaling from lipid rafts, *Immunity*, **14**(2), 169–179.

38. Minskoff, S. A., Matter, K., and Mellman, I. (1998) Fc gamma RII-B1 regulates the presentation of B cell receptor-bound antigens, *J. Immunol.*, **161**, 2079–2083.

39. Weintraub, R. C., Jun, J. E., Bishop, A. C., et al. (2000) Entry of B cell receptor into signaling domains is inhibited in tolerant B cells, *J. Exp. Med.*, **191**, 1443–1448.

40. Germain, R. N. (2002) T-cell development and the CD4-CD8 lineage decision, *Nat. Rev. Immunol.*, **2**, 309–322.

41. Carding, S. R. and Egan, P. J. (2002) Gamma delta T cells: functional plasticity and heterogeneity, *Nat. Rev. Immunol.*, **2**, 336–345.

42. Rosmalen, J. G. M., van Ewijk, W., and Leenen, P. J. M. (2002) T-cell education in autoimmune diabetes: teachers and students, *Trends. Immunol.*, **23**, 40–46.

43. Mombaerts, P., Iacomini, J., Johnson, R. S., Herrup, K., Tonegawa, S., et al. (1992) RAG-1-deficient mice have no mature B and T lymphocytes, *Cell*, **68**, 869–877.

44. Shinkai, Y., Koyasu S., Nakayama K.-I., et al. (1993) Restoration of T cell development in RAG-2 deficient mice by functional ICR transgenes, *Science*, **259**, 822–825.

45. McGargill, M. A., Derbinski, J. M., and Hogquist, K. A. (2000) Receptor editing in developing T cells, *Nat. Immunol.*, **1**, 336–341.

46. Buch, T., Rieux-Laucat, F., Forster, I., and Rajewsky, K. (2002) Failure of HY- specific thymocytes to escape negative selection by receptor editing, *Immunity*, **16**, 707–718.

47. Kurts, C., Miller, J. F., Subramaniam, R. M., Carbone, F. R., and Heath, W. R. (1998) Major histocompatibility complex class I-restricted cross-presentation is biased towards high dose antigens and those released during cellular destruction, *J. Exp. Med.*, **188**, 409–414.

48. Savino, W., Mendes-da-Cruz, D. A., Silva, J. S., Dardenne, M., and Cotta-de- Almeida, V. (2002) Intrathymic T-cell migration: a combinatorial interplay of extracellular matrix and chemokines, *Trends Immunol.*, **23**, 305–313.

49. Yagi, J. and Janeway, C. A., Jr. (1990) Ligand thresholds at different stages of T cell development, *Int. Immunol.*, **2**, 83–89.

50. Pircher, H., Rohrer, U. H., Moskophidis, D., Zinkernagel, R. M., and Hengartner, H. (1991) Low receptor avidity for thymic clonal deletion than for effector T-cell function, *Nature*, **351**, 482–485.

51. Sebzda, E., Mariathasan, S., Ohteki, T., Jones, R., Bachmann, M. F., and Ohashi, P. S. (1999) Selection of the T cell repertoire, *Annu. Rev. Immunol.*, **17**, 829–874.

52. Mariathasan, S., Zakarian, A., Bouchard, D., et al. (2001) Duration and strength of extracellular signal-regulated kinase signals are altered during positive versus negative thymocyte selection, *J. Immunol.*, **167**, 4966–4973.

53. Schild, H. J., Rötzschke, O., Kalbacher, H., Rammensee, H.-G. (1990) Limit of T cell tolerance to self proteins by peptide presentation, *Science*, **247**, 1587–1589.

54. Lohmann, T., Leslie, R. D., and Londei, M. (1996) T cell clones to epitopes of glutamic acid decarboxylase 65 raised from normal subjects and patients with insulin-dependent diabetes, *J. Autoimmun.*, **9**, 385–389.

55. Semana, G., Gausling, R., Jackson, R. A., and Hafler, D. A. (1999) T cell autoreactivity to proinsulin epitopes in diabetic patients and healthy subjects, *J. Autoimmun.*, **12**, 259–267.

56. Walker, L. S. K. and Abbas, A. K. (2002) The enemy within: keeping self-reactive T cells at bay in the periphery, *Nat. Rev. Immunol.*, **2**, 11–19.

57. Garza, K. M., Chan, V. S. F., and Ohashi, P. S. (2000) T cell tolerance and autoimmunity, *Rev. Immunogenet.*, **2**, 217.

58. Lechner, O., Lauber, J., Franzke, A., Sarukhan, A., von Boehmer, H., and Buer, J. (2001) Fingerprints of anergic T cells, *Curr. Biol.*, **11**, 587–595.

59. Kearney, E. R., Pape, K. A., Loh, D. Y. et al. (1994) Visualization of peptide-specific T cell immunity and peripheral tolerance induction in vivo, *Immunity*, **1**, 327–339.

60. Alferink, J., Tafuri, A., Vestweber, D., et al. (1998) Control of neonatal tolerance to tissue antigens by peripheral T cell trafficking, *Science*, **282**, 1338–1341.

61. Bromley, S. K., Peterson, D. A., Gunn, M. D., and Dustin, M. L. (2000) Cutting edge: hierarchy of chemokine receptor and TCR signals regulating T cell migration and proliferation, *J. Immunol.*, **165**, 15–19.

62. Maeda, Y., Noda, S., Tanaka, K., et al. (2001) The failure of oral tolerance induction is functionally coupled to the absence of T cells in Peyer's patches under germfree conditions, *Immunobiology*, **204**, 442–457.

63. Mackay, C. R. (2001) The chemokines: immunology's high impact factors, *Nat. Immunol.*, **2**, 95–101.

64. Sharpe, A. H. and Freeman, G. J. (2002) The B7-CD28 superfamily, *Nat. Rev. Immunol.*, **2**, 116–126.

65. Linsley, P. S., Greene, J. L., Brady, W., Bajorath, J., Ledbetter, J. A., and Peach, R. (1994) Human B7-1 (CD80) and B7-2 (CD86) bind with similar avidities but distinct kinetics to CD28 and CTLA-4 receptors, *Immunity*, **1**, 793–781.

66. Sansom, D.M. (2000) CD28, CTLA-4 and their ligands: who does what and to whom? *Immunology*, **101**, 169–177.

67. Freeman, G. J., Gribben, J. G., Boussiotis, V. A., et al. (1993) Cloning of B7-2: a CTLA-4 counter-receptor that costimulates human T cell proliferation, *Science*, **262**, 909–911.

68. Lenschow, D. J., Walunas, T. L., and Bluestone, J. A. (1996) CD28/B7 system of T cell costimulation, *Annu. Rev. Immunol.*, **14**, 233–258.

69. Thompson, C. B., Lindsten, T., Ledbetter, J. A., et al. (1989) CD28 activation pathway regulates the production of multiple T-cell-derived lymphokines/cytokines, *Proc. Natl. Acad. Sci. U.S.A.*, **86**, 1333–1337.

70. Sperling, A. I., Auger, J. A., Ehst, B. D., Rulifson, I. C., Thompson, C. B., and Bluestone. J. A. (1996) CD28/B7 interactions deliver a unique signal to naive T cells that regulates cell survival but not early proliferation, *J. Immunol.*, **157**, 3909–3917.

71. Krummel, M. and Allison, J. (1995) CD28 and CTLA-4 have opposing effects on the response of T cells to stimulation, *J. Exp. Med.*, **182**, 459–465.

72. Brunet, J. F., Denizot, F., Luciani, M. F., Roux-Dosseto, M., Suzan, M., Mattei, M. F., and Golstein, P. (1987) A new member of the immunoglobulin superfamily CTLA-4, *Nature*, **328**, 267–270.

73. Linsley, P., Brady, W., Urnes, M., et al. (1991) CTLA-4 is a second receptor for the B cell activation antigen B7, *J. Exp. Med.*, **174**, 561–569.

74. Chambers, C. A., Kuhns, M. S., Egen, J. G., and Allison, J. P. (2001) CTLA-4- mediated inhibition in regulation of T cell responses: mechanisms and manipulation in tumor immunotherapy, *Annu. Rev. Immunol.*, **19**, 565–594.

75. Hutloff, A., Dittrich, A. M., Beier, K. C., et al. (1999) ICOS is an inducible T-cell co-stimulator structurally and functionally related to CD28, *Nature*, **397**, 263–266.

76. Yoshinaga, S.K., Whoriskey, J. S., Khare, S. D., et al. (1999) T-cell co-stimulation through B7RP-1 and ICOS, *Nature*, **402**, 827–832.

77. Beier, K. C., Hutloff, A., Dittrich, A. M., et al. (2000) Induction, binding specificity and function of human ICOS, *Eur. J. Immunol.*, **30**, 3707–3717.

78. Coyle, A. J., Lehar, S., Lloyd, C., et al. (2000) The CD28-related molecule ICOS is required for effective T cell-dependent immune responses, *Immunity*, **13**, 95–105.

79. Aicher, A., Hayden-Ledbetter, M., Brady, W. A., et al. (2000) Characterization of human inducible costimulator ligand expression and function, *J. Immunol.*, **164**, 4689–4696.

80. Ling, V., Wu, P. W., Finnerty, H. F., Bean, K. M., Spaulding, V., et al. (2000) Cutting edge: identification of GL50, a novel B7-like protein that functionally binds to ICOS receptor, *J. Immunol.*, **164**, 1653–1657.

81. Agata, Y., Kawasaki, A., Nishimura, H., et al. (1996) Expression of the PD-1 antigen on the surface of stimulated mouse T and B lymphocytes, *Int. Immunol.*, **8**(5), 765–772.

82. Latchman, Y., Wood, C. R., Chernova, T., et al. (2001) PD-L2 is a second ligand for PD-1 and inhibits T cell activation, *Nat. Immunol.*, **2**, 261–268.

83. Freeman, G. J., Long, A., Iwai, Y., et al. (2000) Engagement of the PD-1 immunoinhibitory receptor by a novel B7 family member leads to negative regulation of lymphocyte activation, *J. Exp. Med.*, **192**, 1–9.

84. Chapoval, A., Ni, J., Lau, J. S., et al. (2001) B7-H3: a costimulatory molecule for T cell activation and IFN-gamma production, *Nat. Immunol.*, **2**, 269–274.

85. Sakaguchi, S., Sakaguchi, N., Asano, M., Itoh, M., and Toda, M. (1995) Immunologic self-tolerance maintained by activated T

cells expressing IL-2 receptor α-chains, *J. Immunol.*, **155**, 1151–1164.

86. Thornton, A. M. and Shevach, E. M. (2000) Suppressor effector function of CD4+CD25+ immunoregulatory T cells is antigen nonspecific, *J. Immunol.*, **164**, 183–190.

87. Shevach, E.M. (2002) CD4+CD25+ suppressor T cells: more questions than answers, *Nat. Rev. Immunol.*, **2**, 389–400.

88. Piccirillo, C. and Shevach, E. M. (2001) Cutting edge: control of CD8+ T cell activation by CD4+CD25+ immunoregulatory cells, *J. Immunol.*, **167**, 1137–1140.

89. Thornton, A.M. and Shevach, E. M. (1998) CD4+CD25+ immunoregulatory T cells suppress polycolonal T-cell activation in vitro by inhibiting interlukin-2 production, *J. Exp. Med.*, **188**, 287–296.

90. Takahashi, T., Tagami, T., Yamazaki, S., Uede, T., Shimizu, J., Sakaguchi, N., et al. (2000) Immunologic self-tolerance maintained by CD25+CD4+ regulatory T cells constitutively expressing cytotoxic T lymphocyte-associated antigen 4, *J. Exp. Med.*, **192**, 303–310.

91. Nakamura, K., Kitani, A., and Strober, W. (2001) Cell contact-dependent immunosuppression by CD4(+)CD25(+) regulatory T cells is mediated by cell surface-bound transforming growth factor beta, *J. Exp. Med.*, **194**, 629–644.

92. Suri-Payer, E. and Cantor, H. (2001) Differential cytokine requirements for regulation of autoimmune gastritis and colitis by CD4+CD25+ T cells, *J. Autoimmun.*, **16**, 115–123.

93. Asano, M., Toda, M., Sakaguchi, N., and Sakaguchi, S. (1996) Autoimmune disease as a consequence of developmental abnormality of a T cell subpopulation, *J. Exp. Med.*, **184**, 387–396.

94. Takahashi, T., Kuniyasu, Y., Toda, M., et al. (1998) Immunologic self-tolerance maintained by CD4+CD25+ naturally anergic and suppressive T cells, *Int. Immunol.*, **10**, 1969–1980.

95. Papiernik, M., Leite de Moraes, M., Ponteux, C., Vasseur, F., and Pénit, C. (1998) Regulatory CD4 T cells: expression of IL-2Rα chain, resistance to clonal deletion and IL-2 dependency, *Int. Immunol.*, **10**, 371–378.

96. Groux, H., O'Garra, A., Rouleau, M., et al. (1997) A CD4+ T-cell inhibits antigen- specific T-cell responses and prevents colitis, *Nature*, **389**, 737–742.

97. Jonuleit, H., Schmitt, E., Schuler, G., Knop, J., and Enk, A. H. (2000) Induction of interleukin 10-producing, nonproliferating CD4+ T cells with regulatory properties by repetitive stimulation with allogeneic immature human dendritic cells, *J. Exp. Med.*, **192**, 1213–1222.

98. Kurts, C., Heath, W. R., Carbone, F. R., Allison, J., Miller, J. F., and Kosaka, H. (1996) Constitutive class I-restricted exogenous presentation of self antigens in vivo, *J. Exp. Med.*, **184**, 923–930.

99. Adler, A. J., Marsh, D. W., Yochum, G. S., et al. (1998) CD4+ T cell tolerance to parenchymal self-antigens requires presentation by bone marrow-derived antigen- presenting cells, *J. Exp. Med.*, **187**, 1555–1564.

100. Banchereau, J. and Steinman, R. M. (1998) Dendritic cells and the control of immunity (review), *Nature*, **392**, 245–252.

101. Huang, F. P., Platt, N., Wykes, M., Major, J. R., Powell, T. J., Jenkins, C. D., and MacPherson, G. G. (2000) A discrete subpopulation of dendritic cells transports apoptotic intestinal epithelial cells to T cell areas of mesenteric lymph nodes, *J. Exp. Med.*, **191**, 435–444.

102. Dhodapkar, M.V., Steinman, R. M., Krasovsky, J., Munz, C., and Bhardwaj, N. (2001) Antigen-specific inhibition of effector T cell function in humans after injection of immature dendritic cells, *J. Exp. Med.*, **193**, 233–238.

103. Steinman, R. M. and Nussenzweig, M. C. (2002) Avoiding horror autotoxicus: the importance of dendritic cells in peripheral T cell tolerance, *Proc. Natl. Acad. Sci. U.S.A.*, **99**, 351–358.

104. Janeway, C. A., Jr. (1992) The immune system evolved to discriminate infectious nonself from noninfectious self, *Immunol. Today*, **13**, 11–16.

105. Medzhitov, R., Preston-Hurlburt, P., and Janeway, C. A., Jr. (1997) A human homologue of the *Drosophila* Toll protein signals activation of adaptive immunity, *Nature*, **388**, 394–397.

106. Aderem, A. and Ulevitch, R. J. (2000) Toll-like receptors in the induction of the innate immune response, *Nature*, **406**, 782–787.

107. Basu, S., Binder, R. J., Suto, R., Anderson, K. M., and Srivastava, P. K. (2000) Necrotic but not apoptotic cell death releases heat shock proteins, which deliver a partial maturation signal to dendritic cells and activate the NF-κB pathway, *Int. Immunol.*, **12**, 1539–1546.

108. Larsson, M., Fonteneau, J. F., and Bhardwaj, N. (2001) Dendritic cells resurrect antigens from dead cells, *Trends Immunol.*, **22**, 141–148.

109. Haynes, B. F. and Fauci, A. S. (2005) Chapter 295: Introduction to the immune system. Immune tolerance and autoimmunity. In: *Harrison's Internal Medicine*, 16th ed., (Kasper, D. L., Braunwald, E., Fauci, A. S., Hauser, S. L., Longo, D. L., Jameson, J. L., and Isselbacher, K. J., eds.) (http://www.accessmedicine.com/content.aspx?aID=93538).

110. Mackay, I. R. (2001) Tolerance and autoimmunity, *West J. Med.*, **174**(2), 118–123.

111. Jacobson, D. L., Gange, S. J., Rose, N. R., and Graham, N. M. H. (1997) Epidemiology and estimated population burden of selected autoimmune diseases in the United States, *Clin. Immunol. Immunopathol.*, **84**, 223–243.

112. Rotrosen D., Matthews, J. B., and Bluestone, J. A. (2002) The immune tolerance network: a new paradigm for developing tolerance-inducing therapies, *J. Allergy Clin. Immunol.*, **110**(1), 17–23.

113. Van Parijs, L. and Abbas, A. K. (1998) Homeostasis and self-tolerance in the immune system: turning lymphocytes off, *Science*, **280**, 243–248.

114. Goodnow, C. (1996) Balancing immunity and tolerance: deleting and tuning lymphocyte repertoires, *Proc. Natl. Acad. Sci. U.S.A.*, **93**, 2264–2271.

115. Stockinger, B. (1999) T lymphocyte tolerance: from thymic deletion to peripheral control mechanisms, *Adv. Immunol.*, **71**, 229–265.

116. Tarlinton, D. (1997) Germinal centers: a second childhood for lymphocytes, *Curr. Biol.*, **7**, R155–R159.

117. Nepom, G. T. (1998) Major histocompatibility complex-directed susceptibility to rheumatoid arthritis, *Adv. Immunol.*, **68**, 325–332.

118. Mackay, C. R. (1993) Homing of naive, memory and effector lymphocytes, *Curr. Opin. Immunol.*, **5**, 423–427.

119. Quill, H. (1996) Anergy as a mechanism of peripheral T cell tolerance, *J. Immunol.*, **156**, 1325–1327.

120. Greenfield, E. A., Nguyen, K. A., and Kuchroo, V. K. (1998) CD28/B7 costimulation: a review, *Crit. Rev. Immunol.*, **18**, 389–418.

121. Marelli-Berg, F. M, and Lechler, R. I. (1999) Antigen presentation by parenchymal cells: a route to peripheral tolerance? *Immunol. Rev.*, **172**, 297–314.

122. Seddon, B. and Mason, D. (2000) The third function of the thymus, *Immunol. Today*, **21**, 95–99.

123. Granville, D. J., Carthy, C. M., Hunt, D. W.E., and McManus, B. M. (1998) Apoptosis: molecular aspects of cell death and disease, *Lab. Invest.*, **78**, 893–913.

124. Korb, L. C. and Ahearn, J. M. (1997) C1q binds directly and specifically to surface blebs of apoptotic human keratinocytes:

complement deficiency and systemic lupus erythematosus revisited, *J. Immunol.*, **158**, 4525–4528.

125. Vaishnaw, A. K., Toubi, E., Ohsako, S., et al. (1999) The spectrum of apoptotic defects and clinical manifestations, including systemic lupus erythematosus, in humans with CD95 (Fas/APO-1) mutations, *Arthritis Rheum.*, **42**, 1833–1842.

126. Rizzi, M., Ferrera, M., Filaci, G., and Indiveri, F. (2006) Disruption of immunological tolerance: role of AIRE gene in autoimmunity, *Autoimmune Rev.*, **5**(2), 145–147.

127. Nagamine, K., Peterson, P., Scott, K. S., Kudoh, J., Minoshima, S., et al. (1997) Positional cloning of the APECED gene, *Nat. Genet.*, **17**(4), 393–398.

128. T.F.-G.A. Consortium (1997) An autoimmune disease, APECED, caused by mutations in a novel gene featuring the PHD-type zinc-finger domains, *Nat. Genet.*, **17**(4), 399–403.

129. Uchida, D., Hatakeyama, S., Matsushima, A., Han, H., Ishido, S., Hotta, H., et al. (2004) AIRE functions as an E3 ubiquitin ligase, *J. Exp. Med.*, **199**(2), 167–172.

130. Kogawa, K., Nagafuchi, S., Katsuta, H., Kudoh, J., et al. (2002) Expression of AIRE gene in peripheral monocyte/dendritic cell lineage, *Immunol. Lett.*, **80**, 195–198.

131. Kuroda, N., Mitani, T., Takeda, N., Ishimaru, N., Arakaki, R., Hayashi, Y., et al. (2005) Development of autoimmunity against transcriptionally unrepressed target antigen in the thymus of Aire-deficient mice, *J. Immunol.*, **174** (4), 1862–1870.

132. Anderson, M. S., Venanzi, E. S., Klein, L., Chen, Z., Berzins, S. P., et al. (2002) Projection of an immunological self shadow within the thymus by the AIRE protein, *Science*, **298**, 1395–1401.

133. Liston, A., Gray, D. H., Lesage, S., Fletcher, A. L., Wilson, J., et al. (2004) Gene dosage-limiting role of Aire in thymic expression, clonal deletion, and organ- specific autoimmunity, *J. Exp. Med.*, **200** (8), 1015–1026.

134. Tait, K. F. and Gough, S. C. (2003) The genetics of autoimmune endocrine disease, *Clin. Endocrinol. (Oxford)*, **59** (1), 1–11.

135. Torok, H. P., Tonenchi, L., Glas, J., Schiemann, U., and Folwaczny, C. (2004) No significant association between

mutations in exons 6 and 8 of the autoimmune regulator (AIRE) gene and inflammatory bowel disease, *Eur. J. Immunogenet.*, **31**(2), 83–86.

136. Cavadini, P., Vermi, W., Facchetti, F., Fontana, S., Nagafuchi, S., et al. (2005) AIRE deficiency in thymus of 2 patients with Omenn syndrome, *J. Clin. Invest.*, **115**(3), 728–732.

137. Tazi-Ahnini, R., Cork, M. J., Gawkrodger, D. J., Birch, M. P., Wengraf, D., et al. (2002) Role of the autoimmune regulator (AIRE) gene in alopecia areata: strong association of a potentially functional AIRE polymorphism with alopecia universalis, *Tissue Antigens*, **60**(6), 489–495.

138. Fuchtenbusch, M., Vogel, A., Achenbach, P., Gummer, M., Ziegler, A. G., et al. (2003) Lupus-like panniculitis in a patient with autoimmune polyendocrinopathy-candidiasis-ectodermal dystrophy (APECED), *Exp. Clin. Endocrinol. Diabetes*, **111**(5), 288–293.

139. Kawai, T., Cosimi, A. B., Spitzer, T. R., et al. (2008) HLA-mismatched renal transplantation without maintenance immunosuppression, *N. Engl. J. Med.*, **358**(4), 353–361.

140. Alexander, S. I., Smith, N., Hu, M., et al. (2008) Chimerism and tolerance in a recipient of a deceased-donor liver transplant, *N. Engl. J. Med.*, **358**(4), 369–374.

141. Scandling, J. D., Busque, S., Dejbakhsh-Jones, S., et al., (2008) Tolerance and chimerism after renal and hematopoietic-cell transplantation, *N. Engl. J. Med.*, **358**(4), 362–368.

142. Nicholas, M. W., Dooley, M. A., Hogan, S. L., et al. (2008) A novel subset of memory B cells is enriched in autoreactivity and correlates with adverse outcomes in SLE, *Clin. Immunol.*, **126**, 189–201.

143. Li, X., Xiao, B.-G., Xi, J-Y., Lu, C.-Z., and Lu, J.-H. (2008) Decrease of CD4+CD25^{high} Foxp3$^+$ regulatory T cells and elevation of CD19+BAFF-R+ B cells and soluble ICAM-1 in myasthenia gravis, *Clin. Immunol.*, **126**, 180–188.

144. Lim, D. G., Joe, I. Y., Park, Y. H., et al. (2007) Effect of immunosuppressants on the expansion and function of naturally occurring regulatory T cells, *Transplant Immunol.*, **18**, 94–100.

Chapter 41

Autoimmune Diseases

The immune system is essential to survival, and even a modest decrease in immune function can leave a person susceptible to infection. But the immune system itself can also cause disease, by inappropriately attacking the body's own organs, tissues, or cells (http://www3.niaid.nih.gov/research/topics/autoimmune/introduction.htm).

More than 80 clinically distinct autoimmune diseases have been described to date. In the United States, autoimmune diseases collectively affect between 14 and 22 million people (http://www.immunetolerance.org/; ITN 2007 Annual Research Report). Some, such as type 1 diabetes, attack specific organs, whereas others, such as systemic lupus erythematosus (SLE), involve multiple organs. Although many autoimmune diseases are rare, collectively they affect approximately 5% to 8% of the U.S. population. A disproportionate number of people with autoimmune disorders are women. For unknown reasons, the prevalence of autoimmune diseases is increasing.

Although there has been considerable progress in understanding the immune mechanisms mediating tissue injury in autoimmune diseases, much remains to be learned, such as the causes of these diseases and the genetic factors that make humans susceptible to them, as well as the regulatory mechanisms that control autoantibody production (http://www3.niaid.nih.gov/research/topics/autoimmune/introduction.htm).

Apart from their clinical heterogeneity, the autoimmune diseases present a number of particular challenges in seeking to reestablish self-tolerance. In contrast with transplant setting, in autoimmune diseases, the memory T- and B-cells are key mediators, and in some cases, the pathology of the disease involves both the humoral and cellular responses (http://www.immunetolerance.org/; ITN 2007 Annual Research Report).

Autoimmune diseases (1), with the exception of rheumatoid arthritis and autoimmune thyroiditis, are individually rare, but together they affect approximately 5% of the population in Western countries (2,3). They are a fascinating but poorly understood group of diseases that are usually defined as a clinical syndrome caused by the activation of T cells or B cells, or both, in the absence of an ongoing infection or other discernible cause (1).

For many years, the central dogma of immunology focused on the clonal deletion of autoreactive cells, leaving a repertoire of T- and B-cells that recognize specific foreign antigen. However, the current understanding is that a low level of autoreactivity is physiologic (4) and crucial to normal immune function. To this end, autoantigens are helping to form the repertoire of mature lymphocytes, and the survival of naïve T cells (5) and B cells (6) in the periphery would require a continuous exposure to autoantigens. Because there is no fundamental difference between the structure of self-antigens (or autoantigens) and that of foreign antigens, lymphocytes had evolved not to distinguish self from foreign antigens, as some have speculated, but to respond to antigen only in certain microenvironments, generally in the presence of inflammatory cytokines (7). Because autoreactivity is a physiologic phenomenon, the challenge is to understand how it becomes a pathologic process and how T- and B-cells contribute to tissue injury (1).

41.1 Classification of Autoimmune Diseases

For clinicians, autoimmune diseases appear to be either systemic (as in the case of systemic lupus erythematosus) or organ-specific (as in the case of type 1 diabetes mellitus). This classification, although clinically useful, does not necessarily correspond with a difference in causation (1).

A more useful division distinguishes between diseases in which there is a general alteration in the selection, regulation, or death of T- or B-cells and those in which an aberrant response to a particular antigen, self or foreign, causes autoimmunity (1). An example of a general defect is the absence of the Fas protein or its receptor—proteins involved in cell death—and a representative antigen-specific disorder is the demyelination syndrome that follows enteric infection with Campylobacter jejuni. This classification is useful in deciding on therapy, which may differ according to the pathogenic mechanism. Although this mechanistic classification can be used for animal models, it is often difficult to determine whether a human disease is due to a global

V. St. Georgiev, *National Institute of Allergy and Infectious Diseases, NIH: Impact on Global Health*, vol. 2, DOI 10.1007/978-1-60327-297-1_41, © Humana Press, a part of Springer Science+Business Media, LLC 2009

abnormality in lymphocyte function or an antigen-specific abnormality *(1)*.

Alterations that lower the threshold for the survival and activation of autoreactive B cells often cause the production of multiple autoantibodies, as in the case of the antinuclear and anti-DNA antibodies in systemic lupus erythematosus *(8–33)*. Low levels of these autoantibodies are the rule in all people *(1)*. Other autoantibody-mediated diseases seem to reflect a loss of B-cell tolerance to a particular antigen. For example, the antiganglioside antibodies that cause the Guillain-Barré syndrome appear to arise in the face of intact general tolerance of self by B cells *(34)*. Genetic alterations with global effects on the function of regulatory T cells or cytokine production often lead to inflammatory bowel disease *(35–37)*. This process may reflect enhanced activation of T cells with an exuberant response to gut flora. Changes in the repertoire of T cells may cause a systemic illness or organ-specific abnormalities. For example, thymectomy in neonatal mice eliminates a subgroup of critical regulatory cells and causes a wasting disease or an autoimmune attack on the thyroid, gastric parietal cells, or ovaries, depending on the genetic background of the mouse *(38)*. This example illustrates why the distinction between systemic and organ-specific disease is not always useful for understanding the mechanisms of autoimmunity *(1)*.

In some organ-specific diseases, autoreactivity against a ubiquitous autoantigen develops, but the disease is restricted to a particular organ *(1)*. For example, the ribonucleoprotein antigens targeted in Sjögren's syndrome and the transfer RNA synthetases in polymyositis are ubiquitous intracellular proteins *(39)*, yet the pathologic effects of these diseases are relatively restricted. Presumably, the antigen has greater accessibility in affected tissues, although the patterns of lymphocyte migration may also determine sites of inflammation *(40)*. The differential expression of transport molecules on various subgroups of T cells was well documented *(41)*. The expression of many antigens is also developmentally regulated, making autoreactivity hazardous only at certain stages of growth *(1)*. For example, the antibodies against the Ro (SSA) antigen in Sjögren's syndrome and systemic lupus erythematosus bind to the conducting system in the fetal heart, causing complete heart block, but they do not affect the adult heart *(42)*. Antibodies against desmoglein cause pemphigus in adults but not in neonates, because only one of the two desmogleins in neonatal skin is a target of these antibodies *(43)*.

41.2 Risk Factors in Autoimmune Diseases

The autoimmune responses can draw on a formidable immunologic arsenal *(44)*. A subject of growing interest is the relation between T-lymphocyte responses and chronic inflammation, which depends less on the effects of the inducing agent than on the immune responses directed to its elimination. Unfortunately, when a self-molecule becomes immunogenic, it cannot (in contrast with a pathogen) be eliminated; accordingly, autoimmune inflammation becomes persistent and destructive. The division of CD4 helper T-cells (Th) into two functional subsets, Th1 and Th2, although not as clear in humans as in mice, is a paradigm for understanding how autoimmune and allergic inflammation is orchestrated by cytokines and chemokines *(45,46)*. The cytokines interleukin 12 (IL-12) and interferon-γ (IFN-γ), secreted particularly by antigen-presenting cells, promote proinflammatory and cytodestructive Th1 responses through secretion of IFN-γ and tumor necrosis factor-α (TNF-α), whereas interleukin 4 (IL-4) promotes Th2 responses with the activation of B cells *(44)*. Chemokines are chemotactic proteins secreted by various cell types that, through their interaction with specific receptors, direct the selective traffic of leukocytes throughout the lymphoid system and into inflammatory sites *(46,47)*. Thus, polarization toward a Th1 or Th2 response has been associated with the upregulation of chemokine receptors on Th1 or Th2 cells, respectively *(46)*.

Environmental Risk Factors. Although environmental agents can cause autoimmunity, it is highly unlikely *(44)*. Infection has been strongly implicated because it can readily disrupt peripheral tolerance in ways that include exposure of self to the immune system through a breakdown of vascular or cellular barriers; the occurrence of cell death by necrosis rather than the bland process of apoptosis; "bystander" activation of macrophages and T lymphocytes, which can then provide costimulatory signals; and superantigen effects of bacterial products. Experimental evidence has indicated that mice infected with coxsackievirus that has a tropism for either pancreatic islets *(48)* or heart *(49)* did develop, despite viral clearance, an autoimmune response to breakdown products of islet cells or myocardium, resulting in chronic autoimmune inflammation *(44)*.

In addition, there is the alternative, or perhaps complementary, process of molecular (antigenic) mimicry, whereby an antigen of a microorganism or a constituent of food that sufficiently resembles a self-molecule can induce a cross-reactive autoimmune response *(44)*. The mimicry idea has an attractive logic and supporting experimental evidence *(50)*, but clear examples are lacking for the more common human autoimmune diseases and their animal models.

Other environmental initiators of autoimmunity that break tolerance can act like infections by causing tissue damage, such as sunlight in lupus erythematosus, or alter a host molecule sufficiently that it becomes immunogenic, as in chemical- or drug-induced autoimmune syndromes. In all these examples, a predisposing genetic background is also needed *(44)*.

Autoimmunity might arise entirely from within, by an intracellular self-molecule becoming in some way aberrantly expressed at the cell surface. The "internal" environment accounts for paraneoplastic autoimmune associations of cancers of the ovary, lung, and breast in which an antigen associated with the tumor provokes remarkable autoimmune responses that damage structures, such as cerebellar, motor, or sensory neurons; nerve terminals, as in the Lambert-Eaton myasthenic syndrome; or retinal cells *(51)*. These syndromes reflect a misguided immune defense against the cancer because they usually precede overt expression of the cancer and even limit dissemination *(44)*.

The internal environment is also indirectly relevant because hormones influence female predisposition to autoimmunity and autoimmune thyroid disease and type 1 diabetes mellitus may erupt in the postpartum period. Less well defined are the claimed effects of psychological stress that may act through neuroendocrine pathways *(44)*.

Genetic Risk Factors. All autoimmune diseases probably have some genetic components. Susceptibility genes for autoimmunity may act along two tracks. One track determines tissue and disease specificity by directing the response to particular autoantigens. For example, genes that encode molecules of the major histocompatibility complex can determine which autoantigens are presented to the immune system; genes that encode the specificity of antigen receptors on T- and B-lymphocytes may influence which molecules are attacked; and genes may influence the susceptibility of a particular target tissue to autoimmune attack. The other track is a general susceptibility to autoimmunity through genes that influence tolerance, apoptosis, or inflammatory responses. These genes explain the well-known tendency for autoimmunity to run in families, with multiple and variable expressions of disease in affected individuals. The genes involved are not all wrong; some alleles of the major histocompatibility complex may confer protection against autoimmunity, and the absence of these genes causes susceptibility, as for type 1 diabetes and rheumatoid arthritis *(44)*.

Genetic susceptibility to autoimmune disease is now being investigated in highly informative ways *(52)*. Procedures include genome-wide scanning of individuals from affected families using DNA microarrays to identify specific genetic elements. Variant alleles and their gene products have been identified by linkage analysis and positional cloning. Thus, studies of pairs of siblings in families with autoimmune disease can reveal susceptibility loci by sharing or otherwise of alleles at a known marker locus. Selected breeding of autoimmune strains of mice (such as nonobese diabetic mice or NZB lupus mice) were able to identify susceptibility loci for autoimmunity homologous to those identified in these human diseases *(53)*. Comparison of results from genome-wide scanning of autoimmune humans and mice and use of the database of the Human Genome Project should provide a "blueprint" in the next few years for the estimated 20 (or perhaps more) genetic determinants for autoimmune disease. The protein products encoded by these genes will then be related to particular autoimmune syndromes. These newly acquired genetic data can then be used by clinicians to analyze complex autoimmune syndromes like rheumatoid arthritis, multiple sclerosis, and type 1 diabetes to understand their heterogeneity of expression *(44)*.

Loss of Regulatory Cells. Several kinds of regulatory cells are important in controlling autoreactivity: CD1-restricted T cells, T cells with γ/δ receptors, $CD4^+CD25^+$ T cells, and T cells that produce cytokines that suppress pathogenic autoreactive cells *(1)*. Some of these regulatory cells—for example, $CD4^+CD25^+$ T cells—must mature in the thymus *(38)*; others require activation by autoantigens in the periphery.

Alterations in the number and function of regulatory cells may contribute to autoimmunization. In monozygotic twins who are discordant for diabetes, for instance, levels of CD1-restricted T cells are greatly diminished in the affected twin *(54)*. The antigens that activate regulatory T cells in the body are unknown, and the way in which these cells exert their pressure on immune responses is only partly understood. Most important, the reason for their reduced numbers in patients with diabetes or other autoimmune diseases is unknown *(1)*.

41.3 Genetic Susceptibility

Epidemiologic studies have demonstrated that genetic factors are crucial determinants of susceptibility to autoimmune disease *(1)*. There is familial clustering, and the rate of concordance for autoimmune disease is higher in monozygotic twins than in dizygotic twins *(55–57)*. A few autoimmune diseases, such as autoimmune lymphoproliferative syndrome and the syndrome of autoimmune polyglandular endocrinopathy with candidiasis and ectodermal dysplasia (APECED), are due to mutations in a single gene. Even in these conditions, other genes modify the severity of disease, and not all who possess the mutant gene manifest the disease. Autoimmune lymphoproliferative syndrome is an autosomal dominant disorder involving a defect in the Fas protein or its receptor. The Fas pathway mediates apoptosis, which downregulates immune responses *(58)*. The autoreactivity in this syndrome results from an inability to trigger apoptosis of activated immune cells after encounters with microbial antigens. APECED is caused by a mutation in the gene encoding the autoimmune regulator protein (AIRE), which occurs predominately in the thymic medulla but also in other tissues *(59)* (see Section 40.2.2 in Chapter 40). This protein, presumably a transcriptional regulator, has a role in the selection of T cells in the thymus *(60)* or in their peripheral regulation. The disease is characterized by both autoimmunity and immunodeficiency. These two abnormalities also coexist in other disorders, acquired or inherited, that are characterized by a loss of function of T- or B-cells, such as the acquired immunodeficiency syndrome, complement deficiencies, and IgA deficiency *(1)*.

Most autoimmune diseases are multigenic, with multiple susceptibility genes working in concert to produce the abnormal phenotype. In general, the polymorphisms also occur in normal people and are compatible with normal immune function. Only when present with other susceptibility genes they do contribute to autoimmunity *(61,62)*. Some of these genes confer a much higher level of risk than do others; for example, the major histocompatibility complex makes an important contribution to disease susceptibility *(1)*.

Furthermore, most autoimmune diseases are linked to a particular class I or class II HLA molecule *(63)*, but this association may require linkage with another gene such as the one that encodes tumor necrosis factor-α or complement. In the case of ankylosing spondylitis, diabetes, and rheumatoid arthritis, however, the reproduction of the disease in transgenic animals expressing particular human HLA antigens strongly indicated that the class I or class II molecule itself conferred susceptibility to disease *(64,65)*.

Some HLA alleles protected against disease even when a susceptibility allele is present *(61,62)*. For example, the HLA-DQB1*0602 allele protects against type 1 diabetes even if the HLA-DQB1*0301 or DQB1*0302 susceptibility gene is present *(56)*, and the presence of this protective allele is an exclusion criterion for current diabetes-prevention trials. The mechanism of this protection is not understood *(1)*. Finally, the association of HLA alleles with a particular disease may vary among different populations. The class II HLA-DRB1*0401 and DRB1*0404 alleles are strongly associated with rheumatoid arthritis in persons of Northern European ancestry *(66)*, but not in black or Hispanic populations *(67,68)*.

Genetic engineering of mice has led to the identification of at least 25 genes that can contribute to an autoimmune diathesis when they are deleted or overexpressed. These genes encode cytokines, antigen coreceptors, members of cytokine- or antigen-signaling cascades, costimulatory molecules, molecules involved in pathways that promote apoptosis and those that inhibit it, and molecules that clear antigen or antigen-antibody complexes *(1)*. Two critical lessons have been learned from these models. First, whether a particular gene or mutation causes a disease depends on the overall genetic background of the host: both disease susceptibility and the disease phenotype that result from an alteration of a single gene depend on other genes. Second, some genetic defects can predispose patients to more than one autoimmune disease, so that several diseases may share common pathogenic pathways. This observation suggests the possibility of using common therapeutic strategies in different autoimmune diseases *(1)*.

The findings of genetic studies in humans are consistent with these ideas. There are, for example, allelic variants of the gene encoding cytotoxic T-lymphocyte–associated protein 4 (CTLA-4), a T-cell surface molecule that downregulates activated T cells. One such polymorphism caused a small decrease in the inhibitory signal mediated by CTLA-4 and was associated with type 1 diabetes, thyroid disease, and primary biliary cirrhosis *(69–71)*. More often, however, a genetic locus rather than a single gene has been linked to a susceptibility to autoimmune disease, and many loci have been emerging as potentially important in more than one disease *(61,62)*. The clinical observation that different autoimmune diseases often coexisted within a family has strongly suggested that some genes at these loci predispose patients to more than one disease *(72,73)*.

It is also possible that vulnerability of the target organ to immune-mediated damage would be genetically determined. Thus, a variable threshold to renal and cardiac damage has been clearly demonstrated in animal models *(74,75)*. Genetic variation in vulnerability to autoimmune-induced damage may underlie the clinical observation that persons with the same serologic abnormality do not necessarily have the same tissue abnormality *(1)*.

41.4 Disease Progression and Therapeutic Strategies

Epitope Spreading. As an autoimmune disease progresses from initial activation to a chronic state, there has often been an increase in the number of autoantigens targeted by T cells and antibodies ("epitope spreading") *(76,77)* and, in some cases, a change in participating cells, cytokines, and other inflammatory mediators *(1)*. Both autoreactive T- and B-cells contribute to epitope spreading. Activated autoreactive B cells function as antigen-presenting cells; they present novel (cryptic) peptides of autoantigens *(78,79)* and express costimulatory molecules. They also generate peptides that have not previously been presented to T cells; thus, T cells will not have become tolerant to such cryptic peptides. Over time, multiple novel peptides within a molecule can activate T cells *(1)*.

Furthermore, if a B cell binds and takes in not a single protein but a complex of multiple proteins, epitopes from each protein in the complex will be processed and presented to naïve T cells. The cascade continues, with T cells activating additional autoreactive B cells and B cells presenting additional self-epitopes, until there is autoreactivity to numerous autoantigens. By then, the identity of the initiating antigen can no longer be determined *(1)*.

Tissue Injury. Both autoreactive T cells and autoantibodies can damage tissues. T-cell cytolysis of target cells can be mediated through perforin-induced cellular necrosis or through granzyme B–induced apoptosis *(80)*. It has been suggested that Th1 cells were critical to the induction of autoimmune disease through the recruitment of inflammatory cells and mediators, whereas Th2 cells protect against disease *(81)*. However, it is now clear that cytokines produced by Th1 or Th2 cells and even transforming growth factor-β can cause tissue injury *(82–84)*.

Autoantibodies also cause damage through mechanisms that include the formation of immune complexes, cytolysis or phagocytosis of target cells, and interference with cellular physiology *(1)*. Interference with cellular physiology, first identified in connection with antibodies against acetylcholine in patients with myasthenia gravis *(85)* and antibodies against the receptor for thyrotropin in patients with Graves' disease *(86)*, is a common pathway to tissue injury. In patients with pemphigus, antibodies against desmoglein induce the release of a protease that mediates the formation of blisters *(87)*. In patients with the antiphospholipid-antibody syndrome, antibodies bind to soluble factors in blood that prevent the activation of the clotting cascade, thus triggering coagulation *(88–89)*. Moreover, some autoantibodies that bind to surface receptors are taken up by living cells *(90,91)*. The issue whether such antibodies then interfere with cellular physiology has been controversial *(1)*.

41.4.1 Therapeutic Strategies for Autoimmune Diseases

During the past 10 years or so, the NIAID expanded its capacity for translational and clinical research that included research on immune-mediated diseases. For example, the Non-Human Primate Tolerance Cooperative Research Study Group and several clinical research networks now support preclinical studies and clinical trials in asthma, allergic and autoimmune diseases, and transplantation. Many of those programs benefit from the support and expertise of multiple NIH institutes and are funded in part through special government appropriations of funds (http://www.niddk.nih.gov/fund/diabetesspecialfunds/about.htm) as well as by a variety of public-private partnerships. Each of those programs involves cross-disciplinary efforts, with a focus on the underlying basis of disease and mechanisms of therapeutic efficacy. They provide a framework for "bench-to-bedside" and "bedside-back-to-bench" research that is yielding new therapeutic and preventive approaches and fresh insights into basic processes. Although the challenges are considerable,

scientific opportunities abound, including the potential for breakthroughs that could dramatically alter existing treatment paradigms.

Selective Immunotherapies for Autoimmune Diseases. The goal of replacing blanket immunosuppression by selective immunotherapy for autoimmune diseases seems now attainable, with the many possible "points of engagement" *(44)*. The agents in use or under development include (i) monoclonal antibodies or blocking antagonists against the T-cell synapse (represented by the binding site for the major histocompatibility complex, T-cell receptor, and autoantigen), interactions between costimulatory molecules and ligands, or interactions between cytokines or chemokines with their receptors; (ii) counterregulatory cytokines such as interleukin 10 (IL-10); and (iii) the T-cell downregulatory molecule CTLA-4. Examples in current practice include glatiramer acetate (copolymer-1, Copaxone), which interferes with the interaction between the major histocompatibility complex and a neural autoantigen to prevent relapses in multiple sclerosis *(92)*; monoclonal antibodies or soluble receptor for TNF-α, which block the inflammatory effects of TNF-α in rheumatoid arthritis *(93)* and inflammatory bowel disease; and CTLA-4, which limits graft-versus-host disease in patients with bone marrow transplantation and alleviates psoriasis *(94)*.

An alternative approach is to "rewire" the immune system for tolerance *(44)*. First, antigen-based desensitization (oral tolerance), by repetitive mucosal administration of autoantigens, can prevent or reverse autoimmune disease in animal models. To date, results for human diseases are not encouraging (multiple sclerosis, rheumatoid arthritis, uveitis) or not yet available (type 1 diabetes) *(95)*. The problem may be that long-standing autoimmune disease is maintained by memory-type T-lymphocytes that are difficult to render tolerant. Second, immune ablation by intensive immunosuppression and replacement by the infusion of peripheral blood CD34 stem cells is proving successful in severe refractory autoimmune diseases, lupus erythematosus, rheumatoid arthritis, systemic sclerosis, and multiple sclerosis *(96,97)*, but whether this is simply due to heavy immunosuppression or indicates reprogramming for tolerance as well remains uncertain. Third, for the more distant future, gene therapy for autoimmune disease has been considered for type 1 diabetes *(98)*, but the principles would be applicable to other autoimmune diseases *(61)*.

Rheumatoid Arthritis. The treatment of rheumatoid arthritis has been markedly improved by the recognition that bone erosions occur early in the disease and that therapy should be instituted promptly in many patients *(1)*. Although methotrexate remains the first-line disease-modifying agent, there are some promising new drugs. The fact that activated macrophages contribute to synovial inflammation in this disease has led to the development of modulators of macrophage-derived cytokines. Blockade of TNF-α by a soluble p75 TNF-α receptor-IgG1 fusion protein (etanercept) or a monoclonal antibody against TNF-α (infliximab) was found to be highly effective in preventing erosions when it was used in combination with methotrexate. Etanercept can also be used alone, because it is not immunogenic in humans *(99,100)*. Blockade of TNF-α was also effective in Crohn's disease *(101)* and was useful in refractory psoriatic arthritis *(102)* and ankylosing spondylitis *(103)*, a disease for which no other disease-modifying therapy has been available *(1)*.

Leflunomide, a pyrimidine antagonist that blocks the enzyme dihydroorotate dehydrogenase, thereby blocking the synthesis of DNA, has an efficacy similar to that of methotrexate and can be used either alone or in combination with methotrexate *(104,105)*. Blockade of interleukin-1 receptors with a recombinant interleukin-1-receptor antagonist is less effective than blockade of TNF-α in patients with rheumatoid arthritis, but it may retard the development of bone erosions *(99)*. The long-term safety of these new agents, particularly with respect to the risk of infections, cancer, and other autoimmune diseases, remains to be ascertained *(1)*.

Multiple Sclerosis. Progress has been made in the treatment of multiple sclerosis with the use of interferon-β1a (IFN-β1a) and copolymer 1 *(106)*. Although the indications for and timing of the use of these agents are still debated, a recent study did suggest that IFN-β1a can delay the onset of frank disease when given after a first episode of optic neuritis *(107)*. Copolymer 1 is a nonspecific inhibitor of T cells *in vitro (108)*, although it may also act by immune deviation from Th1 to Th2 cells *(109)*. Treatment with altered peptide ligands derived from myelin basic protein was efficacious in murine models of the disease, but two recent Phase I studies of such peptides have been associated clinically with significant toxicity: one caused hypersensitivity reactions *(110)*, and the second resulted in exacerbations of multiple sclerosis *(111)*. Hence, studies using animal models of disease cannot substitute for clinical trials, and these must proceed with caution *(1)*.

A number of studies have previously demonstrated that blockade of CD28 or CD40 costimulatory signals can suppress experimental autoimmune encephalitis (EAE), the experimental model of multiple sclerosis *(112)*. In a recently completed Phase I dose-escalating study of CTLA4Ig in relapsing-remitting multiple sclerosis, all doses (from 2.0 to 35 mg/kg) were well-tolerated and posed no significant safety risk. Furthermore, mechanistic studies performed in parallel with the clinical evaluations found that the antigen-specific responses to human myelin basic protein were reduced after CTLA-4 administration, whereas expression of CD25 was increased (http://www.immunetolerance.org/; ITN 2007 Annual Research Report).

Psoriasis. Blockade of TNF-α, with or without methotrexate, has been effective in refractory psoriasis *(1)*. Psoriasis

responded to treatment with interleukin-10 in several small and short-term clinical trials *(113)*. Benefit was also achieved with the use of CTLA-4/Ig, a recombinant fusion protein in which the extracellular domain of CTLA-4 is linked to the constant region of IgG1. CTLA-4/Ig is blocking the activation of most naïve T cells as well as both primary and secondary antibody responses *(114)*. However, CTLA-4/Ig exacerbated diabetes in a mouse model in which activation of regulatory cells is thought to prevent initiation of the disease *(115)*.

A number of other biologic agents have also been successfully used to treat psoriasis in small pilot studies *(1)*. These include antibodies against CD4 *(116)*, antibodies against the high-affinity IL-2 receptor CD25 (daclizumab) *(117)*, and antibodies against the CD11a component of the adhesion molecule leukocyte function-associated antigen type 1 (also referred to as $\alpha_1\beta_2$ integrin and CD11aCD18) that mediates migration of T cells into the skin *(118,119)*. A humanized antibody against CD11a is currently being evaluated in a clinical trial in a large cohort of patients with psoriasis *(1)*.

Type 1 Diabetes. Targeting early intervention with disease-modifying therapies is a major goal aimed at preserving the estimated 15% to 40% of beta cells that generally remain capable of insulin production at the time of clinical presentation. The feasibility of this approach has been demonstrated in a 6-week course in which the nonmitogenic anti-CD3 monoclonal antibody hOKT3γ1(Ala-Ala) has been able, at least partially, to arrest autoimmunity and prolong the "honeymoon" phase in newly diagnosed type 1 diabetes patients for up to 2 years *(120,121)*.

In addition, therapeutic efforts in type 1 diabetes have focused on prevention *(1)*. Relatives of patients with diabetes who are at risk for the disease can be identified with near certainty; however, screening of the general population is associated with high false-positive rates that preclude intervention studies *(56)*. Prevention trials are currently assessing the efficacy of inducing antigen-specific immune tolerance through the intravenous or subcutaneous administration of insulin in persons at risk who have evidence of decreased beta-cell mass or through the oral administration of insulin in those who have antibodies against insulin but in whom insulin secretion is normal. Initial results with oral insulin have been disappointing *(122)*, whereas the results of systemic insulin are still unavailable *(1)*.

Systemic Lupus Erythematosus. Clinical trials in patients with systemic lupus erythematosus are significantly complicated by (i) the wide range of disease manifestations; (ii) the relapsing-remitting nature of the disease, which results in high rates of response in groups given a placebo; and (iii) the lack of standardized criteria for remission *(1)*. Whether or not abnormal serologic results should prompt treatment in the absence of clinical signs of the disease still remains debatable. Blockade with CTLA-4/Ig or antibodies against CD40 ligand has been highly effective in the prevention or treatment of nephritis in murine models *(123,124)* but not in humans. Two recent clinical trials of monoclonal antibodies against CD40 ligand were unsuccessful *(1)*: one did not show efficacy, and the other found unexpected toxicity *(125,126)*.

Polymorphisms of the IL-10 gene are associated with systemic lupus erythematosus; a pilot study suggests that treatment of active disease with antibodies against IL-10 may be effective *(127)*.

References

1. Davidson, A. and Diamond, B. (2001) Autoimmune diseases, *N. Engl. J. Med.*, **345**(5), 340–350.
2. Sinha, A. A., Lopez, M. T., and McDevitt, H. O. (1990) Autoimmune diseases: the failure of self tolerance, *Science*, **248**, 1380–1388.
3. Jacobson, D. L., Gange, S. J., Rose, N. R., and Graham N. M. (1997) Epidemiology and estimated population burden of selected autoimmune diseases in the United States, *Clin. Immunol. Immunopathol.*, **84**, 223–243.
4. Dighiero, G. and Rose, N. R. (1999) Critical self-epitopes are key to the understanding of self-tolerance and autoimmunity, *Immunol. Today*, **20**, 423–428.
5. Goldrath, A. W. and Bevan, M. J. (1999) Selecting and maintaining a diverse T-cell repertoire, *Nature*, **402**, 255–262.
6. Gu, H., Tarlinton, D., Muller, W., Rajewsky, K., and Forster, I. (1991) Most peripheral B cells in mice are ligand selected, *J. Exp. Med.*, **173**, 1357–1371.
7. Silverstein, A. M. and Rose, N. R. (2000) There is only one immune system! The view from immunopathology, *Semin. Immunol.*, **12**, 173–178; 257.
8. Takahashi, T., Tanaka, M., Brannan, C. I., et al. (1994) Generalized lymphoproliferative disease in mice, caused by a point mutation in the Fas ligand, *Cell*, **76**, 969–976.
9. Zhou, T., Edwards, C. K., III, Yang, P., Wang, Z., Bluethmann, H., and Mountz, J. D. (1996) Greatly accelerated lymphadenopathy and autoimmune disease in lpr mice lacking tumor necrosis factor receptor I, *J. Immunol.*, **156**, 2661–2665.
10. Dang, H., Geiser, A. G., Letterio, J. J., et al. (1005) SLE-like autoantibodies and Sjogren's syndrome-like lymphoproliferation in TGF-beta knockout mice, *J. Immunol.*, **155**, 3205–3212.
11. Kontoyiannis, D. and Kollias, G. (2000) Accelerated autoimmunity and lupus nephritis in NZB mice with an engineered heterozygous deficiency in tumor necrosis factor, *Eur. J. Immunol.*, **30**, 2038–2047.
12. Napirei, M., Karsunky, H., Zevnik, B., Stephan, H., Mannherz, H. G., and Moroy, T. (2000) Features of systemic lupus erythematosus in Dnase1-deficient mice, *Nat. Genet.*, **25**, 177–181.
13. Bickerstaff, M. C., Botto, M., Hutchinson, W. L., et al. (1999) Serum amyloid P component controls chromatin degradation and prevents antinuclear autoimmunity, *Nat. Med.*, **5**, 694–697.
14. Botto, M. (1998) C1q knock-out mice for the study of complement deficiency in autoimmune disease, *Exp. Clin. Immunogenet.*, **15**, 231–234.
15. Nishizumi, H., Taniuchi, I., Yamanashi, Y., et al. (1995) Impaired proliferation of peripheral B cells and indication of autoimmune disease in lyn-deficient mice, *Immunity*, **3**, 549–560.
16. Westhoff, C. M., Whittier, A., Kathol, S., et al. (1997) DNA-binding antibodies from viable motheaten mutant mice: implications for B cell tolerance, *J. Immunol.*, **159**, 3024–3033.
17. O'Keefe, T. L., Williams, G. T., Davies, S. L., and Neuberger, M.S. (1996) Hyperresponsive B cells in CD22-deficient mice, *Science*, **274**, 798–801.
18. Tanabe-Fukunaga, R., Brannan, C. I., Copeland, N. G., Jenkins, N. A., and Nagata, S. (1992) Lymphoproliferation disorder in mice explained by defects in Fas antigen that mediates apoptosis, *Nature*, **356**, 314–317.
19. Gross, J. A., Johnson, J., Mudri, S., et al. (2000) TACI and BCMA are receptors for a TNF homologue implicated in B-cell autoimmune disease, *Nature*, **404**, 995–999.
20. Mandik-Nayak, L., Nayak, S., Sokol, C., et al. (2000) The origin of anti-nuclear antibodies in bcl-2 transgenic mice, *Int. Immunol.*, **12**, 353–364.
21. Nishimura, H., Nose, M., Hiai, H., Minato, N., and Honjo, T. (1999) Development of lupus-like autoimmune diseases by disruption of the PD-1 gene encoding an ITIM motif-carrying immunoreceptor, *Immunity*, **11**, 141–151.
22. Iizuka, J., Katagiri, Y., Tada, N., et al. (1998) Introduction of an osteopontin gene confers the increase in B1 cell population and the production of anti-DNA autoantibodies, *Lab. Invest.*, **78**, 1523–1533.
23. Cornall, R. J., Cyster, J. G., Hibbs, M. L., et al. (1998) Polygenic autoimmune traits: Lyn, CD22, and SHP-1 are limiting elements of a biochemical pathway regulating BCR signaling and selection, *Immunity*, **8**, 497–508.
24. Seery, J. P., Carroll, J. M., Cattell, V., and Watt, F. M. (1997) Antinuclear autoantibodies and lupus nephritis in transgenic mice expressing interferon gamma in the epidermis, *J. Exp. Med.*, **186**, 1451–1459.
25. Lopez-Hoyos, M., Carrio, R., Merino, R,, et al. (1996) Constitutive expression of bcl-2 in B cells causes a lethal form of lupuslike autoimmune disease after induction of neonatal tolerance to H-2b alloantigens, *J. Exp. Med.*, **183**, 2523–2531.
26. Bolland, S. and Ravetch, J. V. (2000) Spontaneous autoimmune disease in Fc(gamma) RIIB-deficient mice results from strain-specific epistasis, *Immunity*, **13**, 277–285.
27. Balomenos, D., Martin-Caballero, J., Garcia, M. I., et al. (2000) The cell cycle inhibitor p21 controls T-cell proliferation and sex-linked lupus development, *Nat. Med.*, **6**, 171–176.
28. Bouillet, P., Metcalf, D., Huang, D. C., et al. (1999) Proapoptotic Bcl-2 relative Bim required for certain apoptotic responses, leukocyte homeostasis, and to preclude autoimmunity, *Science*, **286**, 1735–1738.
29. Chen, Z., Koralov, S. B., and Kelsoe, G. (2000) Complement C4 inhibits systemic autoimmunity through a mechanism independent of complement receptors CR1 and CR2, *J. Exp. Med.*, **192**, 1339–1352.
30. Sato, S., Ono, N., Steeber, D. A., Pisetsky, D. S., and Tedder, T. F. (1996) CD19 regulates B lymphocyte signaling thresholds critical for the development of B-1 lineage cells and autoimmunity, *J. Immunol.*, **157**, 4371–4378.
31. Gorelik, L. and Flavell, R. A. (2000) Abrogation of TGFbeta signaling in T cells leads to spontaneous T cell differentiation and autoimmune disease, *Immunity*, **12**, 171–181.
32. Di Cristofano, A., Kotsi, P., Peng, Y. F., Cordon-Cardo, C., Elkon, K. B., and Pandolfi, P. P. (1999) Impaired Fas response and autoimmunity in Pten+/−mice, *Science*, **285**, 2122–2125.
33. Majeti, R., Xu, Z., Parslow, T. G., et al. (2000) An inactivating point mutation in the inhibitory wedge of CD45 causes lymphoproliferation and autoimmunity, *Cell*, **103**, 1059–1070.
34. Yuki, N. (1999) Pathogenesis of Guillain-Barré and Miller-Fisher syndromes subsequent to *Campylobacter jejuni* enteritis, *Jpn. J. Infect. Dis.*, **52**, 99–105.
35. Bhan, A. K., Mizoguchi, E., Smith, R. N., and Mizoguchi, A. (1999) Colitis in transgenic and knockout animals as models

of human inflammatory bowel disease, *Immunol. Rev.*, **169**, 195–207.

36. Blumberg, R. S., Saubermann, L. J., and Strober, W. (1999) Animal models of mucosal inflammation and their relation to human inflammatory bowel disease, *Curr. Opin. Immunol.*, **11**, 648–656 [Erratum: *Curr. Opin. Immunol.*, **12**, 226 (2000)].

37. Boismenu, R. and Chen, Y. (2000) Insights from mouse models of colitis, *J. Leukoc. Biol.*, **67**, 267–278.

38. Shevach, E. M. (2000) Regulatory T cells in autoimmunity, *Annu. Rev. Immunol.*, **18**, 423–449.

39. Targoff, I. N. (2000) Update on myositis-specific and myositis-associated autoantibodies, *Curr. Opin. Rheumatol.*, **12**, 475–481.

40. Austrup, F., Vestweber, D., Borges, E., et al. (1997) P- and E-selectin mediate recruitment of T-helper-1 but not T-helper-2 cells into inflamed tissues, *Nature*, **385**, 81–83.

41. von Andrian, U. H. and Mackay, C. R. (2000) T-cell function and migration: two sides of the same coin, *N. Engl. J. Med.*, **343**, 1020–1034.

42. Buyon, J. P., Tseng, C. E., Di Donato, F., Rashbaum, W., Morris, A., and Chan, E. K. (1997) Cardiac expression of 52beta, an alternative transcript of the congenital heart block-associated 52-kd SS-A/Ro autoantigen, is maximal during fetal development, *Arthritis Rheum.*, **40**, 655-660.

43. Edelson, R. L. (2000) Pemphigus - decoding the cellular language of cutaneous autoimmunity, *N. Engl. J. Med.*, **343**, 60–61.

44. Mackay, I. R. (2001) Tolerance and autoimmunity, *West J. Med.*, **174**(2), 118–123.

45. Romagnani, S. (1997) The Th1/Th2 paradigm, *Immunol. Today*, **18**, 263–266.

46. Sallusto, F., Lanzavecchia, A., and Mackay, C. R. (1999) Chemokines and chemokine receptors in T-cell priming and Th1/Th2-mediated responses, *Immunol. Today*,**19**, 568–574.

47. Luster, A.D. (1998) Chemokines - chemotactic cytokines that mediate inflammation, *N. Engl. J. Med.*, **338**, 436–445.

48. Horwitz, M. S., Bradley, L. M., Harbertson, J., Krahl, T., Lee, J., and Sarvetnick, N. (1998) Diabetes induced by Coxsackie virus: initiation by bystander damage and not molecular mimicry, *Nat. Med.*, **4**, 781–785.

49. Neumann, D. A., Rose, N. R., Ansari, A. A., and Herskowitz, A. (1994) Induction of multiple heart autoantibodies in mice with coxsackievirus B3- and cardiac myosin-induced autoimmune myocarditis, *J. Immunol.*, **152**, 343–350.

50. Oldstone, M. B. A. (1998) Molecular mimicry and immune-mediated diseases, *FASEB J.*, **12**, 1255–1265.

51. Darnell, R. B. (1999) The importance of defining the paraneoplastic neurologic disorders [editorial], *N. Engl. J. Med.*, **340**, 1831–1833.

52. Todd, J. A. (1999) From genome to aetiology in a multifactorial disease, type 1 diabetes, *Bioessays*, **21**, 164–174.

53. Griffiths, M. M., Encinas, J. A., Remmers, E. F., Kuchroo, V. K., and Wilder, R. L. (1999) Mapping autoimmunity genes, *Curr. Opin. Immunol.*, **11**, 689–700.

54. Wilson, S. B., Kent, S. C., Patton, K. T., et al. (1998) Extreme Th1 bias of invariant Valpha24JalphaQ T cells in type 1 diabetes, *Nature*, **391**, 177–181 [Erratum: *Nature*, **399**, 84 (1999)].

55. Ortonne, J. P. (1999) Recent developments in the understanding of the pathogenesis of psoriasis, *Br. J. Dermatol.*, **140**(Suppl. 54), 1–7.

56. Kukreja, A, and Maclaren, N. K. (1999) Autoimmunity and diabetes, *J. Clin. Endocrinol. Metab.*, **84**, 4371–4378.

57. Gregersen, P. K. (1997) Genetic analysis of rheumatic diseases. In: *Textbook of Rheumatology*, vol. 1, 5th ed. (Kelley, W. N., Harris, E. D., Jr., Ruddy, S., and Sledge, C. B., eds.), W. B. Saunders, Philadelphia, pp. 209–227.

58. Drappa, J., Vaishnaw, A. K., Sullivan, K. E., Chu, J.-L., and Elkin, K. B. (1996) Fas gene mutations in the Canale-Smith syndrome,

an inherited lymphoproliferative disorder associated with autoimmunity, *N. Engl. J. Med.*, **335**, 1643–1649.

59. Pitkanen, J., Vahamurto, P., Krohn, K., and Peterson, P. (2001) Subcellular localization of the autoimmune regulator protein: characterization of nuclear targeting and transcriptional activation domain, *J. Biol. Chem.*, **276**(22), 19597–19602.

60. Wang, C. Y., Davoodi-Semiromi, A., Huang, W., Connor, E., Shi, J. D., and She, J. X. (1998) Characterization of mutations in patients with autoimmune polyglandular syndrome type 1 (APS1), *Hum. Genet.*, **103**, 681–685.

61. Encinas, J. A. and Kuchroo, V. K. (2000) Mapping and identification of autoimmunity genes, *Curr. Opin. Immunol.*, **12**, 691–697.

62. Becker, K. G. (1999) Comparative genetics of type 1 diabetes and autoimmune disease: common loci, common pathways? *Diabetes*, **48**, 1353–1358.

63. Klein, J. and Sato, A. (2000) The HLA system, *N. Engl. J. Med.*, **343**, 782–786.

64. Taneja, V. and David, C. S. (1999) HLA class II transgenic mice as models of human diseases, *Immunol. Rev.*, **169**, 67–79.

65. Khare, S. D., Luthra, H. S., and David, C. S. (1998) Animal models of human leukocyte antigen B27-linked arthritides, *Rheum. Dis. Clin. North Am.*, **24**, 883–894 [Erratum: *Rheum. Dis. Clin. North Am.*, **25**: xi-xii (1999)].

66. Gregersen, P. K., Silver, J., and Winchester, R. J. (1987) The shared epitope hypothesis: an approach to understanding the molecular genetics of susceptibility to rheumatoid arthritis, *Arthritis Rheum.*, **30**, 1205–1213.

67. McDaniel, D. O., Alarcon, G. S., Pratt, P. W., and Reveille, J. D. (1995) Most African-American patients with rheumatoid arthritis do not have the rheumatoid antigenic determinant (epitope), *Ann. Intern. Med.*, **123**, 181–187.

68. Teller, K., Budhai, L., Zhang, M., Haramati, N., Keiser, H. D., and Davidson, A. (1996) HLA-DRB1 and DQB typing of Hispanic American patients with rheumatoid arthritis: the "shared epitope" hypothesis may not apply, *J. Rheumatol.*, **23**, 1363–1368.

69. Kouki, T., Sawai, Y., Gardine, C. A., Fisfalen, M. E., Alegre, M. L., and DeGroot, L. J. (2000) CTLA-4 gene polymorphism at position 49 in exon 1 reduces the inhibitory function of CTLA-4 and contributes to the pathogenesis of Graves' disease, *J. Immunol.*, **165**, 6606–6611.

70. Agarwal, K., Jones, D. E., Daly, A. K., et al. (2000) CTLA-4 gene polymorphism confers susceptibility to primary biliary cirrhosis, *J. Hepatol.*, **32**, 538–541.

71. Awata, T., Kurihara, S., Iitaka, M., et al. (1998) Association of CTLA-4 gene A-G polymorphism (IDDM12 locus) with acute-onset and insulin-depleted IDDM as well as autoimmune thyroid disease (Graves' disease and Hashimoto's thyroiditis) in the Japanese population, *Diabetes*, **47**, 128–129.

72. Ginn, L. R., Lin, J. P., Plotz, P. H., et al. (1998) Familial autoimmunity in pedigrees of idiopathic inflammatory myopathy patients suggests common genetic risk factors for many autoimmune diseases, *Arthritis Rheum.*, **41**, 400–405.

73. Henderson, R. D., Bain, C. J., and Pender, M. P. (2000) The occurrence of autoimmune diseases in patients with multiple sclerosis and their families, *J. Clin. Neurosci.*, **7**, 434–437.

74. Coelho, S. N., Saleem, S., Konieczny, B. T., Parekh, K. R., Baddoura, F. K., and Lakkis, F. G. (1997) Immunologic determinants of susceptibility to experimental glomerulonephritis: role of cellular immunity, *Kidney Int.*, **51**, 646–652.

75. Liao, L., Sindhwani, R., Rojkind, M., Factor, S., Leinwand, L., and Diamond, B. (1995) Antibody-mediated autoimmune myocarditis depends on genetically determined target organ sensitivity, *J. Exp. Med.*, **181**, 1123–1131.

76. Moudgil, K. D. and Sercarz, E. E. (1994) The T cell repertoire against cryptic self determinants and its involvement in autoimmunity and cancer, *Clin. Immunol. Immunopathol.*, **73**, 283–289.

77. Lanzavecchia, A. (1995) How can cryptic epitopes trigger autoimmunity? *J. Exp. Med.*, **181**, 1945–1948.

78. Vanderlugt, C. L., Neville, K. L., Nikcevich, K. M., Eagar, T. N., Bluestone, J. A., and Miller, S. D. (2000) Pathologic role and temporal appearance of newly emerging autoepitopes in relapsing experimental autoimmune encephalomyelitis, *J. Immunol.*, **164**, 670–678.

79. Liang, B. and Mamula, M. J. (2000) Molecular mimicry and the role of B lymphocytes in the processing of autoantigens, *Cell. Mol. Life Sci.*, **57**, 561–568.

80. Thomas, H. E. and Kay, T. W. (2000) Beta cell destruction in the development of autoimmune diabetes in the non-obese diabetic (NOD) mouse, *Diabetes Metab. Res. Rev.*, **16**, 251–261.

81. O'Garra, A., Steinman, L., and Gijbels, K. (1997) CD4+ T-cell subsets in autoimmunity, *Curr. Opin. Immunol.*, **9**, 872–883.

82. Juedes, A. E., Hjelmstrom, P., Bergman, C. M., Neild, A. L., and Ruddle, N. H. (2000) Kinetics and cellular origin of cytokines in the central nervous system: insight into mechanisms of myelin oligodendrocyte glycoprotein-induced experimental autoimmune encephalomyelitis, *J. Immunol.*, **164**, 419–426.

83. Genain, C. P., Abel, K., Belmar, N., et al. (1996) Late complications of immune deviation therapy in a nonhuman primate, *Science*, **274**, 2054–2057.

84. Saoudi, A., Bernard, I., Hoedemaekers, A., et al. (1999) Experimental autoimmune myasthenia gravis may occur in the context of a polarized Th1- or Th2-type immune response in rats, *J. Immunol.*, **162**, 7189–7197.

85. Balasa, B. and Sarvetnick, N. (2000) Is pathogenic humoral autoimmunity a Th1 response? Lessons from (for) myasthenia gravis, *Immunol. Today*, **21**, 19–23.

86. Takasu, N., Oshiro, C., Akamine, H., et al. (1997) Thyroid-stimulating antibody and TSH-binding inhibitor immunoglobulin in 277 Graves' patients and in 686 normal subjects, *J. Endocrinol. Invest.*, **20**, 452–461.

87. Seishima, M., Iwasaki-Bessho, Y., Itoh, Y., Nozawa, Y., Amagai, M., and Kitajima, Y. (1999) Phosphatidylcholine-specific phospholipase C, but not phospholipase D, is involved in pemphigus IgG-induced signal transduction, *Arch. Dermatol. Res.*, **291**, 606–613.

88. Salemink, I., Blezer, R., Willems, G. M., Galli, M., Bevers, E., and Lindhout, T. (2000) Antibodies to beta2-glycoprotein I associated with antiphospholipid syndrome suppress the inhibitory activity of tissue factor pathway inhibitor, *Thromb. Haemost.*, **84**, 653–656.

89. Merrill, J. T., Zhang, H. W., Shen, C., et al. (1999) Enhancement of protein S anticoagulant function by beta2-glycoprotein I, a major target antigen of antiphospholipid antibodies: beta2-glycoprotein I interferes with binding of protein S to its plasma inhibitor, C4b-binding protein, *Thromb. Haemost.*, **81**, 748–757.

90. Madaio, M. P. and Yanase, K. (1998) Cellular penetration and nuclear localization of anti-DNA antibodies: mechanisms, consequences, implications and applications, *J. Autoimmun.*, **11**, 535–538.

91. Reichlin, M. (1998) Cellular dysfunction induced by penetration of autoantibodies into living cells: cellular damage and dysfunction mediated by antibodies to dsDNA and ribosomal P proteins, *J. Autoimmun.*, **11**, 557–561.

92. Johnson, K. P., Brooks, B. R., Cohen, J. A., et al. (1998) Extended use of glatiramer acetate (Copaxone) is well tolerated and maintains its clinical effect on multiple sclerosis relapse rate and degree of disability: Copolymer I Multiple Sclerosis Study Group, *Neurology*, **50**, 701–708.

93. Feldmann, M., Charles, P., Taylor, P., and Maini, R. N. (1998) Biological insights from clinical trials with anti-TNF therapy, *Springer Semin. Immunopathol.*, **20**, 211–228.

94. Sayegh, M. H. (1999) Finally, CTLA4Ig graduates to the clinic, *J. Clin. Invest.*, **103**, 1223–1225.

95. Tian, J., Olcott, A., Hanssen, L., Zekzer, D., and Kaufman, D. L. (1999) Antigen-based immunotherapy for autoimmune disease: from animal models to humans? *Immunol. Today*, **20**, 190–195.

96. Tyndall, A., Fassas, A., Passweg, J., et al. (1999) Autologous haematopoietic stem cell transplants for autoimmune disease - feasibility and transplant-related mortality: Autoimmune Disease and Lymphoma Working Parties of the European League Against Rheumatism and the International Stem Cell Project for Autoimmune Disease, *Bone Marrow Transplant.*, **24**, 729–734.

97. Potter, M., Black, C., and Berger A. (1999) Bone marrow transplantation for autoimmune diseases [editorial], *Br. Med. J.*, **318**, 750–751.

98. Giannoukakis, N., Rudert, W. A., Robbins, P. D., and Trucco, M. (1999) Targeting autoimmune diabetes with gene therapy, *Diabetes*, **48**, 2107–2121.

99. Maini, R. N. and Taylor, P. C. (2000) Anti-cytokine therapy for rheumatoid arthritis, *Annu. Rev. Med.*, **51**, 207–229.

100. Kremer, J. M. (2001) Rational use of new and existing disease-modifying agents in rheumatoid arthritis, *Ann. Intern. Med.*, **134**, 695–706.

101. Bell, S. and Kamm, M. A. (2000) Antibodies to tumour necrosis factor alpha as treatment for Crohn's disease, *Lancet*, **355**, 858–860.

102. Mease, P. J., Goffe, B. S., Metz, J., VanderStoep, A., Finck, B., and Burge, D. J. (2000) Etanercept in the treatment of psoriatic arthritis and psoriasis: a randomised trial, *Lancet*, **356**, 385–390.

103. Brandt, J., Haibel, H., Cornely, D., et al. (2000) Successful treatment of active ankylosing spondylitis with the anti-tumor necrosis factor alpha monoclonal antibody infliximab, *Arthritis Rheum.*, **43**, 1346–1352.

104. Emery, P., Breedveld, F. C., Lemmel, E. M., et al. (2000) A comparison of the efficacy and safety of leflunomide and methotrexate for the treatment of rheumatoid arthritis, *Rheumatology (Oxford)*, **39**, 655–665.

105. Weinblatt, M. E., Kremer, J. M., Coblyn, J. S., et al. (1999) Pharmacokinetics, safety, and efficacy of combination treatment with methotrexate and leflunomide in patients with active rheumatoid arthritis, *Arthritis Rheum.*, **42**, 1322–1328.

106. Noseworthy, J. H., Lucchinetti, C., Rodriguez, M., and Weinshenker, B. G. (2000) Multiple sclerosis, *N. Engl. J. Med.*, **343**, 938–952.

107. Jacobs, L. D., Beck, R. W., Simon, J. H., et al. (2000) Intramuscular interferon beta-1a therapy initiated during a first demyelinating event in multiple sclerosis, *N. Engl. J. Med.*, **343**, 898–904.

108. Fridkis-Hareli, M., Neveu, J. M., Robinson, R. A., et al. (1999) Binding motifs of copolymer 1 to multiple sclerosis- and rheumatoid arthritis-associated HLA-DR molecules, *J. Immunol.*, **162**, 4697–4704.

109. Duda, P. W., Schmied, M. C., Cook, S. L., Krieger, J. I., and Hafler, D. A. (2000) Glatiramer acetate (Copaxone) induces degenerate, Th2-polarized immune responses in patients with multiple sclerosis, *J. Clin. Invest.*, **105**, 967–976.

110. Kappos, L., Comi, G., Panitch, H., et al. (2000) Induction of a non-encephalitogenic type 2 T helper-cell autoimmune response in multiple sclerosis after administration of an altered peptide ligand in a placebo-controlled, randomized phase II trial, *Nat. Med.*, **6**, 1176–1182.

111. Bielekova, B., Goodwin, B., Richert, N., et al. (2000) Encephalitogenic potential of the myelin basic protein peptide (amino acids 83–99) in multiple sclerosis: results of a phase II clinical trial with an altered peptide ligand, *Nat. Med.*, **6**, 1167–1175.

112. Gallon, L., Chandraker, A., Issazadeh, S., et al. (1997) Defferential effects of B7-1 blockade in the rat experimental autoimmune encephalomyelitis model, *J. Immunol.*, **159**(9), 4212–4216.

113. Asadullah, K., Docke, W. D., Sabat, R. V., Volk, H. D., and Sterry, W. (1999) The treatment of psoriasis with IL-10: rationale and review of the first clinical trials, *Expert Opin. Investig. Drugs*, **9**, 95–102.

114. Abrams, J. R., Lebwohl, M. G., Guzzo, C. A., et al. (1999) CTLA4Ig-mediated blockade of T-cell costimulation in patients with psoriasis vulgaris, *J. Clin. Invest.*, **103**, 1243–1252.

115. Salomon, B., Lenschow, D. J., Rhee, L., et al. (2000) B7/CD28 costimulation is essential for the homeostasis of the CD4$^+$CD25$^+$ immunoregulatory T cells that control autoimmune diabetes, *Immunity*, **12**, 431–440.

116. Gottlieb, A. B., Lebwohl, M., Shirin, S., et al. (2000) Anti-CD4 monoclonal antibody treatment of moderate to severe psoriasis vulgaris: results of a pilot, multicenter, multiple-dose, placebo-controlled study, *J. Am. Acad. Dermatol.*, **43**, 595–604.

117. Krueger, J. G., Walters, I. B., Miyazawa, M., et al. (2000) Successful in vivo blockade of CD25 (high-affinity interleukin 2 receptor) on T cells by administration of humanized anti-Tac antibody to patients with psoriasis, *J. Am. Acad. Dermatol.*, **43**, 448–458.

118. Krueger, J., Gottlieb, A., Miller, B., Dedrick, R., Garovoy, M., and Walicke, P. (2000) Anti-CD11a treatment for psoriasis concurrently increases circulating T-cells and decreases plaque T-cells, consistent with inhibition of cutaneous T-cell trafficking, *J. Invest. Dermatol.*, **115**, 333 [abstract].

119. Gottlieb, A., Krueger, J. G., Bright, R., et al. (2000) Effects of administration of a single dose of a humanized monoclonal antibody to CD11a on the immunobiology and clinical activity of psoriasis, *J. Am. Acad. Dermatol.*, **42**, 428–435.

120. Herold, K. S., Hagopian, W., Auger, J. A., et al. (2002) Anti-CD3 monoclonal antibody in new-onset type 1 diabetes mellitus, *N. Engl. J. Med.*, **346**(22), 1692–1698.

121. Herold, S. K. and Taylor, L. (2003) Treatment of type 1 diabetes with CD3 monoclonal antibody. Induction of immune regulation? *Immunol. Res.*, **28**(2), 141–150.

122. Pozzilli, P., Pitocco, D., Visalli, N., et al. (2000) No effect of oral insulin on residual beta-cell function in recent-onset type I diabetes (the IMDIAB VII), *Diabetologia*, **43**, 1000–1004.

123. Mohan, C., Shi, Y., Laman, J. D., and Datta, S. K. (1995) Interaction between CD40 and its ligand gp39 in the development of murine lupus nephritis, *J. Immunol.*, **154**, 1470–1480.

124. Daikh, D. I. and Wofsy, D. (2001) Reversal of murine lupus nephritis with CTLA4Ig and cyclophosphamide, *J. Immunol.*, **166**, 2913–2916.

125. Kawai, T., Andrews, D., Colvin, R. B., Sachs, D. H., and Cosimi, A. B. (2000) Thromboembolic complications after treatment with monoclonal antibody against CD40 ligand, *Nat. Med.*, **6**, 114–114.

126. Kalunian, K., Davis, J., Merrill, J. T., et al. (2000) Treatment of systemic lupus erythematosus by inhibition of T cell costimulation, *Arthritis Rheum.*, **43**(Suppl.), S271–S271 [abstract].

127. Llorente, L., Richaud-Patin, Y., Garcia-Padilla, C., et al. (2000) Clinical and biologic effects of anti-interleukin-10 monoclonal antibody administration in systemic lupus erythematosus, *Arthritis Rheum.*, **43**, 1790–1800.

Chapter 42

Mucosal Immune System

Protecting mucosal tissues from infection and inflammation is one of the most important challenges to immunology research today *(1,2)*. Vaccines against pathogens that enter or target the mucosa include those for poliomyelitis, influenza, rotavirus, and genital papillomavirus, demonstrating the enormous benefits of protecting those complex tissues and using their potential as effective barriers against the entry of pathogenic microbes into the host. Among the mucosally spread diseases in urgent need of protective vaccines are HIV-AIDS and a potential pandemic influenza; however, many scientific hurdles still must be overcome in the development of such vaccines *(3)*.

Immunity at mucosal surfaces must conform to a spectrum of demands, from maintaining strict sterility in the lungs and upper genital tract to achieving a dynamic coexistence with more than 10^{14} bacteria in the intestines *(4,5)*. Because aberrant hyperreactivity of the mucosal immune system to commensal organisms, foods, or even pathogens can be lethal or very debilitating, the innate immune detection of microbes is highly adapted to the specific mucosal tissue. For example, for recognition of bacterial lipopolysaccharide by Toll-like receptor 4 (TLR4) it uses the coreceptors CD14 and MD-2 systemically but not in mucosal epithelial cells; such a restriction most likely prevents continuous triggering by minute amounts of lipopolysaccharide. Instead, data indicate that bacterial adhesion receptors may serve as obligate TLR4 coreceptors in the mucosa, triggering TLR activation only when there is a threat of colonization or invasion by pathogens *(6)*. Restriction of TLR expression to certain cells is an important strategy for protecting mucosal tissues. "Preferential" expression of TLR5, specific for flagellin present in most motile bacteria, occurs on lamina propria cells of the mouse intestine, and those cells do not express TLR4 *(7)*. An emerging paradigm in mucosal immunity is the requirement for bacterial stimulation to achieve normal immune system development. For example, intestinal immune homeostasis depends on TLR signaling; unexpectedly, in a study of intestinal colonization in mice, that requirement for microbial stimulation extended to normal T-cell maturation by means of a bacterial sugar presented by major histocompati-

bility complex class II *(8,9)*. Those and other studies present unexpected yet credible explanations regarding the requirements for the development of a competent mucosal immune system. Continued progress on a fundamental level should enable the rational development of distinct but conceptually linked capabilities, such as safe and effective mucosal adjuvants and immunotherapeutics for a wide range of mucosal diseases, including asthma and autoimmune diseases of the digestive tract *(3)*.

42.1 The Mucosal Surface

The mucous membranes are one of the largest organs of the body. Collectively, they cover a surface area of more than 400 m^2 (equivalent to one and a half tennis courts) and comprise the linings of the gastrointestinal, urogenital, and respiratory tracts *(1,2,10)*. The mucosal surfaces of the gastrointestinal and respiratory tracts represent the principal portals of entry for most human pathogens. Direct inoculation of pathogens into the bloodstream and sexual contact are other important routes of infection. Most external mucosal surfaces are replete with organized follicles and scattered antigen-reactive or sensitized lymphoid elements, including B cells, T lymphocytes, T-cell subsets, plasma cells, and a variety of other cellular elements involved in the induction and maintenance of immune response.

The mucosal surfaces represent a critical component of the mammalian immunologic repertoire *(1)*. The major antibody isotype in external secretions is secretory immunoglobulin A (S-IgA). Approximately 40 mg of IgA per kilogram of body weight is secreted daily, especially from the gastrointestinal tract, and the total amount of IgA synthesized is almost twice the amount of IgG produced daily in humans. It is, however, interesting that the major effector cells in the mucosal surfaces are not IgA B-cells, but T lymphocytes of CD4$^+$ as well as CD8$^+$ phenotypes. It is estimated that T lymphocytes may represent up to 80% of the entire mucosal lymphoid cell population *(11)*.

These mucosal surfaces, while located inside the body, are actually a physical barrier between the outside and the sterile interior cavity of the body known as the "systemic" environment. Critical nutrients, oxygen, and other molecules are constantly taken up across these mucosal barriers; however, another important function of the mucus is to keep invading pathogens out. Daily these mucous membranes are bombarded by outside elements, and it is up to the unique immune system of the mucus to determine what is potentially harmful and what is beneficial (1,2,10).

The immunologic network operating on external mucosal surfaces consists of gut-associated lymphoid tissue (GALT), the lymphoid structures associated with bronchoepithelium and lower respiratory tract (BALT), ocular tissue, upper airway, salivary glands, tonsils and nasopharynx (NALT), larynx (LALT), middle ear cavity, male and female genital tracts, mammary glands, and the products of lactation (1). The organized lymphoid follicles in the GALT and BALT are considered the principal inductive sites of mucosal immune response (12). It appears that the appendix, peritoneal precursor lymphoid cells, and rectal lymphoepithelial tissue (rectal tonsils) also serve as inductive sites of local immune responses.

GALT and BALT. A substantial body of information has been generated with Peyer's patches and other organized lymphoid follicles in the GALT, including the appendix (13), and the BALT concerning the induction of mucosal immune responses and the development of systemic hyporesponsiveness after oral exposure to an antigen (oral tolerance) (14–16).

The common features of all inductive mucosal sites include an epithelial surface containing *M cells* (cells with microfold) overlying organized lymphoid follicles (1). Mucosal epithelium is a unique structure, and in addition to M cells, it contains mucin-producing glandular cells, lymphocytes, plasma cells, dendritic cells, and macrophages. The mucosal epithelial cells express the polymeric immunoglobulin receptor (pIgR) and secretory component, major histocompatibility complex (MHC) class I and II molecules, other adhesion molecules, and a variety of cytokines and chemokines (17).

The dendritic cells are present in different components of the common mucosal immune system, including the organized lymphoid tissue and the mucosal epithelium (1). These cells can be strongly associated with potentiation of immune response and promote development of active immunity (18,19). However, other recent studies have suggested that dendritic cells may also enhance the induction of mucosal tolerance in *in vivo* settings (20). Recent observations have suggested that dendritic cells are potent antigen-presenting cells (APCs) and are critical in initiating primary immune responses, graft rejection, autoimmune disease, and generation of T-cell–dependent B-cell responses. The func-

tion of APCs is attributed in part to their ability to express costimulatory molecules (CD80 and CD86) and other accessory ligands necessary for upregulation or induction of tolerance (21).

The M cells are important in luminal uptake, transport, processing, and, to a smaller extent, presentation of mucosally introduced antigens (1). The M cells appear to be critical in the transport of luminal antigens and entry of organisms such as reovirus, poliovirus, rotavirus, and salmonellae into the human host (22). M-cell–mediated antigen uptake is characteristically associated with the development of an S-IgA response (23).

The luminal appearance of S-IgA in mucosal secretions results from transcytosis of polymeric IgA (pIgA) across mucosal epithelium via binding to the pIgR. The receptor is eventually cleaved resulting in association of pIgA with a substantial part of pIgR. The complex of IgA and pIgR is referred to as S-IgA (1).

After exposure to an antigen and its uptake via the M cells, there is a variable degree of activation of T cells, dendritic cells, and B cells, especially of the IgA isotype (1). The interaction of lymphocytes with mucosal epithelium is important in differentiation of some segments of mucosal epithelium into M cells (23).

Activation of T cells results in the release of a number of distinct cytokines or chemokines from different T-cell subsets and recognition of antigenic epitopes involving MHC class 1 or 2 molecules. Both T-cell activation and release of specific cytokines are involved in the eventual process of B-cell activation, isotype switch, and specific integrin expression on antigen-sensitized B cells (1). Both Th1 and Th2 cells appear to benefit the development of S-IgA responses (24). Th2 cytokines (IL-4, IL-5, IL-6, IL-9, IL-10, and IL-13) are thought to be of significant help in antibody production. S-IgA antibody response is also enhanced by immunologic adjuvants, such as cholera toxin, which results in polarized Th2 cell response (25). S-IgA antibody response may also be induced through Th1 cytokines (IL-2 and IFN-γ), as shown with studies on intracellular pathogens such as *Salmonella* (26).

It appears that the process of isotype switching of B cells to pIgA-producing plasma cells begins in the mucosal inductive sites. Such switching requires specific signals by costimulating molecules, including cytokines and T-helper cells. However, Th1- and Th2-type cytokines do not contribute significantly to the switching of B cells to surface IgA-positive B cells. However, such switching is greatly enhanced by transforming growth factor beta (TGF-β) (1).

After activation and acquisition of antigen specificity, the IgA-producing cell migrates to the lamina propria of the effector sites in the mucosal tissues, regardless of the site of initial antigen exposure. There is, however, a preponderance of homing to the original site of antigenic exposure (27).

The migration of antigen-sensitized cells is preferentially determined by the concurrent expression of homing-specific adhesion molecules in the tissue endothelium, especially the mucosal addressin cell adhesion molecule-1 (MAdCAM-1) and the specific receptors (integrins) expressed on the activated lymphoid cells. Oral (intestinal) mucosal exposure to antigen seems to favor expression of L-selectin as well as $\alpha_4\beta_7$ integrins. However, systemic immunization is generally restricted to the expression of L-selectin (28,29). The antigen-sensitized B cells undergo terminal differentiation in the mucosal lamina propria to IgA-producing plasma cells. Such differentiation involves interaction with a variety of cytokines and T-cell subsets (1).

Locally produced IgA consists mainly of J-chain–containing dimers and larger p-IgA that is selectively transported through epithelial cells by the pIgR, the secretory component. The resulting S-IgA molecules are designed to participate in immune exclusion and other immunologic functions at the mucosal surface (1). IgG also contributes to such surface defense. Its proinflammatory properties render IgG antibodies of potential immunopathologic importance when IgA-mediated mucosal elimination of antigens is unsuccessful (1).

T-helper cells activated locally, mainly by a Th2 cytokine profile, promote persistent mucosal inflammation with extravasation and priming of inflammatory cells, including eosinophils. This development may be considered "pathologic enhancement" of local defenses (1). It appears to be part of the late-phase allergic reaction, perhaps initially driven by IL-4 released from mast cells subjected to IgE-mediated or other types of degranulation, and subsequently maintained by further Th2 cell stimulation (30).

Eosinophils are potentially tissue damaging, particularly after priming with IL-5. Various cytokines upregulate adhesion molecules on endothelial and epithelial cells, thereby enhancing accumulation of eosinophils and, in addition, resulting in aberrant immune regulation within the epithelium (31–33). It would seem that soluble antigens available at the epithelial surfaces normally appear to induce various immunosuppressive mechanisms, but such homeostasis seems to be less potent in the airways than the induction of systemic hyporesponsiveness to dietary antigens operating in the gastrointestinal tract (1).

Numerous cytokines and chemokines have been shown to be intimately involved in the induction and maintenance of mucosal immune responses and the level of mucosal inflammation during infections and exposure to environmental agents (29,34,35).

NALT. Recent studies in the rat, mouse, and hamster have shown the presence of organized lymphoid tissue at the entrance of the nasopharyngeal duct (1). This phenomenon represents an important component of mucosal lymphoid tissue in the rodents (36). It bears a striking morphologic and functional resemblance to other central lymphoid tissues, such as GALT or BALT. However, NALT appears to have better-developed lymphoid follicles, with marked intraepithelial infiltration by lymphocytes. The follicular areas are organized into B cells and intrafollicular (T cell) areas of approximately similar size. The lymphoid follicles are covered by ciliated epithelium containing few goblet cells and numerous M cells (1). The NALT M-cells appear to be identical to those in Peyer's patches and BALT and are involved in similar immunologic functions, including antigen uptake and subsequent mucosal immune responses to specific antigens (37).

In humans, the nasopharyngeal lymphoid tissue is represented by the salivary glands and other glandular tissue in the Waldeyer's ring, which consists of paired palatine and tubal tonsils and unpaired pharyngeal and lingual tonsils. There is increasing evidence to suggest that human tonsillar and adenoidal tissues are important components of mucosal immunity and function in a manner similar to those of GALT or BALT (38). The tonsils consist of several lymphoid elements. These include follicular germinal centers, mantle zones of lymphoid follicles, the extrafollicular areas, and the reticular crypt epithelium on the surface in constant contact with the external environment. The tonsillar epithelium contains a significant number of dendritic cells, M cells, memory B cells, and scattered B cells and T cells. The formation of the germinal center takes place shortly after birth, secondary to the activation by environmental antigens, and plasma cells appear in tonsils by 2 to 3 weeks of age (1).

Unlike Peyer's patches, tonsils exhibit considerable *in situ* differentiation to plasma cells. The germinal centers (which typically arise during T-cell–dependent B-cell responses) generate plasma blasts and plasma cells of both IgG and IgA isotypes. There is, however, a predominance of IgG isotype (60% to 70% IgG versus 15% to 20% IgA). The follicular germinal centers are often associated with clonal expansion of B cells, somatic hypermutation in the B-cell immunoglobulin variable-region gene, positive selection of B cells, and eventual B-cell differentiation to memory cells and isotype-specific plasma cells (1).

The tonsils, nasal and bronchial mucosa, and salivary glands exhibit similar distribution of IgA and IgD immunocytes. In addition, scattered areas in the crypt epithelium of nasopharyngeal tonsils (but not palatine tonsils) express secretory component (1).

Another important feature of mucosal lymphoid tissue and the follicular germinal center is induction of the J-chain gene in some B-cell subsets. Tonsillar germinal centers express a very high percentage of extrafollicular immunocytes with J-chain expression. More than 90% of these immunocytes are of the IgA isotype (39).

LALT. Some evidence suggest the existence of organized lymphoid tissue in the larynx in humans (1). Lymphoid aggregates have been observed at the laryngeal side of the epiglottis in >80% of infants and children younger than 22 months of age. In the follicular areas of the aggregates, most cells appear to be B lymphocytes, with some CD4$^+$ lymphocytes in the germinal centers, and the interfollicular areas contain equal numbers of B- and T-cells. Other experiments have shown also scattered lymphocytes in the laryngeal epithelium. It remains to be determined whether LALT is a distinct physiologic entity or a pathologic reaction in response to local infections or other environmental insults (1). Many children in whom LALT was identified postmortem had died because of sudden infant death syndrome (40,41). Little or no information is available regarding the role of LALT in antigen processing or presentation or the development of immunologic reactivity in the upper airway (1).

42.1.1 Strategies to Enhance Mucosal Tolerance

The current knowledge has provided ample evidence that mucosal exposure to environmental macromolecules, infectious agents, and dietary antigens can result in immunologic outcomes ranging from the induction of specific immune responses in mucosal and/or systemic sites (infectious agents) to the development of systemic immunologic hyporesponsiveness (mucosal tolerance). The implications of some of these observations have been successfully applied to the development of vaccines against infectious diseases. Currently, efforts are under way to apply the principles of mucosal tolerance to development of vaccines against autoimmune diseases (1).

Several human diseases are attributed to the impairment of immunologic tolerance and enhanced reactivity to autoantigens or environmental agents. These diseases involve a wide range of human tissues and organ systems. Human diseases include multiple sclerosis, rheumatoid arthritis, autoimmune uveitis, type 1 diabetes, thyroiditis, systemic lupus erythematosus, inflammatory bowel disease, and possibly other ill-defined disease syndromes (1).

It is believed that the presence and extent of immunologic hyporesponsiveness, in particular the existence of oral tolerance, is an essential determinant of protection against hypersensitivity reactions to food proteins, normal bacterial flora, and other common environmental macromolecules (42).

Oral tolerance to dietary proteins in normal mice can be abrogated by regulatory T cells and by activation of APCs. It has been shown that oral tolerance cannot be induced after administration of very low doses of dietary antigens and in the neonatal or weaning period after birth. Interestingly, however, subsequent oral challenge in such animals with the antigen has been shown to result in the development

of mucosal pathology, accompanied by local cell-mediated immune response in the draining lymph nodes (43,44). The mucosal pathology observed has been similar to that seen in food hypersensitivity or early in the course of inflammatory bowel disease (45,46). Studies have suggested that rodents and humans are relatively tolerant to the inactive "normal" flora in the intestine. A breakdown in the state of tolerance is associated with the development of IL-12- and IFN-γ–dependent inflammatory bowel disease.

It has been proposed that the role of mucosal tolerance is to provide immunologic homeostasis in the gastrointestinal tract and possibly in the respiratory tract, which would prevent the development of immune response to otherwise harmful dietary and bacterial antigens present constantly and often in large quantities in external mucosal surfaces. The breakdown of tolerance may thus lead to systemic or mucosal immunopathology directed against environmental or autoantigens in the mammalian host (42).

Several possible approaches have been explored to prevent or alter the course of autoimmune disease in humans (21,47–50). These include induction of mucosal tolerance employing specific antigens or peptides, immune deviation by directing T-cell responsiveness from Th1 to Th2 or Th3, suppression of immunologic reactivity by the use of regulatory peptides derived from T-cell receptors, use of specific treatment modalities directed against specific cytokines or receptors, and use of gene therapy using viral receptor–carrying genes coding for specific antigen products and/or cytokines and chemokines (1).

Administration of antigens via the nasal, aerosol, or oral route has been explored in several recent studies involving experimentally induced diseases in animal models or naturally occurring autoimmune diseases in humans (1).

Experimental Autoimmune Encephalomyelitis and Multiple Sclerosis. The clinical manifestation of acute experimental autoimmune encephalomyelitis (EAE) in mice and rats can be effectively suppressed by oral administration of high doses of myelin basic protein (MBP) (14,51,52). Tolerance induction in such a situation appeared to be mediated by clonal anergy. Tolerance can also be induced by low doses of antigen and is mediated in part by downregulation of tumor necrosis factor (TNF)-α and IFN-γ and upregulation of TGF-β (1).

EAE can be suppressed in animals transgenic for an MBP-specific TCR after feeding with MBP (53). Induction of tolerance for EAE has also been achieved with administration of MBP and MBP-peptides via the nasal route (54).

In human multiple sclerosis, clinical trials employing oral treatment with bovine myelin preparations are under way (1). Use of bovine myelin in such patients has been shown to result in the appearance of MBP and proteolipid protein-specific TGF-β–secreting T cells. However, no increase in IFN-γ–secreting cells was noted in myelin-treated patients.

Analysis of magnetic resonance imaging data has revealed significant changes in such patients *(55)*. In a small pilot study, myelin-treated patients, especially responders with similar HLA-DR gene profiles, exhibited positive clinical effects from such treatment. However, a subsequent larger study has failed to confirm the observation of the pilot study *(42)*.

Insulin-Dependent Diabetes. The non-obese diabetic (NOD) mouse spontaneously develops an autoimmune syndrome similar to human insulin-dependent diabetes mellitus *(56)*. In this disease, the development of autoimmunity against B cells is believed to require the predisposition of both genetic and environmental factors. The activation of lymphocytes recognizing B-cell determinants may therefore be triggered by environmental antigens, possibly via molecular mimicry *(57–59)*. In the NOD mouse model, the use of oral insulin delays and in some cases prevents onset of diabetes. Such suppression is transferable by $CD4^+$ T cells. These animals also exhibit decreased IFN-γ and increased expression of TNF-α, IL-4, IL-10, TGF-β, and prostaglandin E_2. Experimental evidence has suggested that the mucosal vascular addressin (MAdCAM-1) was constitutively expressed at low levels on the pancreatic vasculature *(1)*. In conjunction with the appearance of lymphocyte infiltrates (insulitis) in pancreatic islets, MAdCAM-1 has also been strongly induced on islet vessels. This integrin has recently been shown to be necessary for the development of diabetes in such mice. MAdCAM-1 may be required during two distinct steps in an early phase of diabetes development: (i) for the entry of naïve lymphocytes into the lymphoid tissues in which diabetes-causing lymphocytes were originally primed; and (ii) for the subsequent homing of these lymphocytes into the pancreas. Nasal administration of the insulin β-chain or aerosol insulin also suppressed the onset of diabetes in NOD mice *(1)*. Feeding of insulin has been shown to suppress diabetes in an LCMV-induced diabetes model *(60)*. Thus, it is suggested that mucosal lymphoid tissues may be significantly involved in the initiation of pathologic immune responses in NOD mice *(61,62)*.

Clinical trials have also been initiated with recombinant human insulin administered orally in subjects at risk of developing type 1 diabetes. A double-blind study involving oral feeding of insulin in newly diagnosed immune-mediated type 1 diabetes has suggested possible beneficial effects. Results of detailed long-term studies are not yet available to determine the effect of mucosal exposure to insulin on the outcome of type 1 diabetes *(63)*.

Uveitis. Oral administration of S-antigen, a retinal autoantigen, prevented or significantly reduced the clinical severity of experimental autoimmune uveitis (EAU) in experimental animal models *(1)*. In other studies, feeding of interphotoreceptor binding protein (IRBP) has been shown to suppress IRBP-induced retinal disease in humans *(64,65)*.

In human uveitis, feeding of bovine S-antigen and S-antigen mixtures with retinal antigens has been examined for benefits on the outcome of the disease. Oral feeding of peptides derived from the patient's own HLA antigens and oral feeding of bovine S-antigen appeared to provide some benefit against the clinical symptoms. These patients appeared to need reduced doses of steroids and had a significantly reduced intraocular inflammation. The effects seem to be mediated by induction of oral tolerance *(65)*.

Arthritis. The course of experimental models of arthritis induced with collagen, adjuvants, and other antigens can be significantly altered by oral feeding of type II collagen, immunodominant human collagen peptides, and mycobacterial 65-kDa heat shock protein. Suppression of arthritis and induction of tolerance in these animals have also been achieved by nasal administration of collagen *(66,67)*.

Clinical trials with chicken type II collagen in suppression of disease in human rheumatoid arthritis have been encouraging. Oral administration of the collagen in doses ranging from 20 to 2,500 μg have thus far demonstrated significant beneficial effects. Of particular importance is the observation that oral administration of the type II collagen was not associated with any major toxicity. Currently, several multicenter clinical trials are under way to determine the long-term efficacy of oral collagen in the treatment of rheumatoid arthritis *(68–70)*.

Other Disease Models. The use of desensitization has been a long-standing and frequently controversial practice in allergic disorders for many decades. However, as early as the 1960s, a sufficient database was available to suggest that oral tolerance could be induced in humans to contact-sensitizing agents. During the past decade, it has become clear that oral or nasal exposure can mediate tolerance to a variety of allergens or antigens. It has been shown in experimental models that oral or nasal administration of keyhole limpet hemocyanin decreased subsequent cell-mediated immune responses *(1)*.

Factors that favor Th1 response can be expected to abrogate mucosal tolerance. Conventional immunotherapy for allergens is being re-explored with new therapeutic modalities that will direct Th response toward the Th3 type of T-cell reactivity and favor induction or persistence of tolerance *(71–74)*. In this regard, oral DNA vaccines and boosting of tolerogenic responses with specific adjuvants are two possible approaches *(1)*.

It has also been shown that oral administration of nickel induces nickel-specific T cells and such desensitization is effective against nickel allergy and beneficial to patients with nickel-associated cutaneous eczema *(75)*. Finally, gene therapy using virus vectors has been proposed as a localized short-term but potent mechanism to modulate autoimmune disease states *(76,77)*.

References

1. Ogra, P. L., Faden, H., and Welliver, R. C. (2001) Vaccination strategies for mucosal immune responses, *Clin. Microbiol. Revs.*, **14**(2), 430–445.

2. Seipp, R. (2003) Mucosal immunity and vaccines, *The Science Creative Quarterly*, September 07–April 08 (http://www.scq.ubc.ca/mucosal-immunity-and-vaccines/).

3. Hackett, C. J., Rotrosen, D., Auchincloss, H., and Fauci, A. S. (2007) Immunology research: challenges and opportunities in a time of budgetary constraint, *Nat. Immunol.*, **8**, 114–117.

4. Gill, S. R., Pop, M., DeBoy, R. T., et al. (2006) Metagenomic analysis of the human distal gut microbiome, *Science*, **312**(5778), 1355–1359.

5. Lefrancois, L. and Puddington, L. (2006) Intestinal and pulmonary mucosal T cells: local heroes fight to maintain the status quo, *Annu. Rev. Immunol.*, **24**, 681–704.

6. Fischer, H., Yamamoto, M., Akira, S., Beutler, B., and Svanborg, C. (2006) Mechanism of pathogen-specific TLR4 activation in the mucosa: fimbriae, recognition receptors and adaptor protein selection, *Eur. J. Immunol.*, **36**, 267–277.

7. Uematsu, S., Jang, M. H., Chevrier, N., et al. (2006) Detection of pathogenic intestinal bacteria by Toll-like receptor 5 on intestinal CD11c+ lamina propria cells, *Nat. Immunol.*, **7**, 868–874.

8. Rakoff-Nahoum, S., Paglino, J., Eslami-Varzaneh, F., Edberg, S., and Medzhitov, R. (2004) Recognition of commensal microflora by Toll-like receptors is required for intestinal homeostasis, *Cell*, **118**, 229–241.

9. Mazmanian, S. K., Liu, C. H., Tzianabos, A. O., and Kasper, D. L. (2005) An immunomodulatory molecule of symbiotic bacteria directs maturation of the host immune system, *Cell*, **122**, 107–118.

10. Rosenthal, K. L. and Gallichan, W. S. (1997) Challenges for vaccination against sexually-transmitted diseases: induction and long-term maintenance of mucosal immune responses in the female genital tract, *Semin. Immunol.*, **9**(5), 303–314.

11. Conley, M. E. and Delacroix, D. L. (1987) Intravascular and mucosal immunoglobulin A: two separate but related systems of immune defense, *Ann. Intern. Med.*, **106**, 892–899.

12. Staats, H. F., Jackson, R. J., Marinaro, M., Takahashi, I., Kiyono, H., and McGhee, J. R. (1994) Mucosal immunity to infection with implications for vaccine development, *Curr. Opin. Immunol.*, **6**, 572–583.

13. Dasso, J. F. and Howell, M. D. (1997) Neonatal appendectomy impairs mucosal immunity in rabbits, *Cell. Immunol.*, **182**, 29–37.

14. Javed, N. H., Gienapp, I. E., Cox, K. L., and Whitacre, C. C. (1995) Exquisite peptide specificity of oral tolerance in experimental autoimmune encephalomyelitis, *J. Immunol.*, **155**, 1599–1605.

15. Mestecky, J., Moro, I., and Underdown, B. J. (1999) Mucosal immunoglobulins. In: *Mucosal Immunology*, 2nd ed. (Ogra, P. L., Mestecky, J., Lamm, M. E., Strober, W., Bienenstock, J., and McGhee, J. R., eds.), Academic Press, New York, pp. 133–152.

16. Viney, J. L., Mowat, A. M., O'Malley, J. M., Williamson, E., and Fanger, N. A. (1998) Expanding dendritic cells in vivo enhances the induction of oral tolerance, *J. Immunol.*, **160**, 5815–5825.

17. McGhee, J. R., Lamm, M, E., and Strober, W. (1999) Mucosal immune responses: an overview. In: *Mucosal Immunology*, 2nd ed. (Ogra, P. L., Mestecky, J., Lamm, M. E., Strober, W., Bienenstock, J., and McGhee, J. R., eds.), Academic Press, New York, pp. 485–506.

18. Liu, L. M. and MacPherson, G. G. (1991) Lymph-borne (veiled) dendritic cells can acquire and present intestinally administered antigens, *Immunology*, **73**, 281–286.

19. Liu, L. M. and MacPherson, G. G. (1993) Antigen acquisition by dendritic cells: intestinal dendritic cells acquire antigen adminis-tered orally and can prime naive T cells in vivo, *J. Exp. Med.*, **177**, 1299–1307.

20. van Ginkel, F. W., Nguyen, H. H., and McGhee, J. R. (2000) Vaccines for mucosal immunity to combat emerging infectious diseases, *Emerg. Infect. Dis.*, **6**, 123–132.

21. Steinbrink, K., Wölfl, M., Jonuleit, H., Knop, J., and Enk, A. H. (1997) Induction of tolerance by IL 10-treated dendritic cells, *J. Immunol.*, **159**, 4772–4780.

22. Neutra, M. R. and Kraehenbuhl, J.-P. (1999) Cellular and molecular basis for antigen transport across epithelial barriers. In: *Mucosal Immunology*, 2nd ed. (Ogra, P. L., Mestecky, J., Lamm, M. E., Strober, W., Bienenstock, J., and McGhee, J. R., eds.), Academic Press, New York, pp. 101–114.

23. Kerneis, S., Bogdanova, A., Kraehenbuhl, J.-P., and Pringault, E. (1997) Conversion by Peyer's patch lymphocytes of human enterocytes into M cells that transport bacteria, *Science*, **277**, 949–952.

24. Kelsall, B. and Strober, W. (1999) Gut-associated lymphoid tissue: antigen handling and T-lymphocyte responses. In: *Mucosal Immunology*, 2nd ed. (Ogra, P. L., Mestecky, J., Lamm, M. E., Strober, W., Bienenstock, J., and McGhee, J. R., eds.), Academic Press, New York, pp. 293–317.

25. Elson, C. O. and Dertzbaugh, M. T. (1999) Mucosal adjuvants. In: *Mucosal Immunology*, 2nd ed. (Ogra, P. L., Mestecky, J., Lamm, M. E., Strober, W., Bienenstock, J., and McGhee, J. R., eds.), Academic Press, New York, pp. 817–838.

26. Nataro, J. P. and Levine, M. M. (1999) Enteric bacterial vaccines: *Salmonella*, shigella, cholera, *Escherichia coli*. In: *Mucosal Immunology*, 2nd ed. (Ogra, P. L., Mestecky, J., Lamm, M. E., Strober, W., Bienenstock, J., and McGhee, J. R., eds.), Academic Press, New York, pp. 851–865.

27. McIntyre, T. M. and Strober, W. (1999) Gut-associated lymphoid tissue: regulation of IgA B-cell development. In: *Mucosal Immunology*, 2nd ed. (Ogra, P. L., Mestecky, J., Lamm, M. E., Strober, W., Bienenstock, J., and McGhee, J. R., eds.), Academic Press, New York, pp. 319–356.

28. Quiding-Järbrink, M., Nordström, I., Granström, G., Kilander, A., Jertborn, M., Butcher, E. C., Lazarovits, A. I., Holmgren, J., and Czerkinsky, C. (1997) Differential expression of tissue-specific adhesion molecules on human circulating antibody-forming cells after systemic, enteric, and nasal immunizations, *J. Clin. Invest.*, **99**, 1281–1286.

29. Reyes, V., Ye, G., Ogra, P. L., and Garofalo, R. (1997) Antigen presentation of mucosal pathogens: the players and the rules, *Int. Arch. Allergy. Immunol.*, **112**, 103–114.

30. Yoshikawa, T., Gon, Y., Matsui, M., and Yodoi, J. (1999) IgE-mediated allergic responses in the mucosal immune system. In: *Mucosal Immunology*, 2nd ed. (Ogra, P. L., Mestecky, J., Lamm, M. E., Strober, W., Bienenstock, J., and McGhee, J. R., eds.), Academic Press, New York, pp. 575–586.

31. Husband, A. J., Beagley, K. W., and McGhee, J. R. (1999) Mucosal cytokines. In: *Mucosal Immunology*, 2nd ed. (Ogra, P. L., Mestecky, J., Lamm, M. E., Strober, W., Bienenstock, J., and McGhee, J. R., eds.), Academic Press, New York, pp. 541–557.

32. McGee, D. W. (1999) Inflammation and mucosal cytokine production. In: *Mucosal Immunology*, 2nd ed. (Ogra, P. L., Mestecky, J., Lamm, M. E., Strober, W., Bienenstock, J., and McGhee, J. R., eds.), Academic Press, New York, pp. 559–573.

33. Yamamoto, M., Fujihashi, K., Kawabata, K., McGhee, J. R., and Kiyono, H. (1998) A mucosal intranet: intestinal epithelial cells down-regulate intraepithelial, but not peripheral, T lymphocytes, *J. Immunol.*, **160**, 2188–2196.

34. Ogra, P. L. (1996) Summary: *European Science Foundation Meeting on Immunology of Infection: Mucosal Infections, Castelvecchio, Pascoli, Italy*, September 30, 1995 [*Mucosal Immunol. Update*, **4**(2),17–21 (1996)].

35. Saito, T., Deskin, R., Casola, A., Haeber, H., Olzewska, B., et al. (1997) Respiratory syncytial virus induces selective production of the chemokine of RANTES by upper airway epithelial cells, *J. Infect. Dis.*, **175**, 497–504.

36. Small, P. A., Smith, G. L., and Moss, B. (1985) Intranasal vaccination with a recombinant vaccinia virus containing influenza hemagglutinin prevents both influenza virus pneumonia and nasal infection: intradermal vaccination prevents only viral pneumonia. In: *Vaccines'85* (Lerner, R. A., Chanock, R. M, and Brown, F., eds.), Cold Spring Harbor Laboratory, Cold Spring Harbor, NY, p. 175.

37. Sminia, T. and Kraal, G. (1999) Nasal-associated lymphoid tissue. In: *Mucosal Immunology*, 2nd ed. (Ogra, P. L., Mestecky, J., Lamm, M. E., Strober, W., Bienenstock, J., and McGhee, J. R., eds.), Academic Press, New York, pp. 357–379.

38. Bernstein, J. M., Gorfien, J., and Brandtzaeg, P. (1999) The immunobiology of the tonsils and adenoids. In: *Mucosal Immunology*, 2nd ed. (Ogra, P. L., Mestecky, J., Lamm, M. E., Strober, W., Bienenstock, J., and McGhee, J. R., eds.), Academic Press, New York, pp. 1339–1362.

39. Yagi, M. and Koshland, M. E. (1981) Expression of the J chain gene during B cell differentiation is inversely correlated with DNA methylation, *Proc. Natl. Acad. Sci. U.S.A.*, **78**(8), 4907–4911.

40. Kracke, A., Hiller, A. S., Tschernig, T., et al. (1997) Larynx-associated lymphoid tissue (LALT) in young children, *Anat. Rec.*, **248**, 413–420.

41. Tschernig, T., Kleemann, W. J., and Pabst R. (1995) Bronchus-associated lymphoid tissue (BALT) in the lungs of children who had died from sudden infant death syndrome and other causes, *Thorax*, **50**, 658–660.

42. Mowat, A. M. and Weiner, H. L. (1999) Oral tolerance: physiological basis and clinical applications. In: *Mucosal Immunology*, 2nd ed. (Ogra, P. L., Mestecky, J., Lamm, M. E., Strober, W., Bienenstock, J., and McGhee, J. R., eds.), Academic Press, New York, pp. 587–618.

43. Mowat, A. M. (1997) Intestinal graft-versus-host disease. In: *Intestinal Graft-Versus-Host Disease* (Ferrara, J. M., Deeg, J. H., and Burakoff, S. J., eds.), Marcel Dekker, New York, pp. 337–384.

44. Mowat, A. M. and Ferguson, A. (1981) Hypersensitivity in the small intestinal mucosa. V. Induction of cell mediated immunity to a dietary antigen, *Clin. Exp. Immunol.*, **43**, 574–582.

45. Duchmann, R., Kaiser, I., Hermann, E., Mayet, W., Ewe, K., and Meyer zum Büschenfelde, K. H. (1995) Tolerance exists towards resident intestinal flora but is broken in active inflammatory bowel disease (IBD), *Clin. Exp. Immunol.*, **102**, 448–455.

46. Duchmann, R., Schmitt, E., Knolle, P., Meyer zum Büschenfelde, K. H, and Neurath, M. (1996) Tolerance towards resident intestinal flora in mice is abrogated in experimental colitis and restored by treatment with interleukin-10 or antibodies to interleukin-12, *Eur. J. Immunol.*, **26**, 934–938.

47. Barone, K. S., Tolarova, D. D, Ormsby, I., Doetschman, T., and Michael, J. G. (1998) Induction of oral tolerance in TGF-β1 null mice, *J. Immunol.*, **161**, 154–160.

48. Gonnella, P. A., Chen, Y., Inobe, J., Komagata, Y., Quartulli, M., and Weiner, H. L. (1998) In situ immune response in gut-associated lymphoid tissue (GALT) following oral antigen in TCR-transgenic mice, *J. Immunol.*, **160**, 4708–4718.

49. Ke, Y., Pearce, K., Lake, J. P., Ziegler, H. K., and Kapp, J. A. (1997) γδ T lymphocytes regulate the induction and maintenance of oral tolerance, *J. Immunol.*, **158**, 3610–3618.

50. Chandy, A. G., Hultkrantz, S., Raghavan, S. et al. (2006) Oral tolerance induction by mucosal administration of cholera toxin B-coupled antigen involves T-cell proliferation in vivo and is not affected by depletion of CD25$^+$ T cells, *Immunology*, **118**(3), 311–320.

51. Chen, Y., Inobe, J.-I., Kuchroo, V. K., Baron, J. L., Janeway, C. A., and Weiner, H. L. (1996) Oral tolerance in myelin basic protein T-cell receptor transgenic mice: suppression of autoimmune encephalomyelitis and dose-dependent induction of regulatory cells, *Proc. Natl. Acad. Sci. U.S.A.*, **93**, 388–391.

52. Kelly, K. A. and Whitacre, C. C. (1996) Oral tolerance in EAE: reversal of tolerance by T helper cell cytokines, *J. Neuroimmunol.*, **66**, 77–84.

53. Chen, Y., Inobe, J.-I., and Weiner, H. L. (1997) Inductive events in oral tolerance in the TcR transgenic adoptive transfer model, *Cell. Immunol.*, **178**, 62–68.

54. Al-Sabbagh, A., Nelson, P. A., Akselband, Y., Sobel, R. A., and Weiner, H. L. (1996) Antigen-driven peripheral immune tolerance: suppression of experimental autoimmune encephalomyelitis and collagen-induced arthritis by aerosol administration of myelin basic protein or type II collagen, *Cell. Immunol.*, **171**(1), 111–119.

55. Weiner, H. L., Mackin, G. A, Matsui, M., et al. (1993) Double-blind pilot trial of tolerization with myelin antigens in multiple sclerosis, *Science*, **259**, 1321–1324.

56. Atkinson, M. A. and Maclaren, N. K. (1994) The pathogenesis of insulin-dependent diabetes mellitus, *N. Engl. J. Med.*, **331**, 1428–1436.

57. Briskin, M. J., McEvoy, L. M., and Butcher, E. C. (1993) MadCAM-1 has homology to immunoglobulin and mucin-like adhesion receptors and to IgA1, *Nature*, **363**, 461–464.

58. Fynan, E. F., Webster, R. G., Fuller, D. H., Haynes, J. R., Santoro, J. C., and Robinson, H. L. (1993) DNA vaccines: protective immunizations by parenteral mucosal, and gene-gun inoculations, *Proc. Natl. Acad. Sci. U.S.A.*, **90**, 11478–11482.

59. Oldstone, M. B. A. (1987) Molecular mimicry and autoimmune disease, *Cell*, **50**, 819–820.

60. von Herrath, M. G., Dyrberg, T., and Oldstone, M. B. A. (1996) Oral insulin treatment suppresses virus-induced antigen-specific destruction of β cells and prevents autoimmune diabetes in transgenic mice, *J. Clin. Invest.*, **98**, 1324–1331.

61. Hänninen, A., Jaakkola, I., and Jalkanen, S. (1998) Mucosal addressin is required for the development of diabetes in nonobese diabetic mice, *J. Immunol.*, **160**, 6018–6025.

62. Hänninen, A., Taylor, C., Streeter, P. R., et al. (1993) Vascular addressins are induced on islet vessels during insulitis in nonobese diabetic mice and are involved in lymphoid cell binding to islet endothelium, *J. Clin. Invest.*, **92**, 2509–2515.

63. Coutant, R., Zeidler, A., Rappaport, R., et al. (1998) Oral insulin therapy in newly-diagnosed immune mediated (type I) diabetes: preliminary analysis of a randomized double-blind placebo-controlled study, *Diabetes*, **47**(Suppl. 1), A97.

64. Ogra, P. L., Fishaut, M., and Gallagher, M. R. (1980) Viral vaccination via the mucosal route, *Rev. Infect. Dis.*, **2**, 352–369.

65. Nussenblatt, R. B., Gery, I., Weiner, H. L., et al. (1997) Treatment of uveitis by oral administration of retinal antigens: results of a phase I/II randomized masked trial, *Am. J. Ophthalmol.*, **123**, 583–592.

66. Haque, M. A., Yoshino, S., Inada, S., Nomaguchi, H., Tokunaga, O., and Kohashi, O. (1996) Suppression of adjuvant arthritis in rats by induction of oral tolerance to mycobacterial 65-kDa heat shock protein, *Eur. J. Immunol.*, **26**, 2650–2656.

67. Khare, S. D., Krco, C. J., Griffiths, M. M., Luthra, H. S., and David, C. S. (1995) Oral administration of an immunodominant human collagen peptide modulates collagen-induced arthritis, *J. Immunol.*, **155**, 3653–3659.

68. Barnett, M. L., Combitchi, D., and Trentham, D. E. (1996) A pilot trial of oral type II collagen in the treatment of juvenile rheumatoid arthritis, *Arthritis Rheum.*, **39**, 623–628.

69. Barnett, M. L., Kremer, J. M., St. Clair, E. W., et al. (1998) Treatment of rheumatoid arthritis with oral type II collagen: results

of a multicenter, double-blind, placebo-controlled trial, *Arthritis Rheum.*, **41**, 290–297.

70. Trentham, D. E., Dynesius-Trentham, R. A., Orav, E. J., et al. (1993) Effects of oral administration of collagen on rheumatoid arthritis, *Science*, **261**, 1727–1730.

71. Husby, S., Foged, N. A., Host, A., and Svehag, S.-E. (1987) Passage of dietary antigens into the blood of children with coeliac disease: quantification and size distribution of absorbed antigens, *Gut*, **28**, 1062–1072.

72. Husby, S., Jensenius, J. C., and Svehag, S.-E. (1986) Passage of undergraded dietary antigen into the blood of healthy adults: further characterization of the kinetics of uptake and the size distribution of the antigen, *Scand. J. Immunol.*, **24**, 447–452.

73. Husby, S., Mestecky, J., Moldoveanu, Z., Holland, S., and Elson, C. O. (1994) Oral tolerance in humans: T cell but not B cell tolerance after antigen feeding, *J. Immunol.*, **152**, 4663–4670.

74. Jackson, J., Mestecky, J., Childers, N. K., and Michalek, S. M. (1990) Liposomes containing anti-idiotypic antibodies: an oral vaccine to induce protective secretory immune responses specific for pathogens of mucosal surfaces, *Infect. Immun.*, **58**, 1932–1936.

75. Bagot, M., Charue, D., Flechet, M. L., Terki, N., Toma, A., and Revuz, J. (1995) Oral desensitization in nickel allergy induces a decrease in nickel-specific T-cells, *Eur. J. Dermatol.*, **5**, 614–617.

76. Roy, K., Mao, H. Q., Huang, S. K., and Leong, K. W. (1999) Oral gene delivery with chitosan-DNA nanoparticles generates immunologic protection in a murine model of peanut allergy, *Nat. Med.*, **5**(4), 387–391.

77. Spiegelberg, H. L., Orozco, E. M., Roman, M., and Raz, E. (1997) DNA immunization: a novel approach to allergen-specific immunotherapy, *Allergy*, **52**, 964–970.

Chapter 43

The Role of B Cells

Antibodies provide much of the protection afforded by the vaccines in the current arsenal; however, only recently has an in-depth understanding emerged of the molecular basis of B-cell development, selection, and effector function that may allow more strategic manipulation of the B-cell compartment *(1)*.

The B cells are responsible for humoral immunity. They arise from a separate population of stem cells of the bone marrow than that which gives rise to the T cells. The B cells undergo multiplication and processing in lymphoid tissue elsewhere than in the thymus gland. In birds, the lymphoid tissue concerned has been located in the gut and called the bursa of Fabricius. In humans, the site is unknown although there is some evidence to suggest that such processing occurs in the bone marrow itself or in the fetal liver.

43.1 Genealogy of B Cells

Many fundamental concepts about immune system development have changed substantially in the past few years, and rapid advances with animal models are presenting prospects for further discovery. However, continued progress requires a clearer understanding of the relationships between hematopoietic stem cells and the progenitors that replenish each type of lymphocyte pool. Blood-cell formation has traditionally been described in terms of discrete developmental branch points, and a single route is given for each major cell type. However, recent findings suggest that the process of B-cell formation is much more dynamic *(2)*.

The B cells, like T cells, have surface receptors that enable them to recognize the appropriate antigen but do not themselves interact to neutralize or destroy the antigen. On recognition of the antigen, they take up residence in secondary lymphoid tissue and proliferate to form daughter lymphocytes, processed in the same way as themselves. These B cells then develop into short-lived plasma cells. The plasma cells produce antibodies and release them into the circulation at the lymph nodes *(2)*.

Some of the activated B cells do not become plasma cells; instead, they turn into memory cells, which continue to produce small amounts of the antibody long after the infection has been overcome. As with T cells, millions of B cells are produced, each with a different antigen-binding specificity. If the B cell comes into contact with the specific type of antigen to which it is targeted, it divides rapidly to form a clone of identical cells.

This antibody is circulating as part of the gamma globulin fraction of the blood plasma. Should the same antigen enter the body again, this circulating antibody will act quickly to destroy it. At the same time, memory cells quickly divide to produce new clones of the appropriate type of plasma cell *(2)*.

It has long been a goal of immunologists to identify and characterize the "earliest" lymphoid progenitors in the adult bone marrow, but there have been conflicting claims about the properties of such cells. However, microarray, quantitative RT-PCR, and multiplex PCR analyses have generated a wealth of information about patterns of early gene expression *(2)*. For example, many genes commonly associated with T- and B-cells, such as those encoding $CD3\delta$, pre-T-cell receptor (TCR) α-chain (pTCRα), the pre-B-cell receptor (BCR) surrogate light chains VpreB and Vλ5, and the paired box protein 5 (PAX5), were not found active in the path of hemapoietic stem cells (HSCs) (http://stemcells.nih.gov/info/scireport/chapter5.asp) becoming B cells *(3,4)*. However, stem cells do contain detectable mRNA transcripts that correspond with genes that are expressed in multiple other hematopoietic lineages. This may reflect the general availability of developmental options or chromatin status at key genetic loci and does not necessarily presage the fate of individual cells *(5)*. Indeed, this phenomenon has been referred to as "priming" or "promiscuity" of lymphoid and myeloid progenitors *(3)*. Almost all early cell progenitors that express lymphoid-related genes are also positive for granulocyte/macrophage-related transcripts *(4)*.

Given this background, lymphopoietic cells might be called "lymphoid specified" when they express detectable amounts of proteins that are normally restricted to lymphocytes. Evidence has been presented that the expression of terminal deoxynucleotidyltransferase (TdT), an enzyme that diversifies antibody combining sites, is a defining feature of what is referred to as early pro-B cells *(6)*. A series of subsequent studies confirmed the use of this marker to define B-, natural killer (NK)-, and T-lymphoid-specified progenitors, which have been termed *early lymphoid progenitors (ELPs)* *(7,8)*. However, only polyclonal antibodies are available to detect TdT, which is present at quite low levels and can only be visualized in fixed cells. Fortunately, gene-reporter mice and characteristic patterns of cell-surface antigen expression now make it possible to isolate highly enriched populations of lymphoid-specified cells. Although not irrevocably committed to the lymphoid lineage, ELPs appear to have a high probability of becoming lymphocytes and can do so experimentally with remarkable efficiency *(2)*.

Other important issues in lymphopoiesis relate to the nurturing environments for hematopoietic stem cell (HSCs) and the nature of extracellular signals that regulate the earliest events. The pool of subendosteal osteoblasts (cells that line the inner bone surface) has long attracted attention as a potential "niche" to support early lympho-hematopoiesis, but most HSCs are more centrally located in the bone marrow and near perivascular stromal cells *(9)*. It will be a challenge to define such niches because cells with the same mesenchymal origin may assume different functions and produce factors that vary in response to their location. For example, stromal cell lines commonly used to support lympho-hematopoiesis are multipotent and can be induced in culture to become osteoblasts or fat cells *(2)*.

Lymphoid progenitors are scattered throughout the bone marrow, and the earliest ones preferentially interact with VCAM1$^+$ CXC-chemokine ligand 12 (CXCL12)-producing reticular cells *(10,11)*. Although it is clear that CXCL12 has been important for attracting and retaining lymphoid progenitors in the bone marrow, the nature of other important factors produced by reticular cells was also undefined. Thus, distinctly different from reticular cells, VCAM1$^+$ stromal cells produce IL-7, which is needed to support the survival and expansion of progenitors, as well as for immunoglobulin gene recombination. A possibly comparable situation has been found in human bone marrow, where a series of lymphoid progenitors were aligned in close association with VCAM1$^{+/--}$CD10$^+$ stromal cells *(12)*. In addition to these components of the bone marrow, knockout studies indicate that endothelial cells and osteoclasts can also contribute somehow to hematopoiesis *(13,14)*. Morover, HSCs can also develop, reside, and/or traffic in other organs *(15,16)*.

Given the complexity and uncertainty about cells that comprise niches in the bone marrow, it is surprising that progress is being made in the identification of molecules they produce that control the survival, mitotic activity, and differentiation of hematopoietic cells *(17,18)*. The Notch ligands, stem-cell factor (SCF), thrombopoietin, IL-3, IL-11,

IL-6, insulin-like growth factor 2, fibroblast growth factor, and the wingless-type MMTV integration site family, member 3A (WNT3A) have all been used to support modest expansion of long-term self-renewing HSC (LT-HSC) without loss of self-renewal potential *(19–22)*. However, gene-targeting experiments have yet to demonstrate that any of these molecules or their receptors are absolutely essential for lympho-hematopoiesis *(2)*.

The LSK cell subset is defined by high levels of expression of the transmembrane protein tyrosine-kinase receptor KIT, and ELPs are responsive to its corresponding ligand, SCF. Although it is clear that this pair of molecules maintains HSC homeostasis, an important role in B-cell lymphopoiesis for KIT–SCF–associated signals is only obvious many weeks after birth *(23)*. Upregulation of the structurally related protein tyrosine kinase FLT3 parallels the formation of ELPs, however, targeting this receptor protein kinase has only modest effects on B-cell–lineage development *(24)*.

In addition to these positive regulators, there are many factors that constrain clonal expansion and lineage progression at this early stage. Nearly all adult bone-marrow HSCs and most ELPs spend a considerable amount of time in a quiescent, G_0 state of cell-cycle arrest *(25–27)*. This status may be important for controlling population sizes and the lifelong integrity of cells that replenish the immune system *(2)*.

Some mechanisms by which this regulation may occur have been proposed *(2)*. Angiopoietins and osteopontin are thought to regulate stem-cell numbers *(28–30)*, but information is lacking about their effects on very early lymphoid cells. The formation of ELPs from HSCs is blocked by IL-6, and progenitors seem to be redirected to a myeloid-cell fate by this cytokine *(31,32)*. Interestingly, IL-6 has no negative influence and in fact enhances the proliferation of ELPs. Stage-specific action may also be a feature of prostaglandins, which, although long known to induce apoptosis in B-cell–lineage progenitors, have been recently described as stimulants for HSC self-renewal *(33,34)*. There is also substantial evidence to suggest that steroid hormones selectively inhibit B-cell lymphopoiesis under steady-state conditions *(35)*.

More controversial are the functions associated with members of the complex WNT family of molecules. Thus, there have been conflicting reports concerning the physiologic importance of WNT3A in maintaining HSCs *(21,36,37)*. One recent report concluded that although WNT signaling is at least needed for normal T-cell lymphopoiesis, it is accomplished without dependence on its canonical signaling partners β- or γ-catenin *(38)*. However, artificial stimulation of the canonical signaling pathway frequently used by WNT3A dramatically inhibited, and even reversed lineage progression. That is, it caused lymphoid- or myeloid-restricted progenitors to become multipotent *(39,40)*. Furthermore, WNT5A appeared to limit the expansion of B-lineage cells at a later stage *(41)*.

The progeny of ELPs are known by a variety of names, but they represent a series of progenitors that are progressively more likely to become lymphocytes *(2)*. In landmark research in mouse bone marrow, LSK IL-7Rα$^+$ have been identified as *common lymphoid progenitors (CLPs)* and shown that at least some individual cells with these characteristics had the potential to differentiate into both T cells and B cells *(42)*. The same fraction has also generated NK cells when transplanted, but no signs of nonlymphoid differentiation were observed at the time. Subsequent studies established that CLPs represent major intermediates in the B-cell–lineage and NK-cell–lineage pathways but are not totally dedicated to those fates *(10)*. For example, several studies have found that highly purified CLPs can transiently produce small numbers of dendritic cells (DCs) and myeloid cells *(43–45)*. Importantly, there is near consensus that CLPs did not contribute substantially to T-cell–lineage development *(46)*. Although T-cell–lineage lymphocytes can be generated when IL-7Rα$^+$ progenitors are injected into the thymus or cultured with the stromal-cell line OP9 that expresses the Notch ligand delta-like ligand 1 (DLL1; a process known as the *OP9-DLL1 system*), they were unlikely to do so under normal circumstances *(42,44,47,48)*.

Stem Cells Express Toll-like Receptors. Antigen-specific receptors are expressed by maturing lymphocytes and used as checkpoints to choose cells that will be most effective for the adaptive immune system, whereas cells of the innate immune system recognize bacterial and viral products through Toll-like receptors (TLRs) *(2)*. Hematopoietic progenitors were long thought to be incapable of discrimination between self and nonself, but it is now known that they have expressed functional TLRs *(49)*. Moreover, exposure of highly purified stem cells to TLR2 or TLR4 ligands has driven them to proliferate and encourage their differentiation, whereas myeloid progenitors rapidly generated macrophages with similar stimulation *(2)*. CLPs are also responsive to TLR ligands, and more recent studies revealed that TLR9 can mediate their redirection to DC lineages during viral infection *(2)*. These findings have demonstrated that commitment was not irreversible at the pro-lymphocyte/CLP stage and progenitors were still responsive to environmental cues *(2)*.

43.2 BlyS and B Cells Homeostasis

Strides made over the past 5 to 10 years that may allow new strategies for B-cell vaccination include an understanding of B-cell receptor antigen recognition, receptor editing, and growth factors involved in the chief transitions in B-cell maturation before, during, and after antigen selection. For example, the tumor necrosis factor–related cytokines BLyS (also called BAFF) and APRIL target three receptors on B cells: BR3, which responds to BLyS to support primary B-cell survival and growth; BCMA, which promotes memory B-cell development in response to APRIL; and TACI, which is important in B-cell responses to bacterial capsular polysaccharides *(50,51)*. Additional developmental signals may also derive from the stimulation of innate immune receptors on human B cells *(51)*. Those findings raise the possibility that coadministration of critical cytokines or their triggers along with vaccine immunogens may constitute a new vaccine strategy to expand the capabilities of responding B cells beyond those now appreciated. The prospects for a new approach to B-cell manipulation seem to be near; however, studies are needed to address whether new approaches might also bring new problems, such as induction of autoimmunity.

The BLyS family of receptors includes two cytokines, BLyS and APRIL, and three receptors, BR3, BCMA, and TACI. Together, these regulate the size and composition of peripheral B-cell pools *(50–58)*. The multiplicity of ligand-receptor sets, in conjunction with differential receptor expression, alternative binding partners, and disparate downstream signaling characteristics, affords the potential to establish independently regulated homeostatic niches among primary and antigen-experienced B-cell subsets. Thus, BLyS signaling via BR3 is the dominant homeostatic regulator of primary B-cell pools, whereas APRIL interactions with BCMA likely govern memory B-cell populations. Short-lived antibody-forming cell populations and their proliferating progenitors express a TACI-predominant signature. Further, within each niche, relative fitness to compete for available cytokine is determined by exogenous inputs via adaptive and innate receptor systems, affording intramural hierarchies that determine clonotype composition *(50)*.

The B-lymphocyte stimulator (BLyS) and the proliferation-inducing ligand (APRIL) are both members of the tumor necrosis factor (TNF) superfamily. They play diverse roles in regulating the activities of both resting and activated lymphocytes *(59)* and are now recognized as being of central importance in B-cell development and homeostasis *(50)*. Through differential interactions with several receptors, these two ligands profoundly influence multiple aspects of B-cell biology. Their activities include mediating the selection, differentiation, and homeostasis of primary B cells; influencing the differentiation of activated B cells; and controlling the generation and longevity of memory B cells. These broad and largely B-lineage–specific activities, coupled with clear relevance to both autoimmunity and neoplasia, have focused intense scrutiny on BLyS, APRIL, and their corresponding receptors. This concerted activity has already yielded considerable insight into fundamental aspects of B-cell biology and has revealed several promising therapeutic targets, prompting extensive review and commentary *(57–84)*.

Currently, the most extensively studied biological activities of BLyS family members are those associated with developing and primary B cells. This focus reflects the striking phenotypic impact that knockouts and transgenics for certain BLyS family members have on primary B-cell pools, as well as the presumed relevance of these activities to tolerance and autoimmune disease *(50)*.

In contrast, the nature and mechanisms through which BLyS family members influence antigen-experienced B-cell populations remain less extensively explored. Nonetheless, several mechanistic features drawn from studies to date are likely common to all of these interactions. Foremost, the notion of interclonal competition underpins the current perception of how this family controls B-cell survival and selection. According to this notion, pool sizes can be controlled by limiting the amount or availability of cytokine, such that when cytokine consumption equals availability, steady-state pool size is achieved. Further, such competition implies that populations occupying independent homeostatic niches can coexist in the same physical space, so long as each population relies upon and competes for a different cytokine (e.g., APRIL vs. BLyS). A second important feature of the current understanding is that a B-cell's ability to capture these signals is coupled to other cell-intrinsic signaling systems, including innate and adaptive immune receptors. Accordingly, signals via these exogenous sensing systems in aggregate determine a cell's relative fitness compared with others competing for occupation of the same niche *(50)*.

Finally, differential receptor binding activities, in combination with changing expression levels influenced by differentiation or cross-talk with other surface receptors, specifies the cytokine-delineated niche within which each B cell competes *(50)*.

Although these general features of BLyS family activities have been revealed through studies of newly formed and primary B cells, only now are analogous properties being defined within activated and antigen-experienced B-cell populations *(50)*.

The BLyS Family of Receptors and Cytokines. Because of simultaneous initial reports, BLyS is also known as BAFF, TALL-1, zTNF4, and THANK *(85–88)*. Likewise, APRIL has several aliases: TRDL-1, TALL-2, and TNFSF13A *(87–89)*.

Similar to other TNF members, BLyS and APRIL are type II transmembrane proteins that are proteolytically cleaved to generate active soluble forms *(50)*. In fact, APRIL appeared to be available only in soluble form because cleavage occurred in the Golgi apparatus *(90)*, although alternative splice forms with different properties are now being described *(91)*. BLyS also has at least two splice isoforms, one of which can remain membrane bound and appeared to inhibit the activity of soluble BLyS *(92,93)*. Although homotrimers are thought to be the predominant active forms, BLyS and APRIL can also form biologically active heterotrimers both *in vitro* and *in vivo*; however, a differential function for such composites remains to be identified *(94)*.

BLyS was found to bind three receptors: the transmembrane activator and cyclophilin ligand interactor (TACI), the B-cell maturation antigen (BCMA), and the BAFF receptor 3 (BR3) *(56,95–98)*. Two of these receptors, TACI and BCMA, can also bind APRIL *(56,99)*. These receptors are all type III transmembrane proteins possessing extracellular cysteine-rich domains (CRDs) that mediate ligand binding. Whereas TACI possesses two CRDs, BCMA and BR3 have only a single or a partial CRD, respectively *(100,101)*. This variation, along with key charge differences in binding site residues, did allow widely differing affinities for the respective ligands *(50)*. For example, BR3 interacted solely and strongly with BLyS *(102)*, as evidenced by affinity measurements as well as extensive biological findings. By comparison, BCMA had up to 1,000 times greater affinity for APRIL than for BLyS, making APRIL the more physiologically relevant ligand for this receptor *(103,104)*. Between these two extremes, TACI interacted appreciably with both cytokines, albeit with a somewhat higher apparent affinity for APRIL *(56,105)*. Finally, sulfated proteoglycans have been shown to bind APRIL, and although some forms of signaling occurred through this interaction, the physiologic role of this relationship is still not clarified *(106)*. These binding characteristics, coupled with the diverse receptor expression profiles in various B-cell subsets, provide a mechanism for establishing non-overlapping niches of independent homeostatic control via BLyS–BR3 versus APRIL-BCMA interactions *(50)*.

Enabling additional permutations of independent but overlapping control, the downstream mediators of each receptor are distinct but interrelated and involve intersecting pathways used by other key B-lineage receptors. Thus, TACI interacted with TRAFs 2, 5, and 6 and signaled through nuclear factor of activated T-Cells (NF-AT) and AP-1 (activator factor 1 (a transcription factor)) *(56,95,101,107)*; and BCMA associated with TNF receptor associated factors (TRAFs) 1, 2, and 3 and activated Elk-1, JNK, and p38 MAP kinase *(101,108)*. Both of these receptors also induced elements of the classic NF-κB pathway. In contrast, BR3 appeared restricted to using TRAF 3 and preferentially activated the alternative NF-κB pathway *(109–112)*. Thus, in addition to the differential expression of receptors and the varying strength of each ligand-receptor pair, even the same cytokine binding to different receptors will yield alternative outcomes *(50)*.

These properties offer multiple levels at which BLyS signaling can be controlled and refined *(50)*. Certainly, receptor expression and ratio affect outcome, as might cross-talk between BLyS receptors themselves or with other cell surface molecules. Levels of the cytokines themselves may allow further manipulation of the system, however both APRIL and BLyS are expressed ubiquitously *(99,113–117)*, making it unlikely that system-wide variations in cytokine levels will differentially control local niche selection. Nonetheless, localized concentration differences in specialized anatomic sites may allow focal control of different populations. Inasmuch as both APRIL and BLyS are produced by inflammatory cells, such local gradients are an appealing possibility but are difficult to interrogate. In contrast, the expression of BLyS family receptors is clearly differentially regulated in terms of developmental stages and subsets, as well as following exogenous activation cues, making this a clear route of control (50).

BLyS-Dependent Survival Signaling. The B-cell lymphopenia in A/WySn mice resulting from a mutation in BR3 is essentially corrected by the ectopic expression of the anti-apoptotic protein BCL-x_L (118). It has also been repeatedly shown that stimulation with BLyS significantly retards the spontaneous death of B cells *ex vivo* by apoptosis (119,120). These results have been used to support the conclusion that the primary function of BLyS-dependent signaling is to suppress apoptosis in B cells. The BLyS stimulation of both normal and transformed B cells, in the absence of other inducers, is leading to the induction of transcription factors, the activation of survival serine/threonine kinase-dependent signal cascades, and the production and/or modification of proapoptotic and antiapoptotic proteins, thereby accounting for both the growth and survival functions attributed to BLyS (53). Establishing a direct correlation between the activation of a particular signal pathway and apoptosis protection and/or B-cell growth is complicated by three factors. Most studies of BLyS signaling in primary B cells used test populations expressing multiple BLyS receptors, used other activators in addition to BLyS, and/or failed to correlate a signal pathway with a discrete biological effect. Given these considerations, the signal cascades induced by BLyS stimulation that promote the survival of primary follicular B cells *ex vivo* have been examined in an attempt to identify the pathways important for survival irrespective of the receptor that transmits the BLyS dependent signal, and a model that explains the survival signaling mediated by BLyS has been proposed (53).

43.2.1 BlyS and Disease

Owning to BLyS support of the homeostasis of naïve B cells as well as the survival of both malignant and autoreactive B cells, several hematologic malignancies (multiple myeloma, lymphoma, and non–Hodgkin's leukemia) have all been shown to use BLyS for their survival (53,75,77,121–124). Moreover, many transformed B cells were shown capable of synthesizing and secreting BLyS, thereby establishing a pathologic autocrine loop frequently associated with poor disease prognosis (122,123,125).

Dysregulated BLyS expression is also a feature of numerous autoimmune diseases including arthritis, lupus erythematosus, and Sjögren's disease (76,79,126–128). The survival-enhancing property of BLyS is likely to facilitate the autoimmune responses by circumventing tolerance induction to self-antigens, rescuing autoreactive B cells targeted for elimination through anergy or deletion (129,130).

The role of BLyS in these pathologic conditions has provided the impetus for a therapeutic approach targeting BLyS using monoclonal antibodies or recombinant decoy receptors for the treatment of both autoimmune disease and B-cell cancers (131–133).

The identification of the signal pathways mediating BLyS-dependent survival did suggest an alternative treatment strategy targeting these signal cascades (53). The pharmacologic inhibition of B-cell survival signaling may be a necessary adjunct to the current approach that neutralizes BLyS in the host. BLyS is expressed as a membrane-bound ligand on myeloid cells, released by furin cleavage, and both membrane-bound and soluble BLyS are biologically active (14,117). Inhibition of membrane-bound ligand usually requires higher concentrations of competitor and is less efficient than the inhibition of soluble ligands, and this general principle would apply to BLyS. The identification of only two pathways, Akt/mTOR and Pim 2, mediating BLyS-induced survival would provide defined pharmacologic targets for both malignant and autoimmune B cells. The mTOR inhibitor rapamycin is a well tolerated and highly efficient inhibitor that can effectively suppresses BLyS-dependent B-cell survival in the absence of Pim 2 (134). Inhibitors of Pim 2 may be equally efficient and well tolerated because Pim 2–deficient mice have no phenotype (135), and most biological processes mediated by Pim 2, other than B-cell survival, can be effected by other members of the Pim family. A combination therapy targeting mTOR and Pim 2 could have a significant clinical efficacy for the control of autoimmune and neoplastic B cells (53).

References

1. Hackett, C. J., Rotrosen, D., Auchincloss, H., and Fauci, A. S. (2007) Immunology research: challenges and opportunities in a time of budgetary constraint, *Nat. Immunol.*, **8**, 114–117.
2. Welner, R. S., Pelayo, R., and Kincade, P. W. (2008) Evolving genealogy of B cells, *Nat. Rev. Immunol.*, **8**, 95–106.
3. Miyamoto, T., Iwasaki, H., Reizis, B., Ye, M., Graf, T., Weissman, I., and Akashi, K. (2002) Myeloid or lymphoid promiscuity as a critical step in hematopoietic lineage commitment, *Dev. Cell*, **3**, 137–147.
4. Mansson, R., Hultquist, A., Luc, S., et al. (2007) Molecular evidence for hierarchical transcriptional lineage priming in fetal and adult stem cells and multipotent progenitors, *Immunity*, **26**, 407–419.
5. Hu, M., Krause, D., Greaves, D., et al. (1997) Multilineage gene expression precedes commitment in the hematopoietic system, *Genes Dev.*, **11**, 774–785.

6. Park, Y.-H. and Osmond, D. G. (1989) Dynamics of early B lymphocyte precursor cells in mouse bone marrow: proliferation of cells containing terminal deoxynucleotidyl transferase, *Eur. J. Immunol.*, **19**, 2139–2144.

7. Medina, K. L., Garrett, K. P., Thompson, L. F., et al. (2001) Identification of very early lymphoid precursors in bone marrow and their regulation by estrogen, *Nat. Immunol.*, **2**, 718–724.

8. Igarashi, H., Gregory, S. C., Yokota, T., Sakaguchi, N., and Kincade, P. W. (2002) Transcription from the RAG1 locus marks the earliest lymphocyte progenitors in bone marrow, *Immunity*, **17**, 117–130.

9. Kiel, M. J., Yilmaz, Ö., Iwashita, T., Yilmaz, O., Terhorst, C., and Morrison, S. (2005) SLAM family receptors distinguish hematopoietic stem and progenitor cells and reveal endothelial niches for stem cells, *Cell*, **121**, 1109–1121.

10. Hirose, J., Kouro, T., Igarashi, H., Yokota, T., Sakaguchi, N., and Kincade, P. W. (2002) A developing picture of lymphopoiesis in bone marrow, *Immunol. Rev.*, **189**, 28–40.

11. Tokoyoda, K., Egawa, T., Sugiyama, T., Choi, B. I., and Nagasawa, T. (2004) Cellular niches controlling B lymphocyte behaviour within bone marrow during development, *Immunity*, **20**, 707–718.

12. Torlakovic, E., Tenstad, E., Funderud, S., and Rian, E. (2005) CD10$^+$ stromal cells form B-lymphocyte maturation niches in the human bone marrow, *J. Pathol.*, **205**, 311–317.

13. Yao, L., Yokota, T., Xia, L., Kincade, P. W., and McEver, R. P. (2005) Bone marrow dysfunction in mice lacking the cytokine receptor gp130 in endothelial cells, *Blood*, **106**, 4093–4101.

14. Walkley, C. R., Shea, J. M., Sims, N. A., Purton, L. E., and Orkin, S. H. (2007) Rb regulates interactions between hematopoietic stem cells and their bone marrow microenvironment, *Cell*, **129**, 1081–1095.

15. Taniguchi, H., Toyoshima, T., Fukao, K., and Nakauchi, H. (1996) Presence of hematopoietic stem cells in the adult liver, *Nat. Med.*, **2**, 198–203.

16. Bhattacharya, D., Rossi, D. J., Bryder, D., and Weissman, I. L. (2006) Purified hematopoietic stem cell engraftment of rare niches corrects severe lymphoid deficiencies without host conditioning, *J. Exp. Med.*, **203**, 73–85.

17. Wilson, A. and Trumpp, A. (2006) Bone-marrow haematopoietic-stem-cell niches, *Nat. Rev. Immunol.*, **6**, 93–106.

18. Suda, T., Arai, F., and Hirao, A. (2005) Hematopoietic stem cells and their niche, *Trends Immunol.*, **26**, 426–433.

19. Varnum-Finney, B., Brashem-Stein, C., and Bernstein, I. D. (2003) Combined effects of Notch signalling and cytokines induce a multiple log increase in precursors with lymphoid and myeloid reconstituting ability, *Blood*, **101**, 1784–1789.

20. Zhang, C. C. and Lodish, H. F. (2005) Murine hematopoietic stem cells change their surface phenotype during ex vivo expansion, *Blood*, **105**, 4314–4320.

21. Reya, T., Duncan, A. W., Ailles, L., et al. (2003) A role for Wnt signalling in self-renewal of haematopoietic stem cells, *Nature*, **423**, 409–414.

22. Sauvageau, G., Iscove, N. N., and Humphries, R. K. (2004) In vitro and in vivo expansion of hematopoietic stem cells, *Oncogene*, **23**, 7223–7232.

23. Waskow, C., Paul, S., Haller, C., Gassmann, M., Rodewald, H. R. (2002) Viable c-Kit$^{W/W}$ mutants reveal pivotal role for c-kit in the maintenance of lymphopoiesis, *Immunity*, **17**, 277–288.

24. Mackarehtschian, K., Hardin, J. D., Moore, K. A., et al. (1995) Targeted disruption of the flk2/flt3 gene leads to deficiencies in primitive hematopoietic progenitors, *Immunity*, **3**, 147–161.

25. Passegue, E., Wagers, A. J., Giuriato, S., Anderson, W. C., and Weissman, I. L. (2005) Global analysis of proliferation and cell cycle gene expression in the regulation of hematopoietic stem and progenitor cell fates, *J. Exp. Med.*, **202**, 1599–1611.

26. Cheshier, S. H., Morrison, S. J., Liao, X., and Weissman, I. L. (1999) In vivo proliferation and cell cycle kinetics of long-term self-renewing hematopoietic stem cells, *Proc. Natl Acad. Sci. U.S.A.*, **96**, 3120–3125.

27. Pelayo, R., Miyazaki, K., Huang, J., et al. (2006) Cell cycle quiescence of early lymphoid progenitors in adult bone marrow, *Stem Cells*, **24**, 2703–2713.

28. Arai, F., Hirao, A., Ohmura, M., et al. (2004) Tie2/angiopoietin-1 signalling regulates hematopoietic stem cell quiescence in the bone marrow niche, *Cell*, **118**, 149–161.

29. Zhang, C. C., Kaba, M., Ge, G., et al. (2006) Angiopoietin-like proteins stimulate ex vivo expansion of hematopoietic stem cells, *Nat. Med.*, **12**, 240–245.

30. Stier, S., Ko, Y., Forkert, R., et al. (2005) Osteopontin is a hematopoietic stem cell niche component that negatively regulates stem cell pool size, *J. Exp. Med.*, **201**, 1781–1791.

31. Maeda, K., Baba, Y., Nagai, Y., et al. (2005) IL-6 blocks a discrete early step in lymphopoiesis, *Blood*, **106**, 879–885.

32. Nakamura, K., Kouro, T., Kincade, P. W., et al. (2004) Src homology 2-containing 5-inositol phosphatase (SHIP) suppresses an early stage of lymphoid cell development through elevated interleukin-6 production by myeloid cells in bone marrow, *J. Exp. Med.* **199**, 243–254.

33. Kouro, T., Medina, K. L., Oritani, K., and Kincade, P. W. (2001) Characteristics of early murine B lymphocyte precursors and their direct sensitivity to negative regulators, *Blood*, **97**, 2708–2715.

34. North, T. E., Goessling, W., Walkley, C. R., et al. (2007) Prostaglandin E2 regulates vertebrate haematopoietic stem cell homeostasis, *Nature*, **447**, 1007–1011.

35. Kincade, P. W., Igarashi, H., Medina, K. L., et al. (2002) Lymphoid lineage cells in adult murine bone marrow diverge from those of other blood cells at an early, hormone-sensitive stage, *Semin. Immunol.*, **14**, 385–394.

36. Koch, U., Wilson, A., Cobas, M., et al. (2007) Simultaneous loss of β- and γ-catenin does not perturb hematopoiesis or lymphopoiesis, *Blood*, **111**(1), 160–164.

37. Nemeth, M. J., Topol, L., Anderson, S. M., Yang, Y., and Bodine, D. M. (2007) Wnt5a inhibits canonical Wnt signalling in hematopoietic stem cells and enhances repopulation, *Proc. Natl. Acad. Sci. U.S.A.*, **104**, 15436–15441.

38. Jeannet, G., Scheller, M., Scarpellino, L., et al. (2007) Long-term, multilineage hematopoiesis occurs in the combined absence of β-catenin and γ-catenin, *Blood*, **111**(1), 142–149.

39. Baba, Y., Garrett, K. P., and Kincade, P. W. (2005) Constitutively active β-catenin confers multilineage differentiation potential on lymphoid and myeloid progenitors, *Immunity*, **23**, 599–609.

40. Baba, Y., Yokota, T., Spits, H., et al. (2006) Constitutively active β-catenin promotes expansion of multipotent hematopoietic progenitors in culture, *J. Immunol.*, **177**, 2294–2303.

41. Liang, H., Chen, Q., Coles, A., et al. (2003) Wnt5a inhibits B cell proliferation and functions as a tumor suppressor in hematopoietic tissue, *Cancer Cell*, **4**, 349–360.

42. Kondo, M., Weissman, I. L., and Akashi, K. (1997) Identification of clonogenic common lymphoid progenitors in mouse bone marrow, *Cell*, **91**, 661–672.

43. Kondo, M., Weissman, I. L., and Akashi, K. (1997) Identification of clonogenic common lymphoid progenitors in mouse bone marrow, *Cell*, **91**, 661–672.

44. Perry, S. S., Wang, H., Pierce, L. J., et al. (2004) L-selectin defines a bone marrow analogue to the thymic early T-cell-lineage progenitor, *Blood*, **103**, 2990–2996.

45. Kondo, M., Weissman, I. L., and Akashi, K. (1997) Identification of clonogenic common lymphoid progenitors in mouse bone marrow, *Cell*, **91**, 661–672.

46. Bhandoola, A., Von Boehmer, H., Petrie, H. T., and Zúñiga-Pflücker, J. C. (2007) Commitment and developmental potential of extrathymic and intrathymic T cell precursors: plenty to choose from, *Immunity*, **26**, 678–689.

47. Allman, D., Sambandam, A., Kim, S., et al. (2003) Thymopoiesis independent of common lymphoid progenitors, *Nat. Immunol.*, **4**, 168–174.

48. Huang, J., Garrett, K. P., Pelayo, R., et al. (2005) Propensity of adult lymphoid progenitors to progress to DN2/3 stage thymocytes with Notch receptor ligation, *J. Immunol.*, **175**, 4858–4865.

49. Nagai, Y., Garrett, K., Ohta, S., et al. (2006) Toll-like receptors on hematopoietic progenitor cells stimulate innate immune system replenishment, *Immunity*, **24**, 801–812.

50. Treml, L. S., Crowley, J. E., and Cancro, M. P. (2006) BLyS receptor signatures resolve homeostatically independent compartments among naïve and antigen- experienced B cells, *Semin. Immunol.*, **18**(5), 297–304.

51. Ruprecht, C. R. and Lanzavecchia, A. (2006) Toll-like receptor stimulation as a third signal required for activation of human naive B cells, *Eur. J. Immunol.*, **36**(4), 810–816.

52. Bossen, C. and Schneider, P. (2006) BAFF, APRIL and their receptors: structure, function and signaling, *Semin. Immunol.*, **18**(5), 263–275.

53. Woodland, R. T., Schmidt, M. R., and Thompson, C. B. (2006) BLyS and B cell homeostasis, *Semin. Immunol.*, **18**(6), 318–326.

54. Do, R. K. and Chen-Kiang, S. (2002) Mechanism of BLyS action and B cell immunity, *Cytokine Growth Factor Revs.*, **13**(1), 19–25.

55. Baker, K. P. (2004) BLyS – an essential survival factor for B cells: basic biology, links to pathology and therapeutic target, *Autoimmune Revs.*, **3**(5), 368–375.

56. Marsters, S. A., Yan, M., Pitti, R. M., Haas, P. E., Dixit, V. M., and Ashkenazi, A. (2000) Interaction of the TNF homologues BLyS and APRIL with the TNF receptor homologues BCMA and TACI, *Curr. Biol.*, **10**(13), 785–788.

57. Crowley, J. E., Treml, L. S., Stadanlick, J. E., Carpenter, E., and Cancro, M. P. (2005) Homeostatic niche specification among naïve and activated B cells: a growing role for the BLyS family of receptors and ligands, *Semin. Immunol.*, **17**(3), 193–199.

58. Yan, M., Ridgway, J., Chan, B., et al. (2001) Identification of a novel receptor for B lymphocyte stimulator that is mutated in a mouse strain with severe B cell deficiency, *Curr. Biol.*, **11**(19), 1547–1552.

59. Locksley, R. M., Killeen, N., and Lenardo, M. J. (2001) The TNF and TNF receptor superfamilies: integrating mammalian biology, *Cell*, **104**, 487–501.

60. Ware, C. F. (2000) APRIL and BAFF connect autoimmunity and cancer, *J. Exp. Med.*, **192**, F3–F38.

61. Ambrose, C. M. (2002) Baff-R, *J. Biol. Regul. Homeost. Agents*, **16**, 211–213.

62. Kalled, S. L. (2002) BAFF: a novel therapeutic target for autoimmunity, *Curr. Opin. Investig. Drugs*, **3**, 1005–1010.

63. Mackay , F. and Browning, J. L. (2002) BAFF: a fundamental survival factor for B cells, *Nat. Rev. Immunol.*, **2**, 465–475.

64. Nardelli, B., Moore, P. A., Li, Y., and Hilbert, D. M. (2002) B lymphocyte stimulator (BLyS): a therapeutic trichotomy for the treatment of B lymphocyte diseases, *Leuk. Lymphoma.*, **43**, 1367–1373.

65. Stohl, B. (2002) B lymphocyte stimulator protein levels in systemic lupus erythematosus and other diseases, *Curr. Rheumatol. Rep.*, **4**, 345–350.

66. Cancro, M. P. and Smith, S. H. (2003) Peripheral B cell selection and homeostasis, *Immunol Res.*, **27**, 141–148.

67. Carter, R. H. (2003) A role for BLyS in tissue inflammation? *Arthritis Rheum.*, **48**, 882–885.

68. Smith, S. H. and Cancro, M. P. (2003) BLyS: the pivotal determinant of peripheral B cell selection and lifespan, *Curr. Pharm. Des.*, **9**, 1833–1847.

69. Smith, S. H. and Cancro, M. P. (2003) Integrating B cell homeostasis and selection with BLyS, *Arch. Immunol. Ther. Exp. (Warsz)*, **51**, 209–218.

70. Mackay, F. and Ambrose, C. (2003) The TNF family members BAFF and APRIL: the growing complexity, *Cytokine Growth Factor Rev.*, **14**, 311–324.

71. Medema, J. P., Planelles-Carazo, L., Hardenberg, G., and Hahne, M. (2003) The uncertain glory of APRIL, *Cell Death Differ.*, **10**, 1121–1125.

72. Schneider, P. and Tschopp, J. (2003) BAFF and the regulation of B cell survival, *Immunol. Lett.*, **88**, 57–62.

73. Cancro, M. P. (2004) The BLyS family of ligands and receptors: an archetype for niche-specific homeostatic regulation, *Immunol. Rev.*, **202**, 237–249.

74. Cancro, M. P. (2004) Peripheral B-cell maturation: the intersection of selection and homeostasis, *Immunol. Rev.*, **197**, 89–101.

75. Mackay, F. and Tangye, S. G. (2004) The role of the BAFF/APRIL system in B cell homeostasis and lymphoid cancers, *Curr. Opin. Pharmacol.*, **4**, 347–354.

76. Stohl, W. (2004) Targeting B lymphocyte stimulator in systemic lupus erythematosus and other autoimmune rheumatic disorders, *Expert Opin. Ther. Targets*, **8**, 177–189.

77. Jelinek, D. F. and Darce, J. R. (2005) Human B lymphocyte malignancies: exploitation of BLyS and APRIL and their receptors, *Curr. Dir. Autoimmun.*, **8**, 266–288.

78. Kalled, S. L. (2005) The role of BAFF in immune function and implications for autoimmunity, *Immunol Rev.*, **204**, 43–54.

79. Mackay, F., Sierro, F., Grey, S. T. and Gordon, T. P. (2005) The BAFF/APRIL system: an important player in systemic rheumatic diseases, *Curr. Dir. Autoimmun.*, **8**, 243–265.

80. Noelle, R. J. and Erickson, L. D. (2005) Determinations of B cell fate in immunity and autoimmunity, *Curr. Dir. Autoimmun.*, **8**, 1–24.

81. Salzer, U. and Grimbacher, B. (2005) TACItly changing tunes: farewell to a yin and yang of BAFF receptor and TACI in humoral immunity? New genetic defects in common variable immunodeficiency, *Curr. Opin. Allergy Clin. Immunol.*, **5**, 496–503.

82. Schneider, P. (2005) The role of APRIL and BAFF in lymphocyte activation, *Curr. Opin. Immunol.*, **17**, 282–289.

83. Stohl, W. (2005) BlySfulness does not equal blissfulness in systemic lupus erythematosus: a therapeutic role for BLyS antagonists, *Curr. Dir. Autoimmun.*, **8**, 289–304.

84. Szodoray, P. and Jonsson, R. (2005) The BAFF/APRIL system in systemic autoimmune diseases with a special emphasis on Sjogren's syndrome, *Scand. J. Immunol.*, **62**, 421–428.

85. Moore, P. A., Belvedere, O., Orr, A., et al. (1999) BLyS: member of the tumor necrosis factor family and B lymphocyte stimulator, *Science*, **285**, 260–263.

86. Mukhopadhyay, A., Ni, J., Zhai, Y., Yu, G. L., and Aggarwal, B. B. (1999) Identification and characterization of a novel cytokine, THANK, a TNF homologue that activates apoptosis, nuclear factor-kappaB, and c-Jun NH2-terminal kinase, *J. Biol. Chem.*, **274**, 15978–15981.

87. Shu, H. B., Hu, W. H., and Johnson, H. (1999) TALL-1 is a novel member of the TNF family that is down-regulated by mitogens, *J. Leukoc. Biol.*, **65**, 680–683.

88. Schneider, P., MacKay, F., Steiner, V., et al. (1999) BAFF, a novel ligand of the tumor necrosis factor family, stimulates B cell growth, *J. Exp. Med.*, **189**, 1747–1756.

89. Kelly, K., Manos, E., Jensen, G., Nadauld, L., and Jones, D. A. (2000) APRIL/TRDL-1, a tumor necrosis factor-like ligand, stimulates cell death, *Cancer Res.*, **60**, 1021–1027.

90. Lopez-Fraga, M., Fernandez, R., Albar, J. P., and Hahne, M. (2001) Biologically active APRIL is secreted following intracellular processing in the Golgi apparatus by furin convertase, *EMBO Rep.*, **2**, 945–951.

91. Bossen, C., Ingold, K., Tardivel, A., et al. (2006) Interactions of tumor necrosis factor (TNF) and TNF receptor family members in the mouse and human, *J. Biol. Chem.*, **281**, 13964–13971.

92. Gavin, A. L., Duong, B., Skog, P., et al. (2005) DeltaBAFF, a splice isoform of BAFF, opposes full-length BAFF activity in vivo in transgenic mouse models, *J. Immunol.*, **175**, 319–328.

93. Gavin, A. L., Ait-Azzouzene, D., Ware, C. F., and Nemazee, D. (2003) DeltaBAFF, an alternate splice isoform that regulates receptor binding and biopresentation of the B cell survival cytokine, BAFF, *J. Biol. Chem.*, **278**, 38220–38228.

94. Roschke, V., Sosnovtseva, S., Ward, C. D., et al. (2002) BLyS and APRIL form biologically active heterotrimers that are expressed in patients with systemic immune-based rheumatic diseases, *J. Immunol.*, **169**, 4314–4321.

95. Yan, M., Marsters, S. A., Grewal, N., Wang, H., Ashkenazi, A., and Dixit, V. M. (2000) Identification of a receptor for BLyS demonstrates a crucial role in humoral immunity, *Nat. Immunol.*, **1**, 37–41.

96. Moreaux, J., Cremer, F. W., Reme, T., et al. (2005) The level of TACI gene expression in myeloma cells is associated with a signature of microenvironment dependence versus a plasmablastic signature, *Blood*, **106**(3), 1021–1030.

97. Yan, M., Brady, J. R., Chan, B., et al. (2001) Identification of a novel receptor for B lymphocyte stimulator that is mutated in a mouse strain with severe B cell deficiency, *Curr. Biol.*, **11**, 1547–1552.

98. Schiemann, B., Gommerman, J. L., Vora, K., et al. (2001) An essential role for BAFF in the normal development of B cells through a BCMA-independent pathway, *Science*, **293**, 2111–2114.

99. Hahne, M., Kataoka, T., Schroter, M., et al. (1998) APRIL, a new ligand of the tumor necrosis factor family, stimulates tumor cell growth, *J. Exp. Med.*, **188**, 1185–1190.

100. Hymowitz, S. G., Patel, D. R., Wallweber, H. J., et al. (2005) Structures of APRIL-receptor complexes: like BCMA, TACI employs only a single cysteine-rich domain for high affinity ligand binding, *J. Biol. Chem.*, **280**, 7218–7227.

101. von Bulow, G. U. and Bram, R. J. (1997) NF-AT activation induced by a CAML-interacting member of the tumor necrosis factor receptor superfamily, *Science*, **278**, 138–141.

102. Day, E. S., Cachero, T. G., Qian, F., et al. (2005) Selectivity of BAFF/BLyS and APRIL for binding to the TNF family receptors BAFFR/BR3 and BCMA, *Biochemistry*, **44**, 1919–1931.

103. Patel, D. R., Wallweber, H. J., Yin, J., et al. (2004) Engineering an APRIL-specific B cell maturation antigen, *J. Biol. Chem.*, **279**, 16727–16735.

104. Pelletier, M., Thompson, J. S., Qian, F., et al. (2003) Comparison of soluble decoy IgG fusion proteins of BAFF-R and BCMA as antagonists for BAFF, *J. Biol. Chem.*, **278**, 33127–33133.

105. Wu, Y., Bressette, D., Carrell, J. A., et al. (2000) Tumor necrosis factor (TNF) receptor superfamily member TACI is a high affinity receptor for TNF family members APRIL and BLyS, *J. Biol. Chem.*, **275**, 35478–35485.

106. Ingold, K., Zumsteg, A., Tardivel, A., et al. (2005) Identification of proteoglycans as the APRIL-specific binding partners, *J. Exp. Med.*, **201**, 1375–1383.

107. Xia, X. Z., Treanor, J., Senaldi, G., et al. (2000) TACI is a TRAF-interacting receptor for TALL-1, a tumor necrosis factor family member involved in B cell regulation, *J. Exp. Med.*, **192**, 137–143.

108. Hatzoglou, A., Roussel, J., Bourgeade, M. F., et al. (2000) TNF receptor family member BCMA (B cell maturation) associates with TNF receptor-associated factor (TRAF) 1, TRAF2, and TRAF3 and activates NF-kappa B, elk-1, c-Jun N-terminal kinase, and p38 mitogen-activated protein kinase, *J. Immunol.*, **165**, 1322–1330.

109. Claudio, E., Brown, K., Park, S., Wang, H., and Siebenlist, U. (2002) BAFF-induced NEMO-independent processing of NF-kappa B2 in maturing B cells, *Nat. Immunol.*, **3**, 958–965.

110. Kayagaki, N., Yan, M., Seshasayee, D., et al. (2002) BAFF/BLyS receptor 3 binds the B cell survival factor BAFF ligand through a discrete surface loop and promotes processing of NF-kappaB2, *Immunity*, **17**, 515–524.

111. Gordon, N. C., Pan, B., Hymowitz, S. G., et al. (2003) BAFF/BLyS receptor 3 comprises a minimal TNF receptor-like module that encodes a highly focused ligand-binding site, *Biochemistry*, **42**, 5977–5983.

112. Hatada, E. N., Do, R. K., Orlofsky, A., et al. (2003) NF-kappa B1 p50 is required for BLyS attenuation of apoptosis but dispensable for processing of NF-kappa B2 p100 to p52 in quiescent mature B cells, *J. Immunol.*, **171**, 761–768.

113. Roth, W., Wagenknecht, B., Klumpp, A., et al. (2001) APRIL, a new member of the tumor necrosis factor family, modulates death ligand-induced apoptosis, *Cell. Death Differ.*, **8**, 403–410.

114. Nardelli, B., Belvedere, O., Roschke, V., et al. (2001) Synthesis and release of B- lymphocyte stimulator from myeloid cells, *Blood*, **97**, 198–204.

115. Scapini, P., Nardelli, B., Nadali, G., et al. (2003) G-CSF-stimulated neutrophils are a prominent source of functional BLyS, *J. Exp. Med.*, **197**, 297–302.

116. Gorelik, L., Gilbride, K., Dobles, M., Kalled, S. L., Zandman, D., and Scott, M. L. (2003) Normal B cell homeostasis requires B cell activation factor production by radiation-resistant cells, *J. Exp. Med.*, **198**, 937–945.

117. Craxton, A., Magaletti, D., Ryan, E. J., and Clark, E. A. (2003) Macrophage- and dendritic cell-dependent regulation of human B-cell proliferation requires the TNF family ligand BAFF, *Blood*, **101**, 4464–4471.

118. Amanna, I. J., Dingwall, J. P., and Hayes, C. E. (2003) Enforced bcl-xL gene expression restored splenic B lymphocyte development in BAFF-R mutant mice, *J. Immunol.*, **170**(9), 4593–4600.

119. Schneider, P., Mackay, F., Steiner, V., et al. (1999) BAFF a novel ligand of the tumor necrosis factor family, stimulates B cell growth, *J. Exp. Med.*, **189**(11), 1747–1756.

120. Do, R. K., Hatada, E., Lee, H., Tourigny, M. R., Hilbert, D., and Chen-Kiang, S. (2000) Attenuation of apoptosis underlies B lymphocyte stimulator enhancement of humoral immune response, *J. Exp. Med.*, **192**(7), 953–964.

121. Chiu, A., Xu, W., He, B., et al. (2007) Hodgkin lymphoma cells express TACI and BCMA receptors and generate survival and proliferation signals in response to BAFF and APRIL, *Blood*, **109**(2), 729–739.

122. Fu, L., Lin-Lee, Y.-C., Pham, L. V., Tamayo, A., Yoshimura, L., and Ford, R. J. (2006) Constitutive NF-κB and NFAT activation leads to stimulation of the BLyS survival pathway in aggressive B-cell lymphomas, *Blood*, **107**, 4540–4548.

123. Novak, A. J., Grote, D. M., Stenson, M., et al. (2004) Expression of BLyS and its receptors in B-cell non Hodgkin lymphoma: correlation with disease activity and patient outcome, *Blood*, **104**(8), 2247–2253.

124. Moreaux, J., Legouffe, E., Jourdan, E., et al. (2004) BAFF and APRIL protect myeloma cells from apoptosis induced by interleukin 6 deprivation and dexamethasone, *Blood*, **103**(8), 3148–3157.

125. Ng, L. G., Sutherland, A. P., Newton, R., et al. (2004) B cell-activating factor belonging to the TNF family (BAFF)-R is the

principal BAFF receptor facilitating BAFF costimulation of circulating T and B cells, *J. Immunol.*, **173**(2), 807–817.

126. Groom, J., Kalled, S. L., Cutler, A. H., et al. (2002) Association of BAFF/BLyS overexpression and altered B cell differentiation with Sjogren's syndrome, *J. Clin. Invest.*, **109**(1), 59–68.

127. Zhang, J., Roschke, V., Baker, K. P., et al. (2001) Cutting edge: a role for B lymphocyte stimulator in systemic lupus erythematosus, *J. Immunol.*, **166**(1), 6–10.

128. Zhang, M., Ko, K. H., Lam, Q. L., et al. (2005) Expression and function of TNF family member B cell-activating factor in the development of autoimmune arthritis, *Int. Immunol.*, **17**(8), 1081–1092.

129. Lesley, R., Xu, Y., Kalled, S. L., et al. (2004) Reduced competitiveness of autoantigen-engaged B cells due to increased dependence on BAFF, *Immunity*, **20**(4), 441–453.

130. Thien, M., Phan, T. G., Gardam, S., et al. (2004) Excess BAFF rescues self-reactive B cells from peripheral deletion and allows them to enter forbidden follicular and marginal zone niches, *Immunity*, **20**(6), 785–798.

131. Liu, W., Szalai, A., Zhao, L., et al. (2004), Control of spontaneous B lymphocyte autoimmunity with adenovirus-encoded soluble TACI, *Arthritis Rheum.*, **50**(6), 1884–1896.

132. Riccobene, T. A., Miceli, R. C., Lincoln, C., et al. (2003) Rapid and specific targeting of 125I-labeled B lymphocyte stimulator to lymphoid tissues and B cell tumors in mice, *J. Nucl. Med.*, **44**(3), 422–433.

133. Baker, K. P., Edwards, B. M., Main, S. H., et al. (2003) Generation and characterization of LymphoStat-B, a human monoclonal antibody that antagonizes the bioactivities of B lymphocyte stimulator, *Arthritis Rheum.*, **48**(11), 3253–3265.

134. Hernando, E., Charytonowitz, E., Dudas, M. E., et al. (2007) The AKT-mTOR pathway plays a critical role in the development of leiomyosarcomas, *Nat. Med.*, **13**, 748–753.

135. Berns, A., van der Lugt, N., Alkema, M., et al. (1994) Mouse model systems to study multistep tumorigenesis, *Cold Spring Harb. Symp. Quant. Biol.*, **59**, 435–447.

Chapter 44

Transplantation

Transplantation of organs, tissues, and cells has become a powerful mode of treatment for dozens of life-threatening diseases affecting millions of people. Today, transplant surgeons routinely transplant more than 25 different organs and tissues to treat kidney failure, type 1 diabetes, leukemia, end-stage pulmonary disease, liver disorders, cardiovascular disease, and many other disorders (http://www3.niaid. nih.gov/research/topics/transplantation/introduction.htm).

However, two major impediments to successful transplantation still remain. The first of these is rejection by the host immune system. In this regard, recent research advances have provided a much clearer understanding of the immune mechanisms that cause graft rejection. These insights have, in turn, led to better therapies to suppress the immune system and thereby allow a graft to survive and function. As a result, 1-year graft survival rates have increased for all organs and tissues and, in many cases, now exceed 80%. But despite this improvement, long-term graft survival rates have not increased nearly as much (http://www3.niaid.nih. gov/research/topics/transplantation/introduction.htm).

The second barrier to wider use of transplantation is a critical shortage of donor organs and tissues. In the limited states alone, according to 2006 data (*The Organ Procurement and Transplantation Network* [Internet]; data available from www.optn.org/data), there are more than 90,000 candidates on waiting lists for organ transplantation: 66,200 for kidneys; 17,500 for livers; 2,500 for pancreas or combined kidney/pancreas transplants; 3,200 for hearts or heart-lung transplants; and 3,000 for lung transplants. This demand far outstrips the supply of donor organs in the United States. In 2005, 14,492 individuals were organ donors. Unfortunately, many candidates die while awaiting a suitable organ (http://www3.niaid.nih.gov/research/topics/transplantation/introduction.htm).

Immune-mediated graft rejection has a significant impact on the more than 20,000 patients in the United States who receive organ transplants each year. While newer immunosuppressive medications have significantly reduced the incidence of acute allograft rejection, chronic rejection and the risk of infection and malignancies continue to be a major impediment of clinical transplantation (http://www.immunetolerance.org/; ITN 2007 Annual Research Report).

Antigen Processing and Presentation in Transplantation. For many years, the *direct stimulation of T cells* in response to donor major histocompatibility complex (MHC) antigens expressed on donor antigen-presenting cells has been the focus of transplantation immunology *(1)*. Defined as the stimulation of T cell by the allogeneic MHC antigens on allogeneic antigen-presenting cells (APCs), direct T-cell stimulation will occur because of the similarity of allogeneic and self MHC molecules *(2)*. Because of this similarity, allogeneic MHC molecules are nearly unique among foreign proteins in that they do not require processing and presentation as peptides in order to stimulate a T-cell response *(3)*.

In contrast with direct T-cell stimulation, the natural physiologic mechanism for T-cell stimulation is for the T-cell receptors (TCRs) to recognize peptides of foreign proteins that have been processed by self APCs and presented by self MHC molecules *(1)*. In transplantation immunology, this physiologic response is known as *indirect presentation* even though this term fails to convey that this is the normal mechanism for T-cell stimulation.

The indirect recognition in response to peptides of donor antigens presented by self MHC molecules on recipient APCs has not generally been considered an important feature of graft rejection. However, further evidence has suggested that indirect responses may be more important than previously considered, and the new emphasis on indirect pathways in allograft rejection has raised new issues, many of which are still unresolved *(4)*.

The major histocompatibility antigens have the special feature that they can be recognized directly by TCRs, as well as to cause rapid graft rejection. As foreign proteins, however, their peptides can also be processed and presented by the MHC molecules on recipient APCs, thereby generating an indirect response *(1)*. Alternatively, the minor histocompatibility antigens represent peptides of donor proteins that can be processed and presented by self MHC molecules and recognized as foreign by the recipient APCs *(2, 3)*. As

V. St. Georgiev, *National Institute of Allergy and Infectious Diseases, NIH: Impact on Global Health*, vol. 2, DOI 10.1007/978-1-60327-297-1_44, © Humana Press, a part of Springer Science+Business Media, LLC 2009

compared with MHC antigens, however, the minor histocompatibility antigens cause much slower graft rejection. The difference in graft rejection between the MHC antigens and the minor histocompatibility antigens is still not well understood *(1)*. Nonetheless, the evidence of the importance of the indirect pathway for graft rejection and the evidence that matching for MHC antigens is important for graft survival have led to a concept: that MHC matching may be important primarily because of the importance of the MHC proteins in stimulating indirect T-cell responses rather than because of the importance of the direct recognition of intact MHC molecules *(1)*.

To study the role of the direct and indirect pathways in achieving tolerance, genetically altered mouse strains have been used in two ways: (i) MHC class II–deficient mice were used as donors of skin and cardiac grafts to eliminate the direct CD4$^+$ T-cell response; and (ii) B6 II-4^4 mice, which are MHC class II–deficient mice expressing an MHC class II transgene only on thymic epithelium, were used as recipients of normal grafts; these mice cannot mount an indirect response *(5)*. Eliminating the indirect pathway made it more difficult to achieve prolonged allograft survival when costimulatory blockade was used than when both pathways were available. Moreover, the costimulatory blockade was ineffective even when CD4$^+$ T-cells from normal animals were transferred into recipients that lacked MHC class II molecules. These results have suggested that an active CD4$^+$ response through the indirect pathway is necessary for the costimulatory blockade to be effective in prolonging allograft survival *(5)*.

The Importance of an Additional Gene in Matching Bone Marrow Transplants. Thousands of people are diagnosed each year with blood diseases, some of which may be deadly, such as leukemia, a form of cancer. The only cure for many people with leukemia is a bone marrow transplant from a genetically matched donor. Bone marrow contains blood stem cells that are the source of the body's blood and immune systems. The better matched the bone marrow, the greater the chance that the body will accept the transplant and the less likely the recipient will develop a common complication of bone marrow transplantation known as graft-versus-host disease (GVHD) in which the immune cells from the donor react to the recipient's cells and tissues. Unfortunately, finding genetically matched donors is very difficult (http://www3.niaid.nih.gov/healthscience/healthtopics/transplantation/additionalGene.htm).

Improved Criteria for Matching Donor and Recipient Tissue Type. Substantial progress has been made in defining the criteria for matching the donor and recipient tissue type for a successful bone marrow transplant. Modern tissue typing methods allow matching of the precise DNA sequence of human leukocyte antigen (HLA) genes (alleles) that play a major role in the immune system. When a transplant recip-

ient and donor share the same HLA alleles, the recipient is less likely to develop severe GVHD.

A fully matched bone marrow donor is an individual genetically matched for five specific alleles: human leukocyte antigen (HLA) -A, -B, -C, -DRB1, and -DQB1. In this regard, a study supported by NIAID has shown that knowing the matching status of an additional, sixth allele at HLA-DPB1 would provide additional information that will allow for more accurate assessment of the risks and benefits of the bone marrow transplant procedure *(6)*. The extent to which transplantation outcome may be improved with donor matching for HLA-DP is not well defined. The risks of acute GVHD (aGVHD), relapse, and mortality associated with HLA-DPB1 allele mismatching were determined in 5,929 patients who received a myeloablative hematopoietic stem cell transplantation (HCT) from an HLA-A-, HLA-B-, HLA-C-, HLA-DRB1-, and HLA-DQB1-matched or -mismatched donor. There was a statistically significantly higher risk of both grades 2 to 4 aGVHD [odds ratio (OR) = 1.33; $p < 0.001$] and grades 3 to 4 aGVHD (OR = 1.26; $p < 0.001$) after HCT from an HLA-DPB1-mismatched donor compared with a matched donor. The increased risk of aGVHD was accompanied by a statistically significantly decrease in disease relapse [hazard ratio (HR) = 0.82; $p = 0.01$]. HLA-DPB1 functions as a classic transplantation antigen. The increased risk of GVHD associated with HLA-DPB1 mismatching is accompanied by a lower risk of relapse. Knowledge of the DPB1 matching status prior to transplantation will aid in more precise risk stratification for the individual patient *(7)*.

44.1 Islet Transplantation

The goal of current treatments for type 1 diabetes is to establish a normalization of blood glucose levels—efficient glycemic control reduces the long-term risk of diabetes complications. Islet transplantation offers the prospect of efficient glycemic control without major surgical risks.

The Diabetes Control and Complications Trial (DCCT) *(8)*, the most definitive study to date, clearly showed that intensive insulin therapy may significantly reduce the risk of microvascular complications. However, the same therapy was found to be associated with a threefold increased risk of severe hypoglycemia. This study, and others, therefore provide the rationale for the development of improved methods to achieve glucose control (http://www.immunetolerance.org/research/islet/).

Whole-pancreas transplantation has become accepted as an alternative therapy for subjects who are undergoing simultaneous kidney transplants. Although rates of rejection are generally low—about 14% *(9,10)*—the significant risks associated with whole organ transplantation limit its use to co-transplantation with other organs. In addition to improving the ability of the medical community to control glycemia in patients with diabetes, the DCCT also provided a stronger rationale for the use of pancreas transplantation *(11)*. Worldwide, the 3-year organ-survival rate for simultaneous kidney and pancreas transplantation has been approximately 70% to 80% *(12)*, which is similar to the rates for most other types of organ transplantation. When successful, pancreas transplantation is particularly effective in patients with type 1 diabetes and autonomic insufficiency, who struggle with glycemic control, postural hypotension, gastroparesis, and diarrhea and have a dramatically shortened life span *(13,14)*. Pancreas transplantation is more likely to result in normal glycosylated hemoglobin levels than is the intensive insulin-based approach to management prescribed in the DCCT. Long-term studies of motor, sensory, and autonomic neuropathy have demonstrated that these complications stabilize after pancreas transplantation *(15)*, and native-kidney biopsies have shown a dramatic reversal of mesangial accumulation and basement-membrane thickening 10 years after the establishment of normal glucose levels by pancreas transplantation *(16)*. Macrovascular complications are also stabilized by pancreas transplantation *(17–19)*. Quality-of-life studies indicate that patients who undergo successful pancreas transplantation believe that the normalization of glucose levels and the freedom from daily insulin injections outweigh the problems caused by transplantation and its attendant immunosuppression *(20–24)*.

A report of allogenic islet cell transplantation in humans appeared in 1980, with the recipient achieving insulin independence with normal glucose levels at 9 months follow-up *(25)*. Reports of successful islet cell transplantation using conventional immunosuppression have appeared since, but insulin independence at 1 year was less than 10%. Interest in islet cell transplantation was reawakened in 2000 after a successful outcome in seven patients with type 1 diabetes mellitus using a glucocorticoid-free immunosuppression regimen *(26)*. The novel approach used fresh islets from multiple donors injected into the main portal vein on size-restricted, C-peptide–negative type 1 diabetic patients with hypoglycemic unawareness, using a steroid-free immunosuppression regimen that included daclizumab, sirolimus, and low-dose tacrolimus.

Islet transplantation is a much simpler and less costly procedure—it is a much less invasive procedure than whole-pancreas transplantation, and offers the hope that if performed earlier it will result in excellent glucose control and prevent long-term complications *(27, 28)*. Over the years, the technique has had a poor record of accomplishment in achieving independence from exogenous insulin—approximately 10% of subjects were off insulin at 1 year, although 37% may have continued C-peptide production *(29)*.

The Edmonton Protocol. In June 2000, the field of islet transplantation took a remarkable leap forward with the publication of the Edmonton Protocol, which resulted in 8 of 8 patients with stable islet function and no evidence of rejection, some more than a year posttransplant *(26)*. Although this method relies upon the use of life-long maintenance immunosuppression, the effectiveness of this protocol remains a significant advance over previous methods and is currently the gold-standard for beta-cell replacement therapies.

The Immune Tolerance Network (ITN) is currently conducting a multicenter clinical trial of the Edmonton Protocol at nine centers around the world *(30)*. The purposes of the trial have been several, namely, (i) to validate the technique in a multicenter environment; (ii) to establish a network of clinical centers well-trained in the techniques for islet isolation and preparation; and (iii) to provide a baseline measure to which trials of new tolerance therapies may be compared. Results from the trial have shown that of the 36 subjects, 16 (44%) met the primary end-point (insulin independence with adequate glycemic control 1 year after the final transplantation), 10 (28%) had partial function, and 10 (28%) had complete graft loss 1 year after the final transplantation. A total of 21 (58%) subjects attained insulin independence with good glycemic control at any point throughout the trial. Of these subjects, 16 (76%) required insulin again at 2 years; 5 of the 16 (31%) subjects who reached the primary end-point remained insulin-independent at 2 years. Taken as a whole, the results of the international trial have confirmed previous experiences with the Edmonton Protocol at single centers and demonstrated the reproducibility and benefits of islet-alone transplantation in patients who have type 1 diabetes mellitus with unstable glycemic control *(26,31–35)*. The trial succeeded in standardizing pancreas selection, islet processing, product-release criteria, recipient selection, and posttransplantation care under a Food and Drug Administration Investigational New Drug submission *(30)*.

The interpretation of these results has been complicated by the fact that the Edmonton trial design did not include a similar and concurrent control cohort *(11, 34)*. Because the observation period before transplantation was not as long or as intense as the observation period after transplantation, extensive paired analyses of pretransplantation and posttransplantation clinical data were not possible. Whether two islet infusions a month apart were essential is unresolved, as recipients were not randomly assigned to receive either one infusion or two. Relevant data from studies of autologous islet transplantation suggested that islets continually regain function up to 3 months after infusion *(36)*. Nonetheless, one can conclude that in the hands of the Edmonton group, islet transplantation was relatively safe and efficacious in eliminating the need for exogenous insulin and in preventing recurrent hypoglycemia, albeit at a cost of a roughly

10% incidence of liver bleeding related to the procedure. The initial graft survival rate of 80% with the use of islets from multiple donors compares favorably with that of successful pancreas transplantation *(37)* and successful autologous islet transplantation *(38)*. Whether or not the long-term survival of allografts will equal that of autologous grafts is still unknown. Autologous grafts can function successfully for many years after transplantation. A recipient of one such autologous graft was reported to have normal fasting glucose and glycosylated hemoglobin levels 13 years after transplantation *(39)* and is still remaining insulin-independent 16 years later. However, recipients of islet allografts face the additional risk of recurrent autoimmune diabetes *(40, 41)*, as well as of side effects from treatment with immunosuppressive drugs that are potentially lethal to beta cells.

While islet transplantation with the use of the Edmonton Protocol can successfully restore long-term endogenous insulin production and glycemic stability in subjects with type 1 diabetes mellitus and unstable control, the insulin independence was usually not sustainable. However, persistent islet function even without insulin independence provided both protection from severe hypoglycemia and improved the levels of glycated hemoglobin *(30)*.

Tolerance Protocols in Islet Transplantation. Whereas the Edmonton Protocol appears to be less nephrotoxic than standard cyclosporine and higher-dose tacrolimus-based regimens, even low-dose tacrolimus should be used with caution in the face of significant impairment in baseline renal reserve (as evidenced by an increased serum creatinine level). As well, the long-term effects of maintenance immunosuppression remain ill-defined, although it is generally believed to carry increased risks of infection and certain types of cancer. For this reason, the ITN has been actively pursuing protocols that seek to investigate tolerogenic protocols in islet transplantation. As an initial foray into tolerance protocols, the ITN is placing its current emphasis on protocols that use novel tolerogenic agents combined with short-term immunosuppressive therapy that will be withdrawn after approximately 1 year, should circumstances prove efficacious (http://www.immunetolerance.org/research/islet/).

Optimal Sites for Islet Infusion. The liver, spleen, kidney capsule, testes, brain, peritoneal cavity, and omentum have all been considered as potential sites of islet infusion *(11)*. The liver is by far the most commonly used site because of the early successes with autologous islet transplants. However, although autologous islets have been infused intraoperatively directly into the hepatic portal venous circulation under direct view, islet allografts are being infused percutaneously into the portal vein. Potential complications of an infusion into the liver include bleeding, portal venous thrombosis, and portal hypertension. Although portal blood pressure is monitored during the procedure and anticoagulant agents are used to prevent clotting, anticoagulation can

promote hepatic bleeding at the sites of the percutaneous needle punctures. Furthermore, intrahepatic islets may be exposed to environmental toxins and potentially toxic prescribed medications absorbed from the gastrointestinal tract and delivered into the portal vein. To this end, all commonly used immunosuppressive drugs have been reported to have adverse effects on pancreatic beta cells *(37,42–59)*. In addition, the antiproliferative effects of sirolimus may theoretically be disadvantageous both for angiogenesis in newly transplanted islets *(60, 61)* and for islet neogenesis from ductal stem cells *(62)*. Finally, intrahepatic islets are unable to release glucagon during hypoglycemia *(63–66)*. Yet, though intrahepatic islets fail to respond to hypoglycemia, they appear to contain healthy alpha cells that process and secrete glucagon, as indicated by their response to intravenous arginine *(63–65)*. Because not all recipients remain insulin-independent for the rest of their lives, they may become at risk for hypoglycemia and thus would benefit from having a glucagon response *(11)*.

In view of these problems, it is reasonable to consider the use of nonhepatic sites. It might also be possible to infuse unpurified islet preparations into nonhepatic sites, which would eliminate the trauma to and losses of islets caused by purification *(11)*. Potential alternative sites include the peritoneal cavity and omentum, both of which have been used successfully in animal models and shown to be safe for humans *(67, 68)*.

Immunosuppression in Islet Transplantation. The current success in whole-organ transplantation has been based on combination immunosuppression using calcineurin inhibitors and steroids *(69)*. The development of a steroid-free immunosuppression protocol using a combination of sirolimus and tacrolimus by the Edmonton Protocol group resulted in a notably improved outcome of islet cell transplantation and led to many transplant centers using this regimen. Whereas the combination of sirolimus and low-dose tacrolimus has helped move islet cell transplantation forward, these drugs are not ideal. Both drugs are acting by binding to FK binding protein (FKBP) receptors, have similar targets of distribution, and as a result have a number of adverse effects in islet recipients, including painful mouth ulceration, peripheral edema, proteinuria (sirolimus exerts an antiproliferative effect in renal tubular cells and may hinder recovery of an injured kidney), hypercholesterolemia, and hypertension *(70)*.

Although the majority of patients are being managed long-term on the sirolimus and tacrolimus combination, some may require conversion to mycophenolate mofetil (MMF) for side effects. Successful MMF conversion from sirolimus has resulted in improvements in pedal edema, mouth ulcers, and nephrotoxicity without compromising graft function. With anticipated progress in current clinical trials, it is likely that these immunosuppressive agents will be replaced by less toxic and more potent therapies in the future (69).

Although recurrent autoimmunity may play a role, results have shown that autoantibody levels did not correlate with the loss of insulin independence (30). Other studies have revealed a relationship between outcome and autoantibody status in both islet and whole-pancreas transplantation with previous, less potent immunosuppressive regimens (71–73). Most immunosuppressive drugs, including tacrolimus and sirolimus, are known to impair islet function (74–76). Prolonged exposure to these compounds, particularly in the portal-hepatic site, may enhance diabetogenic toxic effects (77, 78), underscoring a need for alternative islet delivery sites (79–81) and for more potent and less diabetogenic immunosuppressive therapy, including drugs with tolerance-inducing potential (80,82–85).

Role of Autoimmunity in Islet Allograft Destruction. Although it has often been assumed that transplanted allogeneic islets can be destroyed by recurrent autoimmunity in recipients with type 1 diabetes, until recently definitive evidence has been lacking, and the settings in which this may occur have not been defined. In experiments to address these issues, the survival of islet transplants (subject to tissue-specific autoimmunity) were compared with cardiac transplants (not subject to tissue-specific autoimmunity) from major histocompatibility complex (MHC)-matched and -mismatched donors transplanted into autoimmune NOD mice recipients (86). The results have shown that when recipients have been treated with combined B7 and CD154 T-cell costimulatory blockade, hearts survived best with better MHC matching, whereas islet survived worst when the donor and the recipient shared MHC class antigens. In the absence of full or MHC class II matching, there was no difference in the survival of islet and cardiac allografts. Furthermore, the tendency of the NOD mice to resist tolerance induction by costimulation blockade has been mediated by both $CD4^+$ and $CD8^+$ T-cells, not directly linked to the presence of autoimmunity, and conferred by non-MHC background genes. Taken together, these findings would have clinical importance because under certain circumstances, avoiding MHC class II sharing may provide better islet allograft survival in recipients with autoimmune diabetes because mismatched allogeneic islets may be resistant to recurrent autoimmunity (86).

Current Clinical Results. After the success of the Edmonton steroid-free immunosuppression protocol, more than 43 institutions worldwide have transplanted at least 470 patients up to May 2005 (69). The American Transplant Congress in June 2003 reported on these patients with a median follow-up of 9 months (31, 32). A 90% insulin-free rate was demonstrated in three centers (Edmonton, Minneapolis, and Miami) with long-standing experience in the field, and the average rate of insulin independence among the remaining six sites

was 23%. Twelve patients achieved insulin independence (five achieving insulin independence after one infusion, five after two infusions, and two patients required three infusions). The overall success rate, in terms of insulin independence, was 52% (69).

The rates of insulin independence achieved currently vary widely, with experienced centers achieving insulin independence in more than 80% of recipients while those with less experience have achieved insulin independence in 0 to 63% at a short-term follow-up (69).

During the posttransplant period, there appeared to be a progressive loss of insulin independence over time, leaving 50% of patients insulin-free at 3 years. A recent report suggested that although insulin independence wanes with time, 83% of patients demonstrated islet function at 5 years when assessed by C-peptide secretion (87). Furthermore, the HbA1c level was well controlled in those patients off insulin (6.4%; range, 6.1% to 6.7%) and in those back on insulin but C-peptide-positive (6.7%, range, 5.9% to 7.5%), and higher in those patients who lost all graft function (9.0%, range, 6.7% to 9.3%) ($p < 0.05$). Those patients who resumed insulin therapy did not appear more insulin-resistant compared with those off insulin and required half their pretransplant insulin dose. However, they had a lower increment of C-peptide to a standard meal challenge [mean (SD) 0.44 (0.06) vs. 0.76 (0.06) nmol/L, $p < 0.001$] (87).

Furthermore, there has been clear improvement in symptom control and metabolic stability. Thus, in a recent report of islet transplantation compared with whole-pancreas transplantation in renal transplant recipients, diabetic control was no different at 3 years between the groups, despite return to insulin therapy in many of the islet recipients (88).

Potential reasons for the decay in rates of insulin independence include chronic allograft rejection, undiagnosed acute rejection, local islet cell toxicity from immunosuppressive drugs, recurrent autoimmunity, intercurrent infection, and failure of islet cells to regenerate (69).

With the momentum created by the Edmonton Protocol, currently islet cell transplantation is being performed more widely (89–91). The challenge is to continue to improve early results and to try to sustain cell function long term. An in-depth study of factors influencing the decay in islet function is looking at serial islet graft biopsies, serologic analysis of donor sensitization, cytokine gene activity (granzyme B), and changes in autoantibody status and T-lymphocyte function, and should provide valuable information over time (69).

The inability to diagnose early rejection in cell transplantation remains a problem, particularly with islets (92–94). The relatively small mass of cells transplanted means that there is a small functional reserve, and it is unlikely that sufficient islets survive a single episode of acute rejection. Newer immunosuppressive therapies may help to suppress acute rejection, such as LEA29Y, a costimulatory signal blocker found to be highly effective in primate trials that is currently being evaluated *(94)*. FTY720, a lymphocyte homing agent, is effective in controlling autoimmunity in NOD mice and in promoting marginal mass islet transplants in primates and is due for evaluation in several centers shortly *(95)*.

The ultimate goal, however, remains *the induction of tolerance*. Current regimens *(96)* are using a combination of anti-thymocyte globulin and rituximab (anti-CD20). The non–Fc-binding HOKT3γ1(Ala-Ala) antibody *(97)* has been effective in abrogating autoimmunity in new-onset diabetes and has facilitated single-donor islet transplant success in ongoing trials *(69)*. A potent, diphtheria-conjugated anti-CD3 immunotoxin combined with deoxyspergualin has also shown robust tolerance induction in a series of primates; the results of these experiments are awaiting evaluation in humans *(69)*.

44.1.1 Xenotransplantation

The shortage of human islets for transplantation is likely to become even more dramatic, as success in clinical protocols and the number of procedures performed increases *(98, 99)*. Alternative sources of insulin-producing tissue are needed, and xenogeneic islets might represent a viable alternative to human islets. Although there has been substantial progress in the current knowledge of the mechanisms of xenogeneic islet recognition and rejection, there are many immunologic hurdles that still need to be addressed *(99)*. Thus, recent studies have shown that pig islets are rejected by CD4$^+$ T-lymphocytes activated via the indirect pathway of antigen recognition *(100)*, and that pig islets were protected from autoimmune recognition in NOD mice after treatment with anti-CD4 antibodies, contributing to elucidation of the mechanisms of islet-specific autoimmune aggression in a xenogeneic combination *(101)*. It was further suggested that encapsulation might work in a remarkable manner, as it does in allografts, in xenogeneic islet transplantation *(102)*. In support of this report has been the observation that pig islet function and survival did improve after encapsulation and culture preconditioning *(103)*. In another study, the transplant of encapsulated pig islets into dogs was carried out using an agarose-polystyrene mixed gel for prolonged graft survival in the absence of immunosuppression and was successful in a sizable percentage of pancreatectomized recipients *(104)*.

Although there is still debate on the impact of the α-galactosyltransferase (α-Gal) epitope on occurrence of islet xenograft rejection, the recent availability of α-Gal knockout pigs will help to definitively address its role *(105)*.

In all patients who had received xenografts, these experiments have been failures in the sense that long-term organ survival was not achieved, although they were able to show that xenogeneic tissue is able to support human life for a period of time. Rejection of xenogeneic tissue was both humoral and cellular and was more difficult to control than allograft rejection, although in the short term, it could be controlled with conventional immunosuppressants, albeit in large doses *(99)*.

Over and above the immunologic and physiologic barriers to xenotransplantation, clinical xenotransplantation raised a number of other issues. They include the rights of humans to use animals to suit their best interests, particularly in the case of primate donors; concerns about the possibility of transmission of xenotransplant-associated zoonoses to recipients under immunosuppression; ethical questions regarding the rights of patients, and the performance of extreme medical interventions, in those with reduced life expectancy. Although it is important that these concerns be addressed when considering clinical xenotransplantation, there are however other fundamental reasons for not yet performing this procedure. These include a lack of sufficient data in support of long-term engraftment, the considerable immunosuppression required to prevent rejection of xenogeneic tissue, and the inability to select appropriate recipients from those currently awaiting allotransplantation *(99)*. Thus, the obstacles to clinical xenotransplantation remain primarily scientific and logistical, rather than ethical.

At present, the greatest barrier to successful xenotransplantation in humans is early and aggressive rejection, which appears to be mediated by humoral mechanisms *(106)*.

Xenogeneic transplants may be classified as either concordant or discordant. Concordant species are those that are phylogenetically closely related; recipients do not have natural antibodies against donor antigens. Nonetheless, organs from concordant species are rejected more rapidly than allogeneic organs, apparently by humoral mechanisms. Discordant species are phylogenetically widely removed and are characterized by the presence of natural antibodies in the recipient serum that act against donor antigens, even in the absence of prior sensitization. These natural antibodies cause hyperacute rejection to occur in most primarily vascularized organs within minutes of transplantation *(107)*.

Natural antibodies appear to be derived primarily from a population of CD5-expressing B cells *(106)*. The reason for their presence in recipient serum is not entirely clear, but they are probably directed against bacterial epitopes that cross-react with antigens present on discordant donor endothelium. They may also help prevent autosensitization or aid in the clearing of senescent cells from the circulation *(108)*.

Rejection by Humoral Mechanisms. Humoral mechanisms in xenotransplantation result in either hyperacute or acute (also called accelerated or vascular) rejection. Hyperacute rejection is characterized by vascular thrombotic occlusion in discordant xenografts in which natural antibody is present. Accelerated rejection occurs in concordant grafts after antibody production is induced in the recipient and is characterized by an occlusive endothelialitis *(106)*.

The vascular endothelium is the target for most humoral rejection. Therefore, immediately vascularized organs, such as kidney and heart, are more susceptible to this response than are neovascularized organs (e.g., skin and pancreatic islets), which have an ingrowth of recipient endothelium *(106)*.

Cell-Mediated Xenograft Rejection. Progress in overcoming hyperacute and delayed xenograft rejection makes it important to understand the mechanisms of cell-mediated rejection in xenogeneic transplantation *(109)*. In this regard, studies in small animals did confirm that the strength of this rejection depended on a CD4-mediated indirect response. Although these studies have generally shown the similarity of this xenogeneic response to a human allogeneic response, molecular incompatibilities between humans and pigs that have an effect on the nature of the xeno-reaction have been identified. Research aimed to genetically engineer pigs to correct these molecular incompatibilities or to achieve supraphysiologic downregulation of cell-mediated immunity has been initiated but is in an early stage of development *(109)*.

44.2 Solid-Organ Transplantation

Currently, transplantation of a solid organ incurs a lifelong burden of immunosuppression for the recipient. In spite of many advances including the development of new agents, the basic premises of immunosuppression strategies remain unchanged and, as such, substantial metabolic, infectious, and neoplastic complications continue to threaten the recipient's life and well-being.

Several reports have, however, shown that a significant proportion of liver recipients (19% to 42%) can maintain normal allograft function without immunosuppression (i.e., the definition of functional tolerance). Although drug weaning in these studies did precipitate rejection in some recipients, the vast majority of episodes were graded as mild or moderate, were easily reversed, and did not result in long-term consequences *(110)*.

Clinical trials in liver and renal transplantation are closely related to those performed in islet transplant recipients (http://www.immunetolerance.org/). Efforts by the Immune Tolerance Network (ITN) and supported by the NIH/NIAID (http://www.nature.com/nm/journal/v5/n5/full/nm0599_470. html) are under way to test potential tolerance induction strategies against the backdrop of maintenance immunosuppression that does not include calcineurin inhibitors. Combination therapies including the use of hematopoietic stem cells chimerization are a key focus of the ITN (http://www.immunetolerance.org/).

44.2.1 *Immune Tolerance in Solid-Organ Transplantation*

Long-term results of organ transplantation remain unsatisfactory, mainly because of chronic rejection and complications associated with immunosuppressive medications *(111, 112)*. Immune tolerance, which has been achieved in animal models, might provide a means for avoiding both of these problems. However, the results of attempts to extend such studies from laboratory animals to humans have been disappointing *(113–117)*.

Immune tolerance of organ transplants has been induced in laboratory animals when persistent mixed blood and immune-cell chimerism has been achieved by infusing hematopoietic cells from the organ donor before or after transplantation of the organ *(118–130)*. The continued presence of the organ donor's immune cells in the recipient's thymus and peripheral lymphoid tissue promotes and maintains immune tolerance by eliminating T-cell clones that can react to alloantigens of the graft *(118–130)*.

Tolerance of allografts has been induced in mice *(118, 119)* and larger animals *(119)* by first transplanting hematopoietic stem cells from the prospective donor into the recipient, thereby creating a *lymphohematopoietic chimera* in which donor and recipient hematopoiesis coexist ("*mixed chimera*") *(120, 131)*.

Complete hematopoietic chimerism classically occurs in bone marrow transplantation, during which all bone marrow–derived cells in the recipient are eliminated and replaced by donor cells *(132)*. Partial or mixed chimerism in bone marrow transplantation occurs when milder forms of preconditioning are used, which initially do not completely ablate the host hematopoietic system *(132)*. Microchimerism, or donor T-cell chimerism, is common after liver transplantation, but it usually disappears within the first 3 weeks *(133)*. The effect of microchimerism in recipients of solid-organ transplants is uncertain, with reported findings ranging from correlation with graft acceptance and tolerance *(134)* to no influence on either tolerance *(132, 135)* or the prevention of rejection *(136, 137)*. Complete hematopoietic chimerism and tolerance of a liver allograft from a deceased male donor developed in a 9-year-old girl, with no evidence of graft-versus-host disease 17 months after transplantation *(138)*. The tolerance was preceded by a period of severe hemolysis, reflecting partial chimerism that was refractory to standard therapies. The hemolysis resolved after the gradual withdrawal of all immunosuppressive therapy. The patient remains well 5 years after transplantation without receiving any immunosuppressive therapy for 4 years, and liver-function tests are normal. A repeat liver biopsy has not been performed because it has not been indicated clinically. The patient has never had any dermatologic or gastrointestinal symptoms to suggest graft-versus-host disease *(138)*.

The achievement of central tolerance has been a major goal of transplantation research, but in clinical practice, it has been limited by the development of severe graft-versus-host disease and complications related to induction regimens *(138)*. In a patient who had received an HLA-identical bone marrow transplant, subsequent successful liver transplantation from the same donor, with discontinuation of immunosuppressive therapy, was reported *(139)*. The use of non-myeloablative conditioning and stem-cell infusion, followed by receipt of a liver transplant from a living related donor, has also resulted in various levels of chimerism and tolerance after transplantation, although graft-versus-host disease usually precludes the withdrawal of immunosuppressive therapy *(140)*. Graft-versus-host disease has also been reported to be a major complication of donor hematopoiesis occurring spontaneously after liver transplantation, resulting in either death of the patient *(140)* or disease requiring ongoing immunosuppressive therapy *(141–143)*. Furthermore, certain immune changes in peripheral blood may predispose liver-transplant recipients to "operational tolerance" *(144)*.

It has been proposed that all outcomes of organ or bone marrow transplantation are determined by the balance between the number of leukocytes that travel to lymphoid organs and the number of donor-specific T cells produced at those sites *(145, 146)*. The movement of donor leukocytes between lymphoid and nonlymphoid compartments in the recipient would govern both the responsiveness and unresponsiveness to the allograft *(145–147)*. Furthermore, it has been proposed that the mechanisms of immune reactivity and nonreactivity, their regulation by leukocyte migration and localization, and potential means of therapeutic manipulation can be generalized *(146, 147)*. The relationship of transplantation to the immunologic aspects of infection, oncology, and other fields has been obscured, however, by the characteristic double-immune reaction of transplantation. In this reaction, the responses of donor and recipient immune cells, each to the other, result in reciprocal clonal expansion followed by mutual clonal deletion *(145–147)*. If this process does not occur, the result is rejection or graft-versus-host disease *(145)*.

44.2.2 Liver Transplantation

Liver transplantation is among the more permissive indications for tolerance, and the risk of failure is diminished by the liver's inherent ability to regenerate and the lack of long-term implications of acute rejection episodes. It has been estimated that perhaps 20% to 30% of liver transplant recipients

might be safely withdrawn from immunosuppression without graft rejecting (http://www.immunetolerance.org/).

Total withdrawal of immunosuppression (TIW) without causing rejection has been reported in some stable liver recipients *(148–150)*. Patient characteristics that predict this clinical tolerance have not been determined. Ursodeoxycholic acid (UDCA) has been reported to reduce the risk of early graft rejection after hepatic and cardiac transplantation *(151)*. A double-blind controlled trial of UDCA therapy followed by TIW in 26 liver recipients has been conducted to determine whether UDCA would facilitate TIW; to assess the safety of attempting TIW; and to determine predictors of success of TIW *(152)*. All patients had been free of rejection for a minimum of 2 years, and on single or double drug immunosuppression, with transaminase levels <1.5 times the upper limit of normal. UDCA (15 mg/kg) or identical placebo capsule was administered, followed by sequential withdrawal of azathioprine (AzA) or prednisone and then graded reduction in cyclosporin A (CyA) dose. End-points were defined as graft dysfunction (alanine aminotransferase >2 times normal) with biopsy confirmation of abnormalities, or 6 months of no immunosuppression and no rejection on repeated biopsy. Rescue therapy for rejection was reinstitution of previous treatment, bolus steroid treatment with tapering, or conversion to tacrolimus-based therapy. The UDCA and placebo groups had similar baseline characteristics. Rejection episodes occurred in 6 of 14 (43%) patients in the UDCA group and in 9 of 12 (75%) of those on placebo ($p = 0.09$). Time to rejection, degree of rejection (blind biopsy review), and immunosuppression at the time rejection developed were similar in the two groups. All patients responded to rescue therapy; none developed chronic rejection. All rejection episodes developed during CyA tapering, with a mean daily dose of 105 mg with whole blood levels <50 ng/mL in all patients. The trial results have shown that late total immunosuppression withdrawal in stable liver transplant recipients is safe but seldom successful and most useful for patients transplanted for alcoholic liver disease and not for patients transplanted for autoimmune liver disease. It has been suggested that the search for an accurate means of identifying allograft tolerance among immunosuppressed recipients should become a priority in liver transplantation *(152)*.

Liver and Kidney Transplantations in HIV-Infected Patients. Organ failure is a significant problem for patients with human immunodeficiency virus infection in the current era of effective highly active antiretroviral therapy (HAART) *(153–155)*. Improvements in HIV-associated morbidity and mortality have made it difficult to deny solid-organ transplantation to this population based on futility arguments alone *(156)*. However, concerns that posttransplant immunosuppression may result in accelerated HIV disease progression have limited the availability to a small number of transplant centers. Despite the need for transplantation, the safety and efficacy of this intervention in HIV-infected recipients is still not known *(157)*.

Transplantation outcomes in the pre-HAART era were generally poor *(158–162)*. More contemporary retrospective analyses, case reports, and small prospective studies have suggested that patient and graft survival in selected HIV-infected patients may be similar to those seen in HIV-uninfected patients *(163–169)*. Although there have been no reports of significant HIV disease progression, allograft rejection rates have been unexpectedly high *(167, 170)*.

A recent prospective, nonrandomized study has described the patient, graft, and HIV-related outcomes of a prospective cohort of both kidney and liver recipients followed for over 3 years in the HAART era *(157)*. Eleven liver and 18 kidney transplant recipients were followed for a median of 3.4 years [interquartile range (IQR) 2.9 to 4.9]. One- and 3-year liver recipients' survival was 91% and 64%, respectively; kidney recipients' survival was 94%. One- and 3-year liver graft survival was 82% and 64%, respectively; kidney graft survival was 83%. Kidney patient and graft survival were similar to the general transplant population, and liver survival was similar to the older population, based on 1999–2004 transplants in the national database (The Organ Procurement and Transplantation Network Survival Database). CD4 T-cell counts and HIV RNA levels were stable; and there were two opportunistic infections. The 1- and 3-year cumulative incidence [95% confidence intervals (CI)] of rejection episodes for kidney recipients was 52% (28% to 75%) and 70% (48% to 92%), respectively. Two-thirds of hepatitis C virus–infected patients, but no patient with hepatitis B virus infection, recurred. Good transplant and HIV-related outcomes among kidney transplant recipients, and reasonable outcomes among liver recipients have indicated that transplantation is an option for selected HIV-infected patients cared for at centers with adequate expertise *(157)*.

Pediatric Liver Transplantation. A study of gradual and complete immunosuppression withdrawal *(171, 172)* is being conducted in a highly selected subgroup of liver transplant recipients: those who underwent living donor liver transplantation as a child (<18 years of age) 4 or more years ago for diseases other than viral hepatitis and autoimmune liver disorders and who continue to have excellent graft function *(173)* (http://www.immunetolerance. org/research/solidorgan/trials/feng.html). For selection, candidates had been meticulously assessed for willingness and appropriateness to participate. Consent was then obtained from both the liver donor and the liver recipient. It is anticipated that enrollees will typically enter on a minimalistic regimen, such that gradual withdrawal according to protocol can be achieved over 6 to 12 months. During and immediately after the weaning, recipients will be closely monitored to ensure expeditious recognition, diagnosis, and, if

necessary, treatment of liver dysfunction. The primary clinical end-points of the trial have been the efficacy and safety of immunosuppression withdrawal in this select subgroup of liver transplant recipients. Therefore, analyses will target the success rate of primary or secondary withdrawal, the duration for which recipients remain off of immunosuppression, the overall incidence of rejection, the incidence of severe and/or refractory rejection, and the timing of rejection.

This study would also encompass a complementary scientific effort to identify, quantify, and characterize donor-specific immune responses and immunologic interactions that may predict or correlate with functional tolerance. The clinical protocol, which did segregate study recipients into tolerant and intolerant groups, has been designed to provide serial cell and tissue specimens before, during, and after withdrawal for immediate as well as future mechanistic testing through ITN core facilities *(173)*.

To examine outcomes and identify prognostic factors affecting survival after pediatric liver transplantation, data from 246 children who underwent a second liver transplantation (rLT) between 1996 and 2004 were analyzed from the SPLIT registry, a multicenter database currently composed of 45 North American pediatric liver transplant programs *(174)*. The main causes for loss of primary graft necessitating rLT were primary nonfunction, vascular complications, chronic rejection, and biliary complications. Three-month, 1- and 2-year patient survival rates were inferior after rLT (74%, 67%, and 65%) compared with primary LT (92%, 88%, and 85%, respectively). Multivariate analysis of pretransplant variables revealed donor age less than 1 year, use of a technical variant allograft, and international normalized ratio (INR) at time of rLT as independent predictive factors for survival after rLT. Survival of patients who underwent early rLT (ErLT, <30 days after LT) was poorer than for those who received rLT >30 days after LT (late rLT, LrLT): 3-month, 1- and 2-year patient survival rates 66%, 59%, and 56% versus 80%, 74%, and 61%, respectively, log-rank $p = 0.0141$. Taken together, the results of the study have indicated that liver retransplantation in children is associated with decreased survival compared with primary LT, particularly in the clinical settings of those patients requiring ErLT *(174)*.

Rejection and infection are important adverse events after pediatric liver transplantation with infection risk far exceeding that of rejection, which causes limited harm to the patient or graft, particularly in infants *(175)*. In this regard, an aggressive infection control, attention to modifiable factors such as pretransplant nutrition and donor organ options, and rigorous age-specific review of the risk/benefit of choice and intensity of immunosuppressive regimes is warranted. Analysis of data, derived from the largest cumulative data set of pediatric liver transplants available, has described outcomes and risk factors in relation to rejection and infection, both being important and potentially inter-related adverse events after liver transplantation. There is no similar concurrent analysis with which to compare these data, which provide a broad view of outcomes across centers in North America, although earlier less focused analyses from the same database stimulated this concurrent study *(175)*.

Rejection has rarely contributed to and was not a risk factor in mortality, and the risk of graft failure from rejection was low, limited to chronic or recurrent rejection, which in itself was uncommon. Single episodes of rejection and rejection in the first 6 months were not predictors of graft failure, suggesting that acute cellular rejection was almost always treatable. In contrast, infection was the most common cause of death and clearly caused much more morbidity than rejection. Young age was an important risk factor for infections, but a negative risk factor for rejection, and infants had half the rate of rejection, three times the rate of bacterial or fungal infection, and 10 times the rate of Epstein-Barr virus–related posttransplant lymphoproliferative disease (PTLD) compared with those for adolescents *(175)*.

44.2.3 Kidney Transplantation

Research experiments have shown that a nonmyeloablative perioperative regimen induced mixed chimerism and tolerance of renal allografts in MHC-mismatched cynomolgus monkeys *(120–123)*. Subsequent studies have demonstrated the clinical feasibility of this approach in recipients of HLA-matched kidneys *(124–126)*. Later, when extended to HLA-mismatched donor-recipient combinations, the outcome has been the first report of a stable renal-allograft function for 2.0 to 5.3 years after complete withdrawal of immunosuppressive drugs in four recipients *(127)*. Though the mechanism responsible for stable graft function without exogenous immunosuppressive therapy in these four recipients is still under investigation, in studies in mice the immune tolerance that followed the induction of chimerism by bone marrow transplantation has been associated with elimination of cells in the thymus that are reactive to donor antigen (called "*central deletion*"). The specific loss of *in vitro* reactivity of the recipient's T cells against the donor's cells in all four of these patients has been consistent with this mechanism, but several other mechanisms are also possible *(127)*.

A recent report has described a recipient of combined kidney and hematopoietic-cell transplants from an HLA-matched donor *(176)*. A posttransplantation conditioning regimen of total lymphoid irradiation and antithymocyte globulin allowed engraftment of the donor's hematopoietic cells. The patient had persistent mixed chimerism, and the function of the kidney allograft has been normal for more than 28 months since discontinuation of all immunosuppressive drugs. Adverse events requiring hospitalization were limited to a 2-day episode of fever with neutropenia. The patient has had neither rejection episodes nor clinical manifestations of graft-versus-host disease *(176)*.

44.3 NIAID Involvement in Transplantation

44.3.1 Immune-Mediated Graft Rejection

To further improve both short- and long-term graft survival, NIAID is supporting a broad portfolio of basic research in transplantation immunology, as well as preclinical evaluation and clinical trials of promising posttransplant therapies (http://www3.niaid.nih.gov/research/topics/transplantation/research_areas/immune-mediated.htm).

The major goals of the NIAID transplantation research program are

- To understand the pathways whereby the immune system recognizes transplanted organs, tissues, and cells; to characterize the cellular and molecular components of acute rejection and chronic graft failure
- To evaluate novel therapies for treating rejection and prolonging graft survival in preclinical models
- To develop and implement strategies for immune tolerance induction
- To conduct clinical trials of new therapies to improve graft survival while minimizing the toxic side effects of immunosuppressive drugs

Kidney transplantation, which is the preferred therapy for end-stage renal disease, accounts for 59% of all solid-organ transplants. *The Cooperative Clinical Trials in Pediatric Transplantation (CCTPT)* program was established in 1994 to support multicenter clinical trials of new ways to prevent graft rejection in pediatric kidney transplant patients, evaluate changes in drug regimens intended to limit side effects of immunosuppression, and assess pretransplant immunotherapies. Ongoing CCTPT clinical trials include an evaluation of the immunosuppressive drug sirolimus for chronic graft failure and a study of the effects of steroid withdrawal in pediatric transplant recipients. CCTPT also conducts immunologic studies to determine how these various interventional approaches affect the immune system.

In a recent development, NIAID collaborated with the National Institute of Diabetes and Digestive and Kidney Diseases (NIDDK) and the National Heart, Lung, and Blood Institute (NHLBI) to establish a clinical consortium intended to improve the success of organ transplants. The goals of the consortium are to identify genetic factors in patients that could help clinicians: (i) to predict transplant outcomes, as well as responses to posttransplant therapy; (ii) to develop diagnostic tests that enable early detection and ongoing monitoring of immune-related processes; and (iii) to test the safety and effectiveness of new, less toxic immunosuppressive drugs.

NIAID and NIDDK also cooperatively established the *Genomics of Transplantation Cooperative Research Program* to support interdisciplinary, large-scale genomic studies in clinical transplantation. The goals of the program are to understand the genetic factors that affect immune-mediated graft rejection and to provide a rational basis for the development of more effective strategies for long-term graft survival (http://www3.niaid.nih.gov/research/topics/ transplantation/research_areas/immune-mediated.htm).

Patients with HIV infection are at high risk for end-stage organ disease. Before the advent of highly active antiretroviral therapy (HAART), patients with HIV were generally not considered for transplants because of their poor prognosis. HAART, however, has improved the outlook for HIV-positive patients so that many more HIV-positive patients with end-stage kidney and liver disease are potential transplant candidates. In 2003, NIAID has launched a clinical trial of the safety and efficacy of kidney and liver transplantation in patients with HIV (see Section 44.2.2).

44.3.2 Induction of Immune Tolerance

The drug regimens that suppress a patient's immune system usually can prevent graft rejection, but they also cause serious side effects such as infections and malignancies. Transplant immunologists, therefore, hope to develop treatments that can both reduce these risks and improve graft survival. One promising alternative is to selectively modify the immune response to establish tolerance to the graft while leaving protective immune responses intact. In 2003, in collaboration with NIDDK, NIAID renewed and expanded the *Nonhuman Primate Immune Tolerance Cooperative Study Group*. This program is evaluating novel regimens intended to induce transplant tolerance in animal models. Scientists working in the study group have already demonstrated that kidney and islet transplant patients given tolerogenic regimens have increased long-term graft acceptance. In 2005, the program has been expanded to include heart and lung transplantation. To accelerate the research conducted through this program, NIAID is also supporting breeding colonies of rhesus and cynomolgus monkeys (http://www3.niaid.nih.gov/research/topics/transplantation/research_areas/induction.htm).

With cosponsorship from NIDDK and the Juvenile Diabetes Research Foundation International (JDRF), NIAID supports the *Immune Tolerance Network (ITN)*, an international consortium of more than 80 investigators in the United States, Canada, Europe, and Australia. Since its inception, ITN has established a variety of state-of-the-art core facilities, initiated more than 20 clinical protocols, and funded several basic science studies of the mechanisms of induced immune tolerance (www.immunetolerance.org).

44.3.3 Shortage of Donor Organs

The number of organ transplants performed in the United States has increased dramatically, from 12,619 in 1988 to 28,110 in 2005. These numbers would be even higher if more donor organs were available; the waiting list for transplants has quadrupled since 1988 (http://www3.niaid.nih.gov/research/topics/transplantation/introduction.htm).

NIAID is addressing this problem by supporting efforts to improve donor registries that identify potential donors and by developing educational initiatives to increase public understanding of organ donation, especially among minority populations (http://www3.niaid.nih.gov/research/topics/transplantation/research_areas/donor_organs.htm).

In 2005, NIAID, with cosponsorship from the National Institute of Neurological Disease and Stroke (NINDS), started funding research cooperative agreements under the new program *Human Leukocyte Antigen (HLA) Region Genetics in Immune-Mediated Diseases*. This program, which is the successor to the *International Histocompatibility Working Group (IHWG)*, will look to define the association between HLA region genes or genetic markers and immune-mediated diseases, including risk and severity of disease and organ and cell transplantation outcomes (http://www3.niaid.nih.gov/research/topics/transplantation/research_areas/donor_organs.htm).

The use of non-human organs, tissues, or cells in human transplantation, called xenotransplantation, is another strategy NIAID is pursuing to increase the supply of transplantable organs and tissues (see Section 44.1.1). The potential of xenotransplantation, however, is severely limited by the violent response of the human immune system to non-human tissues; concerns have also been expressed that infectious agents might inadvertently be introduced from animal donors into humans. The NIAID-supported xenotransplantation research is focused on increasing the current understanding of the human immune response to antigens present on cells from non-human species and on the development of methods for rapid identification and treatment of any infectious diseases that might be caused by organisms present in animal donor tissue.

References

1. Auchincloss, H., Jr. and Sultan, H. (1996) Antigen processing and presentation in transplantation, *Curr. Opin. Immunol.*, **8**(5), 681–687.

2. Auchincloss, H., Jr. and Sachs, D. H. (1993) Transplantation and graft rejection. In: *Fundamental Immunology*, (Paul, W. E., ed.), Raven Press, New York, pp. 1099–1142.

3. Warrens, A. N., Lombardi, G., and Lechler, R. I. (1994) MHC and alloreactivity: presentation and recognition of major and minor histocompatibility antigens, *Transplant Immunol.*, **2**, 102–107.

4. Sayegh, M. H., Watschinger, B., and Carpenter, C. B. (1994) Mechanisms of T cell recognition of alloantigen: the role of peptides, *Transplantation*, **57**, 1295–1302.

5. Yamada, A., Chandraker, A., Laufer, T. M., Gerth, A. J., Sayegh, M. H., and Auchincloss, H., Jr. (2001) Citting edge: Recipient MHC class II expression is required to achieve long-term survival of murine cardiac allograft after costimulatory blockade, *J. Immunol.*, **167**, 5522–5526.

6. Shaw, B., Gooley, T., Malkki, T., et al. (2007) The importance of HLA-DPB1 in unrelated donor haematopoietic cell transplantation, *Blood*, **110**(13), 4560–4565.

7. Matricardi, P. M., Rosmini, F., Panetta, V., et al. (2002) Hay fever and asthma in relation to markers of infection in the United States. *J. Allergy Clin. Immunol.*, **110**, 381–387.

8. Ryan, E. A., Lakey, J. R. T., Rajotte, R. V., et al. (2001) Clinical outcomes and insulin secretion after islet transplantation with the Edmonton Protocol, *Diabetes*, **50**, 710–719.

9. Farney, A. C., Cho, E., Schweitzer, E. J., Dunkin, B., Philosophe, B., et al. (2000) Simultaneous cadaver pancreas living-donor kidney transplantation: a new approach for the type 1 diabetic uremic patient, *Ann. Surg.*, **232**, 696–703.

10. Humar, A., Kandaswamy, R., Granger, D., Gruessner, R. W., Gruessner, A. C., and Sutherland, D. E. (2000) Decreased surgical risks of pancreas transplantation in the modern era, *Ann. Surg.*, **231**, 269–275.

11. Robertson, R. P. (2004) Islet transplantation as a treatment for diabetes – a work in progress, *N. Engl. J. Med.*, **350**(7), 694–705.

12. Gruessner, A. C. and Sutherland, D. E. (2002) Analysis of United States (US) and non-US pancreas transplants reported to the United Network for Organ Sharing (UNOS) and the International Pancreas Transplant Registry (IPTR) as of October 2001. In: *Clinical Transplants 2001*, (Cecka, J. M. and Terasaki, P. I. eds.), UCLA Immunogenetics Center, Los Angeles, pp. 41–72.

13. Robertson, R. P. (1992) Pancreatic and islet transplantation for diabetes – cures or curiosities? *N. Engl. J. Med.*, **327**, 1861–1868.

14. Navarro, X., Kennedy, W. R., Loewenson, R. B., and Sutherland, D. E. (1990) Influence of pancreas transplantation on cardiorespiratory reflexes, nerve conduction, and mortality in diabetes mellitus, *Diabetes*, **39**, 802–806.

15. Navarro, X., Sutherland, D. E., and Kennedy, W. R. (1997) Long-term effects of pancreatic transplantation on diabetic neuropathy, *Ann. Neurol.*, **42**, 727–736.

16. Fioretto, P., Steffes, M. W., Sutherland, D. E. R. , Goetz, F. C., and Mauer, M. (1998) Reversal of lesions of diabetic nephropathy after pancreas transplantation, *N. Engl. J. Med.*, **339**, 69–75.

17. Fiorina, P., La Rocca, E., Venturini, M., et al. (2001) Effects of kidney-pancreas transplantation on atherosclerotic risk factors and endothelial function in patients with uremia and type 1 diabetes, *Diabetes*, **50**, 496–501.

18. Larsen, J. L., Ratanasuwan, T., Burkman, T., et al. (2002) Carotid intima media thickness decreases after pancreas transplantation, *Transplantation*, **73**, 936–940.

19. Jukema, J. W., Smets, Y. F., van der Pijl, J. W., et al. (2002) Impact of simultaneous pancreas and kidney transplantation on progression of coronary atherosclerosis in patients with end-stage renal failure due to type 1 diabetes, *Diabetes Care*, **25**, 906–911.

20. Piehlmeier, W., Bullinger, M., Nusser, J., et al. (1991) Quality of life in type 1 (insulin-dependent) diabetic patients prior to and after pancreas and kidney transplantation in relation to organ function, *Diabetologia*, **34**(Suppl. 1), S150–S157.

21. Milde, F. K., Hart, L. K., and Zehr, P. S. (1992) Quality of life of pancreatic transplant recipients, *Diabetes Care*, **15**, 1459–1463.

22. Gross, C. R. and Zehrer, C. L. (1993) Impact of the addition of a pancreas to quality of life in uremic diabetic recipients of kidney transplants, *Transplant. Proc.*, **25**, 1293–1295.

23. Barrou, B., Baldi, A., Bitker, M. O., Squifflet, J. P., Gruessner, R. W., and Sutherland, D. E. (1995) Pregnancy after pancreas transplantation: report of four new cases and review of the literature, *Transplant. Proc.*, **27**, 303–304.

24. Kairaitis, L. K., Nankivell, B. J., Lawrence, S., et al. (1999) Successful obstetric outcome after simultaneous pancreas and kidney transplantation, *Med. J. Aust.*, **170**, 368–370.

25. Largiader, F., Kolb, E., and Binswanger, U. (1980) A long-term functioning human pancreatic islet allotransplant, *Transplantation*, **29**, 76–77.

26. Shapiro, A. M. J., Lakey, J. R. T., Ryan, E. A., Korbutt, G. S., Toth, E. L., Warnock, G. L., Kneteman, N. N., and Rajotte, R. V. (2000) Islet transplantation in seven patients with type 1 diabetes mellitus using a glucocorticoid-free immunosuppressive regimen, *N. Engl. J. Med.*, **343**, 230–238.

27. Sutherland, D. E., Gruessner, A. C., and Gruessner, R. W. (1998) Pancreas transplantation: a review, *Transplant. Proc.*, **30**, 1940–1943.

28. Ryan, E. A. (1998) Pancreas transplants: for whom? *Lancet*, **351**, 1072–1073.

29. Brendel, M., Hering, B., Schulz, A., and Bretzel, R. (1999) *International Islet Transplant Registry Report*, Justus-Liebis University of Giessen, pp. 1–20.

30. Shapiro, A. M. J., Ricordi, C., Hering, B. J., Auchincloss, H., et al. (2006) International trial of the Edmonton Protocol for islet transplantation, *N. Engl. J. Med.*, **355**(13), 1318–1330.

31. Ault A. (2003) Edmonton's islet success tough to duplicate elsewhere, *Lancet*, **361**(9374), 2054.

32. Shapiro, A. M., Ricordi, C., and Hering, B. (2003) Edmonton's islet success has indeed been replicated elsewhere, *Lancet*, **362**(9391), 1242.

33. Ryan, E. A., Lakey, J. R., Rajotte, R. V., et al. (2001) Clinical outcomes and insulin secretion after islet transplantation with the Edmonton protocol, *Diabetes*, **50**, 710–719.

34. Ryan, E. A., Lakey, J. R., Paty, B. W., et al. (2002) Successful islet transplantation: continued insulin reserve provides long-term glycemic control, *Diabetes*, **51**, 2148–2157.

35. Froud, T., Ricordi, C., Baidal, D. A., et al. (2005) Islet transplantation in type 1 diabetes mellitus using cultured islets and steroid-free immunosuppression: Miami experience, *Am. J. Transplant.*, **5**, 2037–2046.

36. Robertson, R. P. and Kendall, D. (2003) Islet transplantation 2003: questions about its future, *Curr. Opin. Endocrinol. Diabetes*, **10**, 128–132.

37. Gold, G., Qian, R. L., and Grodsky, G. M. (1988) Insulin biosynthesis in HIT cells: effects of glucose, forskolin, IBMX, and dexamethasone, *Diabetes*, **37**, 160–165.

38. Wahoff, D. C., Papalois, B. E., Najarian, J. S., et al. (1995) Autologous islet transplantation to prevent diabetes after pancreatic resection, *Ann. Surg.*, **222**, 562–579.

39. Robertson, R. P., Lanz, K. J., Sutherland, D. E., and Kendall, D. M. (2001) Prevention of diabetes for up to 13 years by autoislet transplantation after pancreatectomy for chronic pancreatitis, *Diabetes*, **50**, 47–50.

40. Jaeger, C., Brendel, M. D., Hering, B. J., Eckhard, M., and Bretzel, R. G. (1997) Progressive islet graft failure occurs significantly earlier in autoantibody-positive than in autoantibody-negative IDDM recipients of intrahepatic islet allografts, *Diabetes*, **46**, 1907–1910.

41. Bosi, E., Braghi, S., Maffi, P., et al. (2001) Autoantibody response to islet transplantation in type 1 diabetes, *Diabetes*, **50**, 2464–2471.

42. Billaudel, B. and Sutter, B. C. (1982) Immediate in-vivo effect of corticosterone on glucose-induced insulin secretion in the rat, *J. Endocrinol.*, **95**, 315–320.

43. Robertson, R. P. (1986) Cyclosporin-induced inhibition of insulin secretion in isolated rat islets and HIT cells, *Diabetes*, **35**, 1016–1019.

44. Nielsen, J. H., Mandrup-Poulsen, T., and Nerup, J. (1986) Direct effects of cyclosporin A on human pancreatic beta-cells, *Diabetes*, **35**, 1049–1052.

45. Draznin, B., Metz, S. A., Sussman, K. E., and Leitner, J. W. (1988) Cyclosporin- induced inhibition of insulin release: possible role of voltage-dependent calcium transport channels, *Biochem. Pharmacol.*, **37**, 3941–3945.

46. Chandrasekar, B. and Mukherjee, S. K. (1988) Effect of prolonged administration of cyclosporin A on (pro)insulin biosynthesis and insulin release by rat islets of Langerhans, *Biochem. Pharmacol.*, **37**, 3609–3611.

47. Gillison, S. L., Bartlett, S. T., and Curry, D. L. (1989) Synthesis-secretion coupling of insulin: effect of cyclosporine, *Diabetes*, **38**, 465–470.

48. Philippe, J. and Missotten, M. (1990) Dexamethasone inhibits insulin biosynthesis by destabilizing insulin messenger ribonucleic acid in hamster insulinoma cells, *Endocrinology*, **127**, 1640–1645.

49. Gillison, S. L., Bartlett, S. T., and Curry, D. L. (1991) Inhibition by cyclosporine of insulin secretion – a beta cell-specific alteration of islet tissue function, *Transplantation*, **52**, 890–895.

50. Ricordi, C., Zeng, Y. J., Alejandro, R., et al. (1991) In vivo effect of FK506 on human pancreatic islets, *Transplantation*, **52**, 519–522.

51. Strasser, S., Alejandro, R., Shapiro, E. T., Ricordi, C., Todo, S., and Mintz, D. H. (1992) Effect of FK506 on insulin secretion in normal dogs, *Metabolism*, **41**, 64–67.

52. Ishizuka, J., Gugliuzza, K. K., Wassmuth, Z., et al. (1993) Effects of FK506 and cyclosporine on dynamic insulin secretion from isolated dog pancreatic islets, *Transplantation*, **56**, 1486–1490.

53. Fabian, M. C., Lakey, J. R., Rajotte, R. V., and Kneteman, N. M. (1993) The efficacy and toxicity of rapamycin in murine islet transplantation: in vitro and in vivo studies, *Transplantation*, **56**, 1137–1142.

54. Redmon, J. B., Olson, L. K., Armstrong, M. B., Greene, M. J., and Robertson, R. P. (1996) Effects of tacrolimus (FK506) on human insulin gene expression, insulin mRNA levels, and insulin secretion in HIT-T15 cells, *J. Clin. Invest.*, **98**, 2786–2793.

55. Meredith, M., Li, G., and Metz, S. A. (1997) Inhibition of calcium-induced insulin secretion from intact HIT-T15 or INS-1 beta cells by GTP depletion, *Biochem. Pharmacol.*, **53**, 1873–1882.

56. Davani, B., Khan, A., Hult, M., et al. (2000) Type 1 11-beta-hydroxysteroid dehydrogenase mediates glucocorticoid activation and insulin release in pancreatic islets, *J. Biol. Chem.*, **275**, 34841–34844.

57. Paty, B. W., Harmon, J. S., Marsh, C. L., and Robertson, R. P. (2002) Inhibitory effects of immunosuppressive drugs on insulin secretion from HIT-T15 drugs and Wistar rat islets, *Transplantation*, **73**, 353–357.

58. Oetjen, E., Baun, D., Beimesche, S., et al. (2003) Inhibition of human insulin gene transcription by the immunosuppressive drugs cyclosporin A and tacrolimus in primary, mature islets of transgenic mice, *Mol. Pharmacol.*, **63**, 1289–1295.

59. Oetjen, E., Grapentin, D., Blume, R., et al. (2003) Regulation of human insulin gene transcription by the immunosuppressive drugs cyclosporin A and tacrolimus at concentrations that inhibit calcineurin activity and involving the transcription factor CREB, *Naunyn Schmiedebergs Arch. Pharmacol.*, **367**, 227–236.

60. Carlsson, P. O., Palm, F., and Mattsson, G. (2002) Low revascularization of experimentally transplanted human pancreatic islets, *J. Clin. Endocrinol. Metab.*, **87**, 5418–5423.

61. Hirshberg, B., Mog, S., Patterson, N., Leconte, J., and Harlan, D. M. (2002) Histopathological study of intrahepatic islets transplanted in the nonhuman primate model using Edmonton protocol immunosuppression, *J. Clin. Endocrinol. Metab.*, **87**, 5424–5429.

62. Bonner-Weir, S., Taneja, M., Weir, G. C., et al. (2000) In vitro cultivation of human islets from expanded ductal tissue, *Proc. Natl. Acad. Sci. U.S.A.*, **97**, 7999–8004.

63. Pyzdrowski, K. L., Kendall, D. M., et al. (1992) Preserved insulin secretion and insulin independence in recipients of islet autografts, *N. Engl. J. Med.*, **327**, 220–226.

64. Kendall, D. M., Teuscher, A. U., and Robertson, R. P. (1997) Defective glucagon secretion during sustained hypoglycemia following successful islet allo- and autotransplantation in humans, *Diabetes*, **46**, 23–27.

65. Gupta, V., Wahoff, D. C., Rooney, D. P., et al. (1997) The defective glucagon response from transplanted intrahepatic pancreatic islets during hypoglycemia is transplantation site-determined, *Diabetes*, **46**, 28–33.

66. Paty, B. W., Ryan, E. A., Shapiro, A. M., Lakey, J. R., and Robertson, R. P. (2002) Intrahepatic islet transplantation in type 1 diabetic patients does not restore hypoglycemic hormonal counter-regulation or symptom recognition after insulin independence, *Diabetes*, **51**, 3428–3434.

67. Kin, T., Korbutt, G. S., and Rajotte, R. V. (2003) Survival and metabolic function of syngeneic rat islet grafts transplanted in the omental pouch, *Am. J. Transplant.*, **3**, 281–285.

68. Robertson, R. P., Lafferty, K. J., Haug, C. E., and Weil, R., III (1987) Effect of human fetal pancreas transplantation on secretion of C-peptide and glucose tolerance in type I diabetics, *Transplant Proc.*, **19**, 2354–2356.

69. Srinivasan, P., Huang, G. C., Amiel, S. A., and Heaton, N. D. (2007) Islet cell transplantation, *Postgrad. Med. J.*, **83**, 224–229.

70. Tsujimura, T., Kuroda, Y., Avila, J. G., et al. (2004) Influence of pancreas preservation on human islet isolation outcomes: impact of the two-layer method, *Transplantation*, **78**, 96–100.

71. Braghi, S., Bonifacio, E., Secchi, A., Di Carlo, V., Pozza, G., and Bosi, E. (2000) Modulation of humoral islet autoimmunity by pancreas allotransplantation influences allograft outcome in patients with type 1 diabetes, *Diabetes*, **49**, 218–224.

72. Jaeger, C., Brendel, M. D., Hering, B. J., Eckhard, M., and Bretzel, R. G. (1997) Progressive islet graft failure occurs significantly earlier in autoantibody-positive than in autoantibody-negative IDDM recipients of intrahepatic islet allografts, *Diabetes*, **46**, 1907–1910.

73. Vantyghem, M. C., Fajardy, I., Pigny, P., et al. (2003) Kinetics of diabetes-associated autoantibodies after sequential intraportal islet allograft associated with kidney transplantation in type 1 diabetes, *Diabetes Metab.*, **29**, 595–601.

74. Hyder, A., Laue, C., and Schrezenmeir, J. (2005) Effect of the immunosuppressive regime of Edmonton protocol on the long-term in vitro insulin secretion from islets of two different species and age categories, *Toxicol. In Vitro*, **19**, 541–546.

75. Nanji, S. A. and Shapiro, A. M. (2004) Islet transplantation in patients with diabetes mellitus: choice of immunosuppression, *BioDrugs*, **18**, 315–328.

76. Lopez-Talavera, J. C., Garcia-Ocana, A., Sipula, I., Takane, K. K., Cozar-Castellano, I., and Stewart, A. F. (2004) Hepatocyte growth factor gene therapy for pancreatic islets in diabetes: reducing the minimal islet transplant mass required in a glucocorticoid-free rat model of allogeneic portal vein islet transplantation, *Endocrinology*, **145**, 467–474.

77. Desai, N. M., Goss, J. A., Deng, S., et al. (2003) Elevated portal vein drug levels of sirolimus and tacrolimus in islet transplant recipients: local immunosuppression or islet toxicity? *Transplantation*, **76**, 1623–1625.

78. Shapiro, A. M. J., Gallant, H. L., Hao, E. G., et al. (2005) The portal immunosuppressive storm: relevance to islet transplantation? *Ther. Drug Monit.*, **27**, 35–37.

79. Hering, B. and Ricordi, C. (1999) Islet transplantation for patients with type 1 diabetes, *Graft*, **2**, 12–27.

80. Ricordi, C. and Strom, T. B. (2004) Clinical islet transplantation: advances and immunological challenges, *Nat. Rev. Immunol.*, **4**, 259–268.

81. Robertson, R. P. (2004) Islet transplantation as a treatment for diabetes – a work in progress, *N. Engl. J. Med.*, **350**, 694–705.

82. Adams, A. B., Shirasugi, N., Durham, M. M., et al. (2002) Calcineurin inhibitor-free CD28 blockade-based protocol protects allogeneic islets in nonhuman primates, *Diabetes*, **51**, 265–270.

83. Adams, A. B., Shirasugi, N., Jones, T. R., et al. (2005) Development of a chimeric anti-CD40 monoclonal antibody that synergizes with LEA29Y to prolong islet allograft survival, *J. Immunol.*, **174**, 542–550.

84. Hering, B. J., Kandaswamy, R., Harmon, J. V., et al. (2004) Transplantation of cultured islets from two-layer preserved pancreases in type 1 diabetes with anti-CD3 antibody, *Am. J. Transplant.*, **4**, 390–401.

85. Alejandro, R., Cutfield, R. G., Shienvold, F. L., et al. (1986) Natural history of intrahepatic canine islet cell autografts, *J. Clin. Invest.*, **78**, 1339–1348.

86. Makhlouf, L., Kishimoto, K., Smith, R. N., Abdi, R., Koulmanda, M., Winn, H. J., Auchincloss, H., Jr., and Sayegh, M. H. (2002) The role of autoimmunity complex class II matching is necessary for autoimmune destruction of allogeneic islet transplants after T-cell costimulatory blockade, *Diabetes*, **51**, 3202–32010.

87. Ryan, E. A., Paty, B. W., Senior, P. A., et al. (2005) Five-year follow-up after clinical islet transplantation, *Diabetes*, **54**, 2060–2069.

88. Gerber, P. A., Pavlicek, V., Zuellig, R., et al. (2006) Which to prefer: simultaneous islet-kidney or pancreas-kidney transplantation in type1 diabetes mellitus: a six year single center follow-up, *Diabetologia*, **49**(Suppl. 1), OP 42.

89. Frank, A., Deng, S., Huang, X., et al. (2004) Transplantation for type 1 diabetes: comparison of vascularized whole-organ pancreas with isolated pancreatic islets, *Ann. Surg.*, **240**(4), 631–643.

90. Hering, B. J., Kandaswamy, R., Ansite, J. D., et al. (2005) Single-donor, marginal- dose islet transplantation in patients with type 1 diabetes, *J. Am. Med. Assoc.*, **293**, 30–35.

91. Rother, K. I. and Harlan, D. M. (2004) Challenges facing islet transplantation for the treatment of type 1 diabetes mellitus, *J. Clin. Invest.*, **114**, 877–883.

92. Couzin, J. (2004) Diabetes. Islet transplants face test of time, *Science*, **306**, 34–37.

93. Shapiro, A. M. J., Geng Hao, E., Lakey, J. R. T., et al. (2001) Novel approaches toward early diagnosis of islet allograft rejection, *Transplantation*, **71**, 1709–1718.

94. Ryan, E. A., Paty, B. W., Senior, P. A., et al. (2005) Beta-score: an assessment of beta-cell function after islet transplantation, *Diabetes Care*, **28**, 343–348.

95. Shapiro, A. M., Lakey, J. R., Paty, B. W., et al. (2005) Strategic opportunities in clinical islet transplantation, *Transplantation*, **79**, 1304–1307.

96. Matthews, J. B., Ramos, E., and Bluestone, J. A. (2003) Clinical trials of transplant tolerance: slow but steady progress, *Am. J. Transplant.*, **3**, 794–803.

97. Herold, K. C., Gitelman, S. E., Masharani, U., Hagopian, W., et al. (2005) A single course of anti-CD3 monoclonal antibody hOKT3gamma1(Ala-Ala) results in improvement in C-peptide responses and clinical parameters for at least 2 years after onset of type 1 diabetes, *Diabetes*, **54**, 1763–1769.

98. Inverardi, L., Kenyon, N. S., and Ricordi, C. (2003) Islet transplantation: immunological perspectives, *Curr. Opin. Immunol.*, **15**(5), 507–511.

99. Steele, D. J. R. and Auchincloss, H., Jr. (1995) The application of xenotransplantation in humans – reasons to delay, *ILAR J.*, V37(1).

100. Olack, B. J., Jaramillo, A., Benshoff, N. D., et al. (2002) Rejection of porcine islet xenografts mediated by CD4$^+$ T cells activated through the indirect antigen recognition pathway, *Xenotransplantation*, **9**, 393–401.

101. Koulmanda, M., Qipo, A., Smith, R. N., and Auchincloss, H. (2003) Pig islet xenografts are resistant to autoimmune destruction by non-obese diabetic recipients after anti-CD4 treatment, *Xenotransplantation*, **10**, 178–184.

102. Omer, A., Duvivier-Kali, V. F., Trivedi, N., et al. (2003) Survival and maturation of microencapsulated porcine neonatal pancreatic cell clusters transplanted into immunocompetent diabetic mice, *Diabetes*, **52**, 69–75.

103. Sato, H., Kobayasi, T., Murakami, M., et al. (2002) Improving function and survival of porcine islet xenografts using microencapsulation and culture preconditioning, *Pancreas*, **25**, 42–49.

104. Kin, T., Iwata, H., Aomatsu, Y., et al. (2002) Xenotransplantation of pig islets in diabetic dogs with use of a microcapsule composed of agarose and polystyrene sulfonic acid mixed gel, *Pancreas*, **25**, 94–100.

105. Phelps, C. J., Koike, C., Vaught, T. D., et al. (2003) Production of alpha 1,3- galactosyltransferase-deficient pigs, *Science*, **299**, 411–414.

106. Steele, D. J. R. and Auchincloss, H., Jr. (1995) Xenotransplantation, *Annu. Rev. Med.*, **46**, 345–360.

107. Calne, R. Y. (1970) Organ transplantation between widely disparate species, *Transplant. Proc.*, **2**(4), 550–553.

108. Platt, J. L., Vercellotti, G. M., and Dalmasso, A. P. (1990) Transplantation of discordant xenografts. A review of progress, *Immunol. Today*, **11**(12), 450–458.

109. Yamada, A. and Auchincloss, H., Jr. (1999) Cell-mediated xenograft rejection, *Curr. Opin. Organ Transplant.*, **4**(1), 90.

110. Feng, S., Thistlethwaite, R., Sukru, E., and Langnas, A. (2007) Immunosuppression withdrawal for stable pediatric living donor liver transplant recipients, *Clinical Trial Research Summary* (http://www.immunetolerance.org/research/solidorgan/trials/feng.html).

111. Pascual, M., Theruvath, T., Kawai, T., Tolkoff-Rubin, N., and Cosimi, A. B. (2002) Strategies to improve long-term outcomes after renal transplantation, *N. Engl. J. Med.*, **346**, 580–590.

112. Sayegh, M. H. and Carpenter, C. B. (2004) Transplantation 50 years later – progress, challenges, and promises, *N. Engl. J. Med.*, **351**, 2761–2766.

113. Murray, J. E., Merrill, J. P., Dammin, G. J., et al. (1960) Study on transplantation immunity after total body irradiation: clinical and experimental investigation, *Surgery*, **48**, 272–284.

114. Barber, W. H., Mankin, J. A., Laskow, D. A., et al. (1991) Long-term results of a controlled prospective study with transfusion of donor-specific bone marrow in 57 cadaveric renal allograft recipients, *Transplantation*, **51**, 70–75.

115. Millan, M. T., Shizuru, J. A., Hoffmann, P., et al. (2002) Mixed chimerism and immunosuppressive drug withdrawal after HLA-

mismatched kidney and hematopoietic progenitor transplantation, *Transplantation*, **73**, 1386–1391.

116. Shapiro, R., Basu, A., Tan, H., et al. (2005) Kidney transplantation under minimal immunosuppression after pretransplant lymphoid depletion with thymoglobulin or campath, *J. Am. Coll. Surg.*, **200**, 505–515.

117. Kirk, A. D., Mannon, R. B., Kleiner, D. E, et al. (2005) Results from a human renal allograft tolerance trial evaluating T-cell depletion with alemtuzumab combined with deoxyspergualin, *Transplantation*, **80**, 1051–1059.

118. Sharabi, Y. and Sachs, D. H. (1989) Mixed chimerism and permanent specific transplantation tolerance induced by a nonlethal preparative regimen, *J. Exp. Med.*, **169**, 493–502.

119. Fuchimoto, Y., Huang, C. A., Yamada, K., et al. (2000) Mixed chimerism and tolerance without whole body irradiation in a large animal model, *J. Clin. Invest.*, **105**, 1779–1789.

120. Kawai, T., Cosimi, A. B., Colvin, R. B, et al. (1995) Mixed allogeneic chimerism and renal allograft tolerance in cynomolgus monkeys, *Transplantation*, **59**, 256–262.

121. Kimikawa, M., Sachs, D. H., Colvin, R. B., Bartholomew, A., Kawai, T., and Cosimi, A. B. (1997) Modifications of the conditioning regimen for achieving mixed chimerism and donor-specific tolerance in cynomolgus monkeys, *Transplantation*, **64**, 709–716.

122. Kawai, T., Poncelet, A., Sachs, D. H., et al. (1999) Long-term outcome and alloantibody production in a non-myeloablative regimen for induction of renal allograft tolerance, *Transplantation*, **68**, 1767–1775.

123. Kawai, T., Sogawa, H., Boskovic, S., et al. (2004) CD154 blockade for induction of mixed chimerism and prolonged renal allograft survival in nonhuman primates, *Am. J. Transplant.*, **4**, 1391–1398.

124. Spitzer, T. R., Delmonico, F., Tolkoff-Rubin, N., et al. (1999) Combined histocompatibility leukocyte antigen-matched donor bone marrow and renal transplantation for multiple myeloma with end stage renal disease: the induction of allograft tolerance through mixed lymphohematopoietic chimerism, *Transplantation*, **68**, 480–484.

125. Bühler, L. H., Spitzer, T. R., Sykes, M., et al. (2002) Induction of kidney allograft tolerance after transient lymphohematopoietic chimerism in patients with multiple myeloma and end-stage renal disease, *Transplantation*, **74**, 1405–1409.

126. Fudaba, Y., Spitzer, T. R., Shaffer, J., et al. (2006) Myeloma responses and tolerance following combined kidney and non-myeloablative marrow transplantation: in vivo and in vitro analyses, *Am. J. Transplant.*, **6**, 2121–2133.

127. Kawai, T., Cosimi, A. B., Spitzer, T. R., et al. (2008) HLA-mismatched renal transplantation without maintenance immunosuppression, *N. Engl. J. Med.*, **358**(4), 353–361.

128. Sykes, M. and Sachs, D. H. (2001) Mixed chimerism, *Philos. Trans. R. Soc. Lond. B Biol. Sci.*, **356**, 707–726.

129. Field, E. H. and Strober, S. (2001) Tolerance, mixed chimerism and protection against graft-versus-host disease after total lymphoid irradiation, *Philos. Trans. R. Soc. Lond. B Biol. Sci.*, **356**, 739–748.

130. Sykes, M. (2001) Mixed chimerism and transplant tolerance, *Immunity*, **14**, 417–424.

131. Wekerle, T. and Sykes, M. (2001) Mixed chimerism and transplantation tolerance, *Annu. Rev. Med.*, **52**, 353–370.

132. Wekerle, T. and Sykes, M. (1999) Mixed chimerism as an approach for the induction of transplantation tolerance, *Transplantation*, **68**, 459–467.

133. Domiati-Saad, R., Klintmalm, G. B., Netto, G., Agura, E. D., Chinnakotla, S., and Smith, D. M. (2005) Acute graft versus host disease after liver transplantation: patterns of lymphocyte chimerism, *Am. J. Transplant.*, **5**, 2968–2973.

134. Starzl, T. E., Demetris, A. J., Murase, N., Ildstad, S., Ricordi, C., and Trucco, M. (1992) Cell migration, chimerism, and graft acceptance, *Lancet*, **339**, 1579–1582.

135. Schlitt, H. J. (1997) Is microchimerism needed for allograft tolerance? *Transplant. Proc.*, **29**, 82–84.

136. Sivasai, K. S., Alevy, Y. G., Duffy, B. F., et al. (1997) Peripheral blood microchimerism in human liver and renal transplant recipients: rejection despite donor-specific chimerism, *Transplantation*, **64**, 427–432.

137. Schlitt, H. J., Hundrieser, J., Ringe, B., and Pichlmayr, R. (1994) Donor-type microchimerism associated with graft rejection eight years after liver transplantation, *N. Engl. J. Med.*, **330**, 646–647.

138. Alexander, S. I., Smith, N., Hu, M., et al. (2008) Chimerism and tolerance in a recipient of a deceased-donor liver transplant, *N. Engl. J. Med.*, **358**(4), 369–374.

139. Andreoni, K. A., Lin, J. I., and Groben, P. A. (2004) Liver transplantation 27 years after bone marrow transplantation from the same living donor, *N. Engl. J. Med.*, **350**, 2624–2625.

140. Donckier, V., Troisi, R., Toungouz, M., et al. (2004) Donor stem cell infusion after non-myeloablative conditioning for tolerance induction to HLA mismatched adult living-donor liver graft, *Transplant. Immunol.*, **13**, 139–146.

141. Collins, R. H., Jr., Anastasi, J., Terstappen, L. W., et al. (1993) Donor-derived long- term multilineage hematopoiesis in a liver-transplant recipient, *N. Engl. J. Med.*, **328**, 762–765.

142. Whitington, P. F., Rubin, C. M., Alonso, E. M., et al. (1996) Complete lymphoid chimerism and chronic graft-versus-host disease in an infant recipient of a hepatic allograft from an HLA-homozygous parental living donor, *Transplantation*, **62**, 1516–1519.

143. Gilroy, R. K., Coccia, P. F., Talmadge, J. E., et al. (2004) Donor immune reconstitution after liver-small bowel transplantation for multiple intestinal atresia with immunodeficiency, *Blood*, **103**, 1171–1174.

144. Li, Y., Koshiba, T., Yoshizawa, A., et al. (2004) Analyses of peripheral blood mononuclear cells in operational tolerance after pediatric living donor liver transplantation, *Am. J. Transplant.*, **4**, 2118–2125.

145. Starzl, T. E. (2008) Immunosuppressive therapy and tolerance of organ allograft, *N. Engl. J. Med.*, **358**(4), 407–411.

146. Starzl, T. E. and Zinkernagel, R. M. (1998) Antigen localization and migration in immunity and tolerance, *N. Engl. J. Med.*, **339**, 1905–1913.

147. Starzl, T. E. and Zinkernagel, R. M. (2001) Transplantation tolerance from a historical perspective, *Nat. Rev. Immunol.*, **1**, 233–239.

148. Pons, J. A., Yelamos, J., Ramirez, P., et al. (2003) Endothelial cell chimerism does not influence allograft tolerance in liver transplant patients after withdrawal of immunosuppression, *Transplantation*, **75**, 1045–1047.

149. Ramos, H. C., Reyes, J., Abo-Elmagd, K., et al. (1995) Weaning of immunosuppression in long term liver transplant recipients, *Transplantation*, **59**, 212–217.

150. Sandborn, W. J., Hay, J. E., Porayko, M. K., et al. (1994) Cyclosporin withdrawal for nephrotoxicity in liver transplant recipients does not result in sustained improvement in kidney function and causes cellular and ductopenic rejection, *Hepatology*, **19**, 925–932.

151. Presson, H., Friman, S., Schersten, T., et al. (1990) Ursodeoxycholic acid for prevention of acute rejection in liver transplant recipients, *Lancet*, **336**, 52–53.

152. Assy, N., Adams, P. C., Myers, P., Simon, V., and Ghent, C. N. (2007) A randomised controlled trial of total immunosuppression withdrawal in stable liver transplant recipients, *Gut*, **56**, 304–306.

153. Rodriguez, R. A., Mendelson, M., O'Hare, A. M., Hsu, L. C., and Schoenfeld, P. (2003) Determinants of survival among

HIV-infected chronic dialysis patients, *J. Am. Soc. Nephrol.*, **14**, 1307–1313.

154. Martin-Carbonero, L., Soriano, V., Valencia, E., et al. (2001) Increasing impact of chronic viral hepatitis on hospital admissions and mortality among HIV-infected patients, *AIDS Res. Hum. Retroviruses*, **17**, 1467–1471.

155. Rosenthal, E., Poiree, M., Pradier, C., et al. (2003) Mortality due to hepatitis C- related liver disease in HIV-infected patients in France (Mortavic 2001 study), *AIDS*, **17**, 1803–1809.

156. Halpern, S. D., Ubel, P. A., and Caplan, A. L. (2002) Solid-organ transplantation in HIV-infected patients, *N. Engl. J. Med.*, **347**, 284–287.

157. Roland, M. E., Barin, B., Carlson, L., et al. (2008) HIV-infected kidney and liver transplant recipients: 1- and 3-year outcome, *Am. J. Transplant.*, **8**(2), 355–365.

158. Dummer, J. S., Erb, S., Breinig, M. K., et al. (1989) Infection with human immunodeficiency virus in the Pittsburgh transplant population. A study of 583 donors and 1043 recipients, 1981–1986, *Transplantation*, **47**, 134–140.

159. Poli, F., Scalamogna, M., Pizzi, C., Mozzi, F., and Sirchia, G. (1989) HIV infection in cadaveric renal allograft recipients in the North Italy Transplant Program, *Transplantation*, **47**, 724–725.

160. Tzakis, A. G., Cooper, M. H., Dummer, J. S., Ragni, M., Ward, J. W., and Starzl, T. E. (1990) Transplantation in HIV+ patients, *Transplantation*, **49**, 354–358.

161. Erice, A., Rhame, F. S., Heussner, R. C., Dunn, D. L., and Balfour, H. H., Jr. (1991) Human immunodeficiency virus infection in patients with solid-organ transplants: report of five cases and review, *Rev. Infect. Dis.*, **13**, 537–547.

162. Bouscarat, F., Samuel, D., Simon, F., Debat, P., Bismuth, H., and Saimot, A. G. (1994) An observational study of 11 French liver transplant recipients infected with human immunodeficiency virus type 1, *Clin. Infect. Dis.*, **19**, 854–859.

163. Ragni, M. V., Dodson, S. F., Hunt, S. C., Bontempo, F. A., and Fung, J. J. (1999) Liver transplantation in a hemophilia patient with acquired immunodeficiency syndrome, *Blood*, **93**, 1113–1114.

164. Calabrese, L. H., Albrecht, M., Young, J., et al. (2003) Successful cardiac transplantation in an HIV-1-infected patient with advanced disease, *N. Engl. J. Med.*, **348**, 2323–2328.

165. Neff, G. W., Bonham, A., Tzakis, A. G. et al. (2003) Orthotopic liver transplantation in patients with human immunodeficiency virus and end-stage liver disease, *Liver Transpl.*, **9**, 239–247.

166. Ragni, M. V., Belle, S. H., Im, K., et al. (2003) Survival of human immunodeficiency virus-infected liver transplant recipients, *J. Infect. Dis.*, **188**, 1412–1420.

167. Stock, P. G., Roland, M. E., Carlson, L., et al. (2003) Kidney and liver transplantation in human immunodeficiency virus-infected patients: a pilot safety and efficacy study, *Transplantation*, **76**, 370–375.

168. Abbott, K. C., Swanson, S. J., Agodoa, L. Y., and Kimmel, P. L. (2004) Human immunodeficiency virus infection and kidney transplantation in the era of highly active antiretroviral therapy and modern immunosuppression, *J. Am. Soc. Nephrol.*, **15**, 1633–1639.

169. Kumar M. S., Sierka D. R., Damask A. M. et al. (2005) Safety and success of kidney transplantation and concomitant immunosuppression in HIV-positive patients, *Kidney Int.*, **67**, 1622–1629.

170. Roland, M. E. and Stock, P. G. (2003) Review of solid-organ transplantation in HIV-infected patients, *Transplantation*, **75**, 425–429.

171. Takatsuki, M., Uemoto, S., Inomata, Y., et al. (2001) Weaning of immunosuppression in living donor liver transplant liver recipients, *Transplantation*, **72**(3), 449–454.

172. Devlin, J., Doherty, D., Thomson, L., et al. (2003) Defining the outcome of immunosuppression withdrawal after liver transplantation, *Hepatology*, **27**(4), 926–933.

173. Feng, S., Thistlethwaite, R., Sukru, E., and Langnas, A. (2007) Immunosuppression withdrawal for stable pediatric living donor liver transplant recipients, *Clinical Trial Research Summary* (http://www.immunetolerance.org/research/solidorgan/ trials/feng.html).

174. Ng, V., Anand, R., Martz, K., and Fecteau, A. (2008) Liver retransplantation in children: a SPLIT database analysis of outcome and predictive factors for survival: in 246 children who underwent a second liver transplant, survival was decreased compared to primary liver transplants, especially for those who required early retransplantation, *Am. J. Transplant.*, **8**(2), 386–395.

175. Shepherd, W., Turmelle, Y., Nadler, M., et al. (2008) Risk factors for rejection and infection in pediatric liver transplantation, *Am. J. Transplant.*, **8**(2), 396–403.

176. Fudaba, Y., Spitzer, T. R., Shaffer, J., et al. (2006) Myeloma responses and tolerance following combined kidney and non-myeloablative marrow transplantation: in vivo and in vitro analyses, *Am. J. Transplant.*, **6**, 2121–2133.

Chapter 45

Asthma and Allergic Diseases

45.1 Pathophysiology of Allergic Diseases

Although not all cases of asthma or rhinitis are clearly attributable to atopy, it is accepted that atopy does play an etiologic role in the pathophysiology of these conditions *(1)*. The reported proportion of asthma and rhinitis cases attributed to atopy varies among studies and populations. The attributable risk is also highly dependent on whether researchers use a more or less conservative definition of atopy. Researchers who have reviewed this literature to calculate the weighted mean population attributable risk suggest that approximately 40% of asthma cases and 50% of noninfectious rhinitis cases can be attributed to atopy *(2, 3)*. Additionally, atopy is one of the strongest currently identified predisposing factors for the development of asthma *(4, 5)*. In light of the common pathophysiologic basis for allergic asthma and allergic rhinitis, it is not surprising that these conditions often coexist. This has led researchers to postulate that these conditions may actually be manifestations of one syndrome *(1, 6)*.

Discussion of the pathophysiology of allergic conditions begins with exposure of an allergen to antigen-presenting cells (macrophages, dendritic cells) *(1)*. These cells engulf the allergen, process it, and display the peptide epitope of the allergen on its cell surface for presentation to T- and B-lymphocytes. This is followed by direct interactions between T- and B-lymphocytes, which initiate B-lymphocyte activation and subsequent allergen-specific IgE production *(7)*. During the progression from an inactive B-lymphocyte to an IgE-secreting plasma cell, the B lymphocytes express membrane-bound IgE (mIgE), which assists in antigen processing and the transduction of signals that drive this progression *(8)*. Plasma cells may then secrete IgE that is available for binding to its receptors on other cells *(1)*.

IgE binds to high-affinity (Fc-epsilon-RI) and low-affinity (Fc-epsilon-RII; also known as CD23) receptors on several immune system cells. The site whereby IgE binds to Fc-epsilon-RI is located on the Fc fragment in the area where the C-epsilon-3 region (or domain) adjoins the C-epsilon-2 domain *(9, 10)*. Although distinct from the Fc-epsilon-RI binding site, the IgE Fc-epsilon-RII binding site is also on the C-epsilon-3 domain *(11)*. During subsequent antigen exposure, there is cross-linking of antigen by multiple Fc-epsilon-RI-bound IgE molecules on basophils and mast cells (basophil-like cells located in tissues) *(1)*.

This triggers degranulation of these cells, resulting in the release of preformed inflammatory mediators (histamine, tryptase) and the synthesis and release of newly generated mediators (prostaglandins, leukotrienes) and cytokines (tumor necrosis factor-α, interleukin [IL]-4, IL-5, IL-6) *(1)*. Released mediators initiate an early-phase response within minutes after allergen exposure. In the bronchial mucosa, this manifests as an asthmatic exacerbation (mucosal edema, mucus production, bronchial smooth muscle spasm); in the nasal mucosa, sneezing, itching, rhinorrhea, and nasal congestion are observed *(4,12–15)*. Some mediators released during the acute-phase response act as chemoattractants and promote the infiltration of mucosal surfaces with immune cells, particularly eosinophils *(12,14,16)*. With subsequent release of eosinophil and newly generated mast cell products, a second wave of allergic symptoms can be observed over the 6 to 12 hours after the early-phase response. Persisting late-phase inflammatory responses may then be responsible for the clinical and histologic findings reported in chronic allergic diseases *(1)*.

In addition to activating basophils through Fc-epsilon-RI binding, IgE may interact with other immune cells in less defined ways *(17)*. IgE binds to Fc-epsilon-RI on antigen-presenting cells and eosinophils. Such interactions appear to facilitate antigen presentation by antigen-presenting cells. Although the effect on eosinophils is less clear, it is postulated that such interactions may regulate local tissue IgE concentrations *(15)*. The other IgE receptor, Fc-epsilon-RII, is found on B lymphocytes; binding to this receptor may augment antigen presentation by these cells *(13, 18)*.

45.2 Characteristics of Asthma

In the United States, asthma, a respiratory disease of the lungs, affects more than 20 million people, including 9 million children, making it the most common serious chronic disease of childhood. It is characterized by episodes of inflammation and narrowing of the lower airways in response to asthma "triggers." These triggers include infectious agents, stress, pollutants such as cigarette smoke, and common allergens such as cat dander, dust mites, and pollen (http://www3.niaid.nih.gov/healthscience/healthtopics/asthma/treatingAsthma.htm).

When a person with allergic asthma is exposed to an allergen for the first time, the immune system responds by *making IgE antibodies to the antigen*. These antibodies then bind to the surface of mast cells. The person is now sensitized to the allergen, and upon re-exposure, the allergen binds to the antibody, and the mast cells release chemical mediators that cause an asthma attack. During an asthma attack, the airways will narrow almost immediately due to contractions of the surrounding smooth muscle; excess mucus is produced; and eosinophils and other inflammatory cells begin to accumulate, giving rise to the classic asthma symptoms of wheezing, coughing, chest tightness, and difficulty breathing. During a severe asthma attack, the airways may constrict so tightly that in rare cases, the individual dies.

The airway inflammatory response in asthma is characterized by inducible expression of multiple genes encoding cytokines, chemokines, and adhesion molecules, which are associated with recruitment of eosinophils and Th2 lymphocytes *(19)*. The changes that occur during acute inflammation of the lower airways usually resolve as repair processes restore normal structure and function. However, in addition to the characteristic Th2-mediated eosinophilic inflammatory response found in the airway during *acute asthma* episodes, a person with *chronic asthma* who is repeatedly exposed to an allergen and goes through many cycles of inflammation and repair may develop permanent changes in the airways, called *airway remodeling (19, 20)*. Remodeling-associated changes in the airway include peribronchial fibrosis with increased deposition of collagen (types I, III, and V), smooth muscle hypertrophy/hyperplasia, and mucus secretion *(19, 20)*. Repeated cycles of inflammation and repair in the airway in chronic asthma are considered to be the driving force for airway remodeling.

Recent studies in mice *(21, 22)* and humans *(23)* have supported an important role for eosinophilic inflammation in allergen-induced airway remodeling. In allergen-challenged IL-5–deficient mice, depletion of eosinophils resulted in significantly reduced levels of eosinophilic airway inflammation, reduced eosinophil TGF-β1 expression, and less airway remodeling *(21)*. Similarly, in humans with mild chronic asthma, depletion of eosinophils with anti-IL-5 antibody did reduce the levels of airway eosinophils, eosinophil TGF-β1 expression, and airway remodeling *(23)*.

In addition to inflammatory cells (eosinophils and Th2 cells), structural cells such as epithelial cells were also hypothesized to contribute to airway remodeling in asthma *(24)*. In asthma, the bronchial epithelium is abnormal, with structural changes including separation of columnar cells from their basal membrane attachments and functional changes including increased expression and release of proinflammatory cytokines, growth factors, and mediator-generating enzymes *(24)*.

45.2.1 Role of the Transcription Factor NF-κB in Airway Remodeling

To start understanding whether genes expressed by the airway epithelium contribute to allergen-induced airway remodeling, the Cre/*loxP* approach *(25)* was used to selectively inactivate in airway epithelium the gene encoding IκB kinase β (IKKβ), which is required for activation of transcription factor NF-κB *(26, 27)*. Because NF-κB regulates the epithelial expression of multiple genes that may be important to airway remodeling, including genes encoding cytokines, chemokines, and adhesion molecules *(28)*, this approach would allow to determine both the role of IKKβ and NF-κB regulated genes in mediating airway remodeling, as well as gain insight into the contribution of the airway epithelium to remodeling response *(29)*.

Dimeric NF-κB transcription factors regulate gene transcription by binding to specific κB elements in the promoter regions of target genes *(28, 30)*. In unstimulated cells, most NF-κB dimers are retained in the cytoplasm by means of association with specific inhibitors termed IκBs *(28, 30)*. Upon cell stimulation, the IκBs are phosphorylated and degraded, and liberated NF-κB dimers enter the nucleus to upregulate genes containing κB elements in their regulatory regions. This pathway of NF-κB activation depends on the *IKK complex*, whose activity is stimulated by proinflammatory stimuli such as TNF *(28, 30)*, a cytokine expressed in the airway in asthma *(31)*, as well as by viruses and bacteria that activate Toll-like receptors *(30)*.

IKK is a multisubunit kinase complex composed of the catalytic subunits IKK-α and IKK-β and the regulatory subunit IKK-γ [also known as *NF-κB essential modulator (NEMO) (28, 30)*]. One of the major functions of the IKK complex is to phosphorylate IκB molecules, thereby triggering their degradation and the activation of NF-κB. Although both IKK-α and IKK-β can phosphorylate all three IκB proteins *in vitro*, studies in mice that are deficient in IKK subunits show that, in most cells, IKK-β has the dominant role in signal-induced phosphorylation and degradation *(28, 30)*.

Gene-disruption experiments have indicated that the IKK activity and classic NF-κB activation were absolutely dependent on the integrity of IKK-γ *(32)*. Interestingly, however, IKK-γ was not required for activation of the alternative NF-κB signaling pathway, which leads to the nuclear translocation of p52-RelB dimers *(33)*. Of the two catalytic subunits, the most important for activation of the classic NF-κB signaling pathway is IKK-β *(34, 35)*. Interestingly, cells that were lacking IKK-α have shown normal induction of the NF-κB DNA-binding activity in response to most stimuli *(36, 37)*. Nonetheless, IKK-α has been required for activation of the NF-κB DNA-binding activity in response to the engagement of the receptor activator of NF-κB (RANK), a member of the tumor-necrosis factor receptor (TNFR) family *(38)*. Recent experiments have indicated that IKK-α might also contribute to the induction of NF-κB–dependent gene expression in fibroblasts stimulated with TNF-α, by acting as a histone H3 kinase *(39)*. However, mice that were lacking IKK-α kinase activity did not show any major defects that were consistent with aberrant activation of NF-κB target genes in response to TNF-α cell types, such as fibroblasts *(40)*. The inhibition of IKK-α activity did not have the same pathophysiologic outcomes as did the inhibition of IKK-β activity. The IKK-α kinase activity, however, has been indispensable for activation of the alternative NF-κB signaling pathway, as it was essential for the inducible p100 processing *(33, 41, 42)*. This function of IKK-α cannot be provided by IKK-β despite the close structural similarity between the two catalytic subunits. Another unique function of IKK-α has been its role in the induction of keratinocyte differentiation *(37)*. This function, however, did not depend on the protein kinase activity of IKK-α, its ability to bind IKK-γ or the activation of NF-κB *(37)*.

The activation of most forms of NF-κB, especially the most common form—the p50-RelA dimer—depends on the phosphorylation-induced ubiquitination of the IκB proteins. This sequential modification depends on two protein complexes: the IκB kinase complex and the E3^{IκB}ubiquitin ligase complex *(43)*. Once poly-ubiquitinated, the IκBs would undergo rapid degradation through the 26S proteasome, and the liberated NF-κB dimers translocate to the nucleus, where they participate in transcriptional activation of specific target genes *(28, 42)*.

Evidence that NF-κB may have an important role in asthma has been derived from both animal models of asthma in which components of NF-κB have been inactivated *(44–46)*, as well as from human studies showing that airway epithelial cells in bronchial biopsies have increased nuclear levels of the RelA (p65) NF-κB subunit compared with specimens from normal subjects *(47)*. Electrophoretic mobility-shift assays and immunohistochemical studies have also suggested a greater activation of RelA-containing NF-κB dimers in severe asthmatics *(48)*. In mouse models of asthma, mice deficient in either the p50 *(44, 45)* or the c-Rel *(46)* NF-κB subunits, or mice treated with inhibitors of epithelial NF-κB activity *(49)*, have significantly reduced levels of eosinophilic lung inflammation when challenged with inhaled allergen.

Results from subsequent studies investigating the contribution of epithelial genes regulated by NF-κB to allergen-induced airway remodeling after chronic ovalbumin (OVA) challenge have shown evidence for a critical role of the epithelial NF-κB in airway remodeling caused by chronic inflammation in asthma *(29)*. To determine the contribution of epithelial cell NF-κB activation to the remodeling response, *CC10-Cre^{tg}/Ikkβ$^{Δ/Δ}$* mice were generated in which NF-κB signaling through IκB kinase β (IKKβ) is selectively ablated in the airway epithelium by conditional Cre-recombinase expression from the Clara cell (CC10) promoter. Repetitive ovalbumin challenge of mice deficient in airway epithelial IKKβ prevented nuclear translocation of the RelA NF-κB subunit only in airway epithelial cells, resulting in significantly lower peribronchial fibrosis in *CC10-Cre^{tg}/Ikkβ$^{Δ/Δ}$* mice compared with littermate controls as assessed by peribronchial trichrome staining and total lung collagen content. Levels of airway mucus, airway eosinophils, and peribronchial CD4$^+$ T-cells in ovalbumin-challenged mice were also reduced significantly upon airway epithelial *Ikkβ* ablation. The diminished inflammatory response was associated with reduced expression of NF-κB–regulated chemokines, including eotaxin-1 and thymus- and activation-regulated chemokine, which attract eosinophils and Th2 cells, respectively, into the airway. The number of peribronchial cells expressing TGF-β1, as well as TGF-β1 amounts in bronchoalveolar lavage, were also significantly reduced in mice deficient in airway epithelium IKKβ. Overall, these studies have demonstrated an important role for NF-κB regulated genes in airway epithelium in allergen-induced airway remodeling, including peribronchial fibrosis and mucus production. Blocking the activity of NF-κB, perhaps by using an inhaled inhibitor of the protein, may be an effective strategy for treating asthma and other lung diseases *(29)*.

45.2.2 Strategies for Inhibiting NF-κB

Several different strategies for inhibiting NF-κB activation or function have been suggested *(50)*. One such possibility is to interfere with the binding of NF-κB to DNA. Although this can be accomplished through the use of decoy κB sites or their analogues, such molecules are quite large and polar, properties that are likely to hinder their cellular uptake and bioavailability. Given the large interaction surface mediating the binding of NF-κB to DNA, it would be very unlikely that small, nonpolar molecules that specifically block NF-κB DNA binding can be found. The same logic applies for molecules that inhibit the dimerization of NF-κB proteins *(50)*.

Another strategy that is more likely to succeed would be to interfere with the process of NF-κB activation. Indeed, inhibitors of the 26S proteasome were shown to inhibit IκB degradation and NF-κB nuclear translocation *(36)*, as well as inducible p100 processing *(37)*. At least one proteasome inhibitor, bortezomib (Velcade), has entered clinical development and received FDA approval for the treatment of multiple myeloma *(51)*. Nonetheless, it is not clear whether the therapeutic effects of bortezomib were due to inhibition of IκB degradation (and NF-κB activation) or to inhibition of other targets *(50)*. After all, the proteasome is involved in the degradation of all polyubiquitinated proteins. A higher degree of specificity might be expected from inhibitors of the E3 ubiquitin ligases and the E2 ubiquitin-conjugating enzymes responsible for the phosphorylation-dependent poly-ubiquitination of IκBs and p100 *(52)*. However, even these enzymes have been involved in the poly-ubiquitination of several targets, and their inhibition is unlikely to result in very specific inhibition of NF-κB activation. For instance, the $E3^{IκB}$ complex has also been implicated in the degradation of β-catenin *(53–55)*. As accumulation of β-catenin can promote neoplastic transformation *(56, 57)*, inhibition of $E3^{IκB}$ activity might not offer the best approach for inhibiting NF-κB activation *(50)*.

Given the genetic analysis described above, the most effective and selective approach for inhibition of NF-κB activation might be offered by inhibitors of IKK activity. To date, there is little evidence that either IKK-α or IKK-β would phosphorylate proteins that are not involved in the NF-κB signaling. In addition, with the exception of the involvement of IKK-α in keratinocyte differentiation, all of the phenotypes caused by loss of IKK-α or IKK-β function can be attributed to defective activation of either the alternative or the classic NF-κB signaling pathway. Therefore, both IKK-α and IKK-β have been pursued by many groups as targets for the development of therapeutic agents to be used for the treatment of cancer, as well as inflammatory and metabolic diseases *(50)*. A number of agents found to specifically inhibit IKK enzymatic activity included nonsteroidal anti-inflammatory drugs (NSAIDs), which as recent data indicated function as nonspecific IKK inhibitors.

Nonsteroidal Anti-inflammatory Drugs. With the growing understanding of the importance of NF-κB in regulating the inflammatory process, the function of conventionally used anti-inflammatory agents has been reevaluated and shown to be due, at least partially, to interference with the IKK-NF-κB system *(50)*.

Several NSAIDs have been capable of inhibiting NF-κB activation. These agents include aspirin and salicylates *(58–60)*, sulindac and its analogues *(61–63)*, and sulfasalazine and its metabolites *(64–66)*. The most commonly accepted mechanism by which NSAIDs exert their anti-inflammatory activities is by inhibition of cyclooxygenases (COX), which are essential for the production of prostaglandins. However, the effects of these agents on the NF-κB pathway are independent of COX inhibition, as suggested by the fact that indomethacin, a potent inhibitor of prostaglandin synthesis, did not inhibit the NF-κB pathway *(60, 61)*. Aspirin and sodium salicylate inhibited TNF-α–induced endothelial expression of the adhesion molecules, the vascular cell adhesion molecule-1 (VCAM-1) and the intercellular adhesion molecule-1 (ICAM-1) *(59)*, which are encoded by the NF-κB target genes. Treatment of endothelial monolayers with sodium salicylate also inhibited the transendothelial migration of leukocytes *(59)*, which depends on the VCAM-1 and ICAM-1 expression. Such findings did indicate that part of the anti-inflammatory properties of the salicylates can be accounted for by inhibition of the NF-κB pathway *(50)*. Furthermore, aspirin and sodium salicylate are known competitive inhibitors of the ATP-binding site of IKK-β, thereby impairing the phosphorylation of IκBs and subsequent activation of NF-κB *(60)*.

Sulindac, which is structurally related to indomethacin, and its derivatives (sulindac sulfide and sulindac sulfone) have also been reported capable of binding IKK-β and inhibiting its catalytic activity and thereby preventing NF-κB activation in response to TNF-α stimulation *(61)*. In the colon cancer cell line HCT-15, which is defective in prostaglandin synthesis, sulindac, and to a lesser extent aspirin, enhanced the TNF-α–mediated apoptosis, suggesting that the proapoptotic response seen in these cells has been independent of COX inhibition *(64)*. Sulindac also blocked TNF-α–induced NF-κB DNA binding, potentiates TNF-α–mediated cell killing in pulmonary carcinoma cell lines *(62)*, and suppresses tumor growth of gastric carcinoma cells in nude mice *(63)*. These data indicate that treatment with sulindac in combination with cytokines that both induce apoptosis and activate the NF-κB pathway might result in enhanced cell death *(50)*.

Sulfasalazine, another NSAID that is widely used to treat inflammatory bowel disease, is cleaved after oral administration to 5-amino-salicylic acid (5-ASA) and sulfapyridine. The treatment of human colonic epithelial cells with sulfasalazine, but not 5-ASA or sulfapyridine, prevented the NF-κB activation through blocking IκB phosphorylation and degradation in response to TNF-α, lipopolysaccharide (LPS), or phorbol esters *(64)*. However, in a more recent study, 5-ASA was shown to block NF-κB activation by inhibiting both IKK-α and IKK-β kinase activity in mouse colonic cells *(65)*. This discrepancy might have simply resulted from different permeability or uptake of 5-ASA in different cells. Mesalamine, a related aminosalicylate, can block the phosphorylation of p65 without affecting IκB degradation *(66)*. Although the effects of sulfasalazine and its metabolites have been contradictory, these data did indicate that these agents can block the NF-κB activation pathway at multiple steps *(50)*.

Immunomodulatory Drugs. Thalidomide and its analogues, which are known as immunomodulatory drugs (IMiDs), have anticancer, anti-inflammatory, antiangiogenic, and immunosuppressive effects that are achieved by modulating the levels of cytokines, including TNF-α, interleukin-6, IL-12, and vascular endothelial growth factor (VEGF). Subsequently, these agents, including IMiD CC-5013 and IMiD CC-4047 *(67)*, have shown promise in clinical trials for the treatment of different cancers. Among several different hypotheses, the inhibition of NF-κB activation has been proposed to explain the therapeutic activity of thalidomide and related agents *(68)*.

In endothelial cells, thalidomide prevented the degradation of IκB-α by inhibiting IKK-β, which is consistent with its role in inhibiting the cytokine-induced NF-κB activation *(68)*. The inhibitory effect of thalidomide on TNF-α and H_2O_2-induced NF-κB activation is also seen in other cell types, including T lymphocytes, and myeloid and epithelial cells *(69)*. IMiD-induced apoptosis in multiple myeloma cells was associated with downregulation of NF-κB DNA-binding activity, as well as the reduced expression of NF-κB–dependent proteins, including the cellular inhibitor of apoptosis protein 2 (c-IAP-2) and the FLICE inhibitory protein (c-FLIP) *(70)*. Therefore, a portion of the immunosuppressive effects of thalidomide might be due to inhibition of NF-κB activation *(50)*.

Cyclopentenone prostaglandins (cyPGs) are naturally occurring prostaglandin metabolites *(71)*. These molecules are synthesized during the late phase of an inflammatory response and are thought to be key regulators in the resolution of inflammation. The anti-inflammatory activity of CyPGs has been attributed to their ability to inhibit NF-κB activation or activity *(50)*. This effect could be partly due to the ability of cyPGs to activate the peroxisome proliferation-activated receptor-γ (PPAR-γ), which has been shown to antagonize NF-κB transcriptional activity *(72)*. The treatment of peritoneal macrophages with the cyPG 15-deoxy-$\Delta^{12,14}$-prostaglandin J_2 (15d-PGJ$_2$) did inhibit the expression of inducible nitric oxide synthase (iNOS), as well as the NF-κB activity in a PPAR-γ–dependent manner. The synthetic PPAR-γ ligand BRL-49653 can also inhibit NF-κB activity. However, cyPGs can directly inhibit activation of NF-κB pathway by blocking the IKK-β activity *(73)*.

Both 15d-PGJ$_2$ and PGA$_1$ inhibited the IκB-α degradation through inhibition of the IKK activity by direct covalent modification of IKK-β at cysteine 179 within its activation loop. The cysteine residues in the DNA-binding domain of p50 and p65 may also be targets of cyPGs *(74)*. The substitu-

tion of these cysteines with serines did abolish the inhibitory effects of 15d-PGJ$_2$ on NF-κB DNA binding, suggesting that modification of p50 and/or p65 by cyPGs might be important for the inhibition of NF-κB activation. Interestingly, NF-κB may be involved not only in the onset of inflammation but also in its resolution by being able to activate genes encoding both pro- and anti-inflammatory mediators *(75)*. For example, the NF-κB activity has been associated with increased iNOS expression during the onset of inflammation, whereas in the late phase of this process, the NF-κB activation was associated with expression of COX2, which is directing the synthesis of the anti-inflammatory cyPGs *(75)*. As such, the inhibition of NF-κB by cyPGs may be part of a negative-feedback loop that contributes to the resolution of inflammation *(50)*.

Dietary supplements and herbs are commonly used to reduce the risk of atherosclerosis, neurodegenerative disorders, and cancer *(50)*. Several studies have recently suggested that the potential benefits of these agents might have resulted from inhibition of the NF-κB signaling pathways along one or several steps in their activation cascade. Antioxidants, including vitamin C *(76, 77)*, and flavonoids *(78, 79)* are examples of such agents. Antioxidants can reduce the balance of reactive oxygen species (ROS) generated by phagocytic leukocytes during chronic and acute inflammatory diseases or by environmental stresses *(80)*. It was initially reported that oxidative stress did enhance the expression of proinflammatory genes regulated by NF-κB, and that NF-κB activation can also increase the levels of intracellular ROS. However, recent studies have shown that inhibition of the NF-κB activation actually promotes the ROS production *(81)* and that ROS may not play a crucial role in NF-κB activation *(82)*. Therefore, the mechanism of antioxidant action is far from being clearly understood *(50)*.

Nevertheless, the administration of the antioxidant *N*-acetyl-L-cysteine (NAC) suppressed the LPS-induced NF-κB activity and neutrophilic alveolitis in rats *(83)*.

Furthermore, vitamin C has inhibited the TNF-α– and IL-1β–induced IKK phosphorylation of IκB-α and subsequent NF-κB DNA binding in endothelial cell lines *(76)*. The inhibitory effect of vitamin C is relieved by treatment with a p38 mitogen-activated protein kinase (MAPK) inhibitor, suggesting that vitamin C is enhancing the activity of p38 MAPK and apparently exerting an indirect negative regulatory effect that acts between the TNF-α receptor and IKK complex *(76)*. In a study of dehydroascorbic acid (DHA), which is the oxidized form of ascorbic acid generated in the biosynthetic pathway of vitamin C, suppression of TNF-α–induced NF-κB activation was proposed to result from the direct inhibition of IKK-β kinase activity independent of p38 MAPK *(77)*. It is important to realize that antioxidants can also inhibit the activity of other components of NF-κB signaling pathways, including TNF receptors and the proteasome, without exerting any direct effect on IKK *(81)*.

Flavonoids are naturally occurring phenolic compounds that are ubiquitous in plants and that have been used to suppress inflammation, prevent the development of cancer, and protect against vascular disease *(50)*. Several studies have demonstrated that flavonoids mediated their effects by inhibiting NF-κB signaling *(78, 79)*. For example, resveratrol inhibited the expression of iNOS and decreased the nitric oxide production in activated macrophages, which has been associated with inhibition of the LPS-induced IκB-α phosphorylation and the NF-κB DNA-binding activity *(78)*. Resveratrol has also been able to induce apoptosis in Rat-1 cells by inhibiting the Ras-mediated activation of NF-κB *(79)*. These results have demonstrated that at least some of the biological activities of flavonoids have been mediated by inhibition of NF-κB pathways. In this regard, however, it remains to be examined whether the flavonoids could act as direct IKK inhibitors *(50)*.

The reevaluation of the function of commonly used anti-inflammatory and dietary agents did illustrate that the inhibition of the NF-κB pathway could be an important part of their therapeutic efficacy, as well as their potential toxicity *(50)*. A better understanding of the target specificity, and the determination of the serum levels of these agents required for inhibition of NF-κB signaling, will allow a more rational use of these agents. In addition, greater knowledge of the molecular determinants used by these compounds to inhibit IKK or other components of the NF-κB pathway should provide clues for the development of more specific and efficacious NF-κB inhibitors *(50)*.

Development of Selective IKK Inhibitors. A major effort toward the development of selective IKK or NF-κB inhibitors has been undertaken by the pharmaceutical industry *(50)*. Much of this effort entails the screening of large compound libraries, or the use of combinational chemistry to identify inhibitors of IKK-α and/or IKK-β catalytic activities. The unique role of IKK-α in the activation of the alternative pathway, which is important for B-cell–mediated responses, and the recent demonstration of the auxiliary role of IKK-α in the classic pathway, indicate that IKK-α might be an attractive target for therapeutic intervention in autoimmune diseases and cancer *(38, 39, 41, 84)*. It is therefore anticipated that recent developments in the understanding of the IKK-α–dependent alternative pathway *(42)* will provide better cell-based assays for the identification of IKK-α–selective inhibitors *(50)*.

By comparison, the development of specific IKK-β inhibitors has progressed rather rapidly *(50)*. A number of novel small-molecule inhibitors of IKK-β have been disclosed. For example, *SPC-839*, a member of a series of quinazoline analogues *(85–87)*, is one of the more extensively studied IKK-β inhibitors. Thus, SPC-839 has inhibited

IKK-β with an IC_{50} of 62 nM and has a 200-fold selectivity for IKK-β over IKK-α (IC_{50} = 13 μM). This compound also inhibited IL-6 and IL-8 production in Jurkat T cells. When tested in animal models, SPC-839 blocked TNF-α production in LPS-challenged rats at 10 mg/kg and reduced paw edema in a rat arthritis model at 30 mg/kg *(86, 87)*.

Several groups have reported the inhibition of IKK-β activity by β-carboline derivatives *(88–90)*. Of these, *PS-1145*, which was developed from a β-carboline natural product known to inhibit several different kinases *(89)*, has been extensively evaluated in various *in vitro* assays *(88–90)*. Furthermore, PS-1145 inhibited the IKK complex with an IC_{50} of 150 nM, blocked the TNF-α–induced IκB phosphorylation and degradation in HeLa cells, and reduced the production of TNF-α in LPS-challenged mice *(89)*. In a separate study, PS-1145 was shown to interfere with the NF-κB activation, abrogated the cytokine production and secretion, and inhibited the cell proliferation when tested in multiple myeloma cells *(87)*.

Another well-studied molecule that inhibited IKK-β has been *BMS-345541*, along with its related analogues *(91, 92)*. BMS-345541 has shown greater than 10-fold selectivity for IKK-β (IC_{50} = 0.3 μM) over IKK-α (IC_{50} = 4 μM) but failed to inhibit a panel of 15 other cellular protein kinases at concentrations as high as 100 μM. Unlike other reported IKK inhibitors, BMS-345541 was found to bind at an allosteric site of IKK-β, thereby behaving as an ATP-noncompetitive inhibitor *(92)*. In addition, this molecule inhibited the LPS-induced production of several cytokines, including TNF-α, IL-1, IL-6, and IL-8 in THP-1 monocytic cells, with IC_{50} values in the range 1 to 5 μM *(92)*. When tested in LPS-challenged mice, BMS-345541 blocked TNF-α production, measured in the serum of animals, with an EC_{50} of approximately 10 mg/kg *(50)*. BMS-345541 has also shown dose-dependent efficacy in terms of reducing disease severity in a murine model of collagen-induced arthritis *(93)*. The histopathologic evaluation of various tissues, including liver, heart, lung, and bone marrow of the mice treated with BMS-345541 (6 weeks of dosing at 100 mg/kg), revealed no toxicologic changes *(3)*.

Recently, another IKK-β–selective inhibitor, *SC-514*, has been reported *(94)*. SC-514 is similar to a group of amino-thiophenecarboxamides reported previously *(95)*. This compound inhibited various forms of recombinant IKK-β with IC_{50} values of 3 to 12 μM *(94)*. Unlike BMS-345541, SC-514 is a reversible ATP competitive inhibitor. Although it did bind IKK-β at the conserved ATP-binding pocket, SC-514 has demonstrated good selectivity, in that it did not inhibit about 30 cellular protein kinases tested and had little effect on other members of the IKK family, including IKK-α, IKK-ε, and TBK1 *in vitro* *(94)*. It is interesting to note that SC-514 inhibited the expression of NF-κB–dependent cytokines, such as IL-6 and IL-8, through the inhibition of IKK-β–

mediated phosphorylation of IκB-α and p65 (94). Although SC-514 has limited bioavailability (2%) and a poor half-life (0.2 hours), it has been efficacious in acute inflammation model and blocked TNF-α production in LPS-challenged rats (94).

In addition, several other compounds have been reported as nanomolar-range inhibitors of IKK-β kinase activity and have demonstrated inhibitory activity in functional cell-based assays and shown efficacy in experimental models. It is noteworthy that a group of ureidocarboxamido thiophenes (96–98), some of which inhibited IKK-β with an IC_{50} as low as 18 nM, were found to reduce paw edema in a rat arthritis model by 100% at a dose of 30 mg/kg (99), indicating a potential use in the treatment of inflammatory disorders (50).

In a recent study, the development of a group of 2-amino-3-cyano-4,6,-diarylpyridines as selective IKK-β inhibitors has been described (100–102). For example, one of these compounds has shown an IC_{50} of 0.6 μM and 20 μM against the IκB-α kinase activity of IKK-β and IKK-α, respectively (102). When tested in an acute cytokine-release model (LPS-induced TNF-α in mice), this inhibitor demonstrated in vivo efficacy with an ED_{50} of 2 mg/kg (102). In addition, a number of anilinopyrimidine derivatives were reported to inhibit IKK-β–mediated IκB phosphorylation and block LPS-induced TNF-α production in mice with ED_{50} values in the range of 1 to 30 mg/kg (103).

Recently, a group of optically active pyridine analogues were reported to inhibit IKK-β activity showing IC_{50} values as low as 4 nM (104). A number of other small molecules with diversified structures have also been found to inhibit IKK-β (105–110); however, no detailed information has been discussed in these disclosures (50).

It is interesting to note that one compound, CHS-828, and a group of related pyridyl cyanoguanidines were reported in a recent patent as IKK inhibitors (111, 112). CHS-828 was originally identified and evaluated as an antitumor agent in clinical trials (113–115). It is possible that CHS-828 and its analogues have acted by inhibiting IKK activity and blocking NF-κB activation. These studies, taken together with results obtained with PS-1145 discussed above, provide a framework for considering the potential use of IKK-β inhibitors in cancer treatment. However, the safety and efficacy profiles of these compounds remain to be determined, and until then it is not clear whether they can be used in the treatment of chronic inflammatory disorders (50).

Other Aproaches. In addition to efforts that focus on the design of specific small-molecule inhibitors, the use of macromolecules to block the activity or expression of IKKs has also been explored (50). These approaches include the use of antisense oligonucleotides that target the nucleic acid sequence of IKK-β to inhibit its expression, and thereby prevent NF-κB activation (116). Numerous recent reports have described the use of small interfering RNAs (siRNA) that modulate the expression of IKK proteins through RNA interference (RNAi); however, these approaches seem to be more suitable for mechanistic and target-validation studies than for therapeutic applications (117). In addition to antisense oligonucleotides and RNAi approaches, the development of cell-permeable peptides containing the IKK-γ–binding motif, which is located at the C-termini of IKK-α and IKK-β, has also been reported (116, 117). These peptides compete with IKK-α and IKK-β for binding to IKK-γ, thereby preventing assembly of the IKK complex and blocking the activation of the canonical pathway. As expected, these peptides were shown to inhibit TNF-α–induced NF-κB activation and reduce the expression of NF-κB–dependent genes in human endothelial cells (118, 119).

In summary, given the recent progress in the development of IKK inhibitors, there is much hope that one or several of these inhibitors will enter clinical testing and prove useful in either cancer therapy as an apoptosis-sensitizing drug or in the therapy of inflammatory and autoimmune diseases (50).

45.3 Treatment of Asthma

Treatment for asthma, both acute and chronic, involves two main types of drugs that control asthma symptoms. Quick-relief medicines taken at the first signs of an asthma attack, such as inhaled bronchodilators, relax the smooth muscles surrounding the airways; for effective long-term control, individuals use corticosteroids, which reduce airway inflammation. Moreover, current treatments only control asthma symptoms without providing cure.

Immunotherapy as Asthma Prevention. The development of antigen-specific T-cell memory commonly occurs during the preschool years and is responsible for the development of atopic disease, and perhaps its severity, during adulthood. Thus, there has been an increasing interest in prevention of asthma by reducing allergic sensitization during childhood. To date, however, most attempts employing anti-inflammatory drugs or strict avoidance measures have been disappointing (www.immunetolerance.org).

Sublingual immunotherapy, however, in which repeated doses of allergen are administered via the oral mucosa, has been shown in several studies to be a safe, effective treatment for certain allergies, even in children as young as 2 years old (www.immunetolerance.org).

45.3.1 Anti-IgE Treatment of Asthma

Since the discovery of immunoglobulin (Ig)E or reaginic antibody, it has been appreciated that any means of reducing circulating levels of IgE could be beneficial in the treatment of allergic diseases. Levels of IgE are highly correlated with the development of asthma and bronchial hyperresponsiveness. Elevated serum levels of allergen-specific IgE directed toward environmental or aeroallergens characterize allergic diseases, such as rhinitis and asthma, whereas those against foods are associated with food allergy and eosinophilic disorders of the gastrointestinal tract (http://www.medscape.com/viewarticle/530088).

The Role of IgE. The predominant role played by IgE is in type I hypersensitivity reactions, binding to *high-affinity IgE receptors (Fc-epsilon-RI)* on mast cells and basophils. Binding to the receptor occurs via the C-epsilon-3 domain on the Fc fragment. Levels of Fc-epsilon-RI expression correlate with serum levels of IgE *(120)*; a number of studies have shown a close association between serum levels of IgE so that any reduction can result in significant decreases in expression of this key receptor *(121)* (http://www.medscape.com/viewarticle/530088). High-affinity Fc-epsilon-RI receptors are also expressed on dendritic cells (DCs), especially type II DCs that promote Th2 responses. IgE occupancy of the Fc-epsilon-RI on DCs is associated with enhanced allergen uptake and the ensuing allergic responses.

In addition, IgE has also been found to bind to *low-affinity receptors (Fc-epsilon-RII, CD23)* also expressed on dendritic cells and other antigen-presenting cells. Occupancy of this receptor resulted in amplification of the immune response *(122, 123)*. In the absence of this receptor in mice, lower responses to antigen have been described, including the response to allergen sensitization and challenge *(124)*.

45.3.1.1 Omalizumab

Omalizumab (Xolair) is a recombinant humanized monoclonal antibody directed against IgE to inhibit the immune response to allergen exposure. Omalizumab has been identified through conventional somatic cell hybridization techniques *(125)*. Through this process, researchers identified a murine monoclonal anti-human IgE antibody, MAE11, whose paratope was directed toward the site that binds Fc-epsilon-RI on basophils and mast cells *(9, 10)*. MAE11 was humanized in a process involving transplantation of the *complementarity-determining regions* (CDRs; specific areas within the paratope that interact with an antigen—in this instance, human IgE) onto a human IgG1 antibody framework *(126)*. Additional MAE11 amino acid sequences were also incorporated into the humanized antibody to maintain the proper CDR spatial arrangement. This process resulted in a humanized monoclonal antihuman IgE antibody, rhuMAb-E25 (later named omalizumab), which contained approximately 5% non-human amino-acid residues *(1)*.

The anti-IgE antibody activity of omalizumab is directed against the binding site of IgE (C-epsilon-3 domain) for the high-affinity receptor, and as a result, it iprevents free-serum IgE from attaching to mast cells and other IgE receptor-expressing cells thereby preventing IgE-mediated responses *(1,127–131)*. Following allergen cross-linking of mast cell–bound IgE, these cells are activated and virtually immediately would release a granule-associated substance, such as histamine. Within minutes, *de novo* synthesis of important lipid mediators (*cysteinyl leukotrienes*) is initiated from membrane phospholipids. After a few hours, the activated mast cells are also capable of the transcription, translation, synthesis, and release of a large number of cytokines, including interleukin (IL)-4, IL-6, IL-9, IL-13, and tumor necrosis factor-α. This sequential and programmed cascade of events has been implicated in the development of both early- and late-phase allergic responses.

Dosage Range. The exact dosage of omalizumab is determined by body weight and pretreatment serum total IgE levels *(130)*. Doses greater than 150 mg are to be divided among more than one injection site. The medication is absorbed slowly after subcutaneous administration. With a mean elimination half-life of 26 days, omalizumab [0.016 mg/kg/IgE (IU/mL) per 4 weeks] can be administered every 2 weeks or monthly. The bioavailability of omalizumab is 62% after subcutaneous administration. It reaches a peak concentration within 7 to 8 days after subcutaneous administration. Omalizumab is eliminated by the liver through the reticuloendothelial system (www.clevelandclinicmeded. com/medical_info/ pharmacy/janfeb2004/omalizumab.htm).

Clinical Studies of Omalizumab. Omalizumab treatment is known to result in a marked reduction in serum levels of free IgE and a downregulation of IgE receptors on circulating basophils (http://www.medscape.com/viewarticle/530088). Omalizumab may also be associated with a downregulation of IgE receptors on DCs, indicating that reducing free IgE may inhibit more chronic aspects of allergic inflammation involving T-cell antigen presentation and activation.

From the initial studies in patients with mild allergic asthma, omalizumab demonstrated clinical effects with inhibition of allergen-induced lung function changes in both the early- and late-phase bronchoconstrictor responses *(132, 133)*. In patients with moderate-to-severe allergic asthma, omalizumab reduced asthma exacerbations and corticosteroid requirements *(134–136)* when given subcutaneously at doses of 150 to 1,375 mg. The effectiveness of the antibody was shown in children, adolescents, and adults *(134–136)* with a dose of omalizumab to provide at least 0.016 mg/kg/IgE (IU/mL) per 4 weeks *(137)*. In these studies, omalizumab was added on to inhaled corticosteroid (ICS) for 16 weeks, and during a 12-week steroid-reduction phase, ICS was decreased to establish the lowest optimal dose required for optimal control. The primary end-point was reduction in asthma exacerbations, and in all studies, both the incidence and frequency of exacerbations were significantly reduced in the omalizumab versus the placebo-treated groups *(134–136)*. A greater reduction in ICS requirements as well as a substantially greater proportion of patients discontinuing ICS were seen in the omalizumab-treated group (http://www.medscape.com/viewarticle/530088). Furthermore, a reduction in serious asthma exacerbations after omalizumab treatment has also been described as well as a reduction in hospitalizations *(138)*. In a double-blind, parallel, multicenter study of inadequately controlled severe persistent asthma, omalizumab was shown to be an effective add-on therapy for difficult-to-treat patients *(139)*; the results have been confirmed in additional studies *(140)*.

Several studies have shown that in asthmatics, omalizumab reduces airway eosinophilia and can alter cytokine levels *(141, 142)* as well as the numbers of Fc-epsilon-RI$^+$ or IL-4$^+$ cells *(142)*. Despite these changes, however, changes in lung function or bronchial hyperresponsiveness were not seen (http://www.medscape.com/viewarticle/530088).

In one meta-analysis *(143)*, the annualized rate of significant asthma exacerbation episodes was defined as a doubling of baseline ICS dose or use of systemic steroids. Analysis of the annualized asthma exacerbation episodes showed a statistically significant difference in favor of omalizumab over placebo (0.69 episodes vs. 1.56 episodes). The benefit of omalizumab was most apparent in high-risk patients.

A recent Cochrane Review examined eight randomized controlled trials *(144)*.

Treatment with intravenous and subcutaneous omalizumab reduced free IgE and inhaled steroid consumption and increased the number of participants who were able to reduce steroids by more than 50% or completely withdraw their daily steroid intake. Participants treated with omalizumab were also less likely to suffer an asthma exacerbation with treatment as an adjunct to steroids or as a steroid-tapering agent.

The development of a humanized, selective anti-IgE monoclonal antibody is a major clinical advance in interrupting the allergic cascade. The most obvious impact is in cases of severe, difficult-to-treat asthmatics. The mechanisms defining how omalizumab influences the pathophysiologic responses in the allergic lung still remain to be defined despite some evidence for alterations in cytokine levels, inflammatory cell accumulation, and expression of Fc-epsilon-RI and IL-4 receptors. Unlike allergic rhinitis, the effects of omalizumab anecdotally appeared to take much longer (4 to 6 months) to emerge. Understanding the mechanisms of action will allow more specific studies to be designed and which would take maximum advantage of this new avenue of therapy *(145)*.

45.3.2 *Allergic Rhinitis*

Seasonal allergic rhinitis (hayfever) as the sixth leading cause of chronic illness affects an estimated 40 million people (http://www.immunetolerance.org/). Currently, a wide range of drugs offer symptomatic improvement, such as corticosteroids, antihistamines, leukotrienes, and β-2 receptor agonists. Nevertheless, these therapies do little to alter the underlying allergen hypersensitivity characterized by a primarily Th2-driven inflammatory response and the production of allergen-specific IgE immunoglobulin (http://www.immunetolerance.org/).

Allergen immunotherapy is the only known antigen-specific immunomodulatory treatment for seasonal allergic rhinitis *(146)*. Immunotherapy reduces immediate allergen-induced symptoms and concentrations of inflammatory mediators in nasal lavage fluid, including histamine and prostaglandin D$_2$ *(147)*. Successful treatment is associated with blunting of seasonal increases in allergen-specific IgE levels, together with increasing levels of allergen-specific IgG, particularly IgG4 *(148–150)*. Other proposed mechanisms of immunotherapy include immune deviation *(151)* and the induction of regulatory T cells producing suppressive cytokines, such as IL-10 and TGF-β *(151, 152)*.

Allergen-specific immunotherapy (SIT), which involves the administration of low doses of allergen extracts over a prolonged period, has proved able to alter the natural cause of the disease and establish long-term tolerance to a number of allergens. However, even while effective, SIT is often impractical because it will require several months of ramp-up and several years of maintenance doses to complete and has not been effective for food allergies (http://www.immunetolerance.org/).

Rush immunotherapy (RIT) is considered an attractive alternative to SIT providing better compliance and more immediate efficacy with its accelerated dosing schedules (http://www.immunetolerance.org/). On the other hand, rush protocols have been associated with a significantly higher risk of systemic reactions, thought to be the results of early increases in total and specific IgE (http://www.immunetolerance.org/).

Omalizumab in Allergic Rhinitis. Large Phase III studies in allergic rhinitis have also demonstrated the efficacy of omalizumab in reducing symptoms and improving inherent quality of life for patients with intermittent (seasonal) and persistent (perennial) disease *(153–155)*. In patients with rhinitis, initial responses (e.g., ragweed-induced nasal volume) were seen on day 7 and peaked on day 42 *(156)*.

The combination of anti-IgE (omalizumab) therapy with ragweed injection immunotherapy for seasonal allergic rhinitis results in a significant reduction of systemic side effects and enhanced efficacy compared with immunotherapy alone.

One proposed mechanism of immunotherapy is to induce regulatory antibodies that inhibit facilitated antigen presentation. Ragweed allergen immunotherapy with and without omalizumab therapy was tested in a four-arm, double-blind, placebo-controlled study. Flow cytometry was used to detect serum inhibitory activity for IgE-facilitated CD23-dependent allergen binding to B cells as a surrogate marker for facilitated antigen presentation. Serum ragweed-specific IgG4 was measured by means of ELISA *(157)*. Overall, the results of the study have shown that ragweed immunotherapy induced serum regulatory antibodies that partially blocked binding of allergen-IgE complexes to B cells. The addition of anti-IgE to ragweed, by directly blocking IgE binding to CD23, completely inhibited allergen-IgE binding, which might have contributed to the observed enhanced efficacy with the combination therapy. Although the cost of the combination of immunotherapy with anti-IgE treatment is high, this combination should be considered in view of the enhanced benefit/risk ratio and the known long-term benefits of allergen immunotherapy *(158)*. Whether the prolonged inhibition of allergen-IgE binding that was seen after discontinuation of the combination compared with either treatment alone could result in a more prolonged duration of efficacy remains to be determined *(157)*.

Rush immunotherapy presents an attractive alternative to standard immunotherapy; however it carries a much greater risk of acute allergic reactions, including anaphylaxis caused by the relatively large doses of allergen required for efficacy *(159–161)*. In a trial designed to evaluate the safety and clinical efficacy combination of RIT with omalizumab, adult patients with ragweed allergic rhinitis were enrolled in a three-center, four-arm, double-blind, parallel-group, placebo-controlled study *(158)*. Patients received either 9 weeks of omalizumab [0.016 mg/kg/IgE (IU/mL)/month] or placebo, followed by 1-day RIT (maximal dose 1.2 to 4.0 µg Amb a 1) or placebo immunotherapy, then 12 weeks of omalizumab or placebo plus immunotherapy. Of the 159 patients enrolled, 123 completed all treatments. Ragweed-specific IgG levels increased >11-fold in immunotherapy patients, and free IgE levels declined >10-fold in omalizumab patients. Patients receiving omalizumab plus immunotherapy had fewer adverse events than did those receiving immunotherapy alone. *Post hoc* analysis of groups receiving immunotherapy demonstrated that addition of omalizumab resulted in a fivefold decrease in risk of anaphylaxis caused by RIT (odds ratio, 0.17; $p = 0.026$). On an intent-to-treat basis, patients receiving both omalizumab and immunotherapy showed a significant improvement in severity scores during the ragweed season compared with those receiving immunotherapy alone (0.69 vs. 0.86; $p = 0.044$) *(158)*.

AIC Vaccine. Standard immunotherapy is generally performed with crude allergen extracts that contain a mixture of different allergenic and nonallergenic components. The extracts can vary significantly in both concentration of the major allergens and in *de novo* immune responses to new epitopes and allergens present in the extract. To circumvent these problems, conjugating immunostimulatory sequences of DNA to specific allergens offers a new approach to allergen immunotherapy that reduces acute allergic responses. Thus, Amb a 1, the major epitope of the ragweed allergen, has been conjugated to a phosphorothioate oligodeoxyribonucleotide immunostimulatory sequence of DNA containing a CpG motif (AIC) *(162)*. The resulting conjugate has been shown to be more immunogenic than Amb a 1 and more effective in inhibiting and reversing the Th2-based allergic responses (http://www.immunetolerance.org/). The immunostimulatory sequence binds to Toll-like receptor 9 (TLR9), which is predominately expressed in plasmacytoid dendritic cells, and this interaction is associated with the inhibition of immune responses mediated by type 2 helper T (Th2) cells *(162, 163)*. In addition, when peripheral-blood mononuclear cells from patients who are allergic to ragweed are exposed to the Amb a 1–immunostimulatory oligodeoxyribonucleotide conjugate (AIC) *in vitro*, production of the Th2 cytokines interleukin-4 and interleukin-5 is decreased *(164)*, suggesting a potential therapeutic role for AIC in these patients.

In a randomized, double-blind, placebo-controlled Phase II clinical trial, 25 adults who were allergic to ragweed received six weekly injections of the AIC vaccine or vaccine before the first ragweed season and were monitored during the next two ragweed seasons *(158)*. The results of the study have shown no pattern of vaccine-associated systemic reactions or clinically significant laboratory abnormalities. AIC did not alter the primary endpoint, the vascular permeability response (measured by the albumin level in nasal-lavage fluid) to nasal provocation. During the first ragweed season, the AIC group had better peak-season rhinitis scores on the visual analog scale ($p = 0.006$), peak-season daily nasal symptom diary scores ($p = 0.02$), and midseason overall quality-of-life scores ($p = 0.05$) than did the placebo group. Furthermore, AIC induced a transient increase in Amb a 1–specific IgG antibody but suppressed the seasonal increase in Amb a 1–specific IgE antibody. A reduction in the number of interleukin-4–positive basophils in AIC-treated patients correlated with lower rhinitis visual analog scores (r = 0.49, $p = 0.03$). Clinical benefits of AIC were again observed in the subsequent ragweed season, with improvements over placebo in peak-season rhinitis visual analog scores ($p = 0.02$) and peak-season daily nasal symptom diary scores ($p = 0.02$). The seasonal specific IgE antibody response was again suppressed, with no significant change in IgE antibody titer during the ragweed season ($p = 0.19$). Overall, the results of this pilot study demonstrated that a 6-week regimen of the AIC vaccine appeared to offer long-term clinical efficacy in the treatment of ragweed allergic rhinitis *(58)*.

45.3.3 Peanut Allergy

In Western countries like the United States and the United Kingdom, peanut allergy is a growing health problem affecting nearly 1 in 70 individuals. In order to stem its growth, government agencies have issued recommendations that peanut and peanut protein be avoided in the first 3 years of life, particularly in high-risk children. Despite these recommendations, however, the prevalence of peanut allergy has doubled in the past 10 years. The situation in the Westernized countries sharply contrasts with other often less developed nations where peanut allergy remains relatively uncommon. Low rates of peanut allergy are observed in places such as Southeast Asia, Africa, and Israel, despite the fact that high levels of peanut protein are generally consumed during infancy (http://www.immunetolerance.org/).

Food-induced anaphylaxis is primarily a clinical diagnosis and is often mistaken for severe status asthmaticus or an acute cardiovascular event *(165)*. People who have life-threatening reactions usually have asthma and frequently have a history of atopy, including atopic dermatitis and food allergy as young children *(166)*. Symptoms may develop within minutes to a few hours after ingestion of the food, and in life-threatening cases, symptoms include severe bronchospasm. Although similar to anaphylaxis due to other causes, early symptoms of food-induced anaphylaxis often include oral pruritus and "tingling," pharyngeal pruritus and a sensation of tightening of the airways, colicky abdominal pain, nausea and vomiting, and cutaneous flushing, urticaria, and angioedema *(165)*. Progressive respiratory symptoms, hypotension, and dysrhythmias typically develop in fatal and near-fatal cases. Obstructive laryngeal edema is uncommon, and cutaneous symptoms may be absent in severe cases. Surveys of fatal and near-fatal reactions have suggested that a delay in the initiation of therapy such as injectable epinephrine has been associated with a poorer prognosis, although about 10% of patients who receive epinephrine early still die *(167, 168)*. Biphasic reactions have been noted in up to one third of patients with fatal or near-fatal reactions. These patients seemed to have fully recovered when severe bronchospasm suddenly recurs; the recurrence is typically more refractory to standard therapy and often requires intubation and mechanical ventilation. The mechanism underlying this phenomenon is unknown, but it appears to be more common when therapy has been initiated late and symptoms at presentation have been more severe. Secondary pneumothoraxes have been a fairly common consequence of the high airway pressures generally required to overcome the obstruction *(165)*.

Although the relative epidemic of peanut allergy appears to be a phenomenon of the past two decades, peanuts were first cultivated in South America about 2000–3000 BC, and the practice has spread throughout the world *(169)*. After the Civil War, peanuts became increasingly popular throughout the United States. The United States now ranks third only to China and India in peanut production, with more than 40% of the U.S. peanut crop consumed as peanut butter. Whereas the per capita consumption of peanuts in China is similar to that of the United States *(170)*, peanut allergy is extremely rare in China *(171)*.

In a cohort of U.S. children referred for the evaluation of moderate-to-severe atopic dermatitis between 1990 and 1994, the prevalence of allergic reactivity to peanuts was nearly twice as high as that in a similar group evaluated between 1980 and 1984 *(172)*. Data from the third National Health and Nutrition Examination Survey (collected from 1988 to 1994) indicated that about 6% of people living in the United States have serologic evidence of sensitivity to peanuts (i.e., the presence of IgE antibodies specific for peanut proteins) *(173)*, although the majority of these people will not have an allergic reaction when they eat peanuts *(165)*.

There appears to be something unique about the peanut that is not shared by other members of the legume family or most other food proteins. The three major allergenic proteins in peanuts are Ara h 1, 2, and 3 *(174)*. Although other legumes contain similar proteins and most patients with peanut allergy have IgE antibodies against these proteins, fewer than 15% of such patients react to other members of the legume family *(175)*. In addition, other legumes rarely provoke severe anaphylactic reactions or result in a lifelong allergy. However, in 25% to 35% of patients with peanut allergy, an allergic reaction to tree nuts (such as walnuts, cashews, and pistachios) will develop even though tree nuts are from a different botanical family *(165, 176)*.

Peanut allergy generally develops at an early age and, unlike many other food allergies in children, is often a lifelong disorder. In a registry of 4,685 patients with peanut allergy, the first reaction to peanuts occurred at a median age of 14 months *(177)*. Infants who have peanut allergy tend to have more severe allergic reactions as they get older. However, recent studies suggest that about 20% of young infants who have allergic reactions to peanuts will outgrow their allergy, especially if they have low levels of peanut-specific serum IgE antibodies in infancy (less than 5 kU/L) *(178)*. Therefore, children with low levels of peanut-specific IgE antibodies should be reevaluated periodically to determine whether they have outgrown their allergy. A conversion of the skin-prick test from positive to negative generally indicates that a patient has outgrown his or her peanut allergy.

However, skin-prick tests often remain positive for many years in children who have outgrown their peanut allergy and are therefore not as useful as the measurement of peanut-specific IgE antibodies for assessing clinical reactivity *(165)*.

The diagnosis of an acute allergic reaction is based on clinical symptoms and a history of exposure to an allergen. Laboratory studies are not helpful in distinguishing food-induced anaphylaxis from severe asthma, because serum β-tryptase levels, a hallmark of mast-cell activation that is associated with anaphylactic reactions, usually remain normal in patients with food-induced anaphylaxis *(167, 179)*.

Avon Longitudinal Study. The Avon Longitudinal Study of Parents and Children, a geographically defined cohort study of 13,971 preschool children, has been designed to identify those with a convincing history of peanut allergy and the subgroup that reacted to a double-blind peanut challenge *(180)*. Researchers had first prospectively collected data on the whole cohort and then collected detailed information retrospectively by interview from the parents of children with peanut reactions and of children from two groups of controls (a random sample from the cohort and a group of children whose mothers had a history of eczema and who had had eczema themselves in the first 6 months of life). The results of the study have shown that 49 children had a history of peanut allergy; peanut allergy was confirmed by peanut challenge in 23 of 36 children tested. There was no evidence of prenatal sensitization from the maternal diet, and peanut-specific IgE was not detectable in the cord blood. Peanut allergy was independently associated with intake of soy milk or soy formula (odds ratio, 2.6; 95% confidence interval, 1.3 to 5.2), rash over joints and skin creases (odds ratio, 2.6; 95% confidence interval, 1.4 to 5.0), and oozing, crusted rash (odds ratio, 5.2; 95% confidence interval, 2.7 to 10.2). The analysis of interview data demonstrated a significant independent relation of peanut allergy with the use of skin preparations containing peanut oil (odds ratio, 6.8; 95% confidence interval, 1.4 to 32.9). Based on data from the study, it is thought that sensitization to peanut protein may occur in children through the application of peanut oil to inflamed skin. The association with soy protein could arise from cross-sensitization through common epitopes. Confirmation of these risk factors in future studies could lead to new strategies to prevent sensitization in infants who are at risk for subsequent peanut allergy *(180)*.

Treatment of Peanut Allergy. Currently, the preventive treatment of peanut allergy consists of teaching patients and their families how to avoid the accidental ingestion of peanuts, how to recognize early symptoms of an allergic reaction, and how to manage the early stages of an anaphylactic reaction *(181)*.

Patients who have an anaphylactic reaction to peanuts should be treated aggressively with intramuscular epinephrine *(182)*; oral, intramuscular, or intravenous histamine H_1- and H_2-receptor antagonists; oxygen; inhaled albuterol; and systemic corticosteroids *(165)*. Because more than 90% of biphasic responses will occur within 4 hours after the initial reaction, patients should be observed for at least 4 hours before being discharged from the emergency department *(167)*. The administration of corticosteroids does not appear to reduce the risk of a biphasic response. A subsequent 3-day course of oral prednisone (1 mg/kg of body weight per day; maximum, 75 mg per day) and an antihistamine is often recommended, although there have been no studies demonstrating that this practice decreases the risk of recurrent symptoms *(165)*.

Unlike traditional immunotherapy for allergic reactions to inhalants and bee stings, injections of peanut extracts have an unacceptable risk-benefit ratio *(183)*. However, novel therapeutic agents are being investigated for the treatment of peanut allergy *(184)*.

One approach being evaluated in Phase I and Phase II trials is monthly injections of humanized recombinant anti-IgE antibodies, which may reduce the levels of IgE bound to mast cells and basophils sufficiently to prevent the activation of allergic responses, at least to small amounts of peanut protein *(165)*. For traditional desensitizing therapy another approach has used engineered (mutant) recombinant peanut proteins, in which substitutions of critical amino acids within the IgE-binding epitopes would prevent the activation of IgE-mediated reactions *(165)*. Both engineered recombinant proteins and a series of overlapping peptides comprising T-cell epitopes of peanut reversed sensitivity to peanuts in a murine model of peanut-induced anaphylaxis without triggering IgE-mediated acute reactions *(184)*. However, the clinical usefulness of these approaches has not been established *(165)*.

45.4 NIAID Involvement in Asthma and Allergic Diseases

The causes, pathogenesis, diagnosis, treatment, and prevention of asthma and allergic diseases are major areas of emphasis for NIAID. The institute vigorously pursues research on asthma and allergic diseases by supporting investigator-initiated projects, cooperative clinical studies, a national network of research centers, and demonstration and education research projects. The goal of NIAID's asthma and allergic diseases research program is to develop more effective treatments and prevention strategies (http://www3.niaid.nih.gov/research/topics/allergies/Introduction.htm).

Allergies are the result of inappropriate immune responses to normally harmless substances. Allergy symptoms vary widely, from the sneezing, watery eyes, and nasal congestion of mild "hay fever" to severe rashes, swelling, and shock. Asthma is a chronic inflammation of the lungs that airborne allergens can trigger in susceptible people; tobacco smoke, air pollution, viral respiratory infections, or strenuous exercise can also contribute (http://www3.niaid. nih.gov/research/topics/allergies/Introduction.htm).

Allergies are the sixth leading cause of chronic disease in the United States and cost the health care system $18 billion annually [American Academy of Allergy, Asthma and Immunology (AAAAI): The Allergy Report (http://www.aaaai.org/ar/default.stm)]. About half of all Americans test positive for at least 1 of the 10 most common allergens *(185)*:

Ragweed	White oak	Cat
Bermuda grass	Russian thistle	House dust mite
Rye grass	Alternaria mold	German cockroach
Peanut		

Food allergy occurs in 6% to 8% of children age 6 years or younger and in 2% of adults *(186)*. Common food allergens include:

Cow's milk

Eggs

Shellfish

Nuts: peanuts and tree nuts are the leading causes of fatal and near-fatal food allergy reactions

The prevalence of asthma is also high. For reasons that are still unclear, the prevalence of both allergy and asthma in the United States is increasing (http://www3.niaid.nih.gov/research/topics/allergies/Introduction.htm). For example:

- In 2005, 30 million people living in the United States had asthma, resulting in more than 480,000 hospitalizations and approximately 4,200 deaths

- In 2002, the asthma prevalence among non-Hispanic African-Americans was approximately 30% higher than among non-Hispanic whites and approximately double the level among Hispanics

- Among individual race/ethnic groups, Puerto Ricans have the highest levels of asthma prevalence and asthma attack prevalence

45.4.1 Research Activities

Allergen and T-Cell Reagent Resources for the Study of Allergic Diseases. The NIAID developed this new program in response to a 2005 NIAID-sponsored workshop on the future of immunotherapy. It has been recognized that there is a great need to identify and characterize allergen-specific T-cell epitopes for use in the development of novel immune-based therapeutics, including those that

may induce immune tolerance against clinically important allergens. The goal of this program is to identify and characterize novel allergen-specific T-cell epitopes that would activate both effector and regulatory T-cell subsets. This initiative is expected to contribute significantly to the current understanding of the mechanisms that underlie allergic disease and will lead to the development of new peptide-based immunotherapies. Epitopes identified by the investigators supported through this 2007 funding initiative will be deposited in the publicly accessible *NIAID Immune Epitope Database and Analysis Resource* (http://www3.niaid.nih.gov/research/topics/allergies/research_activities.htm).

Asthma and Allergic Diseases Cooperative Research Centers. The NIAID has established the first *Asthma and Allergic Diseases Centers* in 1971, and the program is now in its fourth decade of continuous funding. *The Asthma and Allergic Diseases Cooperative Research Centers* have been responsible for many important basic science discoveries and clinical advances in the fields of asthma and allergy and have trained many of today's academic leaders in these fields. The program currently supports 15 centers located throughout the United States. These centers conduct basic and clinical research on the mechanisms, diagnosis, treatment, and prevention of asthma and allergic diseases. Several of the centers are preparing to launch clinical studies, including the study of anti-IgE therapy on airway responsiveness to allergen challenge, interaction of endotoxin- and allergen-induced inflammation on airway physiology, penicillin desensitization and its effects on mast cells, the interaction between allergen-induced chronic hyperplastic eosinophilic airway disease and asthma, the effect of nasal provocation with atmospheric particulate matter on allergic sensitization, and the use of oral immunotherapy to treat cow's milk allergy (http://www3.niaid.nih.gov/research/topics/allergies/research_activities.htm).

Consortium of Food Allergy Research. The NIAID established this program in 2005 to study the natural history of food allergy and develop new approaches to treat and prevent food allergies. The consortium is currently conducting an observational study in young children at high risk of developing peanut allergy. This study will correlate biologic markers and immunologic changes associated with the development of peanut allergy and the resolution of egg and cow's milk allergy. Another study is evaluating the capacity of oral egg administration, in egg-allergic children, to induce immune tolerance to this food. The consortium is also developing a clinical trial of sublingual immunotherapy for peanut allergy, as well as a "first-in-man" mucosal immunotherapy clinical trial that will attempt to induce T-cell tolerance in peanut-allergic subjects using recombinant and genetically modified peanut allergen proteins, administered rectally within killed *Escherichia coli* (http://www3.niaid.nih.gov/research/topics/allergies/research_activities.htm).

Exploratory Investigations on Food Allergy. Cosponsored by the NIAID, the Food Allergy and Anaphylaxis Network, the Food Allergy Project, and the United States Environmental Protection Agency, this initiative will support innovative exploratory and developmental research on the mechanisms of food allergy and associated comorbid conditions, including atopic dermatitis, asthma, and eosinophilic gastroenteritis, using *ex vivo* specimens from human subjects or animal models of food allergy. One important goal of this initiative is to attract additional investigators to the field of food allergy research (http://www3.niaid. nih.gov/research/topics/allergies/research_activities.htm).

Atopic Dermatitis and Vaccinia Immunization Network (ADVN). The NIAID established the ADVN in 2004 with the goal of reducing the risk of eczema vaccinatum, a potentially life-threatening complication of immunization with smallpox vaccine. Eczema vaccinatum occurs almost exclusively in persons with atopic dermatitis. Smallpox vaccination in the United States was halted in 1972 due to the eradication of smallpox, but the ADVN was launched because of the potential use of smallpox as an agent of bioterrorism and the possibility of vaccinating large numbers of people with vaccinia-based vaccine. The ADVN includes both clinical studies and studies in mouse models of atopic dermatitis. ADVN investigators have shown that subjects with atopic dermatitis have diminished cutaneous innate immune responses. Moreover, subsets of atopic dermatitis patients with a history of eczema herpeticum have been found to have a more profound defect in their capacity to mount an innate immune response. Lessons learned from studies of patients with eczema herpeticum are expected to provide important information about the risk of eczema vaccinatum in persons with atopic dermatitis (http://www3.niaid.nih.gov/ research/topics/allergies/research_activities.htm).

Inner-City Asthma Consortium (ICAC). Since 1991, the NIAID has funded research on asthma in inner-city areas with the goal of improving the treatment of children living in environments where the prevalence and severity of asthma is particularly high. The current program consists of 10 academic clinical centers, an administrative center, and a statistical and data coordinating center. The goals of the ICAC are to evaluate the safety and efficacy of promising immune-based therapies to reduce the severity of asthma and prevent disease onset, to investigate the mechanisms of action of immune-based therapies developed to treat this disease, as well as to develop diagnostic and prognostic biomarkers (http://www3.niaid. nih.gov/research/topics/allergies/research_activities.htm).

Recently completed and ongoing clinical studies include (i) evaluation of the use of exhaled nitric oxide as a biomarker to supplement a guidelines-based approach to the management of children with asthma; (ii) a clinical trial of the effectiveness of anti-IgE therapy in asthmatic children; (iii) a

Phase I study of sublingual cockroach immunotherapy; and (iv) a birth cohort study of children at high risk of developing asthma with the goal of identifying immunologic characteristics that will predict the development and the severity of asthma at a later age.

Immune Tolerance Network (ITN). First funded in 1999, the ITN is an international consortium of investigators in the United States, Canada, Europe, and Australia dedicated to the development and evaluation of novel, tolerance-inducing therapies in immune-mediated disorders, including asthma and allergic disease. Cosponsored by NIAID, the National Institute of Diabetes and Digestive and Kidney Diseases (NIDDK), and the Juvenile Diabetes Research Foundation International, the ITN (http://www.immunetolerance.org/) recently completed a proof-of-principle clinical trial using a recombinant ragweed allergen chemically conjugated to immunostimulatory DNA to treat allergic rhinitis *(187)*. Just six injections of this allergen-DNA conjugate, given to ragweed allergic patients prior to seasonal exposure to ragweed pollen, markedly reduced rhinitis symptoms during both that year's and the following year's ragweed season. An ongoing ITN clinical trial is testing whether regular consumption of a peanut snack by high-risk children enrolled between 4 and 10 months of age will prevent the later development of peanut allergy (http://www3.niaid.nih.gov/ research/topics/allergies/research_activities.htm).

45.4.2 Resources for Researchers

NIAID supports 13 *Asthma and Allergic Diseases Research Centers (AADRCs)*, which are the cornerstone of the pathobiology component of the NIAID asthma and allergy research portfolio (http://www3.niaid.nih. gov/research/topics/allergies/resources.htm). The AADRCs conduct basic and clinical research on the mechanisms, diagnosis, treatment, and prevention of asthma and allergic diseases.

45.4.3 Clinical Trials

The Inner-City Asthma Study, cofunded by NIAID and the National Institute of Environmental and Health Sciences (NIEHS), has been carried out in seven inner cities (http://www3.niaid.nih.gov/research/topics/allergies/ clinicaltrials.htm). The multicenter, randomized controlled trial tested the effectiveness of two interventions in reducing the asthma morbidity among inner-city children with moderate to severe asthma. One intervention provided physicians with more detailed and up-to-date information on participants' recent asthma symptoms and medication use. The other intervention aimed at reducing exposure to environmental triggers such as tobacco smoke, allergens derived from cockroaches, house dust mites, mold, furry pets, and rodents. Participants were evaluated during both the 1-year intervention period and a 1-year follow-up period. The study included 937 children between the ages of 5 and 10 years *(188)*. The objective of the study was to determine whether an environmental intervention tailored to each child's allergic sensitization and environmental risk factors could improve asthma-related outcomes. The results demonstrated that among inner-city children with atopic asthma, an individualized, home-based, comprehensive environmental intervention will decrease the exposure to indoor allergens, including cockroach and dust-mite allergens, resulting in reduced asthma-associated morbidity *(188)*.

The cost-effectiveness of the environmental intervention of the Inner-City Asthma Study has been assessed by calculating incremental cost-effectiveness ratios for a 2-year study period. The health outcome was measured as symptom-free days. The resource used measures included ambulatory visits, hospitalizations, and pharmaceutical use. The overall results did indicate that targeted home-based environmental intervention improved health and reduced service use in inner-city children with moderate-to-severe asthma. The intervention is cost-effective when the aim is to reduce asthma symptom days and the associated costs *(189)*.

One project within the Inner-City Asthma Study evaluated the impact of indoor and outdoor fine particles and co-pollutants on respiratory illnesses. Recently published data from this study, which was funded by NIAID, NIEHS, and the U.S. Environmental Protection Agency, demonstrated that approximately 25% of indoor particle concentration has been contributed by outdoor particles. These data have also demonstrated that smoking has been the major source of indoor particles and that indoor concentrations of fine particles peak in the late evening in homes where smoking did occur, perhaps reflecting the influence of after-dinner smoking. Analysis of data pertaining to the effects of particle concentrations on asthma symptoms is currently under way (http://www3.niaid.nih.gov/research/topics/allergies/clinicaltrials.htm).

An important NIAID intramural study is examining how allergen immunotherapy (AIT) is reducing or preventing reactions to allergens such as pollen, dust, or cat dander (http://www3.niaid.nih.gov/research/topics/allergies/clinicaltrials.htm). Although the efficacy of AIT in asthma is modest, it is nonetheless the only disease-modifying therapy for allergic asthma currently known. Certain types of white blood cells, called Th2 cells, produce substances that contribute to the development of allergies, whereas others (Th1 cells) produce substances that can inhibit the development of allergies. This study will determine whether AIT is changing the immune response to allergens by reducing the number of Th2 cells or by converting them into Th1 cells (http://www3.niaid.nih.gov/research/topics/allergies/clinicaltrials.htm).

References

1. Belliveau, P. P. (2005) Omalizumab: a monoclonal anti-IgE antibody, *Med. Gen. Med.*, **7**(1), 27.
2. Pearce, N., Pekkanen, J., and Beasley, R. (1999) How much asthma is really attributable to atopy? *Thorax*, **54**, 268–272.
3. Zacharasiewicz, A., Douwes, J., and Pearce, N. (2003) What proportion of rhinitis symptoms is attributable to atopy? *J. Clin. Epidemiol.*, **56**, 385–390.
4. National Asthma Education and Prevention Program. Expert panel report: Guidelines for the diagnosis and management of asthma. Updated selected topics-2002, *J. Allergy Clin. Immunol.*, **110**(Part 2), S141–S219.
5. Baroody, F. M. (2003) Allergic rhinitis: broader disease effects and implications for management, *Otolaryngol. Head Neck Surg.*, **128**, 616–631.
6. Togias, A. (2003) Rhinitis and asthma: evidence for respiratory system integration, *J. Allergy Clin. Immunol.*, **111**, 1171–1183.
7. Goldsby, R. A., Kindt, T. J., Osborne, B. A., and Kuby, J. (eds.) (2003) *Immunology*, 5th ed., W. H. Freeman and Company, New York.
8. Tarlinton, D. (1997) Enhanced: antigen presentation by memory B cells – the sting is in the tail, *Science*, **276**, 374–375.
9. Hook, W. A., Zinsser, F. U., Berenstein, E. H., and Siraganian, R. P. (1991) Monoclonal antibodies defining epitopes on human IgE, *Mol. Immunol.*, **28**, 631–639.
10. Presta, L., Shields, R., O'Connell, L., et al. (1994) The binding site on human immunoglobulin E for its high affinity receptor, *J. Biol. Chem.*, **269**, 26368–26373.
11. Nissim, A., Schwarzbaum, S., Siraganian, R., and Eshhar, Z. (1993) Fine specificity of the IgE interaction with the low and high affinity Fc receptor, *J. Immunol.*, **150**, 1365–1374.
12. Bousquet, J., Van Cauwenberge, P., Khaltaev, N. (2001) Aria Workshop Group. Allergic rhinitis and its impact on asthma, *J. Allergy Clin. Immunol.*, **108**(Suppl), S147–S334.
13. Oettgen, H. C. and Geha, R. S. (1999) IgE in asthma and atopy: cellular and molecular connections, *J. Clin. Invest.*, **104**, 829–835.
14. Broide, D. H. (2001) Molecular and cellular mechanisms of allergic disease, *J. Allergy Clin. Immunol.*, **108**, S65–S71.
15. Kay, A. B. (2001) Allergy and allergic diseases, *N. Engl. J. Med.*, **344**, 30–37.
16. Pearlman, D. S. (1999) Pathophysiology of the inflammatory response, *J. Allergy Clin. Immunol.*, **104**, S132–S137.
17. Novak, N., Kraft, S., and Bieber, T. (2001) IgE receptors, *Curr. Opin. Immunol.*, **13**, 721–726.
18. Gustavsson, S., Hjulstrom, S., Tianmin, L., and Heyman, B. (1994) CD23/IgE- mediated regulation of the specific antibody response in vivo, *J. Immunol.*, **152**, 4793–4800.
19. Cohn, L., Elias, J. A., and Chupp, G. L. (2004) Asthma: mechanisms of disease persistence and progression, *Annu. Rev. Immunol.*, **22**, 789–815.
20. Davies, D. E., Wicks, J., Powell, R. M., Puddicombe, S. M., and Holgate, S. T. (2003) Airway remodeling in asthma: new insights, *J. Allergy Clin. Immunol.*, **111**, 215–225.

21. Cho, J. Y., Miller, M., Baek, K. J., Han, J. W., Nayar, J., Lee, S. Y., McElwain K., McElwain, S., Friedman, S., and Broide, D. H. (2004) Inhibition of airway remodeling in IL-5-deficient mice, *J. Clin. Invest.*, **113**, 551–560.

22. Humbles, A. A., Lloyd, C. M., McMillan, S. J., Friend, D. S., Xanthou, G., et al. (2004) A critical role for eosinophils in allergic airways remodeling, *Science*, **305**, 1776–1779.

23. Flood-Page, P., Menzies-Gow, A., Phipps, S., Ying, S., et al. (2003) Anti-IL-5 treatment reduces deposition of ECM proteins in the bronchial subepithelial basement membrane of mild atopic asthmatics, *J. Clin. Invest.*, **112**, 1029–1036.

24. Holgate, S. T., Davies, D. E., Lackie, P. M., Wilson, S. J., Puddicombe, S. M., and Lordan, J. L. (2000) Epithelial-mesenchymal interactions in the pathogenesis of asthma, *J. Allergy Clin. Immunol.*, **105**, 193–204.

25. Marth, J. D. (1996) Recent advances in gene mutagenesis by site-directed recombination, *J. Clin. Invest.*, **97**, 1999–2002.

26. Maeda, S., Chang, L., Li, Z. W., Luo, J. L., Leffert, H., and Karin, M. (2003) IKK beta is required for prevention of apoptosis mediated by cell-bound but not by circulating TNFalpha, *Immunity*, **19**, 725–737.

27. Li, Z. W., Omori, S. A., Labuda, T., Karin, M., and Rickert, R. C. (2003) IKK beta is required for peripheral B cell survival and proliferation, *J. Immunol.*, **170**, 4630–4637.

28. Gilmore, T. D. (2006) Introduction To NF-κB: players, pathways, perspectives, *Oncogene*, **25**, 6680–6684.

29. Broide, D., Lawrence, T., Doherty, T., et al. (2005) Allergen-induced peribronchial fibrosis and mucus production mediated by IκB kinase β-dependent genes in airway epithelium, *Proc. Natl. Acad. Sci. U.S.A.*, **102**(49), 17423–17727.

30. Bonizzi, G. and Karin, M. (2004) The two NF-kappaB activation pathways and their role in innate and adaptive immunity, *Trends Immunol.*, **25**, 280–288.

31. Broide, D. H., Lotz, M., Cuomo, A. J., Coburn, D. A., Federman, E. C., and Wasserman, S. I. (1992) Cytokines in symptomatic asthma airways, *J. Allergy Clin. Immunol.*, **89**, 958–967.

32. Makris, C., Godfrey, G., Krähn-Senftleben, T., et al. (2000) Female mice heterozygous for IKK-γ/NEMO deficiencies develop a dermatopathy similar to the human X-linked disorder incontinentia pigmenti, *Mol. Cell*, **5**, 969–979.

33. Dejardin, E., Droin, N., Delhase, M., et al. (2002) The lymphotoxin-β receptor induces different patterns of gene expression via two NF-κB pathways, *Immunity*, **17**, 525–535.

34. Li, Z. W., Chu, W., Hu, Y., et al. (1999) The IKKβ subunit of IκB kinase (IKK) is essential for nuclear factor κB activation and prevention of apoptosis, *J. Exp. Med.*, **189**, 1839–1845.

35. Chen, L. W., Egan, L., Li, Z.-W., et al. (2003) The two faces of IKK and NF-κB inhibition: prevention of systemic inflammation but increased local injury following intestinal ischemia-reperfusion, *Nat. Med.*, **9**, 575–581.

36. Hu, Y., Baud, V., Delhase, M., et al. (1999) Abnormal morphogenesis but intact activation in mice lacking the IKKα subunit of IκB kinase, *Science*, **284**, 316–320.

37. Hu, Y., Baud, V., Oga, T., et al. (2001) IKKα controls formation of the epidermis independently of NF-κB, *Nature*, **410**, 710–714.

38. Cao, Y., Bonizzi, G., Seagroves, T., et al. (2001) IKKα provides an essential link between RANK signaling and cyclin D1 expression during mammary gland development, *Cell*, **107**, 763–775.

39. Yamamoto, Y., Verma, U. N., Prajapati, S., Kwak, Y. T., and Gaynor, R. B. (2003) Histone H3 phosphorylation by IKK-α is critical for cytokine-induced gene expression, *Nature*, **423**, 655–659.

40. Israel, A. (2003) Signal transduction: a regulator branches out, *Nature*, **423**, 596–597 (2003).

41. Senftleben, U., Cao, Y., Xiao, G., et al. (2001) Activation by IKKα of a second, evolutionary conserved, NF-κB signaling pathway, *Science*, **293**, 1495–1499.

42. Ghosh, S. and Karin, M. (2002) Missing pieces in the NF-κB puzzle, *Cell*, **109**, S81–S96.

43. Karin, M. and Ben-Neriah, Y. (2000) Phosphorylation meets ubiquitination: the control of NF-κB activity, *Annu. Rev. Immunol.*, **18**, 621–663.

44. Yang, L., Cohn, L., Zhang, D. H., Homer, R., Ray, A., and Ray, P. (1998) Essential role of nuclear factor kappaB in the induction of eosinophilia in allergic airway inflammation, *J. Exp. Med.*, **188**, 1739–1750.

45. Das, J., Chen, C. H., Yang, L., Cohn, L., Ray, P., and Ray, A. (2001) A critical role for NF-kappa B in GATA3 expression and TH2 differentiation in allergic airway inflammation, *Nat. Immunol.*, **2**, 45–50.

46. Donovan, C. E., Mark, D. A., He, H. Z., Liou, H. C., Kobzik, L., et al. (1999) NF- kappa B/Rel transcription factors: c-Rel promotes airway hyperresponsiveness and allergic pulmonary inflammation, *J. Immunol.*, **163**, 6827–6833.

47. Hart, L. A., Krishnan, V. L., Adcock, I. M., Barnes, P. J., and Chung, K. F. (1998) Activation and localization of transcription factor, nuclear factor-kappaB, in asthma, *Am. J. Respir. Crit. Care Med.*, **158**, 1585–1592.

48. Gagliardo, R., Chanez, P., Mathieu, M., Bruno, A., Costanzo, G., et al. (2003) Persistent activation of nuclear factor-kappaB signaling pathway in severe uncontrolled asthma, *Am. J. Respir. Crit. Care Med.*, **168**, 1190–1198.

49. Poynter, M. E., Cloots, R., van Woerkom, T., Butnor, K. J., Vacek, P., et al. (2004) NF-kappa B activation in airways modulates allergic inflammation but not hyperresponsiveness, *J. Immunol.* **173**, 7003–7009.

50. Karin, M., Yamamoto, Y., and Wang, Q. M. (2004), The IKK NF-κB system: a treasure trove for drug development, *Nat. Rev. Drug Discov.*, **3**, 17–26.

51. Lenz, H. J. (2003) Clinical update: proteasome inhibitors in solid tumors, *Cancer Treat. Rev.*, **29** (Suppl. 1), 41–48.

52. Li, Q., Van Antwerp, D., Mercurio, F., Lee, K. F., and Verma, I. M. (1999) Severe liver degeneration in mice lacking the IκB kinase 2 gene, *Science*, **284**, 321–325.

53. Kitagawa, M., Hatekeyama, S., Shirane, M., et al. (1999) An F-box protein, FWD1, mediates ubiquitin-dependent proteolysis of β-catenin, *EMBO J.*, **18**, 2401–2410.

54. Winston, J. T., Strack, P., Beer-Romero, P., Chu, C., Elledge, S. J., and Harper, J. W. (1999) The SCF-β-TRCP ubiquitin ligase complex associates specifically with phosphorylated destruction motifs in IκBβ and B-catenin and stimulates IκBα ubiquitination in vitro, *Genes Dev.*, **13**, 270–283.

55. Fuchs, S. Y., Chen, A., Xiong, Y., Pan, Z. Q., and Ronai, Z. (1999) HOS, a human homolog of Slimb, forms an SCF complex with Skp1 and Cullin1 and targets the phosphorylation-dependent degradation of IκB and β-catenin, *Oncogene*, **18**, 2039–2046.

56. Rubinfeld, B., Robbins, P., El-Gamil, M., et al. (1997) Stabilization of β-catenin by genetic defects in melanoma cell lines, *Science*, **275**, 1790–1792.

57. Morin, P. J., Sparks, A. B. Korinek, V., et al. (1997) Activation of β-catenin-Tcf signaling in colon cancer by mutations in β-catenin or APC, *Science*, **275**, 1787–1790.

58. Kopp, E. and Ghosh, S. (1994) Inhibition of NF-κB by sodium salicylate and aspirin, *Science*, **265**, 956–959.

59. Pierce, J. W., Read, M. A., Ding, H., Luscinskas, F. W., and Collins, T. (1996) Salicylates inhibit IκBα phosphorylation, endothelial-leukocyte adhesion molecule expression, and neutrophil transmigration, *J. Immunol.*, **156**, 3961–3969.

60. Yin, M.-J., Yamamoto, Y., and Gaynor, R. B. (1998) The anti-inflammatory agents aspirin and salicylate inhibit the activity of IκB kinase-β, *Nature*, **396**, 77–80.

61. Yamamoto, Y., Yin, M.-J., Lin, K.-M., and Gaynor, R. B. (1999) Sulindac inhibits activation of the NF-κB pathway, *J. Biol. Chem.*, **274**, 27307–27314.

62. Berman, K. S., Verma, U. N., Harburg, G., et al. (2002) Sulindac enhances tumor necrosis factor-α-mediated apoptosis of lung cancer cell lines by inhibition of nuclear factor-κB, *Clin. Cancer Res.*, **8**, 354–360.

63. Yasui, H., Adachi, M., and Imai, K. (2003) Combination of tumor necrosis factor-α with sulindac augments its apoptotic potential and suppresses tumor growth of human carcinoma cells in nude mice, *Cancer*, **97**, 1412–1420.

64. Wahl, C., Liptay, S., Adler, G., and Schmid, R. M. (1997) Sulfasalazine: a potent and specific inhibitor of NF-κB, *J. Clin. Invest.*, **101**, 1163–1174.

65. Yan, F. and Polk, D. B. (1999) Aminosalicylic acid inhibits IκB kinase-α phosphorylation of IκBαI in mouse intestinal epithelial cells, *J. Biol. Chem.*, **274**, 36631–36636.

66. Egan, L. J., Mays, D. C., Huntoon, C. J., et al. (1999) Inhibition of interleukin-1- stimulated NF-κB RelA/p65 phosphorylation by mesalamine is accompanied by decreased transcriptional activity, *J. Biol. Chem.*, **274**, 26448–26453.

67. Dredge, K., Dalgleish, A. G., and Marriott, J. B. (2003) Thalidomide analogs as emerging anti-cancer drugs, *Anticancer Drugs* **14**, 331–335.

68. Keifer, J. A., Guttridge, D. C., Ashburner, B. P., and Baldwin, A. S., Jr. (2001) Inhibition of NF-κB activity by thalidomide through suppression of IκB kinase activity, *J. Biol. Chem.*, **276**, 22382–22387.

69. Majumdar, S., Lamothe, B., and Aggarwal, B. B. (2002) Thalidomide suppresses NF-κB activation induced by TNF and H_2O_2, but not that activated by ceramide, lipopolysaccharides, or phorbol ester, *J. Immunol.*, **168**, 2644–2651.

70. Mitsiades, N., Mitsiadis, C. S., Poulaki, V., et al. (2002) Apoptotic signaling induced by immunomodulatory thalidomide analogs in human multiple myeloma cells: therapeutic implications, *Blood*, **99**, 4525–4530.

71. Gilroy, D. W., Colville-Nash, P. R., Willis, D., et al. (1999) Inducible cyclooxygenase may have anti-inflammatory properties, *Nat. Med.*, **5**, 698–701.

72. Ricote, M., Li, A. C., Willson, T. M., Kelly, C. J., and Glass, C. K. (1998) The peroxisome proliferator-activated receptor-γ is a negative regulator of macrophage activation, *Nature*, **391**, 79–82.

73. Rossi, A., Kapahi, P., Natoli, G., et al. (2000) Anti-inflammatory cyclopentenone prostaglandins are direct inhibitors of IκB kinase, *Nature*, **403**, 103–108.

74. Straus, D. S., Pascual, G., Li, M., et al. (2000) 15-deoxy-$\Delta^{12,14}$-prostaglandin J2 inhibits multiple steps in the NF-κB signaling pathway, *Proc. Natl Acad. Sci. U.S.A.*, **97**, 4844–4849.

75. Lawrence, T., Gilroy, D. W., Colville-Nash, P. R., and Willoughby, D. A. (2001) Possible new role for NF-κB in the resolution of inflammation, *Nat. Med.*, **7**, 1291–1297.

76. Bowie, A. G. and O'Neill, L. A. (2000) Vitamin C inhibits NF-κB activation by TNF via the activation of p38 mitogen-activated protein kinase, *J. Immunol.*, **165**, 7180–7188.

77. Carcamo, J. M., Pedraza, A., Borquez-Ojeda, O., and Golde, D. W. (2002) Vitamin C suppresses TNF-α-induced NF-κB activation by inhibiting IκBα phosphorylation, *Biochemistry*, **41**, 12995–13002.

78. Tsai, S. H., Liang, Y. C., Lin-Shiau, S. Y., and Lin, J. K. (1999) Suppression of TNFα-mediated NF-κB activity by myricetin and other flavonoids through downregulating the activity of IKK in ECV304 cells, *J. Cell Biochem.*, **74**, 606–615.

79. Holmes-McNary, M. and Baldwin, A. S., Jr. (2000) Chemopreventive properties of trans-resveratrol are associated with inhibition of activation of the IκB kinase, *Cancer Res.*, **60**, 3477–3483.

80. Berlett, B. S. and Stadtman, E. R. (1997) Protein oxidation in aging, disease, and oxidative stress, *J. Biol. Chem.*, **272**, 20313–20316.

81. Hayakawa, M., Miyashita, H., Sakamoto, I., et al. (2003) Evidence that reactive oxygen species do not mediate NF-κB activation, *EMBO J.*, **22**, 3356–3366.

82. Sakon, S., Xue, X., Takekawa, M., et al. (2003) NF-κB inhibits TNF-induced accumulation of ROS that mediate prolonged MAPK activation and necrotic cell death, *EMBO J.*, **22**, 3898–3909.

83. Blackwell, T. S., Blackwell, T. R., Holden, E. P., Christman, B. W., and Christman, J. W. (1996) *In vivo* antioxidant treatment suppresses nuclear factor-κB activation and neutrophilic lung inflammation, *J. Immunol.*, **157**, 1630–1637.

84. Anest, V., Hanson, J. L., Cogswell, P. C., et al. (2003) A nucleosomal function for IκB kinase-α in NF-κB-dependent gene expression, *Nature*, **423**, 659–663.

85. Signal Pharmaceuticals, Inc. (1999) Quinazoline analogs and related compounds and methods for treating inflammatory conditions. WO 199901441.

86. Leisten, J. C. et al. (2002) Identification of a disease modifying IKK2 inhibitor in rat adjuvant arthritis, *Inflamm. Res.*, **51**(Suppl. 2), A25.

87. Palanki, M. S., Gayo-Fung, L.M., Shevlin, G. I., et al. (2002) Structure–activity relationship studies of ethyl 2-[(3-methyl-2,5-dioxo(3-pyrrolinyl))amino]-4-(trifluoromethyl)pyrimidine-5-carboxylate: an inhibitor of AP-1 and NF-κB mediated gene expression, *Bioorg. Med. Chem. Lett.*, **12**, 2573–2577.

88. Aventis Pharma (2002) Preparation of substituted β-carbolines as potential therapeutics in diseases associated with increased IB kinase activity. WO 2001068648.

89. Castro, A. C., Dang, L. C., Soucy, F., et al. (2003) Novel IKK inhibitors: β- carbolines, *Bioorg. Med. Chem. Lett.*, **13**, 2419–2422.

90. Hideshima, T., Chauhan, D., Richardson, P., et al. (2003) NF-κB as a therapeutic target in multiple myeloma, *J. Biol. Chem.*, **277**, 16639–16647.

91. Bristol-Myers Squibb Co. (2002) Method of treating inflammatory and immune diseases using 4-amino substituted imidazoquinoxaline, benzopyrazoloquinazoline, benzoimidazoquinoxaline and benzoimidazoquinoline inhibitors of IκB kinase (IKK). WO 2002060386.

92. Burke, J. R., Pattoli, M. A., Gregor, K. R., et al. (2003) BMS-345541 is a highly selective inhibitor of IκB kinase that binds at an allosteric site of the enzyme and blocks NF-κB-dependent transcription in mice, *J. Biol. Chem.*, **278**, 1450–1456.

93. McIntyre, K. W., Shuster, D. J., Gillooly, K. M., et al. (2003) A highly selective inhibitor of IκB kinase, BMS-345541, blocks both joint inflammation and destruction in collagen-induced arthritis in mice, *Arthritis Rheum.*, **48**, 2652–2659.

94. Kishore, N., Sommers, C., Mathialagan, S., et al. (2003) A selective IKK-2 inhibitor blocks NF-κB-dependent gene expression in IL-1β stimulated synovial fibroblasts, *J. Biol. Chem.*, **278**, 32861–32871.

95. SmithKline Beecham Corp. (2002) Preparation of 2-aminothiophene-3-carboxamides as NF-κB inhibitors. WO 2002030353.

96. SmithKline Beecham Corp. (2003) NF-κB inhibitors. WO 2003029242.

97. AstraZeneca (2003) Preparation of ureido–carboxamido thiophene as inhibitors of IKK2 kinase. WO 2003010163.

98. AstraZeneca (2001) Preparation of thiophenecarboxamides as inhibitors of the enzyme IKK-2. WO 2001058890.

99. Roshak, A. K, Callahan, J. F., and Blake, S. M (2002) A small molecule inhibitor of IκB kinase β (IKKβ) blocks inflammation and protects joint integrity in *in vivo* models of arthritis, *Inflamm. Res.* **51**(Suppl. 2), S4.

100. Bayer (2002) Preparation of 2,4-diarylpyridines as IκB kinase β inhibitors useful as antiinflammatories. WO 2002044153.

101. Bayer (2002) Preparation of hydroxyarylpyridines with IκB kinase β (IKK) inhibiting activity. WO 2002024679.

102. Murata, T., Shimada, M., Sakakibara, S., et al. (2003) Discovery of novel and selective IKK-β serine-threonine protein kinase inhibitors. Part 1, *Bioorg. Med. Chem. Lett.*, **13**, 913–918.

103. Signal Pharmaceuticals, Inc. (2003) Preparation of anilinopyrimidines as IKK inhibitors. WO 2002046171.

104. Bayer (2003) Preparation of optically active pyridooxazinones as antiinflammatory agents. WO 2003076447.

105. Aventis Pharma (2001) Preparation of amino acid indolecarboxamides as modulators of NF-κB activity. WO 2001030774.

106. Aventis Pharma (2001) Preparation of benzimidazolecarboxylic acid amino acid amides as IκB kinase inhibitors. WO 2001000610.

107. Pharmacia Corp. (2003) Preparation of pyrazolo [4,3-c] quinolines, chromeno[4,3-c]pyrazoles, and analogs for treatment of inflammation. WO 2003024936.

108. Pharmacia Corp. (2003) Preparation of 4,5-dihydro-1H-benzo[g]indazole-3-carboxamides for treatment of inflammation. WO 2003024935.

109. Tularik Inc. (2002) Preparation of imidazolylquinolinecarboxaldehyde semicarbazones as IKK modulators. WO 2002041843.

110. SmithKline Beecham Corp. (2002) Preparation of 5-amino-1H-imidazole-4-carboxamides as NF-κB inhibitors. WO 200230423.

111. Leo Pharma (2002) A method using cyanoguanidine compounds for modulating NF-κB activity and use for the treatment of cancer. WO 2002094265.

112. Leo Pharma (2002) Antitumor drug–cyanoguanidine IKK inhibitor combination. WO 2002094322.

113. Schou, C., Ottose, E. R., Petersen H. J., et al. (1997) Novel cyanoguanidines with potent oral antitumour activity, *Bioorg. Med. Chem. Lett.*, **7**, 3095–3100.

114. Hjarnaa, P. J., Jonsson, E., Latini, S., et al. (1999) CHS 828, a novel pyridyl cyanoguanidine with potent antitumor activity *in vitro* and *in vivo*, *Cancer Res.* **59**, 5751–5157.

115. Martinsson, P., Ekelund, S., Nygren, P., et al. (2002) The combination of the antitumoural pyridyl cyanoguanidine CHS 828 and etoposide *in vitro* – from cytotoxic synergy to complete inhibition of apoptosis, *Br. J. Pharmacol.*, **137**, 568–573.

116. Isis Pharmaceuticals, Inc. (2000) Antisense modulation of inhibitor-κ B kinase-β gene expression. WO 2000031105.

117. Takaesu, G., Sarabhi, R. M., Park, K.-J., et al. (2003) TAK1 is critical for IκB kinase-mediated activation of the NF-κB pathway, *J. Mol. Biol.*, **326**, 105–115.

118. May, M. J. and Ghosh, S. (2002) Anti-inflammatory compounds and uses thereof. A cell-permeable peptide encompassing NEMO binding domain of IκB kinase was able to not only inhibit TNFα-induced NF-κB activation but also reduce expression of E-selectin, an NF-κB-dependent target gene, in primary human endothelial cells. WO 2002156000.

119. May, M., D'Acquisto, F., Madge, L. A., et al. (2000) Selective inhibition of NF-κB activation by a peptide that blocks the interaction of NEMO with the IκB kinase complex, *Science*, **289**, 1550–1554.

120. Malveaux, F. J., Conroy, M. C., Adkinson, N. F., Jr., and Lichtensterin, L. M. (1978) IgE receptors on human basophils. Relationship to serum IgE concentration, *J. Clin. Invest.*, **62**, 176–181.

121. MacGlashan, D., McKenzie-White, J., Chichester, K., et al. (1998) In vitro regulation of FcepsilonRIalpha expression on human basophils by IgE antibody, *Blood*, **91**, 1633–1643.

122. Stingl, G. and Maurer, D. (1997) IgE-mediated allergen presentation via Fc epsilon RI on antigen-presenting cells, *Intl. Arch. Allergy Immunol.*, **113**, 24–29.

123. Maurer, D., Ebner, C., Reininger, B., et al. (1995) The high affinity IgE receptor (Fc epsilon RI) mediates IgE-dependent allergen presentation, *J. Immunol.*, **154**, 6285–6290.

124. Haczku, A., Takeda, K., Hamelmann, E., et al. (1997) CD23 deficient mice develop allergic airway hyperresponsiveness following sensitization with ovalbumin, *Am. J. Respir. Crit. Care Med.*, **156**, 1945–1955.

125. Breedveld, F. C. (2000) Therapeutic monoclonal antibodies, *Lancet*, **355**, 735–740.

126. Presta, L. G., Lahr, S. J., Shields, R. L., et al. (1993) Humanization of an antibody directed against IgE, *J. Immunol.*, **151**, 2623–2632.

127. Casale, T. B. (2001) Anti-immunoglobulin E (omalizumab) therapy in seasonal allergic rhinitis, *Am. J. Respir. Crit. Care Med.*, **164**(8), S18–S21.

128. Scheinfeld, N. (2005) Omalizumab: a recombinant humanized monoclonal IgE- blocking antibody, *Dermatol. Online J.*, **11**(2), 2.

129. D'Amato, G. (2006) Role of anti-IgE monoclonal antibody (omalizumab) in the treatment of bronchial asthma and allergic respiratory diseases, *Eur. J. Pharmacol.*, **533**(1–3), 302–307.

130. Bang, L. M. and Plosker, G. L. (2004) Omalizumab: a review of its use in the management of allergic asthma, *Treat. Respir. Med.*, **3**, 183–199.

131. Belliveau, P. P. (2005) Omalizumab: a monoclonal anti-IgE antibody, *Med. Gen. Med.*, **7**(1), 27.

132. Fahy, J. V., Fleming, H. E., Wong, H. H., et al. (1997) The effect of an anti-IgE monoclonal antibody on the early- and late-phase responses to allergen inhalation in asthmatic subjects, *Am. J. Respir. Crit. Care Med.*, **155**, 1828–1834.

133. Boulet, L. P., Chapman, K. R., Cote, J., et al. (1997) Inhibitory effects of an anti- IgE antibody E25 on allergen-induced early asthmatic response, *Am. J. Respir. Crit. Care Med.*, **155**, 1835–1840.

134. Milgrom, H., Berger, W., Nayak, A., et al. (2001) Treatment of childhood asthma with anti-immunoglobulin E antibody (omalizumab), *Pediatrics*, **108**, E36.

135. Busse, W., Corren, J., Lanier, B. Q., et al. (2001) Omalizumab, anti-IgE recombinant humanized monoclonal antibody, for the treatment of severe allergic asthma, *J. Allergy Clin. Immunol.*, **108**, 184–190.

136. Soler, M., Matz, J., Townley, R., et al. (2001) The anti-IgE antibody omalizumab reduces exacerbations and steroid requirement in allergic asthmatics, *Eur. Respir. J.*, **18**, 254–261.

137. Hochhaus, G., Brookman, L., Fox, H., et al. (2003) Pharmacodynamics of omalizumab: implications for optimised dosing strategies and clinical efficacy in the treatment of allergic asthma, *Curr. Med. Res. Opin.*, **19**, 491–498.

138. Corren, J., Casale, T., Deniz, Y., and Ashby, M. (2003) Omalizumab, a recombinant humanized anti-IgE antibody, reduces asthma-related emergency room visits and hospitalizations in patients with allergic asthma, *J. Allergy Clin. Immunol.*, **111**, 87–90.

139. Humbert, M., Beasley, R., Ayres, J., et al. (2005) Benefits of omalizumab as add-on therapy in patients with severe persistent asthma who are inadequately controlled despite best available therapy (GINA 2002 step 4 treatment): INNOVATE, *Allergy*, **60**, 309–316.

140. Bousquet, J., Cabrera, P., Berkman, N., et al. (2005) The effect of treatment with omalizumab, an anti-IgE antibody, on asthma exacerbations and emergency medical visits in patients with severe persistent asthma, *Allergy*, **60**, 302–308.

141. Noga, O., Hanf, G., and Kunkel, G. (2003) Immunological changes in allergic asthmatics following treatment with omalizumab, *Intl. Arch. Allergy Immunol.*, **131**, 46–52.

142. Djukanovic, R., Wilson, S., Kraft, M., et al. (2004) Effects of treatment with anti- immunoglobulin E antibody omalizumab on airway inflammation in allergic asthma, *Am. J. Respir. Crit. Care Med.*, **170**, 583–593.

143. Holgate, S. T., Bousquet, J., Wenzel, S., Fox, H., Liu, J., and Castellsague, J. (2001) Efficacy of omalizumab, an anti-immunoglobulin E antibody in patients with allergic asthma at high risk of serious asthma-related morbidity and mortality, *Curr. Med. Res. Opin.*, **17**, 233–240.

144. Walker, S., Monteil, M., Phelan, K., Lasserson, T. J., and Walters, E. H. (2005) Anti-IgE for chronic asthma in adults and children (Cochrane Review), *The Cochrane Library Issue*, vol. 2, Wiley, Chichester, UK.

145. Casale, T. B., Busse, W. W., Kline, J. N., et al. (2006) Immune Tolerance Network Group. Omalizumab pretreatment decreases acute reactions after rush immunotherapy for ragweed-induced seasonal allergic rhinitis, *J. Allergy Clin. Immunol.*, **117**, 134–140.

146. Bousquet, J., Lockey, R., and Malling, H. J. (1998) Allergen immunotherapy: therapeutic vaccines for allergic diseases. A WHO position paper, *J. Allergy Clin. Immunol*, **102**, 558–562.

147. Creticos, P. S., Reed, C. E., Norman, P. S., Khoury, J., Adkinson, N. F., Jr., et al. (1996) Ragweed immunotherapy in adult asthma, *N. Engl. J. Med.*, **334**, 501–506.

148. Gehlhar, K., Schlaak, M., Becker, W., and Bufe, A. (1999) Monitoring allergen immunotherapy of pollen-allergic patients: the ratio of allergen-specific IgG4 to IgG1 correlates with clinical outcome, *Clin. Exp. Allergy*, **29**, 497–506.

149. Jutel, M., Akdis, M., Budak, F., et al. (2003) IL-10 and TGF-beta cooperate in the regulatory T cell response to mucosal allergens in normal immunity and specific immunotherapy, *Eur. J. Immunol.*, **33**, 1205–1214.

150. Nouri-Aria, K. T., Wachholz, P. A., Francis, J. N., et al. (2004) Grass pollen immunotherapy induces mucosal and peripheral IL-10 responses and blocking IgG activity, *J. Immunol.*, **172**, 3252–3259.

151. Hamid, Q. A., Schotman, E., Jacobson, M. R., Walker, S. M., and Durham, S. R. (1997) Increases in IL-12 messenger RNA+ cells accompany inhibition of allergen- induced late skin responses after successful grass pollen immunotherapy, *J. Allergy Clin. Immunol.*, **99**, 254–260.

152. Francis, J. N., Till, S. J., and Durham, S. R. (2003) Induction of IL- 10+CD4+CD25+ T cells by grass pollen immunotherapy, *J. Allergy Clin. Immunol.*, **111**, 1255–1261.

153. Adelroth, E., Rak, S., Haahtela, T., et al. (2001) Recombinant humanized mAb-E25, an anti-IgE mAb, in birch pollen-induced seasonal allergic rhinitis, *J. Allergy Clin. Immunol.*, **106**, 253–259.

154. Casale, T, B., Condemi, J., LaForce, C., et al. (2001) Effect of omalizumab on symptoms of seasonal allergic rhinitis, *J. Am. Med. Assoc.*, **286**, 2956–2967.

155. Chervinsky, P., Casale, T., Townley, R., et al. (2003) Omalizumab, an anti-IgE antibody, in the treatment of adults and adolescents with perennial allergic rhinitis, *Ann. Allergy Asthma Immunol.*, **91**, 160–167.

156. Lin, H., Boesel, K. M., Griffith, D. T., et al. (2004) Omalizumab rapidly decreases nasal allergic response and FceRI on basophils, *J. Allergy Clin. Immunol.*, **113**, 297–302.

157. Klunker, S., Saggar, L. R., Seyfert-Margolis, V., Asare, A. L., Casale, T. B., Durham, S. R., Francis, J. N., and the Immune Tolerance Network Group (2007) Combination treatment with omalizumab and rush immunotherapy for ragweed-induced allergic

158. rhinitis: inhibition of IgE-facilitated allergen binding, *J. Allergy Clin. Immunol.*, **120**(3), 688–695.

158. Casale, T. B., Busse, W. W., Kline, J. N., et al., and the Immune Tolerance Network Group (2006) Omalizumab pretreatment decreases acute reactions after rush immunotherapy for ragweed-induced seasonal allergic rhinitis, *J. Allergy Clin. Immunol.*, **117**, 134–140.

159. Lockey, R. F., Benedict, L. M., Turkeltaub, P. C., and Bukantz, S. C. (1987) Fatalities from immunotherapy (IT) and skin testing (ST), *J. Allergy Clin. Immunol.*, **79**, 660–677.

160. Du Buske, L. M., Ling, C. J., and Sheffer, A. L. (1992) Special problems regarding allergen immunotherapy, *Immunol. Allergy Clin. North Am.*, **12**, 145–175.

161. Bukantz, S. C. and Lockey, R. F. (2004) Adverse effects and fatalities associated with subcutaneous allergen immunotherapy, *Clin. Allergy Immunol.*, **18**, 711–727.

162. Tighe, H., Takabayashi, K., Schwartz, D., et al. (2000) Conjugation of immunostimulatory DNA to the short ragweed allergen Amb a 1 enhances its immunogenicity and reduces its allergenicity, *J. Allergy Clin. Immunol.*, **106**, 124–134.

163. Tighe, H., Takabayashi, K., Schwartz, D., et al. (2000) Conjugation of protein to immunostimulatory DNA results in a rapid, long-lasting and potent induction of cell-mediated and humoral immunity, *Eur. J. Immunol.*, **30**, 1939–1947.

164. Marshall, J. D., Abtahi, S., Eiden, J. J., et al. (2001) Immunostimulatory sequence DNA linked to the Amb a 1 allergen promotes T(H)1 cytokine expression while downregulating T(H)2 cytokine expression in PBMCs from human patients with ragweed allergy, *J. Allergy Clin. Immunol.*, **108**, 191–197.

165. Sampson, H. A (2002) Peanut allergy, *N. Engl. J. Med.*, **346**(17), 1294–1299.

166. Sampson, H. A. (1998) Fatal food-induced anaphylaxis, *Allergy*, **53**(Suppl.), 125–130.

167. Sampson, H. A., Mendelson, L., and Rosen, J. P. (1992) Fatal and near-fatal anaphylactic reactions to food in children and adolescents, *N. Engl. J. Med.*, **327**, 380–384.

168. Bock, S. A., Munoz-Furlong, A., and Sampson, H. A. (2001) Fatalities due to anaphylactic reactions to foods, *J. Allergy Clin. Immunol.*, **107**, 191–193.

169. Saavedra-Delgado, A. (1989) The many faces of the peanut, *Allergy Proc.*, **10**, 291–294.

170. Beyer, K., Morrow, E., Li, X. M., et al. (2001) Effects of cooking methods on peanut allergenicity, *J. Allergy Clin. Immunol.*, **107**, 1077–1081.

171. Hatahet, R., Kirch, F., Kanny, G., and Moneret-Vautrin, D. A. (1994) Sensibilisation aux allergènes d'arachide chez les nourrissons de moins de quatre mois: à propos de 125 observations, *Rev. Fr. Allergol. Immunol. Clin.*, **34**, 377–381.

172. Sampson, H. A. (1996) Managing peanut allergy, *Br. Med. J.*, **312**, 1050–1051.

173. Chiu, L., Sampson, H. A., and Sicherer, S. H. (2001) Estimation of the sensitization rate to peanut by prick skin test in the general population: results from the National Health and Nutrition Examination Survey 1988–1994 (NHANES III), *J. Allergy Clin. Immunol.*, **107**(Suppl.), S192–S192 [abstract].

174. Burks, W., Sampson, H. A., and Bannon, G. A. (1998) Peanut allergens, *Allergy*, **53**, 725–730.

175. Bernhisel-Broadbent, J. and Sampson, H. A. (1989) Cross-allergenicity in the legume botanical family in children with food hypersensitivity, *J. Allergy Clin. Immunol.*, **83**, 435–440.

176. Sicherer, S. H., Burks, A. W., and Sampson, H. A. (1998) Clinical features of acute allergic reactions to peanut and tree nuts in children, *Pediatrics*, **102**, 131–131 [abstract].

177. Sicherer, S. H., Furlong, T. J., Munoz-Furlong, A., Burks, A. W., and Sampson, H. A. (2001) A voluntary registry for peanut

and tree nut allergy: characteristics of the first 5149 registrants, *J. Allergy Clin. Immunol.*, **108**, 128–132.

178. Skolnick, H. S., Conover-Walker, M. K., Koerner, C. B., Sampson, H. A., et al. (2001) The natural history of peanut allergy, *J. Allergy Clin. Immunol.*, **107**, 367–374.

179. Lin, R. Y., Schwartz, L. B., Curry, A., et al. (2000) Histamine and tryptase levels in patients with acute allergic reactions: an emergency department-based study, *J. Allergy Clin. Immunol.*, **106**, 65–71.

180. Lack, G., Fox, D., Northstone, K., and Golding, J., for the Avon Longitudinal Study of Parents and Children Study Team (2003) Factors associated with the development of peanut allergy in childhood, *N. Engl. J. Med.*, **348**(11), 977–985 [comments: *J. Fam. Pract.*, **52**(7), 516–517 (2003); *N. Engl. J. Med.*, **348**(11), 975–976 (2003); *N. Engl. J. Med.*, **348**(11), 1946–1048 (2003); *N. Engl. J. Med.*, **349**(3), 301–303 (2003)].

181. Sampson, H. A. (1999) Food allergy. 2. Diagnosis and management, *J. Allergy Clin. Immunol.*, **103**, 981–989.

182. Simons, F. E., Gu, X., and Simons, K. J. (2001) Epinephrine absorption in adults: intramuscular versus subcutaneous injection, *J. Allergy Clin. Immunol.*, **108**, 871–873.

183. Oppenheimer, J. J., Nelson, H. S., Bock, S. A., Christensen, F., and Leung, D. Y. M. (1992) Treatment of peanut allergy with rush immunotherapy, *J. Allergy Clin. Immunol.*, **90**, 256–262.

184. Sampson, H. A. (2001) Immunological approaches to the treatment of food allergy, *Pediatr. Allergy Immunol.*, **12**(Suppl.), **14**, 91–96.

185. Matricardi, P. M., Rosmini, F., Panetta, V., et al. (2002) Hay fever and asthma in relation to markers of infection in the United States, *J. Allergy Clin. Immunol.*, **110,** 381–387.

186. Sampson H. (2002) Peanut allergy, *N. Engl. J. Med.*, **346,** 1294–1299.

187. Creticos, P. S., Schroeder, J. T., Hamilton, R. G. (2006) Immunotherapy with a ragweed-Toll-like receptor 9 agonist vaccine for allergic rhinitis, *N. Engl. J. Med.*, **355**(14), 27–37.

188. Cohn, L., Elias, J. A., and Chupp, G. L. (2004) Asthma: mechanisms of disease persistence and progression, *Annu. Rev. Immunol.*, **22**, 789–815.

189. Davies, D. E., Wicks, J., Powell, R. M., Puddicombe, S. M., and Holgate, S. T. (2003) Airway remodeling in asthma: new insights, *J. Allergy Clin. Immunol.*, **111**, 215–225.

Index